Metabolic Medicine and Surgery

Metabolic Medicine and Surgery

Edited by

Michael M. Rothkopf, MD, FACP, FACN
Metabolic Medicine Center
Atlantic Health System
Morristown, New Jersey, USA

Clinical Assistant Professor of Medicine
Icahn School of Medicine at Mount Sinai
Mount Sinai Health System
New York, New York, USA

Michael J. Nusbaum, MD, FACS, FASMBS
Metabolic Medicine Center
Atlantic Health System
Morristown, New Jersey, USA

Lisa P. Haverstick, RDN, CNSC, FAND
Metabolic Medicine Center
Atlantic Health System
Morristown, New Jersey, USA

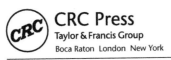

CRC Press
Taylor & Francis Group
Boca Raton London New York

CRC Press is an imprint of the
Taylor & Francis Group, an **informa** business

CRC Press
Taylor & Francis Group
6000 Broken Sound Parkway NW, Suite 300
Boca Raton, FL 33487-2742

First issued in paperback 2017

© 2015 by Taylor & Francis Group, LLC
CRC Press is an imprint of Taylor & Francis Group, an Informa business

No claim to original U.S. Government works

ISBN-13: 978-1-4665-6711-5 (hbk)
ISBN-13: 978-1-138-03388-7 (pbk)

Library of Congress Cataloging-in-Publication Data

Metabolic medicine and surgery / editors, Michael M. Rothkopf, Michael J. Nusbaum, Lisa P. Haverstick.
    p. ; cm.
    Includes bibliographical references and index.
    Summary: "Health practitioners who deal with disease by attempting to restore normal metabolism are said to practice metabolic medicine. This book is intended to be the first comprehensive overview in the field of metabolic medicine, which is dedicated to controlling the epidemic of obesity and preventing obesity's consequences. It introduces metabolic medicine and surgery, and covers metabolic syndrome as an epidemic, metabolic approaches to diabetes and obesity, and metabolic management in chronic disease states"--Provided by publisher.
    ISBN 978-1-4665-6711-5 (hardcover : alk. paper)
    I. Rothkopf, Michael M., editor. II. Nusbaum, Michael J., editor. III. Haverstick, Lisa P., editor.
    [DNLM: 1. Metabolic Syndrome X--surgery. 2. Bariatric Surgery. 3. Malnutrition. 4. Nutritional Support. 5. Obesity--surgery. WK 820]

RD540.5
617.4'3--dc23

2014032603

Visit the Taylor & Francis Web site at
http://www.taylorandfrancis.com

and the CRC Press Web site at
http://www.crcpress.com

We dedicate this book to our mentors, colleagues, and patients. We have learned much from all of you and treasure your ongoing support.

Michael M. Rothkopf
Michael J. Nusbaum
Lisa P. Haverstick

To Amy, Rebecca, Zachary, Max, Ariel, and Jacob. You have witnessed the determination needed to forge a new specialty. Be bold in your lives. Be creative. Don't let others define you. Find out what you love to do and pursue it with tenacity and courage.

Michael M. Rothkopf
Michael J. Nusbaum

As senior editor, I have the privilege of offering a personal dedication to my wife Gail who has been a constant source of clarity and virtue—thank you for renewing my contract, year after year.

Michael M. Rothkopf

Contents

SECTION I   Metabolic Medicine and Surgery—A New Paradigm in Healthcare

SECTION II   Metabolic Syndrome, Insulin Resistance, and Obesity—An Opportunity to Prevent, Control, and Reverse Disease

SECTION III   Diseases of Undernutrition and Absorption

SECTION IV   A Nutritional Relationship to Neurological Diseases

Surgical Foreword

This book edited by Michael M. Rothkopf, Michael J. Nusbaum, and Lisa P. Haverstick is a gem, encompassing chapters on metabolic medicine and surgery and associated sciences. It crystallizes the efforts of a multitude of physicians and scientists trying to control a pandemic of type 2 diabetes worldwide. The World Health Organization (WHO) has recorded that noncommunicable diseases (NCDs) kill more than 36 million people each year, mostly under the age of 60. The goal of the United Nations Millennium is to lessen those estimates; however, it appears impossible in the near future as NCDs are rising rapidly in populous countries such as India and China. All efforts are needed to limit NCDs, and since the WHO is expanding comprehensive global monitoring prevention and control of NCDs, surgical interventions, the only effective long-term cure, should be expanded.

Just a few years short of the 100-year anniversary of the discovery of insulin and Nobel Prize of Medicine by Banting and Best, let's recall this collaboration between the mentor and the medical student during a summer project in Toronto, Canada. It is also one of the best examples on how observations on surgical effects led to the discovery of diabetes treatment, a surgical ligature around the pancreatic duct, followed by isolation of the islets extracts. On July 27, 1921, a pancreatectomized dog (Marjorie) was kept alive the whole summer by injection of those extracts.[1] The first American patient was Elizabeth Hughes Gossett, daughter of Charles Evans Hughes, the governor of New York. She had been treated on a strict 400 calories a day diet and lost a dangerous amount of weight to 45 pounds (age 14), but her diabetes persisted until she received insulin extracts from Dr. Banting in 1922 and survived to the age of 73. The rest, as we say, is history.

More than 15 years ago, after creating the bariatric surgical unit at Mount Sinai School of Medicine, I had the fortunate assistance of Francesco Rubino who accepted my offer to do another year of research and fellowship in laparoscopic surgery.

This is actually where the idea of diabetes surgery began.[2] The observation of rapid resolution of diabetes after gastric bypass was confirmed (which had been known for several decades by other bariatric and digestive surgeons), and a search for a specific hormone had led to systematic serum determination in postgastric bypass patients of all GI hormones known at the time, including GIP.[3] Our human protocol on a randomized study looking at the best medical treatment versus Roux-en-Y gastric bypass for type 2 diabetes was rejected by the local Institutional Review Board. However, several experiments on Goto-Kakizaki rats were initiated, and the concept of metabolic surgery emerged.[2]

The future, just like the discovery of insulin, lies in the collaboration between our colleagues in the medical and biological sciences to unlock the secret of this disease and get a cure for all patients. This book is a real attempt at doing so, and I congratulate the editors and authors for their efforts.

REFERENCES

1. Krishnamurthy K. *Pioneers in Scientific Discoveries*. New Delhi, India: Mittal Publications, 2002:266.
2. Rubino F, Gagner M. Potential of surgery for curing type 2 diabetes mellitus. *Ann Surg*. 2002;236(5):554–9.
3. Rubino F, Gagner M, Gentileschi P, Kini S, Fukuyama S, Feng J, Diamond E. The early effect of the Roux-en-Y gastric bypass on hormones involved in body weight regulation and glucose metabolism. *Ann Surg*. 2004;240(2):236–42.

Michel Gagner, MD, FRCSC, FACS, FASMBS, FICS, AFC (Hon.)
Clinical Professor of Surgery, FIU
Senior Consultant, Hopital du Sacre Coeur, Montreal
President, IFSO 2014—19th World Congress of International Federation
for the Surgery of Obesity and Metabolic Disorders

Metabolist Foreword

Cardiometabolic is an adjective that relates heart disease and metabolic disorders. This is a new term that, in less than a decade, has found a place in science and medicine. Perhaps the name was a result of concerns that cardiovascular disease (CVD) risk was more than family history, smoking, cholesterol, and blood pressure. In 1998, the World Health Organization began a process to capture this added CVD risk by defining a number of contributing risk factors that they named the metabolic syndrome. Subsequently, a number of organizations have modified the definition with some additions and omissions from the original definition.

Looking back, the metabolic syndrome is not a new concept. In 1923, Swedish physician scientist Eskil Kylin described the association of hyperglycemia with hypertension and gout. Then in the late 1940s, Jean Vague drew attention to the relationship of upper body adiposity as an obesity phenotype that commonly occurred with metabolic abnormalities associated with type 2 diabetes and CVD. Perhaps most noteworthy is the Banting Lecture of Gerald Reaven in 1988 that connected the dots between insulin resistance in glucose metabolism and alterations in lipid and lipoprotein metabolism.

Although a consensus for the precise definition of metabolic syndrome is still developing, experts agree that it has multiple components, and those to be included in the definition may be arbitrary. What is universally recognized is that a significant link exists between aberrant metabolism and CVD. In fact, the term "metabolic syndrome" is extremely well founded, having been referenced in the scientific literature over 50,000 times, mostly within the past 15 years. Moreover, reference to the metabolic syndrome is found in high-impact basic science journals such as *Nature, Science*, and *Cell*.

Editors Michael M. Rothkopf, Michael J. Nusbaum, and Lisa P. Haverstick are to be congratulated for taking on a topic that relates cardiometabolic epidemiology to pathophysiology, prevention, and therapeutics including lifestyle, medical, and surgical. If one uses the metabolic syndrome to represent cardiometabolic, then the chapters herein cover the waterfront. Included in all definitions are central obesity, glucose intolerance, dyslipidemia, and hypertension; however, nonalcoholic liver disease, inflammation, disturbances in coagulation and fibrinolysis, cancer, PCOS, infertility, microalbuminuria, and hyperuricemia have also been included. Insulin resistance relates to all of these disturbances, and it may be the mechanism linking the major underlying metabolic disturbances to CVD. Because obesity, especially central obesity, is the global issue that has led to what we now call cardiometabolic, the book importantly focuses on nutritional, medical, and surgical approaches to deal with this most important contributor to insulin resistance. However, all of the aspects of insulin resistance in the expanded metabolic syndrome are not covered in the book, and that reflects the need to address additional topics that represent the background and experience of the editors.

In particular, the background of the editors makes nutrition a central focus, both in therapeutics and prevention including that of type 2 diabetes. Moreover, nutritional issues related to short bowel syndrome, enteral and total parenteral nutrition, inflammatory bowel disease, neurological diseases, and immunity are covered. Exemplary here is the fact that many of the risk factors for CVD are those for Alzheimer's disease. That of course does not equate downstream mechanisms of diseases in two different organ systems but does provide a systems biology scenario that could very much relate to nutrition.

Metabolic medicine is more than a trending science that has recently grabbed the attention of health care providers. It exists as a foundation for the prevention and therapeutics of many of the disorders we face in an ever-expanding and complex environment. The science of nutrition can be confusing, and the chapters within this text provide some of the validated science needed to apply within clinical practice. Happy reading and enjoy!

Robert H. Eckel, MD
Professor of Medicine
Division of Endocrinology, Metabolism and Diabetes
Division of Cardiology
Professor of Physiology and Biophysics
Charles A. Boettcher II Chair in Atherosclerosis
University of Colorado Anschutz Medical Campus
Director Lipid Clinic, University Hospital
Denver, Colorado

Preface

Let us start with a fresh slate. And, for arguments sake, let us forget the current boundaries between the traditional specialties. Our task is to design a new specialty to serve patients with obesity, metabolic syndrome, cardiovascular risk, prediabetes, maldigestion, malabsorption, malnutrition, nutritional deficiencies, and other diseases in which nutritional factors clearly play a role. How would you do it?

Metabolic medicine and metabolic surgery responded to this challenge by creating a multidisciplinary, comprehensive approach to patient management, with synergies between the specialists. Each member is responsible for a set of diagnostic and therapeutic processes.

This approach was initiated by the three editors of this text in 1998, when we effectively integrated our clinical activities in the management of patients with obesity. Sixteen years and thousands of patients later, we feel we have proven the value of the methodology. The dynamic flow between our separate disciplines has allowed us to learn much from each other's perspectives. It has made us each more engaged and complete practitioners, with obvious benefit to our delivery of care. Having created a successful model, we want to share it with others, expecting them to embellish and improve upon it. We offer this book as an example for the framework of our integrated approach to patient care.

The book is intended for physicians, residents, medical students, nurse practitioners, dietitians, physician assistants, and other practitioners who care for patients with metabolic illnesses. Since these conditions have now been shown to affect large percentages of our population, it is likely that most clinicians will see patients with metabolic conditions throughout their careers. This is certainly the case for those in primary care settings, where two thirds of all patients are overweight or obese. A large percentage of the general population also has metabolic syndrome and is at risk for the development of diabetes and cardiovascular disease.

This book could also be used as a text for those preparing to practice as specialists in the field or those who wish to expand their scope of practice to include management of metabolic patients. Furthermore, we hope this text will be seen as a useful reference for those already practicing in the fields of metabolic medicine, metabolic surgery, obesity, diabetes, and nutrition.

The volume is presented in four sections. Section I is an overview of the field and outlines our vision for the future of metabolic medicine and surgery. Each chapter is written collectively by the editors. In Chapter 1, "An Overview of Metabolic Medicine," we review the history of the field and its recent developments. In Chapter 2, "Practice of Metabolic Medicine," we attempt to delineate the structure of our day-to-day activities. In Chapter 3, "Concept of Metabolic Surgery," we review the history and scope of the surgical approaches to metabolic diseases.

Section II includes 17 chapters on metabolic syndrome, insulin resistance, and obesity. We begin with an overview of "Metabolic Syndrome" and "Nonalcoholic Fatty Liver Disease" in Chapters 4 and 5, written by our current fellows, Dr. Amrita Sawhney and Dr. Olga Melzer, with help from Drs. Rothkopf and Ganjhu (on Chapter 5). These are followed by a discussion of "Insulin, the Glycemic Index, and Carcinogenesis" by Dr. David Jenkins and his colleagues, Dr. Augustin, Dr. Kendall, Dr. Mirrahimi, and Dr. Nishi, at the Department of Nutritional Sciences at the University of Toronto, in Chapter 6.

Next, we explore the diet–heart hypothesis by two remarkable groups of experts with unique perspectives. In Chapter 7, "Nutrition and Cardiovascular Disease," Dr. Miquel Angel Martinez and his associate Dr. Bes-Rastrollo explore the epidemiological evidence for the connection between food patterns and cardiovascular disease. The reader will recall that Dr. Martinez and his colleagues in Spain have recently published the results of their groundbreaking Predimed Study. Predimed is the first study to report level 1 evidence of a significant reduction in cardiovascular disease among individuals following a Mediterranean diet. In Chapter 8, Dr. Amalia Gastadelli and her colleagues Dr. Del Turco and Dr. Sicari in Pisa, Italy, explore a biochemical and endocrine pathogenesis of cardiovascular disease in "Risk Relationship between Insulin Resistance, Diabetes, and Atherosclerotic Cardiovascular Disease."

Chapter 9, "Strategies for the Prevention of Type 2 Diabetes," by Drs. Preuss and Preuss is the most comprehensive review of the subject we have seen anywhere. From Rome's Catholic University, Dr. Mingrone and Dr. Castagneto present their pioneering work on "Bariatric Surgery for Type 2 Diabetes Mellitus Resolution" in Chapter 10. Their studies have been widely published in major medical journals. They are certainly among the most distinguished experts in this rapidly developing field, and we are fortunate to have their input. To further this stimulating discussion, we have a very thorough contribution from Dr. Dutia and Dr. Laferrère in Chapter 11 on "Incretin Response after Bariatric Surgery." The readers will note that Dr. Laferrère has published extensively on this topic and is a renowned thought leader in the field.

In Chapter 12, we begin our specific attention to obesity with "Medical Obesity Management" by Dr. DeRosimo of the American Society of Bariatric Physicians. Next, Dr. Sumithran and Dr. Proietto from Melbourne, Australia, discuss their fascinating research into "Peripheral Endocrine Response to Weight Loss" in Chapter 13. This chapter helps explain the challenges of medical weight loss and is a natural segue into "An Overview of Surgical Weight Loss Options" in Chapter 14 by Dr. Sawhney and Dr. Fishman. Dr. Francesco Rubino (now of London) and his associates, Dr. Shukla and Dr. Patel, complete this focus with an excellent review of "Diabetes Surgery" in Chapter 15.

Beginning with Chapter 16, we present a concentration on bariatric postoperative surgical care. Dr. Simonetti and Dr. Apovian from Boston describe the "Metabolic Changes Post-Bariatric Surgery." Next, Dr. Sasha Stiles of Hawaii (by way of Colorado and New York University) reviews "Metabolic Monitoring of the Bariatric Surgery Patient" in Chapter 17. Then we move on to a look at some of the rarer complications of bariatric surgery. This includes "Hypoglycemia after Roux-en-Y Gastric Bypass Surgery" in Chapter 18 by Shannon Roque, Drs. Sridhar Nambi, and Michael M. Rothkopf, "Micronutrient-Deficient Encephalopathy after Bariatric Surgery" in Chapter 19 by Dr. Melzer and Dr. Rothkopf, and "Hyperammonemic Encephalopathy after Roux-en-Y Gastric Bypass Surgery" by Dr. Fenves and Dr. Shchelochkov in Chapter 20.

Section III contains six chapters on diseases of undernutrition, each of which represents a wealth of experience and perspective in the field. In Chapter 21, Dr. Arthur Heller gives us his approach to "Bedside Diagnosis of Malnutrition." The chapter is illustrated with photographs of his own patients as well as a patient from his fellowship with Dr. Maurice Shils. Dr. Shils' early research in nutritional sciences provides the underpinnings of much of what we practice today. Dr. Heller's chapter lets us all honor Dr. Shils' legacy and gain from his experience. Next, we are very fortunate to have the input of another giant in nutrition, Dr. Stanley Dudrick, who (along with two devoted colleagues) takes us through "Nutritional Support: Enteral and Parenteral Nutrition" in Chapter 22. The reader will recall that Dr. Dudrick is widely recognized for having pioneered the concept of total parenteral nutrition (TPN) in the 1960s. Rounding out this focus on nutritional support, Dr. Beverly Teter teaches us about the "Metabolic Effects of Omega-3 Fatty Acids" in Chapter 23. Dr. Teter is a lipid biochemist from the University of Maryland and has conducted extensive research in this area.

Chapters 24, 25, and 26 deal with the bowel–nutrient interface. First, Dr. Kudsk and Dr. Pierre discuss "Nutrition and Gut Immunity" from the standpoint of bowel flora adaptive and innate mucosal immunity. Next, Dr. Leo Galland describes his approach to "Nutrition Therapy for Inflammatory Bowel Disease." Dr. Galland has extensive experience in this field and has widely published on his concept of the "specific carbohydrate diet." Finally, Dr. Grovit, Dr. Ferbas, and Dr. Slonim provide us with special insight on the "Nutritional Management of Short Bowel Syndrome in the Adult with Crohn's Disease." Dr. Grovit's observations are particularly noteworthy as he has applied them successfully to his own personal health challenges.

Section IV contains six outstanding chapters exploring the new developments in the area of nutrition and neurologic disease. The section starts with an exhaustive overview of "Neurologic Disease of Metabolism" by Dr. Guha Venkatraman in Chapter 27. Next, Dr. Politsky and Dr. Karbinovskaya provide us with their valuable insights on the "Nutritional Approaches to Epilepsy." In Chapter 29, Dr. Kolb, Dr. Faheem, and Dr. Weinstock-Guttman illustrate "Role of Nutritional Factors in Multiple Sclerosis," while in Chapter 30, Dr. Pollock explores the "Micromineral Considerations in Alzheimer's Dementia."

The section on neurology is completed by the contributions of two more titans of nutritional science: Dr. George Brewer and Dr. Ananda Prasad. Dr. Brewer is best known for his lifetime of research into the role of copper in health and disease. Dr. Prasad is famous for his pioneering work on zinc deficiency and malnutrition. Dr. Brewer and his colleague Dr. Kaur state that "Ingestion of Inorganic Copper from Drinking Water and Supplements Is a Major Causal Factor in the Epidemic of Alzheimer's Disease" in Chapter 31. Dr. Prasad finishes with his insights on "Zinc, Health, and Immunity" in Chapter 32.

This book has taken us countless hours to complete. More than that, it represents our life's work in the field and our efforts on behalf of our many patients. We hope readers will appreciate our efforts and value the result.

Michael M. Rothkopf
Michael J. Nusbaum
Lisa P. Haverstick

Acknowledgments

The editors acknowledge the American College of Nutrition, whose members include many of the contributors to this volume.

The initial concept for this book was based on a symposium entitled "Metabolic Medicine/ Metabolic Surgery" presented at the 52nd Annual Meeting of the American College of Nutrition on November 17, 2011 in Morristown, New Jersey.

A number of individuals provided important editorial assistance in the preparation of this manuscript. They are worthy of our gratitude and deserve special mention for their help. Kelly Iorillo assisted with reviewing the manuscript and made valuable recommendations for Chapters 1–3. Dr. Joseph Proietto reviewed the manuscript and made valuable recommendations for Chapter 4. Zachary Simon Rothkopf assisted with the drafting of figures and tables, as well as obtaining permissions for images from outside publishers for Chapters 1–5, 14, 17, and 21.

Editors

The editors have worked collaboratively for two decades and have cared for thousands of metabolic patients during that period. Dr. Michael Rothkopf is the medical director of the Atlantic Health Metabolic Medicine Center, Morristown, New Jersey. Dr. Michael Nusbaum is the surgical director and Lisa Haverstick is the nutrition and research coordinator.

Early in their careers, each of them benefitted from the tutelage of pioneers and was fortunate to witness many important developments in the field. Dr. Rothkopf trained under Dr. John Kinney at the Surgical Metabolic Unit of Columbia Presbyterian Medical Center in New York and was mentored in functional biochemistry by Dr. Eric Newsholme of Merton College, Oxford University. Dr. Nusbaum trained under Dr. Michel Gagner of Weill Cornell Medical Center in New York and Dr. Ludymr Kusmack, inventor of the adjustable gastric band. Lisa Haverstick trained with Dr. George Blackburn and Dr. Bruce Bistrian at the New England Deaconness Hospital in Boston. Collectively, they have published more than 125 scientific papers, chapters, and abstracts and coedited three previous texts.

Dr. Rothkopf is a fellow of the American College of Nutrition, the American College of Physicians, and the Obesity Society. He is a director of the American College of Nutrition and the National Board of Physician Nutrition Specialists. He is a member of the examination committee of the Certifying Board of Nutrition Specialists. Dr. Rothkopf is a clinical assistant of medicine at the Icahn School of Medicine at Mount Sinai and a director of the Pediatric Angel Network.

Dr. Nusbaum is a fellow of the American College of Surgeons and the American Society for Metabolic and Bariatric Surgery (ASMBS). He previously served as president of the NJ Chapter of ASMBS. Dr. Nusbaum is the chairman of the Pediatric Angel Network, a charitable organization that provides financial support and medical supplies to families of underprivileged pediatric patients.

Ms. Haverstick was among the earliest nutrition support clinicians certified by the American Society of Parenteral and Enteral Nutrition. She is a fellow of the Academy of Nutrition and Dietetics, and has served on the American College of Nutrition programs committee. Her work on identifying patients at nutritional risk has been utilized throughout the US Department of Veterans Affairs medical system.

Contributors

Caroline Apovian
Nutrition and Weight Management Center
and
Nutrition and Support Service
Boston Medical Center
Boston University
Boston, Massachusetts

Livia S.A. Augustin
Clinical Nutrition and Risk Factor
    Modification Center
Toronto, Ontario, Canada

Maira Bes-Rastrollo
Department of Preventive Medicine and
    Public Health
School of Medicine
University of Navarra
Pamplona, Spain

George J. Brewer
University of Michigan
Ann Arbor, Michigan

Marco Castagneto
Department of Surgery
Catholic University
Rome, Italy

Serena Del Turco
National Research Council
Institute of Clinical Physiology
Pisa, Italy

Lisa Marie DeRosimo
American Board of Obesity Medicine
Denver, Colorado

Stanley J. Dudrick
Misericordia University
Dallas, Pennsylvania

and

The Commonwealth Medical College
Scranton, Pennsylvania

and

Yale University Medical School
New Haven, Connecticut

Roxanne Dutia
New York Obesity Nutrition Research Center
Columbia University
and
St. Luke's Roosevelt Hospital Center
New York, New York

Sheikh M. Faheem
Jacobs MS Center
Jacobs Neurological Institute
SUNY University at Buffalo
Buffalo, New York

Andrew Z. Fenves
Massachusetts General Hospital
Harvard Medical School
Boston, Massachusetts

Kathie Grovit Ferbas
UCLA AIDS Institute
David Geffen School of Medicine at UCLA
Los Angeles, California

Michael Fishman
Metabolic Medicine Center
Morristown, New Jersey

Leo Galland
Foundation for Integrated Medicine
New York, New York

Lisa Ganjhu
Division of Gastroenterology and Liver
    Diseases
St. Luke's Roosevelt Hospital Center
and
Columbia University College of Physicians and
    Surgeons
and
Touro College of Osteopathic Medicine
New York, New York

Amalia Gastaldelli
National Research Council
Institute of Clinical Physiology
Pisa, Italy

Melvyn Grovit
Metabolism Program
Division of Molecular Genetics
Department of Pediatrics
Columbia University Medical Center
New York, New York

Lisa P. Haverstick
Metabolic Medicine Center
Morristown, New Jersey

Arthur D. Heller
Division of Gastroenterology and Liver
    Diseases
Department of Medicine
New York Presbyterian Hospital
Weill Cornell Medical College
New York, New York

David J.A. Jenkins
Clinical Nutrition and Risk Factor
    Modification Center
and
Keenan Research Center of the Li Ka Shing
    Knowledge Institute
and
St. Michael's Hospital
and
Department of Nutritional Sciences
Faculty of Medicine
University of Toronto
Toronto, Ontario Canada

Yelena Karbinovskaya
Department of Pediatrics
Jacobi Medical Center
Albert Einstein College of Medicine
Bronx, New York

Sukhvir Kaur
Monmouth University
West Long Branch, New Jersey

Cyril W.C. Kendall
Clinical Nutrition and Risk Factor
    Modification Center
Toronto, Canada

and

Department of Nutritional Sciences
Faculty of Medicine
University of Toronto
Ontario, Canada

and

College of Pharmacy and Nutrition
University of Saskatchewan
Saskatoon, Saskatchewan, Canada

Channna Kolb
Jacobs MS Center
Jacobs Neurological Institute
SUNY University at Buffalo
Buffalo, New York

Kenneth A. Kudsk
University of Wisconsin-Madison School of
Medicine and Public Health
and
Veterans Administration Surgical Services
William S. Middleton Memorial Veterans
Hospital
Madison, Wisconsin

Blandine Laferrère
Department of Medicine
New York Obesity Nutrition Research Center
St. Luke's Roosevelt Hospital Center
and
Division of Endocrinology and Diabetes
Columbia University College of Physicians
and Surgeons
New York, New York

Miguel A. Martinez-Gonzalez
Department of Preventive Medicine and
Public Health
School of Medicine
University of Navarra
Pamplona, Spain

Olga A. Melzer
Morristown Medical Center
Morristown, New Jersey

Geltrude Mingrone
Department of Internal Medicine
Catholic University
Rome, Italy

Arash Mirrahimi
Clinical Nutrition and Risk Factor
Modification Center
Toronto, Ontario, Canada

Sridhar Nambi
St. Barnabas Medical Center
Livingston, New Jersey

Stephanie Nishi
Clinical Nutrition and Risk Factor
Modification Center
and
Department of Nutritional Sciences
Faculty of Medicine
University of Toronto
Toronto, Ontario, Canada

Michael J. Nusbaum
Metabolic Medicine Center
Morristown, New Jersey

Rajesh T. Patel
Weill Cornell Medical College
New York, New York

Joseph F. Pierre
Section of Gastroenterology, Hepatology, and
Nutrition
Department of Medicine
University of Chicago
Chicago, Illinois

Jeffrey M. Politsky
Overlook Medical Center
Summit, New Jersey

Diana Pollock
Madonna Ptak Alzheimer Research Center
Clearwater, Florida

Ananda Prasad
Department of Oncology
Wayne State University School of Medicine
Barbara Ann Karmanos Cancer Center
Detroit, Michigan

Harry G. Preuss
Georgetown University Medical Center
Washington, DC

Jeffrey M. Preuss
Emergency Department
Lewis-Gale Medical Center
Roanoke, Virginia

Joseph Proietto
Department of Medicine (Austin Health)
University of Melbourne
Melbourne, Australia

Shannon Roque
Metabolic Medicine Center
Morristown, New Jersey

Michael M. Rothkopf
Morristown Medical Center
Morristown, New Jersey

Francesco Rubino
King's College London
King's College Hospital
London, United Kingdom

Amrita G. Sawhney
Metabolic Medicine Center
Morristown, New Jersey

Oleg A. Shchelochkov
Division of Genetics
Department of Pediatrics
University of Iowa Hospitals and Clinics
Iowa City, Iowa

Alpana Shukla
Center for Weight Management and Metabolic
    Clinical Research
Division of Endocrinology, Diabetes, and
    Metabolism
Weill Cornell Medical College
New York, New York

Rosa Sicari
Institute of Clinical Physiology
National Research Council
Pisa, Italy

Juliana S. Simonetti
Division of Diabetes, Nutrition and Weight
    Management
Department of Endocrinology
Boston University School of Medicine
Boston, Massachussetts

Alfred E. Slonim
Division of Molecular Genetics
Department of Pediatrics: Metabolism
Columbia University Medical Center
New York, New York

L.E. Sasha Stiles
Comprehensive Weight Management Program
Queens Medical Center
Honolulu, Hawaii

Priya Sumithran
Department of Medicine (Austin Health)
University of Melbourne
Melbourne, Australia

Beverly B. Teter
Animal and Avian Science Department
University of Maryland
College Park, Maryland

Guha K. Venkatraman
Institute of Neurology and Neurosurgery at
    St. Barnabas
and
St. Barnabas Medical Center
Livingston, New Jersey

Bianca Weinstock-Guttman
Jacobs MS Center
Jacobs Neurological Institute
SUNY University at Buffalo
Buffalo, New York

Section I

Metabolic Medicine and
Surgery—A New Paradigm in Healthcare

1 An Overview of Metabolic Medicine

Michael M. Rothkopf, Lisa P. Haverstick,
and Michael J. Nusbaum

CONTENTS

HISTORICAL FACTORS LEADING TO THE DEVELOPMENT OF METABOLIC MEDICINE

The field of metabolic medicine has evolved into a unique discipline that requires both clinical acumen and biochemical expertise to master. Metabolic specialists treat conditions from the very common to those that are exceedingly rare. In a single day's work, a metabolic physician can go from seeing patients with obesity or metabolic syndrome (MetS) to those with mitochondrial diseases or micronutrient deficiencies.

What these diverse patients have in common is that each suffers from an illness in which their metabolism is a major factor and where specialized nutrition serves as a mainstay of therapy.

Metabolic medicine can be thought of as applied biochemistry. Therefore, a thorough understanding of biochemical metabolic pathways is imperative. This is obvious when it comes to a case of an inborn error of metabolism. But the truth is that it is just as relevant for the common patient with diabetes or dyslipidemia.

This chapter will provide the historical context and scientific principles relevant to metabolic medicine. The authors have been fortunate in being present to observe many of these developments first hand and to learn from some of the true masters of the field. Our focus in providing this overview will be for the purpose of introducing the specialty to those who are contemplating practicing metabolic medicine as a career. The subjects covered in this introduction will be analyzed in greater detail throughout the chapters of this textbook. While it is beyond the scope of this chapter to provide a detailed review of the important biochemical concepts, an introduction of the most salient points will be presented.

The metabolic physician must have strong clinical skills in the area of physical examination and bedside diagnosis. In particular, he or she must develop techniques for accurate assessment of the skeletal muscular system, cardiovascular system, gastrointestinal system, liver, thyroid, adrenals, skin, hair, and nails. A strong working knowledge of endocrine physiology and dysfunction is also necessary.

It is also imperative for the metabolic physician to have some background in the behavioral sciences. Although the issues that the patient faces are pathophysiological, the treatment demands will certainly include major changes in food consumption and exercise patterns. The clinician must be prepared to guide a patient through this lifestyle change with effective behavioral modification techniques.

Given the complex array of medical conditions and the detailed biochemistry required to comprehend them, a demanding training program is required to obtain the expertise needed to practice metabolic medicine. Globally, metabolic medicine training programs vary in their depth and complexity. The field is very dynamic, with significant changes frequently occurring. In addition, differences in the health care systems from country to country put different demands on metabolic physicians. Therefore, the curriculum for training varies slightly in each country where specialty training for metabolic medicine has been developing.

In the United States, metabolic medicine is generally focused on three major areas: malnutrition, obesity, and the MetS. In other countries, more attention is given to the long-term management of patients with inborn errors of metabolism (IEM) as many of these individuals are living well into adulthood. Furthermore, better diagnostic techniques are permitting the diagnosis of mild, previously unrecognized forms of these diseases.

The field of metabolic medicine can be seen as paralleling the evolution of nutritional science. It began with the management of hospital malnutrition and the need to have the expertise available for the provision of complex therapies such as total parenteral nutrition (TPN). This created a platform for training physicians in nutritional biochemistry. The obesity epidemic and the understanding of the MetS as a precursor to diabetes and cardiovascular disease have broadened metabolic medicine from a niche practice to a comprehensive specialty.

MALNUTRITION

Modern diagnosis and management of malnutrition started with the critically ill and other nutritionally compromised hospital patients. The clear recognition of this phenomenon began as post-World War II medical care became increasingly technical and patients remained in the hospital for longer and more complex illness courses.

Most physicians of that era were unfamiliar with nutritional concepts and approaches. They were ill-prepared to deal with the challenges of a severely malnourished patient. Furthermore, there were few treatment options or recognized techniques for the delivery of nutritional therapy to these metabolically compromised individuals [1,2].

Transformative developments occurred in the late 1960s when Dr. Stanley Dudrick and colleagues at the University of Pennsylvania and Dr. Arvid Wretlind at the Karolinska Institute of Sweden demonstrated the first practical methods of intravenous nutritional support therapy, which was termed "hyperalimentation" [3,4]. Following the realization that this therapy could be universally applied, a practice focus developed to offer specialized management of parenteral and enteral nutrition to hospitalized malnourished patients [3–7]. Although many advancements and refinements have occurred, the essence of nutritional support remains very close to the model first described by Dudrick and Wretlind nearly half a century ago.

The initial function of the early metabolic physician was as the leader of a multidisciplinary team referred to as the nutrition support team (NST). The NST consisted of a physician, dietitian, pharmacist, and IV nurse [8]. These teams were supported by each hospital's administration since it was necessary to provide this complex form of expertise in order to safely administer hyperalimentation.

However, as cost restrictions developed, hospitals sought to reduce the overhead related to the NST or eliminate them entirely.

In its heyday, the NST functioned as a consulting service for the diagnosis of malnutrition, a therapeutic service for the management of malnourished patients, and a care delivery service for the insertion of central venous catheters. The NST monitored all TPN patients, performing routine tasks such as sterile catheter dressing changes and monitoring laboratory data. The NST would routinely recommend or perform adjustments to the TPN formula based on the patient's progress. With the reduction or elimination of full-time equivalent positions on the NST, the metabolic physician was left with the choice of either incorporating the various roles of the NST or stopping to provide nutritional support services.

Although some physicians discontinued their involvement in nutritional support when these constraints occurred, others took on the challenge of amalgamating the roles of the physician, dietitian, pharmacist, and IV access expert to become a metabolic consultant within the hospital. In this new type of practice, a physician consultation for nutritional support would expect the metabolic physician to diagnose the state of malnutrition, outline a course of therapy, insert a central venous catheter, order parenteral nutrition, and monitor the clinical course of therapy. Therefore, the cost-control measures that eliminated financial support for the NST caused a consolidation of clinical duties that can be seen as one of the defining moments of metabolic medicine. In effect, the absence of the NST made the metabolic physician an essential component to the hospital.

At roughly the same time interval as cost constraints in hospitals were being brought to the fore, advances in the science of intravenous nutrition permitted the simplification of TPN formulas and improved the safety of their administration.

Paramount among these advances was the development of efficacious forms of intravenous lipid emulsion. An early form of intravenous fat emulsion had been found to be toxic and was withdrawn from the market [9]. But Wretlind and colleagues realized that if fat emulsion was to be safe for intravenous administration, it would need to mimic the natural way in which fat is transported within the body. This led them to conceptualize the artificial chylomicron, which became the product Intralipid [10].

The newly formed intravenous lipid emulsions proved to be a successful means of administering calories as fat to critically ill patients. Furthermore, the use of intravenous lipid emulsion permitted a reduction in the provision of calories in the form of glucose. Intravenous nutrition could now become a more balanced formula delivering physiologic levels of the macronutrients—protein, carbohydrate, and fat.

This physiologically balanced approach to nutritional support became incongruous with the concept of "hyper" alimentation. A more appropriate term denoting this balanced concept emerged, and the modality became thereafter known as total parental nutrition (TPN) [11].

Another factor for change was developing in the late 1970s: a movement for more patient independence and self-reliance. This movement envisioned that patients would want to be looked upon as health care consumers rather than passive recipients of care.

When the patient independence and cost-control movements converged in the 1980s, long-term hospitalized nutritional support patients with complex illnesses became home TPN patients [12]. The transition from hospital care to home became another facet of the practice of metabolic medicine. Home care techniques became more standardized and routine, allowing hospital-level care to transition into outpatient settings.

With the knowledge gained from the routine monitoring of nutritionally impaired individuals, the field experienced a natural extension to include other disorders of the undernourished, such as vitamin and mineral deficiencies. These previously esoteric conditions were seen commonly in the supervision of patients with short bowel syndrome or enterocutaneous fistulae. As we will see later, the additional role of metabolic monitoring in bariatric surgery further enhanced practical knowledge in the area of micronutrient deficiency.

OBESITY AND BARIATRICS

The practice of obesity medicine also came into reality in the postwar era, roughly at the same time as the field of nutritional support was emerging. Yet, most of the practitioners of obesity and weight loss medicine could not have considered themselves more different from their colleagues in the TPN arena.

The former were mostly composed of endocrinologists, noninvasive cardiologists, and internists. They were mainly office-based practitioners. The latter were surgeons, anesthesiologists, and intensivists. These doctors were primarily hospital-based specialists.

Yet there were some unifying features between the underweight and overweight. Both were suffering from an imbalance of energy stores, albeit on opposite ends of the spectrum. Both had an abnormal body composition, and both required a return to a more balanced healthy equilibrium.

As the obesity problem reached epidemic proportions, the need to treat it more scientifically also grew. Could the growing community of physician nutrition experts created to manage hospital malnutrition apply the knowledge of energy metabolism to the control of body weight and obesity? A scientific method for this was still lacking.

A platform for unification between nutrition support and obesity physicians was created by the development of the protein sparing modified fast (PSMF) by Dr. George Blackburn of Harvard University in the 1970s [13,14]. Dr. Blackburn's earlier work was on the metabolic assessment of the hospitalized patient. His work on energy and nitrogen balance in malnutrition was highly regarded. He was widely seen as a leader in the field of nutritional support.

Blackburn's use of scientific nutritional concepts in the management of obesity created an opportunity for the TPN community to realize a role in obesity management. Many followed Blackburn's lead to open PSMF programs. This created a two-tiered practice environment in which physicians could complement their in-patient nutritional support services with outpatient obesity management.

With this development, doctors who previously thought of their nutritional support work as an adjunct to their medical or surgical practices saw that the field of nutrition and metabolism could become an all-encompassing entity that might stand on its own. In many ways, this recognition can be seen as a watershed moment, which fostered the birth of metabolic medicine as an independent specialty.

The growth of bariatric surgery and the recognition of the metabolic effects of procedures such as the Roux-en-Y gastric bypass and the biliopancreatic diversion further cemented a role for the metabolic physician [15]. These patients faced an array of micronutrient disturbances, which became progressively more severe with the passage of postoperative time. The diagnosis and management of these deficiencies were generally outside the scope of the bariatric surgeon. In fact, most internists were also ill-prepared to accurately diagnose and treat these conditions. But the metabolic physician, flush with experience in the management of the chronically malnourished, was ideally suited to this clinical challenge.

In addition to monitoring, preventing, and managing micronutrient deficiencies, the metabolic physician was called upon to help bariatric patients withdraw from diabetic, hypertensive, and lipid medications. The metabolic physician would also be expected to help wean patients from CPAP devices as the weight loss progressed.

When complications of bariatric surgery occurred, the metabolic physician would be called upon to use his or her nutritional therapeutic skills to support a bariatric patient that could not maintain their intake. A particularly worrisome subset of these patients includes those who become pregnant within a year of surgery and are still rapidly losing weight while supporting a pregnancy. TPN may be required in these settings, completing a conceptual circle that links the historical developments of the field.

The metabolic physician's skills with medical weight loss will also be useful for those bariatric patients who experience weight loss failure (WLF) prior to reaching their goal. Some 20–40% of bariatric surgery patients experience WLF, particularly those who undergo less intense procedures such as the laparoscopic adjustable gastric band (LAGB) [16].

METABOLIC SYNDROME AND CARDIOVASCULAR DISEASE PREVENTION

Another important historical event in metabolic medicine was to take place roughly a decade after the clinical adoption of PSMF programs. In 1988, Dr. Gerald Reaven [17] took the podium to deliver the annual Banting Lecture at Stanford University. In this lecture, he proposed that associated conditions of obesity, impaired glucose tolerance, hyperlipidemia, and hypertension were connected by a common thread: insulin resistance (IR). This concept became known as "Syndrome X" and has since been recognized as MetS. MetS has also been referred to as the cardiometabolic syndrome, IR syndrome, and Reaven's syndrome.

There are differing criteria for the diagnosis of MetS, but most agree that MetS is a constellation of conditions that includes central abdominal adiposity (increased waist circumference), hypertension, dyslipidemia (especially with elevated triglycerides and a low high-density lipoprotein), and impaired glucose tolerance [18]. This subject will be covered in greater detail elsewhere in the textbook.

The presence of IR with some or all of these conditions creates the diagnosis of MetS. Recently, inflammatory biomarkers such as high-sensitivity c-reactive protein have been considered as part of the syndrome [19]. In addition, the development of nonalcoholic fatty liver disease is believed to affect many individuals with IR and MetS [20].

Using this type of criteria, the CDC has estimated that more than 25% of the US population is affected [21]. MetS is a component of 75% of type II diabetes mellitus cases and 50% of patients with coronary artery disease [22]. Furthermore, MetS has been shown to precede both diabetes and cardiovascular disease. Therefore, its early identification can be considered an important tool for the prevention of disease.

The importance of MetS and its prevalence in the general population provided the third significant foundational component to the specialty of metabolic medicine. It created the opportunity for metabolic physicians to differentiate themselves from endocrinologists, cardiologists, and others.

Endocrinologists were involved in the treatment of diabetes and its complications. But the treatment of MetS could be seen as a path to circumventing the development of diabetes. Thus, the metabolic physician was not in the practice of treating diabetes, but preventing it.

Similarly, cardiologists were involved in the treatment of coronary artery disease, atherosclerosis, and hypertension. Instead, metabolic physicians are focused on preventing them.

ADJUNCTIVE THERAPY

The emergence of disease-specific nutritional approaches promises a future in which there is a "metabolic component" of nearly every medical specialty. Similar trends are evident in neurology, nephrology, urology, rheumatology, ophthalmology, immunology, pulmonology, gastroenterology, hepatology, and dermatology. In this regard, metabolic medicine has a potential interaction with the growing specialty of integrative medicine.

AN INTRODUCTION TO NUTRITIONAL BIOCHEMISTRY

PROTEIN

We will begin our overview of nutritional biochemistry with what many consider the most essential of the daily nutritional requirements: protein. Of the three macronutrients, protein is the only one for which the body has no storage form. Therefore, to meet the body's daily needs, protein must either be consumed or administered.

If an exogenous source of protein is not available, the body will initiate a catabolic process to break down intact proteins found in the muscle, solid organs, and circulating plasma. This will liberate amino acids from the structure of otherwise functional proteins. As existing and functional structures are sacrificed for their component amino acids, the health of the individual deteriorates, leading to malnutrition. Therefore, the provision of a source of exogenous protein must be considered a primary goal of nutritional support.

But how to provide the protein, in what form, and how much to give remain areas of controversy. Most experts consider the requirement for protein to be roughly 1 g/kg of ideal body weight (IBW) per day, with a range of 0.5–2.0 g/kg/day. However, the precise protein intake requirements may vary based on the growth rate, physical activity, and the presence of illness or injury.

In general, protein requirements increase during childhood, pregnancy, and breast-feeding. Protein requirements also increase during catabolic states such as infection and trauma when additional protein turnover is occurring. The recovery of protein depletion from malnutrition will also usually require higher than normal amounts of protein intake. On the other hand, protein requirements are generally decreased in patients who cannot adequately metabolize or excrete urea, ammonia, and other waste products of protein metabolism, i.e., patients with renal and/or hepatic insufficiency [23].

Another important concept about protein intake has to do with the value of the form of protein being ingested or administered. Protein foods vary in terms of their amino acid content. The extent with which a protein food's amino acid content differs from that of a standard animal protein source such as a whole egg is referred to as its biological value (BV). The BV also depends on the digestability of the protein source. These factors can be used to assign a numeric BV. For example, by this method, soy protein has been reported to have a BV of 74, whereas whey protein has a BV of 96 [24].

The BV can be used to modify the range of acceptable protein intake. Using this approach, plant-based proteins would require a higher total intake to meet nutritional needs than animal-based proteins. However, in a meta-analysis of nitrogen balance studies to estimate protein requirements in healthy adults, Rand et al. [25] found that the variance was actually quite small. The median requirement for protein in healthy adults ranged from 105 to 132 mg of nitrogen per kilogram per day. This equates to roughly 0.65 to 0.83 g of good-quality protein per kilogram per day [25].

The traditional method of determining the adequacy of protein intake has been the nitrogen (N+) balance. This is a simple concept in which the protein balance is evaluated in terms of N+ intake minus N+ loss. A positive value indicates that more protein was consumed than excreted. A negative value means the opposite. In this method, protein intake is converted to its nitrogen content. This is roughly 16% of the protein content. Therefore, N+ intake is estimated as the protein intake in grams/6.25.

The N+ loss is primarily urinary urea nitrogen. A small amount of urine nitrogen is represented by creatinine, ammonia, hippuric acid, free amino acids, and other nitrogenous waste. Approximately 1 g of nitrogen is lost via the stool and roughly 500 mg through perspiration. Thus, the formula for nitrogen balance is nitrogen intake (total protein intake/6.25) − nitrogen loss (urine nitrogen + fecal nitrogen + dermal nitrogen losses). In practical terms, the urine urea nitrogen alone can be used as a rough estimate for total nitrogen loss. In studies using this method, the 24-h urine urea nitrogen is multiplied by 1.25 to correct for other nitrogenous losses. But some authors feel that this method is error-prone and prefer traditional nitrogen balance studies [26].

ENERGY

Once the body's protein needs are met, the energy requirements can be considered. A number of classic studies have resulted in mathematical derivations to predict the total energy expenditure (TEE). The most well recognized of these is the Harris–Benedict equation (HBE) [27]. A number of others, including the Ireton-Jones equation, have gained favor recently [28].

Many clinicians use a simple estimate based on kilocalories per kilogram of IBW An average person requires 20–40 kcal/kg/day. A rule of thumb estimate of the midrange value, 30 kcal/kg/day, works in most cases. But fuel requirements vary broadly based on growth, physical activity, and the presence of illness or injury.

In 1963, Dr. John Kinney began his studies on the effects of stress on energy requirements. This work, performed over the course of two decades in the famed surgical metabolic unit (SMU) of the Columbia-Presbyterian Medical Center, delineated the concept of stress metabolism [29]. Under this framework, we have come to understand that energy needs increase incrementally with increasing levels of stress.

Energy expenditure can be measured by a number of techniques including direct calorimetry, indirect calorimetry, and stable isotope techniques. But from a practical point of view, indirect calorimetry is the standard method. This can be obtained through the use of a simple bedside oxygen consumption (VO2) device, which uses a modified Weir equation to convert VO2 into a resting metabolic rate (RMR) [30]. More complex forms of indirect calorimetry devices also measure CO_2 production (VCO2) and yield a respiratory quotient (RQ). In the latter example, data from VO2 and VCO2 can be used to provide information on substrate utilization in addition to energy expenditure.

The total daily expenditure or TEE is composed of three major components. The basal metabolic rate (BMR) represents the amount of fuel needed for organ function at rest. The major fuel consumers under basal conditions are the liver, brain, resting skeletal muscle, kidneys, and heart. Because it is difficult to ensure a true basal state in which the sympathetic nervous system is not stimulated, we generally substitute a more practical method known as the RMR for the BMR.

The RMR represents about 70% of the daily TEE. The daily activity energy expenditure (AEE) contributes approximately 20% of the TEE. Thermogenesis, also referred to as the thermic effect of food (TEF), contributes the remaining 10% of the TEE.

Energy can be provided by carbohydrates, lipids, and protein. The requirement for protein has been reviewed above. But clinicians often forget that one of the uses of dietary protein is to provide the backbone for glucose production during gluconeogenesis. Roughly a third of dietary protein is ultimately utilized as fuel, not protein synthesis. Therefore, the protein intake's energy value must be considered as part of the total daily energy intake.

It is useful to consider the fuel intake in terms of separate nonprotein calorie and protein intakes. The ratio of these components can vary based on the patient's requirements. Nutritional science has traditionally referred to protein intake by way of the nitrogen content provided. So the relationship of nonprotein calories to protein intake is expressed as the nonprotein-calorie-to-nitrogen ratio (NPC/N).

The more stressed an individual is, the more protein they are likely to require. This is due to the increased gluconeogenesis that accompanies catabolism. Since protein (i.e., nitrogen) is the denominator of the NPC/N ratio equation, a higher protein intake automatically means a smaller NPC/N ratio. The recognized desirable NPC/N ratios are as follows: 80:1 for patients under severe stress, 100:1 for patients under moderate stress, and 150:1 for patients without additional stress [31].

Another concept worthy of mention here is that more nonprotein calories, especially in the form of carbohydrates, tend to enhance N+ balance. This is referred to as the nitrogen (protein) sparing effect of glucose. Under this concept, studies with a fixed amount of nitrogen (protein) showed progressively increased N+ balance when the nonprotein calories (glucose) were increased [32].

CARBOHYDRATES

Humans require roughly 3 g of glucose per kilogram of IBW. For an average 70-kg male, this is around 200 g/day. Glucose requirement can also be expressed in terms of milligrams per kilogram per minute. Most authors use a value of 2–3 mg/kg/min for this approach. Interestingly, for the same average 70-kg male, the latter formula yields a glucose requirement of roughly 200 g/day. Therefore, there is near unity between the two formulas. A more precise estimate can be obtained if a metabolic cart measurement is available with an RQ. Using this information, a calculated value for carbohydrate oxidation can be derived [33].

Dietary carbohydrates are available in the form of simple sugars, oligosaccharides, and polysaccharides or complex carbohydrates. The latter are composed of glycogen, starches, and fiber. Fibers are further subdivided into soluble and insoluble forms.

Simple sugars, oligosaccharides, and polysaccharides are rapidly digested by the human gastrointestinal tract, beginning in the mouth with salivary alpha amylase. In the gut, pancreatic alpha amylase completes the digestion of glycogen and the starches amylose and amylopectin. Simple sugars such as glucose and fructose are directly absorbed. Disaccharides such as lactose, sucrose, and maltose are digested by their corresponding brush border enzymes. Other disaccharides also exist on the brush border.

Dietary fibers are polysaccharides whose chemical bonds are not susceptible to breakdown by alpha-amylase. Therefore, they are indigestible by the human gut and pass into the colon unprocessed. Bacteria of the colon digest these fiber polysaccharides as fuel and may yield important byproducts such as short-chain fatty acids. Undigested fiber also plays important roles in water-holding capacity, which assists in stool elimination, bowel cleansing, and toxin adsorption.

LIPIDS

Dietary lipids are almost entirely composed of long-chain triglycerides (LCT), either of animal or plant origin. There is a very small daily requirement for lipids, roughly 10 g/day. Most of this is the requirement for linoleic acid to form prostaglandins and leukotrienes. There is also a requirement for intake of the fat-soluble vitamins (A, D, E, and K).

LCTs are digested through pancreatic lipase and a complex brush border process that de-esterifies and re-esterifies them to be transported via the gut lymphatics in the form of chylomicrons. Dietary fats can be subdivided into saturated and unsaturated. The unsaturated portion is then further subdivided into monounsaturated and polyunsaturated fats. Among the polyunsaturated fats, a differentiation between omega-6 fatty acids and omega-3 fatty acids has proven to be of clinical significance. This subject will be addressed in greater detail elsewhere in the text.

STARVATION METABOLISM

The metabolic machinery of the human body uses energy continuously. To protect the fuel source, the body preserves energy balance very carefully and defends itself from becoming depleted. Our biological machines are kept at the ready so that we can respond to a challenge quickly. Organ function and skeletal muscle maintain a high energy use even at rest.

When food is not available for an extended period, and we enter starvation, the body shifts fuel utilization and substrate production. This is mostly designed to protect ongoing function for the central nervous system and erythrocytes (Figure 1.1) [34].

Since the erythrocytes are glucose dependent, the loss of exogenous glucose presents a metabolic challenge. This is first met by depleting stored carbohydrates in the form of glycogen. However, hepatic glycogen stores are generally only capable of sustaining glucose output for 1–2 days.

As the glycogen stores become depleted, gluconeogenesis must serve as the source for glucose. The liver and kidneys perform this function through the catabolism of alanine and glutamate.

The liver performs roughly 60% of the necessary gluconeogenesis using alanine derived from muscle catabolism as its carbon source. The kidneys degrade glutamine for the remainder. In both instances, the amino acids are cleaved of their nitrogen and the remaining carbon skeletons are utilized to form glucose. The liberated amino groups are then converted to urea or excreted as free ammonia (Figure 1.2) [35].

However, gluconeogenesis cannot continue to be the source for a fuel substrate for the brain and RBCs indefinitely. If it were, the body would consume so much muscle that long-term survival of the entire organism would be dramatically compromised.

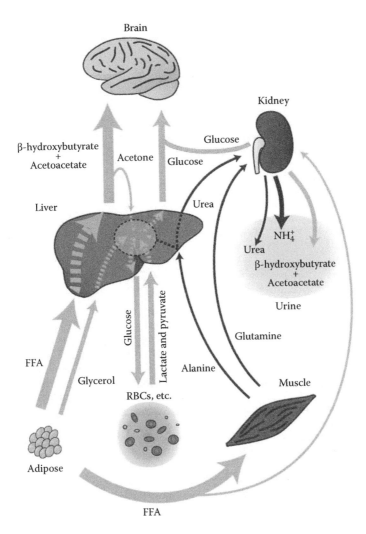

FIGURE 1.1 **(See color insert.)** Overall scheme of starvation fuel metabolism. The liver derives its major energy by partial oxidation of free fatty acids (FFAs) to beta-hydroxybutyrate and acetoacetate; muscle and kidney by complete oxidation of FFA to CO_2 and H_2O. The brain utilizes beta-hydroxybutyrate, acetoacetate, and glucose. Erythrocytes (RBC) require glucose. (Reprinted from Cahill GF, *Ann Rev Nutr* 2006;26:1–22. With permission.)

To compensate, a key adaptation for starvation metabolism must occur in order to spare the muscle protein [36]. This concept is often referred to as "nitrogen sparing." In order to permit long-term maintenance of substrate provision, this adaptation must find an alternative source of substrate for the body's major fuel consuming organ, the brain; for the most part, that alternate substrate is ketone bodies released from fatty tissue.

Studies by Owen, Felig, and Cahill in the late 1960s demonstrated that two-thirds of brain substrate consumption during starvation could be attributed to beta-hydroxybutyrate and acetoacetate [37,38]. A normal adult could survive for 2 months of starvation with this adapted metabolism. An obese individual could survive much longer (Figure 1.3).

The production of ketone bodies begins to occur within 3–4 days of starvation and has an immediate effect on reducing gluconeogenesis and sparing muscle protein. Plasma levels of

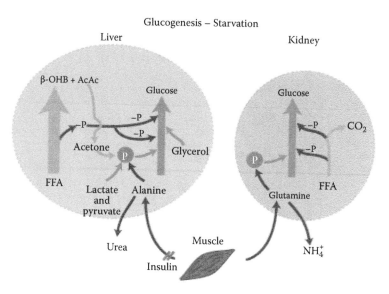

FIGURE 1.2 **(See color insert.)** Glucogenesis in starvation in liver and kidney. Precursors in liver via mitochondrial pyruvate carboxylation (white "P" in blue circle) are acetone, recycling lactate and pyruvate, and pyruvate from deaminated alanine from muscle. Glycerol from adipose tissue enters the glucogenic pathway at triose phosphate. Precursors in kidney are from deamidated and deaminated glutamine with the alpha-ketoglutarate residue made into glucose via the classical mitochondrial and glucogenic intermediates. The energy (–P) in kidney is derived from FFAs to CO_2 and H_2O. In liver, it is mainly from ketogenesis. Nitrogen is returned to blood by liver urea synthesis for renal excretion and in kidney by synthesis and excretion of NH_4. The latter titrates the renal loss of acetoacetate and beta-hydroxybutyrate. (Reprinted from Cahill GF, *Ann Rev Nutr* 2006;26:1–22. With permission.)

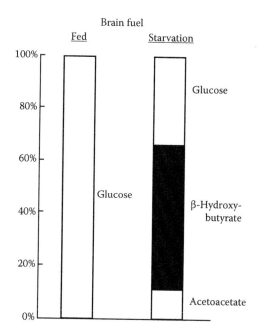

FIGURE 1.3 Brain substrate utilization in three fasting obese volunteers after several weeks of starvation. Many studies suggest that human brain cells can survive with little to no glucose, but proving the point is difficult as well as experimentally difficult and ethically questionable. (Reprinted from Cahill GF, *Ann Rev Nutr* 2006;26:1–22. With permission.)

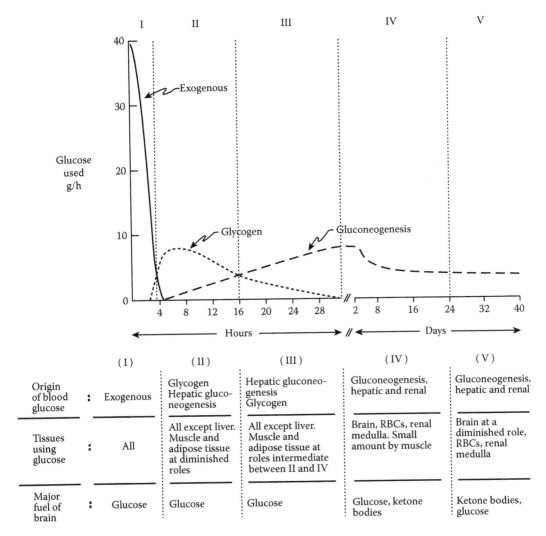

FIGURE 1.4 The five metabolic stages between the postabsorptive state and the near-steady state of prolonged starvation. (Reprinted from Cahill GF, *Ann Rev Nutr* 2006;26:1–22. With permission.)

acetoacetate rise by more than 100%, whereas the beta hydroxybutyrate rises by more than three orders of magnitude.

Levels of FFAs are also elevated to provide fuel for the nonglucose-dependent tissues. A small amount of glucose production continues through recycled lactate and pyruvate. There is also a small amount of ongoing glucose synthesis from fat-derived glycerol and ketone bodies (Figure 1.4) [34].

STRESS METABOLISM

The baseline resting metabolic rate runs at around 1 cal/min or roughly 1500 cal/day. We are capable of increasing this by multiples of our basal metabolism (Mets) for short requirements like exercise. But it is very unusual to see the daily metabolic expenditure increase by more than twice the baseline. Stress increases the metabolic rate by means of sympathetic nervous system activation, endocrine changes, and immunohematological changes occurring in response to injury, infection, trauma, etc.

Some of the metabolic rate changes are direct consequences of the underlying condition. For example, an infection will cause an increased temperature, heart rate, and cardiac output. There will also be a cytokine and neutrophil response along with lymphocyte activation. The immunologic system will have initiated a cascade of events leading to eliminating foreign organisms, toxins, injured tissue, etc.

On the other hand, the changes in metabolic rate and fuel utilization in stress are directed to providing protein and energy requirements to repair injured tissues and maintain homeostatic function in support systems.

Kinney et al. [39] described three distinct levels of stress response: mild, moderate, and severe. This correlated with increased nitrogen loss and negative nitrogen balances. He and Elwyn postulated that this phenomenon was due to various degrees of elevation in the stress response hormones from the hypothalamus, pituitary, thyroid, adrenals, and pancreas. This was referred to as the neuroendocrine stress response (NESR) (Figures 1.5 through 1.7). Chernow and others later correlated the stress degree to actual hormone levels in ICU patients [40–43].

The principal hormonal responses to stress include growth hormone, adrenocorticotrophic hormone, thyroid-stimulating hormone, follicle-stimulating hormone, luteinizing hormone, vasopressin, cortisol, aldosterone, epinephrine, norepinephrine, insulin, glucagon, thyroxine, and triiodothyronine [40,44,45]. The net effect of the NESR is to increase catabolism and to alter fuel utilization. The same hormonal signaling that increases glucose production through gluconeogenesis provokes lipolysis and the release of FFAs. Simultaneously, insulin resistance limits the use of the newly manufactured glucose by muscle and adipocytes [46].

As in starvation, glucose production during stress metabolism is initially supported through glycogenolysis. But glycogen will be more quickly depleted in stress than in starvation because the metabolic rate has been increased. Fortunately, the biochemical effect of cyclic AMP signaling by elevated hormones will be translated into ongoing gluconeogenesis.

This process utilizes amino acids from tissue breakdown (primarily muscle), lactate and pyruvate from tissue glycolysis, and glycerol from fatty acids [44]. Patients in stress metabolism may increase the glucose production from a normal of 200 g/day to as much as 400 g/day [47]. The process of obtaining the amino acids needed for gluconeogenesis requires catabolization of intact protein from functional structures. Catabolic cytokines like TNF-alpha appear to be essential to the activation of this process [48]. Protein is then catabolized via several pathways, including lysosomal, cytosolic, and mitochondrial systems. But the ubiquitin–proteosome pathway appears to be responsible for the bulk of intracellular protein degradation [49].

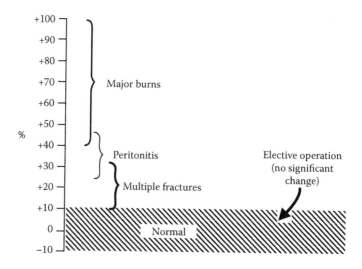

FIGURE 1.5   Effects of injury and sepsis on resting energy expenditure. (Based on Kinney JM et al., *J Clin Path* 1970;4(Suppl 23):65–72. Reproduced from Long CL, *Am J Clin Nutr* 1977;30(8):1301–10.)

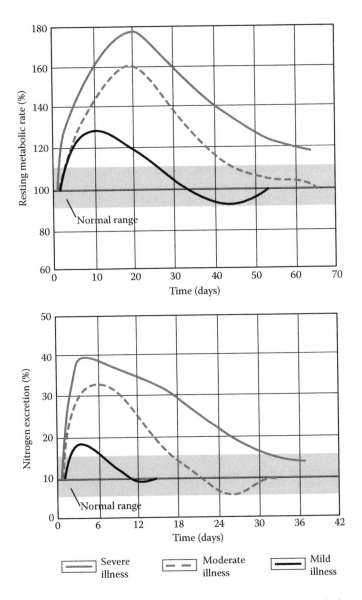

Severe illness ———   **Moderate illness** – – –   **Mild illness** ———

FIGURE 1.6 Increased resting metabolic activity (hypermetabolism) and increased nitrogen loss are closely related during critical surgical illness. Both correlate with the severity of illness and return to normal as the patient recovers. Patients with severe illness are represented by the solid gray line, those with moderate illness by the broken gray line, and those with mild illness by the solid black line; the normal range is shown by the light-gray bar. (Reproduced from Bessey PQ, *Metabolic Response to Critical Illness*, Chapter 25. ACS Surgery, WebMD, Inc, 2004. Available at http://www.acssurgery.com. With permission.)

The free amino acids released must then be deaminated so that the carbon skeletons can be converted into fuel. The glucogenic amino acids are converted to alpha ketoacids via hepatic transaminases and then to pyruvate, alpha ketoglutarate, succinyl CoA, or fumarate. The final Krebs cycle step is the conversion to oxaloacetate and then to glucose.

On the other hand, ketogenic amino acids are converted to acetoacetate and acetyl CoA. Most of the ketogenic amino acids can also be used for gluconeogenesis. But two, lysine and leucine, can only be converted to ketones (Figures 1.8 and 1.9) [50].

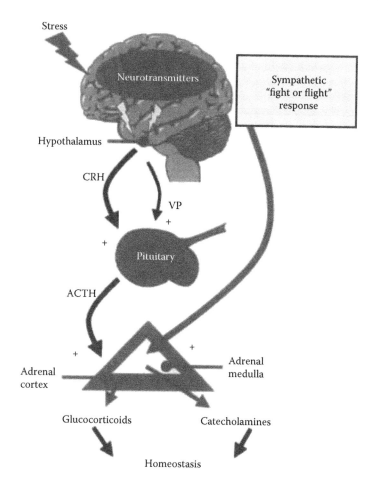

FIGURE 1.7 The NESR. The hypothalamic–pituitary axis can be stimulated by either neural impulses or humoral agents released by circulating inflammatory cells. (From Matteri RL et al., *Biology of Animal Stress: Basic Principles and Implications for Animal Welfare.* CAB International, Wallingford, UK, 2000. With permission.)

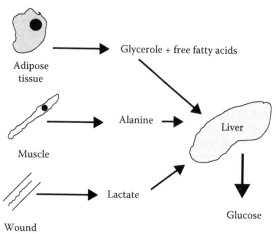

FIGURE 1.8 Hepatic gluconeogenesis is increased during stress. Sources of substrate include glycerol from lipolysis, alanine from proteolysis, and lactate from anaerobic glycolysis. (From Weissman C, *Crit Care* 1999;3:R67–R75. With permission.)

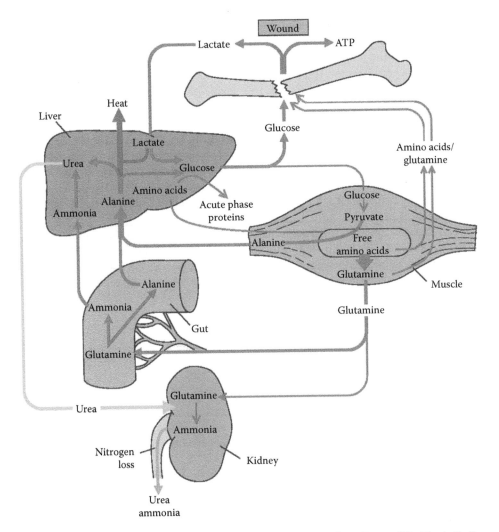

FIGURE 1.9 (See color insert.) Metabolic response to critical illness. (From Bessey PQ, *Metabolic Response to Critical Illness*, Chapter 25. ACS Surgery, WebMD, Inc, 2004. Available at http://www.acssurgery.com. With permission.)

The deamination of glucogenic amino acids results in nitrogen disposal via the urea cycle, ammonia, and other pathways. Ureagenesis accounts for roughly 85% of the body's nitrogen elimination. Therefore, the degree of amino acid catabolism occurring is reflected by the amount of urea excretion. The 24-h urine urea nitrogen thus provides a valuable insight to this phenomenon.

The biochemical sequences outlined above result in increased energy expenditure and fuel requirements. Furthermore, there is an alteration in fuel utilization toward glucose uptake. The NESR helps address the need for increased fuel by promoting glucose production through gluconeogenesis. The same pathways are responsible for inducing lipolysis and releasing FFAs.

We lack the metabolic processes to efficiently convert the fatty acids into glucose. But the stress metabolic state helps promote fatty acid oxidation. Therefore, we have two fuel systems running during stress metabolism: glucose and fatty acids. The remaining issue to delineate in our understanding of fuel utilization during stress is: which fuel goes where.

During stress metabolism, the body is going to great effort and expense to liberate energy sources. It is breaking down structural protein to support gluconeogenesis, sacrificing function to make fuel. It would not be logical to allow glucose produced in this manner to be used indiscriminately. This is especially true because certain essential cells are obligate glucose metabolizers while others are not.

It would be ideal if the glucose produced by the stress metabolic state could be restricted to use by the glucose-dependent tissues. In particular, there should be a filter that blocks the significant body cell mass of adipose tissue and muscle from using glucose produced during stress metabolism. This would, in effect, ensure that glucose manufactured through the process of catabolism is shunted to the cells that need it most.

The method by which the body directs glucose uptake is the glucose transport protein (GLUT) system. The GLUT, or SLC2A, are a family of transmembrane proteins that facilitate the transport of glucose and related sugars. Different glucose transporters are expressed in certain cell types. GLUT1 is found in erythrocytes and at the blood–brain barrier. GLUT2 is found in the liver, pancreatic beta cells, and kidney. GLUT3 is found in neurons and many other tissues. GLUT4 is found in muscle and fat [51,52].

GLUTs 1–3 are independent of insulin and can facilitate the diffusion of glucose without it. When insulin binds to the insulin receptors on the surface of muscle and fat cells, it initiates a cascade of events involving the insulin receptor substrate (IRS-1) system and intracellular enzymes such as PI-3 kinase. This results in the exocytosis of GLUT4 vesicles and the surface expression of GLUT4, leading to facilitated diffusion of glucose into the cells [53].

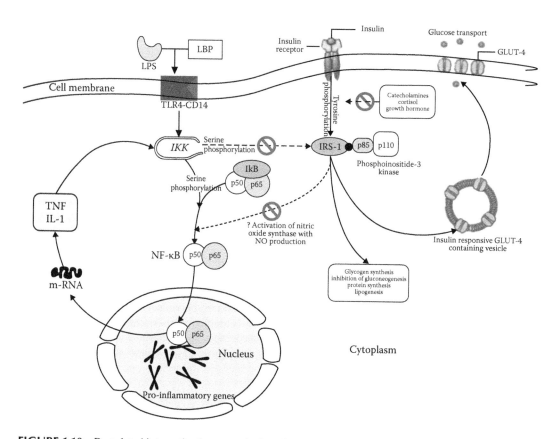

FIGURE 1.10 Postulated interaction between the insulin signaling pathway and activation of the proinflammatory cascade in the pathogenesis of stress hyperglycemia of sepsis. LPS: lipopolysaccharide; LBP: lipopolysaccharide binding protein; TLR4: Toll-like receptor 4; IkB: inhibitor; IKK: inhibitor kB kinase; IRS-1: insulin receptor substrate-1; IL-1: interleukin-1; TNF: tumor necrosis factor; NFκB: nuclear factor-kappa B. (Marik PE, Raghavan M, *Intensive Care Med* 2004;30:748–756. With permission.)

If we examine the distribution of glucose transporters from the perspective of their dependence on insulin, an interesting dichotomy emerges. It is apparent that the obligate glucose metabolizers (the CNS and erythrocytes) do not need insulin to facilitate glucose transport because they have GLUTs 1–3 expression. But, without insulin, muscle and adipose cannot activate their glucose transporter (GLUT4) sufficiently to adequately uptake glucose. This implies that the level of insulin or the sensitivity of the insulin receptor would play an important role in restricting the uptake of glucose into nonglucose-dependent cells during stress metabolism (Figure 1.10) [54].

Stress metabolic states, such as sepsis, are characterized by IR. As was shown by the early work of Kinney, Chernow, and others, the counterregulatory hormone levels and IR increase proportionately with the level of the stress response. The biochemistry of the IR in stress conditions has now been elucidated to reveal that insulin-induced tyrosine phosphorylation of IRS-1 and activation of PI-3 kinase are impaired in this state [54]. This contributes to the blocking of glucose uptake by non-obligate glucose metabolizers during stress, thereby conserving the glucose produced through gluconeogenesis for the tissues that need it most.

Understanding this complex sequence of events has led us to a more complete comprehension of energy and protein metabolism during stress. The NESR appears to have developed a masterful set of mechanisms to preserve energy delivery while minimizing the necessary sacrifices it creates. It is crucial that physicians caring for patients in stress metabolism recognize this homeostatic balance and avoid disrupting it inappropriately.

SUMMARY

This chapter has provided an overview of a newly emerging specialty, metabolic medicine. We have reviewed its historical development and highlighted its key points of evolution. Particular attention was given to the development of scientific approaches in three major clinical areas: malnutrition, obesity management, and the MetS.

The proper assessment and management of patients suffering from malnutrition can be a complex and challenging undertaking. Astute observation, skilled physical examination, and a thorough understanding of the biochemistry involved are the prerequisites for the clinician managing these difficult cases. The metabolic physician must fully appreciate the clinical impact of the many biochemical pathways involved in the patient's illness. He or she must be prepared to integrate this knowledge for the patient's benefit at the bedside.

In taking on this role, the clinician should be aware of the awesome responsibility that it involves. This is particularly true with the administration of central TPN, as this therapy artificially replaces posthepatic nutrient delivery to the central circulation. Therefore, the metabolic physician should project his or her thinking in terms of what would be expected from the gut and liver if normal nutrition were possible under the clinical circumstances.

If they are willing to take on the responsibility of this role, the metabolic physician can play a vital part in assisting with the care of complex patients, particularly during their hospital stay and critical illness. Appropriate attention to the patient's nutritional requirements may make the difference between a favorable and unfavorable outcome. But the "metabolist" must be cautious not to overwhelm the patient's physiology and attempt to rapidly correct malnutrition. As in any specialty, the effective clinician walks a fine line between providing benefit and managing risk.

The natural extension of TPN and enteral therapies into the home care environment for patients who need ongoing nutritional support is another valuable service performed by practitioners in our specialty. Once again, there is a high degree of responsibility incumbent on this type of management. The metabolic physician should establish methods and protocols within his/her practice to appropriately supervise the members of the home care team and protect the patient from the potential metabolic and infectious complications of home infusion.

The provision of compassionate, comprehensive management of obesity and its related diseases provides an important opportunity for the metabolic physician to utilize his or her clinical expertise for the benefit of the patient. This extends from those patients seeking medical management of obesity to those who undergo weight-loss surgeries and require ongoing metabolic monitoring. Once again, the application of scientific biochemical principles can distinguish the metabolic physician from other members of the obesity management team and provide crucial support for a favorable outcome.

The appropriate evaluation and aggressive treatment of patients with the MetS has the potential to prevent the development of diabetes and cardiovascular disease. This process is likely to be too time-consuming for the primary care physician. The metabolic physician has a significant opportunity to improve the health of the community at large by utilizing the diagnosis and management of MetS to prevent disease.

We have briefly examined some of the fundamental scientific concepts that underlie the clinical aspects of the field. We have also summarized some of the fundamental biochemistry involved in metabolism, such as protein and energy requirements, starvation metabolism, and stress metabolism. Most of the subjects described in this introduction will be discussed in greater detail throughout this volume. For more specific information on the biochemistry involved, the reader is referred to the recent textbook, *Functional Biochemistry*, by our late mentor, Dr. Eric Newsholme of Oxford University [23].

The field of metabolic medicine represents a paradigm shift in health care. Unlike other specialties that are based on a single organ system or a particular set of practitioner skills, metabolic medicine addresses a broad array of conditions that are linked by their biochemistry. As has been shown above, the historical need to develop the specialty was driven by a clinical imperative to manage patients whose problems required knowledge that was generally outside of the scope of standard medical approaches. Therefore, the patient's needs were not being adequately addressed by existing medical specialties. What has emerged is a practice entity that cuts across the traditional borderlines of our health care system's hierarchical structure.

As the field coalesces, metabolic physicians will find themselves called upon by a wide variety of their colleagues to assist in the management of patients whose conditions have their roots in, or are affected by, unique aspects of their metabolism. Furthermore, patients may directly seek out a metabolic physician, after realizing that standard medical care cannot adequately address their conditions.

The authors hope that this textbook will provide a reliable reference point as the readers undertake the intricate work of evaluating and caring for the complex individuals who require metabolic support. This can often be an arduous and intimidating process. But we believe that the metabolic physician will find gratification and fulfillment in the performance of a vital and unique service for the benefit of their patients, colleagues, and the community.

ACKNOWLEDGMENTS

The authors thank Kelly Iorillo for reviewing the manuscript and Zachary Simon Rothkopf for his editorial assistance in its preparation.

REFERENCES

1. Bistrian BR, Blackburn GL, Vitale J, Cochran D, Naylor J. Prevalence of malnutrition in general medical patients. *JAMA* 1979;235:1567–1570.
2. Weinsier RL, Hunker EM, Krumdieck CL, Butterworth CE Jr. Hospital malnutrition. A prospective evaluation of general medical patients during the course of hospitalization. *Am J Clin Nutr* 1979;32:418–426.
3. Dudrick SJ, Wilmore DW, Vars HM, Rhoads JE. Long-term total parenteral nutrition with growth, development and positive nitrogen balance. *Surgery* 1968;64:134–142.
4. Dudrick SJ. History of parenteral nutrition. *J Am Coll Nutr* 2009;28:243–251.
5. Dudrick SJ, Rhoads JE. New horizons for intravenous feedings. *JAMA* 1971;215:939–949.
6. Dudrick SJ, Long JM, Steiger E, Rhoads JE. Intravenous hyperalimentation. *Med Clin N Am* 1970;54:577–589.

7. Dudrick SJ, Ruberg TL. Principles and practice of parenteral nutrition. *Gastroenterology* 1971;61:901–910.

8. Skoutakis VA, Martinez DR, Miller WA. Team approach to total parenteral nutrition. *Am J Hosp Pharm* 1975;32:693–697.

9. Brown RO, Minard G. Parenteral nutrition. In Shils ME, Shike M (eds.), *Modern Nutrition in Health and Disease*. Lippincott Williams & Wilkins, Ambler, PA, 2006.

10. Schuberth O, Wretlind A. Intravenous infusion of fat emulsions, phosphatides and emulsifying agents. *Acta Chir Scand* 1961;278(Suppl):1–21.

11. Vinnars E, Wilmore D. Jonathan Roads Symposium Papers. History of parenteral nutrition. *JPEN J Parenter Enteral Nutr* 2003;27:225–231.

12. Rothkopf MM. Concept and scope of intensive homecare. In Rothkopf MM, Askanazi J (eds.). *Intensive Homecare*. Lippincott Williams & Wilkins, Baltimore, MD, 1992.

13. Blackburn GL, Greenberg I. Multidisciplinary approach to adult obesity therapy. *Int J Obesity* 1978;2:133–142.

14. Bistrian BR. Clinical use of a protein-sparing modified fast. *JAMA* 1978;2401:2299–2302.

15. Fujioka K. Follow-up of nutritional and metabolic problems after bariatric surgery. *Diabetes Care* 2005;28:481–484.

16. Bessler M, Daud A, DiGiorgi MF, Schrope BA, Inabnet WB, Davis DG. Frequency distribution of weight loss percentage after gastric bypass and adjustable gastric banding. *Surg Obes Relat Dis* 2008;4:486–491.

17. Reaven GM. Banting Lecture 1988. Role of insulin resistance in human disease. *Diabetes* 1988;37:1595–1607.

18. Grundy SM, Brewer HB Jr, Cleeman JI, Smith SC Jr, Lenfant C; American Heart Association; National Heart, Lung, and Blood Institute. Definition of metabolic syndrome: Report of the National Heart, Lung, and Blood Institute/American Heart Association conference on scientific issues related to definition. *Circulation* 2004;109:433–438.

19. Ridker PM, Wilson PWF, Grundy SM. Should C-reactive protein be added to metabolic syndrome and to assessment of global cardiovascular risk? *Circulation* 2004;109:2818–2825.

20. Marchesini G, Brizi M, Bianchi G, Tomassetti S, Bugianesi E, Lenzi M, McCullough AJ, Natale S, Forlani G, Melchionda N. Nonalcoholic fatty liver disease: A feature of the metabolic syndrome. *Diabetes* 2001;50:1844–1850.

21. Ervin RB. Prevalence of metabolic syndrome among adults 20 years of age and over, by sex, age, race and ethnicity, and body mass index: United States, 2003–2006. *Natl Health Stat Report* 2009;(13):1–7.

22. Chung EH, Curran PJ, Sivasankaran S, Manish S, Chauhan DE, Grossman CT, Pyne TC, Piemonte JW, Bilazarian S. Prevalence of metabolic syndrome in patients < or = 45 years of age with acute myocardial infarction having percutaneous coronary intervention. *Am J Cardiol* 2007;100:1052–1055.

23. Newsholme EA, Leech A. *Functional Biochemistry in Health and Disease*. John Wiley and Sons, West Sussex, UK, 2010.

24. Chick H, Boas-Fixsen MA, Hutchinson JCD, Jackson HM. The biological value of proteins. *Biochem J* 1935;29:1712–1719.

25. Rand WM, Pellett PL, Young VR. Meta-analysis of nitrogen balance studies for estimating protein requirements in healthy adults. *Am J Clin Nutr* 2003;77:109–127.

26. Konstantinides FN, Konstantinides NN, Li JC, Myaya ME, Cerra FB. Urinary urea nitrogen: Too insensitive for calculating nitrogen balance studies in surgical clinical nutrition. *JPEN J Parenter Enteral Nutr* 1991;15:189–193.

27. Harris JA, Benedict FG. *Biometric Studies of Basal Metabolism in Man*. Publication No 279. Carnegie Institute of Washington, Washington, DC, 1919.

28. Ireton-Jones CS, Turner WW Jr, Liepa GU, Baxter CR. Equations for the estimation of energy expenditures in patients with burns with special reference to ventilatory status. *J Burn Care Rehabil* 1992;13: 330–333.

29. Kinney JM et al. *Nutrition and Metabolism in Patient Care*. Saunders, Philadelphia, 1988.

30. Weir JB. New methods for calculating metabolic rate with special reference to protein metabolism. *J Physiol* 1949;109:1–9.

31. Skipper A, Tupesis N. Is there a role for nonprotein calories in developing and evaluating the nutrient prescription? *Nutr Clin Prac* 2005;20:321–324.

32. Elwyn DH, Gump FE, Iles M, Long CL, Kinney JM. Protein and energy sparing of glucose added in hypocaloric amounts to peripheral infusions of amino acids. *Metabolism* 1978;27:325–331.

33. Burstein S, Elwyn DH, Askanazi J, Kinney JM, Kvetan V, Rothkopf MM, Weissman C. *Energy Metabolism, Indirect Calorimetry, and Nutrition*. Lippincott Williams & Wilkins, Baltimore, MD, 1989.

34. Cahill GF. Fuel metabolism in starvation. *Ann Rev Nutr* 2006;26:1–22.

35. Kerndt PR, Naughton JL, Driscoll CE, Loxterkamp DA. Fasting: The history, pathophysiology and complications (medical progress). *West J Med* 1982;137:379–399.
36. Edens NK, Gil KM, Elwyn DH. The effects of varying energy and nitrogen intake on nitrogen balance, body composition, and metabolic rate. *Clin Chest Med* 1986;7:3–17.
37. Owen OE, Felig P, Morgan AP, Wahren J, Cahill GF. Liver and kidney metabolism during prolonged starvation. *J Clin Invest* 1969;48:574–583.
38. Owen OE, Morgan AP, Kemp HG, Sullivan JM, Herrera MG, Cahill GF. Brain metabolism during fasting. *J Clin Invest* 1967;46:1589–1595.
39. Kinney JM, Duke JH Jr, Long CL, Gump FE. Tissue fuel and weight loss after injury. *J Clin Path* 1970;4(Suppl 23):65–72.
40. Chernow B, Anderson DM. Endocrine responses to critical illness. *Semin Respir Med* 1985;7:1–10.
41. Long CL. Energy balance and carbohydrate metabolism in infection and sepsis. *Am J Clin Nutr* 1977;30:1301–1310.
42. Bessey PQ. *Metabolic Response to Critical Illness*, Chapter 25. ACS Surgery, WebMD, Inc, New York, NY, 2004.
43. Matteri RL, Carrol JA, Dyer CJ. *Biology of Animal Stress: Basic Principles and Implications for Animal Welfare*. CAB International, Wallingford, UK, 2000.
44. Weissman C. The metabolic response to stress: An overview and update. *Anesthesiology* 1990;73:308–327.
45. Desborough JP, Hall GM. Endocrine response to surgery. In Kaufman L (ed.), *Anaesthesia Review*, Vol. 10. Churchill Livingstone, Edinburgh, 1993;131–148.
46. Goldstein SA, Elwyn DH. The effects of injury and sepsis on fuel utilization. *Ann Rev Nutr* 1989;9:445–473.
47. Black PR, Brooks DC, Bessey PQ, Wolfe RR, Wilmore DW. Mechanisms of insulin resistance following injury. *Ann Surg* 1982;196:420–435.
48. Cooney RN, Kimball SR, Vary TC. Regulation of skeletal muscle protein turnover during sepsis: Mechanisms and mediators. *Shock* 1997;7:1–16.
49. Lecker SH, Solomon V, Mitch WE, Goldberg AL. Muscle protein breakdown and the critical role of the ubiquitin-proteasome pathway in normal and disease states. *J Nutr* 1999;129:227S–237S.
50. Weissman C. Nutrition in the intensive care unit. *Crit Care* 1999;3:R67–R75.
51. Wright PA. Nitrogen excretion: Three end products, many physiological roles. *J Exp Biol* 1995;198:273–281.
52. Wright EM, Turk E. The sodium/glucose cotransport family SLC5. *Pflügers Archiv* 2004;447:510–518.
53. Saltiel AR, Kahn CR. Insulin signalling and the regulation of glucose and lipid metabolism. *Nature* 2001;414:799–806.
54. Marik PE, Raghavan M. Stress-hyperglycemia, insulin and immunomodulation in sepsis. *Intensive Care Med* 2004;30:748–756.

2 Practice of Metabolic Medicine

Michael M. Rothkopf, Lisa P. Haverstick,
and Michael J. Nusbaum

CONTENTS

In this chapter, we will outline the day-to-day activities of the metabolic physician as taken from our own experience within the field over the last 25 years. Our metabolic approach to the patient will be presented as an example of the type of evaluations we routinely perform. This review is intended to provide insight into the actual processes of functioning as a metabolic physician. We believe that it also provides a structural framework or primer for those contemplating entering the field.

PRACTICE COMPONENTS

The specialty of metabolic medicine contains six main components and practice focus regions. Most practitioners in the field balance a mixture of these functions within each day of the practice. Additional components may surface over the course of time that can become important aspects of the practitioner's individual activities.

For example, we were recently asked to begin routine consultations of patients admitted to the hospital with fragility fractures. These patients generally have osteoporosis and would benefit from a metabolic bone disease evaluation and treatment of the underlying condition. The large number of patients admitted with fragility fracture has required us to commit significant resources to these consultations and office follow-up. On the other hand, consultations for conditions such as AIDS wasting syndrome, which was a major component of our work in the early days of the epidemic, have practically disappeared with advances in antiviral therapy.

Hospital Consultations for Malnutrition and Monitoring of Nutritional Support

The specialty of metabolic medicine had its roots in addressing the challenges of providing nutritional support to the malnourished and metabolically stressed hospital patient. Most of our colleagues practicing in the field continue to see such patients as part of their regular day's schedule.

A metabolic medicine consultation is generally called if the patient has evidence of malnutrition and is unable to eat. The consult may be generated by the hospitalist, internist, oncologist, surgeon, or any other member of the medical staff. In some hospitals, the metabolic medicine consultation is triggered by the registered dietitian's assessment of the patient's depleted nutritional status and risk of malnutrition. In others, the metabolic medicine consultation may be a hospital requirement to order total parenteral nutrition (TPN).

The metabolic medicine consultation is a comprehensive overview of the patient's case, including the current and past medical history, review of systems (ROS), physical examination (PE), a review of laboratory data, and other testing, assessment, and plan of treatment. The difference is that each of these elements is focused on the question of the patient's current nutritional status and their ability to recover from a metabolically depleted state. In our practice, we utilize a system called "metabolic mapping" to summarize the assessment and plan for patients with malnutrition (see below).

Within the assessment section of the consultation, the metabolic physician should determine the type of malnutrition (calorie, protein, protein–calorie, stress metabolism, etc.) and its degree (mild, moderate, severe). Any electrolyte disturbances and suspected micronutrient deficiencies should also be enumerated. An estimate of the patient's nutritional requirements should be calculated and included within the consultation report.

The consultation's treatment plan should lay out the manner intended to further delineate and eventually restore the patient's nutritional status. The need for additional testing such as micronutrient levels and resting metabolic rate (RMR) should be explained. The likelihood of using the GI tract to accommodate nutritional intake should be considered. In the event that the GI tract is found to be compromised, parenteral nutrition should be recommended.

In general, the use of the GI tract is always favored over intravenous nutrition. This follows the common sense dogma that, "if the gut works, use it." Enteral feeding entails the use of a premixed formula, which is administered via a nasogastric, gastrostomy, or jejunostomy tube.

The enteral formula may be complex (polymeric) or elemental. Polymeric formulas are composed of intact protein, oligosaccharides, and long-chain triglycerides. These formulas require both digestion and absorption. Elemental formulas are composed of amino acids and peptides, glucose, and medium-chain triglycerides. Elemental formulas do not require pancreatic and luminal enzymatic digestion, but still require an intact absorptive gut surface. The caloric density of an enteral formula may range from 0.5 to 2.0 kcal/mL.

The metabolic physician is expected to be knowledgeable in the specific differences between the various commercial enteral formulas. When enteral feeding is chosen, the role of the metabolic physician includes monitoring the patient for complications of tube feeding such as aspiration of the formula and symptoms of intolerance, especially diarrhea.

If parenteral nutrition is chosen, the route and rate of the formula must be specified (see Chapter 22). Peripheral IV lines cannot accommodate a solution with an osmolarity much above 700. Therefore, central venous access is often necessary to deliver full intravenous nutritional support. This is especially true in the patient who requires volume restriction because of cardiac, renal, or hepatic disease.

The initiation of nutritional support in a malnourished patient is not without its caveats. The first phase of nutrition infusion is generally associated with significant electrolyte, vitamin, and micromineral shifts between the extracellular and intracellular spaces. If not done judiciously, this can lead to dangerous imbalances, often referred to as "refeeding syndrome." Therefore, the first step in providing nutritional support should almost always begin with infusion of saline, electrolytes, and multivitamins.

In a typical metabolic medicine practice, the day usually begins with nutritional support rounds at the hospital. Each patient on service is seen, examined, and monitored for progress and complications. The visit is similar to that of a hospital internist but with a focus on the patient's nutritional care. We query the patient and the nursing staff about the ability to resume oral intake, tolerance of differing diet consistencies, safety of swallowing, risk of aspiration, postdigestive reactions such as nausea, vomiting, diarrhea, etc. Part of this subjective information is intended to assess the continued requirement for artificial feedings. Once this is established, the patient's tolerance to the current nutritional support regimen is assessed.

The patient is then examined to determine if he or she is tolerating the volume of infusion and reacting favorably to the various components of the nutritional formula. The labs are reviewed to ensure that glycemia is well controlled, fluid and electrolytes are balanced, and protein levels are slowly improving. More details on the metabolic evaluation of the malnourished patient are covered in the following sections and in other chapters throughout this book.

HOME TPN MANAGEMENT

The revolutionary concept of home care emerged in the early 1980s as the powerful trends for both cost containment and patient independence converged [1]. Discharge of a patient who requires long-term TPN at home requires considerable preparation and counseling. The patient must be prepared to appropriately administer, monitor, and dispose of TPN materials. They must also be committed to communicating regularly with the home care team.

Once the patient is discharged, the metabolic physician will be responsible for renewing TPN orders and certifying the ongoing need for at-home nutritional support. Just as in the hospital, a multidisciplinary team is best prepared to assist in managing these patients in the home care setting. The home care nurse, dietitian, and pharmacist will communicate with the metabolic physician's office regularly. In our practice, a dedicated certified nutrition support dietitian serves as the home TPN coordinator.

Inpatient Hospital Consultations for Metabolic Monitoring of the Bariatric Surgery Patient

Bariatric surgery dates back to the 1950s with the development of effective procedures such as various forms of the jejunoileostomy or JI bypass (JIB) [2]. Unfortunately, this procedure was fraught with medical risks including severe vitamin deficiencies and blind loop syndrome. Hepatic dysfunction and even liver failure occurred, resulting in the procedure's discontinuation [3]. This was followed by the development of the Roux-en-Y gastric bypass (RYGB) by Mason and Ito in 1966 [4] and the biliopancreatic diversion (BPD) by Scopinaro et al. in 1979 [5].

Research into gastric restriction through devices placed around the stomach culminated in 1986 with the development of the silicon adjustable gastric band (AGB) by our departed colleague, Lubomyr Kuzmak [6]. Further breakthroughs occurred with the development of laparoscopic techniques for the AGB in 1992 [7] and the RYGB in 1994 [8].

The laparoscopic sleeve gastrectomy (LSG) was initially developed as a staging procedure for supermorbid patients preparing for BPD. But Regan et al. [9] realized that many of their patients lost sufficient weight with this first-stage procedure, which obviated the need for additional surgery. The popularity of the LSG has steadily grown, and it is now the leading bariatric procedure at our center [10].

The value of the laparoscopic approach was more than a matter of convenience and reduction of postoperative pain. The challenges of open abdominal surgery in the morbidly obese are significant. We saw many patients who underwent successful bariatric procedures only to suffer complications related to closure of the abdominal wound. A laparoscopic approach all but eliminated this disadvantageous aspect of bariatric surgery.

With the troublesome hurdle of abdominal wound dehiscence and infection all but overcome, bariatric surgery became a much more practical and popular option. Bariatric surgery has grown significantly as a result. The need for trained metabolic physicians to perform metabolic monitoring grew along with the growth in surgeries.

The in-hospital consultation for metabolic monitoring of a bariatric surgery patient starts with a thorough medical evaluation for postoperative care including cardiac and pulmonary monitoring (encompassing continuous positive airway pressure [CPAP], if appropriate), fluid and electrolyte balance, blood pressure control, glucose control, infection, deep vein thrombosis (DVT), and atelectasis prophylaxis.

The immediate postsurgical hospital stay is an opportune moment to review the patient's prior medications and adjust them for the postbariatric conditions. We often find that diabetic and hypertensive meds can be significantly reduced or even discontinued. For example, diuretics should generally be avoided until the patient has advanced to stage 4 of the bariatric diet.

The postoperative stay is also an excellent time to consider the patient's micronutrient status. We routinely provide double-dose intravenous multivitamins during this period. Intravenous iron replacement therapy is also administered, if necessary. For patients with excessive post-op vomiting, we recommend infusions of thiamine prior to discharge.

The patient is counseled about the importance of following up with a metabolic physician to avoid the metabolic complications of bariatric surgery. The bariatric dietary progression is carefully reviewed by a bariatric dietitian with special attention to the need to take vitamin and mineral supplements postoperatively. The patient should be forewarned about the symptoms of dumping syndrome and other types of food intolerances. All team members should stress the patient's need for lifelong commitment to diet, exercise, and compliance to the bariatric protocol.

If there is a personal or family history of thromboembolism, we generally recommend short-term anticoagulation prophylaxis following discharge. In some cases, a full hypercoagulability workup should be considered.

All postoperative medications should be modified to comply with the limitations of the gastric restriction. Therefore, we generally convert oral meds to liquid, dissolvable, or topical forms if possible. If not, tablets should be crushed and capsules opened with their contents mixed in water.

We recommend that postoperative bariatric patients take a proton pump inhibitor for at least 6 months after surgery to minimize the effects of hyperacidity after gastric surgery. A dissolvable antiemetic is also advisable for the initial weeks after discharge.

OUTPATIENT FOLLOW-UP METABOLIC MONITORING OF THE BARIATRIC SURGERY PATIENT

The function of monitoring the postoperative bariatric surgery patient has become an important part of the metabolic physician's daily clinical activity. It can be summarized as encompassing four significant functions: (1) monitoring for medical and metabolic complications; (2) ensuring ongoing compliance to protocol; (3) continued medication adjustment and/or discontinuation; and (4) addressing weight loss failure (WLF).

The monitoring of medical and metabolic complications can be divided into early, midterm, and late events. They are further subdivided by the type of procedure and other unique factors such as the individual surgeon's methodology.

The first postoperative visit for metabolic monitoring is intended to focus on the immediate medical and metabolic complications. The patient should undergo a thorough post-op examination by the metabolic physician. The metabolic physician should be cognizant of the surgical complications and be able to recognize them quickly. These include dehydration, arrhythmia, stomal stenosis, incisional hernia, internal hernia, cholecystitis, small bowel obstruction, marginal ulcer, wound infection, bleeding, anastomotic leak, and DVT/pulmonary embolus. The physical exam should document the absence of signs of such complications and include a statement on the status of the wound site, the absence of pain and distention, and the adequacy of bowel sounds.

The patient should be evaluated for compliance to the protocol elements of adequate fluid intake, as well as protein, vitamin, and mineral supplementation. The patient should be taught about the nature of dumping syndrome and other food intolerances.

In our practice, we provide an order for laboratory measurement of baseline micronutrient status as part of the hospital discharge package. Therefore, most patients arrive for their first visit with these values already obtained. The labs are reviewed with the patient in detail and any deficiencies are noted and discussed. If necessary, nutritional supplements are ordered. We generally provide a copy of these labs for the patients so that they can share them with the surgeon and their primary care provider.

The first outpatient bariatric visit provides another opportunity to adjust the patient's preexisting medications. The rapid weight loss, change in diet, and exercise favorably affect the need for diabetic, antihypertensive, or antihyperlipidemic pharmaceuticals. Similarly, patients with pre-op sleep apnea often are able to reduce their CPAP or discontinue use of their devices entirely.

Subsequent visits are used to follow up on vitamin and mineral deficiencies identified at baseline and to make certain that new problems do not develop. We pay particular attention to the levels of the major electrolytes (Na, K, Ca, PO_4, Mg), major metals (iron, zinc, copper), and major vitamins (A, D, K, B1, B6, folate, B12). Many of these deficiencies will not manifest until 12, 18, or 24 months after surgery.

The late metabolic complications of bariatric surgery become more apparent as the postoperative interval increases. Iron deficiency with or without anemia is a common problem. Hyperparathyroidism and metabolic bone disease resulting from inadequate calcium absorption are also commonly seen. Kidney stones may develop due to hyperoxaluria. Renal failure is uncommon. Similarly, hepatitis and cirrhosis are not commonly seen.

Our group previously reported on the neurological complications of bariatric surgery [11]. These are believed to be the result of one or more micronutrient deficiencies. Among those at greatest risk are deficiencies of thiamine, B12, vitamin A, vitamin D, and copper.

A small number of patients may develop protein–calorie malnutrition if they are unable to advance their diet or if surgical complications interfere with their progress. For these patients, TPN will likely be needed as a bridge therapy until oral intake can resume.

Another rare but disturbing late complication of gastric bypass is the syndrome of profound reactive hyperinsulinemic hypoglycemia [12,13]. In our practice, we see one or two cases of this syndrome per year. Most can be managed with strict adherence to a low-carbohydrate diet. A small number require medication with alpha-glucosidase inhibitors, somatostatin or diazoxide. Few of these patients will require bypass reversal. But some patients have even required partial pancreatectomy.

It is useful to check on the rate of weight loss and discuss goal weight with the patient. The concepts of excess body weight (EBW) and adjusted body weight (ABW) are often very enlightening teaching points for the patient at this stage of their journey.

WLF occurs in roughly 25% of gastric bypass patients and 40% of patients after a gastric band [14]. The causes are mechanical, dietary, behavioral, and metabolic. The common mechanical causes include enlarged gastric pouch, suboptimal gastric restriction, and a dilated anastomosis. These should be addressed by the surgeon, with consideration for revision of the procedure.

The dietary causes of WLF are related to noncompliance to the bariatric protocol. For example, maladaptive eating occurs when patients choose soft or liquefied food because they report it "goes down easier." These foods do not require a large gastric volume to accommodate their consumption. Therefore, caloric intake remains high. These dietary issues are best addressed by experienced bariatric dietitians and psychologists.

The behavioral causes of WLF can be very difficult to manage as they often include disorders of compulsivity [15]. Binge eating behavior, sweet eating, cravings, etc. should be identified prior to surgery by the psychological screening. However, these are often missed in the patient's enthusiasm to move ahead in the surgical preparation [15]. They require ongoing behavioral modification counseling and may benefit from pharmaceuticals.

The metabolic components of WLF can be summarized into effects on reduced energy expenditure, hormonal imbalance, mesolimbic reward system, and weight control center (WCC) defense of set point. We have previously shown that a pharmaceutical approach to these conditions can be helpful in addressing WLF after bariatric surgery [15].

MEDICAL OBESITY MANAGEMENT

Medical management of obesity is a complex field, which includes lifestyle modification, behavior modification, pharmaceutical therapy, and protein sparing modified fasts (PSMF). The individual components generally depend on the degree of obesity based on the body mass index (BMI), with more aggressive therapy employed for higher degrees of obesity.

In addition to the BMI, an assessment of the patient's comorbidities of obesity such as the Edmonton Obesity Staging System (EOSS) may be useful. This system approaches the patient's obesity from a functional perspective. Such an approach can be helpful in determining the need for aggressive therapy and setting the appropriate motivational aspects of care for the patient [16].

A comprehensive weight management program should begin with a thorough review of the patient's weight history and factors contributing to obesity. The examination should be focused on signs of hormonal imbalance and manifestations of obesity-related disease. Laboratory tests and metabolic measurements complete the initial analysis.

In our practice, we utilize a system called "metabolic mapping" (see Metabolic Mapping of the Malnourished Patient) in which the data collected from the history, physical, lab, and metabolic testing are entered into a treatment algorithm that matches the management approach to the patient's individualized needs.

DIAGNOSIS AND MANAGEMENT OF THE METABOLIC SYNDROME

Patients who present with obesity and increased abdominal adiposity must be considered potential candidates for the diagnosis of metabolic syndrome. The diagnosis of this condition can be thought of as a method to identify patients at risk for the development of diabetes and cardiovascular disease. The metabolic syndrome is a constellation of obesity, abdominal adiposity, hypertension, insulin resistance (IR), dyslipidemia, and abnormal glucose tolerance. There is still some disagreement on the exact diagnostic ranges for each of the components.

A waist circumference at the umbilicus of greater than 35 in. in women and 40 in. in men defines abdominal adiposity [17]. The hypertension criteria should extend into the prehypertension range in order to identify all patients at possible risk. The diagnosis of dyslipidemia would encompass the familiar hypercholesterolemias. But it should also include hypertriglyceridemias and syndromes of low high-density lipoprotein (HDL). With the recent advancements in lipid laboratory analysis, even patients with abnormal low-density lipoprotein (LDL) particle size and quantity should be considered [18].

By the same token, a spectrum of glucose abnormalities should be considered in the diagnostic criterion of metabolic syndrome. Impaired glucose metabolism is generally defined as an elevated fasting glucose. But patients with elevated postprandial glucoses or mildly elevated hbA1C should also be considered.

As noted in Chapter 1, the metabolic syndrome is a constellation of conditions linked to the common thread of IR. So, the logical question must be asked about how to best diagnose IR. Various numeric formulas have been proposed for this function [19]. Perhaps the most popular of these formulas is the HOMA-IR, a formula that takes into account the fasting glucose and insulin together. The formula for HOMA-IR is [fasting glucose (mg/dL) × fasting insulin (uU/mL)]/405.

However, many authors have pointed out the limitations of the HOMA-IR in diagnosing IR [19]. For this reason, we prefer to use the glucose tolerance test with paired insulin responses to judge the degree of IR.

Since the diagnosis of metabolic syndrome is a known risk factor for the onset of diabetes, more must be understood about our ability to reverse the trend and prevent diabetes. This has been demonstrated by the diabetes prevention program [20] and the diabetes prevention program outcomes study [21]. These large-scale population studies showed that lifestyle intervention of diet, exercise, and weight loss could prevent diabetes in 58% of at-risk individuals. Lifestyle intervention was effective in both sexes and through all racial and ethnic groups in this study.

Despite these impressive results, the application of diabetes prevention as a clinical program has failed to achieve significant traction among primary care physicians [22]. Therefore, the great majority of individuals with the metabolic syndrome are unaware of their condition or the risks that it poses to their long-term health.

Diabetes prevention program components include intensive counseling on diet, behavior, food patterns, snacking, emotional eating, exercise, stress reduction, sleep quality, etc. Most primary care physicians do not have sufficient resources to provide the vast array of therapies necessary to manage this complex care. Furthermore, there is little financial incentive for reimbursement of such services in the primary care physician (PCP) office.

The metabolic medicine practice provides an important service to the community health by addressing diabetes prevention in a systematic and thorough manner. This is one of the primary benefits of obesity management in susceptible patients. The uncovering of factors suggesting prediabetes is crucial to the recognition of patients who require aggressive diabetes prevention efforts.

METABOLIC PATIENT EVALUATION

The metabolic consultation follows many of the guidelines of a comprehensive history and physical with all of the usual elements including history of present illness (HPI), ROS, family and social history (FSH), past medical and surgical history (PMSH), and PE. However, elements are added to further elucidate the metabolic condition. These added elements can be considered as metabolic or nutritional components to the HPI, ROS, and PE. They are further subdivided based on whether the patient is undernourished or overnourished. In the case of the undernourished, the HPI and

ROS components follow the logical sequence of food seeking, ingestion, mastication, swallowing, digestion, and elimination. In the overnourished, these factors deal more with the type, timing, and quantity of food ingested.

METABOLIC EVALUATION OF THE UNDERNOURISHED

Body Weight

If a patient presents with weight loss or malnutrition, or appears undernourished for any reason, a metabolic history should be obtained. This begins with a detailed analysis of the patient's weight history including the usual body weight (UBW), the amount of weight lost, and the period of time during which the weight loss occurred. It is important to determine the velocity of the weight loss. Ask if it appears to have stabilized, is decelerating, or is accelerating.

Patients are often forgetful about the precise details of their weight changes, so it may be helpful to have some objective measure of weight, for example, from a past work physical or doctor's visits. Family members can be reliable observers of weight changes and will relate information on clothing size and physical appearance.

Calculate the ideal body weight (IBW) and see how this conforms to the patient's UBW. Determine if the patient was overweight, normal weight, or underweight before the weight loss occurred. Had the UBW been stable for some time or did their weight often fluctuate?

Food Intake

Assess the patient's nutritional intake prior to the onset of weight loss. Were they a picky eater, normal eater, or overeater? Did the patient take a vitamin supplement regularly? What other supplements does the patient take routinely?

Next we want to query the patient regarding the initiation of food intake. Does the patient feel physical hunger? Is there a desire to eat? When foods are offered do they look appealing to the patient? These questions may seem similar, but there are slight differences between the three features of hunger, desire, and appeal [23].

Once food is taken, can the patient taste and smell it normally? Many patients describe a change in taste or flavor with illness (dysgeusia). This makes the eating experience less meaningful and suppresses intake. Often the taste or smell dyscrasia involves a heightened sense of one taste region over another. For example, gastrectomy patients often complain of foods tasting too sweet. Cancer patients may complain of foods tasting too salty or not salty enough [23]. Hyperemesis patients may complain of a heightened sense of smell (hyperosmia) such that flavors are too intense to be pleasurable.

Spector [23] described three taste domains in understanding a person's response to eating. The first is sensory. The question here is whether or not the patient can perceive taste from each of the four main sensory groups: sweet, sour, bitter, and salt. The second domain is pleasure or a hedonistic response to tasting. It asks the question of whether or not the patient likes what he or she has eaten. The third domain is physiologic response. How does eating a certain food make the patient feel? Do they become nauseated or vomit? Do they feel fullness quickly?

Each of these three domains, and indeed many more, can be considered in asking a patient the simple question of what they perceive as the reason they are eating less. Very often, the process of asking these questions allows the patient to focus clearly on this issue for the first time. Some insight may be realized in this process that was not present before.

There may also be a psychological condition, such as depression, which diminishes the desire to eat. Medications may have affected interest and/or pleasure in food. There may be a fear of eating because of difficulty swallowing, acting as a negative feedback. All of these factors need to be considered within the context of the nutritional history.

Chewing and Swallowing

In order to ingest solid food, a process of mastication is required. The teeth are often affected by illness, and this may limit the patient's ability to chew. Similarly, the muscles of mastication may be dysfunctional; saliva production can be inadequate. Mouth sores, wounds, or infections may make it impossible to hold food in the mouth or on the tongue. All of these can alter intake.

Once the food is masticated, or if it is presented in a puréed or liquid form, which obviates the need for chewing, it must be properly swallowed. There are three phases of swallowing: oral, pharyngeal, and esophageal [24]. Insight can be gained by asking about the process based on the physiologic phases and the responses to different food consistencies such as solids and liquids.

The oral phase begins with moistening and mastication and proceeds to formation of a trough for food to pass over the back of the tongue. As the tongue is pushed against the hard palate from front to back, it forces the food bolus posteriorly, and coordinated contractions of mouth muscles propel the bolus into the pharynx.

The pharyngeal phase involves closure of the nasopharynx, opening of the auditory tube, closure of the oropharynx and larynx, and hyoid bone elevation. The food bolus transits the pharynx, passing over the closed glottis to avoid aspiration.

In the esophageal phase, the upper esophageal sphincter relaxes and constrictor muscles of the pharynx push the bolus of food into the esophagus. A peristaltic wave of striated upper esophageal muscle is then followed by smooth lower esophageal muscle contraction, which propels the food at a rate of 3–5 cm/s [24]. The lower esophageal sphincter then relaxes, allowing food to enter the stomach. A relaxation phase follows in which the larynx, pharynx, and hyoid return to their basal positions [25].

Swallowing is a complex coordinated process involving many different nerves, muscles, reflexes, and structures. While the initiation of swallowing is under voluntary control, the process becomes involuntary as the food bolus advances. Despite this, patients often have an insight about the location or reasons for their dysphasia. The metabolic history should include a detailed account of any difficulty with chewing and/or swallowing.

Stomach Factors

The stomach is a hollow vessel that acts as a simple reservoir, holding the contents of a meal and preparing it for digestion. The stomach also secretes pepsin, hydrochloric acid for decontamination, and hormones (i.e., ghrelin), which have a role in hunger and satiety. It has recently become clear that the stomach has receptors that can "taste" the presence of glutamic acid, protein, carbohydrates, and fats [26]. Therefore, the stomach acts as a part of the feedback system to inform the central nervous system of the nutritive value of a meal.

Food enters the stomach at the cardia and fills the body until it reaches the fundus. The mechanical churning of the food and its mixing with gastric secretions creates chyme, which is then propelled in small aliquots through the pylorus for digestion by the gut.

The metabolic history should include reference to the stomach's capacity to retain food and process it adequately. Information on the quantity of food ingested before a sense of fullness can elucidate conditions in which the volume of the stomach is compromised or the muscular function delayed. Symptoms of recurrent nausea and/or vomiting may provide insight to the stomach's capacity.

Digestion

Once the chyme enters the duodenum, full digestion of the nutrients can occur. Complex foods in the form of glycogen, starch, intact proteins, and fats are broken down to simpler components by the pancreatic enzymes amylase, trypsin, and lipase. Luminal brush border enzymes complete the process. Carbohydrates are converted to glucose, proteins to peptides and amino acids and fats to free fatty acids. The nutrients are then actively absorbed by the thick villi of the duodenum with a small amount remaining to be absorbed by the rest of the gut.

Foods that are not digested or absorbed normally will produce symptoms. As they are propelled through the bowel by peristalsis, cramping, bloating, and intestinal gurgling may be reported by the patient. Dumping symptoms may occur. If undigested food reaches the distal bowel, which is rich in bacterial flora, excessive gas production will result. Diarrhea with evidence of fat or protein maldigestion will be evident.

Physical Examination Findings of Malnutrition

The unique components of the PE in an undernourished patient are aimed at documenting the degree of nutritional deficiency. The first determination should be about the muscle mass. As we have already described, the muscle mass will be sacrificed if protein intake is inadequate.

Muscle mass is easily evaluated through examination of the face, chest, and extremities. Make note of temporal and masseter muscle wasting in the face. The intercostal muscles, biceps, triceps, quadriceps, and interosseous muscles of the hands and feet are also particularly useful indicators. The degree of muscle wasting (sarcopenia) should be quantified by the examiner as mild, moderate, or severe. Some have used a 1–4+ grading system. Either method is considered acceptable.

The presence of "nutritional edema" because of reduced colloid osmotic pressure is an important observation. This is indistinguishable from the pitting edema of congestive heart failure or the ascites of portal hypertension. However, it presents in the absence of these underlying conditions.

Fat mass can be observed in the abdomen, buttocks, and thighs of both genders. However, loss of subcutaneous fat can also be a useful indicator in young and middle-aged women.

Examining the patient for micronutrient deficiency can be complex. A careful analysis of the hair, eyes, oral mucosa, and tongue surface should be part of the head, eyes, ears, nose, and throat (HEENT) exam. This may yield information on vitamin deficiencies. The skin should be examined for signs of excessive dryness and hornification. If present, ichthyosis should be documented. The neurological exam may yield important clues about vitamin and mineral deficiencies. We have found the tuning fork test for vibratory sensation to be of particular value.

Anthropometric measurements can also be performed to document the degree of malnutrition. These should be considered specialized forms of the PE in an undernourished patient. They have fallen out of favor because of technical issues and interoperator variability. Furthermore, new techniques such as bioimpedance and x-ray absorptiometry have emerged as replacements for the anthropometric exam. Still, some clinicians find it useful to measure a mid-upper arm circumference (MUAC) and caliper triceps skin fold (TSF) thickness. A number of derivative equations exist to obtain mid-upper arm muscle area, mass, and fat mass through this measurement [27].

Specialized Metabolic Testing

The metabolic physician should be prepared to utilize an RMR and body composition analysis if the patient's status requires it. Considerable expertise is needed to interpret the results.

Metabolic rate measurement is a complex science and can be performed at various levels of intensity. The test should be performed with the patient nil per os (NPO) for at least 4 h, but preferably overnight. In its simplest form, the information is obtained by a handheld VO2 monitor that performs a breath-by-breath analysis and gives an averaged VO2 over 5–10 min. This information is then extrapolated to the 1440 min of the day to give a daily RMR estimate.

A more accurate RMR is obtained by equipment that measures both the VO2 and VCO2. Such equipment can be utilized to also obtain the respiratory quotient (RQ) and derivative information on carbohydrate, lipid, and protein oxidation. This more complex equipment can also be used to obtain metabolic data during exercise. There are full-scale, room-sized versions of this equipment that also allow for a subject to stay under study conditions for an extended period of time.

Body composition analysis can be performed through bedside techniques such as the mid-arm circumference and skin fold calipers noted above. The previous gold standard of underwater weighing has now been replaced by computerized devices that use dual photon x-ray absorptiometry (DEXA) or bioimpedance (BIA) [28].

Nitrogen (N+) balance can be very helpful in interpreting the degree of catabolism. This can further refine the estimate for protein needs. N+ balance studies require an accurate estimate of total protein intake, along with an accurate collection of nitrogen output from urine and stool. To calculate nitrogen intake, grams of protein consumed are divided by 6.25 to convert the protein to grams of nitrogen. The nitrogen output (urine, stool, and skin) is subtracted from nitrogen intake to yield a positive or negative result (positive or negative N+ balance).

Many facilities lack the equipment to perform the necessary urine, stool, and skin nitrogen analysis. Because the majority of the nitrogen output is represented by urea, the urinary urea nitrogen (UUN) has been routinely substituted for measurement of nitrogen output. In this method, the UUN is multiplied by a factor to compensate for the absence of other urine nitrogen. Another factor is used to estimate stool and skin losses [29].

Metabolic Laboratory Data

A full metabolic evaluation of a malnourished patient would not be complete without examination of certain biochemical parameters. This may overlap with some of the standard testing but should still be considered as part of the specialized exam. The labwork should include serum glucose and lipids as well as measurements of circulating proteins (total protein, albumin, and prealbumin), major electrolytes (sodium, potassium, chloride, bicarbonate, calcium, phosphorus, and magnesium), microminerals (iron, zinc, copper, selenium, and manganese), major vitamins (A, D, E, C, B1, B6, folate, and B12), and some special items such as carnitine, etc. The use of N+ balance studies has been limited but is still in clinical use.

Metabolic Mapping of the Malnourished Patient

Once the patient evaluation is complete, a listing of the abnormalities detected can provide a guide for the correction of the metabolic disturbances. We refer to this type of list as a "metabolic map" because it delineates the areas of concern and focuses attention on their restoration. This reduces the risk that an important metabolic aspect of the malnourished patient's case will be overlooked.

The metabolic map can be used to delineate the degree of penetrance for each nutritional aspect of the patient's case. It can also be used as a repository for the various pieces of data that return to the patient's chart at different times. In this way, the metabolic map provides a complete overview of the patient's metabolic status.

Once the metabolic problems have been outlined and delineated and the data amassed, a corrective action plan can be formulated. This final aspect should be thought of as the mirror image to the problem list. Each problem of metabolism with significant penetrance is matched to a potential solution. If a solution cannot be found for the delineated condition, the metabolic map helps to identify areas requiring further evaluation (Table 2.1).

Example Case of Metabolic Mapping for Malnutrition

We have prepared an example case to demonstrate the utility of metabolic mapping in patients with malnutrition.

GS is a 70-year-old male who presented for a new patient visit for unplanned weight loss. He was 5'8" tall and weighed 132 lbs. His BMI was 20.06. His UBW was 150 lbs. He had lost 18 lbs. in 1 month. He had a complicated medical history. As a young man, he was diagnosed with Hodgkin's disease and underwent extensive radiation therapy to the chest and abdomen. As a result, he developed avascular necrosis of the hips and aortic valve disease. He was status post aortic valve/mitral

TABLE 2.1
Metabolic Map in Malnutrition

	Metabolic Parameter	Present/Absent (Yes/No) (Results)	Degree of Penetration (Mild/Moderate/Severe)	Details	Corrective Action Plan
History	Unintended weight loss				
	Weight loss quantity				
	Weight loss period				
	Inadequacy for food intake				
	Decreased hunger				
	Decreased appetite				
	Decreased interest in food				
	Decreased desire for food				
	Olfactory disturbances				
	Taste disturbances				
	Chewing difficulty				
	Mouth pain				
	Tongue pain				
	Swallowing difficulty				
	Esophageal dysfunction				
	Reduced gastric capacity				
	Nausea				
	Vomiting				
	Delayed gastric emptying				
	Gastric dumping				
	Delayed bowel motility				
	Accelerated bowel motility				
	Maldigestion				
	Malabsorption				
	Postprandial pain				
	Postprandial bloating				
	Excessive gas				
	Diarrhea				
	Constipation				
	Floating stools				
	Fat streaked stool				
	Mucous in stool				
	Orange-colored stool				
	Undigested food in stool				
	Foul smelling stools				
	Toilet bowl coating				
	Other				

(continued)

TABLE 2.1 (Continued)
Metabolic Map in Malnutrition

	Metabolic Parameter	Present/Absent (Yes/No) (Results)	Degree of Penetration (Mild/Moderate/Severe)	Details	Corrective Action Plan
Physical	Muscle wasting				
	Fat depletion				
	Body composition data				
	Resting metabolic rate				
	Physical findings of micronutrient deficiency				
	Other				
Labs	Circulating proteins				
	Electrolyte status				
	Fluid balance				
	Vitamin status				
	Micromineral status				
	Nitrogen balance				
	D-Xylose absorption test				
	Fecal fat				
	Other				

valve (AV/MV) replacement and status post coronary artery bypass grafting (CABG). He had a history of pericarditis and pleural effusion and had a defibrillator for atrial fibrillation, and he was on chronic amiodarone therapy. He had chronic anemia and renal insufficiency, which prevented him from being fully anticoagulated. He had also had a thyroidectomy and a total colectomy for adenomatous polyposis in November 2012. After the total colectomy in November 2012, he developed diarrhea. Cultures were negative for *Clostridium difficile*. He complained of anorexia, nausea, abdominal pain, and diarrhea. He denied any problem with chewing or swallowing, or altered taste/smell sensation. On exam, he had overt muscle wasting and fat depletion. His labs at that time showed a BUN of 37 mg/dL, a creatinine of 1.8 mg/dL, and a serum albumin of 2.8 g/dL.

He was started on megestrol acetate, oral iron supplements, and cholestyramine. A low-fat, high-protein diet with MCT oil supplements and small frequent feedings were prescribed.

He required hospitalization for continued diarrhea leading to further weight loss and dehydration. He had a positive fecal fat test. He was subsequently diagnosed with a villous adenoma of the duodenum on upper gastrointestinal (UGI) endoscopy. Biopsy results revealed an infiltrating, poorly differentiated adenocarcinoma. He was discharged on home TPN in an attempt to maximize his nutritional status prior to a Whipple procedure and surgery to resolve a partial small bowel obstruction.

The metabolic map of this example case is shown in Table 2.2. The first column defines the general region of interest. In the second column, we see a list of the metabolic parameters detected by the patient evaluation. The third column provides the degree of penetrance of each condition noted in column 2. The fourth column allows for the recording of further details on the conditions listed, which have significant penetrance. This can also be thought of as a repository for data returning to the chart during the course of the patient's hospitalization. The final column of the metabolic map lists the definitive solutions, which match the problems. Some problems may not have matching definitive solutions and must be recognized as unaddressable at the current time.

TABLE 2.2
Metabolic Map of Patient GS

	Metabolic Parameter	Present/Absent (Yes/No) (Results)	Degree of Penetration (Mild/Moderate/Severe)	Details	Corrective Action Plan
History	Unintended weight loss	Yes	Severe		Appetite stimulant
	Weight loss quantity		Severe	18 lbs.	Appetite stimulant
	Weight loss period		Severe	1 month	Appetite stimulant
	Inadequacy for food intake	Yes	Severe		Appetite stimulant
	Decreased hunger	Yes	Severe		Appetite stimulant
	Decreased appetite	Yes	Severe		Appetite stimulant
	Decreased interest in food	Yes	Severe		Appetite stimulant
	Decreased desire for food	Yes	Severe		Appetite stimulant
	Olfactory disturbances	No			
	Taste disturbances	No			
	Chewing difficulty	No			
	Mouth pain	No			
	Tongue pain	No			
	Swallowing difficulty	No			
	Esophageal dysfunction	No			
	Reduced gastric capacity	Yes	Moderate		Promotility agents contraindicated
	Nausea	Yes	Severe		Antiemetics
	Vomiting	Yes	Severe		Antiemetics
	Delayed gastric emptying	No			
	Gastric dumping	No			
	Delayed bowel motility	No			
	Accelerated bowel motility	Yes	Severe		Antidiarrheal therapy
	Maldigestion	No			
	Malabsorption	Yes	Severe		Digestive enzymes
	Postprandial pain	No			
	Postprandial bloating	Yes	Moderate		Digestive enzymes
	Excessive gas	Yes	Moderate		Probiotics
	Diarrhea	Yes	Severe		Antidiarrheals
	Constipation	No			

(*continued*)

TABLE 2.2 (Continued)
Metabolic Map of Patient GS

	Metabolic Parameter	Present/Absent (Yes/No) (Results)	Degree of Penetration (Mild/Moderate/Severe)	Details	Corrective Action Plan
	Floating stools	Yes	Moderate		Digestive enzymes
	Fat streaked stool	Yes	Moderate		Digestive enzymes
	Mucous in stool	No			
	Orange-colored stool	No			
	Undigested food in stool	No			
	Foul smelling stools	No			
	Toilet bowl coating	No			
	Other				
Physical	Muscle wasting	Yes	Severe		Protein supplements
	Fat depletion	Yes	Severe		MCT oil
	Body composition data				
	Resting metabolic rate				
	Physical findings of micronutrient deficiency				
	Other				
Labs	Circulating proteins	Abnormal	Mild	Albumin 2.8	Consider TPN if no improvement
	Electrolyte status	NL			
	Fluid balance	NL			
	Vitamin status	NL			
	Micromineral status	Abnormal	Moderate	Iron = 18	Iron supplementation
	Nitrogen balance				
	D-Xylose absorption test				
	Fecal fat	Abnormal	Moderate	Positive	Digestive enzymes
	Other				

METABOLIC EVALUATION OF THE OVERNOURISHED

Body Weight

In a patient that presents for medical weight loss, the metabolic history has a different goal than in the undernourished. But it still begins with a detailed analysis of the patient's weight history.

We find it important to establish the patients' maximum body weight. Often this is their weight at the time of their first visit to the metabolic center. Ask how long the patients were at the maximum weight and what their prior stable weight had been. How long did it take to increase from their previous stable weight to the maximum figure? Determine the velocity of the weight gain. Ask if it appears to have stabilized, or if it is decelerating or accelerating.

As in the malnourished patient, it is often helpful to have some objective measure of weight. This information is particularly important if the patient is seeking the option of weight loss surgery. Often, insurance companies require such documentation in the surgical preapproval process.

Calculate the IBW and derive the ABW. Ask the patient for their goal weight. The goal should roughly coincide with the ABW.

Factors Contributing to Weight Gain

We begin the process of gathering dietary information though a nutrition questionnaire. The following areas are addressed in the questionnaire.

1. Duration: Patients are asked how long they have had a problem with their weight.
2. Etiology: Was there a specific trigger (depression, pregnancy, following emotional stress or injury, medication use, etc.)?
3. Amount of weight gain
4. Physiologic contributing factors: Is there a family history of diabetes, obesity, or cardiovascular disease? A personal history of diabetes, including gestational diabetes, hyperlipidemia, hypothyroidism, carbohydrate cravings?
5. Diet history: What type of diets have they tried? How many meals a day are consumed? How many meals are eaten outside the home?
6. Eating pattern: Do they skip meals? Choose large portions? Eat quickly? Fail to stop eating when full? Drink inadequate water with meals?
7. Snack pattern: How often do they snack? When do they snack? What foods do they snack on?
8. Behavior pattern: Do they eat for stress, comfort, or reward? Is there compulsive eating or late night eating?
9. Exercise methods: What kind of exercise is done?
10. Exercise pattern: How often do they exercise?

After reviewing the questionnaire with the patient, we can identify the specific concerns that need to be addressed in order to formulate an appropriate treatment plan.

An important subset of this area is asking the patient what initiates eating a meal and what completes it. It is important to begin to create a structure in which food intake has a beginning and an end. This concept can be introduced with the very first interview as a means of information gathering.

Determine if they begin a meal because of a physiologic stimulus such as hunger, stomach pain, a hollow feeling, emptiness, etc. Do they begin because of social pressures such as family or work schedule. Another common statement is that the patient keeps to a certain pattern or habit, regardless of the other factors.

We then ask what completes the meal. Ideally, it should be the opposite of what initiates it. So hunger would be balanced by the absence of hunger, stomach pain balanced by the absence of pain, hollowness or emptiness by fullness, etc. But often patients state they stop when the plate is clean or when the other family members stop or when there is no more in the serving dish. Furthermore, many patients report that they routinely eat past the point of fullness.

Nonnutritive Eating Patterns

This component refers to the consumption of snacks. Do they snack? How often and when do they snack? What type of foods do they snack on? This is distinguished from meal eating and is generally a process that the patient does alone or in the context of a social event. Snacking is not initiated because of hunger or other physiologic stimulus. It does not conform to a structure of portion size or time constraints. Therefore its initiation is completely nonnutritive. Similarly, the end point of snacking is not based on the reversal of the initiating circumstance. It is not controlled by lack of hunger, desire, fullness, etc. Here again, snack consumption proves to be nonnutritive.

These factors would be problematic in their own right, since initiating food intake for reasons other than the need for nutrition will certainly provide calories when the body does not need them. But the situation is exacerbated by the fact that many snack foods are simple carbohydrates that are rapidly digested and therefore not filling. In essence, these foods present the option of limitless consumption. Flavor enhancements, color, packaging, and media promotion often make snack foods nearly irresistible to the average person.

A patient may be eating a perfectly acceptable diet at three well organized meals a day and then consume a vast amount of calories during snacks. Our experience is that snacking may account for up to 1000 cal/day. Therefore, snacking patterns must be carefully evaluated.

Eating Behaviors

A separate category is included for the evaluation of abnormal eating due to behavioral issues. This is not precisely the same as snacking, as it has its origin in the perceived need to use food in relation to an emotional or psychological state. Are they eating because of stress, as a reward, or for comfort? Is there any compulsive or late-night eating? Similar to snacking, behavioral eating has a nonnutrition initiation point and no obvious stopping point. Also, similar to snacking, behavioral eating often involves refined carbohydrates that have an addictive component. Therefore, massive calorie consumption is possible when this behavior is triggered.

Goal Setting

Another important component to the initial metabolic evaluation of an overweight patient has to do with goal setting. Patients often have unrealistic goals for the rate and extent of weight loss. These are driven by personal desires for social acceptance and fed by a culture that allows irresponsible promotion of weight loss products and services. A common subset of this is the patient who is trying to lose weight in preparation for a life event such as a wedding, family celebration, or change of season.

These types of motivations tend to be detrimental because they are too short term. Furthermore, the focus on social issues rather than health as the motivation for weight loss does not provide sufficient impetus for commitment to change long-standing behaviors.

Patients often have an unrealistic goal for their weight loss. They seek to achieve the body image that they may have had earlier in life. Alternatively, many patients have been told they should be able to achieve an IBW based upon height/weight tables, or they may have seen a picture in a textbook or magazine. Recently, the promotion of the concept of a healthy BMI has led patients to focus on this number as a means of attaining their goal weight.

We prefer to take a longer view and to counsel patients on an achievable and sustainable weight, which can be maintained lifelong. We tend to use the ABW formula as our guide for the goal weight. If the patient's ABW can be achieved through weight reduction of 30% or less from their current weight, we believe that medical therapy is appropriate for weight loss. If the ABW goal requires a weight loss of greater than 30%, we routinely open a discussion regarding bariatric surgery.

Physical Examination Findings of Overnutrition

The examination of an overweight and obese patient follows the guidelines of a comprehensive physical exam, but with some significant additions. The purpose of the additional components are to identify risk factors related to the overweight status of the patient and to make sure etiologies of obesity are eliminated.

The skin of an overweight or obese individual may provide important clues to metabolic processes, especially IR. The most telling of these signs is *Acanthosis nigricans*, which is often detected at the base of the neck and in the folds of the axilla and inguinal areas. The face exam should rule out signs of Cushing's syndrome and acromegaly. The eye exam should include evaluations to eliminate signs of hypothyroidism and hyperthyroidism. The neck exam should include an evaluation of the carotids for atherosclerosis, and the thyroid should be carefully examined to eliminate thyroiditis and thyroid nodules. The abdomen should be examined for aortic bruits and striae. The lower extremities should be examined for edema and stasis dermatitis.

Metabolic Laboratory Data

There are a variety of metabolic lab evaluations for the overweight and obese patient. Most programs employ a basic panel of hematology and chemistry with additional studies of cardiometabolic risk such as lipids, C-reactive protein (CRP), urine microalbumin, and hemoglobin A1C. Many also perform a glucose tolerance and insulin response study. Endocrine studies should be performed to evaluate the pituitary, thyroid, and adrenal function. The patient should also be evaluated for major nutrient deficiencies, including iron and vitamins A, D, and B12.

Metabolic Mapping of the Overnourished Patient

As with the malnourished evaluation, we use the "metabolic mapping" concept to organize our findings and plans in obesity management. Obesity is a very complex, multifactorial condition. While diet and exercise play key roles, we have found that other factors such as eating behaviors, lifestyle habits, metabolic conditions, and endocrine disorders are frequently involved.

The metabolic map provides a means to organize these multifactorial aspects of the patient's obesity management. Just as was described in the section on Metabolic Mapping of the Malnourished Patient, this system can be used to delineate the degree of penetrance for each nutritional aspect of the patient's case. We have found this aspect of penetrance to be extremely valuable in the management of obesity. This is because it permits us to understand the patient's unique situation. By delineating the problems and their degree of contribution to the patients' obesity, we can help the patients to see the roots of their condition more clearly.

Once the metabolic problems have been outlined and delineated and the data amassed, a corrective action plan can be developed and shared with the patient as well as other members of the multidisciplinary team. This corrective action plan should be thought of as a reverse image to the problem list. Each problem of metabolism with significant penetrance is matched to a potential solution. If no immediate solution can be found for the delineated condition, the metabolic map helps to identify areas requiring further evaluation.

Since the metabolic map has provided a degree of severity for each problem, the intensity of each aspect of the corrective action plan can also be varied accordingly.

Example Case of Metabolic Mapping for Overnutrition

We have prepared an example case to demonstrate the utility of metabolic mapping in obesity management (Table 2.3).

LC is a 55-year-old female who presented for medical weight loss management. She is 5′9″ tall and had an initial weight of 237 lbs. Her BMI was 34.99.

Her nutrition history revealed that her obesity had been present for several years after moving from New York City. She had a history of depression and was on serotonin uptake inhibitor medication, which she believed contributed to her weight gain. She had recently undergone smoking cessation.

She consumed three meals a day, but 10 meals per week were eaten outside the home. She ate quickly, chose large portions of food, and failed to stop eating when full. She reported that she rarely snacked between meals. She did not participate in any form of exercise on a regular basis.

On physical examination, she was found to be hypertensive with a blood pressure of 140/90. Her BMI was 35. Her waist circumference was 41 inches. There was no evidence of moon facies, buffalo hump, striae, or peripheral edema. Her thyroid was normal.

TABLE 2.3

Metabolic Map in Overnutrition

	Metabolic Parameter	Present/Absent (Yes/No) (Results)	Degree of Penetration (Mild/Moderate/Severe)	Details	Corrective Action Plan
Baseline Data	Maximum BW				
	Optimal BW				
	IBW				
	ABW				
	BMI				
	Edmonton stage				
	% WL needed to achieve ABW				
	Other				
History	Weight gain quantity				
	Weight gain velocity				
	Weight gain contributors				
	Meal pattern				
	Snack pattern				
	Global diet assessment				
	Meal initiation				
	Meal completion				
	Emotional eating				
	Compulsive eating				
	Eating triggers				
	Night eating				
	Sleep disturbance				
	OSA				
	Exercise				
	Other				
Physical	Weight				
	Height				
	BMI				
	Waist circumference				
	Body composition				
	Metabolic rate				
	Acanthosis				
	Thyroid nodules				
	Buffalo hump				
	Striae				
	Edema				
	Other				
Labs	GTT				
	IR				
	HbA1c				
	uMA				
	Dyslipidemia				
	Pituitary function				
	Adrenal function				
	Thyroid function				

(continued)

TABLE 2.3 (Continued)
Metabolic Map in Overnutrition

Metabolic Parameter	Present/Absent (Yes/No) (Results)	Degree of Penetration (Mild/Moderate/Severe)	Details	Corrective Action Plan
Gonadal function				
Gluten sensitivity				
Iron deficiency				
Vitamin deficiency				
Other				

She was diagnosed with impaired glucose tolerance and IR. She was considered to be prediabetic. She had hypertension, obesity, increased waist circumference, elevated glucose, elevated cholesterol, and CRP. She was therefore felt to have metabolic syndrome. A RMR was measured at 990 cal/day, significantly below the predicted rate of 1751 (based on the Harris–Benedict equation). Her body fat was 40% (Tables 2.4 and 2.5).

She was advised to follow a low-carbohydrate diet and to begin regular exercise. She was referred for evaluation by an exercise physiologist. She was followed monthly and eventually given both metabolic stimulants and insulin sensitizers. She lost 85 lbs. over a period of 24 months. Her hypertension, impaired glucose tolerance, IR, and elevated CRP had resolved. Her medications were discontinued, and she remained on diet and lifestyle therapy.

The metabolic map of this example case is shown in Table 2.6. The first column defines the area. In the second column, we see a list of the conditions detected by the patient evaluation. The third column provides the degree of penetrance of each condition noted in column 2. The fourth column allows for the recording of further details on the conditions listed, which have significant penetrance. The final column of the metabolic map lists the definitive solutions that match the problems. Some problems may not have matching definitive solutions and must be recognized as unaddressable at the current time. The intensity of the corrective action plan is matched to the degree of penetration for each aspect of the patient's obesity.

TABLE 2.4
Glucose Tolerance Test Data for Patient LC

Time	Glucose	Insulin
Fasting	88	12.7
1 h	214	72.9
2 h	183	80.7
3 h	71	21.4

TABLE 2.5
Significant Laboratory Data for Patient LC

hbA1c	5.6
CRP	26.8
Total cholesterol	218
Triglycerides	116
HDL	83
LDL	112

TABLE 2.6
Metabolic Map for Patient LC

	Metabolic Parameter	Present/Absent (Yes/No) (Results)	Degree of Penetration (Mild/ Moderate/Significant)	Details	Corrective Action Plan
Baseline Data	Maximum BW	237			
	Optimal BW	160			
	IBW	145			
	ABW	168			
	BMI	35	Moderate		
	Edmonton stage				
	% WL needed to achieve ABW	30%			Medical weight management
	Other				
History	Weight gain quantity	70 lbs.			
	Weight gain velocity	5 years			
	Weight gain contributors	Move from city, smoking cessation, antidepressants			
	Restaurant meals	Frequent	Significant		Limit restaurant meals
	Portion sizes	Large	Significant		Controlled portions
	Consumption pattern	Eating quickly	Significant		Train on slowing consumption
	Snack pattern	Rarely	Mild		
	Global diet assessment	Uncontrolled	Significant		Low CHO diet
	Meal initiation	Hunger			
	Meal completion	Portion completion	Significant		Train on meal quantity
	Eats past fullness	Yes	Significant		Satiety training
	Emotional eating	Yes	Moderate		Counsel on coping skills
	Compulsive eating	No			
	Eating triggers	Stress	Moderate		Counsel on coping skills
	Night eating	No			
	Sleep disturbance	No			
	OSA	No			
	Exercise	None	Significant		Exercise physiologist
	Other				
Exam	Weight	237			
	Height	69			
	BMI	35			
	Waist circumference	41	Significant		
	Body composition	40% BF	Significant		
	Metabolic rate	990	Significant		Metabolic stimulant
	Acanthosis	No			
	Thyroid nodules	No			
	Buffalo hump	No			
	Striae	No			
	Edema	No			

(continued)

TABLE 2.6 (Continued)
Metabolic Map for Patient LC

	Metabolic Parameter	Present/Absent (Yes/No) (Results)	Degree of Penetration (Mild/ Moderate/Significant)	Details	Corrective Action Plan
	Other				
Labs	GTT	Abnormal	Significant		Metformin
	IR	Abnormal	Significant		Insulin sensitizer
	HbA1c	Normal			
	uMA	Abnormal	Significant		ACE/ARB
	Dyslipidemia	Abnormal	Significant		Statin
	CRP	Abnormal	Significant		Statin
	Pituitary function	Normal			
	Adrenal function	Normal			
	Thyroid function	Normal			
	Gonadal function	Normal			
	Gluten sensitivity	Normal			
	Iron deficiency	Normal			
	Vitamin deficiency	Normal			

SUMMARY

In this chapter, we have detailed many of the practical aspects of a metabolic physician's daily clinical activities, which extend from the hospital to clinic and even home care environments. In general, the metabolic medicine practice involves six key focus areas: in-hospital nutritional support, home care nutritional support, in-hospital monitoring of the postoperative bariatric surgery patient, outpatient/long-term metabolic monitoring after bariatric surgery, medical obesity management, and the diagnosis and management of metabolic syndrome.

Additional unique functions may develop as the metabolic physician is called upon to apply his or her biochemistry knowledge for specific conditions. This can involve the application of metabolic concepts into other specialties such as metabolic bone disease, nutritional aspects of chronic lung disease, and management of adult patients with inborn errors of metabolism. Numerous opportunities to extend our approaches for the care of other patient groups exist, and the metabolic physician must be prepared to creatively tackle these issues.

Superlative clinical skills, advanced clinical judgment, and a detailed understanding of biochemistry is necessary for the metabolic physician to perform his or her role as a specialist in nutritional support. While the metabolic physician must work alongside his or her colleagues, it is essential to differentiate the metabolic role from that of other specialists. The "metabolist" is charged with providing substrates and cofactors to optimize the patient's recovery and functional capacity. We must walk the fine line of supplying these critical nutrients without overwhelming the patient's physiology. Only then can our input play its appropriate and vital part in the favorable outcome of our complex patients.

The metabolic physician has an important collaborative role in assisting with the process of weight loss surgery. This may begin with the preoperative evaluation of potential patients who are seeking a bariatric procedure. Often we are called upon to certify that the patient is medically cleared and properly prepared to undergo the procedure and take on the responsibility of adhering to the postoperative guidelines. In the hospital, we are charged with the responsibility of ensuring that the medical aspects of the immediate postoperative period are properly addressed. Medication adjustment and/or withdrawal will often be required.

In the clinic, long-term metabolic monitoring of the bariatric surgery patient is an imperative component of a favorable outcome. Micronutrient deficiencies must be avoided. Patients must be continuously reminded of the requirements for fluid intake, protein intake, vitamin and mineral supplementation, and proper dietary adherence. Patients who fail to meet their weight loss goal after bariatric surgery will seek out a metabolic physician to utilize his or her expertise in completing their weight loss process.

A small subset of bariatric patients may go on to suffer late complications of their procedures. The metabolic physician plays a critical role in identifying and managing these conditions.

Major developments are occurring in the field of medical obesity management. New concepts and recently released pharmaceuticals offer additional opportunities for patients and clinicians. The metabolic physician is an obesity specialist who can counsel patients on both medical and surgical approaches in the management of this difficult illness. A scientific, biochemically based approach has the best opportunity to produce meaningful and lasting weight loss. The metabolic physician's knowledge of these concepts can distinguish practitioners in our specialty from the multitude of others who claim expertise.

In addition to the treatment of current conditions, the metabolic physician has an important role in the prevention of illness, particularly diabetes and cardiovascular disease. This relates to the diagnosis and management of the metabolic syndrome. As its name implies, the metabolic syndrome is a core component of metabolic medicine. In addition to the opportunity to assist in the care of individual patients, screening programs can uncover asymptomatic patients with metabolic syndrome. In this way, metabolic physicians can play an important role in community-based health initiatives.

In this chapter, we have also provided an overview of our approach to patient evaluation in major metabolic conditions. We have presented our concept of "metabolic mapping" for both, including undernutrition and overnutrition, and provided illustrative cases for each.

Given the scope of the concepts and the complexity of the field, it is impossible to summarize the practical aspects of the entire specialty in a single chapter. Other chapters in this book will explore these and additional subjects in greater detail.

ACKNOWLEDGMENTS

The authors thank Kelly Iorillo for reviewing the manuscript and Zachary Simon Rothkopf for his editorial assistance in its preparation.

REFERENCES

1. Rothkopf MM. Concept and scope of intensive homecare. In Rothkopf MM, Askanazi J (eds.), *Intensive Homecare*, Lippincott Williams and Wilkins, Baltimore, MD, 1992.
2. Payne JH, DeWind LT. Surgical treatment of obesity. *Am J Surg* 1969;118:141–147.
3. Griffen WO, Bivins BA, Bell RM. The decline and fall of the jejunoileal bypass. *Surg Gynecol Obstet* 1983;157:301–308.
4. Mason EE, Ito C. Gastric bypass in obesity. *Surg Clin North Am* 1967;47:1345–1351.
5. Scopinaro N, Gianetta E, Civalleri D, Bonalumi U, Bachi V. Bilio-pancreatic by-pass for obesity: II. Initial experience in man. *Br J Surg* 1979;66:618–620.
6. Kuzmak LI. Silicone gastric banding: A simple and effective operation for morbid obesity. *Cont Surg* 1986;28:13–18.
7. Catona A, Gossenberg M, La Manna A, Mussini G. Laparoscopic gastric banding: Preliminary series. *Obes Surg* 1993;3:207–209.
8. Wittgrove AC, Clark GW, Tremblay LJ. Laparoscopic gastric bypass Roux-en-Y: Preliminary report of five cases. *Obes Surg* 1994;4:353–357.
9. Regan JP, Inabnet WB, Gagner M, Pomp A. Early experience with two-stage laparoscopic Roux-en-Y gastric bypass as an alternative in the super-super obese patient. *Obes Surg* 2003;13:861–864.
10. Sarelx AI, Dexter SPL, O'Kane M, Menon A, McMahon MJ. Long term follow up after laparoscopic sleeve gastrectomy: 8–9 year results. *Surg Obes Relat Dis* 2012;8:679–684.

11. Rothkopf MM, Sobelman JS, Mathis AS, Haverstick LP, Nusbaum MJ. Micronutrient-responsive cerebral dysfunction other than Wernicke's encephalopathy after malabsorptive surgery. *Surg Obes Relat Dis* 2010;6(2):171–180.

12. Patti ME, McMahon G, Mun EC et al. Severe hypoglycaemia post-gastric bypass requiring partial pancreatectomy: Evidence for inappropriate insulin secretion and pancreatic islet hyperplasia. *Diabetologia* 2005;48(11):2236–2240.

13. Service GS, Thompson GB, Service FJ, Andrews JC, Collazo-Clavell ML, Lloyd RV. Hyperinsulinemic hypoglycemia with nesidioblastosis after gastric-bypass surgery. *N Engl J Med* 2005;353(3):249–254.

14. Christou NV, Look D, MacLean LD. Weight gain after short- and long-limb gastric bypass in patients followed for longer than 10 years. *Ann Surg* 2006;244:734–740.

15. Rothkopf MM, Haverstick LP, Nusbaum MJ. A proposed method for categorizing weight loss failure (WLF) after laparoscopic gastric banding (LAGB). Abstract presented at American College of Nutrition 52nd Annual Conference, November 2011.

16. Sharma AM, Kushner RF. A proposed clinical staging system for obesity. *Int J Obes* 2009;33:289–295.

17. Rollinson D, Shikra SA, Saltzman E. Obesity. In Gottschlich MM (ed.), *The ASPEN Nutrition Support Care Curriculum: A Care Based Approach—The Adult Patient*. American Society for Parenteral and Enteral Nutrition, Silver Spring, MD, 2007:695–721.

18. Friedlander Y, Kidron M, Caslake M, Lamb T, Mcconnell M, Baron H. Low density lipoprotein particle size and risk factor of insulin resistance syndrome. *Atherosclerosis* 200;148:141–149.

19. Wallace TM, Levy JC, Mattheus DR. Use and abuse of HOMA modeling. *Diabetes Care* 2004;27(6):1487–1495.

20. Diabetes Prevention Program Research Group. Reduction in the incidence of type 2 diabetes with lifestyle intervention or metformin. *N Engl J Med* 2002;346:393–403.

21. Diabetes Prevention Program Research Group. The 10-year cost-effectiveness of lifestyle intervention or metformin for diabetes prevention: An intent-to-treat analysis of the DPP/DPPOS. *Diabetes Care* 2012;35:723–730.

22. Fradkin JE, Roberts BT, Rodgers GR. What's preventing us from preventing type 2 diabetes? *N Engl J Med* 2012;367:1177–1179.

23. Spector AC. Linking gustatory neurobiology to behavior in vertebrates. *Neurosci Biobehav Rev* 2000;24:391–416.

24. Dodds WJ, Stewart ET, Logermann JA. Physiology and radiology of the normal oral and pharyngeal phase of swallowing. *AJR* 1990;154:953–963.

25. Clave P, De Kraa M, Arreola V, Girvent M, Farre R, Palomera E, Serra-Prat M. The effect of bolus viscosity on swallowing function in neurogenic dysphagia. *Aliment Pharmacol Ther* 2006;24:1385–1394.

26. Trivedi BP. Neuroscience: Hardwired for taste. *Nature* 2012;486:S7–S9.

27. Malone A. Anthropometric assessment. In Malone A, Charney P (eds.), *ADA Pocket Guide to Nutrition Assessment*. American Diabetic Association, Chicago, 2004:142–152.

28. Bolanowzki M, Nilsson BE. Assessment of human body composition using dual energy x-ray absorptiometry and bioelectrical impedance analysis. *Med Sci Monthly* 2001;5:1029–1033.

29. Long CL, Schaffel N, Geiger JA, Schiller WR, Blakemore WS. Metabolic response to injury and illness: Estimation of energy and protein needs from indirect calorimetry and nitrogen balance. *J Parenter Enteral Nutr* 1979;3(6):452–456.

3 Concept of Metabolic Surgery

Michael J. Nusbaum, Michael M. Rothkopf,
and Lisa P. Haverstick

CONTENTS

One of the most significant developments in the field of bariatrics was the recognition that weight loss surgery may be the most effective way to reverse type 2 diabetes [1]. Although this was first observed in 1955 [2], it was not generally appreciated until the 1990s [3] and not completely accepted until 2012 [4].

It is now clear that procedures such as the gastric bypass exert beneficial metabolic effects that extend well beyond simple weight loss. In 2007, this realization led the American Society for Bariatric Surgery to change its name to the American Society for *Metabolic* and Bariatric Surgery [5].

The concept of metabolic surgery involves operations whose actions exceed the anatomical alteration of organ structure. These surgeries are actually performed for their physiologic effects on organ function and the alteration of hormone secretion. Although these procedures appear similar to operations performed for weight loss or gastrointestinal (GI) tract diseases, they are primarily metabolic in intent and should be reclassified as such. In this framework, it is the operation's outcomes, not its anatomical components, that define it.

The delineation of this concept is necessary because our understanding of both the gut and the visceral fat has dramatically changed. It is now clear that the GI tract is actually a significant component in processes well beyond nutrient digestion and absorption. The gut is involved in a multitude of interactions that impact multiple organs and extend throughout the body. We see the gut as a bona fide endocrine organ and also as a secondary modulator of other endocrine glands [6]. We also see the gut and the bowel flora as a source of inflammation and a component in immune modulation [7].

Surgical alteration of the nutrient flow through metabolic procedures changes the intestinal flora [8]. Developments in microbial genetics have led to the recognition of an extensive taxonomic complexity among intestinal microbes. The gut flora are part of a vast array of microorganisms that exceed the mammalian tissue in our body by a factor of 10:1 [9]. Specifically, the GI microbiota is believed to possess a significant impact on human physiology. The bowel flora produce vitamin K, biotin, and pantothenic acid. They help digest nutrients and assist intestinal cells to maintain homeostasis [10].

However, the bowel flora are also considered to be a component in the cause of diseases such as inflammatory bowel disease and obesity [11].

Along with our new knowledge of bowel function and bowel flora, we are likewise experiencing a new comprehension of the metabolic role of visceral adipose tissue (VAT). The VAT has been shown to have a role in disease processes that was not previously imagined. Like the GI tract, the VAT is itself a newly recognized endocrine organ [12]. However, unlike the classical components of the endocrine system, VAT hormones seem to be particularly attuned to exerting detrimental as well as beneficial effects [13]. In addition, the VAT is believed to be in communication with a diffuse array of organs including the cardiovascular, GI, renal, neurologic, and other systems [14].

With this understanding, it has become even clearer that we need effective tools to deal with the VAT and to rebalance its output in favor of its beneficial effects. But removing adipose tissue interwoven within the bowel and positioned around visceral organs is currently a technical impossibility. Therefore, it is the fat-depleting aspect of metabolic surgery that provides the most realistic opportunity for reducing the VAT mass and controlling its harmful effects [15].

The new knowledge of the enteroendocrine system, the bowel microbiota, and the VAT has expanded our understanding of human physiology. It has changed our perspective on prevention and treatment of major illnesses including diabetes, cardiovascular disease, and cancer. These developments have shown us that surgery has a significant role in normalizing aberrant physiology. This, in turn, has led to new ways of utilizing existing procedures and to the development of even more novel approaches.

THE GUT AS A SECRETOR/MEDIATOR OF HORMONES

The gut functions as a hormone secretor and a hormone modulator. In terms of endocrine output, more than 30 hormonal substances are secreted by the gut. These include major hormones such as secretin, gastrin, ghrelin, cholecystokinin (CCK), motolin, glucagon-like peptide-1 and 2 (GLP-1/2), gastric inhibitory polypeptide (GIP), vasoactive intestinal polypeptide (VIP), somatostatin, calcitonin, enteroglucagon, and peptide YY (PYY). But in addition, other less well-known substances such as TGF-beta, neurokinins A and B, neurotensin, enkephalins, substance P, and enterogastrone are also part of the vast GI–endocrine array [16]. This effect is demonstrated in the sleeve gastrectomy, wherein the removal of the fundus of the stomach results in dramatic hormonal modulation on a scale comparable to a Roux-en-Y gastric bypass (RYGB).

Not surprisingly, many of these hormones have to do with signaling a need to obtain food or a response to food consumption. They serve to coordinate the process of digestion and to maximize the recovery of nutrients consumed. These hormones interface with the pancreatic and luminal enzymes of digestion, bile emulsifiers, goblet cells, pit glands, tubular glands, mucous glands, acinous glands, and peristaltic contractions to permit the movement of a food bolus through the stages of digestion.

Another fascinating aspect of the enteroendocrine system has to do with its effects on insulin secretion and satiety signaling. The K and L cells of the intestine and cells of the pancreas itself are primarily involved in this process. They release a number of hormones that signal the postprandial response: an increase in insulin secretion by the beta cells, suppression of glucagon output from the alpha cells, and anorexogenic impact on the hypothalamus. CCK, amylin, PYY, and GLP-1 appear to be the major effectors in creating the postprandial physiology [17].

ROLE OF GUT FLORA IN DIGESTION, IMMUNITY, AND INFLAMMATION

The gut flora contains an enormous variety of microorganisms that play important roles in digestive processes, nutrient balance, immune modulation, and CNS function. In fact, it has been estimated that bacterial cells outnumber human cells in the body by a factor of 10 to 1. The millions of microbial genes, gene interactions, and epigenetics are part of who we all are as individuals [18].

Some of these genes encode for the production of beneficial substances such as vitamin K and pantothenic acid. But it is also now apparent that other genes act to modify gut responses to nutrients and inflammation.

For example, *Helicobacter pylori* has long been recognized for its role in regulating stomach acid and the pathogenesis of peptic ulcer disease. However, it also appears to play a role in modulating the ghrelin response. Francois et al. [19] showed that patients who had *H. pylori* eradication had less postprandial attenuation of ghrelin than those who had *H. pylori* colonization intact. Furthermore, *H. pylori* infection remains the number one cause of gastric ulceration following bariatric surgery, followed closely by smoking.

Of perhaps even greater significance is the realization that microbes such as *Bacteroides fragilis* enhance our immune system. Mazmanian and Kasper [20] showed that expression of polysaccharide A by *B. fragilis* may be necessary for proper maturation of T cell function.

In animal models, transplant of the gut microbiome has had dramatic effects on body weight, hormonal response, and inflammation. Bariatric surgery is known to alter bowel flora significantly. The possibility exists for this to be a major component of the mechanisms behind the beneficial effects of bariatric surgery.

Alteration of the gut structure in a way that favors the beneficial aspects of these parameters and suppresses the detrimental aspects would be highly advantageous. It is now thought that metabolic procedures such as the gastric bypass may accomplish some of these goals. By diverting the flow of nutrients away from the normal path, communication between the VAT and GI tract may be altered in a way that will assist the patient in recovering from not only obesity but also the deranged metabolic processes of obesity-related diseases.

Alteration of the GI tract anatomy also has the potential to exert a profound effect on the bowel flora. This, in turn, may benefit the patient by changing adipose–GI interactions as well as inflammation.

SURGERY TO MEANINGFULLY ALTER THE VAT

The VAT appears to have specific communication axes to the central nervous system (CNS), liver, gut, skeletal muscle, and genitalia. Other axes have also been postulated. In addition to the direct response to its VAT axis, the gut also interacts with adipose tissue to mediate some of the other VAT–end organ axes. In this way, the gut responses assist in regulating energy stores, food intake, nutrient utilization, and inflammation.

Another important concept in understanding the new capacity of metabolic surgery has to do with the recognition of the VAT as an endocrine-like organ. The VAT is capable of producing or modifying a significant array of hormones and modulating chemicals that have far-reaching effects in the body. A short listing of these would include corticoids, estrogens, endocannabinoids, cytokines (such as TNF-a and IL-6), adipokines (such as leptin, adiponectin, resistin, omentin, visfatin, vaspin, apelin), angiotensinogen, plasminogen activator inhibitor 1 (PAI-1), and adipsin [21]. This is in addition to the levels of insulin, C-reactive protein (CRP) and circulating free fatty acids.

Imbedded macrophages in the VAT play a significant role in creating inflammation throughout the body. Evidence shows that such inflammation has a significant role in atherosclerotic disease throughout the cardiovascular system. Because of this, we now consider inflammation as presented by biomarkers such as CRP to be equivalent in risk of atherosclerosis development to low-density lipoprotein cholesterol [22].

Such inflammation is critical not only in the cause of atherosclerosis but also in the remodeling that takes place in the process of healing damaged areas such as in myocardial infarction. In the early phase of healing, proinflammatory monocytes predominate. This removes the dead and dying cells. Later in healing, a less inflammatory subset of monocytes assist in the permanent healing through phagocytosis and angiogenesis. This permits the reconstruction of damaged myocardial tissue [23]. VAT-related inflammation may alter this balance, effecting long-term healing. In addition, VAT-related inflammation also plays a detrimental role in other classic inflammatory diseases such as rheumatoid arthritis and psoriasis [24].

Since the VAT is intertwined within the abdominal viscera and vasculature, its surgical removal is currently impossible. But weight loss surgery has the capacity to induce sufficient disruption in caloric balance to reduce the VAT substantially. This change is associated with a decrease in the detrimental hormones, cytokines, and adipokines. These include insulin, corticoids, estrogens, inflammatory cytokines, adipokines (leptin, resistin, omentin, visfatin, vaspin, and apelin), angiotensinogen, PAI-1, adipsin, CRP, and circulating free fatty acids. At the same time, reduction in VAT increases beneficial secretions of substances such as endocannabinoids and adiponectin [25].

These three concepts, taken together, provide the foundation for recognizing a new type of "metabolic" surgery. Surgery has unique effectiveness in changing VAT axes communicating with the GI tract as well as the CNS, liver, and skeletal muscle. Surgery alters the bowel flora without the need for antibiotics. Surgery can reduce the volume of the VAT and thereby rebalance the output of hormones, cytokines, and adipokines.

METABOLIC SURGERY OVERCOMES WEIGHT LOSS RESISTANCE

Weight loss (the weight-reduced state) creates metabolic challenges that resist further weight reduction. This will often thwart a patient's ability to complete the weight loss process successfully, which leads to frustration and defeat.

The patient's weight loss often seems to slow down or halt around previously maintained weight points. This phenomenon is often referred to as the weight loss plateau or set point. The science behind this condition has recently been elucidated.

THE SET POINT

Our bodies control weight just like every other homeostatic aspect of our physiology. We are designed to defend our weight within a certain weight range and within a certain body mass index (BMI). Current thinking is that weight is controlled between dual intervention points, one at a low weight threshold and another at a high weight threshold [26]. When a patient tries to lose weight and drops his or her BMI, there is a compensatory drop in energy expenditure and a coordinated stimulus to increase energy intake. This creates a positive energy balance that pushes the patient back toward his or her previous weight and BMI. Thus, the patient is defending the set point from a negative effect.

On the opposite side, if the person gains weight, there is a suppression of intake and increase in energy expenditure creating a negative energy balance that pushes the BMI back down toward the baseline. Again, the set point is defended, albeit from the opposite direction. We will learn more about this later. In particular, we will see that the set point defense seems to be much more powerful against the negative influence (i.e., weight loss) than a positive one (weight gain).

But there can be no doubt that we defend our weight around a set point. How is this accomplished? The set point is controlled by the hypothalamus within an area we refer to as the weight control center (WCC). The WCC contains important neurons within the arcuate nucleus, paraventricular nucleus, lateral hypothalamic area, and the nucleus of the tractus solitarius. Sixteen or more different CNS regions are involved [27].

Within the arcuate nucleus, the proopiomelanocortin (POMC), PYY, and agouti peptide neurons receive information from the periphery on food intake and energy stores. This information then creates a balance of signals that is either orexigenic (stimulating food intake) or anorexigenic (suppressing food intake). Similar pathways also create signaling that is either hypermetabolic (increased energy expenditure) or hypometabolic (decreased energy expenditure) [28].

The GI system provides the major afferent signaling to the WCC neurons in response to food intake. Information is provided on the timing from the last meal, the quantity and type of intake, and whether or not the intake was adequate. This information is provided via the GI tract's neuronal and endocrine cells. Further details on this process are discussed in Chapters 11, 13, and 16.

Information on the body's energy stores is also transmitted to the WCC by a hormonal signal. This is primarily via the production of leptin and adiponectin within the adipose tissue. Together with the GI tract hormones, these adipose tissue cytokines transmit complex information to the hypothalamus, which affects the overall metabolism and eating behavior.

As we have said, the body is very good at defending the set point from a negative deflection. This is referred to as the "weight-reduced state" and has been extensively studied by Michael Rosenbaum and colleagues at Columbia and Rockefeller Universities [29]. In these studies, induced weight loss results in a variety of physiologic responses. These responses can be grouped as those that reduce energy needs and those that increase energy intake.

The responses that reduce energy use collectively cause a decrease in total energy expenditure (TEE) of about 300 to 400 kcal/day. This is produced through a variety of functions. There is a decrease in autonomic tone, especially in the sympathetic nervous system. The thyroid responds with a decrease in active T3 and an increase in the inactive hormone, reverse T3. Skeletal muscle metabolism becomes more efficient, which means there is a decrease in the use of fuel by the myocytes.

The combination of metabolic adaptations suppresses the amount of total calories burned. This concept is referred to as "adaptive thermogenesis" [30]. While the term "thermogenesis" may seem arcane, it derives from the fact that energy expenditure is measured in calories. Since calories are units of heat, the amount of calories burned equals an amount of heat generated.

On the other side of the equation, the WCC is also adapted to increase food intake. This orexigenic signaling is initiated by GI hormonal changes that rebalance after weight loss. Hormones such as ghrelin, which stimulates hunger, are increased. Hormones such as PYY, CCK, and amylin, which promote satiety are decreased [31]. The net effect is that the person who loses weight is hungrier and less satisfied by meals than the same individual before weight loss. Therefore, the weight-reduced person will seek more food and larger portions. This, in turn, increases caloric intake. More on this subject is covered in Chapters 13 and 16 of this book.

The combination of adaptive thermogenesis and increased caloric intake provides the necessary changes in caloric balance to set the conditions for weight gain. Once the body weight is restored to the prior set point, the mechanisms for weight-reduced adaptation are satisfied and homeostasis is achieved.

The signal behind this process seems to be the circulating level of leptin [32]. Since leptin is a hormone made by the fat cells, and corresponds to the degree of fat storage, we can see leptin as a type of "current" in the weight control "circuit." This circuit has resistors represented by the hypothalamic receptors, which fire if the current drops or rises. These "resistors" tell the brain whether to increase/decrease energy expenditure or to increase/decrease food intake.

The leptin level is a threshold that the body homeostatically defends. But it appears that the threshold is changed in obesity. It seems that when the threshold is raised, the new leptin level, not the pre-obese level, is the threshold that is defended [33]. Therefore, attempts to lose weight induce weight loss resistance and will be observed by the patient as a weight loss plateau. The metabolic rate will be decreased, and the stimulus for food seeking will be increased. This is why patients have such a hard time losing weight and maintaining meaningful weight loss.

We can summarize the set point phenomenon as containing the following components: a decrease in resting energy expenditure, a decrease in active energy expenditure, an increase in orexigenic signaling, and a decrease in anorexigenic signaling. The decrease in resting energy expenditure is primarily a sympathetic nervous system adaptation. The decrease in active energy expenditure is primarily a skeletal muscle system adaptation. The increase in orexigenic signaling involves increased ghrelin levels from the gastric fundus and hypothalamic signaling provoked by the reduction of leptin below the acceptable threshold. This may represent one of the main mechanisms of weight loss seen with the sleeve gastrectomy. The decrease in anorexigenic signaling involves reduction in gut hormones of meal satisfaction (i.e., PYY, CCK, amylin, etc.) and hypothalamic signaling provoked by the reduction of leptin below the acceptable threshold.

METABOLIC SURGERY EFFECT ON THE SET POINT AND PLATEAU PHENOMENON

Bariatric surgery has proven to be the most effective means of accomplishing meaningful weight loss in morbidly obese patients. Even more, surgical weight loss techniques have been found to be more effective than medical therapy for long-term weight loss success and maintenance in these patients. The reasons for this become clearer when we look at the components of the set point and plateau phenomenon as outlined above and examine how surgery addresses them.

Each surgery has its own set of effects in this approach. But, for simplification, we will examine the RYGB as the standard example of bariatric surgery and point out the differences between it and other procedures as appropriate. As we will see, these surgeries have the capacity to produce conditions that cannot be completely adapted by the WCC.

The RYGB is a complex procedure. It has been described as having at least four separate components. First, it performs an isolation of the gastric cardia while creating a small gastric pouch. Second, the operation creates exclusion of the distal stomach. Third, it creates exclusion of the duodenum and proximal jejunum. Fourth, it exposes the distal intestine to undigested nutrients.

The effect of isolation of the gastric cardia is primarily thought of as a means to achieve a limitation on caloric intake. The gastric volume is reduced by 90%. This creates a so-called "gastric pouch" with a very small capacity of roughly 30 mL. This limited gastric pouch forces the patient to consume a smaller volume of food and to eat at a considerably slower rate. There is a rapid feeling of fullness and often a sense of overfilling in which the food bolus is backed up into the lower esophagus. This is a distinctly uncomfortable sensation, and it induces a negative feedback that creates a food aversion. A similar effect can be created by insertion of a gastric band as well as by other gastric restrictive procedures such as the sleeve gastrectomy and the gastric component of the biliopancreatic diversion.

However, it is now recognized that isolation of the gastric cardia and separation of the gastric pouch from the fundus and body of the stomach may have an additional important metabolic role. The hormone ghrelin, which is an octopeptide secreted by the stomach to signal hunger and induce food seeking, is altered by the RYGB. Korner et al. [34] showed that ghrelin levels were significantly reduced after RYGB. This reduction persisted for many months after surgery. Thus, patients who undergo RYGB not only have less capacity to eat but also have a need to eat more slowly and develop food aversions if they eat too much or too quickly. They also have reduced hunger because of reduced levels of ghrelin.

The gastric band does not appear to share this ghrelin-reducing effect of the RYGB. It appears evident that the sleeve gastrectomy shares this mechanism, but it is unclear if the gastric component of the biliopancreatic diversion has this effect.

The exclusion of the distal stomach produces a slightly different effect than that seen with the isolation of the gastric cardia and creation of the gastric pouch. It certainly contributes to the reduction in gastric volume, essentially eliminating the reservoir capacity of the stomach. But it appears to have a unique additional effect on food preferences and cravings [35]. This is highlighted by the fact that the gastric sleeve and the first stage of the biliopancreatic diversion procedure share an alteration on food preferences with the RYGB. Interestingly, the gastric band does not seem to hold this role.

To elucidate this effect, we must understand the three taste domains as described by Spector [36] in 2000. There are three taste domains: sensory, hedonistic, and physiologic. The sensory domain involves a change in taste perception. We refer here to the major taste bud receptors of sweet, sour, bitter, and salty. These physiologic components can be altered by events such as pregnancy.

Studies by le Roux et al. [37] in London and others [38] have shown that sham-operated animals continue to eat high-fat food but the bypass animals did not. They selected low-fat diets that we know to be paradoxical because weight loss should induce consumption of higher calorie diets.

After gastric bypass, patients describe a heightened sense of sweet perception. In le Roux et al.'s [39] studies, they were shown to perceive sweetness at about half the level of sucrose after surgery than before (7.8 mmol of sucrose vs. 14 mmol). We have observed a similar effect in the clinic as patients routinely complain to us that sugary foods taste "too sweet" after RYGB. Many patients also report an aversion to the smell of cooking of certain foods.

In fact, this phenomenon has been a troublesome aspect of care in the rare patient who has overshot his or her weight loss goal after bypass or develops a medical condition such as cancer and needs to gain weight back. These patients do not tolerate sweetened food supplements such as Ensure® because they complain that they are too sweet.

The hedonistic domain also appears altered by RYGB in that there is evidence of a significant change in food cravings after surgery. Leahey et al. [40] showed a decrease in fast food and sweet cravings along with consumption of these types of foods. Positron emission tomography (PET) scanning before and after gastric bypass has demonstrated a decrease in dopamine receptors after the bypass, suggesting an alteration in the hedonistic response [41].

The physiologic domain is also referred to as the postdigestive effect. It can be altered by reactions to eating such as chemotherapy-induced nausea and vomiting. The development of food aversions after bariatric surgery can create negative postdigestive effects and further food seeking.

The exclusion of duodenum and proximal jejunum appears to be responsible for the increase in TEE. Several studies indicate that the increased TEE is actually primarily due to an increase in the specific dynamic action (SDA), also known as the diet-induced thermogenesis (DIT) or thermic effect of food (TEF). This is essentially the fuel required for digestion. Animal studies and work with experimental procedures such as the endoluminal sleeve seem to support this notion [42].

This fact is among the most compelling aspects of the RYGB because it would be a component of energy metabolism that cannot be easily adapted by the WCC. The WCC knows how to reduce resting energy expenditure (EE) and activity EE. But as far as we know, it does not have a mechanism to reduce TEF.

Perhaps the most exciting and discussed aspect of the RYGB is its exposure of the distal intestine to undigested nutrients. This surgical component was initially designed for its malabsorptive role. But this function has been shown to induce important neuroendocrine changes mediated by the intestinal K and L endocrine cells [43]. There is also an apparent coordinated release of pancreatic hormones [44]. The result is a rapid and substantial release of GIP, CCK, GLP-1/2, PYY, and amylin. These are the same hormones that were previously thought of as the "intestinal brake." They provide feedback to the brain that we have eaten sufficiently so that we are satisfied.

Korner et al. [45] have shown that this effect is not produced by the band. But surprisingly, it has been demonstrated that at least the GLP-1 component does exist for the sleeve [46].

A final aspect to mention is the effect on vagal tone. The RYGB (but not the band or the sleeve) includes a partial vagotomy, which would have the effect of interference with normal transmission of the vagal tone. Vagal blocking has an effect on intake that we know of from the experimental use of the vagal nerve stimulator and other neural regulators that provide a vagal blocking current. The induction of a decreased parasympathetic nervous system condition (and perhaps the compensatory increase in sympathetic nervous system output) appears to favor food avoidance.

WEIGHT LOSS SURGERY REVERSES OBESITY-RELATED DISEASE

The early enthusiasm behind bariatric surgery stemmed from its ability to achieve meaningful and lasting weight loss in morbidly obese individuals. These patients appeared to be resistant to any other form of weight loss or, at least, unable to sustain weight loss in any other way. While the complex science behind weight loss resistance was unknown at the time, the clinical observation that patients with severe obesity could not be expected to succeed with diet, exercise, or pharmaceutical weight loss was well accepted.

Bariatric surgery works with long-term weight loss in most patients. This has subsequently been proven definitively by prospective studies such as the Swedish Obese Subjects (SOS) study [47] and the Utah Bariatric Surgery study [48].

There have been several studies documenting the effectiveness of bariatric surgery on long-term weight loss. The most definitive and widely referenced of these is the SOS study.

The SOS study is an ongoing, nonrandomized, prospective, controlled study conducted at 25 surgical departments and 480 primary care centers. The study tracks the outcomes of 2010 obese participants who underwent bariatric surgery and 2037 matched obese controls who received conventional treatment. In the surgery group, 265 individuals underwent gastric bypass (13.2%), 376 had gastric banding (18.7%), and 1369 underwent vertical banded gastroplasty (68.1%). The controls received usual care in the Swedish primary health care system.

To date, they have reported on follow-up data after 2, 10, 15, and 20 years [49]. The mean changes in body weight in the surgery group were −23% at 2 years, −17% at 10 years, −16% at 15 years, and −18% at 20 years. By comparison, the usual care control group remained weight stable during these same measuring points, at 0%, 1%, −1%, and −1%, respectively. Although the SOS study is powered to yield results on health outcomes and mortality, one thing it definitively proved is that bariatric surgery works over the long term.

The SOS study also reported on the overall reduction in mortality and the development of coronary artery disease and diabetes [50]. Bariatric surgery was associated with a reduction in overall mortality. There were 101 deaths in the surgery group and 129 deaths in the control group. The unadjusted overall hazard ratio was 0.76 in the surgery group ($P = 0.04$) compared with the control group. The adjusted hazard ratio (adjusted for sex, age, and risk factors) was 0.71 ($P = 0.01$). It appeared that the mortality reduction in the surgery group was about 30% in subjects above the median BMI (40.8) and about 20% in subjects below it.

The risk reduction achieved by surgery appeared much larger in older subjects (25%) than in younger subjects (6%).

In earlier reports from the SOS study group, bariatric surgery was also associated with beneficial effects on cardiovascular risk factors, cardiovascular symptoms, progression of carotid artery intima–media thickness, sleep apnea, joint pain, and health-related quality of life. Recently, the SOS study has also shown the value of bariatric surgery in preventing type 2 diabetes mellitus [51].

In the Utah study, long-term mortality was compared between 9949 patients who had undergone gastric bypass surgery and 9628 severely obese persons who applied for driver's licenses. From this pool, 7925 surgical patients and 7925 severely obese control subjects were matched according to age, gender, and BMI. The rates of death were recorded with the use of the National Death Index.

During a 7-year follow-up, all-cause mortality decreased by 40% in the surgery group (37.6 vs. 57.1 deaths per 10,000 person-years, $P < 0.001$). Coronary artery disease-specific mortality decreased by 56% (2.6 vs. 5.9 per 10,000 person-years, $P = 0.006$). Mortality from diabetes decreased by 92% (0.4 vs. 3.4 per 10,000 person-years, $P = 0.005$). Cancer mortality decreased by 60% (5.5 vs. 13.3 per 10,000 person-years, $P < 0.001$).

Even though rates of death from accidents and suicide were 58% higher in the surgery group, the study estimated that 137 lives were saved for every 10,000 surgeries.

In 2004, Buchwald [52] conducted a meta-analysis of the previously published observational and interventional bariatric surgery trials. Their paper screened 2738 citations of which 1777 were rejected. Of the remaining 961 articles, 825 did not meet criteria for further analysis. The remaining 136 fully extracted primary studies (a total of 22,094 patients) were available for meta-analysis and were reviewed for weight loss, operative mortality, and outcomes (diabetes, hyperlipidemia, hypertension, and sleep apnea).

The mean percentage of excess weight loss was 61.2%. Patients who underwent gastric banding lost an average of 47.5% (40.7–54.2%). Gastric bypass patients lost an average of 61.6% (56.7–66.5%). Gastroplasty patients lost an average of 68.2% (61.5–74.8%), and biliopancreatic diversion or duodenal switch patients lost an average of 70.1% (66.3–73.9%). The ≤30 days operative mortality was 0.1% for the gastric band and gastroplasty, 0.5% for gastric bypass, and 1.1% for biliopancreatic diversion or duodenal switch.

Diabetes completely resolved in 76.8% of the patients. In 86% of the patients, diabetes either resolved or was improved. Hyperlipidemia improved in 70% of the patients. Hypertension resolved in 61.7% of the patients. In 78.5% of the patients, hypertension either resolved or improved. Obstructive sleep apnea resolved in 85.7% of the patients.

In a 2004 consensus panel report to the American Society for Bariatric Surgery, Buchwald [52] concluded that, "Bariatric surgery results in marked and long-lasting weight loss and elimination or improvement of most obesity-related medical complications, including diabetes, hypertension, hyperlipidemia, obstructive sleep apnea, gastroesophageal reflux disease, cardiac dysfunction, osteoarthritis and low back pain, nonalcoholic fatty liver disease, intertriginous dermatitis, stress incontinence, symptoms of depression, and eating disorders."

Up until this point, all of the benefits of bariatric surgery were presumed to be due to the weight loss. But we have learned that there was much more involved in the metabolic response to surgery.

METABOLIC SURGERY IMPROVES UNEXPECTED CONDITIONS

It has been fascinating to observe that metabolic surgery improved many related conditions even though they are not thought of as directly related to excess weight gain. This list included conditions such as polycystic ovary syndrome (PCOS), acanthosis nigricans, metabolic syndrome, gout, arthritis, and asthma [53]. The first three of this group are conditions of insulin resistance, whereas the latter three are inflammatory conditions. Resolution of the symptoms of pseudotumor cerebri has also been seen after surgical weight loss procedures. Therefore, the surgical outcomes seemed to have a mechanism involving two distinct etiologies.

Insulin resistance is a complex phenomenon. While it is still incompletely understood, it involves alteration in signaling between the pancreatic beta cells, visceral fat, the liver, and the skeletal muscle. By substantially reducing the VAT, surgical weight loss appears to alter this signaling in a favorable manner [54]. Reductions in adipokines such as leptin and resistin, coupled with increases in beneficial substances such as adiponectin, are thought to reduce insulin resistance. Further, the reduction in circulating free fatty acids and possibly the reduction in glycerol that accompanies fat loss may favor insulin sensitivity. Finally, the effect of reducing glucose delivery by the dietary constraints of weight loss surgery must also be considered as part of the reduction in insulin resistance after surgery.

But the output of beta cell–trophic hormones such as GLP-1 may have a rebalancing effect on pancreatic hormone production, leading to a reduction in glucagon and an elevation in insulin-secreting capacity. Such an effect would be very beneficial in controlling insulin resistance.

Talchai et al. [55] have suggested that beta cells that have lost insulin-secreting capacity are not apoptotic but are rather dedifferentiated. Such dedifferentiated cells behave like alpha cells, secreting glucagon and somatostatin in deference to insulin. If this theory bears out, it would help us understand how gastric bypass reverses diabetes, even after beta-cell function seems to have been lost. It is possible that the trophic hormones released after surgery are able to reprogram beta cells back into normal function.

The diseases of excess inflammation, including the diseases of autoimmunity, can also be influenced by changes in diet. These conditions are accelerated by a proinflammatory diet, which is high in saturated fat. The dietary requirements of weight loss surgery include a reduction in total fat intake, which lowers saturated fat.

But the beneficial effects of surgery on inflammation appear to exceed these dietary changes. They may go to a similar site of origin as the one noted in insulin resistance: reduction of the visceral fat [56]. This is because visceral fat tissue produces proinflammatory cytokines that worsen conditions such as arthritis and asthma.

Increases in visceral fat are associated with higher plasma IL-6, adiponectin, PAI-1, and CRP [57]. Production of these and other cytokines by the VAT is thought to create a low-grade inflammatory condition [58]. Obesity-associated adipose tissue inflammation is characterized by infiltration of macrophages, which are stimulated to increase cytokine and chemokine production. Furthermore, it is possible that proinflammatory T-lymphocytes in the VAT signal the appearance of macrophages and initiate inflammatory cell activation [59]. This apparently gives the VAT a unique inflammatory profile [60]. Given these findings, it is not hard to imagine a link between VAT reduction and inflammatory disease amelioration.

METABOLIC SURGERY REVERSED DIABETES MELLITUS *BEFORE* WEIGHT LOSS

In February 1955, surgeons at a Brooklyn, NY, hospital published a paper on the amelioration of diabetes mellitus in three patients after subtotal gastrectomy [2]. Several additional reports with similar results followed. Large-scale studies on the subject began in the 1980s.

In 1995, Pories et al. [3] presented the first major retrospective review on the results of diabetes resolution in 608 gastric bypass patients. The patients were followed for 14 years, between 1980 and 1994. They showed definitively that the operation provided long-term control of type 2 DM. They found that 82.9% of the patients with type 2 DM and 98.7% with impaired glucose tolerance achieved and maintained normal levels of plasma glucose, glycosylated hemoglobin, and insulin [3].

Dixon et al. reported on a prospective randomized control study on diabetes resolution after gastric banding [61]. Mingrone et al. [62] reported on a prospective randomized controlled trial on diabetes resolution after conventional medical therapy, gastric bypass, and biliopancreatic diversion. Sixty obese patients with a diabetes history of 5 years or more and a glycated hemoglobin level of 7.0% or more were studied. The primary end point was the rate of diabetes remission (DMr) at 2 years. DMr was defined as a fasting glucose level of <100 mg/dL and a glycated hemoglobin level of <6.5% in the absence of pharmacologic therapy.

DMr did not occur in any patient within the medical therapy group. However, 75% of patients in the gastric bypass group and 95% in the biliopancreatic diversion group ($P < 0.001$ for both) achieved DMr. Age, sex, baseline BMI, duration of diabetes, and weight changes were not significant predictors of DMr at 2 years. Glycated hemoglobin level decreased to 7.69% ± 0.57% in the medical therapy group, 6.35% ± 1.42% in the gastric bypass group, and 4.95% ± 0.49% in the biliopancreatic diversion group.

Schauer et al. [63] reported on a prospective randomized, nonblinded, single-center control study on diabetes resolution after intensive medical therapy alone versus medical therapy plus RYGB or sleeve gastrectomy. A total of 150 obese patients with uncontrolled type 2 diabetes (age 49 ± 8 years, 66% women, average glycated hemoglobin level 9.2% ± 1.5%) were enrolled.

The results showed that 12% (5 of 41 patients) in the medical therapy group versus 42% (21 of 50 patients) in the gastric bypass group ($P = 0.002$) and 37% (18 of 49 patients) in the sleeve gastrectomy group ($P = 0.008$) achieved the primary end point of a glycated hemoglobin level of 6.0% or less 12 months after treatment. Weight loss was greater in the gastric bypass group and sleeve gastrectomy group (−29.4 ± 9.0 and −25.1 ± 8.5 kg, respectively) than in the medical therapy group (−5.4 ± 8.0 kg) ($P < 0.001$ for both comparisons).

The use of drugs to lower glucose, lipid, and blood pressure levels decreased significantly after both surgical procedures but increased in patients receiving medical therapy alone. The three data from this study were recently reported [64]. At 36 months of follow-up, the primary end point was met by 5% of the patients in the medical-therapy group, as compared to 24% of those in the sleeve-gastrectomy group and 38% of those in the gastric-bypass group.

Initially, the resolution of type 2 diabetes after bariatric surgery was believed to be a function of the dietary restriction and weight loss. Virtually all of the initial patients studied were obese. The reason for surgery was morbid obesity rather than diabetes. So the major measurable outcome was loss of excess body weight (EBWL).

At the time that this concept was being first explored, EBWL had already been demonstrated to improve glucose tolerance and reduce the need for diabetic medical therapy [65]. This was based on studies conducted using the protein-sparing modified fast (PSMF) [66]. In these medical weight loss studies, diabetic patients greatly benefitted from massive weight loss. The general reduction in body weight and, in particular, the loss of abdominal fat (now understood as VAT) improved fasting and postprandial glucose and reduced insulin resistance.

The PSMF diet was essentially devoid of carbohydrate. Under these conditions, the exogenous delivery of glucose was brought to a bare minimum, practically nil. This was seen as an effective means of controlling postprandial glucose elevations in patients who had intact insulin production.

The combination of improved insulin resistance and restricted glucose delivery was seen as an effective method for diabetes management and one that could be reliably reproduced by bariatric surgery. Surgery would obviate the need for an artificial diet. The diet would be modified by the inherent sugar and starch intolerance built into the procedure.

Many of the early papers on the gastric bypass pointed to its role as a malabsorptive procedure to explain the weight loss [67]. But subsequent studies have shown that this is not really the case. In fact, the degree of malabsorption after a RYGB is quite small [68].

Instead, the mechanisms for diabetic resolution after gastric bypass seem to be multifactorial. First, there are fundamental changes in taste, desire, and response to food, which reduce intake and glucose delivery [69], which are also seen with the sleeve gastrectomy. Second, the significant weight loss improves insulin sensitivity so that the insulin made by the remaining beta cells is enough to match the (diet-reduced) glucose appearance in the serum [70]. Third, significant increases in the incretin hormones after RYGB (such as GLP-1) improve beta-cell stimulation and may play a role in beta-cell recovery and tropism [71].

METABOLIC EFFECTS OF THE GASTRIC BAND, SLEEVE GASTRECTOMY, AND RYGB

A differential of metabolic effects exists between the three major forms of bariatric surgery currently in use. An understanding of this differential is essential for the proper selection of the procedure for each individual patient. In this section, we will delineate the known metabolic effects of each operation and compare the advantages and disadvantages for the various patient scenarios.

Kaplan and Seely [72] have described a differential of effects based on four broad factors: weight loss, food intake, energy expenditure, and glucose metabolism. They compared six procedures: gastric bypass, biliopancreatic diversion, endoluminal sleeve, ileal transposition, gastric banding, and gastric plication.

In our conceptualization, we would limit this grid to the three major existing procedures: gastric band, sleeve gastrectomy, and gastric bypass. We would then add effects on bowel flora, VAT, and enteroendocrine effects of each procedure (Table 3.1).

The three procedures can be seen as having different effects on each component. This opens the door to the use of a logic-based flow diagram for patient–procedure selection. The categories in this grid are weight loss, VAT reduction, microbiota, food intake control, energy expenditure, glucose metabolism, and enteroendocrine stimulation.

TABLE 3.1

Differential of Effects of Three Common Bariatric Procedures on Weight, VAT, Microbiota, Food Intake, Energy Expenditure, Glucose Metabolism, and Enteroendocrine Secretion

	Weight Loss	VAT Loss	Microbiota Effect	Food Intake	Energy Expenditure	Glucose Metabolism	Enteroendocrine
Bypass	4+	4+	4+	4+	4+	4+	4+
Sleeve	3+	4+	2+	3+	?	3+	2+
Band	2+	2+	1+	2+	0	2+	0

Source: Modified from Kaplan LM, Seely RJ. The Biology of Body Weight: Implications for Bariatric Surgery. Metabolic Applied Research Strategy (MARS) eCourse Presentation. Ethicon Endo-surgery, 2010.

EFFECT ON WEIGHT LOSS

Before we begin this discussion it is important to establish the terminology. In the bariatric field (whether medical or surgical), weight loss is usually measured in terms of a reduction in excess weight. This is a different approach than looking at the raw number of overall weight loss or overall percentage of weight loss.

The calculation of excess body weight (EBW) is usually based on the difference in weight between the maximum body weight (MaxBW) of the patient minus their ideal body weight (IBW). The MaxBW is the heaviest reported weight but should not include pregnancy weight in women or states of fluid overload. The IBW is a calculated figure based on the height–weight tables or standard formulae. Thus, EBW = MaxBW − IBW.

The majority of the EBW is due to fat mass (FM). However, a portion of the EBW is assumed to belong to nonfat or lean body mass (LBM) tissues. These include skin, muscle, and bone, which increased in size to accommodate the strain of the added adipose tissue weight. In general, 25% of the EBW is considered to belong to these non-adipose tissues.

From these concepts, the derivation of an appropriate goal weight can be construed. This value is often referred to as the adjusted body weight (ABW); it adjusts the IBW for the fact that obesity has caused an additional LBM as well as FM. In most studies, the ABW is considered the appropriate goal of weight loss management. In others the ABW is implied because the goal of therapy is stated to be 75% loss of the EBW.

The three major forms of weight loss surgery produce different expectations of EBWL. As one would expect, the differential follows the aggressiveness of the procedure. So the band produces less weight loss than the sleeve, whereas the sleeve produces less than the bypass. In terms of the EBW, the band is expected to yield a 50% EBWL. The sleeve is expected to yield a 60% EBWL. The bypass is expected to yield a 75% EBWL.

Patients who do not achieve at least 50% of the expected goal for each procedure can be considered a weight loss failure (WLF) and should be referred for metabolic therapy.

VAT REDUCTION

Surgical weight loss results in improvements in hypertension, dyslipidemia, glucose metabolism, and insulin sensitivity [73]. VAT plays a major role in the development of these metabolic, obesity-associated diseases. Therefore, the reduction of VAT is an important goal of metabolic surgery.

All forms of weight loss surgery are capable of reducing VAT mass through their effects on weight loss as noted above. Evidence from body composition studies have confirmed that VAT is successfully reduced by bariatric surgery [74].

But the reduction in VAT does not appear as intuitive as with simple weight loss. While the gastric band is inferior to either the sleeve or the bypass, the sleeve may be more effective at VAT reduction than RYGB [75]. The reason for the sleeve superiority of laparoscopic sleeve gastrectomy over the bypass is unclear and needs further evaluation.

MICROBIOTA

The distribution of bacterial species in gut microbiota is thought to be a factor in the development of obesity. Manipulation of the gut bacterial flora has been shown to alter body weight experimental models. Therefore, it is possible that pharmaceuticals and procedures that alter the gut microbiota may impact body weight.

An alteration of the gut bacterial microbiota from bariatric surgery begins with the perioperative bowel cleansing and the use of antibiotic prophylaxis. After surgery, patients are instructed to follow a specific dietary protocol. Following dietary advancement, patients often report an altered food selection, thoroughness of mastication, and greater need to consume liquids. In addition, each procedure may have different effects on gastric acid production, pH and bowel motility, enterohepatic circulation, and enterohormone production. All of these conditions may play a role in altering the gut microbiota (Table 3.2).

Two early studies have examined microbiota changes after RYGB. Zhang et al. [76] used large-scale pyrosequencing on a small group of normal weight, morbidly obese and post-RYGB individuals. They found that Firmicutes species were dominant in normal weight and obese individuals but markedly reduced in post-RYGB patients. H2-producing bacterial groups and H2-using methanogenic Archea (which are both involved in energy extraction from indigestible polysaccharides) were found in the obese individuals, but not in lean individuals or those after RYGB. Levels of gamma-proteobacteria were increased after surgery (Figure 3.1).

Furet et al. [77] studied gut microbiota by real-time quantitative polymerase chain reaction in 13 lean control subjects and in 30 obese individuals (seven with type 2 diabetes) before and after RYGB. They found that the *Bacteroides/Prevotella* group was lower in obese subjects preoperatively than in control subjects and increased postoperatively. *Escherichia coli* species increased postoperatively and was inversely correlated with fat mass and leptin levels. The *Lactobacillus/Leuconostoc/Pediococcus* group and *Bifidobacterium* genus decreased postoperatively.

TABLE 3.2
Dietary and Digestive Changes Induced by Different Types of Bariatric Surgery

Changes	LAGB	Sleeve Gastrectomy	RYGB
Rate of eating	↓	↓	↓
Quantity of food consumed	↓	↓↓	↓↓
Acid production		↓	↓
Bowel motility		↑	↑
Ghrelin		↓	↓
GLP-1		↑	↑
PYY			↑

Source: Adapted from Aron-Wisnewsky J. et al., *Nat. Rev. Gastroenterol. Hepatol.*, 9: 590–598, 2012.

Note: GLP-1, glucagon-like peptide-1; LAGB, laparoscopic adjustable gastric band; PYY, peptide YY; RYGB, Roux-en-Y gastric bypass; ↓, decreased; ↑, increased.

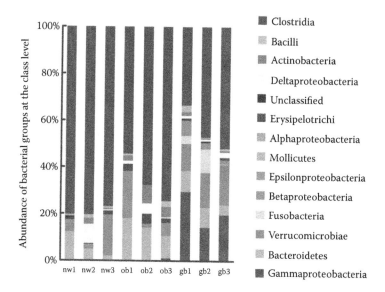

FIGURE 3.1 Taxonomic breakdown of human intestinal bacterial V6 tags obtained by pyrosequencing in the normal-weight (nw1, nw2, and nw3), obese (ob1, ob2, and ob3), and postgastric bypass (gb1, gb2, and gb3) subjects. (From Zhang H. et al., *PNAS*, 106:2365–2370, 2009. With permission.)

FOOD INTAKE CONTROL

Each of the three major bariatric procedures has a component of gastric restriction that leads to a reduction in eating capacity. However, there are significant differences among the procedures, even in this most basic of functions.

The gastric band creates a 30-mL pouch at the cardia of the stomach and a narrow opening (10 mm) between the pouch and the body of the stomach. Eating produces a rapid filling of the pouch. Food eaten after the pouch is filled will back up into the lower esophagus, producing an unpleasant symptom of lower thoracic fullness. If further food is ingested, pharyngeal hypersecretion, nausea, and vomiting may follow.

The negative feedback of this reaction thereby restricts the volume and rate of eating. The patient quickly learns that his or her eating patterns must drastically change in order to avoid the discomfort. The patient must chew slowly, swallow carefully, and avoid drinking and eating at the same time. This negative feedback may produce food aversions that ultimately change the desirability of certain foods.

The band has little to no effect on gastric ghrelin secretion. The octopeptide ghrelin is widely seen as the signal for initiating a sense of hunger. Similarly, the band has little to no effect on stimulating the hormones of satiety, including GIP, PYY, CCK, amylin, and GLP-1. Maintenance of intact ghrelin signaling without stimulation of GIP, PYY, CCK, amylin, or GLP-1 could lead to the initiation of hunger, which the band patient cannot satisfy.

Thus, the band can be thought of as a primarily restrictive device that alters eating patterns and behavior but has little effect on neurochemical and endocrine GI responses.

The sleeve gastrectomy procedure was initially also thought of as a primarily restrictive procedure regarding food intake. However, recent studies by Wilson-Pérez and colleagues [78] have demonstrated that the sleeve produces some unique effects on food selection, taste, and preferences. The sleeve also increases GLP-1 while reducing ghrelin levels.

The bypass restricts food intake by at least three mechanisms. First, the creation of a small gastric pouch reduces food volume and eating rate. Second, the bypass alters taste and food preferences. Third, the bypass alters the enteroendocrine system in ways that would be expected to assist with intake control. The secretion of hunger-inducing ghrelin is reduced. At the same time, the secretion of satiety-inducing hormones such as GIP, PYY, and GLP-1 is increased.

ENERGY EXPENDITURE

The exclusion of the duodenum and proximal jejunum appears to be responsible for the increase in TEE. Several studies indicate that the increased TEE is actually primarily due to an increase in the SDA, also known as DIT. This is essentially the fuel required for digestion. Animal studies and work with experimental procedures such as the endoluminal sleeve seem to support this notion.

This fact is among the most compelling aspects of the RYGB because it would be a component of energy metabolism that cannot be easily adapted by the WCC. The WCC can reduce resting EE and activity EE but, as far as we know, not SDA.

Another interesting aspect of the increase in any energy expenditure after gastric bypass is related to the hormone oxyntomodulin. This is a 37-amino acid peptide, which is a product of the pro-glucagon gene. It is released by the L cells of the small intestine following caloric intake.

Oxyntomodulin exerts a trimodal effect on energy metabolism [79]. First, it provides a satiety signal to the WCC, thereby reducing energy expenditure. This action appears to be mediated through the GLP-1 receptor. Secondly, oxyntomodulin is thought to have an incretin effect similar to GLP-1.

But recent studies have also shown that this hormone can also elevate TEE. According to Wynne et al. [80], oxyntomodulin increases daily activity related energy expenditure by roughly 26%. In their studies, this increased caloric expenditure by an average of 143 kcal/day [80].

According to Laferrère et al. [81], oxyntomodulin is elevated following gastric bypass. In their studies comparing obese women with type 2 diabetes before and after gastric bypass, they found that oxyntomodulin rose significantly after surgery. Thus far, there is no evidence that either the gastric band or the sleeve gastrectomy can produce a similar effect.

GLUCOSE METABOLISM

Bariatric surgery has the capacity to greatly improve glucose metabolism through a number of mechanisms. First and foremost, all forms of bariatric surgery greatly reduce food intake and therefore glucose delivery. In particular, many forms of food-containing sugars and starches become intolerant to the postbariatric patient. It is common for patients who have had all three of the major forms of bariatric surgery to complain of a sense of fullness after consuming foods such as bread, rice, and pasta. This is presumably because these foodstuffs swell in the gastric pouch or gastric sleeve.

Because all forms of bariatric surgery would be associated with weight loss, there is an anticipated improvement in insulin resistance from each of the procedures. This has been demonstrated in prior studies. However, it appears that procedures such as the gastric sleeve and gastric bypass produce more reduction in insulin resistance than that from the gastric band or medical weight loss. Furthermore, the latter two procedures, and in particular the gastric bypass, seem to be able to improve insulin dynamics even before any significant weight loss has occurred.

At least in the bypass, this phenomenon is related to beneficial changes in hepatic, muscle, and adipose tissue insulin sensitivity. There is an increase in high molecular weight adiponectin. There is a decrease in inflammatory cytokines and a decrease in intrahepatic and intramuscular lipids.

However, an important aspect of the improvement in glucose metabolism following bariatric surgery appears to be related to the so-called incretin effect, which will be detailed below. This effect has been shown to be produced by both the gastric sleeve and the gastric bypass procedures. But there is no known incretin effect produced by the gastric band.

Therefore, a differential can be envisioned wherein patients with impaired glucose tolerance and early diabetes (less than 2 years duration) would have significant benefit from all three bariatric procedures. But patients who have more advanced or long-standing diabetes may require more aggressive forms of surgery.

ENTERO-ENDOCRINE STIMULATION

The gastric bypass causes exposure of the distal intestine to undigested nutrients. This phenomenon has been shown to induce neuroendocrine changes mediated by the intestinal K and L endocrine cells. There is also an apparent coordinated release of pancreatic hormones. The result is a rapid and substantial release of GIP, CCK, GLP-1/2, PYY, oxyntomodulin, and amylin. These are the same hormones that were previously thought of as the "intestinal brake." They provide feedback to the brain that we have eaten sufficiently to be satisfied.

Korner et al. [45] have shown that this effect is not produced by the band. But Wilson-Pérez and colleagues [78] have demonstrated that an incretin effect does exist for the sleeve. In animal studies, they showed an increase in insulin secretion after both the gastric bypass and gastric sleeve. Similarly, glucose regulation was enhanced by both procedures. The mechanism for this surprising observation appears to be the sleeve's capability to enhance GLP-1 secretion. Thus, it appears that the gastric sleeve has a similar effect on postprandial GLP-1 as that seen with the bypass.

SUMMARY

The concept of metabolic surgery involves the recognition that certain types of weight loss surgery can be physiologic rather than just anatomic. It is well recognized that bariatric procedures such as the RYGB produce effective, meaningful, and long-lasting weight loss. Therefore, it is not surprising that weight loss surgery reverses obesity-related disease.

But procedures like the RYGB exert powerful effects on the metabolic rate and metabolic signaling of food intake. This overcomes weight loss resistance because it produces conditions to which the body cannot easily adapt. This is not only a matter of restricting intake or even malabsorption of consumed calories. The metabolic aspect of the operation is its ability to lower ghrelin, increase GLP-1, increase energy expenditure, and alter taste domains. Similarly, the increasingly popular sleeve gastrectomy clearly has its benefits in the metabolic signaling of food intake as it completely lacks the malabsorptive component, yet its weight loss effect remains evident.

These operations have been shown to reverse conditions that are not purely weight related. Such conditions are caused by insulin resistance and overstimulation of the inflammatory system. And some bariatric operations can reverse type 2 diabetes even before significant weight loss occurred, often within days.

This has led to an understanding that these operations exert metabolic effects that favorably stimulate GI hormone production, change bowel flora, and reduce the harmful activity of the VAT. The result of these actions is a significant reduction in insulin resistance and inflammation in a way not currently possible by other means.

The concept of metabolic surgery involves procedures that are performed for their physiologic effects on organ function and the alteration of hormone secretion. In this framework, it is the operation's outcomes, not its anatomical components, that define it.

REFERENCES

1. Buchwald H, Avidor Y, Braunwald E et al. Bariatric surgery: A systematic review and meta-analysis. *JAMA* 2004; 13: 1724–1737.
2. Friedman NM, Sancetta AJ, Magovern GJ. The amelioration of diabetes mellitus following subtotal gastrectomy. *Surg Gynecol Obstet* 1955; 100: 201–204.
3. Pories WJ, Swanson MS, MacDonald KG et al. Who would have thought it? An operation proves to be the most effective therapy for adult-onset diabetes mellitus. *Ann Surg* 1995; 222: 339–350.
4. Zimmet P, Alberti KG. Surgery or medical therapy for obese patients with type 2 diabetes? *N Engl J Med* 2012; 366: 1635–1636.
5. Sugerman HJ. ASBS name change/decreased mortality with bariatric surgery. *Surg Obes Relat Dis* 2007; 3: 491.
6. Ahlman H, Nilsson O. The gut as the largest endocrine organ in the body. *Ann Oncol* 2001; 12: S63–S68.

7. O'Hara AM, Shanahan F. The gut flora as a forgotten organ. *EMBO Rep* 2006 7: 688–693.

8. Aron-Wisnewsky J, Doré J, Clement K. The importance of the gut microbiota after bariatric surgery. *Nat Rev Gastroenterol Hepatol* 2012; 9: 590–598.

9. Nicholson JK, Holmes E, Kinross J et al. Host-gut microbiota metabolic interactions. *Science* 2012; 336: 1262–1267.

10. Gerritsen J, Smidt H, Rijkers GT, de Vos WM. Intestinal microbiota in human health and disease: The impact of probiotics. *Genes Nutr* 2011; 6: 209–240.

11. Caesar R, Fak F, Backhed F. Effects of gut microbiota on obesity and atherosclerosis via modulation of inflammation and lipid metabolism. *J Intern Med* 2010; 268: 320–328.

12. Kershaw EE, Flier JS. Adipose tissue as an endocrine organ. *J Clin Endocrinol Metab* 2004; 89: 2548–2556.

13. Drucker DJ. Unraveling the complexities of gut endocrinology. *Nat Clin Pract Endocrinol Metab* 2007; 3: 317.

14. Bays HE, Gonzalez-Campoy JM, Bray GA et al. Pathogenic potential of adipose tissue and metabolic consequences of adipocyte hypertrophy and increased visceral adiposity. *Expert Rev Cardiovasc Ther* 2008; 6: 343–368.

15. Bays HE, Laferrère B, Dixon J et al. Adiposopathy and bariatric surgery: Is 'sick fat' a surgical disease? *Int J Clin Pract* 2009; 63: 1285–1300.

16. Walsh JH. Gastrointestinal hormones. In: *Physiology of the Gastrointestinal Tract*, 3rd ed., edited by Johnson LR, Alpers DH, Christensen J, Jacobson ED, and Walsh JH. Raven Press, New York, 1984; 1–128.

17. Batterham RL, Cowley MA, Small CJ et al. Gut hormone PYY3-36 physiologically inhibits food intake. *Nature* 2002; 418: 650–654.

18. Kinross JM, Darzi AW, Nicholson JK. Gut microbiome-host interactions in health and disease. *Genome Medicine* 2011; 3: 14.

19. Francois F, Roper J, Joseph N et al. The effect of H. pylori eradication on meal-associated changes in plasma ghrelin and leptin. *BMC Gastroenterol* 2011; 11: 37.

20. Mazmanian SK, Kasper DL. The love-hate relationship between bacterial polysaccharides and the host immune system. *Nat Rev Immunol* 2006; 6: 849–858.

21. Trayhurn P, Bing C, Wood SI. Adipose tissue and adipokines—Energy regulation from the human perspective. *J Nutr* 2006; 136: 1935S–1939S.

22. Ridker PM, Danielson E, Fonseca FAH et al. Rosuvastatin to prevent vascular events in men and women with elevated C-reactive protein. *N Engl J Med* 2008; 359: 2195–2207.

23. Selvaraju V, Joshi M, Suresh S et al. Diabetes, oxidative stress, molecular mechanism, and cardiovascular disease—An overview. *Toxicol Mech Methods* 2012; 5: 330–335.

24. O'Rourke RW. Inflammation in obesity-related disease. *Surgery* 2009; 145: 255–259.

25. Kempf K, Hector J, Strate T et al. Immune-mediated activation of the endocannabinoid system in visceral adipose tissue in obesity. *Horm Metab Res* 2007; 39: 596–600.

26. Speakman JR, Levitsky DA, Allison DA et al. Set points, settling points and some alternative models: Theoretical options to understand how genes and environments combine to regulate body adiposity. *Dis Model Mech* 2011; 4: 733–745.

27. Elmquist JK, Elias CF, Saper CB. From lesions to leptin: Hypothalamic control of food intake and body weight. *Neuron* 1999; 22: 221–232.

28. Schwartz MW, Morton GJ. Obesity: Keeping hunger at bay. *Nature* 2002; 418: 595–597.

29. Rosenbaum M, Kissileff HR, Mayer LES, Hirsch J, Leibel RL. Energy intake in weight-reduced humans. *Brain Res* 2010; 2: 95–102.

30. Weinsier RL, Nagy TR, Hunter GR et al. Do adaptive changes in metabolic rate favor weight regain in weight-reduced individuals? An examination of the set-point theory. *Am J Clin Nutr* 2000; 72: 1088–1094.

31. Sumithran P, Prendergast LA, Delbridge E et al. Long-term persistence of hormonal adaptations to weight loss. *N Engl J Med* 2011; 365: 1597–1604.

32. Rosenbaum M, Goldsmith R, Bloomfield D et al. Low-dose leptin reverses skeletal muscle, autonomic, and neuroendocrine adaptations to maintenance of reduced weight. *J Clin Invest* 2005; 115: 579–586.

33. Rosenbaum M, Leibel RL. Brain reorganization following weight loss. *Nestle Nutr Inst Workshop Ser* 2012; 73: 1–20.

34. Korner J, Inabnet W, Conwell IM et al. Differential effects of gastric bypass and banding on circulating gut hormone and leptin levels. *Obesity* 2006; 14: 1553–1561.

35. Tichansky DS, Boughter JD Jr, Madan AK. Taste change after laparoscopic Roux-en-Y gastric bypass and laparoscopic adjustable gastric banding. *Surg Obes Relat Dis* 2006; 2: 440–444.

36. Spector AC. Linking gustatory neurobiology to behavior in vertebrates. *Neurosci Biobehav Rev* 2000; 24: 391–416.

37. le Roux CW, Bueter M, Theis N et al. Gastric bypass reduces fat intake and preference. *Am J Physiol Regul Integr Comp Physiol* 2011; 301: R1057–R1066.

38. Hajnal A, Kovacs P, Ahmed T et al. Gastric bypass surgery alters behavioral and neural taste functions for sweet taste in obese rats. *Am J Physiol Gastrointest Liver Physiol* 2010; 299: G967–G979.

39. Bueter M, Miras AD, Chichger H et al. Alterations of sucrose preference after Roux-en-Y gastric bypass. *Physiol Behav* 2011; 24: 709–721.

40. Leahey TM, Bond DS, Raynor H et al. Effects of bariatric surgery on food cravings: Do food cravings and the consumption of craved foods "normalize" after surgery? *Surg Obes Relat Dis* 2012; 8: 84–91.

41. Dunn JP, Cowan RL, Volkow ND et al. Decreased dopamine type 2 receptor availability after bariatric surgery: Preliminary findings. *Brain Res* 2010; 1350: 123–130.

42. Munoz R, Carmody JS, Stylopoulos N, Davis P, Kaplan LM. Isolated duodenal exclusion increases energy expenditure and improves glucose homeostasis in diet-induced obese rats. *Am J Physiol Regul Integr Comp Physiol* 2012; 303: R985–R993.

43. Fetner R, McGinty J, Russell C, Pi-Sunyer FX, Laferrère B. Incretins, diabetes, and bariatric surgery: A review. *Surg Obes Relat Dis* 2005; 1(6): 589–597.

44. Swarbrick MM, Stanhope IT, Austrheim-Smith T et al. Longitudinal changes in pancreatic and adipocyte hormones following Roux-en-Y gastric bypass surgery. *Diabetologia* 2008; 51: 1901–1911.

45. Korner J, Bessler M, Inabnet W, Taveras C, Holst JJ. Exaggerated GLP-1 and blunted GIP secretion are associated with Roux-en-Y gastric bypass but not adjustable gastric banding. *Surg Obes Relat Dis* 2007; 3: 597–601.

46. Romero F, Nicolau J, Flores L et al. Comparable early changes in gastrointestinal hormones after sleeve gastrectomy and Roux-en-Y gastric bypass surgery for morbidly obese type 2 diabetic subjects. *Surg Endosc* 2012; 26: 2231–2239.

47. Sjöström L, Lindroos AK, Peltonen M et al. Lifestyle, diabetes, and cardiovascular risk factors 10 years after bariatric surgery. *N Engl J Med* 2004; 351: 2683–2693.

48. Adams TD, Davidson LE, Litwin SE et al. Health benefits of gastric bypass surgery after 6 years. *JAMA* 2012; 308: 1122–1131.

49. Sjöström L, Narbro K, Sjöström CD et al. Effects of bariatric surgery on mortality in Swedish obese subjects. *N Engl J Med* 2007; 357: 741–752.

50. Sjöström L. Review of the key results of the Swedish Obese Subjects (SOS) trial: A prospective controlled intervention study of bariatric surgery. *J Intern Med* 2013; 273: 219–234.

51. Carlsson L, Peltonen M, Ahlin S et al. Bariatric surgery and prevention of type 2 diabetes in Swedish Obese Subjects. *N Engl J Med* 2012; 367: 695–704.

52. Buchwald H. 2004 ASBS Consensus Conference, Consensus Conference Statement Bariatric surgery for morbid obesity: Health implications for patients, health professionals, and third-party payers. *Surg Obes Relat Dis* 2005; 1: 371–381.

53. Grundy SM, Barnett JP. Metabolic and health complications of obesity. *Dis Mon* 1990; 36: 641–731.

54. Catalán V, Gómez-Ambrosi J, Ramirez B et al. Proinflammatory cytokines in obesity: Impact of type 2 diabetes mellitus and gastric bypass. *Obes Surg* 2007; 17: 1464–1474.

55. Talchai C, Xuan S, Lin HV, Sussel L, Accili D. Pancreatic β cell dedifferentiation as a mechanism of diabetic β cell failure. *Cell* 2012; 150: 1223–1234.

56. Zhang H, Wang Y, Zhang J et al. Bariatric surgery reduces visceral adipose inflammation and improves endothelial function in type 2 diabetic mice. *Arterioscler Thromb Vasc Biol* 2011; 31: 2063–2069.

57. van den Borst B, Gosker HR, Koster A et al. The influence of abdominal visceral fat on inflammatory pathways and mortality risk in obstructive lung disease. *Am J Clin Nutr* 2012; 96: 516–526.

58. Visser M, Bouter LM, McQuillen GM, Wener MH, Harris TP. Elevated C-reactive protein levels in overweight and obese adults. *JAMA* 1999; 282: 2131–2135.

59. Kintscher U, Hartge M, Hess K et al. T-lymphocyte infiltration in visceral adipose tissue: A primary event in adipose tissue inflammation and the development of obesity-mediated insulin resistance. *Arterioscler Thromb Vasc Biol* 2008; 28: 1304–1310.

60. Alvehus M, Burén J, Sjöström M, Goedecke J, Olsson T. The human visceral fat depot has a unique inflammatory profile. *Obesity* 2010; 18: 879–883.

61. Dixon JB, O'Brien PE, Playfair J et al. Adjustable gastric banding and conventional therapy for type 2 diabetes: A randomized controlled trial. *JAMA* 2008; 299: 316–323.

62. Mingrone G, Panunzi S, De Gaetano A et al. Bariatric surgery versus conventional medical therapy for type 2 diabetes. *N Engl J Med* 2012; 366: 1577–1585.

63. Schauer PR, Kashyap SR, Wolski K et al. Bariatric surgery versus intensive medical therapy in obese patients with diabetes. *N Engl J Med* 2012; 366: 1567–1576.

64. Schauer PR, Bhatt DL, Kirwan JP et al. For the stampede investigators. *N Engl J Med* 2014; 370: 2002–2013.

65. Long SD, O'Brien K, MacDonald KG Jr et al. Weight loss in severely obese subjects prevents the progression of impaired glucose tolerance to type II diabetes. A longitudinal interventional study. *Diabetes Care* 1994; 17: 372–375.

66. Suskind RM, Sothern MS, Andrews RE, Udall JN, Blecker U. The effect of protein-sparing modified fast in obese children with insulin dependent MODY-type diabetes mellitus. *Pediatr Res* 1997; 41: 73.

67. Cummings DE, Overduin J, Foster-Schubert KE. Gastric bypass for obesity: Mechanisms of weight loss and diabetes resolution. *J Clin Endocrinol Metab* 2004; 89: 2608–2615.

68. Cummings DE, Overduin J, Foster-Schubert KE, Carlson MJ. Role of the bypassed proximal intestine in the anti-diabetic effects of bariatric surgery. *Surg Obes Relat Dis* 2007; 3: 109–115.

69. Thaler JP, Cummings DE. Hormonal and metabolic mechanisms of diabetes remission after gastrointestinal surgery. *Endocrinology* 2009; 150: 2518–2525.

70. Mun EC, Blackburn GL, Matthews JB. Current status of medical and surgical therapy for obesity. *Gastroenterology* 2001; 120: 669–681.

71. Drucker DJ. The role of gut hormones in glucose homeostasis. *J Clin Invest* 2007; 117: 24–32.

72. Kaplan LM, Seely RJ. The Biology of Body Weight: Implications for Bariatric Surgery. Metabolic Applied Research Strategy (MARS) eCourse Presentation. Ethicon Endo-surgery, 2010.

73. Strum W, Tschoner A, Engl J et al. Effect of bariatric surgery on both functional and structural measures of premature atherosclerosis. *Eur Heart J* 2009; 30: 2038–2043.

74. Mizrahi I, Grinbaum R, Loubashevsky N et al. A prospective comparison study of visceral and subcutaneous fat reduction in morbidly obese subjects undergoing laparoscopic gastric banding, sleeve gastrectomy and Roux-en-Y gastric bypass. *Obes Surg* 2012; 22: 1315–1419.

75. Gaborit B, Jacquier A, Kober F et al. Effects of bariatric surgery on cardiac ectopic fat: Lesser decrease in epicardial fat compared to visceral fat loss and no change in myocardial triglyceride content. *J Am Coll Cardiol* 2012; 60: 1381–1389.

76. Zhang H, DiBaise JK, Zuccolo A et al. Human gut microbiota in obesity and after gastric bypass. *PNAS* 2009; 106: 2365–2370.

77. Furet JP, Kong LC, Tap J et al. Differential adaptation of human gut microbiota to bariatric surgery-induced weight loss links with metabolic and low-grade inflammation markers. *Diabetes* 2010; 59: 3049–3057.

78. Wilson-Pérez HE, Chambers AP, Ryan KK et al. Vertical sleeve gastrectomy is effective in two genetic mouse models of glucagon-like peptide-1 receptor deficiency. *Diabetes* 2013; 62(7): 2380–2385.

79. Wynne K, Field BC, Bloom SR. The mechanism of action for oxyntomodulin in the regulation of obesity. *Curr Opin Investig Drugs* 2010; 11: 1151–1157.

80. Wynne KW, Park AJ, Small CJ et al. Oxyntomodulin increases energy expenditure in addition to decreasing energy intake in overweight and obese humans: A randomized controlled trial. *Int J Obes* 2006; 30: 1729–1736.

81. Laferrère B, Swerdlow N, Bawa B et al. Rise of oxyntomodulin in response to oral glucose after gastric bypass surgery in patients with type 2 diabetes. *J Clin Endocrinol Metab* 2010; 95: 4072–4076.

Section II

Metabolic Syndrome, Insulin Resistance and Obesity—An Opportunity to Prevent, Control and Reverse Disease

4 Metabolic Syndrome

Amrita G. Sawhney and Michael M. Rothkopf

CONTENTS

INTRODUCTION

Metabolic syndrome predisposes affected individuals to the development of diabetes, cardiovascular disease (CVD), nonalcoholic fatty liver disease (NAFLD), and other serious conditions, including some forms of cancer [1]. Its etiology appears to stem from a lifestyle of excessive consumption and physical inactivity coupled with underlying pathophysiological conditions such as insulin resistance (IR) [2,3].

The clinical manifestations of metabolic syndrome include abdominal adiposity, impaired glucose tolerance (IGT), excessive insulin exposure, atherogenic dyslipidemia, hypertension (HTN), a proinflammatory state, and a prothrombotic state [3]. These components combine to produce a powerful deleterious effect, inducing disease and shortening lifespan [4].

The presence of metabolic syndrome produces a fivefold increase in the risk of developing type 2 diabetes and doubles the risk of cardiovascular disease [5]. It is believed to increase the likelihood of developing NAFLD by 4 to 11 times [6]. Longitudinal studies have shown a 56% increase in the risk of cancer mortality associated with metabolic syndrome [7]. Its impact on life expectancy has been estimated at a cost of between 3 and 11 years [5].

In the United States, 80 million Americans are estimated to have metabolic syndrome [8]. But this is a worldwide phenomenon in which 25% of all adults are thought to be affected [9]. This is particularly true in westernized cultures, but a disturbing trend can be seen in emerging societies as well.

Clinicians, from a wide spectrum of medical specialties, can expect to routinely encounter patients with metabolic syndrome. Therefore, physicians should be prepared to recognize these individuals and provide the appropriate intervention.

This chapter will review the history, definitions, prevalence, and economic impact of metabolic syndrome. We will explore some of the mechanisms for its development. We will also present our approach to the evaluation and management of patients at risk for the condition.

DEFINITION OF METABOLIC SYNDROME

EVOLUTION OF THE CURRENT DEFINITION

The initial recognition of the condition we now refer to as metabolic syndrome first occurred nearly a century ago. However, its widespread acceptance and the definition of its diagnostic criteria have gone through a bumpy process of evolution. Controversies emerged as different specialty groups provided their own unique perspectives. Fortunately, a consensus on its definition now appears to be emerging.

Dr. Eskil Kylin is generally credited with first observing a connection between the development of cardiovascular disease, HTN, hyperglycemia, and gout in 1923 [10]. In 1947, Dr. Jean Vague further contributed when he observed that upper body fat was associated with diabetes, gout, and atherosclerosis [11]. In 1980, Dr. Margaret Albrink tied together the relationship between obesity, low high-density lipoprotein (HDL), and high triglycerides [12].

These advances set the stage for the transformative contribution made by the American endocrinologist, Dr. Gerald M. Reaven. He proposed the link between central obesity, IGT, diabetes, and HTN with IR. Further, he believed that the constellation of these conditions predisposed the patient to the development of cardiovascular disease [13]. He called this clustering of conditions Syndrome X. Reaven presented his theory at the 1988 American Diabetes Association (ADA) Banting Lecture at Stanford University.

The lecture is given in memory of Sir Frederick Banting, physician and Nobel laureate, and a key investigator in the discovery of insulin. The presenter is also honored with the Banting Medal, the highest scientific award of the ADA. Reaven's presentation at such a distinguished forum is now recognized as the landmark event in the widespread recognition of metabolic syndrome. His contribution is deemed so important that many textbooks refer to metabolic syndrome as Reaven's syndrome.

After 1988, medical researchers around the world began to report on the presence of metabolic syndrome in their countries [14]. This was seen predominantly in cultures where calorically dense, processed, and inexpensive food was readily available, and sedentary lifestyles were becoming the norm.

National and international organizations convened expert panels to discuss the growing recognition of metabolic syndrome and agree on its definition. The first of these to gain real traction was from a diabetologist consulting group to the World Health Organization (WHO) in 1998–1999 [15]. IR was viewed as the prevailing underlying risk factor for metabolic syndrome in this report, and evidence of IR was required in the definition. The 1999 WHO definition included IGT or diabetes and/or IR, together with two or more of the following: HTN, elevated triglycerides, low HDL, central obesity, and the presence of microalbuminuria [16]. In the WHO criteria, IR was assessed by insulin clamp studies.

Shortly after the WHO study, the European Group for the study of Insulin Resistance (EGIR) released a modification, primarily for use in a nondiabetic population [17]. The EGIR used impaired fasting glucose (IFG) instead of IGT and fasting insulin levels instead of insulin clamp studies. HTN, central obesity, and dyslipidemia were included, but not microalbuminuria.

In 2001, the National Cholesterol Education Program's Adult Treatment Panel III (NCEP ATP III) offered its own definition. The contributors were primarily cardiologists and lipidologists, and their intent was to utilize easily obtainable clinical data to diagnose metabolic syndrome [18]. The NCEP definition did not require the inclusion of any one single factor to make the diagnosis. Instead, the definition was made by the presence of three or more of any of the following five criteria: central obesity, elevated triglycerides, low HDL, HTN, and elevated fasting glucose (IFG or the presence of diabetes) [19].

However, the existence of multiple criteria for metabolic syndrome led to some confusion, as evidenced by a large Australian study that attempted to utilize all three existing definitions [20]. In this study, the definitions only overlapped in roughly half of the individuals.

In 2002, the American Association of Clinical Endocrinologists (AACE) created a definition for what they termed, insulin resistance syndrome, to focus on the underlying pathophysiology of cardiovascular risk [21]. The components of this definition included obesity, elevated triglycerides, low HDL, elevated blood pressure, and elevated glucose at fasting and/or after a 2-h glucose challenge. Other contributing risk factors included family history of type 2 diabetes, HTN, or CVD, polycystic ovary syndrome, sedentary lifestyle, advancing age, and an ethnicity group with a high risk of type 2 diabetes or CVD.

In 2004, the International Diabetes Federation (IDF) convened a panel to establish a universal definition of metabolic syndrome [15]. The IDF published its definition in 2005 with an emphasis on creating a diagnostic tool that permitted comparison of data across ethnicities [22]. The IDF included central obesity as a required criterion along with hypertriglyceridemia, low HDL, HTN, and elevated fasting blood glucose (FBG). The IDF also recognized that waist circumference measurements should be applied according to ethnic groups. IR was dropped as a required component by the IDF.

Also, in 2005, the American Heart Association/National Heart, Lung, and Blood Institute (AHA/NHLBI) put forth its definition of metabolic syndrome [23]. As with the IDF, NHLBI utilized the ATP III as the basis for its recommendations. However, an important difference between the two was the treatment of waist circumference. While the IDF mandated waist circumference as one of the five required criteria for the diagnosis, the AHA/NHLBI did not make waist circumference an obligatory criterion [15]. The IDF and the AHA/NHLBI also disagreed on the measurement cutoffs to define risk-conferring abdominal girth.

While each of these definitions was useful in their own right, the differences made it challenging for clinicians and scientists alike. A consensus was sought, which appeared in 2009 as, "The Joint Statement of the International Diabetes Federation Task Force on Epidemiology and Prevention; National Heart, Lung, and Blood Institute; American Heart Association; World Heart Federation; International Atherosclerosis Society, and International Association for the Study of Obesity" [15].

Current Definition

Under the joint task force definition, clinicians can diagnose a patient with metabolic syndrome, utilizing five criteria: FBG, triglycerides, HDL cholesterol, blood pressure, and waist circumference [15]. In their paper, Alberti et al. state that by the joint task force definition, any three out of five abnormal findings are sufficient to make the diagnosis of metabolic syndrome. They defined a single set of cutoff points for all components with the exception of waist circumference, which was set according to regional/ethnic criteria. Although waist circumference was not universally agreed upon as a requirement for diagnosis, it was felt to serve as a useful screening tool. Therefore, it was included as a non-obligatory criterion in the task force definition, whereas it had been an obligatory criterion in past definitions.

Table 4.1 shows the definitions for the five criteria currently agreed upon in the diagnosis of metabolic syndrome. Drug treatment for dyslipidemia and HTN is considered to be an alternate indicator for the cut points. This is followed in Table 4.2 by the cut points for waist circumference.

TABLE 4.1

Metabolic Syndrome Criteria

Criteria	Cut Points
Fasting hyperglycemia	≥100 mg/dL (>5.5 mmol/L)
Elevated triglycerides	≥150 mg/dL (1.7 mmol/L)
Low HDL-C	<40 mg/dL (1.0 mmol/L in males)
	<50 mg/dL (1.3 mmol/L in females)
HTN	Systolic ≥ 130 and/or diastolic ≥ 85 mm Hg
Elevated waist circumference	See Table 4.2

Source: Adapted from Alberti KGMM et al., *Circulation*, 20, 1640–1645, 2009.

TABLE 4.2
Current Recommended Waist Circumference Thresholds for Abdominal Obesity by Organization

Population	Organization/Reference	Waist Circumference in Centimeters	
		Men	Women
Europid	IDF	≥94	≥80
Caucasian	WHO	≥94 (poses increased risk)	≥80 (poses increased risk)
		≥102 (poses even greater risk)	≥88 (poses even greater risk)
United States	AHA/NHLBI (ATP III)	≥102	≥88
Canada	Health Canada	≥102	≥88
European	European Cardiovascular Societies	≥102	≥88
Asian (including Japanese)	IDF	≥90	≥80
Asian	WHO	≥90	≥80
Japanese	Japanese Obesity Society	≥85	≥90
China	Cooperative Task Force	≥85	≥80
Middle East, Mediterranean	IDF	≥94	≥80
Sub-Saharan African	IDF	≥94	≥80
Ethnic Central and South American	IDF	≥90	≥80

Source: Adapted from Alberti KGMM et al., *Circulation*, 20, 1640–1645, 2009.

Note: The AHA/NHLBI guidelines suggest that in people/populations with increased IR, men with waist circumference ≥94 cm and women with waist circumference ≥80 cm are at increased risk for CVD and diabetes. These can be considered as optional cut points.

PREVALENCE OF METABOLIC SYNDROME

UNITED STATES

Metabolic syndrome is a significant concern in the United States. Its prevalence in the United States can be estimated at one third of the adult population [8]. This translates into roughly 80 million Americans. These individuals are at twice the risk of CVD and five times the risk of diabetes [9].

The occurrence of metabolic syndrome in the United States appears to be increasing at an alarming rate. This is best demonstrated by data from the National Health and Nutrition Examination Survey (NHANES). NHANES is a cross-sectional, nationally representative sample of data collected from adults 20 years of age and older. Survey results from 1988 to 1994 were compared to results from 2003 to 2006. This showed a rise in the incidence of metabolic syndrome in the United States from 24% to 34% [24].

The 2003–2006 data show that metabolic syndrome increases with age and body mass index (BMI), and it varies by race, ethnicity, and gender. In this survey group, abdominal obesity was present in 53%, hypertension in 40%, hyperglycemia in 39%, hypertriglyceridemia in 31%, and low HDL cholesterol in 25% [24].

Subset analysis further revealed an increase in prevalence with increasing age. For example, the prevalence of metabolic syndrome for those younger than 40 was 20% in males and 16% in females. But for those above age 60, it was 52% in males and 54% in females. Adults over the age of 60 had four times the risk of metabolic syndrome when compared to the youngest group of adults studied [24].

Obesity was also a significant factor. Among males in the population studied, metabolic syndrome was present in 7% of underweight and normal weight males, 30% of overweight males, and 65% of obese males. Among females in the population studied, metabolic syndrome was present in 9% of underweight and normal weight females, 33% of overweight females, and 56% of obese females [24].

There were also associations between metabolic syndrome, race, ethnicity, and gender. Non-Hispanic black males have a lower incidence of metabolic syndrome (25%) than non-Hispanic white males (37%) [24]. In females, non-Hispanic black and Mexican-American females were about 1.5 times more likely to meet the criteria for metabolic syndrome than non-Hispanic white females.

From prior NHANES data, 1988–1994, the highest prevalence of metabolic syndrome was seen in Hispanics. The overall prevalence in Hispanics was 32%, and 35% of Hispanic females were affected [25]. Among Native Americans data from the Strong Heart Study, 1989–1999, metabolic syndrome was present in 35% of the population [26].

INTERNATIONAL

There are 1.1 billion adults classified as overweight with an additional 312 million counted as obese worldwide [27]. Broadly speaking, this would translate into a 20–30% prevalence of metabolic syndrome in adults in most countries [9]. Increasing age is strongly associated with the prevalence of metabolic syndrome [28]. With rising rates of overweight and obese individuals, the prevalence of metabolic syndrome is only likely to increase in the next worldwide analysis, especially when considering that 155 million children are overweight or obese [29].

While a country-by-country-based review of prevalence is beyond the scope of this chapter, it is illustrative to look at data for the world's most populated countries: China and India. The population of China is nearly 1.4 billion, roughly a third of whom are overweight [30]. In a 2000–2001 study, Gu et al. [31] found that metabolic syndrome was present in 9.8% Chinese men and 17.8% of Chinese women. Based upon population data at the time, this would translate to 58 million men and 106 million women with metabolic syndrome in China.

The population of India is roughly 1.2 billion. Metabolic syndrome was observed in 41% of urban Indians between the ages 20 and 75 [32]. A trend was seen toward the increased prevalence of metabolic syndrome as people migrated into urban centers. An increased prevalence of metabolic syndrome was also observed in middle income individuals as opposed to their lower income counterparts [33].

Globally, as countries adopt Western lifestyles, the trend toward obesity increases. In addition to China and India, other high risk populations reside in the Middle East, Pacific Islands, Southeast Asia, Latin America, and the Caribbean [33].

SOCIOECONOMIC IMPACT OF METABOLIC SYNDROME

Metabolic syndrome's socioeconomic impact can be observed on many levels. The clearest of these is the direct health care expenditure of doctor's visits, laboratory testing, pharmaceutical expenses, hospitalizations, surgery, and rehabilitation. But the cost of this condition extends into the workplace with lost productivity and wages. Patients with metabolic syndrome who prematurely exit the workforce take their skills and knowledge with them. This effectively negates the investment an employer has made in time and training. But even those who continue to work are affected. Patients with metabolic syndrome have greater absences from work. In addition, their effectiveness at work is diminished. As we will see below, the concept of presenteeism may be a major factor in metabolic syndrome's economic impact.

Another way to look at the cost of metabolic syndrome is the lost opportunity to prevent significant diseases. The Centers for Disease Control and Prevention (CDC) reported that, in 2010, the total cost of cardiovascular disease was $444 billion and that $1 of every $6 spent on health care in the United States went to CVD [34]. The CDC statistics for the cost of diabetes are also significant. In 2007, the total cost of diabetes was $174 billion [35]. The average medical expense for a person with diabetes is more than twice that for an individual without diabetes. The costs are predicted to rise by 2050 when a third of the population is predicted to become diabetic if current trends are unchecked [35].

Finally there is a personal cost to deteriorating health and shortening lifespan. This cannot be calculated in dollar figures, but the impact is nonetheless significant. We will explore these topics in greater detail below.

HEALTH CARE EXPENDITURE

A number of studies have examined the issue of health care expenditures related to metabolic syndrome. Curtis et al. [25] reviewed medical costs among 3789 elderly individuals. They utilized a log-linear regression model to assess the contributions of metabolic syndrome and its components to 10-year medical costs. Metabolic syndrome was defined using the NCEP ATP III criteria. In this analysis, the health cost for participants was 20% higher among those with metabolic syndrome. Individual components such as abdominal adiposity, low HDL cholesterol, and elevated blood pressure also increased 10-year cost (15%, 16%, and 20%, respectively).

In her doctoral thesis for the University of Michigan, Alyssa Schultz studied metabolic syndrome and workplace outcomes [36]. She reviewed the health risk assessment (HRA) of 4188 participants in a corporate medical plan. Within the study population, 30.2% met the criteria for metabolic syndrome. Her review showed higher rates of arthritis, chronic pain, heartburn, depression, diabetes, heart problems, and stroke in those with metabolic syndrome. Individuals with metabolic syndrome had annual health care costs more than twice as high as those without it. In addition, a higher percentage of employees with metabolic syndrome reported presenteeism, adding further to associated costs.

Nichols and Moler [37] studied the cost of metabolic syndrome among 58,056 patients in Kaiser Permanente Northwest. Their aim was to quantify the cost of metabolic syndrome by the number of risk factors present in an individual. The study population was nonpregnant adults over the age of 30, with metabolic syndrome diagnosed in 2003 or 2004 and no prior evidence of diabetes. Subjects remained in the Kaiser population for at least 5 years following their diagnosis with metabolic syndrome. Cost data from inpatient, outpatient, and pharmacy expenditures were collected. Patients without metabolic syndrome incurred an adjusted annualized cost of $3932. Patients with one risk factor incurred an annualized medical cost of $4282; two risk factors, $4707; three risk factors, $5106; four risk factors, $5286; and all five risk factors, $5677. Hospitalization for CVD incurred an additional annual cost of $5571, and development of diabetes incurred an additional annual cost of $2807.

LOST WAGES

As demonstrated above, the financial impact of metabolic syndrome is enormous for the institutions responsible for paying out on its adverse outcomes. Another way to view the cost is to look at the impact on individuals.

In their paper, Productivity Costs Associated with Cardiometabolic Risk Factor Cluster in the United States, Sullivan and colleagues looked at the loss of productivity in a representative sample of US adults. They utilized data collected in the 2000 and 2002 Medical Expenditure Panel Survey (MEPS) Household Component to analyze the number of work days missed by people with a BMI > 25, and hypertension, hyperlipidemia, and/or diabetes.

The analysis showed an average of 10 days of lost productivity per individual with the cardiometabolic risk factor cluster as opposed to 5 days in individuals without it. This translated into $561 annually per worker in 2005 dollars. For employers, this amounted to an annual total loss of productivity of $10.3 billion [38].

Obesity is associated with employees missing more work days than non-obese employees. These lost days are due to short-term absences, long-term disability, and premature death [39]. This may also be due to obesity leading to lower wages [40].

Data on the financial impact of metabolic syndrome can be gleaned by its outcome as diabetes. Vijan et al. [41] reviewed lost wages due to diabetes from 1992 to 2000. They calculated that diabetes was responsible for a cost to US workers of "$4.4 billion in lost income due to early retirement, $0.5 billion due to increased sick days, $31.7 billion due to disability, and $22.0 billion in lost income due to premature mortality, for a total of $58.6 billion in lost productivity, or $7.3 billion per year."

LONGEVITY

Metabolic syndrome can be explained to patients as a type of precocious aging that is not only self-inflicted in most cases but also can be prevented or reversed. Data from subjects in the Framingham Heart Study were reviewed to evaluate the effects of the overweight and obese states on lifespan. The study revealed that a 40-year-old overweight female (nonsmoker without CVD) lost an average of 3 years of lifespan years compared to normal weight counterparts. If the weight gain resulted in obesity, the total lifespan reduction was 7 years for females and 6 years for males. Obese females were 115% more likely to die before the age of 70. Obese males were 81% more likely to die before the age of 70 [42].

Longevity in metabolic syndrome can also be evaluated in terms of altered life expectancy in patients who have developed DM II and cardiovascular disease. In one study, UK researchers evaluated the life expectancy of patients with type 2 diabetes. A sample of their results showed that a 55-year-old male, 5 years after diagnosis, with the worst risk group (smoker, systolic BP 180 mm Hg, total/HDL cholesterol ratio of 8, HgA1C 10%), could expect to live another 13.2 years. Compared to his nondiabetic counterpart with a life expectancy of an additional 24.7 years, this is a loss of 11.5 years. In a diabetic with the best risk profile (nonsmoker, SBP 120 mm Hg, total/HDL cholesterol ratio of 4, HgA1C 6%), life expectancy would be an additional 21.1 years with a loss of 3.6 years [43].

PATHOGENESIS AND METABOLIC DERANGEMENTS

The pathogenesis of metabolic syndrome is multifactorial. IR and abdominal adiposity are predominant factors [44]. Some researchers view IR as a unifying factor for all components of metabolic syndrome [45]. Lifestyle choices including physical inactivity and poor nutritional choices also contribute. Below, we will discuss the pathophysiology and the underlying metabolic disturbances in metabolic syndrome.

INSULIN RESISTANCE

IR is a physiologic state in which the normal level of insulin is no longer capable of maintaining a euglycemic state within the body. This appears to be occurring due to intracellular, post receptor insulin signaling defect. As postprandial glucose levels rise, the GLUT2 transporter senses the increased level via first-order kinetics. This results in increasing levels of insulin secretion by pancreatic beta cells. Eventually, the degree of insulinemia is inappropriately high, leading to conditions of insulin excess.

IR often occurs prior to the development of hyperglycemia. It may also persist in a euglycemic state [28]. However, the eventual degradation of overstimulated beta cells is thought to be a mechanism for the progression from IR to frank diabetes mellitus.

The target tissues of insulin are primarily skeletal muscle, liver, and adipose tissue, and they are of particular importance to the development of IR. Controversy exists as to which organ system is the originator of the resistant state [46]. Furthermore, the precise biochemical derangements of intracellular insulin signaling remain unclear [46].

But many authors believe that the process of IR starts with an increased visceral adipose tissue (VAT) mass [47]. Under this hypothesis, the expanded VAT releases excessive free fatty acids (FFAs) into circulation. The excess FFAs, in turn, lead to skeletal muscle IR by interfering with insulin receptor substrate-1 (IRS-1) and PI3-kinase [48].

The rate-controlled step in the uptake of glucose into the myocyte by the presence of insulin is the translocation of GLUT-4 to the muscle plasma membrane. Normal signaling activity of intracellular IRS-1/IRS-2 and PI3-kinase is required for GLUT-4 translocation to the myocyte cell surface. Therefore, abnormal signaling of the subunits following insulin-induced tyrosine kinase activity would be expected to alter glucose uptake by the myocyte [49]. Since skeletal muscle comprises nearly 40% of the body cell mass, a reduced glucose uptake by myocytes can be understood to have an immediate effect on whole-body glycemia [50]. This process can then become a vicious cycle wherein reduced skeletal muscle uptake of glucose leads to higher glucose levels, which in turn leads to increased GLUT2 transporter activity in the beta cells and increased insulin secretion.

IR, in turn, increases the level of FFAs in circulation [51]. Under normal physiologic conditions, insulin suppresses FFA mobilization from adipose tissue by inhibiting lipolysis. In insulin-resistant cells, lipolysis is no longer suppressed normally, and the serum levels of FFAs rise [52].

In addition to the lipocentric view of IR, other important factors and mechanisms are proposed. Physical inactivity is one important mechanism. Insulin sensitivity has been shown to improve with exercise independent of weight reductions and body composition changes [53]. The increased glucose uptake observed with exercise is linked to activation of AMP kinase, which, in turn, causes an increase in GLUT-4 translocation to surface membranes [54]. Studies of the offspring of type 2 diabetics with IR demonstrated increased glucose uptake and glycogen synthesis after 6 weeks of physical training [55]. Research is also exploring genetic defects in the receptors responsible for normal insulin signaling pathways. These include genetic defects in the insulin receptor, IRS-1 and IRS-2 mutations, PI3-kinase mutations, and others [55].

The role of chronic low-grade inflammation and release of proinflammatory cytokines and adipokines is another important factor in the development of IR [56]. A detailed presentation of IR is found elsewhere in this text.

VISCERAL ADIPOSITY

Clinicians have long observed that as patients gain weight, the increased adipose tissue volume is distributed in distinct patterns. Jean Vague [57] was one of the first to report his observations in his 1947 paper, which proposed a gender pattern between the males who had "android type" and females who had "gynoid type" obesity and noted that android type obesity adversely affected longevity. Researchers moved away from this gender paradigm in the 1980s and started looking at non-gender-based regional patterns (central vs. peripheral, upper body vs. lower body) [58,59]. Tokunaga et al. [60] furthered this viewpoint by using computed tomography (CT) images to actually see and measure adipose tissue of test subjects and subsequently proposed a classification system of fat into "visceral fat obesity" and "subcutaneous fat obesity."

Understanding the distribution of body fat is important because fat in the visceral compartment behaves differently than that in the subcutaneous compartment. All fat was once thought of simply in terms of an energy reservoir, but more recently, research has revealed that VAT is a metabolically active endocrine organ [61]. In VAT, adipocytes are the predominant cell type; however, other cell types are present, which also contribute to its growth and function. These include preadipocytes, lymphocytes, macrophages, fibroblasts, and vascular cells.

The discovery of cytokines secreted by the VAT, termed adipokines, has led to the view of VAT as an endocrine organ [61,62]. The adipokines have proinflammatory and anti-inflammatory

TABLE 4.3
Key Adipokines

Adipokine	Primary Source(s)	Binding Partner or Receptor	Function
Leptin	Adipocytes	Leptin receptor	Appetite control through the central nervous system
Resistin	Peripheral blood mononuclear cells (human), adipocytes (rodent)	Unknown	Promotes IR and inflammation through IL-6 and TNF secretion from macrophages
RBP4	Liver, adipocytes, macrophages	Retinol (vitamin A), transthyretin	Implicated in systemic insulin resistance
Lipocalin 2	Adipocytes, macrophages	Unknown	Promotes IR and inflammation through TNF secretion from adipocytes
ANGPTL2	Adipocytes, other cells	Unknown	Local and vascular inflammation
TNF	Stromal vascular fraction cells, adipocytes	TNF receptor	Inflammation, antagonism of insulin signaling
IL-6	Adipocytes, stromal vascular fraction cells, liver, muscle	IL-6 receptor	Changes with source and target tissue
IL-18	Stromal vascular fraction cells	IL-18 receptor, IL-18 binding protein	Broad-spectrum inflammation
CCL2	Adipocytes, stromal vascular fraction cells	CCR2	Monocyte recruitment
CXCL5	Stromal vascular fraction cells (macrophages)	CXCR2	Antagonism of insulin signaling through the JAK–STAT pathway
NAMPT	Adipocytes, macrophages, other cells	Unknown	Monocyte chemotactic activity
Adiponectin	Adipocytes	Adiponectin receptors 1 and 2, T-cadherin, calreticulin-CD91	Insulin sensitizer, anti-inflammatory
SFRP5	Adipocytes	WNT5a	Suppression of proinflammatory WNT signaling

Source: Adapted from Ouchi N et al., *Nat Rev Immunol*, 11(2), 85–97, 2011.

Note: ANGPTL2, angiopoietin-like protein 2; CCL2, CC-chemokine ligand 2; CXCL5, CXC-chemokine ligand 5; IL, interleukin; JAK, Janus kinase; NAMPT, nicotinamide phosphoribosyltransferase; RBP4, retinol-binding protein 4; SFRP5, secreted frizzled-related protein 5; STAT, signal transducer and activator of transcription; TNF, tumor necrosis factor.

functions. Central obesity due to expanded VAT causes dysregulation of adipokines, which leads to a predominantly proinflammatory state. Table 4.3 lists adipokines in the VAT [63].

As noted above, visceral adiposity is thought to be linked to IR and the pathogenesis of metabolic syndrome through FFA release and their effect on skeletal muscle insulin signaling. In addition to the development of IR, VAT-induced whole-body inflammation is shown to be elevated in metabolic syndrome. This appears to be part of the explanation for the increases in cardiovascular disease, arthritis, and other conditions associated with metabolic syndrome [64].

INFLAMMATION

Expanded VAT and IR set the stage for chronic low-grade inflammation [65,66] by serving as an endocrine organ that releases proinflammatory and anti-inflammatory adipokines. When the VAT is in a state of dysregulation, a shift toward the secretion of proinflammatory substances appears to dominate. It is likely that much of this activity can be traced to adipose tissue-embedded macrophages, which are themselves responding to signaling from the VAT [67]. Another possibility is that mature adipocytes may undergo a transformation that activates some of the genes classically expressed by macrophages [67]. Tissue hypoxia due to insufficient blood flow to the expanded adipose mass in obesity is thought to be an inciting event resulting in acute and subsequent chronic inflammation [67].

Regardless of the precise mechanisms, there is little doubt that VAT can produce a large variety of inflammatory mediators. The VAT can also induce a cytokine cascade and secrete acute phase reactants [68]. In the overweight and obese state, the adipose tissue mass increases in size. This increased adipose mass leads to an increase in the production of inflammatory mediators. Conversely, when patients lose weight, the decreased adipose tissue mass leads to a decrease in inflammation [69].

Numerous adipokines and cytokines play a role in this process, and pathophysiological mechanisms remain to be fully elucidated. Table 4.3 lists the key adipokines. Several of these including interleukin-6 (IL-6), tumor necrosis factor alpha (TNF-α), adiponectin, and the proinflammatory marker C-reactive protein (CRP) are discussed here.

IL-6 is produced by adipose tissue, endothelial cells, macrophages, lymphocytes, and muscle cells [70]. CRP is synthesized in the liver, largely in response to IL-6. Studies have shown that inflammation when measured by increases in IL-6 and CRP levels predicts cardiovascular events and the development of diabetes [71]. Weight loss leads to reductions in IL-6 and CRP levels [72]. One third of the circulating level of IL-6 is thought to be produced by adipose tissues [73]. The primary cell type is thought to be the macrophages [74].

Several mechanisms by which IL-6 promotes inflammation and IR have been proposed, but more research is warranted. IL-6 stimulates other major proinflammatory cytokines as IL-1 and TNF-α. TNF-α decreases insulin-mediated uptake of glucose and impairs endothelial function. Interference with insulin signaling in hepatocytes may result from IL-6-induced production of suppressors of cytokine signaling (SOCS) family proteins [75]. These proteins can bind to the insulin receptor and interfere with downstream events. In adipose tissue, reduced levels of IL-6 protect against the development of IR through modulation of SOCS-3 expression in the liver [76]. IL-6 has been shown to interfere with the ability of insulin to suppress glucose production by the liver [77]. It is capable of suppressing lipoprotein lipase activity [78].

TNF-α interferes with adipocyte regulation at multiple levels: transcriptional regulation, glucose and fatty acid metabolism, and hormone receptor signaling [79]. Its circulating levels correlate to the degree of adiposity, are decreased in weight loss, and are associated with IR [71,80]. TNF-α-induced IR is linked to its ability to dephosphorylate IRS-1 through activation of protein phosphatases [80]. TNF-α also induces adipocyte apoptosis [81]. It increases proinflammatory IL-6 and reduces anti-inflammatory adiponectin, and was shown to increase its own levels [82].

Adiponectin is an anti-inflammatory adipokine, which is synthesized by adipocytes almost exclusively [83]. Adipokine levels decrease in the obese state [84], and weight loss has been shown to increase its levels [74]. Furthermore, adiponectin levels are negatively correlated with VAT accumulation [84] and are decreased in patients with type 2 diabetes, and high levels of adiponectin are associated with a lower risk for type 2 diabetes [83]. Adiponectin is inhibited by TNF-α and IL-6 [74]. The actions of adiponectin include regulation of lipid and glucose metabolism, increase in insulin sensitivity, and protection from chronic inflammation [85]. When adiponectin levels are diminished, there is associated development of IR, hyperinsulinemia, and type 2 diabetes independent of fat mass [86].

Adiponectin is thought to exert anti-inflammatory effects via macrophages. Ohashi et al. [87] have demonstrated that low levels of adiponectin are associated with changes in macrophages, favoring a proinflammatory macrophage phenotype. They state that high levels of adiponectin favor an anti-inflammatory state, which may deter metabolic and cardiovascular disease.

Glucose Intolerance

IGT is a condition wherein euglycemia cannot be maintained after a glucose challenge. Although this is not the same as IFG, the two are often linked. In fact, it is common for physicians to label patients with IFG as having IGT. While it is true that IGT can eventually lead to IFG, the condition should be thought of as distinct initially. Furthermore, there are occasional cases in which fasting glucose is abnormal but postchallenge glucose is not.

In our experience, the glucose tolerance test is the earliest indicator of beta cell dysfunction. Therefore, we routinely perform a 3-h glucose tolerance test for patients in whom we suspect metabolic syndrome. Published reports have demonstrated the utility of the glucose tolerance test in this regard [88]. In particular, the glucose level at 2 h postglucose challenge has been frequently cited [89].

When beta cells are functioning normally, a glucose challenge will elicit a biphasic response in insulin secretion. The first phase occurs within minutes and is managed by preformed insulin in the beta cells. The second phase occurs later and requires the synthesis of additional insulin. With IGT, the vigorous first-phase insulin response is diminished or lost [90]. Subsequently, the second phase may be reduced or, paradoxically, elevated. When this latter event occurs, reactive hypoglycemia may result.

The precise mechanism by which beta cells become functionally abnormal is not known. But, it is believed that individuals with IGT have a decrease in their pancreatic islets and beta cell mass [91]. There are also reports of a decreased content of insulin within islets of such patients and a decreased sensitivity to release insulin in the presence of glucose [91]. These characteristics may be the result of high levels of beta cell oxidative stress, especially due to the presence of the toxic reactive oxygen species, superoxide, and hydrogen peroxide. Beta cells injured in this manner may possess reduced levels of the enzymes required to inactivate these reactive oxygen species [92].

DYSLIPIDEMIA

Under normal metabolic conditions, the actions of insulin on adipocytes decrease the rate of lipolysis, which leads to lowered plasma FFA levels, stimulates FFA and triacylglycerol synthesis, increases the uptake of triglycerides into adipose tissue and muscle, and decreases the rate of fatty acid oxidation in muscle and liver [93]. In the insulin-resistant state, visceral adipocyte metabolism is dysregulated in favor of lipolytic hormones [94]. Conditions favoring lipolysis in the expanded VAT leads to an increased level of FFAs released by adipocytes into the portal system. This increased FFA load is processed by the liver into triglycerides and triglyceride-rich very low density lipoprotein (VLDL) particles [95].

Low levels of HDL in metabolic syndrome are viewed as a consequence of elevated triglyceride levels [96]. Cholesterol ester transfer protein (CETP) mediates the transfer of cholesterol esters and triglycerides between lipoproteins. When this occurs in the setting of increased levels of triglycerides, the CETP exchange between and HDL particles is thought to lead to triglyceride-rich and cholesterol-depleted HDL. In this state, HDL is more susceptible to catabolization [96]. Another mechanism for reduced HDL in metabolic syndrome may result from the effect of IR, which can decrease the production of Apo A. Apo A is required in the formation of HDL [96]. Additional mechanisms for HDL reduction in IR include altered ATP binding cassette A1 transporter protein, required for the formation of HDL particles and Apo A clearance via the kidneys in response to reduced cholesterol efflux [95].

In addition to elevated triglycerides and low HDL levels, there are other signs of dyslipidemia in metabolic syndrome. The dyslipidemia profile in metabolic syndrome is summarized in Table 4.4.

IR AND HYPERTENSION

The pathophysiology of hypertension in the setting of metabolic syndrome is complex. IR and visceral adiposity are thought to be the major contributors in the development of HTN in metabolic syndrome [97]. Insulin and viscerally active fat affect sympathetic tone and endothelial function and lead to dysregulation of adipokines.

TABLE 4.4

Lipid Abnormalities in Metabolic Syndrome (Fasting State)

Lipids	Lipoproteins	Apolipoprotein	Enzymes, Proteins
Increased FFAs	Increased VLDL	Increased apo B-100 and apo B-48	Decreased lipoprotein lipase
Increased triglycerides	Increased small dense LDL Decreased HDL	Decreased apo A	Increased hepatic lipase Increased CETP

Source: Adapted from Kolovou GD et al., *Postgrad Med J*, 81, 358–366, 2005.

The sympathetic nervous system is frequently thought of in terms of the response to stress, classically as the "flight or fight" response. It is important to remember that it acts on a basal level to maintain homeostasis. Its functions in this capacity include maintenance of blood pressure. Sympathetic tone is regulated to achieve normotension. In patients with metabolic syndrome, hyperinsulinemia, hyperleptinemia, and hyperlipidemia are believed to exacerbate sympathetic tone [98]. Hyperinsulinemia is known to increase circulating levels of noradrenaline leading to an increase in blood pressure [99]. Excessive insulin increases sodium reabsorption, expanding extracellular volume, resulting in hypertension [100,101]. The obese state adds to this by impairment of renal-pressure natriuresis causing sodium retention [102].

The effect of IR on the vascular endothelium also contributes to the development of hypertension in metabolic syndrome. Under normal circumstances, in the vascular system of a normal weight person, the presence of insulin leads to vasodilation [103]. This effect is believed to occur after insulin binds its receptor on the vascular endothelium [104]. Endothelial cells respond to insulin binding by releasing nitric oxide (NO), a potent vasodilator. In the insulin-resistant state, this vasodilatory effect is altered. This is thought to occur due to impaired NO synthase activity [105]. When NO synthase activity is inhibited, the vasodilatory and capillary recruitment is diminished [105,106]. Research has also shown that when NO synthase activity is reduced, insulin can then act on the vascular endothelium by increasing the levels of endothelin-1 (ET-1), a very potent vasoconstrictor [107]. ET-1-mediated vasoconstriction occurs when NO synthase is inhibited [108].

Adipokines that are thought to play a role in hypertension include leptin and adiponectin, and adipocyte-derived prostaglandins, angiotensin II, and ET-1.

Leptin receptors are located on endothelial cells as well as in the hypothalamus [109]. Leptin is a NO-dependent vasodilator, and it also increases peripheral vascular resistance and increases sympathetic nerve activity [110]. Different theories have been proposed on the relationship between increased leptin levels in the obese state and hypertension. While not currently understood fully, the role of leptin in hypertension is thought to be associated with endothelial dysfunction [111].

The presence of adiponectin is associated with improved NO-dependent vasodilation [112]. Adiponectin levels are known to decrease in the presence of increasing body mass [113]. Low levels of adiponectin occur in IR and hyperinsulinemia [98]. Because of its relationship to NO-mediated vasodilation, low levels of adiponectin are thought to be associated with hypertension [101].

Adipocytes are stimulated to release prostaglandins in response to sympathetic activity [98]. Sympathetic stimulation leads to lipolysis during which FFAs and the prostaglandins PGE2 and PGI2 are released by adipocytes [98]. PGI2 is a potent vasodilator [114]. Insulin is an antilipolytic hormone, and its presence reduces the release of prostaglandins [115]. Thus, in hyperinsulinemia and IR, the decreased production of PGI2 is thought to lead to hypertension [116].

Adipocytes synthesize angiotensin II, and angiotensinogen gene production is known to be higher in visceral fat than in other fat depots and other tissues [117]. This correlates with the observation that in the obese state, angiotensin II levels are increased [118]. Adipocytes also produce aldosterone in response to angiotensin II, leading some researchers to dub visceral fat as a "miniature" renin–angiotensin–aldosterone system [98]. This work was confirmed by Giacchetti et al. [119] whose research demonstrated that all components of the RAS are present in both visceral and subcutaneous fat. Goossens et al. [120] state that "components of the RAS produced by adipocytes may play an autocrine, a paracrine and/or an endocrine role in the pathophysiology of obesity and provide a potential pathway through which obesity leads to hypertension and Type 2 Diabetes mellitus."

In the obese state, adipose tissue releases 2.5 times the amount of ET-1 as compared to normal-weight individuals [121]. As stated above, ET-1 is a potent vasoconstrictor, and it is known to be increased in obesity and type 2 diabetes. It is released by the visceral fat and not by the subcutaneous fat [121]. The expanded visceral fat mass in the obese state may provide another explanation for the development of hypertension with this significant increase in ET-1.

THROMBOSIS

One of the most significant hemostatic impairments in patients with metabolic syndrome is prolonged clot lysis time [122]. This is thought to be principally due to increased circulating levels of plasminogen activator inhibitor-1 (PAI-1) [123]. PAI-1 is the major physiologic inhibitor of tissue-type plasminogen activator [124] in plasma, which catalyzes the conversion of plasminogen to plasmin, the major enzyme responsible for clot breakdown. Increased levels of PAI-1 lead to impaired removal of thrombi [125]. High levels are predictors of myocardial infarction [126]. Increased levels of PAI-1 strongly correlate with the presence of metabolic syndrome. In large epidemiological studies, the predictive ability of PAI-1 disappears after adjusting for metabolic syndrome, suggesting that IR and abdominal obesity are prerequisites for increased PAI-1 levels [127].

In addition to hypofibrinolysis due to increased levels of PAI-1, a number of other disruptions to normal hemostasis occur in metabolic syndrome. These include hypercoagulability, platelet hyperactivity, and endothelial dysfunction [127]. Plasma from patients with metabolic syndrome has been shown to form denser clots, which increase with the number of components present [122]. Stiffer and denser clots are associated with premature cardiovascular disease [128]. In addition to cardiovascular disease, the prothrombotic abnormalities and dyslipidemia in metabolic syndrome confer an increased association with the development of venous thromboembolism [129].

VITAMIN D DEFICIENCY

Vitamin D (VD) is a hormone with multiple functions. Its effect ranges from immune regulation to mineral metabolism [130]. Deficiencies in VD have traditionally been viewed as deleteriously affecting bone health. However, more recent data have shown a relationship with metabolic syndrome, type 2 diabetes, and HTN.

The relationship between VD intake (dietary and supplemental) and metabolic syndrome was evaluated by Fung et al. [131] using data from the Coronary Artery Risk Development in Young Adults study, consisting of 4727 18–30 year old US males. Participants were followed out for 20 years. The researchers reported that VD intake was inversely related to the prevalence of abdominal obesity ($P = 0.05$), high glucose ($P = 0.02$), and low HDL ($P = 0.004$). Similar findings were observed in an older study population of nondiabetic men and women aged 40–69 years followed for 10 years. An inverse relationship between baseline serum 25(OH)D and development of dysglycemia, IR, and metabolic syndrome was demonstrated [132]. Other studies including The Women's Health Study and NHANES (2003–2004) also showed an inverse relationship between vitamin D intakes and risk of having metabolic syndrome [17,22,133].

Lim et al. [130] studied the incidence of type 2 diabetes in a population of 1080 nondiabetic Koreans who were considered at high risk for the development of diabetes. They were known to have one or more of the following risk factors: obesity, hypertension, dyslipidemia, and/or a family history of type 2 diabetes [130]. The participants were followed for 5 years. In this study, 10.5% had 25(OH)D deficiency, 51.6% had insufficiency, and 38% had sufficiency. The incidence of type

2 diabetes was 15.9%, 10.2%, and 5.4%, respectively. Therefore, it appeared that the incidence of diabetes was inversely related to VD sufficiency.

Boucher et al. studied the relationship between hypovitaminosis D and IR and beta cell function [134]. They found that in glucose-tolerant individuals, VD concentration had a positive relationship to insulin sensitivity and a negative effect on beta cell function. They concluded that VD deficiency may be a risk factor for both diabetes and metabolic syndrome. Other studies have supported this relationship [134,135].

The VD receptor is located on a wide variety of cells including vascular smooth muscle cells and renal cells, which have implications for blood pressure control. VD has been shown to inhibit renin expression [23,136] and block the proliferation of vascular smooth muscle cells [137]. Studies have shown that skin exposure to UV light, which promotes activation of VD, is associated with lower blood pressure. VD supplementation in VD-deficient patients can decrease systolic blood pressure [133]. Forman looked at the relationship between plasma VD levels and the incidence of HTN in 613 men and 1198 women without HTN at baseline. The relative risk of HTN at 4 years was 6.13 for VD-deficient males and 2.67 for females [138].

Research into the ability of VD to affect beta cell function, insulin sensitivity, and inflammation is underway. Although the mechanism remains elusive, it may relate to the role of VD in the promotion of beta cell calcium influx and insulin secretion [139,140]. It appears that the effect of VD is exerted on the beta cell in response to the presence of glucose as opposed to the basal secretion of insulin [141,142]. The release of insulin from the beta cell is regulated by calcium influx, a process that requires proper calcium homeostasis. Insufficient VD or inadequate calcium intake may derange beta cell calcium channels and lead to abnormal insulin release in the presence of glucose [143]. The presence of sufficient VD may improve IR by stimulating the expression of the insulin receptor or in its role in the beta cell calcium channel regulation. Studies have shown a reduction of GLUT-4 activity due to changes in calcium in insulin target tissues [143].

Zhang et al. [144] examined the role of VD in inflammation. They found that VD-depleted cells produced higher levels of IL-6 and TNF-α than VD-sufficient cells. Their research showed that VD can bind directly to DNA and activates the MKP-1 gene, which interferes with the inflammatory cascade [144].

OBESITY-ASSOCIATED CONDITIONS

CANCER

Certain forms of cancer are believed to be promoted by IR and obesity [94]. As obesity rates rise, a parallel increase in the prevalence of cancer has been observed [94]. The links between metabolic syndrome and cancer are multifactorial and complex and remain to be fully elucidated. These links may include factors such as inflammation, IR, and adipokine dysregulation.

Specific cancer associations with metabolic syndrome were seen in a meta-analysis of 43 articles, which included 38,940 cases [145]. In males, there was a positive association with cancers of the liver, colorectum, and bladder. In females, there was a positive association with cancers of the endometrium, pancreas, postmenopausal breast, and rectum.

Rudolph Virchow, known as the father of pathology, suggested the link between cancer and inflammation in 1863 when he demonstrated leucocytes in neoplastic tissue [146]. Today, it is believed that chronic low-grade inflammation may be linked to a tumor-promoting environment. Obesity and an expanded fat mass, especially in the visceral fat depot, are thought to be of particular significance.

VAT-driven inflammation is due to the production and dysregulation of IL-6, monocyte chemoattractant protein, PAI-1, adiponectin, leptin, and TNF-α [147,148]. PAI-1 expression, for example, is linked to poorer outcomes in breast cancer [149]. IL-6 is known to suppress the ability of the host to mount an antitumor response while it promotes cell proliferation, survival, and invasion [150].

IR and resulting high circulating insulin levels may also contribute to the pro tumor environment. This effect is thought to occur due to insulin-mediated binding of the insulin and insulin-like growth factor (IGF) receptors, which are part of the tyrosine kinase receptor family. These growth factor receptors exist on the cell surfaces of many cancer cells [95]. Downstream signaling pathways can lead to proliferation, evasion of apoptosis, tissue invasion, and metastasis [151]. Indirect effects of hyperinsulinemia add to the pro tumor environment. This occurs when insulin induces the liver to reduce the production of IGF binding protein, leading to increased IGF-1 freely circulating in the blood. The IGF-1 isoform may have an even greater mitogenic and antiapoptotic potential than insulin [152].

Cognitive Decline

Several studies have linked cognitive decline with metabolic syndrome. While this is most prominent in the elderly, the effects of various metabolic derangements on mental function can be seen across the age spectrum. The increased risk of dementia in patients with metabolic syndrome is one of the most disturbing aspects of this association.

Elderly patients with metabolic syndrome were evaluated in the Amsterdam Longitudinal Aging Study. A total of 1183 patients, aged 65–88 years old, were examined. Roughly a third (36.3%) met criteria for metabolic syndrome. The authors found that those with metabolic syndrome had a significantly poorer cognitive function ($P < 0.05$). Hyperglycemia was the most strongly associated metabolic/cognitive function component by a multivariate adjusted model. The presence of inflammation was also negatively associated with cognition ($P < 0.05$) [153].

The Whitehall II prospective cohort study sought to determine if the association of metabolic syndrome and cognition could be identified at an earlier age. They followed 4150 white, British office workers aged 35–55 years over a 10-year period. They assessed the presence of metabolic syndrome using the NCEP ATP III criteria three times during a 10-year follow-up. Cognitive function was assessed using a battery of tests at the end of the study. Cognitive scores for reasoning, vocabulary, semantic fluency, and memory were lower in subjects with persistent metabolic syndrome compared to those who either never had metabolic syndrome or whose metabolic syndrome reversed during the study [154].

Yates et al. [155] performed a meta-analysis of cognitive function and metabolic syndrome components in non-elderly adults and adolescents. Twenty studies were reviewed to determine the impact of metabolic syndrome components on cognitive functioning and brain integrity. Metabolic syndrome in adults was associated with deficits in memory, visuospatial abilities, executive functioning, processing speed, and overall intellectual functioning. In children, components of metabolic syndrome (obesity, hypertension, IFG) were linked to lower IQ and executive functioning. Children with type 2 diabetes were shown to perform worse than their peers in global functioning, memory, and attention.

Yates et al. [155] noted that few reports brain imaging exist in metabolic syndrome. But they reviewed some that reported increased intracranial arteriosclerosis [155], periventricular white matter hyperintensivities (PWMH), and subcortical white matter (WM) lesions [155] in patients with metabolic syndrome. Segura et al. [156] characterized WM abnormalities associated with the presence of metabolic syndrome components, and Haley et al. [157] demonstrated alterations in brain metabolism. Yates, therefore, concluded that, "subclinical alterations in cerebral metabolism may represent early brain compromise associated with peripheral metabolic disturbances."

Stroke

Because of its association with hypertension, dyslipidemia, and inflammation, the relationship between metabolic syndrome and ischemic stroke is not unexpected. In an evaluation of 10,357 subjects of the NHANES III study, metabolic syndrome was strongly associated with myocardial infarction or stroke in both men and women [158].

In a large family study of 4483 subjects with type 2 diabetes in Finland and Sweden [159], cardiovascular risk was associated with the metabolic syndrome. The risk for coronary heart disease and stroke was increased by a factor of 3 in subjects with metabolic syndrome ($P < 0.001$). Of metabolic syndrome components, microalbuminuria conferred the strongest risk of cardiovascular death.

To look specifically at stroke, Kurl et al. [160] followed a Finnish cohort of 1131 middle-aged males for 14.3 years prospectively. None had a history of cardiovascular disease or diabetes at the outset of the study period. Metabolic syndrome was defined according to NCEP ATP III criteria. At the end of the observation period, 65 strokes occurred, 45 of which were ischemic. Subjects with metabolic syndrome were found to have a 2.05-fold increased risk for all stroke ($P = 0.042$) and a 2.41-fold increase in ischemic stroke ($P = 0.025$) compared to those without metabolic syndrome [160].

Milionis et al. [161] evaluated modifiable risk factors in a case-controlled study of 163 elderly patients with first-ever stroke. Components for metabolic syndrome were examined as was the diagnosis of metabolic syndrome by NCEP ATP III criteria. Metabolic syndrome was observed in 46% of stroke patients. Stroke patients showed higher concentrations of metabolic syndrome components, including triglycerides, total cholesterol, and inflammatory markers such as fibrinogen, as well as lower HDL ratios [161].

Wannamethee et al. [162] evaluated the NCEP ATP III metabolic syndrome score as a predictor of CVD, including stroke. They analyzed data from the British Regional Heart Study, a large prospective study of 7735 men, aged 40–59. Metabolic syndrome was a significant predictor of CHD and stroke, although inferior to the Framingham Risk Score.

Nonalcoholic Fatty Liver Disease

NAFLD and metabolic syndrome are considered by some researchers to have a common origin in IR, representing the predominant metabolic disturbance in both cases [163]. NAFLD is also associated with obesity with a central fat distribution, HTN, dyslipidemia, CVD, and diabetes, all features of metabolic syndrome [164].

NAFLD is seen in up to 95% of obese individuals and in up to 70% of patients with type 2 diabetes [165]. Among NAFLD patients, 90% have at least one of the criteria for metabolic syndrome and 33% have all of them [6].

Hamaguchi et al. [166], in a prospective observational study of 4401 people, reported that subjects with metabolic syndrome had 4–11 times higher risk for NAFLD. They also reported that if patients have both metabolic syndrome and NAFLD, the likelihood of disease regression is diminished [166].

Patients with metabolic syndrome have a fourfold increase in the amount of fat in their livers compared to those without metabolic syndrome [167]. The incidence of NAFLD is greater in women than in men, and is present in children with obesity and IR [166,168]. A detailed discussion of NAFLD, including the current view of its pathogenesis, is found elsewhere in the text.

Polycystic Ovarian Syndrome

Polycystic ovarian syndrome (PCOS) and metabolic syndrome share certain features including IR, obesity, and dyslipidemia. Women with PCOS are at greater risk for developing type 2 diabetes and CVD [169,170].

PCOS commonly presents as hirsutism and anovulation. It affects 4% to 12% of women of reproductive age, making it a very common disorder [171,172]. Its prevalence rises to as high as 28% in overweight/obese patients [173]. Its hallmarks are chronic anovulation leading to oligomenorrhea and hyperandrogenism (acne or hirsutism) or hyperandrogenemia (elevated free testosterone or dehydroepiandrosterone-sulfate) [174].

Compared to their weight-matched controls, women with PCOS have a higher prevalence and increased levels of hyperinsulinemia and IR [174]. Among obese women with PCOS, the rate of IGT is 30% and diabetes is 7.5% [174]. Non-obese women with PCOS are also at increased risk for IGT and diabetes, 10.3% and 1.5%, respectively [173]. Long-term (20–30 years) follow-up for women with PCOS reveals that 16% develop diabetes prior to menopause [175].

CVD and PCOS are not currently as well defined. Predictive models based on the combined risks of PCOS and metabolic syndrome suggest a sevenfold increase in myocardial infarction compared to age-matched controls [176,177]. While the rate of events is not clearly established, there is evidence of subclinical CVD [178,179].

Clinicians must be aware of the parallel nature of metabolic syndrome and PCOS. Women who present initially for acne, increased body hair, and menstrual irregularities must be vigorously investigated for signs of both conditions. They should be treated at the earliest opportunity to prevent the sequelae of unchecked IR and the progression to overt diabetes and cardiovascular disease.

OBSTRUCTIVE SLEEP APNEA

Obstructive sleep apnea (OSA) is a significant concern in patients with metabolic syndrome. OSA leads to both fragmented sleep and intermittent hypoxia. Approximately 60% of metabolic syndrome patients are thought to also have OSA [180].

The primary cause of OSA is collapse of the pharyngeal airway. Anatomically, the pharynx is not supported by rigid structures and requires neuromuscular control for patency, leaving it vulnerable to pressure from surrounding tissues, especially during sleep. The expanded adipose mass in the neck of obese patients is thought to narrow the airway by contributing to increased pharyngeal tissue pressure.

Drager et al. [180] also reported physiologic evidence that sympathetic activation, systemic inflammation, and endothelial dysfunction are more prevalent in patients with OSA compared to those without it. They go on to state that the intermittent hypoxia of OSA augments IR and NAFLD [180]. OSA is also associated with inflammation and reduced adiponectin levels [181]. Clinicians should have their metabolic syndrome patients evaluated and treated for OSA. The importance of identification and management of patients with OSA can be seen in another study by Drager et al. [182] on the effects of CPAP. In a 4-month trial with effective CPAP treatment, markers of inflammation and sympathetic activity were reduced, as evidenced by reductions of CRP and catecholamines [182].

PATIENT EVALUATION

Patients who present with abdominal adiposity and more than one of the associated risk factors (hypertension, hyperglycemia, dyslipidemia) should be evaluated for the diagnosis of metabolic syndrome. As was noted above, the diagnostic criteria are now generally accepted based on the consensus literature. But there is still some disagreement on the exact diagnostic ranges for each of the components. Many of the conditions involved are on a spectrum of disease that is progressive. For example, a patient with a normal fasting glucose but abnormal 2-h glucose tolerance cannot be considered to be free of risk. However, the data in this example case would not meet the criteria for metabolic syndrome as outlined in Table 4.1.

Since we intend to utilize the diagnosis of metabolic syndrome as a motivator for the prevention of diabetes and cardiovascular disease, it may be permissible to take a more aggressive stance on its evaluation. The real question for the clinician seeing a patient is, how can I best define the cardiometabolic risk? Within this concept, our approach is to view any measurable abnormality in each category as a reason to suspect the diagnosis. But it is important to stress that we utilize this approach in the context of one-on-one patient care.

On the other hand, we believe that screening programs should maintain adherence to the published criteria of metabolic syndrome. Screening the general public can be an important community health program, and this function has the potential to create a valued niche for the metabolic medicine practice. The goal is to identify patients at cardiometabolic risk who can then be referred for follow-up medical care. Therefore, we feel it is more important to stay within established boundaries for such screening programs.

The criteria for the diagnosis of metabolic syndrome are shown in Table 4.1. In this section, we offer further details for clinicians on our approach to the precise aspects of each category.

WAIST MEASUREMENT

At our center, we initially assess the presence of expanded VAT by measuring the waist circumference of the patient. Waist circumference correlates closely to the amount of VAT and is superior to the correlation between VAT and BMI or body fat percentage [183,184].

The correct position for measuring waist circumference is at the point midway between the uppermost border of the iliac crest and the lower border of the costal margin. In the overweight and the obese individual, it may be difficult to palpate these landmarks. In this case, some practitioners choose to use the level of the umbilicus as a surrogate point [185].

The measurement should be made with the patient standing, the tape measure should be placed directly on the skin, and the patient should be instructed to breathe normally, with the abdomen relaxed in a neutral position. The tape measure should not compress the skin, but it should be snug against the body.

LABORATORY TESTING

Hyperglycemia

Hyperglycemia is a key component of the diagnosis of metabolic syndrome. A blood glucose value ≥100 mg/dL (>5.5 mmol/L) was determined to be the cut point for inclusion as one of the five criteria for diagnosis. There is some controversy among researchers as to whether a "normal" glucose level of 99 mg/dL is too high. Nichols et al. [186] studied the risk of diabetes in 46,578 people with normal FBG levels. The population was divided into five groups according to the FBG levels; the lowest was <85 mg/dl, and the highest was 95–99 mg/dL. The results showed that each 1 mg/dL increase in glucose incurred a 6% increase in the risk of diabetes. In the 95–99 mg/dL group, the risk of developing diabetes was three times higher than in subjects with FBG below 90 mg/dL. Subjects in the 90–94 mg/dL group had a 49% greater risk for diabetes compared to subjects in the <85 mg/dl group. This has led some clinicians to intervene at "normal" glucose levels and advise patients that perhaps 85 mg/dl should be their target.

The controversy regarding what should be accepted as "normal" extends to HgA1C, which is currently defined at <6%. This corresponds to an average blood glucose of 120 mg/dL. Khaw et al. [187] have shown that individuals with an HgA1C below 5% (average blood glucose of 90 mg/dL) had the lowest rates of cardiovascular disease and that each 1% increase (up to 6%) increased CVD significantly. Further evidence for even tighter blood glucose levels was seen in a study by Selvin et al. [188] who showed the risk for coronary heart disease, but higher values rose significantly at an HbA1c level above 4.6% (average blood glucose of 86 mg/dL) ($P < 0.001$).

In current practice, clinicians typically screen patients for hyperglycemia by measuring the FBG, typically as part of the basic metabolic panel. Insulin is usually not measured at all. Cut points for "normal" values are used but, as discussed above, may not utilize the most insightful ranges. Such routine testing patterns may miss a critical opportunity for early intervention in metabolic syndrome. This can rob the patient of a diagnosis at the earliest possible opportunity, when intervention is likely to have its greatest impact.

The underdiagnosis of diabetes is also a significant concern. The DECODE (Diabetes Epidemiology: Collaborative Analysis of Diagnostic Criteria in Europe) study group reported that as many as one third of diabetes cases are missed [189]. Additional studies in Asian, Australian, Micronesian, Polynesian, and Indian populations have concurred with this finding [190,191]. The proportion of underdiagnosed subjects is suspected to increase with age [192].

Glucose values can also be utilized to assess the risk for CVD. Qiao et al. [193] studied the FBG and the 2-h oral glucose tolerance test (OGTT) in 6766 Finnish subjects. After 7–10 years of follow-up, the group showed that the 2-h OGTT proved superior to fasting glucose as a predictor for the incidence of coronary heart disease and cardiovascular mortality compared to fasting glucose [193]. Other studies have shown the increase in cardiovascular events with blood glucose levels below the diabetic range [194,195].

Basal insulin levels are typically not measured in patients, but there is strong evidence that basal hyperinsulinemia is an even earlier metabolic derangement on the path to diabetes. Dankner et al. [196] studied basal rates of insulin in 515 subjects who had undergone a 2-h OGTT 24 years prior to follow-up. The study population group had normal glucose levels at the start of the study. Participants were determined to be hyperinsulinemic based on insulin levels in the uppermost quintile of the study population. At 24 years, 50% developed dysglycemia with 24% becoming diabetic. The authors concluded that basal insulin levels were the strongest predictor for progression to type 2 diabetes.

The homeostatic model assessment (HOMA) is a mathematical method used to quantify IR and beta cell function [197–199]. Mathematical calculation to establish the HOMA score is derived from fasting plasma glucose (FPG) and fasting plasma insulin (FPI) levels. Because the HOMA model requires only a single measurement of glucose and insulin in the basal state, it is considered by some to be superior to the other methods that are more time consuming and invasive. Kang et al. [200] compared the HOMA IR score (HOMA-IR) to the 3-h euglycemic–hyperinsulinemic clamp and found some shortcomings in determining IR among patients with type 2 diabetes. This study showed moderate agreement between the two methods, but it pointed to some limitations with looking at specific factors. This included a decreased magnitude of correlation in patients with a lower BMI, lower beta cell function, and high fasting glucose levels.

Clinicians may therefore consider ordering an OGTT with insulin response, which can give information on both glucose and insulin. The OGTT is administered after an overnight fast of at least 12 h. At time zero, blood is drawn for fasting glucose and insulin levels. A beverage containing a 75-g glucose load is then ingested. Glucose and insulin levels are subsequently measured at 30-min intervals until the conclusion of the test. This dynamic test delivers fasting levels of glucose and insulin and establishes response curves that can help diagnose IR, IGT, and reactive hypoglycemia. Valuable information such as the time to dysregulation and the degree of dysregulation can be established. This knowledge provides an opportunity to teach patients about their individualized response to the ingestion of carbohydrates. It also allows the clinician the potential to intervene earlier in the development of beta cell impairment.

At our center, we routinely perform the 3-h OGTT with insulin response. We have found that patients are willing to undergo the test and have very few complaints regarding any inconvenience it may cause them. In our experience, with thousands of patients, we have encountered numerous episodes in which a patient with a normal fasting glucose becomes hyperglycemic during the OGTT. Because our test extends to 3 h, we are also able to observe a significant number of cases of reactive hypoglycemia, which would have been missed at the 2-h mark. These are patients who develop the tendency for defensive cyclical eating to restore their blood glucose, typically choosing from simple carbohydrate options. This pattern of defensive cyclical eating promotes hyperinsulinemia and weight gain, particularly as visceral fat. Our method of testing with the 3-h OGTT has permitted us to intervene in patients much earlier in the disease process, even before other physicians are typically aware of metabolic disturbances.

DYSLIPIDEMIA

Dyslipidemia accounts for two of the five risks for metabolic syndrome: elevated triglycerides ≥ 150 mg/dL (1.7 mmol/L) and low HDL < 40 mg/dL (1.0 mmol/L) in males and <50 mg/dL (1.3 mmol/L) in females. Current methods used for testing are the standard lipid panel, the vertical auto profile-II (VAP-II), and the nuclear magnetic resonance (NMR) test.

The standard lipid panel measures HDL, triglycerides, and total cholesterol. It utilizes a calculated LDL. The LDL particle number is quantified using apolipoprotein B-100 (apo B-100) as a surrogate marker. Apo B-100 is used because each LDL particle contains only one molecule of apo B-100 on its cell surface [201]. The VLDL is calculated using the Friedewald's equation: VLDL = triglycerides/5 or VLDL = total cholesterol − (HDL + LDL) [202].

The VAP test directly measures total cholesterol, HDL, LDL, triglycerides, and VLDL. HDL is separated into HDL 2 (most protective) and HDL 3 (less protective). LDL is separated into LDL-R, Lp (a), and IDL. Lp(a) is a genetic risk factor for heart disease when elevated. IDL also carries associated risk for coronary artery disease. VLDL is separated into three forms; VLDL 3 is the smallest and most dense and therefore more dangerous than VLDL 1 and 2. The test also measures LDL pattern density. Pattern A consists of large, buoyant particles. Pattern B consists of small, dense particles that are more atherogenic [203].

An alternative is the NMR spectroscopy test. This method measures the amplitude of spectral signals emitted by lipoprotein subclasses based on their size [204] and renders the number and size of LDL and HDL particles as part of the results profile. The amplitude of the spectral analysis is not affected by the chemical composition of the particles and is therefore believed to give a direct measurement of the subclass particle components and their concentrations. A significant difference between the NMR and VAP-II tests is in the ability of the NMR to measure the LDL particle number and its size.

The relationship between the small LDL particle and CVD disease is well established [205,206]. The atherogenicity of small LDL particles may be due in part to their increased ability for transendothelial movement and accumulation in arterial walls [207] and increased oxidative susceptibility [208]. The relevance of the LDL particle number in metabolic syndrome was demonstrated by Koskinen et al. They measured the LDL particle number in 1400 subjects, without established disease. Subjects with the highest LDL particle number were 2.8 times likelier to have metabolic syndrome than those with the lowest level of LDL particles [209]. The Framingham Offspring Study also concluded that the LDL particle number was better at predicting cardiovascular disease events than LDL [210].

At our institution, we typically measure lipids with the NMR test. This allows us to more specifically address dyslipidemia with patients as it relates to metabolic syndrome than the standard lipid profile.

C-REACTIVE PROTEIN

An important goal in the management of metabolic syndrome is the reduction of inflammation. Evaluation of inflammation begins with the waist measurement, which, if increased from the accepted cut points, indicates expanded visceral adiposity. Inflammation can also be measured biochemically by testing for inflammatory markers. One method to do this is by obtaining the serum level of CRP.

The presence of elevated CRP has been shown to positively correlate with BMI, waist circumference, triglyceride levels, blood pressure, serum glucose, and IR and to negatively correlate with HDL cholesterol [211]. CRP is synthesized in the liver, largely in response to IL-6. Studies have shown that inflammation when measured by increases in 70%.

Elevations of CRP levels occur in states of inflammation, infection, trauma, and tissue necrosis. For example, there is a rapid rise (up to 50,000 times within 2 h) in acute infections. Under these circumstances, CRP levels generally peak at 48 h. The half-life of CRP is 19 h [212].

Hepatocytes manufacture CRP in response to cytokines, such as IL-6, released by macrophages and adipocytes. The gene encoding CRP is located on chromosome 1 (1q21-q23). The normal physiological role of CRP is to bind to its target, phosphocholine. Phosphocholine is expressed on the surface of cells that are dead or dying and some types of bacteria. The phosphocholine binding of CRP initiates the phagocytic immune response via the complement system [213].

Laboratory methods to determine CRP levels were initially only qualitative in nature. At that time, CRP measurement was not considered sensitive enough or cost effective enough to be widely used. In the late 1970s, this changed with the introduction of highly sensitive laboratory techniques, which permitted quantification to the pictogram range possible [214].

The landmark Justification for the Use of Statins in Prevention: an Intervention Trial Evaluating Rosuvastatin (JUPITER) study published in 2008 in NEJM firmly established the role of CRP as a biomarker for CVD risk in patients and underscored the role of inflammation in CVD [215]. High-sensitivity assays for CRP stratify CRP levels into three risk groups: CRP < 1 corresponds to low risk, CRP = 1–3 as intermediate risk, and CRP > 3 as high risk for future cardiovascular events [216].

At our center, we use CRP routinely as a biomarker to assess inflammation in our patients with metabolic syndrome. We consider levels at or above 3 as placing patients at high risk for cardiovascular events. As patients progress in our program, we reevaluate CRP levels.

MANAGEMENT OF METABOLIC SYNDROME

Since metabolic syndrome is a known risk factor for the onset of diabetes and cardiovascular disease, there is a clinical imperative to develop effective management of this condition. As data become stronger regarding the link of metabolic syndrome to conditions such as end-stage liver disease, dementia, and certain cancers, we anticipate that the need for metabolic syndrome management will intensify.

The three cornerstones for the management of metabolic syndrome are weight reduction, exercise, and a cardioprotective and anti-inflammatory diet. This triad is often referred to as lifestyle therapy. Because these are treatments that do not necessarily include pharmaceuticals or interventional procedures, they are often thought of a second-class status by both patients and providers alike. But the reality is quite the contrary. Such lifestyle therapy can effectively replace many pharmaceutical approaches. Furthermore, certain components of diet and exercise can surpass standard therapy in many instances.

Yet, lifestyle changes can be daunting for many patients who must redraw long-term patterns of eating, behavior, and activity. The situation is not helped by the fact that most of us live in what is referred to as the "obesogenic environment" [217]. The challenge to clinicians who accept the role of managing metabolic medicine is to overcome these barriers and help the patients navigate to real and meaningful change.

Weight Loss

Weight loss is believed to have a beneficial effect on patients with metabolic syndrome. Reducing total body weight ameliorates IR, decreases abdominal adiposity, lowers LDL cholesterol and triglycerides, increases HDL cholesterol, improves IGT, lowers blood pressure, and decreases low-grade systemic inflammation. The effect of these individual components is well known. But data on the overall effect on metabolic syndrome are not readily available.

Nonetheless, in their report of the AHA/NHLBI/ADA conference proceedings on the clinical management of metabolic syndrome, Grundy et al. [44] stressed the value of 7–10% weight loss on preventing or reversing metabolic syndrome. Case et al. [218] studied the effects of weight loss on metabolic syndrome. They reviewed 125 patients undergoing weight loss management who met the NCEP ATP III definition of metabolic syndrome. A moderate decrease in weight (6.5%) induced by a very low calorie diet (VLCD) resulted in substantial reductions of blood pressure, glucose, triglycerides, and total cholesterol (all $P < 0.001$). They concluded that moderate weight loss can have a marked impact on metabolic syndrome.

Some of the clearest data we have on the effect of weight loss in metabolic syndrome come from outcome studies of bariatric surgery. A long-term population-based retrospective study was performed by the Mayo Clinic on 180 patients who underwent Roux-en-Y gastric bypass surgery. The prevalence of metabolic syndrome preoperatively was 87% (AHA/NHLBI criteria). At the end of the observation period, the prevalence of metabolic syndrome was 29% (a 58% reduction). A comparison cohort of patients undergoing non-operative weight loss management had a reduction of metabolic syndrome prevalence from 85% to 75%. Notably, the patients who did not achieve resolution of metabolic syndrome had higher persistent excess adipose tissue when compared to those whose metabolic syndrome was resolved [219].

In the Swedish Obesity Study, cardiovascular risk characteristics declined in patients who successfully maintained weight loss after undergoing bariatric surgery compared to a nonsurgical cohort who did not lose weight [220]. In the Utah obesity study, hyperglycemia, dyslipidemia, and hypertension all improved in patients who successfully maintained weight loss after undergoing bariatric surgery [221].

Since we lack clear data on a specific effect of medical weight loss on outcomes in metabolic syndrome, it may be informative to rely on data concerning weight loss and diabetes prevention. The Finnish Diabetes Prevention Study provided early information regarding the impact of nutrition and exercise intervention [222]. They studied 522 middle-aged, overweight subjects with IGT who were randomized to either intensive lifestyle intervention or usual care. After 3 years, the intensive lifestyle intervention group lost 4% of the initial body weight compared to 1.1% in the control. Significant improvements in hemoglobin A1 C and dyslipidemia were noted in association with weight loss.

The Diabetes Prevention Program (DPP) followed 2766 individuals to evaluate the progression to diabetes [223]. The subjects were randomly assigned to one of three groups: intensive lifestyle intervention, metformin, or placebo. The goal of the intensive lifestyle group was to achieve and maintain a weight loss of at least 7%. At the 10-year follow-up, the diabetes incidence rates were 4.8 cases per 100 person-years in the intensive lifestyle intervention group, 7.8 in the metformin group, and 11.0 in the placebo group. Therefore, the 10-year incidence of diabetes was reduced by 34% in the intensive lifestyle group.

Other diabetes prevention studies including those reporting from Finland [159], China [224], and Sweden [225] have shown similar benefits from lifestyle intervention in the prevention or delay to type 2 diabetes.

An important weight loss goal is achieving a target waist circumference below the cut points for abdominal obesity. Patients at or below their gender and ethnic cut points indicate an acceptable VAT mass.

However, despite the impressive data on weight loss and diabetes prevention, less than 50% of overweight adults are counseled to lose weight by their health care professionals [226]. More attention to this important aspect of health care will be needed if we are to successfully manage metabolic syndrome in the future.

EXERCISE

Physical activity plays a key role in combating metabolic syndrome because of its ability to improve insulin sensitivity. Insulin sensitivity improves with even a single bout of exercise [227], and the level of improvement is in proportion to the intensity of the exercise [228]. Because increased insulin sensitivity after chronic exercise diminishes after 6 days of exercise cessation [229], physical training must be adapted as a permanent lifestyle change in the treatment of metabolic syndrome.

Physical conditioning is reduced in individuals with the metabolic syndrome and is believed to be an important predictor of mortality. This "deconditioning" is also thought to have a deleterious effect on vascular endothelial function. An increase in physical activity improves the components for metabolic syndrome and may improve endothelial function [230]. This, in turn, would be expected to result in a reduction in mortality.

The specific amounts and forms of exercise may vary by individual, but at least 30 min of daily activity is generally recommended. Some disagreement remains as to the specific benefits of aerobic versus resistive training [230]. But there can be little doubt that any form of exercise is better than none for patients who have metabolic syndrome.

Smutok et al. [231] studied 37 previously untrained middle-aged males before and after 20 weeks of either resistive exercise or aerobic exercise. Lipid profiles, blood pressure, and glycemic control were assessed before and after training. They observed that both interventions resulted in increased glucose tolerance and insulin sensitivity. Katzel et al. [232] studied 21 obese middle-aged men with 9 months of aerobic exercise and weight loss. They found that aerobic exercise improved exercise capacity but not the lipid profile or BP.

One of the largest controlled exercise trials, the health, risk factors, exercise training, and genetics (HERITAGE) study, examined the effects of 20 weeks of aerobic exercise on 675 normolipidemic men and women. They found that HDL-C increased, whereas triglycerides and LDL-C decreased following exercise.

Tjonna et al. [233] studied patients with metabolic syndrome under two levels of aerobic exercise intensity for 16 weeks. The first group underwent moderate continuous aerobic training (CME), whereas the second underwent high-intensity aerobic interval training (AIT). Maximal oxygen uptake, endothelial function, and metabolic syndrome parameters were monitored. Muscle biopsies of the vastus lateralis muscle were obtained before and after training. They found that exercise capacity increased more after AIT than CME and that the more intense exercise method reduced metabolic syndrome parameters more than moderate exercise. AIT was also superior to CME in enhancing endothelial function, insulin signaling in fat and skeletal muscle, skeletal muscle biogenesis, and excitation–contraction coupling.

NHANES data from 1999 to 2004 found that individuals who perform resistive exercise (weight lifting) reduced the development of metabolic syndrome by 37% [158]. A relatively modest number (8.8%) of the total NHANES population (5618) reported weight lifting. Weight lifting was more common in men than women, less common in Hispanics, more common in younger individuals, and more common in individuals from higher socioeconomic groups.

Tibana et al. [234] studied resistance training in middle-aged women with metabolic syndrome. The exercises involved three sets of 8–12 maximal repetitions of 12 exercises, performed on three nonconsecutive days of the week. The results showed a decrease in blood pressure after 8 weeks [234].

In the diabetes aerobic and resistance exercise (DARE) study, Sigal et al. [235] conducted a 26-week trial of resistance training, aerobic training, and combined exercise training in 251 patients with type 2 diabetes. The hemoglobin A1c value decreased by 0.38 in the resistance group, 0.43 in the aerobic group, and 0.9 in the combined exercise group [235]. Dyslipidemia improved only in the combined exercise group. Modest weight loss occurred in all exercise groups, from 1.1 to 2.6 kg. Importantly, waist circumference also decreased in all exercise groups, from 3.1 to 3.3 cm.

Patients in the DARE study also underwent body composition testing with bioimpedance and CT. These data showed a reduction in abdominal visceral fat in all exercise groups, with the greatest reduction after combined exercise. Similarly, there was a reduction in abdominal subcutaneous fat in all exercise groups, with the most pronounced results being after combined. Mid-thigh muscle cross-sectional area was measured and was found to increase in all exercise groups. The most pronounced increase was seen in the combined exercise group.

DIET

The overfed state has been shown to increase overall and especially visceral adiposity, which is considered to be a key causal factor leading to IR, which is viewed as a key component in the development of metabolic syndrome. The typical diet of most Americans tends to be derived from obesogenic foods and beverages that are typically highly processed, rich in simple carbohydrates, and devoid of nutrients.

We have learned a great deal about nutrition intervention form the Nurses' Health Study about the combination of healthy behaviors combined with a cardioprotective diet. Nurses who did not smoke, were physically active, maintained a BMI of <25, drank only moderate amounts of alcohol, and consumed a healthy diet enjoyed an 80% lower rate of coronary events than those who did not.

Salas-Salvado et al. [236] recently reviewed the role of diet in the prevention of type II diabetes. They examined the different effects of carbohydrate and fat intake as well as those of specific foods and whole diets. They concluded that there was no universal dietary strategy to prevent diabetes or delay its onset. The maintenance of ideal body weight and a prudent diet, characterized by more plant-based foods and less red meat, meat products, sweets, high-fat dairy, and refined grains, appeared to be sensible. But they stated that the Mediterranean diet, which is rich in olive oil, fruits and vegetables, whole grains, nuts, low-fat dairy, and red wine may be the best strategy to decrease diabetes risk.

In their review, they presented results from large population studies. These are shown in Table 4.5.

By way of conclusion, Salas-Salvado et al. presented the likely benefits and risks from various food components and dietary patterns. This is reproduced in Table 4.6. Some controversy remains about the specific risks associated with some of the foods, nutrients, and dietary patterns. But the components of this table are the result of evidence from perspective observational studies and randomized trials as well as expert opinions.

The Mediterranean Diet

As was noted above, the Mediterranean diet appears to have value as a treatment modality for individuals at risk for type II diabetes mellitus and CVD [237]. Esposito et al. [238] conducted a randomized prospective trial to understand the specific effects of a Mediterranean style diet on components of the metabolic syndrome.

The study participants included 180 men and women diagnosed with metabolic syndrome according to the ATP III criteria. Each subject had at least three of the five criteria present. All subjects were advised to follow a prudent diet that was composed of 50–60% carbohydrates, 15–20% protein, and less than 30% total fat. Saturated fat was less than 10% and cholesterol consumption less than 300 mg per day. Subjects in the intervention group ($n = 90$) were advised to consume at least 250–300 g of fruits, 125–150 g of vegetables, and 25–50 g of walnuts per day. They were also encouraged to consume 400 g of whole grains daily and to increase their consumption of olive oil. Subjects in the control group ($n = 90$) did not supplement their diet with the Mediterranean style elements. The investigators monitored the number of ATP III components as well as endothelial function, lipid and glucose parameters, insulin sensitivity, CRP, and levels of interleukins.

After 24 months, subjects in the intervention group had significant decreases in body weight, BMI, waist circumference, HOMA score, blood pressure, levels of glucose, insulin, total cholesterol, and triglycerides and a significant increase in levels of HDL cholesterol. At the end of the study, the number of ATP III components decreased in 60 of the intervention group subjects. The extent of this change meant that only 40 intervention group subjects could still be classified as having metabolic syndrome by ATP III criteria. This level of improvement was not seen in the control group, where 78 subjects were still classified as having metabolic syndrome ($P < 0.001$).

The PREDIMED trial (Prevención con Dieta Mediterránea) was a parallel-group, multicenter, randomized study that was designed to determine efficacy of two specific Mediterranean diets on

TABLE 4.5

Observational Studies of Food Patterns and Risk of Type 2 Diabetes

Studies	Number and Follow-Up	Higher-Risk Food Patterns	Lower-Risk Food Patterns
Health Professionals, van Dam et al. 2002	42,504 men (12 years)	Red and processed meats, sweets and desserts, French fries, refined grains, high-fat dairy products	–
Nurses' Health Study, Fung et al. 2004	69,554 women (14 years)	Red and processed meats, sweets and desserts, French fries, refined grains	Fruits, vegetables, whole grains, fish, poultry, low-fat dairy
Finnish Mobile, Montonen et al. 2005	4304 men and women (23 years)	Butter, potatoes, high-fat milk, red and processed meats	Fruits and vegetables
EPIC-Potsdam, EPIC 2005	192 cases and 382 controls	Soft drinks, beer, red and processed meats, poultry, refined breads, legumes	Fresh fruits
Melbourne, Hodge et al. 2007	31,641 men and women (4 years)	Red meats, fried fish, processed meats, fat-cooked potatoes	Salads, cooked vegetables, whole grains
Whitehall II, Brunner et al. 2008	7,731 men and women (15 years)	–	Whole meal bread, fruits and vegetables, PUFA-rich margarine
Multiethnic Study of Atherosclerosis, Nettleton 2008	5011 men and women (5 years)	Tomatoes, beans, refined grains, high-fat dairy, red meat	Whole grains, fruit, nuts/seeds, green leafy vegetables, low-fat dairy
Insulin Resistance Atherosclerosis, Liese et al. 2009	880 men and women (5 years)	Red meats, refined cereals, dried beans, fried potatoes, tomato vegetables, eggs, cheese	–
Nurses Health Study, Hu et al. 2001	84,941 women (16 years)	Glycemic index and trans fats	PUFA/SFA ratio and cereal fiber
GISSI, Mozaffarian et al. 2007	8291 men and women (3.2 years)	–	Mediterranean (cooked or raw vegetables, fruit, fish, olive oil)
SUN, Martinez-Gonzalez 2008	13,380 men and women (4.4 years)	Meats and dairy products	Mediterranean (MUFA/SFA, vegetables, fruit, fish, legumes, cereals, alcohol)
Cardiovascular Health Study, Mozaffarian 2009	4883 men and women (10 years)	Glycemic index and trans fats	PUFA/SFA ratio and fiber

Source: Adapted from Salas-Salvado J et al., *Nutr Metabol Cardiovasc Dis*, 21, B32–B48, 2011.

primary cardiovascular prevention. A total of 7447 individuals were enrolled. The subjects ranged in age from 55 to 80 years; 57% were women. They were considered to be at risk for cardiovascular disease because they had either type 2 diabetes mellitus or at least three major risk factors: smoking, hypertension, dyslipidemia, overweight/obesity, or a family history of premature coronary heart disease.

The Mediterranean diets were supplemented with either extra-virgin olive oil (approximately 150 mL per day) or 30 g of mixed nuts per day. Those in the control group followed a low-fat diet. The study participants are evenly distributed between the three groups (Mediterranean diet +

TABLE 4.6

Foods, Nutrients, and Dietary Patterns in the Prevention of Type 2 Diabetes

Foods, Nutrients, and Dietary Patterns	Increase Risk	Decrease Risk
Foods	Sugar-rich beverages, fruit juices[a]	Whole grains[a]
	Meat and processed meat[a]	Coffee and tea[a]
	Hydrogenated oils and margarines[b]	Low-fat milk and dairy products[a]
	Eggs[b]	Moderate alcohol consumption[b]
		Fruits and vegetables[b]
		Pulses[b]
		Nuts (in women)[b]
Nutrients	Saturated fatty acids[b]	Fiber[a]
	Trans fatty acids[b]	Unsaturated fatty acids[a]
		Antioxidants[b]
		Magnesium[b]
Dietary patterns	High glycemic index diets[a]	Low glycemic index diets[b]
	Western dietary pattern[a]	Mediterranean diet[c]
		Low-fat prudent diet[c]

Source: Adapted from Salas-Salvado J et al., *Nutr Metabol Cardiovasc Dis*, 21: B32–B48, 2011.

[a] Moderate evidence from several prospective observational studies or meta-analysis.

[b] Reasonable evidence from some prospective observational studies or expert opinions.

[c] High level of evidence from several prospective observational studies and randomized trials.

EVOO, $n = 2543$; Mediterranean diet + Nuts, $n = 2454$; Control, $n = 2450$). There was no caloric restriction and no directive on physical activity. After a median of 4.8 years of follow-up, subjects on either Mediterranean diet showed a significant reduction in major cardiovascular risk.

Recently, Ibarrola-Jurado et al. [239] conducted a cross-sectional assessment of the PREDIMED Study to determine the specific effects of nut consumption on metabolic syndrome, obesity, and other cardiometabolic risk factors (*PLoS ONE* 8(2): e573). Metabolic syndrome was defined according to the IDF/AHA/NHLBI joint criteria. Subjects were diagnosed with metabolic syndrome if they had at least three of the five components. After excluding a small number of the total PREDIMED study participants for technical reasons, they evaluated a total of 7210 subjects, 3067 men and 4143 women. Through the use of a 137-item food frequency questionnaire, they determined three average levels of nut consumption: 0.48, 5.88, and 25.48 g per day. This corresponded to less than one serving per week, one to three servings per week, and more than three servings per week. The data were analyzed using analysis of variance (ANOVA), chi-square, and multiple logistic regression models. The study found that, in elderly subjects at high cardiovascular risk, nut consumption was inversely associated with the prevalence of metabolic syndrome, obesity, and diabetes.

Recent findings on the beneficial effect of nut consumption in metabolic syndrome have also been reported in the NHANES 1999 to 2004 cohort [240]. Furthermore, recent data from the SUN cohort showed that participants who consumed more than two servings of nuts per week had a 32% reduction in the risk of developing metabolic syndrome compared to those who almost never consume nuts [241].

The Mediterranean diet can also be considered an alternative to the use of statins. In the above study, participants in the Mediterranean diet group reduced the risk of cardiovascular disease by approximately 30%. This favorably compares to the benefits shown by statin drugs, estimated at 25% reduction in cardiovascular disease events (Tables 4.7 and 4.8) [242].

TABLE 4.7
Therapeutic Goals and Management for Dyslipidemia

Goal of Therapy	Therapeutic Recommendations
Primary target — *LDL*: High-risk patients[a]—<100 mg/dL (2.6 mmol/L) (for very high-risk patients[b] in this category, optional goal <70 mg/dL)	High-risk patients: lifestyle therapies—+ LDL-C-lowering drug to achieve recommended goal – If baseline LDL-C ≥ 100 mg/dL, initiate LDL-lowering drug therapy C6 – If on-treatment LDL-C ≥ 100 mg/dL, intensify LDL-lowering drug therapy (may require LDL-lowering drug combination) – If baseline LDL-C <100 mg/dL, initiate LDL-lowering therapy based on clinical judgment (i.e., assessment that patient is at very high risk)
LDL: Moderately high-risk patients[c]—<130 mg/dL (3.4 mmol/L) (for higher-risk patients; in this category, optional goal is <100 mg/dL [2.6 mmol/L])	Moderately high-risk patients: lifestyle therapies+ LDL-lowering drug if necessary to achieve recommended goal when LDL-C ≥ 130 mg/dL (3.4 mmol/L) after lifestyle therapies. If baseline LDL-C is 100 to 129 mg/dL, LDL-lowering therapy can be introduced if patient's risk is assessed to be in upper ranges of this risk category
LDL: Moderate-risk patients[d]—<130 mg/dL (3.4 mmol/L)	Moderate risk patients: lifestyle therapies + LDL-C lowering drug if necessary to achieve recommended goal when LDL-C ≥ 160 mg/dL (4.1 mmol/L) after lifestyle therapies
LDL: Lower-risk patients[e]: <160 mg/dL (4.9 mmol/L)	Lower-risk patients: lifestyle therapies + LDL-C lowering drug if necessary to achieve recommended goal when LDL-C ≥ 190 mg/dL after lifestyle therapies (for LDL-C 160 to 189 mg/dL, LDL-lowering drug is optional)
Secondary target — *Elevated non-HDL-C*: High-risk patients—<130 mg/dL (3.4 mmol/L) (optional: <100 mg/dL [2.6 mmol/L] for very high-risk patients) *Elevated non-HDL-C*: Moderately high-risk patients—<160 mg/dL (4.1 mmol/L). Therapeutic option: <130 mg/dL (3.4 mmol/L) *Elevated non-HDL-C*: Moderate-risk patients: <160 mg/dL (4.1 mmol/L) *Elevated non-HDL-C*: Lower-risk patients: <190 mg/dL (4.9 mmol/L)	First option to achieve non-HDL-C goal: Intensify LDL-lowering therapy option to achieve non-HDL-C goal—Add fibrate (preferably fenofibrate) or nicotinic acid if non-HDL-C remains relatively high after LDL-lowering drug therapy. Give preference to adding fibrate or nicotinic acid in high-risk patients. Give preference to avoiding addition of fibrate or nicotinic acid in moderately high-risk or moderate-risk patients. All patients: If TG is ≥500 mg/dL, initiate fibrate or nicotinic acid (before LDL-lowering therapy; treat non-HDL-C to goal after TG-lowering therapy)
Tertiary target — *Elevated non-HDL-C*: No specific goal—Raise HDL-C to extent possible with standard therapies for atherogenic dyslipidemia	Maximize lifestyle therapies: weight reduction and increased physical activity. Consider adding fibrate or nicotinic acid after LDL-C-lowering drug therapy as outlined for elevated non-HDL-C

Source: Adapted from Grundy SM et al., *Circulation*, 112(17): 2735–2752, 2005.

[a] High-risk patients are those with established ASCVD, diabetes, or 10-year risk for coronary heart disease > 20%. For cerebrovascular disease, high-risk condition includes TIA or stroke of carotid origin or >50% carotid stenosis.

[b] Very high-risk patients are those who are likely to have major CVD events in next few years, and diagnosis depends on clinical assessment. Factors that may confer very high risk include recent acute coronary syndromes, and established coronary heart disease + any of the following: multiple major risk factors (especially diabetes), severe and poorly controlled risk factors (especially continued cigarette smoking), and metabolic syndrome.

[c] Moderately high-risk patients are those with 10-year risk for coronary heart disease 10% to 20%. Factors that favor therapeutic option of non-HDL-C < 100 mg/dL are those that can raise individuals to upper range of moderately high risk: multiple major risk factors, severe and poorly controlled risk factors (especially continued cigarette smoking), metabolic syndrome, and documented advanced subclinical atherosclerotic disease (e.g., coronary calcium or carotid intimal–medial thickness > 75th percentile for age and sex).

[d] Moderate-risk patients are those with 2+ major risk factors and 10-year risk < 10%.

[e] Lower-risk patients are those with 0 or 1 major risk factor and 10-year risk < 10%.

TABLE 4.8

Therapeutic Goals and Management for Hypertension, Hyperglycemia, Prothrombotic, and Proinflammatory State

Hypertension	Reduce BP to at least achieve BP of <140/90 mm Hg (or <130/80 mm Hg if diabetes is present). Reduce BP further to extent possible through lifestyle changes.	For BP ≥ 120/80 mm Hg: Initiate or maintain lifestyle modification in all patients with metabolic syndrome—weight control, increased physical activity, alcohol moderation, sodium reduction, and emphasis on increased consumption of fresh fruits, vegetables, and low-fat dairy products. For BP ≥ 140/90 mm Hg (or ≥130/80 mm Hg for individuals with chronic kidney disease or diabetes)—As tolerated, add BP medication as needed to achieve goal BP
Elevated glucose	For IFG, delay progression to type 2 diabetes mellitus. For diabetes, hemoglobin A1C < 7.0%.	For IFG, encourage weight reduction and increased physical activity. For type 2 diabetes mellitus, lifestyle therapy, and pharmacotherapy, if necessary, should be used to achieve near-normal HbA1C (<7%). Modify other risk factors and behaviors (e.g., abdominal obesity, physical inactivity, elevated BP, lipid abnormalities)
Prothrombotic state	Reduce thrombotic and fibrinolytic risk factors.	High-risk patients: initiate and continue low-dose aspirin therapy; in patients with ASCVD, consider clopidogrel if aspirin is contraindicated. Moderately high-risk patients: consider low-dose aspirin prophylaxis
Proinflammatory state		Recommendations: no specific therapies beyond lifestyle therapies

Source: Adapted from Grundy SM et al., *Circulation*, 112(17): 2735–2752, 2005.

MEDICATIONS

Despite a commitment to aggressive lifestyle changes, some patients have persistent metabolic abnormalities and remain at risk from the consequences of hyperglycemia, dyslipidemia, inflammation, and a prothrombotic state. In these individuals, the additional option of pharmaceuticals such as hypoglycemics/insulin sensitizers, antidyslipidemics, and antithrombotics should be considered.

HYPOGLYCEMIC AND INSULIN-SENSITIZING AGENTS

Since IGT and IR are fundamental aspects of the metabolic syndrome, pharmaceutical approaches to these underlying conditions are among the most commonly considered therapeutic agents. Metformin, thiazolidinediones (TZDs), and acarbose have each been studied as potential treatments for patients with metabolic syndrome. Lengthy experience with metformin has shown it to be a generally safe, first-line therapy in newly diagnosed diabetes [243,244]. The TZDs, which have a shorter track record and more concerns regarding toxicity, are also considered to be insulin sensitizing. Acarbose, which blocks luminal carbohydrate digestion, slows glucose delivery.

Metformin

Metformin acts on the liver, adipose tissue, muscle, and the small intestine [245]. The major effect of metformin is the reduction of hepatic gluconeogenesis. Its specific mechanism is unknown. Metformin reduces IR, suppresses adipose tissue lipolysis, and increases glucose uptake in muscle and bowel.

Unlike many other antidiabetic medications, metformin generally does not cause hypoglycemia or weight gain. In addition, metformin is thought to have vasoprotective effects [245]. The side effects of low-dose metformin are limited to GI intolerance. In higher doses, metformin can cause metabolic acidosis if used in patients with renal failure.

Metformin has been extensively studied for diabetes prevention. For example, the DPP compared lifestyle (7% weight loss, diet, and exercise) to metformin (850 mg BID) or placebo [223]. Both intervention groups did well as compared to the placebo group. Lifestyle intervention reduced the incidence of type 2 diabetes by 58%, and metformin use decreased the risk by 31%.

The DPP study included a follow-up period of approximately 3 years. To examine if these benefits continued, the Diabetes Prevention Program Outcomes Study (DPPOS) was initiated. The DPPOS study showed that after 10 years, lifestyle intervention decreased the incidence of type 2 diabetes by 34% and metformin by 18% [245].

Thiazolidinediones

TZDs activate the peroxisome proliferator-activated receptors (PPARs), modulating gene transcription. The TZD effect includes decreased IR, decreased vascular endothelial growth factor (VEGF)-induced angiogenesis, decreased IL-6, and increased adiponectin [246,247].

The TZD effect on fat and glucose metabolism results in a reduction of triglycerides, LDL, and FFAs. HDL cholesterol is increased. Goldberg et al. [248] demonstrated that pioglitazone improved LDL particle concentration and LDL particle size. TZDs can decrease inflammation through PPAR gamma receptor binding to proinflammatory KF-KB transcription factors. This binding leads to the decreased expression of a number of proinflammatory genes.

The TRIPOD study showed that treatment with troglitazone can slow the progression to type 2 diabetes in high-risk women with recent gestational diabetes [249]. The DREAM study showed that treatment with rosiglitazone slowed the progression to type 2 diabetes by 60% [250].

However, troglitazone use has been discontinued because of an increased risk of drug-induced hepatitis. Rosiglitazone had been restricted in the United States and withdrawn in Europe due to an increased cardiovascular risk. However, this restriction was removed in November 2013 by the FDA [251]. Pioglitazone use has been suspended in some European countries because of the risk of bladder cancer. But pioglitazone remains available in the United States.

DeFronzo et al. [252] studied the effects of pioglitazone in a randomized, double-blind, placebo-controlled study of 602 patients followed for 2.4 years. The incidence rate of diabetes was significantly lower (2.1%) among patients receiving pioglitazone than placebo (7.6%). Furthermore, conversion to normal glycemia occurred in 48% of patients receiving pioglitazone compared to 28% in the placebo group. Therefore, despite the concerns of possible toxicity with these agents, TZDs may have a role in the management of metabolic syndrome.

Acarbose

Acarbose is an alpha-glucosidase inhibitor that delays the absorption of carbohydrates and glucose delivery to the plasma. Given its mechanism of action, it would not generally be considered to alter IR. But surprisingly, the evidence shows that acarbose has a beneficial effect on insulin homeostasis [253]. In the STOP-NIDDM trial [254], the acarbose study group had a significant reduction in the progression to diabetes compared to placebo (32% vs. 42%).

ANTIATHEROGENIC DYSLIPIDEMIA AGENTS

Atherogenic dyslipidemia is a prominent factor in the diagnosis of metabolic syndrome and is thought to be a significant contributor to the development of cardiovascular disease. Therefore, many of the lipid-lowering drugs have been considered in its management. Prominent among these are the statins, which inhibit HMG co-A reductase and impede the hepatic production of cholesterol. This enzymatic blockade may, in turn, upregulate the LDL receptor.

In addition to their lipid-lowering effect, statins have been shown to have a significant anti-inflammatory capacity. And it is possible that some of the benefits derived from statin therapy are due to this function.

Fibric acid derivatives are also attractive therapeutic options because of their ability to both lower triglycerides and raise HDL. The pharmaceutical potency of certain nutrients such as niacin and omega-3-fatty acids may also have value in this regard.

Statins

The statin group of pharmaceuticals can lower LDL-C from 20% to 50% [255]. They increase HDL by 5–10% and reduce triglycerides by 7–30% [181]. Statin-related increases in HDL-C correlates to the reduction in plasma triglycerides [256]. The effectiveness of statin therapy in reducing cardiovascular death was demonstrated by the Scandinavian Simvastatin Survival Study (4S) [257]. Cholesterol lowering in 4444 patients with coronary heart disease during 5.4 years of follow-up showed that the relative risk of death in the simvastatin group was 0.70 (95% CI 0.58–0.85, $P = 0.0003$). This proved that statins could be utilized as secondary prevention in cardiovascular disease.

The Air Force/Texas Coronary Atherosclerosis Prevention Study (AFCAPS/TexCAPS) was the first trial to demonstrate a significant statin cardioprotective effect in primary prevention. In that study of 6605 men and women, lovastatin use reduced the risk of a first acute major coronary event by 37% ($P = 0.00008$) [258].

In the Heart Protection Study (HPS), 20,536 adults with cardiovascular disease or diabetes were randomized to receive 40 mg simvastatin daily or matching placebo [259]. There was a highly significant (18%) reduction in the coronary death rate among the intervention group. In a subgroup analysis of the 5963 adults with diabetes, there was a 22% reduction of major cardiovascular events [260].

In addition to their ability to alter atherogenic dyslipidemia, the powerful anti-inflammatory effect of statins may have particular value for metabolic syndrome. As we have described above, VAT can release a powerful proinflammatory signal through a number of inflammatory mediators. Therefore, it is possible that a statin-induced anti-inflammatory effect could reverse the risks associated with adipokine-associated cardiovascular risk.

This concept was the subject of the JUPITER study published in the *New England Journal of Medicine* [261]. The study was conducted among healthy adult men and women with no evidence of cardiovascular disease or dyslipidemia. However, all patients enrolled in the study needed to have a high-sensitivity CRP value of >2.0 mg/L. A total of 17,802 subjects from 1315 sites in 26 countries were randomized to receive rosuvastatin, 20 mg daily, or placebo. After a median follow-up of 1.9 years, the rosuvastatin group had significantly fewer major cardiovascular events.

Niacin

Niacin (nicotinic acid, vitamin B3) improves dyslipidemia by increasing HDL cholesterol (15–35%), increasing HDL particle size, lowering triglycerides (20–50%), and lowering LDL cholesterol (5–25%) [262,263]. Niacin has also been shown to increase levels of adiponectin and decrease CRP in patients with metabolic syndrome [264]. When statin and niacin are combined, the effect is better than when either is given alone [265]. However, high doses of niacin can cause mild, reversible hyperglycemia [266]. Some authors have advocated treatment with oral hypoglycemic agents for niacin-related hyperglycemia [267].

Fibrates

Fibrates such as gemfibrozil and fenofibrate can decrease serum triglycerides by 25–50%, increase HDL by 5–15%, and reduce LDL-C by up to 30% [181]. Fibrates have been evaluated in several cardiovascular prevention trials. Gemfibrozil was used for primary prevention in the Helsinki Heart Study, a double-blind 5-year trial of 4081 asymptomatic middle-aged men [268]. Gemfibrozil reduced the incidence of coronary heart disease by 34%. The value of gemfibrozil for secondary prevention was shown in the VA-HIT study of 2531 men with a history of coronary heart disease [269]. The Bezafibrate Infarction Prevention (BIP) trial [270] and Fenofibrate Intervention and Event Lowering in Diabetes (FIELD) study [271] have also shown the potential protective benefits of fibrates. However, in the ACCORD study, the combination of fenofibrate and simvastatin did not reduce the rate of major cardiovascular events [272].

ANTIHYPERTENSIVES

The guideline for hypertension in the diagnosis of metabolic syndrome is a BP > 130/85 or the presence of preexisting antihypertensive medical therapy. Until more research is available on the treatment goals of hypertension in metabolic syndrome, we rely on the guidelines established by The Seventh Report of the Joint National Committee on Prevention, Detection, Evaluation, and Treatment of High Blood Pressure [273]. The goal for antihypertensive therapy in patients without diabetes or chronic renal disease is blood pressure of <140/90 mm Hg. If patients have diabetes or chronic renal disease, the blood pressure goal is <130/80 mm Hg.

The initial approach to blood pressure management is aggressive lifestyle therapy [274]. Mild elevations in blood pressure can be addressed with weight reduction, exercise, and proper nutrition plan. The Dietary Approaches to Stop Hypertension (DASH) diet exemplifies an eating plan whose aim is to reduce blood pressure [275]. The diet emphasizes consumption of fresh fruits, vegetables, and nonfat or low-fat dairy. These provide more key nutrients, including potassium, calcium, and magnesium, which are associated with lower blood pressure. Sodium recommendations follow United States Recommended Daily Allowances (USRDA) guidelines, which for most Americans translate to restriction. The DASH diet also includes lean meats, fish, poultry, nuts, seeds, and legumes. The foods recommended are compatible with a Mediterranean diet. Smoking cessation and alcohol moderation are also recommended [275].

When blood pressure remains elevated after lifestyle management, medications should be considered to protect patients from the consequences of chronic HTN, such as myocardial infarction, stroke, and chronic kidney disease [276]. Some clinicians support the use of angiotensin-converting enzyme (ACE) inhibitors as first-line therapy for hypertension in the metabolic syndrome, especially when diabetes or chronic renal disease is present [277,278]. Another approach is supported by the Antihypertensive and Lipid-Lowering Treatment to Prevent Heart Attack Trial (ALLHAT). This trial showed that treatment with a thiazide diuretic is a better first-line therapy with better outcomes on CVD than calcium channel blockers, α-blockers, or ACE inhibitors [279]. ALLHAT also showed that the combination of a diuretic with a β-blocker lowers the risk of CVD events [280]. There is some evidence that these agents are associated with an increased risk for diabetes [280,281].

ANTITHROMBOTIC AGENTS

Aspirin

Metabolic syndrome is a prothrombotic state associated with a number of abnormalities in hemostasis and thrombosis. Platelet hyperactivity, hypercoagulability, hypofibrinolysis, endothelial dysfunction, and venous thromboembolism have all been observed in association with the condition [282].

Low-dose aspirin prophylaxis has been recommended for patients with the metabolic syndrome [283]. However, there are no primary prevention studies of the use of aspirin or other antiplatelet agents for metabolic syndrome. In the AHA/NHLBI Scientific Statement on the Diagnosis and Management of the Metabolic Syndrome, reduction of thrombotic and fibrinolytic risk factors was recommended [284]. This recommendation was tiered based on risk. Continuous low-dose aspirin therapy was recommended for high-risk patients. Low-dose aspirin prophylaxis was recommended for patients not considered to be high risk. For patients with known cardiovascular disease, clopido-grel should be considered, especially if aspirin is contraindicated.

Patients with metabolic syndrome may have a diminished response to aspirin therapy. Studies have shown that patients with metabolic syndrome demonstrate increased platelet activation compared to controls [285,286]. This may offset the beneficial antiplatelet effect of aspirin in these patients.

ANTI-INFLAMMATORY AGENTS

Omega-3-Fatty Acids

Omega-3 fatty acids are members of the polyunsaturated fatty acid (PUFA) family. PUFAs are characterized by having a double-bond three carbons from the methyl terminus. Omega-3 fatty acids compete for enzymes in prostaglandin and leukotriene biosynthesis. The substitution of omega-3 fatty acids in these pathways results in specific subtypes of prostaglandins and leukotrienes. These subtypes may produce dramatically different effects than prostaglandins and leukotrienes derived from linoleic acid.

Studies have shown that 2–4 g of omega-3 fatty acids can reduce serum triglycerides by 20–40% [287,288]. In a review by Harris [289] at this dose range, omega-3 fatty acids increased HDL-C by 1–3%, but LDL was also increased by 5–10%.

Omega-3 fatty acids can be combined with statins as part of the management of dyslipidemia. A randomized clinical trial was conducted by Durrington et al. [290] in patients with persistent hyper-triglyceridemia. Patients were randomized to receive a statin plus omega-3 fatty acids or a statin plus placebo. The treatment group had 20% to 30% decreases in serum triglyceride concentrations and 30% to 40% decreases in VLDL cholesterol levels compared to the placebo group. In this study, no increase in LDL was observed.

In addition to their triglyceride lowering capacity, omega-3 fatty acids have other effects that might be beneficial to the patient with metabolic syndrome. They are known to be anti-inflammatory [291]. They have a beneficial effect on hemostasis and thrombosis by reducing platelet aggrega-tion [292]. Furthermore, omega-3 fatty acids can enhance endothelial function [276].

Omega-3 fatty acids can lower blood pressure in hypertensive patients [291,293].

The reduction in blood pressure has been evaluated in meta-analyses and trials. These revealed that fish oil at 5.6 g/day reduced blood pressure by 3.4/2.0 mm Hg [294], at least 3 g/day reduced blood pres-sure by 5.5/3.5 mm Hg, and at least 3.7 g/day reduced blood pressure by 2.1/1.6 mm Hg [295].

SURGERY

Bariatric surgery is another treatment modality for metabolic syndrome. Some overweight and obese patients become candidates for bariatric surgery as a result of failure to adapt to exercise and diet intervention. Their persistent metabolic abnormalities and obesity may then require bariatric surgery to prevent CVD and diabetes. For others, bariatric surgery is considered at earlier time points, perhaps even at presentation. These patients may include those whose weight has progressed to a level where lifestyle and medical management will not likely achieve adequate reduction in adipose mass.

The effects of bariatric surgery on metabolic syndrome are encouraging. A long-term (1990–2003) population-based retrospective study was performed by the department of surgery at the Mayo Clinic to analyze the long-term effects of bariatric surgery on metabolic syndrome. Of the 180 patients who underwent Roux-en-Y gastric bypass surgery, the prevalence of metabolic syndrome preoperatively was 87% (AHA/NHLBI criteria). At the end of the observation period, the preva-lence of metabolic syndrome was 29% (a 58% reduction). A comparison cohort of patients under-going non-operative weight loss management meanwhile had a reduction of metabolic syndrome prevalence from 85% to 75%. Notably, the patients who did not achieve resolution of metabolic syndrome after surgery had higher persistent excess adipose tissue when compared to those whose metabolic syndrome resolved [219].

Looking at the individual components of bariatric surgery, studies show that surgery can reduce the prevalence of type 2 diabetes, hypertension, hyperlipidemia, and OSA. A meta-analysis of bariatric surgery patients by Buchwald et al. [296] showed resolution of type 2 diabetes in excess of three quarters of patients. Of those who did not experience complete resolution, greater than 50% showed improvement. Other more recent reviews confirm this finding with diabetes resolution in 83% [297] and 86% [298] of patients.

Diabetes resolution was affected by the type of operation. It was greatest for patients who received a predominantly malabsorptive procedure compared to those receiving mixed malabsorptive/restrictive and purely restrictive operations. The diabetes resolution rate was 98.9% for patients with biliopancreatic diversion or duodenal switch, 83.7% for patients with gastric bypass, 71.6% for patients with gastroplasty, and 47.9% for patients with gastric banding [296]. The time to resolution occurred within days of surgery, before any significant weight loss [299].

Postoperative insulin levels decreased 60% and plasma glucose decreased 20% in the Swedish Obesity Subjects study [220].

Hypertension resolution and improvement are affected by even modest weight reduction (e.g., 10%), regardless of the type of procedure. Meta-analysis by Heneghan et al. [300] of 16,867 patients worldwide revealed resolution or remission of hypertension in 68% of patients and hyperlipidemia resolved or remitted in 71%.

METABOLIC SYNDROME AND THE PEDIATRIC POPULATION

The rate of childhood obesity has more than doubled in children and tripled among adolescents in the past 30 years [301]. Some 32% of children in the United States were either overweight or obese in 2012 [302]. The US census bureau estimates that 24% of the population in the United States is under the age of 18. This means that there are 74.2 million children in the United States and that approximately 23.7 million are overweight or obese.

Like their adult counterparts, children who are overweight and obese see a trend toward increased abdominal adiposity, leading to an increase in IR [303,304]. This, in turn, places overweight and obese children at risk for developing metabolic syndrome.

Metabolic syndrome was observed in 32.1% of children with a BMI ≥ 95th percentile for weight [305]. When the population is stratified for moderate or severe obesity, the prevalence of metabolic syndrome in children was 38.7% and 49.7%, respectively.

According to data from the Fels Longitudinal Study, childhood obesity is linked to the development of metabolic syndrome in adults [306]. The BMI of boys destined to become men with metabolic syndrome were in the 75th percentile for growth. This compared to boys in the 50th growth percentile for participants who did not develop metabolic syndrome as adults. For girls who developed into women with metabolic syndrome, the BMI was in the 60th percentile as compared to the 50th percentile for those girls who did not.

A statistically significant divergence in BMI was observed at age 8 for boys and 13 for girls. Waist circumference diverged at age 6 in boys who went on to develop metabolic syndrome and age 13 in girls. Based on this information, it seems that both BMI and waist circumference in the pediatric population may be useful as predictors for the development of metabolic syndrome in adults.

CONCLUSION

This chapter has reviewed the history, definitions, prevalence, and economic impact of metabolic syndrome. The mechanisms for its development have been elucidated, and our approach to the evaluation and management of patients has been discussed.

Metabolic syndrome is a global epidemic of immense proportions. It strips years from affected individuals and diminishes the quality of already shortened lives. Individuals, employers, and society as a whole are burdened by the cost of this condition. No one is spared. Men, women, and children of all socioeconomic groups are vulnerable.

The causes of metabolic syndrome are multifactorial. But its strong association with abdominal adiposity implies that it is at least partially the result of living in an obesogenic environment. If current trends continue, metabolic syndrome has the potential to bankrupt health care systems as patients progress to the end points of cardiovascular disease, stroke, and diabetes. Therefore, once the diagnosis has been made, there is a clinical imperative to prevent this progression from occurring.

Lifestyle therapy with diet, exercise, and weight loss is the cornerstone of management. Multidisciplinary support should be offered to patients including intervention with nutritionists, behavioral therapists, and exercise physiologists. Despite these efforts, some patients will require additional intervention with pharmaceuticals and perhaps even bariatric surgery.

The savings in terms of human suffering and health care dollars can be tremendous.

ACKNOWLEDGMENT

The authors wish to gratefully acknowledge Dr. Joseph Proietto for his careful review of the manuscript and Zachary Simon Rothkopf for his editorial assistance in its preparation.

REFERENCES

1. Grundy SM. A constellation of complications: The metabolic syndrome. *Clin Cornerstone*. 2005; 7(2–3):36–45.
2. Ford ES, Kohl HW 3rd, Mokdad AH, Ajani UA. Sedentary behavior, physical activity, and the metabolic syndrome among US adults. *Obes Res*. 2005;13(3):608–614.
3. Despres JP, Lemieux I. Abdominal obesity and metabolic syndrome. *Nature*. 2006;444(7121):881–887.
4. Lee YH, Pratley RE. The evolving role of inflammation in obesity and the metabolic syndrome. *Curr Diab Rep*. 2005;5:70–75.
5. Shaw J. Diabetes, the metabolic syndrome, and the epidemic of cardiovascular disease. *Diabetes Voice*. 2006;5:25–27.
6. Paschos P, Paeletas K. Non alcoholic fatty liver disease and metabolic syndrome. *Hippokratia*. 2009;13(1):9–19.
7. Braun S, Bitton-Worms K, LeRoith D. The link between the metabolic syndrome and cancer. *Int J Biol Sci*. 2011;7(7):1003–1015.
8. Steinberg GB, Church BW, McCall CJ et al. Novel predictive models for metabolic syndrome risk: A "big data" analytic. *Am J Manag Care*. 2014;20(6):e221–e228.
9. Grundy SM. Metabolic syndrome pandemic. *Arterioscler Thromb Vasc Biol*. 2008;28:629–636.
10. Kylin E. *Die Hypertoniekrankheiten*, 2nd rev. ed. Berlin: Springer, 1930.
11. Vague J. La differenciation sexuelle, facteur determinant des formes de l'obesité. Presse Medl 1947;53:339–340.
12. Albrink MJ, Krauss RM, Lindgrem FT et al. Intercorrelations among plasma high density lipoprotein, obesity, and triglycerides in a normal population. *Lipids*. 1980;15:668–676.
13. Reaven GM. Role of insulin resistance in human disease. *Diabetes*. 1988;37(12):1595–1607.
14. Zimmet P, Magliano D, Matsuzawa Y et al. The metabolic syndrome: A global health problem and a new definition. *J Artherosc Thromb*. 2005;12(6):295–300.
15. Alberti KGMM, Eckel RH, Grundy SM et al. Harmonizing the metabolic syndrome: A joint interim statement of the International Diabetes Federation Task Force on Epidemiology and Prevention: National Heart, Lung, and Blood Institute; American Heart Association; World Heart Federation; International Atherosclerosis Society; and International Association for the Study of Obesity. *Circulation*. 2009;120:1640–1645.
16. Alberti G. Introduction to metabolic syndrome. *Eur Heart J Suppl*. 2005;7:D3–D5.
17. Liu S, Song Y, Ford ES et al. Dietary calcium, vitamin D and the prevalence of metabolic syndrome in middle-aged and older U.S. women. *Diabetes Care*. 2005;28:2926–2932.

18. Alberti G. Introduction to metabolic syndrome. *Eur Heart J Suppl.* 2005;7(Suppl D):D3–D5.
19. National Cholesterol Education Program (NCEP) Expert Panel on Detection, Evaluation, and Treatment of High Blood Cholesterol in Adults (Adult Treatment Panel III). Third Report of the National Cholesterol Education Program (NCEP) Expert Panel on Detection, Evaluation, and Treatment of High Blood Cholesterol in Adults (Adult Treatment Panel III) final report. *Circulation.* 2002;106:3143–3421.
20. Snijder MB, Zimmet PZ, Visser M et al. Independent and opposite associations of waist and hip circumferences with diabetes, hypertension and dyslipidemia: The AusDiab study. *Int J Obes.* 2004;28:402–409.
21. Grundy SM, Brewer HB, Cleeman JI et al. Definition of metabolic syndrome: Report of the national heart, lung, and blood institute/American heart association conference on scientific issues related to definition. *Circulation.* 2004;109:433–438.
22. Reis JP, von Muhlen D, Miller ER. Relation of 25-hydroxyvitamin D and parathyroid hormone levels with metabolic syndrome among US adults. *Eur J Endocrinol.* 2008;159:41–48.
23. Li YC, Kong J, Wei M et al. 1,25-dihydroxyvitamin D(3) is a negative endocrine regulator of the renin-angiotensin system. *J Clin Invest.* 2002;110:229–238.
24. Ervin BR. Prevalence of metabolic syndrome among adults 20 years of age and over, by sex, age, race and ethnicity, and body mass index: United States, 2003–2006. *Natl Health Stat Rep.* 2009;(13):1–8. Hyattsville, MD: National Center for Health Statistics.
25. Curtis LH, Hammill BG, Bethel MA et al. Cost of metabolic syndrome in elderly individuals—Findings from the cardiovascular health study. *Diabetes Care.* 2007;30:2553–2558.
26. Resnick HE, Jones K, Ruotolo G et al. Insulin resistance, the metabolic syndrome, and risk of incident cardiovascular disease in nondiabetic American Indians. The Strong Heart Study. *Diabetes Care.* 2003;26:861–867.
27. Haslam DW, James WP. Obesity. *Lancet.* 2005;366:1197–1209.
28. Eckel RH, Grundy SM, Zimmet PZ. The metabolic syndrome. *Lancet.* 2005;365:1415–1428.
29. Hossain P, Kawar B, El Nahas M. Obesity and diabetes in the developing world—A growing challenge. *N Engl J Med.* 2007;356:3.
30. Wang Y, Mi J, Shan X et al. Is China facing an obesity epidemic and the consequences? The trends in obesity and chronic disease in China. *Int J Obes.* 2007;31(1):177–188.
31. Gu D, Reynolds K, Wu X et al. Prevalence of the metabolic syndrome and overweight among adults in China. *Lancet.* 2005;365:1398–1405.
32. Ramachandran A, Snehalatha C, Satyavani K et al. Metabolic syndrome in urban Asian Indian adults—A population study using modified ATP III critera. *Diabetes Res Clin Pract.* 2003;60:199–204.
33. Mohan V, Shanthirani S, Deepa R et al. Intra-urban differences in the prevalence of the metabolic syndrome in southern India—The Chennai urban population study (CUPS No. 4). *Diabetic Med.* 18:280–287.
34. CDC. Heart Disease and Stroke Prevention: Addressing the Nation's Leading Killers: At a Glance 2011. Available at http://www.cdc.gov/chronicdisease/resources/publications/AAG/dhdsp.htm.
35. CDC. Diabetes: Successes and Opportunities for Population-Based Prevention and Control: At a Glance 2011. Available at http://www.cdc.gov/chronicdisease/resources/publications/aag/ddt.htm.
36. Schultz AB, Edington DW. Metabolic syndrome in a workplace: Prevalence, co-morbidities, and economic impact. *Metab Syndr Relat Disord.* 2009;7(5):459–468.
37. Nichols GA, Moler EJ. Abstract 18103: Medical costs associated with all components of metabolic syndrome components. *Circulation.* 2010;122:A18103.
38. Sullivan PW, Ghushchyan V, Wyatt HR et al. Productivity costs associated with carsiometabolic risk factor clusters in the United States. *Value Health.* 2007;10(6):443–450.
39. Colditz GA. Economic costs of obesity. *Am J Clin Nutr.* 1992;55:503S–507S.
40. Colditz GW, Wang YC. Economic costs of obesity. In: Hu F (ed.), *Obesity Epidemiology.* New York: Oxford University Press, 2008.
41. Vijan S, Hayward RA, Langs KM. The impact of diabetes on workforce participation: Results from a national household example. *Health Serv Res.* 2004;39(6 Pt 1):1653–1670.
42. Peters A, Barendregt JJ, Willekens F et al. Obesity in adulthood and its consequences for life expectancy: A life-table analysis. *Ann Intern Med.* 2003;138:24–32.
43. Leal J, Gray AM, Clarke PM. Development of life-expectancy tables for people with type 2 diabetes. *Eur Heart J.* 2009;30:834–839.
44. Grundy SM et al. Diagnosis and management of the metabolic syndrome. An American Heart Association/National Heart, Lung, and Blood scientific statement. *Circulation.* 2005;112:2735–2752.
45. Reaven G. The metabolic syndrome or the insulin resistance syndrome? Different names, different concepts, and different goals. *Endocrinol Metab Clin North Am.* 2004;33:283–303.

46. Benito M. Tissue specificity on insulin action and resistance: Past to recent mechanisms. *Acta Physiol.* 2011;201(3):297–312.
47. Bjorntorp P. Regional patterns of fat distribution. *Ann Intern Med.* 1985;103:994–995.
48. Yu C, Cline GW, Zhang D et al. Mechanism by which fatty acids inhibit insulin activation of insulin receptor substrate-1 (IRS-1)-associated phosphatidylinositol 3-kinase activity in muscle. *J Biol Chem.* 2002;277:50230–50236.
49. Lane MD, Flores-Riveros JR, Hresko RC et al. Insulin-receptor tyrosine kinase and glucose transport. *Diabetes Care.* 1990;13(6):565–575.
50. Metabolic syndrome. Levinson RS (ed). Supplement to *Nature Med.* December, 2011. Available at http://www.nature.com/nm/poster/index.html.
51. Kahn BB, Flier JS. Obesity and insulin resistance. *J Clin Invest.* 2000;106:473–481.
52. Wilcox G. Insulin and insulin resistance. *Clin Biochem Rev.* 2005;26(2):19–39.
53. Matthaei S, Stumvoll M, Kellerer M, Haring HU. Pathophysiology and pharmacological treatment on insulin resistance. *Endocrine Rev.* 2000;21(6):585–618.
54. Kurth-Kraczek RJ, Hirshman MF, Goodyear LJ, Winder WW. 5′ AMP-activated protein kinase activation causes GLUT4 translocation in skeletal muscle. *Diabetes.* 1999;48(8):1667–1671.
55. Perseghin G, Price TB, Petersen KF et al. Increased glucose transport-phosphorylation and muscle glycogen synthesis after exercise training in insulin-resistent subjects. *N Engl J Med.* 1996;335:1357–1362.
56. Pickup JC, Mattock MB, Chusny GD et al. Inflammation and activated innate immunity in the pathogenesis of type 2 diabetes. *Diabetes Care.* 2004;27:813–823.
57. Vague J. La différenciation sexuelle-facteur déterminant des formes de l'obésité. *Press Med.* 1947;55:339–340.
58. Enzi G, Gasparo M, Biondetti PR et al. Subcutaneous and visceral fat distribution according to sex, age, and overweight, evaluated by computed tomography. *Am J Clin Nutr.* 1986;44(6):739–746.
59. Kissebah AH, Vydelingum N, Murray R et al. Relation of body fat distribution to metabolic complications of obesity. *J Clin Endocrinol Metab.* 1982;54:254–260.
60. Tokunaga K, Matsuzawa Y, Ishikawa K, Tarui S. Novel technique for the determination of body fat by computed tomography. *Int J Obes.* 1983;7:437–445.
61. Maury E, Brichard SM. Adipokine dysregulation, adipose tissue inflammation and metabolic syndrome. *Mol Cell Endocrinol.* 2010;314:1–16.
62. Ahima RS, Flier JS. Adipose tissue as an endocrine organ. *Trends Endocrinol Metab.* 2000;11:327–332.
63. Ouchi N, Parker JL, Lugus JJ, Walsh K. Adipokines in inflammation and metabolic disease. *Nat. Rev. Immunol.* 2011;11(2):85–97.
64. Gremese E, Ferraccioli G. The metabolic syndrome: The crossroads between rheumatoid arthritis and cardiovascular risk. *Autoimmun Rev.* 2011;10(10):582–589.
65. Hotamisligil GS. Inflammation and metabolic disorders. *Nature.* 2006;444:860–867.
66. Shoelson SE, Lee J, Goldfine AB. Inflammation and insulin resistance. *J Clin Invest.* 2006;116:1793–1801.
67. Cinti S, Mitchell G, Barbatelli B et al. Adipocyte death defines macrophage localization and function in adipose tissue of obese mice and humans. *J Lipid Res.* 2005;46(11):2347–2355.
68. Berh AH, Scherer PE. Adipose tissue, adipokines, inflammation and cardiovascular disease. *Circ Res.* 2005;96:939–949.
69. Heilbronn LK, Noakes M, Clifton PM. Energy restriction and weight loss on very-low-fat diets reduce C-reactive protein concentration in obese, healthy women. *Arterioscler Thromb Vasc Biol.* 2001;21:968–970.
70. Pedersen BK, Febbraio M. Muscle as an endocrine organ: Focus on muscle-derived interleukin-6. *Physiol Rev.* 2008;88:1379–1406.
71. Laaksonen DE, Niskanen L, Punnonen K et al. C-reactive protein and the development of the metabolic syndrome and diabetes in middle-aged men. *Diabetologica.* 2004;47:1403–1410.
72. Esposito K, Pontillo A, Di Palo C et al. Effect of weight loss and lifestyle changes on vascular inflammatory markers in obese women: A randomized trial. *JAMA.* 2003;289:1799–1804.
73. Greenberg AS, Obin MS. Obesity and the role of adipose tissue in inflammation and metabolism. *Am J Clin Nutr.* 2006;83(2):461S–465S.
74. Faloia E, Micheti G, De Robertis M et al. Inflammation as a link between obesity and metabolic syndrome. *J Nutr Metab.* 2012;2012:476380.
75. Senn JJ, Klover PJ, Nowak IA et al. Suppressor of cytokine signaling-3 (SOCS-3), a potential mediator of interleukin-6-dependent insulin resistance in hepatocytes. *J Biol Chem.* 2003;278:13740–13746.
76. Sabio G, Das M, Mora A et al. A stress signaling pathway in adipose tissue regulates hepatic insulin resistance. *Science.* 2008;322:1539–1543.

77. Kim HJ, Higashimori T, Park SY et al. Differential effects of interleukin-6 and-10 on skeletal muscle and liver insulin action in vivo. *Diabetes*. 2004;53:1060–1067.

78. Fried SK, Bunkin DA, Greenberg AS. Omental and subcutaneous adipose tissues of obese subjects release interleukin-6: Depot difference and regulation by glucocorticoid. *J Clin Endocrinol Metab*. 1998;83(3):847–850.

79. Sethi JK, Hotamisligil GS. The role of TNF alpha in adipocyte metabolism. *Semin Cell Dev Biol*. 1999;10(1):19–29.

80. Hotamisligil GS, Shargill NS, Spiegelman BM. Adipose expression of tumor necrosis factor-alpha: Direct role in obesity-linked insulin resistance. *Science*. 1993;259(5091):87–91.

81. Prins JB, Niesler CU, Winterford CM et al. Tumor necrosis factor-α induces apoptosis of human adipose cells. *Diabetes*. 1997;46(12):1939–1944.

82. Wang B, Trayhurn P. Acute and prolonged effects of TNF-α on the expression and secretion of inflammation-related adipokines by human adipocytes differentiated in culture. *Pflugers Archiv Eur J Physiol*. 2006;452(4):418–427.

83. Tilg H, Moschen AR. Adipocytokines: Mediators linking adipose tissue, inflammation and immunity. *Nat Rev Immunol*. 2006;6(10):772–783.

84. Ryo M, Nakamura T, Kihara S et al. Adiponectin as a biomarker of the metabolic syndrome. *Circ J*. 2004;68:975–981.

85. Liu M, Liu F. Transcriptional and post-translational regulation of adiponectin. *Biochem J*. 2009;425:41–52.

86. Fumeron F, Aubert R, Siddiq A et al. Adiponectin gene polymorphisms and adiponectin levels are independently associated with the development of hyperglycemia during a 3-year period: The epidemiologic data on insulin resistance syndrome prospective study. *Diabetes*. 2004;53(4):1150–1157.

87. Ohashi K, Parker JL, Ouchi N et al. Adiponectin promotes macrophage polarization toward an anti-inflammatory phenotype. *J Biol Chem*. 2010;285(9):6153–6160.

88. Gastaldelli A, Ferrannini E, Miyazaki Y et al. Beta-cell dysfunction and glucose intolerance: Results from the San Antonio metabolism (SAM) study. *Diabetologia*. 2004;47(1):31–39.

89. Saaristo T, Peltonen M, Lindström J et al. Cross-sectional evaluation of the Finnish Diabetes Risk Score: A tool to identify undetected type 2 diabetes, abnormal glucose tolerance and metabolic syndrome. *Diabetes and Vascular Disease Research*. 2005;2(2):67–72.

90. Davies MJ, Rayman G, Grenfell A et al. Loss of the first phase insulin response to intravenous glucose in subjects with persistent impaired glucose tolerance. *Diabetes Med*. 1991;11(5):432–436.

91. Donath MY, Halban PA. Decreased beta-cell mass in diabetes: Significance, mechanisms and therapeutic implications. *Diabetologia*. 2004;47(3):581–589.

92. Phillips LS, Rhee MK. The metabolic syndrome and glucose intolerance. *Hosp Physician*. 2006;71:26–38.

93. Dimitriadis G, Mitrou P, Lambadiari V et al. Insulin effects in muscle and adipose tissue. *Diabetes Res Clin Pract*. 2011;93(Suppl 1):S52–S59.

94. McFarlane SI, Banerji M, Sowers JR. Insulin resistance and cardiovascular disease. *J Clin Endocrinol Metab*. 2001;86:713–718.

95. Kolovou GD, Anagnostopoulou KK, Cokkinos DV. Pathophysiology of dyslipidaemia in the metabolic syndrome. *Postgrad Med J*. 2005;81:358–366.

96. Reilly MP, Rader DJ. The metabolic syndrome: more than the sum of its parts? *Circulation*. 2003;108:1546–1551.

97. Congressional Diabetes Caucus. Facts and figures. Available at http://www.house.gov/degette/diabetes/facts.shtml, 4 March 2013.

98. Rowe JW, Young JB, Minaker KL et al. Effect of insulin and glucose infusion in sympathetic nervous system activity in normal man. *Diabetes*. 1981;30:219–225.

99. Mendizabal Y, Llorens S, Nava E. Hypertension in metabolic syndrome: Vascular pathophysiology. *Int J Hypertens*. 2013;2013: Article ID 230868.

100. Horita S, Seki G, Yamada H et al. Insulin resistance, obesity, hypertension, and renal sodium transport. *Int J Hypertens*. 2011: Article ID 391762. Available at http://www.hindawi.com/journals/ijhy/2011/391762/.

101. Ter Maaten JC, Voorburg A, Heine RJ et al. Renal handling of urate and sodium during acute physiological hyperinsulinemia in healthy subjects. *Clin Sci*. 1997;92:51–58.

102. Hall JE. Mechanisms of abnormal renal sodium handling in obesity hypertension. *Am J Hypertens*. 1197;10:49S–55S.

103. Steinberg HO, Brechtel G, Johnson A et al. Insulin-mediated skeletal muscle vasodilation is nitric oxide dependent. A novel action of insulin to increase nitric oxide release. *J Clin Invest*. 1994; 94(3):1172–1179.

104. King GL, Johnson SM. Receptor-mediated transport of insulin across endothelial cells. *Science*. 1985;227(4694):1583–1586.

105. Kashyap SR, Roman LJ, Lamont J et al. Insulin resistance is associated with impaired nitric oxide synthesis in the skeletal muscle of type 2 diabetic subjects. *J Clin Endocrinol Metab*. 1992;90:1100–1105.

106. Calver A, Collier J, Vallance P. Inhibition and stimulation of nitric oxide synthesis in the human forearm arterial bed of patients with insulin-dependent diabetes. *J Clin Invest*. 1992;90:2548–2554.

107. Olivier FJ, De la Rubia G, Feener EP et al. Stimulation of endothelin-1 gene expression by insulin in endothelial cells. *J Biol Chem*. 1991;266:23251–23256.

108. Eringa EC, Stehouwer DA, Merlijn T et al. Physiological concentrations of insulin induce endothelium-mediated vasoconstriction during inhibition of NOS or PI3-kinase in skeletal muscle arterioles. *Cardivasc Res*. 2002;37:328–333.

109. Sierra-Honigmann MR, Nath AK, Murakami C et al. Biological action of leptin as an angiogenic factor. *Science*. 1998;281:1683–1686.

110. Shirasaka T, Takasaki M, Kannan H. Cardiovascular effects of leptin and orexins. *Am J Physiol*. 2003;284:R639–R651.

111. Knidsen JD, Dincer UD, Zhang C et al. Leptin receptors are expressed in coronary arteries, and hyperlipidemia causes significant coronary endothelial dysfunction. *Am J Physiol*. 2005;289:H48–H56.

112. Xi W, Satoh H, Kase K et al. Stimulated HSP90 binding to eNOS and activation of the PI3-akt pathway contribute to globular adiponectin-induced NO production: Vasorelaxation in response to globular adiponectin. *Biochem Biophys Res Commun*. 2005;75:719–727.

113. Takahashi M, Funahashi T, Shimomura I et al. Plasma leptin levels and body fat distribution. *Horm Metab Res*. 1996;28:751–752.

114. Kadowitz PJ, Chapnick BM, Feigen LP et al. Pulmonary and systemic vasodilator effects of the newly discovered prostaglandin, PGI2. *J Appl Physiol Respir Environ Exerc Physiol*. 1978;45(3):408–413.

115. Richelson B, Borglum JD, Sorensen SS. Biosynthetic capacity and regulatory aspects of prostaglandin E2 formation in adipocytes. *Mol Cell Endocrinol*. 1002;83(1–2):73–81.

116. Parker J, Lane J, Axelrod L. Cooperation of adipocytes and endothelial cells required for catecholamine stimulation of PGI2 production by rat adipose tissue. *Diabetes*. 1989;12(9):1123–1132.

117. Rahmouni K, Mark AL, Haynes WG, Sigmind CD. Adipose depot-specific modulation of angiotensinogen gene expression in diet-induced obesity. *Am J Physiol*. 2004;286(6):E891–E895.

118. Boustany CM, Bharadwaj K, Daugherty A et al. Activation of the systemic and adipose renin-angiotensin system in rats with diet-induced obesity and hypertension. *Am J Physiol*. 2004;287(6):R943–R949.

119. Giacchetti G, Faloia E, Mariniello B, Sardu C. Overexpression of the renin-angiotensin system in human visceral adipose tissue in normal and overweight subjects. *AJH*. 2002;15:381–388.

120. Goossens GH, Blaak EE, Van Baak MA. Possible involvement of the adipose tissue renin-angiotensin system in the pathophysiology of obesity and obesity-related disorders. *Obes Rev*. 2003;4(1):43–55.

121. Van Harmelin V, Eriksson A, Astrom G et al. Vascular peptide endothelin-1 links fat accumulation with alterations of visceral adipocyte lipolysis. *Diabetes*. 2008;57(2):378–386.

122. Carter AM, Cymbalista CM, Spector TD et al. Heritability of clot formation, morphology, and lysis: The EuroCLOT study. *Arterioscler Thromb Vasc Biol*. 2007;27:2783–2789.

123. Alessi MC, Juhan-Vague I. PAI-1 and the metabolic syndrome: Links, causes, and consequences. *Arterioscler Thromb Vasc Biol*. 2006;26:2200–2207.

124. Vaughan DE. PAI-1 and atherothrombosis. *J Thromb Haemost*. 2005;3(8):1879–1883.

125. Eren M, Painter CA, Atkinson JB et al. Age-dependent spontaneous coronary arterial thrombosis in transgenic mice that express a stable form of human plasminogen activator inhibitor-1. *Circulation*. 2002;106:491–496.

126. Juhan-Vague I, Pyke SDM, Alessi MC et al. Fibrinolytic factors and the risk of myocardial infarction or sudden death in patients with angina pectoris. *Circulation*. 1996;94:2057–2063.

127. Alessi MC, Juhan-Vague I. Metabolic syndrome, haemostasis and thrombosis. *Thromb Haemost*. 2008;99:995–1000.

128. Collet JP, Allali Y, Lesty C et al. Altered fibrin architecture is associated with hypofibrinolysis and premature coronary atherothrombosis. *Arterioscler Thromb Vasc Biol*. 2006;26:2567–2573.

129. Ageno W, Becattini C, Brighton T et al. Cardiovascular risk factors and venous thromboembolism: A meta-analysis. *Circulation*. 2008;117:93–102.

130. Lim S, Kim MJ, Choi SH et al. Association of vitamin D deficiency with incidence of type 2 diabetes in high-risk Asian subjects. *Am J Clin Nutr*. 2013;97:524–530.

131. Fung GJ, Steffen LM, Zhou X et al. Vitamin D intake is inversely related to risk of developing metabolic syndrome in African American and white men and women over 20 y: The coronary artery risk development in young adults study. *Am J Clin Nutr*. 2012;96(1):24–29.

132. Fourouhi N, Luan J, Cooper A et al. Baseline serum 25-hydroxy vitamin D is predictive of future glycemic status and insulin resistance. *Diabetes*. 2008;57:2619–2625.

133. Ford ES, Ajani UA, McGuire L, Liu S. Concentrations of serum vitamin D and the metabolic syndrome among U.S. adults. *Diabetes Care.* 2005;28:1228–1230.

134. Boucher BJ, Mannan N, Noonan K et al. Glucose intolerance and impairment of insulin secretion in relation to vitamin D deficiency in East London Asians. *Diabetologia.* 1995;38:1239–1245.

135. Lind L, Heanni A, Lithell H et al. Vitamin D is related to blood pressure and other cardiovascular risk factors in middle-aged men. *Am J Hypertens.* 1995;8:894–901.

136. Qiao G, Kong J, Uskovic M, Li YC. Analogs of 1alpha,25-dihydroxyvitamin D(3) as novel inhibitors of renin biosynthesis. *J Steroid Biochem Mol Biol.* 2005;96:59–66.

137. Carthy EP, Yamashita W, Hsu A, Ooi BS. 1,25-Dihydroxyvitamin D3 and rat smooth muscle cell growth. *Hypertension.* 1989;13:954–959.

138. Forman JP, Giovannucci E, Holmes MD et al. Plasma 25-hydroxy D levels and risk of incident hypertension. *Hypertension.* 2007;49:1063–1069.

139. Pérez-López FR. Vitamin D metabolism and cardiovascular risk factors in postmenopausal women. *Maturitas.* 2009;62:248–262.

140. Oh JY, Barrett-Connor E. Association between vitamin D receptor polymorphism and type 2 diabetes or metabolic syndrome in community-dwelling older adults: The Rancho Bernardo Study. *Metabolism.* 2002;51:356–359.

141. Bourlon PM, Billaudel B, Faure-Dussert A. Influence of vitamin D3 deficiency and 1,25 dihydroxy-vitamin D3 on de novo insulin biosynthesis in islets of the rat endocrine pancreas. *J Endocrinol.* 1999;160:87–95.

142. Zaita U, Weber K, Soegiarto DW et al. Impaired insulin secretory capacity in mice lacking a functional vitamin D receptor. *FASEB J.* 2003;17:509–511.

143. Pittas A, Lau J, Hu F, Dawson-Hughes B. The role of vitamin D and calcium in type 2 diabetes. A systematic review and meta-analysis. *J Clin Endocrinol Metab.* 2007;92(6):2017–2029.

144. Zhang Y, Leung DYM, Richers BN et al. Vitamin D inhibits monocyte/macrophage proinflammatory cytokine production by targeting MAPK phosphatase-1. *J Immunol.* 2012;188(5):2127–2135.

145. Esposito K, Chiodini P, Colao A et al. Metabolic syndrome and risk of cancer: A systematic review and meta-analysis. *Diabetes Care.* 2012;35:2401–2411.

146. Macarthur M, Hold GL, El-Omar EM. Inflammation and cancer II. Role of chronic inflammation and cytokine gene polymorphisms in the pathogenesis of gastrointestinal malignancy. *Am J Physiol Gastrointest Liver Physiol.* 2004;286:G515–G520.

147. Harvey AE, Lashinger LM, Hursting SD. The growing challenge of obesity and cancer: An inflammatory issue. *Ann NY Acad Sci.* 2011;1229:45–52.

148. Van Kruijsdijk RC, Van der Wall E, Visceren FL. Obesity and cancer: The role of dysfunctional adipose tissue. *Cancer Epidemiol Biomarkers Prev.* 2009;18:2569–2578.

149. Ulisse S, Baldini E, Sorrenti S, D'Armiento M. The urokinase plasminogen activator system: A target for anti-cancer therapy. *Curr Cancer Drug Targets.* 2009;9:32–71.

150. Yu H, Paerdoll D, Jove R. STATs in cancer inflammation and immunity: A leading role for STAT3. *Nat Rev Cancer.* 2009;9:798–809.

151. Giovannucci E, Harlan DM, Archer AC et al. Diabetes and cancer. A consensus report. *Diabetes Care.* 2010;33:1674–1685.

152. Weinstein D, Simon M, Yehezkel E et al. Insulin analogues display IGF-1-like mitogenic and anti-apoptotic activities in cultured cancer cells. *Diabetes Metab Res Rev.* 2009;25:41–49.

153. Dik MG, Jonker C, Comijs HC et al. Contribution of metabolic syndrome components to cognition in older individuals. *Diabetes Care.* 2007;30(10):2655–2660.

154. Akbaraly TN, Kivimaki M, Shipley MJ et al. Metabolic syndrome over 10 years and cognitive functioning in late midlife: The Whitehall II study. *Diabetes Care.* 2010;33(1):84–89.

155. Yates KF, Sweat V, Yau PL et al. Impact of metabolic syndrome on cognition and brain: A selected review of the literature. *Arterioscler Thromb Vasc Biol.* 2012;32(9):2060–2067.

156. Segura B, Jurado MA, Freixenet N et al. Microstructural white matter changes in metabolic syndrome. *Neurology.* 2009;73(6):438–444.

157. Haley AP, Gonzales MM, Tarumi T et al. Elevated cerebral glutamate and myo-inositol levels in cognitively normal middle-aged adults with metabolic syndrome. *Metab Brain Dis.* 2010;29:397–405.

158. Magyari PM, Churilla JR. Association between lifting weights and metabolic syndrome among U.S. adults: 1999–2004 National Health and Nutrition Examination Survey. *J Strength Cond Res.* 2012;26(11):3113–3117.

159. Tuomilehto J, Lindstrom J, Eriksson JG et al. Prevention of type 2 diabetes mellitus by changes in lifestyle among subjects with impaired glucose tolerance. *N Engl J Med.* 2001;344:1343–1352.

160. Kurl S, Laukkanen A, Niskanen L et al. Metabolic syndrome and the risk of stroke in middle-aged men. *Stroke*. 2006;37:806–811.

161. Milionis HJ, Rizos E, Goudevenos J et al. Components of the metabolic syndrome and risk for first-ever acute ischemic nonembolic stroke in elderly subjects. *Stroke*. 2005;36:1372–1376.

162. Wannamethee SG, Shaper AG, Morris RW, Whincup PH. Measures of adiposity in the identification of metabolic abnormalities in elderly men. *Am J Clin Nutr*. 2005;81:1313–1321.

163. Marchesni G, Brizi M, Morselli Labate AM et al. Association of non-alcoholic fatty liver disease to insulin resistance. *Am G Med*. 1999;107:450–455.

164. Cortez-Pinto H, Camilo ME, Baptista A et al. Non-alcoholic fatty liver: Another manifestation of the metabolic syndrome? *Clin Nutr*. 1999;18:353–356.

165. Bloomgarden ZT. Second World Congress on the insulin resistance syndrome: Insulin resistance syndrome and nonalcoholic fatty liver disease. *Diabetes Care*. 2005;28:1518–1523.

166. Hamaguchi M, Kojima T, Takeda N et al. The metabolic syndrome as a predictor of non alcoholic fatty liver disease. *Ann Intern Med*. 2005;143:722–728.

167. Kotronen A, Westerbacka J, Bergholm R et al. Liver fat in the metabolic syndrome. *J Clin Endocrinol Metab*. 2008;92:3490–3497.

168. Bloomgarden ZT. Nonalcoholic fatty liver disease and insulin resistance in youth. *Diabetes Care*. 2007;30:1663–1669.

169. Ehrmann DA, Barnes RB, Rosenfeld RL et al. Prevalence of impaired glucose tolerance and diabetes on women with polycystic ovarian syndrome. *Diabetes Care*. 1999;22:141–146.

170. Cho LW, Atkin SL. Cardiovascular risk in women with polycystic ovarian syndrome. *Minerva Endocrinol*. 2007;32:263–273.

171. Farah L, Lazenby AJ, Boots LR, Azziz R. Prevalence of polycystic ovary syndrome in women seeking treatment from community electrologists. Alabama Professional Electrology Association Study Group. *J Reprod Med*. 1999;44:870–874.

172. Knochenhauer ES, Key TJ, Kahsar-Miller M et al. Prevalence of the polycystic ovary syndrome in unselected black and white women of the southeastern United States: A prospective study. *J Clin Endocrinol Metab*. 1998;83:3078–3082.

173. Alvarez-Blasco F, Botella-Carretero JI, San Millan JL, Escobar-Morreale HF. Prevalence and characteristics of the polycystic ovary syndrome in overweight and obese women. *Arch Intern Med*. 2006; 166:2081–2086.

174. Sharpless JL. Polycystic ovary syndrome and the metabolic syndrome. *Clinical Diabetes*. 2003;21: 154–161.

175. Dahlgren E, Johansson S, Lindstedt G et al. Women with polycystic ovary syndrome wedge resected in 1956 to 1965: A long-term follow-up focusing on natural history and circulating hormones. *Fertil Steril*. 1992;57:505–513.

176. Dahlgren E, Janson PO, Johansson S et al. Polycystic ovary syndrome and risk for myocardial infarction. Evaluated from a risk factor model based on a prospective population study of women. *Acta Obstet Gynecol Scand*. 1992;71:599–604.

177. Legro RS. Polycystic ovary syndrome and cardiovascular disease: A premature association? *Endocrine Rev*. 2003;24:302–312.

178. Talbott EO, Guzick DS, Sutton-Tyrrell K et al. Evidence for association between polycystic ovary syndrome and premature carotid atherosclerosis in middle-aged women. *Arterioscler Thromb Vasc Biol*. 2000;20:2414–2421.

179. Christian RC, Dumesic DA, Behrenbeck T et al. Prevalence and predictors of coronary artery calcification in women with polycystic ovary syndrome. *J Clin Endocrinol Metab*. 2003;88:2562–2568.

180. Drager LF, Togeiro SM, Polotsky VY, Lorenzi-Filho G. Obstructive sleep apnea a cardiometabolic risk in obesity and the metabolic syndrome. *J Am Coll Cardiol*. 2013;62(7):569–576.

181. Cornier MA, Dabelea D, Hernandez TL et al. The metabolic syndrome. *Endocr Rev*. 2008;29:777–822.

182. Drager LF, Bortolotto LA, Figueiredo AC et al. Effects of continuous positive airway pressure on early signs of atherosclerosis in obstructive sleep apnea. *Am J Respir Crit Care Med*. 2007;176(7): 706–712.

183. Sanches FM, Avesani CM, Kamimura MA et al. Waist circumference and visceral fat in CKD: A cross-sectional study. *Am J Kidney Dis*. 2008;52(1):66–73.

184. Shen W, Punyanitya M, Gallagher D et al. Waist circumference correlates with metabolic syndrome indicators better than percentage fat. *Obesity*. 2006;14(4):727–736.

185. Matsushita Y, Yokoyama T, Mizoue T. Optimal waist circumference measurement site for assessing the metabolic syndrome. *Diabetes Care*. 2009;32(6):e70.

186. Nichols GA, Hillier TA, Brown JB. Normal fasting plasma glucose and risk of type 2 diabetes diagnosis. *Am J Med.* 2008;121:519–524.

187. Khaw KT, Wareham N, Bingham S et al. Association of hemoglobin A1C with cardiovascular disease and mortality in adults: The European prospective investigation into cancer in Norfolk. *Ann Intern Med.* 2004;141(6):413–420.

188. Selvin E, Steffes MW, Zhu H et al. Glycated hemoglobin, diabetes, and cardiovascular risk in nondiabetic adults. *N Engl J Med.* 2010;362: 800–811.

189. The DECODE-Study Group on behalf of the European Diabetes Epidemiology Group. Is fasting glucose sufficient to diagnose diabetes? Epidemiological data from 20 European studies. *Diabetilogica.* 1999;42:647–654.

190. Qiao Q, Nakagami T, Tuomilheto et al. for the DECODE study group in behalf of the international diabetes epidemiology group. Comparison of ADA fasting and WHO 2-hour glucose criteria for diabetes in different Asian populations. *Diabetilogica.* 2000;43:1470–1475.

191. Shaw JE, de Courten M, Boyko EJ, Zimmet PZ. Impact of new diagnostic criteria for diabetes in different populations. *Diabetes Care.* 1999;22:762–766.

192. The DECODE Study Group. Consequences of the new diagnostic criteria for diabetes in older men and women. *Diabetes Care.* 1999;22:1667–1671.

193. Qiao Q, Pyorala A, Nissenen J et al. Two-hour glucose is a better risk predictor for incident coronary heart disease and cardiovascular mortality than fasting glucose. *Eur Heart J.* 2002;23:1267–1275.

194. Coutinho M, Gerstain HC, Wang Y, Yusuf S. The relationship between glucose and incident cardiovascular events. A metaregression analysis of published data from 20 studies of 95,783 individuals followed for 12.4 years. *Diabetes Care.* 1999;22:233–240.

195. Balkau B, Ducimetiere P, Bertrais S, Eschwege E. Is there a glycemic threshold for mortality risk? *Diabetes Care.* 1999;22:696–699.

196. Dankner R, Chetrit A, Shanik MH et al. Basal-state hyperinsulinemia in healthy normoglycemic adults is predictive of type 2 diabetes over a 24-year follow-up, a preliminary report. *Diabetes Care.* 2009;32:1464–1466.

197. Song Y, Manson JE, Tinker L et al. Insulin sensitivity and insulin secretion determined by homeostasis model assessment and risk of diabetes in a multiethnic cohort of women: The Women's Health Initiative Observational Study. *Diabetes Care.* 2007;30(7):1747–1752.

198. Wallace TM, Levy JC, Matthews DR. Use and abuse of HOMA modeling. *Diabetes Care.* 2004;27(6): 1487–1495.

199. Haffner SM, Miettinen H, Stern MP. The homeostasis model in the San Antonio Heart Study. *Diabetes Care.* 1997;20(7):1087–1092.

200. Kang ES, Yun YS, Park SW et al. Limitation of the validity of the homeostasis model assessment as an index of insulin resistance in Korea. *Metabolism.* 2005;54(2):206–211.

201. Mudd JO, Borlaug BA, Johnston PV et al. Beyond low-density lipoprotein cholesterol: Defining the role of low-density lipoprotein heterogeneity in coronary artery disease. *J Am Coll Cardiol.* 2007;50:1735–1741.

202. Friedewald WT, Levy RI, Fredrickson DS. Estimation of the concentration of low-density lipoprotein cholesterol in plasma, without use of the preparative ultracentrifuge. *Clin Chem.* 1972;18:499–502.

203. Kulkarni KR, Marcovina SM, Krauss RM et al. Quantification of HDL2 and HDL3 cholesterol by the Vertical Auto Profile-II (VAP-II) methodology. *Lipid Res.* 1997;38:2353–2364.

204. Blake GJ, Otvos JD, Rifai N, Ridker PM. Low-density lipoprotein particle concentration and size as determined by nuclear magnetic resonance spectroscopy as predictors of cardiovascular disease in women. *Circulation.* 2002;106:1930–1937.

205. Crouse JR, Parks JS, Schey HM, Kahl FR. Studies of low density lipoprotein molecular weight in human beings with coronary artery disease. *Lipid Res.* 1985;26:566–574.

206. Austin MA, Breslow JL, Hennekens CH et al. Low density lipoprotein subclass patterns and risk of myocardial infarction. *JAMA.* 1988;260:1917–1921.

207. Bjornheden T, Babyi A, Bondjers G, Wiklund O. Accumulation of lipoprotein fractions and subfractions in the arterial wall, determined in an in vitro perfusion system. *Atherosclerosis.* 1996;123:43–56.

208. Tribble DL, Rizzo M, Chait A et al. Enhanced oxidative susceptibility and reduced antioxidant content of metabolic precursors of small, dense low-density lipoproteins. *Am J Med.* 2001;110:103–110.

209. Koskinen J, Magnussen CG, Wurtz P et al. Apolipoprotein N, oxidized low-density lipoprotein, and LDL particle size in predicting the incidence of metabolic syndrome: The cardiovascular risk in young Finns. *Eur J Prev Cardiol.* 2012;19(6) 1296–1303.

210. Cromwell WC, Otvos JD, Keyes MJ et al. LDL particle number and risk of future cardiovascular disease in the Framingham offspring study—Implications for LDL management. *J Clin Lipidol.* 2007;1(6):583–592.

211. Lee WY, Park JS, Noh SY et al. C-reactive protein concentrations are related in insulin resistance and metabolic syndrome as defined by the ATP III report. *Int J Cardiol*. 2004;101–106.

212. Ho KW. C-reactive protein as a prognostic indicator in clinical medicine. *Sci Med*. 2009;1(2).

213. Bodman-Smith KB, Melendez AJ, Campbell I et al. C-reactive protein-mediated phagocytosis and phospholipase D signaling through the high-affinity receptor for immunoglobulin G (FcγRI). *Immunology*. 2002;107(2):252–260.

214. Husain TM, Kim DH. C-reactive protein and erythrocyte sedimentation rate in orthopaedics. *UPOJ*. 2002;15:13–16.

215. Ridker PM, Danielson E, Fonseca FAH et al. Rosuvastatin to prevent vascular events in men and women with elevated C-reactive protein. *N Engl J Med*. 2008;359:2195–2207.

216. Ridker PM. Clinical application of C-reactive protein for cardiovascular disease detection and prevention. *Circulation*. 2003;107:363–369.

217. Lake A, Townshend T. Obesogenic environments: Exploring the built and food environments. *J R Soc Promot Health*. 2006;26(6):262–267.

218. Case CC, Jones PH, Nelson K et al. Impact of weight loss on the metabolic syndrome. *Diabetes Obes Metab*. 2002;4(6):407–414.

219. Batsis JA, Romero-Corral A, Collazo-Clavell M et al. Effect of bariatric surgery on the metabolic syndrome: A population-based, long-term controlled study. *Mayo Clin Proc*. 2008;83(8):897–907.

220. Sjostrom CD, Lissner L, Wedel H, Sjostrom L. Reduction in incidence of diabetes, hypertension and lipid disturbances after intentional weight loss induced by bariatric surgery: The SOS intervention study. *Obes Res*. 1999;7:477–484.

221. Adams TD, Avelar E, Cloward T et al. Design and rationale of the Utah obesity study. A study to assess morbidity following gastric bypass surgery. *Contemp Clin Trials*. 2005;26:534–551.

222. Lindstrom J, Louheranta A, Mannelin M et al. The Finnish diabetes prevention study. *Diabetes Care*. 2003;26:3230–3236.

223. Diabetes Prevention Program. Reduction on the incidence of type 2 diabetes with lifestyle intervention or metformin. *N Engl J Med*. 2002;346(6):393–403.

224. Pan XR, Li GW, Hu YH et al. Effects of diet and exercise in preventing NIDDM in people with impaired glucose tolerance: The Da Qing IGT and Diabetes Study. *Diabetes Care*. 1997;20:537–544.

225. Eriksson KF, Lindgarde F. Prevention of type 2 (noninsulin-dependent) diabetes mellitus by diet and physical exercise: The 6-year Malmo feasibility study. *Diabetologia*. 1997;34:891–898.

226. Fontaine KR, Haaz S, Bartlett SJ. Are overweight and obese adults with arthritis being advised to lose weight? *J Clin Rheumatol*. 2007;13:12–15.

227. Fujita S, Rasmussen BB, Cadenas JG et al. Aerobic exercise overcomes the age-related insulin resistance of muscle protein metabolism by improving endothelial function and Akt/mammalian target of Rapamycin signaling. *Diabetes*. 2007;56:1615–1622.

228. Thompson PD, Crouse SF, Goodpaster B et al. The acute versus the chronic response to exercise. *Med Sci Sports Exerc*. 2001;33:S438–S445; discussion S452–S453.

229. Vukovich MD, Arciero PJ, Kohrt WM et al. Changes in insulin action and GLUT-4 with 6 days of inactivity in endurance runners. *J Appl Physiol*. 1996;80:240–244.

230. Rennie KL, McCarthy N, Yazdgerdi S et al. Association of the metabolic syndrome with both vigorous and moderate physical activity. *Int J Epidem*. 2003;32(4):600–606.

231. Smutok MA, Reece C, Kokkinos PF et al. Effects of exercise training modality on glucose tolerance in men with abnormal glucose regulation. *Int J Sports Med*. 1994;15(6):283–289.

232. Katzel LI, Bleecker ER, Colman EG et al. Effects of weight loss vs aerobic exercise training on risk factors for coronary disease in healthy, obese, middle-aged and older men. A randomized control trial. *JAMA*. 1995;274(24):1915–1921.

233. Tjonna AE, Lee SJ, Rognmo O et al. Aerobic interval training vs. continuous moderate exercise as a treatment for the metabolic syndrome—"A Pilot Study". *Circulation*. 2008;118(4):346–354.

234. Tibana RA, Pereira GB, Navalta J et al. Effects of eight weeks of resistance training on the risk factors of metabolic syndrome in overweight/obese women—"A Pilot Study". *Diabetol Metab Syndr*. 2013;5:11.

235. Sigal RJ, Kenny GP, Boule NG et al. Effects on aerobic training, resistance training, or both on glycemic control in type 2 diabetes: A randomized trial. *Ann Int Med*. 2007;147(6):357–369.

236. Salas-Salvado J, Martinez-Gonzalez MA, Bullo M, Ros E. The role of diet in the prevention of type 2 diabetes. *Nutr Metabol Cardiovasc Dis*. 2011;21(2):B32–B48.

237. PRDIMED Study Investigators. Effects of a Mediterranean-style diet on cardiovascular risk factors: A randomized trial. *Ann Intern Med*. 2006;145(1):1–11.

238. Esposito K, Marfella R, Ciotola M et al. Effect of a Mediterranean-style diet on endothelial dysfunction and markers of vascular inflammation in the metabolic syndrome. *JAMA.* 2004;292:1440–1446.

239. Ibarrola-Jurado N, Bulio M, Guash-Ferre M et al. Cross-sectional assessment of nut consumption and obesity, metabolic syndrome and other cardiometabolic risk factors: The PREDIMED study. *PloS one.* 8(2):e57367.

240. O'Neil CE, Keast DR, Nicklas TA, Fulgoni VL 3rd. Nut consumption is associated with decreased health risk factors for cardiovascular disease and metabolic syndrome in U.S. adults: NHANES 1999–2004. *J Am Coll Nutr.* 2011;30(6):502–510.

241. Fernandez-Montero A, Bes-Rastrollo M, Beunza JJ et al. Nut consumption and incidence of metabolic syndrome after 6-year follow-up: The SUN (Seguimiento Universidad de Navarra, University of Navarra follow-up) cohort. *Public Health Nutr.* 2013;16(11):2064–2072.

242. Minder CM, Blumenthal RS, Blaha MJ. Statins for primary prevention of cardiovascular disease: The benefits outweigh the risks. *Curr Opin Cardiol.* 2013;28(5):554–560.

243. Nathan DM, Buse JB, Davidson MB et al. Management of hyperglycemia in type 2 diabetes— A consensus algorithm for the initiation and adjustment of therapy: A consensus statement from the American Diabetes Association and the European Association for the Study of Diabetes. *Diabetes Care.* 2006;29(8):1963–1972.

244. Nathan DM, Buse JB, Davidson MB et al. Medical management of hyperglycemia in type 2 diabetes— A consensus algorithm for the initiation and adjustment of therapy: A consensus statement of the American Diabetes Association and the European Association for the Study of Diabetes. *Diabetes Care.* 2009;32(1):193–203.

245. Bailey CJ. Biguanides and NIDDM. *Diabetes Care.* 1992;15(6):755–772.

246. Hauner H. The mode of action of thiazolidinediones. *Diabetes Metab Res Rev.* 2002;18(2):S10–S15.

247. Consoli A, Devangelio E. Thiazolidinediones and inflammation. *Lupus.* 2005;14(9):794–797.

248. Goldberg RB, Kendall DM, Deeg MA et al. A comparison of lipid and glycemic effects of pioglitazone and rosiglitazone in patients with type 2 diabetes and dyslipidemia. *Diabetes Care.* 2005;28(7):1547–1554.

249. Buchanan TA, Xiang AH, Peters RK et al. Preservation of pancreatic beta-cell function and prevention of type 2 diabetes by pharmaceutical treatment of insulin resistance in high-risk Hispanic women. *Diabetes.* 2002;51:2796–2803.

250. Gerstein HC, Yusuf S, Bosch J et al. Effect of rosiglitazone on the frequency of diabetes in patients with impaired glucose tolerance or impaired fasting glucose a randomized trial. *Lancet.* 2006;368:1096–1105.

251. Available at http://www.fda.gov/Drugs/DrugSafety/PostmarketDrugSafetyInformationforPatientsand Providers/ucm376365.htm.

252. DeFronzo RA, Tripathy D, Schwenke DC et al. Pioglitazone for diabetes prevention in impaired glucose tolerance. *N Engl J Med.* 2011;364:1104–1115.

253. Meneilly GS, Ryan EA, Radziuk J et al. Effect of acarbose on insulin sensitivity in elderly patients with diabetes. *Diabetes Care.* 2000;23(8):1162–1167.

254. Chiasson JL, Josse RG, Gomis R et al. Acarbose for prevention of type 2 diabetes mellitus: The STOP-NIDDM randomised trial. *Lancet.* 2002;359(9323):2072–2077.

255. Laufs U, Weintraub WS, Packard CJ. Beyond statins: What to expect from add-on lipid regulating therapy? *Eur Heart J.* 2013;34(34):2660–2665.

256. Barter PJ, Brandrup-Wognsen G, Palmer MK, Nicholls SJ. Effect of statins on HDL-C—A complex process unrelated to changes in LDL-C: Analysis of the VOYAGER Database. *J Lipid Res.* 2010;51(6):1546–1553.

257. Pedersen T, Kjekshus J, Berg K, Haghfelt T. Randomised trial of cholesterol lowering in 4444 patients with coronary heart disease: The Scandinavian simvastatin survival study (4S). *Lancet.* 1994;344(8934): 1383–1389.

258. Downs JR, Clearfield M, Weis S et al. Primary prevention of acute coronary events with lovastatin in men and women with average cholesterol levels: Results of AFCAPS/TexCAPS. Air Force/Texas Coronary Atherosclerosis Prevention Study. *JAMA.* 1998;279(20):1615–1622.

259. Heart Protection Study Collaborative Group. MRC/BHF Heart Protection Study of cholesterol lowering with simvastatin in 20,536 high-risk individuals: A randomised placebo controlled trial. *Lancet.* 2002;360(9326):7–22.

260. Goldberg RB. Statin treatment in diabetic subjects: What the heart protection study shows. *Clinical Diabetes.* 2003;21(4):151–152.

261. Rao AD, Milbrandt EB. To JUPITER and beyond: Statins, inflammation, and primary prevention. *Critical Care.* 2010;14:310.

262. Kashyap ML, McGovern ME, Berra K et al. Long-term safety of extended-release once-daily niacin/lovastatin formulation for patients with dyslipidemia. *Am J Cardiol.* 2002;89:672–678.

263. Grundy SM et al. Third report of the national cholesterol education program (NCEP) expert panel on detection, evaluation, and treatment of high blood cholesterol in adults (adult treatment panel III) final report. *Circulation.* 2002;106:3142–3421.

264. Vaccari CS, Nagamia S, Thoenes M et al. Efficacy of controlled-release niacin in treatment of metabolic syndrome: Correlation to surrogate markers of atherosclerosis, vascular reactivity, and inflammation. *J Clin Lipidol.* 2007;1(6):605–613.

265. Hunninghake DB, McGovern ME, Koren M et al. A dose-ranging study of a new, once-daily, dual-component drug product containing niacin extended release and lovastatin. *Clin Cardiol.* 2003;26:112–118.

266. Grundy SM, Vega GL, McGovern ME et al. Efficacy, safety, and tolerability of once-daily niacin for the treatment of dyslipidemia associated with type 2 diabetes: Results of the assessment of diabetes control and evaluation of the efficacy of niaspan trial. *Arch Intern Med.* 2002;162:1568–1576.

267. Goldberg RB, Jacobson TA. Effects of niacin on glucose control in patients with dyslipidemia. *Mayo Clin Proc.* 2008;83(4):470–478.

268. Frick MH, Elo O, Haapa K et al. Helsinki heart study: Primary-prevention trial with gemfibrozil in middle-aged men with dyslipidemia. Safety of treatment, changes in risk factors, and incidence of coronary heart disease. *N Eng J Med.* 1987;317:1237–1245.

269. Rubins HB, Robins SJ, Collins D et al. Gemfibrozil for the secondary prevention of coronary heart disease in men with low levels of high-density lipoprotein cholesterol. Veterans Affairs High-Density Lipoprotein Cholesterol Intervention Study Group. *N Eng J Med.* 1999;341:410–418.

270. Bezafibrate Infarction Prevention (BIP) study. Secondary prevention by raising HDL cholesterol and reducing triglycerides in patients with coronary artery disease. *Circulation.* 2000;102:21–27.

271. Keech A, Simes RJ, Barter P et al. Effects of long-term fenofibrate therapy on cardiovascular events in 9795 people with type 2 diabetes mellitus (the FIELD study): Randomised controlled trial. *Lancet.* 2005;366:1849–1861.

272. Ginsberg HN. The ACCORD (Action to Control Cardiovascular Risk in Diabetes) Lipid Trial. What we learn from subgroup analyses. *Diabetes Care.* 2011;34(2):S107–S108.

273. Chobanian AV, Bakris GL, Black HR et al. National Heart, Lung, and Blood Institute Joint National Committee on Prevention, Detection, Evaluation, and Treatment of High Blood Pressure; National High Blood Pressure Education Program Coordinating Committee. The Seventh Report of the Joint National Committee on Prevention, Detection, Evaluation, and Treatment of High Blood Pressure: The JNC 7 report. *JAMA.* 2003;289:2560–2572.

274. Appel Ll, Brands MW, Daniels SR et al. Dietary approaches to prevent and treat hypertension: A scientific statement from the American Heart Association. *Hypertension.* 2006;47:296–308.

275. Available at http://www.dashdiet.org.

276. Meydani M. Omega-3 fatty acids alter soluble markers of endothelial function in coronary heart disease patients. *Nutr Rev.* 2000;58:56–59.

277. Bestermann W, Houston MC, Basile J et al. Addressing the global and cardiovascular risk of hypertension, dyslipidemia, diabetes mellitus, and the metabolic syndrome in the southeastern United States. Part II: Treatment recommendations for management of the global cardiovascular risk of hypertension, dyslipidemia, diabetes mellitus, and the metabolic syndrome. *Am J Med Sci.* 2005;329:292–305.

278. Israili ZH, Lyoussi B, Hernandez-Hernandez R, Velasco M. Metabolic syndrome: Treatment of hypertensive patients. *Am J Ther.* 2007;14:386–402.

279. Wright JT Jr, Harris-Haywood S, Pressel S et al. Clinical outcomes by race in hypertensive patients with and without metabolic syndrome: Antihypertensive and lipid-lowering treatment to prevent heart attack trial (ALLHAT). *Arch Intern Med.* 2008;168:207–217.

280. Black HR, Davis B, Barzilay J et al. Metabolic and clinical outcomes in non-diabetic individuals with metabolic syndrome assigned to chlorthalidone, amlodipine, or lisinopril as initial treatment for hypertension: A report from the antihypertensive and lipid-lowering treatment to prevent heart attack trial (ALLHAT). *Diabetes Care.* 2008;21:353–360.

281. ALLHAT Officers and Coordinators for the ALLHAT Collaborative Research Group. The Antihypertensive and Lipid-Lowering Treatment to Prevent Heart Attack Trial. Major outcomes in high-risk hypertensive patients randomized to angiotensin-converting enzyme inhibitor or calcium channel blocker vs diuretic: The antihypertensive and lipid-lowering treatment to prevent heart attack trial (ALLHAT). *JAMA.* 2002;288:2981–2997.

282. Palomo I, Alarcon M, Moore-Carrasco R, Argiles JP. Hemostasis alterations in metabolic syndrome (review). *Int J Mol Med.* 2006;18:969–974.

283. Franchini M, Lippi G, Manzato F et al. Hemostatic abnormalities in endocrine and metabolic disorders. *Eur J Endocrinol.* 162(3):439–451.

284. Grundy SM, Cleeman JI, Daniels SR et al. Diagnosis and management of the metabolic syndrome: An American Heart Association/National Heart, Lung, and Blood Institute Scientific Statement. American Heart Association; National Heart, Lung, and Blood Institute. *Circulation.* 2005;112(17):2735–2752.

285. Arteaga RB, Chirinos JA, Soriano AO et al. Endothelial microparticles and platelet and leukocyte activation in patients with the metabolic syndrome. *Am J Cardiol.* 2006;98:70–74.

286. Serebruany VL, Malinin A, Ong S et al. Patients with metabolic syndrome exhibit higher platelet activity than those with conventional risk factors for vascular disease. *J Thromb Thrombolysis.* 2008;25:207–213.

287. Weber P, Raederstorff D. Triglyceride-lowering effect of omega-3 LC-polyunsaturated fatty acids—A review. *Nutr Metab Cardiovasc Dis.* 2000;10:28–37.

288. Pownall HJ, Brauchi D, Kilinc C et al. Correlation of serum triglyceride and its reduction by omega-3 fatty acids with lipid transfer activity and the neutral lipid compositions of high-density and low-density lipoproteins. *Atherosclerosis.* 1999;143:285–297.

289. Harris WS. N-3 fatty acids and serum lipoproteins: Human studies. *Am J Clin Nutr.* 1997;65:1645S–1654S.

290. Durrington PN, Bhatnagar D, Mackness MI et al. An omega-3 polyunsaturated fatty acid concentrate administered for one year decreased triglycerides in simvastatin treated patients with coronary heart disease and persisting hypertriglyceridaemia. *Heart.* 2001;85:544–548.

291. Simopoulos AP. Omega-3 fatty acids in inflammation and autoimmune diseases. *J Am Coll Nutr.* 2002;21:495–505.

292. Von Schacky C, Fischer S, Weber PC. Long-term effects of dietary marine omega-3 fatty acids upon plasma and cellular lipids, platelet function, and eicosanoid formation in humans. *J Clin Invest.* 1985;76:1626–1631.

293. Covington MG. Omega-3 fatty acids. *Am Fam Physician.* 2004;70(1):133–140.

294. Morris MC, Sacks F, Rosner B. Does fish oil lower blood pressure? A meta-analysis of controlled trials. *Circulation.* 1993;88:523–533.

295. Appel LJ, Miller ER 3rd, Seidler AJ, Whelton PK. Does supplementation of diet with 'fish oil' reduce blood pressure? A meta-analysis of controlled clinical trials. *Arch Intern Med.* 1993;153:1429–1438.

296. Buchwald H, Avidor Y, Braunwald E et al. Bariatric Surgery: A systematic review and meta-analysis. *JAMA.* 2004;292(14):1724–1737.

297. Schauer PR, Burguera B, Ikramuddin S et al. Effect of laparoscopic Roux-en-Y gastric bypass on type 2 diabetes mellitus. *Ann Surg.* 2003;238:467–484.

298. Sugerman HJ, Wolfe LG, Sica DA, Clore JN. Diabetes and hypertension in severe obesity and effects of gastric bypass-induced weight loss. *Ann Surg.* 2003;237:751–756.

299. Pories WJ, Swanson MS, MacDonald KG et al. Who would have thought it? An operation proves to be the most effective therapy for adult-onset diabetes mellitus. *Ann Surg.* 1995;222:339–352.

300. Heneghan HM, Meron-Eldar S, Brethauer SA et al. Effect of bariatric surgery on cardiovascular risk profile. *Am J Cardiol.* 2011;108(10):1499–1507.

301. Ogden CL, Carroll MD, Kit BK, Flegal KM. Prevalence of obesity and trends in body mass index among US children and adolescents, 1999–2010. *JAMA.* 2012;307:483–490.

302. Ogden CL, Carroll MD, Curtin LR et al. Prevalence of high body mass index in the US children and adolescents, 2007–2008. *JAMA.* 2010;303:242–249.

303. Weiss R, Dufour S, Taksali SE et al. Prediabetes in obese youth: A syndrome of impaired glucose tolerance, severe insulin resistance, and altered myocellular and abdominal fat partitioning. *Lancet.* 2003;352:951–957.

304. Weiss R, Taksali SE, Dufour S et al. The "obese insulin-sensitive" adolescent: Importance of adiponectin and lipid partitioning. *J Clin Endocrinol Metab.* 2005;90:3731–3737.

305. Duncan GE, Li SM, Zhou XH. Prevalence and trends of a metabolic syndrome phenotype among US adolescents, 1999–2000. *Diabetes Care.* 2004;27:2438–2443.

306. Sun SS, Liang R, Huang T et al. Childhood obesity predicts adult metabolic syndrome: The Fels longitudinal study. *J Pediatr.* 2008;152:191–200.

5 Nonalcoholic Fatty Liver Disease

Olga A. Melzer, Michael M. Rothkopf, and Lisa Ganjhu

CONTENTS

DEFINITIONS

Nonalcoholic fatty liver disease (NAFLD) is an umbrella diagnosis that includes isolated fatty liver (IFL) and nonalcoholic steatohepatitis (NASH). Histologically, NAFLD resembles alcoholic liver disease. It is defined by the presence of macrovesicular fat in more than 5% of hepatocytes in patients without a history of excessive alcohol consumption.

IFL is characterized by hepatic steatosis without hepatocellular injury or inflammation. NASH is distinguished from IFL by the presence of hepatocyte injury (ballooning), lobular inflammation, and/or portal and periportal fibrosis.

The natural history of IFL seems to be fairly benign, with only rare cases progressing to end-stage liver disease [1,2]. NASH, on the other hand, has the potential of fully developing into hepatic cirrhosis and, later, hepatocellular carcinoma (HCC). Thus, we view NASH as having the real potential for increasing liver-related morbidity and mortality.

EPIDEMIOLOGY

NAFLD can be considered a hepatic manifestation of metabolic syndrome. Therefore, the prevalence of NAFLD is seen as closely correlated with the rising epidemic of obesity in the Western World. In the United States, almost one third of all children and two thirds of all adults are considered to be either overweight or obese. These individuals are at increased risk of NAFLD. If current trends continue, NAFLD is likely to become the predominant liver disease of the twenty-first century.

The prevalence of NAFLD varies widely depending on population studies and methods used for the diagnosis. Its prevalence rate increases with increasing body mass index (BMI). For example, data from available studies in non-obese persons suggest that the prevalence rate of IFL is approximately 15%. The prevalence rate of NASH is thought to be approximately 3% in the non-obese. But in those with a BMI of 30 to 39.9 kg/m², the rate of IFL was 65%, whereas the rate of NASH was 20%. For patients with a BMI > 40 kg/m², the rate of IFL was 85%, whereas the rate of NASH was 40% [3]. Autopsy studies have placed the prevalence of NASH at 2.7% among lean persons to 18.5% among morbidly obese patients [4].

The Dallas Heart Study assessed 2287 adults for the prevalence of NAFLD by magnetic resonance (MR) spectroscopy. The general prevalence of NAFLD was 31% (range of 24–45%). Most individuals (79%) with fatty liver did not exhibit aminotransferase (ALT) level elevation [5].

In the NHANES III study of 15,676 adults, elevated aminotransferase levels were present in 7.9% of the population. The majority of aminotransferase elevations (69%) was unexplained and was suspected to be caused by NAFLD [6].

Ethnic variations in the prevalence of NAFLD have been suggested. Several studies showed the highest rates of NAFLD in Hispanics (45–58.3%), followed by Caucasians (33–44.4%), and the lowest rates in African-American (24–35.1%). But a recent analysis showed no significant increase in the prevalence of NAFLD in Hispanics when data were controlled for obesity [7]. The reasons for this difference in prevalence of NAFLD in different ethnic groups are not completely defined, although genetic and environmental factors seem to be important contributors.

Another ethnic group with increasing incidence of NAFLD is the Asian population. Asians seem to be more susceptible to developing complications of metabolic syndrome such as diabetes and NAFLD at much lower BMI levels than Caucasians, potentially due to higher visceral fat deposition than subcutaneous adipose tissue [8]. A study of 482 lean, young individuals revealed increased hepatic triglyceride content in Southeast Asians than in men of European descent [9].

NAFLD prevalence also varies by gender, generally being more common in men. This is particularly true among Caucasians. However, postmenopausal women have a similar incidence of NAFLD as men [10]. This suggests that sex hormones may play a role in the pathogenesis of NAFLD.

NAFLD and type 2 diabetes mellitus are both associated with increased insulin resistance (IR). Furthermore, the prevalence of fatty liver disease is much higher in the diabetic population, 69.5–74% for NAFLD and 22.2% for NASH [11,12].

In addition to those with diabetes, patients with hyperlipidemia are also considered to be at increased risk for NAFLD. In a study by Assy et al. [13], hypercholesterolemic, hypertriglyceridemic, and mixed dyslipidemia patients had a 50% prevalence of NAFLD.

NAFLD is becoming more common in the pediatric population as well, with a reported prevalence of up to 13% [14].

CLINICAL FEATURES

NAFLD is usually clinically silent. Sometimes nonspecific symptoms such as fatigue and vague right upper quadrant abdominal discomfort may be present. Hepatomegaly is the most common physical finding [15]. General examination may reveal features of metabolic syndrome, obesity, and diabetes.

Most patients will come to a physician's attention because of incidental findings of abnormal liver enzymes or radiographic findings of steatosis. Usually levels of liver transaminases (ALT and AST) are elevated by less than five times the upper limit of normal. Based on a large retrospective study by Harrison et al. [16], patients with IFL had median serum ALT levels of 69 U/L and serum AST levels of 48 U/L. The patients with NASH had higher median levels of serum aminotransferases, with ALT levels of 83 U/L and AST levels of 62 U/L [16].

Other serum markers can be elevated in NAFLD, such as gamma-glutamyl tranferase (GGT), antinuclear antibodies (ANA), antismooth antibodies, and ferritin levels. When these markers are present, it is usually associated with more advanced liver disease and a worsened prognosis.

COMORBID CONDITIONS

NAFLD patients have many additional cardiovascular risk factors, including obesity, IR, diabetes, and metabolic syndrome. However, NAFLD has been shown to increase the risk of cardiovascular events independently of traditional risk factors. Cardiovascular disease (CVD) is the number one cause of mortality in NAFLD patients. Furthermore, with the development of NASH, the degree and severity of CVD become directly proportional to the amount of inflammation on liver biopsy [17,18].

Approximately one half (46%) of NAFLD patients have symptoms of obstructive sleep apnea (OSA) [19]. By comparison, the estimated prevalence of OSA in the general population is 1–4%. Daltro et al. [20] evaluated 40 obese patients who presented for bariatric surgery. OSA was present in 80%, NAFLD in 82%, and NASH in 80% of the patients [20]. Studies have shown improvement in serum aminotransferase levels in patients with OSA after treatment with continuous positive airway pressure (CPAP) [21]. However, further studies are required to clarify an association between OSA and NAFLD.

PATHOPHYSIOLOGY

Despite all the advances in recent years in the basic and clinical research of the condition, NAFLD pathophysiology remains incompletely understood. The original working theory considered NAFLD to be a disease continuum, evolving from simple steatosis to NASH. According to this traditional view, hepatic fat accumulation is a prerequisite for hepatocyte injury to develop in NAFLD. In this hypothesis, cytokines, adipokines, bacterial endotoxins, mitochondrial dysfunction, and endoplasmic reticulum (ER) stress represent the second hit necessary for the progression to NASH [22].

But longitudinal studies have shown that IFL rarely progresses to NASH. This has led to a challenge to the NAFLD disease continuum theory. It is possible that IFL and NASH are two separate disease entities and not part of progression of fat-induced liver disease. Keeping this perspective in mind, we will now review the current evidence and piece the NAFLD puzzle together.

INSULIN RESISTANCE

Insulin Resistance (IR) seems to be a cornerstone in the pathogenesis of NAFLD (see Figure 5.1). IR will generally result in an excess production of insulin and in excess exposure of insulin's effects across multiple organ systems. With regard to fatty liver disease, we are particularly focused on insulin's actions at the hepatocyte, myocyte, and adipocyte.

In the liver, IR can manifest by attenuating insulin's normal suppression of gluconeogenesis. This results in ongoing glucose production by the liver, despite the possible presence of hyperglycemia. Under these conditions, the liver is actually manufacturing glucose, even though there is adequate glucose available in circulation. Furthermore, excessive insulin may result in excessive triglyceride production and liver lipid deposition.

At the level of skeletal muscle, IR results in decreased glucose uptake via the GLUT4 transport system. This results in a diversion of ingested glucose away from the muscle for oxidation and into the liver where it will likely be converted to triglycerides. Excessive insulin also drives muscle glycogen synthesis and increases intramyocellular lipids in the form of diacylglycerol and ceramides. Increases in acylcarnitines have also been found and are thought to be due to incomplete mitochondrial fatty acid (FA) oxidation.

Development of IR at the level of adipose tissue impairs insulin-mediated suppression of lipolysis. This can lead to increased storage of lipids, with a larger lipid droplet size and an increased amount of larger adipocytes. These changes eventually challenge the adipocyte metabolically, leading to inflammation and abnormal cytokine production.

When an organism is exposed to chronic overfeeding, adipose tissue acts as a protective system to absorb and retain excess nutrients in the form of fat or triglycerides, which is the most economical way to store excess energy. In order for adipocytes to adapt to chronic overfeeding, cells undergo hypertrophy and hyperplasia. However, in this process, several inflammatory pathways become activated and result in development of adipose tissue IR.

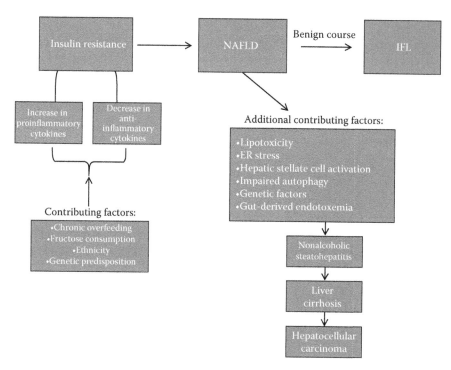

FIGURE 5.1   IR in the pathogenesis of NAFLD.

Adipose tissue is a very metabolically active organ and secretes many cytokines and adipokines that play key roles in the regulation of insulin sensitivity. A greater degree of obesity is expected to yield a greater degree of cytokine and adipokine imbalance. Therefore, more obesity should equal more IR. But not all obese persons develop IR. Despite chronic overfeeding, some individuals can remain metabolically normal.

Adipose tissue–macrophage content appears to be an important differentiator between those obese individuals who do or do not develop IR. These macrophages are responsible for the production of proinflammatory adipokines and cytokines, such as TNF-alpha, IL-6, and resistin. In obese persons with NAFLD, dysfunctional adipose tissue increases the secretion of these proinflammatory substances.

A further metabolic disturbance is seen in obese persons with NAFLD. In addition to the production of proinflammatory adipokines and cytokines, a decrease in the production of metabolically favorable hormones such as adiponectin has been observed. Normal levels of adiponectin are thought to be anti-inflammatory and insulin sensitizing. Low adiponectin levels are associated with the opposite effect, producing inflammation, systemic IR, and ectopic fat accumulation in organs other than subcutaneous tissue.

Therefore, it appears that the obese individual with NAFLD suffers from an imbalance of adipose-derived substances, which favor inflammation and IR.

Biochemically, this proinflammatory state is activated via several different pathways. For example, FAs activate Toll-like receptor TLR-4 in macrophages and adipocytes via the inhibitor kB kinase/nuclear factor kB pathway. In the c-Jun N-terminal kinase/activator protein 1 pathway, insulin signaling is inhibited in the presence of TNF-alpha. In the cyclic adenosine monophosphate pathway, the responsive element binding protein H (CREB-H) pathway results in the secretion of acute-phase proteins such as C-reactive protein and generation of reactive oxygen species. The Janus kinase JAK/signal transducer and activator of transcription (STAT) pathways play important roles in cytokine transduction.

Once adipose tissue becomes insulin resistant, inhibition of lipolysis is diminished. Adipocytes start to release free FAs (FFAs) into the systemic circulation, which ultimately reach the liver. Liver steatosis develops when the rate of FA input (uptake from circulation and de novo synthesis) is greater than the rate of FA output (via oxidation or very low density lipoprotein [VLDL] secretion).

In general, the majority of FFAs are delivered to the liver from subcutaneous adipose tissue via systemic circulation. The contribution of splanchnic lipolysis to hepatic FFA delivery is increased in obese subjects. Visceral fat mass contributes about 6% of all FFAs in lean subjects and 13–17% in obese subjects [23]. The rate of FFA release is proportional to the fat mass and is greater in obese persons than in lean persons. In addition, gene expression of hepatic lipase and hepatic lipoprotein lipase is higher in obese subjects with NAFLD than in those without NAFLD. Gene expression of FAT/CD36, which is an important regulator of tissue FFA uptake, is increased in the liver and skeletal muscle but decreased in adipose tissue in patients with NAFLD. Therefore, we have evidence of increased delivery of FFAs from subcutaneous and visceral adipose tissue, enhanced ability of the liver to extract FAs from circulating triglycerides (TG), and rerouting of FA transport from the adipose tissue to the liver and skeletal muscle in patients with NAFLD.

The liver also actively produces de novo FAs (de novo lipogenesis [DNL]). The pathway of the DNL becomes activated by hyperinsulinemia and by abundance of the substrate acetyl-CoA. Influx of acetyl-CoA is increased in the setting of muscle IR and redelivery of glucose to the liver. Contribution of DNL to the total intrahepatic TG pool accounts for 15–23% in the patients with NAFLD [3].

There are three major routes by which the liver deals with this excess of FA: FA oxidation (FAO), packaging into VLDL particles, and esterifying FAs into TGs and storing them within the hepatocyte as lipid droplets.

Studies have shown that patients with NAFLD have either normal or increased FAO. The rate of VLDL secretion seems to be greater in subjects with NAFLD but not high enough to compensate for excess influx of FAs; thus, they accumulate within hepatocytes, manifesting as steatosis.

The type of food consumption also plays an important role in developing NAFLD. If ingested in excess, the carbohydrates, and particularly fructose, enter the pathway of FA synthesis in the liver. As mentioned above, DNL is activated in the presence of high levels of insulin and substrate availability. Fructose cannot be used to synthesize glycogen and instead is converted to glyceraldehyde-3-phosphate, which becomes a substrate for DNL. Several studies have shown an association between high intakes of fructose, increased DNL, and an increased incidence of NAFLD [24,25]. Abdelmalek et al. [26] were able to demonstrate a higher fibrosis stage in association with daily fructose consumption, as well as increased hepatic inflammation and hepatocyte ballooning in older adults with NAFLD.

PATHOGENESIS OF NASH AND FIBROSIS

There are several mechanisms that have been proposed as being involved in the pathogenesis of NASH. Lipotoxicity, ER stress, skeletal muscle IR, intrahepatic factors, gut microbiota, and genetic risk factors have all been considered. These are suspected of leading to the development of hepatocyte injury, inflammation, and fibrosis.

LIPOTOXICITY

It has been suggested that packaging of excess FAs as TG lipid droplets within hepatocytes is actually a protective mechanism. If an unknown trigger disrupts that process, then lipotoxicity can develop. Deleterious effects of free FAs, and specifically saturated FAs (SFAs), have been seen at the level of ER and the mitochondria of the hepatocyte. In animal models, exposure of hepatocytes to saturated FAs can trigger inflammation by interacting with Toll-like receptors.

In addition to SFA, there is accumulation of lipid byproducts, such as diacylglycerol, long-chain fatty acyl-CoA, ceramide, lysophosphatidic acid, and phosphatidic acid. These substances are thought to interfere with insulin signaling and activate inflammatory pathways. However, the exact lipid intermediate and precise mechanisms are yet unknown.

ENDOPLASMIC RETICULUM STRESS

Under stress conditions, such as hypoxia, alterations in energy and substrates, toxins, viral infections, and exposure to SFAs, unfolded proteins accumulate in the ER and initiate an adaptive response known as the unfolded protein response (UPR). While it serves the protective purpose of leaning out unfolded proteins, it also activates the c-Jun NH2-terminal kinase (JNK) pathway and inhibits insulin signaling through phosphorylation and/or degradation of IRS1. ER stress also may stimulate hedgehog pathway ligands and contribute to the development of fibrogenesis.

SKELETAL MUSCLE INSULIN RESISTANCE

Adipose tissue IR not only promotes downstream liver IR but also can promote skeletal muscle IR. An increase in plasma FFA concentration impairs insulin signaling. The accumulation of intramyocellular lipids in the form of various lipid-derived toxic metabolites can also promote IR. For example, incomplete oxidation products of FAs, such as acylcarnitines, long-chain fatty acyl Co-A, ceramides, and diacylglycerol, can impair insulin signaling. They can also activate inflammatory pathways, including protein kinase C and IkB/nuclear factor kB [27]. Furthermore, skeletal muscle gets attacked by numerous inflammatory cytokines, which are released by dysfunctional adipose tissue. Once skeletal muscle IR becomes evident, it contributes to hepatic steatosis by rerouting glucose back to the liver where it becomes a substrate for DNL. The resultant hyperinsulinemia stimulates hepatic sterol regulatory element binding protein Ic (SREBP-Ic) activity and increases DNL as well.

NALFD AND LIVER FIBROSIS

Several pathways have been implicated in the development of fibrosis in NAFLD. One involves hepatic epithelial progenitor cells. When exposed to a stressful environment, these cells can undergo a hedgehog ligand-mediated process called epithelial-to-mesenchymal transition (EMT), making them less vulnerable to apoptosis and augmenting profibrogenic pathways.

Hedgehog pathway signaling also modulates the conversion of quiescent hepatic stellate cells to myofibroblasts, the accumulation of which leads to abnormal liver repair, fibrosis, and eventual cirrhosis. Inhibition of hedgehog signaling in mice reverses liver fibrosis and even HCC and may be an important therapeutic target [28].

The cellular process of cleaning up damaged structures and organelles, which is called autophagy, is important in preventing cellular injury and apoptosis. SFAs are capable of suppressing autophagy, which leads to accumulation of dysfunctional mitochondria, ER, and enhanced oxidative stress and ultimately can lead to apoptosis.

GUT MICROBIOTA AND NAFLD

Gut microbiota is being increasingly recognized as an important factor in pathogenesis of many diseases, including NAFLD. Most of the data on gut microbiota come from animal studies, but nonetheless, these let us appreciate its importance in many pathways involving obesity, IR, and NAFLD.

It has been shown that obese individuals have a different composition of microbiota than lean controls, with considerably more Firmicutes and less Bacteroidetes. This composition changes with weight loss either through diet [29] or after gastric bypass surgery [30]. The proposed mechanism of contribution of certain gut microbiota to obesity lies in the increased microbial extraction of calories by degrading normally indigestible plant polysaccharides, which can increase caloric intake by 10–15% [31].

Overgrowth of Gram-negative bacteria and gut-derived endotoxemia are involved in the development of NASH. Intestinal microbiota produces a number of potentially toxic substances, such as ammonia, ethanol, acetaldehyde, phenols, and lipopolysaccharide (LPS). Animal models of NAFLD have shown that endotoxin LPS activates the pattern recognition receptor, Toll-like receptor 4, on Kupffer cells, and this results in upregulation of several inflammatory pathways including JNK and nuclear factor kB. Proinflammatory cytokines such as TNF-alpha and IL-1beta as well as direct effects of LPS subsequently promote hepatic stellate cell activation and fibrogenesis. Modification of intestinal flora with probiotics results in decreased IR [32].

A higher prevalence of small intestinal bacterial overgrowth and elevated levels of TNF have been reported in patients with NASH compared to controls [33]. NASH occurred frequently after jejunoileal bypass surgery, used in the past as a weight loss procedure. Administration of metronidazole or resection of the bypassed section of the intestine resulted in improvement of steatohepatitis [31].

GENETIC RISK FACTORS

Although we know that obesity, IR, lipotoxicity, and activation of proinflammatory and fibrogenic pathways play important roles in the pathogenesis of NAFLD, not all subjects with obesity develop NAFLD. Several genes have been identified as predisposing factors for NAFLD.

One genetic variant is a missense mutation (I148M) in patatin-like phospholipase domain-containing gene PNPLA3 (also called adiponutrin). The frequency of this variant in different ethnic groups correlates with prevalence of NAFLD. The physiological role of PNPLA3 and the mechanism by which I148M isoform causes NAFLD are yet unknown. Recent study by Sookoian and Pirola [34] showed that this gene variant exerts a strong influence on liver fat accumulation, susceptibility to a more aggressive necroinflammation, and fibrosis.

Other genetic mutations that potentially could be linked to NAFLD are apolipoprotein C3 (APOC3) mutation, NCAN, glucokinase regulatory protein, and LYPLAL1.

DIAGNOSIS

The diagnosis of NAFLD requires the presence of hepatic steatosis by imaging or histology in the absence of significant alcohol consumption, as well as the exclusion of other secondary causes of hepatic steatosis. Significant alcohol consumption is defined as >21 drinks per week in men and >14 drinks per week in women over a 2-year prior to baseline testing (10 g of alcohol per one drink unit) [35]. Establishing a proper history of alcohol use is an important step in evaluating a patient for suspected NAFLD. If clinical suspicion of alcohol use is high and inconsistent with patient-reported history, consider confirmation from a family member.

Patients also should be evaluated for the presence of metabolic syndrome and diabetes mellitus. Similarly, a history of hyperlipidemia and OSA can be important.

Exclusion of other causes of hepatic steatosis, in addition to alcohol liver disease, is necessary. Common alternative causes are hepatitis C, medications (i.e., amiodarone, methotrexate, tamoxifen, and corticosteroids), Wilson's disease, starvation, and parenteral nutrition. It is important to evaluate a patient for the presence of coexisting chronic liver conditions, such as viral hepatitis, autoimmune liver disease, hemochromatosis, and Wilson's disease.

When evaluating a patient with NAFLD, it is important to determine if a patient has IFL or NASH for prognostic and therapeutic decision-making purposes. This may require a liver biopsy. The diagnosis of steatosis can be suspected noninvasively by laboratory and available imaging modalities. These tests are able to detect fatty liver infiltration with good accuracy. However, there is no laboratory or imaging test that can distinguish IFL from NASH.

LABORATORY TESTS

Liver transaminases (ALT and AST) are typically modestly elevated, no more than five times the upper level of normal. In contrast to those with alcohol liver hepatitis, most patients with NAFLD have a ratio of AST/ALT of less than 1. As the disease progresses, levels of AST increase more than ALT, and the ratio can become more than 1. Presence of elevated liver enzymes does not confirm the diagnosis of NASH, and many patients with biopsy-proven NASH have normal liver enzymes.

Elevated GGT levels are also common in patients with NAFLD and have been reported to be associated with increased mortality. Other laboratory abnormalities that have been reported in association with NAFLD include hyperuricemia, increased ferritin, vitamin D deficiency and positive serum autoantibodies.

In addition to the laboratory tests outlined above, tests used to exclude other causes of fatty liver should be considered. With this in mind, it may be important to obtain negative results for viral hepatitis, autoimmune hepatitis, primary biliary cirrhosis, hereditary hemochromatosis, Wilson's disease, and alpha 1-antitrypsin deficiency.

Different biomarkers and scoring systems have been developed to identify the patients at risk for NASH and fibrosis, and can be used to identify patients who would benefit from diagnostic liver biopsy.

The NAFLD fibrosis score has been studied most extensively out of all scoring systems [36]. It does require a calculator, which is available online (http://nafldscore.com). It is based on six readily available variables: age, BMI, hyperglycemia, platelet count, albumin, and AST/ALT ratio. A NAFLD fibrosis score of <–1.455 has negative predictive value of 88%, and the score above

0.676 has positive predictive value of 82% to identify advance fibrosis [37]. Unfortunately, up to one fourth of patients fall into an intermediate range and cannot be classified by this scoring system [38].

The FibroTest FibroSURE (Bioprotective, Paris, France) is based on alpha2-macroglobulin, apolipoprotein A1, haptoglobin, total bilirubin, and GGT levels. It was reported to have a 90% negative predictive value and 70% positive predictive value for advanced fibrosis [39]. In general, these types of scoring systems are better at predicting patients who do not have advanced fibrosis [40].

The BARD score (BMI, AST/ALT ratio, diabetes) reliably predicts significant fibrosis by combining BMI of 28 kg/m² or higher (1 point), AST/ALT ratio of 0.8 or higher (2 points), and diabetes (1 point). A score of two or more is considered a positive score and was associated with an odds ratio for advanced fibrosis of 17, and has a negative predictive value of 96% [16].

Other scoring systems exist that require use of specific biomarkers of matrix turnover.

The Enhanced Liver Fibrosis Panel (ELF) combines three matrix turnover proteins: hyaluronic acid, tissue inhibitor of metalloproteinase 1, and aminoterminal peptide of procollagen III (P3NP), and had AUROC of 0.90 with 80% sensitivity and 90% specificity for detecting advanced fibrosis [35,39].

Circulating levels of cytokeratin-18 (CK-18) fragments have been investigated as novel biomarkers for the presence of steatohepatitis in patients with NAFLD. Plasma CK-18 fragments are markedly elevated in patients with NASH as compared with patients with IFL or normal controls [35]. This assay is not commercially available and cutoff values for diagnosing steatohepatitis have yet to be established.

IMAGING MODALITIES

A number of radiologic tests are available that show good accuracy in diagnosing hepatic steatosis. Ultrasound (US) is the most commonly used modality in evaluating patients with suspected NAFLD. US is easy to perform, widely available, and not associated with radiation exposure. US can pick up liver steatosis with a degree of fat infiltration of more than 30%. The sensitivity is decreased in obese patients and in cases of fat infiltration of less than 30%. It cannot differentiate between simple steatosis and steatohepatitis.

Computed tomography (CT) scan is another modality that can detect liver steatosis and has similar accuracy as US. Steatosis is best detected with noncontrast CT. Its use is limited by radiation exposure.

MR imaging (MRI) can detect steatosis starting at minimal levels of 3% fat infiltration. MR spectroscopy can identify signals from fat and water separately, therefore providing accurate information on the extent of liver fat infiltration. However, it is expensive and not widely available.

Several imaging modalities have tried to evaluate the degree of liver fibrosis. US-based transient elastography (TE) or FibroScan has been used successfully in Europe and Canada to identify liver fibrosis in patients with chronic hepatitis C. TE measures the velocity of a low-amplitude shear wave that is propagated through the liver to determine tissue stiffness and to estimate hepatic fibrosis. This technology has been tested in application to patients with NAFLD with variable success. Initially it failed to provide accurate results in obese patients [41], and for that reason, a different probe (XL probe) was developed to overcome the limitations of this test in patients with a BMI greater than 30. XL probe has shown better accuracy [42].

HISTOLOGY

Percutaneous liver biopsy remains the gold standard for diagnosis of NAFLD and the only way to reliably distinguish between IFL and NASH. Hepatic steatosis is histologically defined when 5% or more of hepatocytes contain visible intracellular TGs.

The Brunt criteria are the most commonly used to make the diagnosis of NASH [43]. The histological grade indicates the activity of steatohepatitic lesions, and the histological stage reflects the degree of fibrosis. NASH is defined by a pattern of hepatocyte ballooning, lobular inflammation, and macrovesicular steatosis. Mallory–Denk bodies may or may not be present. Microvesicular steatosis is seen in 10% of liver biopsies and has been shown to correlate with a higher grade of steatosis, cell injury, and fibrosis.

NAFLD Activity Score (NAS) is used in clinical trials and provides a composite score based on the degree of steatosis, lobular inflammation, and hepatocyte ballooning. Fibrosis is reported separately [39].

Liver biopsy has its own limitations. It is invasive and can result in complications such as bleeding and even death. In addition, correct diagnosis can be missed due to sample variability, since lesions of NASH may not be distributed evenly, and there are intraobserver variations [38].

Given the high prevalence of obesity and NAFLD, it is impractical to subject all patients to liver biopsy for diagnosis. Several guidelines by different medical associations have been published on criteria for liver biopsy.

The European Association for the Study of Liver Diseases recommend liver biopsy when noninvasive markers suggest advanced fibrosis and in indeterminate cases when the suspicion of fibrosis remains high [44,45].

Practice guidelines by the American Gastroenterological Association, American Association for the Study of Liver Diseases, and American College of Gastroenterology recommend obtaining liver biopsy in the following situations:

1. Liver biopsy should be considered in patients with NAFLD who are at increased risk to have steatohepatitis and advanced fibrosis (strength: 1, evidence: B).
2. The presence of metabolic syndrome and the NAFLD Fibrosis Score may be used for identifying those patients who are at risk for steatohepatitis and advanced fibrosis.
3. Liver biopsy should be considered in patients with suspected NAFLD in whom competing etiologies for hepatic steatosis and coexisting chronic liver diseases cannot be excluded without a liver biopsy.

Researchers at the Cleveland Clinic consider liver biopsy in patients with NAFLD who have persistently elevated liver enzymes despite interventions to reverse conditions associated with metabolic syndrome [46]. Others have suggested performing liver biopsy in all patients who have diabetes and/or metabolic syndrome and elevated transaminases [44].

NATURAL HISTORY

IFL carries a benign prognosis and rarely progresses to NASH or end-stage liver disease. On the other hand, NASH can be progressive and lead to liver cirrhosis, HCC, and liver-related death.

Patients with NAFLD have an increased cardiovascular mortality compared to a control population, and patients with NASH have increased liver-related mortality rate.

Longitudinal studies report that about 32–41% of patients with newly diagnosed NASH had histological progression of the disease over a median follow-up of 4.3–13.7 years [46]. NASH with fibrosis has been shown to carry a worse prognosis than NASH without fibrosis. Fibrosis progression has been associated with DM, severe IR, elevated BMI, weight gain of more than 5 kg, and rising ALT and AST. Progression to NASH cirrhosis has been reported at a rate of 11% over a 15-year period.

There is also indirect evidence that patients with cryptogenic cirrhosis might in fact have a "burnt out" NASH cirrhosis. Those patients typically have high prevalence of NAFLD risk factors, such as metabolic syndrome, diabetes, and obesity. Several studies have shown that loss of histological features of NASH might happen with progression to NASH cirrhosis [35].

NASH is also a risk factor for developing HCC. Recent studies suggest that about 7% of patients with NASH cirrhosis will develop HCC over a 6.5-year period. The data range from 2.4% to 12.8% during 3.2–10 years of follow-up [7]. However, there are case reports and small case series of diagnosis of HCC in NASH patients without cirrhosis.

Patients typically have large, well-differentiated tumors at the time of presentation, which may be secondary to a delayed diagnosis. Older age, iron deposition, obesity, diabetes, and advanced fibrosis were the strongest risk factors for the development of HCC [47].

The estimated yearly incidence of HCC among NASH cirrhosis patients is 2.7% [48]. These data suggest that NASH patients with cirrhosis should be screened for HCC [46].

LIVER TRANSPLANTATION

For NASH patients with advanced liver disease, liver transplantation is an available option. According to the 2011 United Network for Organ Sharing Registry database for liver transplant recipients, NASH is the fourth most common cause of liver transplantation. Considering the increasing number of patients with obesity and metabolic syndrome, there will be an even greater number of transplantations performed for NASH-related liver failure.

The evaluation of recurrence rate on NAFLD in the post-transplant setting is complicated by the potential presence of transplant rejection, post-transplant idiopathic chronic hepatitis, side effects of antirejection medications, and post-transplant infections. Unlike patients with alcohol-related liver failure, who are required to be abstinent from alcohol before transplantation, many patients with NASH-related end-stage liver disease may have persistent risk factors for NAFLD, such as obesity, metabolic syndrome, and diabetes mellitus. These conditions could actually worsen after the transplantation.

The recurrence rates for steatosis, steatohepatitis, and fibrosis vary widely, depending on the individual studies. The rates of recurrence for steatosis reported to range 8.2–62.5% over 4 months to 10 years of follow-up, the rates for steatohepatitis ranged from 4% to 33% over 6 weeks to 20 years, and the rates of advanced fibrosis are infrequent, 0% to 33%, and occurring later in the follow-up course. In one study, patients with BMI > 30 kg/m^2 had higher recurrence of the steatosis, steatohepatitis, and fibrosis.

Potential reasons for this variability include difference in study population, clinical features, biopsy protocols, and histological criteria used [49]. However, graft and patient survival rates are comparable for these patients and patients undergoing transplantation for other liver disease.

Another problem related to liver transplantation and NAFLD is the high frequency of NAFLD in potential liver donors. Steatosis is currently detected in approximately one third to one half of potential living and deceased donors. Livers with less than 30% steatosis are considered optimal for transplantation, and are typically rejected if more than 60% of fat infiltration is present.

TREATMENT

Management of patients with NAFLD should include not only treatment of liver disease but also optimization of other components of metabolic syndrome, such as obesity, diabetes, hyperlipidemia, and hypertension. It is important to remember that CVD is still a number one cause of mortality in these patients and should be addressed.

Patients with suspected or confirmed NASH should be treated aggressively to prevent liver-associated morbidity and mortality. There is no ideal established treatment for NASH, and most of the information comes from small trials (Figure 5.2). Histological improvement is the ultimate goal of treatment, whereas most studies used surrogate markers of improvement, such as liver enzymes and/or the degree of steatosis based on radiological data, and should be interpreted with caution, as it may not correlate with histological changes.

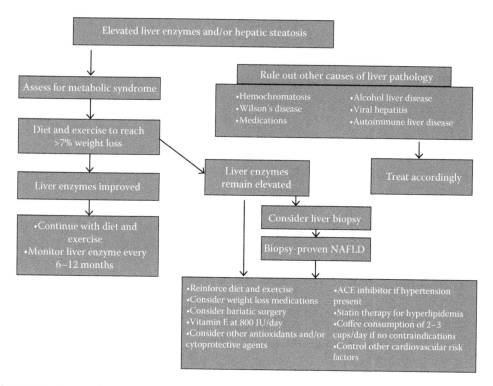

FIGURE 5.2   Proposed treatment algorithm for NASH.

LIFESTYLE MODIFICATIONS

Diet, weight loss, and exercise are mainstay therapeutic approaches for patients with NAFLD. Multiple studies showed a benefit of weight loss through diet and combination of diet and exercise. The best results were seen after loss of 7% or more of body weight. A landmark study by Promrat et al. [50] of lifestyle interventions (diet and exercise) in patients with NASH showed histological improvement by liver biopsy in those who lost more than 7% of body weight. Significant results were seen in attenuation of lobular inflammation, ballooning, and hepatic steatosis. However, the fibrosis score was unchanged [50].

Most studies focused on general calorie restriction rather than specific diet composition. Kirk et al. [51] explored differences in effects of low-carbohydrate diet versus high-carbohydrate diet (with calorie restriction in both arms) and showed greater improvement in hepatic insulin sensitivity in the low-carbohydrate group, although the degree of steatosis regression was similar after 7% of weight loss [51].

Based on comparative review of diets by Zivkovic et al. [52], it can be recommended that patients with NAFLD decrease the intake of saturated fats and simple carbohydrates, including fructose consumption, and increase the intake of monounsaturated and polyunsaturated fats and high-fiber foods, in addition to restricting caloric intake [52].

Interestingly, coffee caffeine consumption has been associated with lower rates of fibrosis progression in patients with liver cirrhosis due to hepatitis C, especially high intakes of two to three cups a day. Molloy et al. [53] have seen similar results in patients with NASH as well.

Degree of weight loss should not exceed more than 1 kg/week, since rapid weight loss can exacerbate steatosis [39].

Several studies explored the effect of exercise alone without calorie restriction and also showed positive results with decrease in intrahepatic triglyceride content by MR spectroscopy without overall change in body weight [7,35].

Adjunct Weight Loss Pharmacotherapy

Orlistat was evaluated by Harrison et al. [54] as adjunct pharmacotherapy for weight loss in patients with biopsy-proven NASH. Patients were randomized to receive either orlistat/diet/vitamin E or diet/vitamin E. Those patients who achieved 5% or more of weight loss had improvement in IR and steatosis, and those subjects with more than 9% weight loss had improvement in hepatic necroinflammation, regardless of orlistat intake.

No other weight loss medications were evaluated in clinical trials specifically for patients with NAFLD. However, it seems that just the degree of weight loss itself is the major contributor to NALFD improvement, and other approved medications for weight loss can be reasonably used to achieve a weight loss goal.

Bariatric Surgery

Surgical therapy for weight loss is an invaluable option since, for a majority of patients, weight loss is difficult to achieve and even more so difficult to sustain over time. Weight loss surgery has been shown to significantly improve and even resolve features of metabolic syndrome, such as obesity, diabetes, and hypertension [55].

There are no randomized controlled trials that evaluated a type of bariatric surgery specifically for treatment of NALFD, but there are data available from retrospective and prospective studies that compared liver histologies before and after the surgery. Mathurin et al. [56] reported liver biopsy results in patients with NALFD and severe obesity before, 1 year, and 5 years after bariatric surgery. Gastric band, bilio-intestinal bypass, and gastric bypass were done in 56%, 23%, and 21% of cases, respectively. Compared to baseline, there was definite improvement in steatosis and hepatocyte ballooning following bariatric surgery. Patients with refractory IR had persistent histological features of NALFD [56].

However, a recent Cochrane review was unable to confirm these benefits because of a lack of randomized trials that used bariatric surgery for treatment of NASH [57]. It does remain a reasonable approach in patients with NAFLD and other indications for bariatric surgery.

INSULIN SENSITIZERS AND OTHER DIABETES MEDICATIONS

Metformin

Several studies investigated the effects of metformin on liver histology in NAFLD patients. Although initially, small trials showed some benefit of metformin [58], most recent studies failed to prove any improvement in aminotransferases or liver histology and cannot be recommended as treatment for NALFD [59,60]. Metformin does remain valuable in patients with concurrent glucose intolerance and diabetes mellitus.

Thiazolidinediones

Thiazolidinediones (TZDs) are a unique class of insulin-sensitizing medications. Only one drug remains as approved on the market without restriction—pioglitazone. The main target of TZDs is a peroxisome proliferator-activated receptor (PPAR)-gamma, which can be found in skeletal muscle, adipose tissue, and the liver. Acting as a PPAR-gamma agonist, pioglitazone improves insulin sensitivity at the level of those tissues and is associated with increase in plasma adiponectin levels (an anti-inflammatory adipose tissue hormone). Many studies have proven that pioglitazone decreases liver steatosis and necroinflammation with improvement in NAS score and even possible improvement in fibrosis [61,62].

The effect of TZDs does not last after discontinuation of drug therapy [63], and there have been many concerns regarding the long-term safety of pioglitazone. Weight gain, congestive heart failure, bone loss, and a recently reported increased incidence of bladder cancer limit the widespread use of this medication.

GLP-1 ANALOGUES

Pharmacologic agents that mimic the effects of endogenous incretins, such as glucagone-like peptide-1 (GLP-1) analogues (exenatide and liraglutide), have been used extensively in patients with diabetes mellitus. In addition to lower glucose levels, they have been shown to improve hepatocyte macro- and chaperone-mediated autophagy and ER stress [27]. Available studies on use of exenatide in treatment of NAFLD are small and do not provide conclusive evidence of benefit on histological improvement [64].

ANTIOXIDANTS AND CYTOPROTECTIVE AGENTS

Vitamin E

Oxidative stress is considered to be one of the pathological pathways leading to development of necroinflammation and cell death in NASH. Vitamin E has been known for its antioxidative properties and has been studied as a therapeutic approach in patients with NASH [65]. Sanyal et al. [66] conducted the largest randomized controlled trial. This showed a significant improvement in steatosis and lobular inflammation, but not fibrosis with 96 weeks of therapy with 800 IU/day of alpha-tocopherol compared to placebo and pioglitazone 30 mg/day [66]. For unclear reasons, similar results with use of vitamin E were not seen on pediatric population [67].

Although vitamin E therapy is generally seen as benign, some concerning side effects such as increased mortality and intracranial hemorrhage have been reported [7,39].

Betaine

Another antioxidant that has been studied primarily in animals for NAFLD treatment is betaine. It works by increasing levels of S-adenosylmethionine. A randomized controlled trial of betaine use in patients with biopsy-proven NASH did not show improvement of liver enzymes or histology as compared to placebo [68]. Further studies are needed before it can be recommended for use in patients with NAFLD.

Ursodeoxycholic Acid

Ursodeoxycholic acid (UDCA) is one of the agents considered to have cytoprotective properties and has been studied in patients with NASH. But the majority of trials failed to show definite benefit of UDCA in improving histology, and it cannot be recommended for the treatment of NAFLD at this point [7,35].

Pentoxifylline

Pentoxifylline (PTX) has been shown to have anti-inflammatory properties by inhibiting proinflammatory cytokines, such as TNF-alpha, and reducing production of free radicals. Available data from small studies, investigating the use of PTX in NASH patients, are promising, with reported improvement in liver enzymes, IR, hepatic steatosis, inflammation, and ballooning. The latest trial by Zein et al. [69] even showed improvement in histological features of NASH compared to placebo and even trends toward improvement in fibrosis, although this was not statistically significant. Therapy with this medication is well tolerated, but because of the lack of large-scale trials, it is not one of the recommended drug therapy agents yet.

Other Agents

Angiotensin-receptor blockers (ARBs) have been evaluated for their antifibrotic properties. In animal studies, ARBs have shown to inhibit hepatic stellate cell activity, leading to decrease in hepatic fibrosis. ARBs can be considered for use in patients with NASH and coexisting hypertension.

Lipid-lowering medications, such as statins and ezetimibe, have been studied in patients with NASH and appear to improve aminotransferase levels, but results on histological improvement are inconclusive. Many patients with NASH also have other indications for lipid-lowering therapy, and such drugs can be used safely to control hyperlipidemia.

SUMMARY

NAFLD is becoming the most common cause of incidental elevation of liver enzymes in the Western world, including the United States. It is considered to be a manifestation of metabolic syndrome, and its prevalence parallels that of obesity.

NAFLD's course can take one of two pathways: it can remain as simple steatosis without inflammation or cellular damage (IFL) or progress to NASH, with development of lobular inflammation, hepatocyte injury, and fibrosis. Patients with NASH are also at risk for developing liver cirrhosis and HCC.

Chronic overfeeding, including high fructose consumption, can lead to IR. This is a cornerstone in the pathogenesis of fat accumulation in the liver, leading to IFL. In some patients, presence of other triggers of inflammation and cell damage leads to development of NASH, liver cirrhosis, and possibly HCC.

Most patients will present with incidental findings of liver enzyme elevation and/or presence of fatty liver on imaging studies. Evaluation of patients with NAFLD involves ruling out other causes of liver pathology, as well as screening for other manifestations of metabolic syndrome. While many imaging studies are available to detect the presence of liver steatosis (US, CT, MRI), liver biopsy is required to rule out NASH. Different serum markers and scoring systems have been developed to predict NASH or cirrhosis, but to date, there is no method to diagnose NASH other than liver biopsy.

Weight loss through diet, exercise, use of weight loss medications, and bariatric surgery are currently the mainstay therapeutic approaches for patients with NAFLD. Loss of 7% or more of weight was shown to improve not only biochemical parameters but also the histological features of NASH.

Among various pharmacological agents, which were explored in the treatment of NALFD, only vitamin E and TZDs showed a consistent positive effect on histology. Unfortunately, they do have significant side effects or potential complication in certain populations. If other indications exist, agents such as statins, ACE inhibitors, pentoxifylline, and metformin can be of benefit.

None of the above-mentioned treatments are FDA-approved, and a continuous search for effective therapy is needed. Given the high prevalence of NAFLD and potential increased morbidity and mortality, efforts also should be aimed at obesity prevention at the population level.

ACKNOWLEDGMENT

The authors express their appreciation to Zachary S. Rothkopf for his assistance in preparing the figures.

REFERENCES

1. Mehta R, Younossi ZM. Natural history of nonalcoholic fatty liver disease. *Clin Liver Dis* 2012; 1(4): 111–112.
2. Vernon G, Baranova A, Younossi ZM. Systematic review: The epidemiology and natural history of non-alcoholic fatty liver disease and non-alcoholic steatohepatitis in adults. *Aliment Pharmacol Ther* 2011; 34(3): 274–285.
3. Fabbrini E, Sullivan S, Klein S. Obesity and nonalcoholic fatty liver disease: Biochemical, metabolic and clinical implications. *Hepatology* 2010; 51(2): 679–689.
4. Wanless IR, Lentz JS. Fatty liver hepatitis (steatohepatitis) and obesity: An autopsy study with analysis of risk factors. *Hepatology* 1990; 12: 1106–1110.
5. Browning JD, Szczepaniak LS, Dobbins R, Nuremberg P, Hotron JD, Cohen JC, Grundy SM, Hobbs HH. Prevalence of hepatic steatosis in an urban population in the United States: Impact of ethnicity. *Hepatology* 2004; 40: 1387–1395.

6. Clark JM, Brancati FL, Diehl AM. The prevalence and etiology of elevated aminotransferase levels in the United States. *Am J Gastroenterol* 2003; 98(5): 960–967.

7. Torres DM, Williams CD, Harrison SA. Features, diagnosis, and treatment of nonalcoholic fatty liver disease. *Clin Gastroenterol Hepatol* 2012; 10: 837–858.

8. Despres JP. Body fat distribution and risk of cardiovascular disease: An update. *Circulation* 2012; 126: 1301–1313.

9. Cohen JC, Horton JD, Hobbs HH. Human fatty liver disease: Old questions and new insights. *Science* 2011; 332(6037): 1519–1523.

10. Lavoie JM, Pighon A. NAFLD, estrogens, and physical exercise: The animal model. *J Nutr Metab* 2012; article ID 914938.

11. Targher G, Bertolini L, Padovani R, Rodella S, Tessari R, Zenari L, Day C, Arcaro G. Prevalence of nonalcoholic fatty liver disease and its association with cardiovascular disease in type 2 diabetic patients. *Diabetes Care* 2007; 30: 1212–1218.

12. Williams CD, Stengel J, Asike MI, Torres DM, Shaw J, Contreras M, Landt CL, Harrison SA. Prevalence of nonalcoholic fatty liver disease and nonalcoholic steatohepatitis among a largely middle-aged population utilizing ultrasound and liver biopsy: A prospective study. *Gastroenterology* 2011; 140: 124–131.

13. Assy N, Kaita K, Mymin D, Levy C, Rosser B, Minuk G. Fatty infiltration of liver in hyperlipidemic patients. *Dig Dis Sci* 2000; 45: 1929–1934.

14. Schwimmer JB, Deutsch R, Kahen T, Lavine JE, Stanley C, Behling C. Prevalence of fatty liver in children and adolescents. *Pediatrics* 2006; 118: 1388–1393.

15. Puri P, Sanyal AJ. Nonalcoholic fatty liver disease: Definitions, risk factors, and workup. *Clin Liver Dis* 2012; 1(4): 99–103.

16. Harrison SA, Oliver D, Arnold HL, Gogia S, Neuschwander-Tetri BA. Development and validation of a simple NAFLD clinical scoring system for identifying patients without advanced disease. *Gut* 2008; 57: 1441–1447.

17. Monsour HP Jr, Frenette CT, Wayne K. Fatty liver: A link to cardiovascular disease—its natural history, pathogenesis, and treatment. *MDCVJ* 2012; VIII(3): 21–25.

18. Treeprasersuk S, Lopez-Jimenez F, Lindor KD. Nonalcoholic fatty liver disease and the coronary artery disease. *Dig Dis Sci* 2011; 56: 35–45.

19. Singh H, Pollock R, Uhanova J, Fryger M, Hawkins K, Minuk GY. Symptoms of obstructive sleep apnea in patients with nonalcoholic fatty liver disease. *Dig Dis Sci* 2005; 50(12): 2338–2343.

20. Daltro C, Cotrim HP, Alves E, de Freitas LA, Araujo L, Boente L, Leal R, Portugal T. Nonalcoholic fatty liver disease associated with obstructive sleep apnea: Just a coincidence? *Obes Surg* 2010; 20(11): 1536–1543.

21. Chin K, Nakamura T, Takahashi K, Sumi K, Ogawa Y, Masuzaki H, Muro S, Hattori N, Matsumoto H, Niimi A, Chiba T, Nakao K, Mishima M, Ohi M, Nakamura T. Effects of obstructive sleep apnea syndrome on serum aminotransferase levels in obese patients. *Am J Med* 2003; 114(5): 370–376.

22. Yilmaz Y. Review article: Is non-alcoholic fatty liver disease a spectrum, or are steatosis and non-alcoholic steatohepatitis distinct conditions? *Aliment Pharmacol Ther* 2012; 36(9): 815–823.

23. Nielsen S, Guo Z, Johnson CM, Hensrud DD, Jensen MD. Splanchnic lipolysis in human obesity. *J Clin Invest* 2004; 113(11): 1582–1588.

24. Stanhope KL, Havel PJ. Fructose consumption: Considerations for future research on its effects on adipose distribution, lipid metabolism, and insulin sensitivity in humans. *J Nutr* 2009; 139(6): 1236S–1241S.

25. Stanhope KL, Schwarz JM, Havel PJ. Adverse metabolic effects of dietary fructose: Results from the recent epidemiological, clinical and mechanistic studies. *Curr Opin Lipidol* 2013; 24(3): 198–206.

26. Abdelmalek MF, Suzuki A, Guy C, Unalp-Arida A, Colvin R, Johnson RJ, Diehl AM. Increased fructose consumption is associated with fibrosis severity in patients with nonalcoholic fatty liver disease. *Hepatology* 2010; 51(6): 1961–1971.

27. Cusi K. Role of obesity and lipotoxicity in the development of nonalcoholic steatohepatitis: Pathophysiology and clinical implications. *Gastroenterology* 2012; 142: 711–725.

28. Philips GM, Chan IS, Swiderska M, Schroder VT, Guy C, Karaca GF, Moylan C, Venkatraman T, Feuerlein S, Syn WK, Jung Y, Witek RP, Choi S, Michelotti GA, Rangwala F, Merkle E, Lascola C, Diehl AM. Hedgehog signaling antagonist promotes regression of both liver fibrosis and hepatocellular carcinoma in a murine model of primary liver cancer. *PLoS ONE* 2011; 6(9): e23943.

29. Ley RE, Turnbaugh PJ, Klein S, Gordon JI. Microbial ecology: Human gut microbes associate with obesity. *Nature* 2006; 444(7122): 1022–1023.

30. Zhang H, DiBaise JK, Zuccolo A, Kudrna D, Braidotti M, Yu Y, Parameswaran P, Crowell MD, Wing R, Rittmann BE, Krajmalnik-Brown R. Human gut microbiota in obesity and after gastric bypass. *Proc Natl Acad Sci USA* 2009; 106(7): 2365–2370.

31. Abu-Shanab A, Quigley EMM. The role of the gut microbiota in nonalcoholic fatty liver disease. *Gastroenterol Hepatol* 2010; 7: 691–701.

32. Li Z, Yang S, Lin H, Huang J, Watkins PA, Moser AB, Desimone C, Song XY, Diehl AM. Probiotics and antibodies to TNF inhibit inflammatory activity and improve nonalcoholic fatty liver disease. *Hepatology* 2003; 37(2): 343–350.

33. Wigg AJ, Roberts-Thomson IC, Dymock RB, McCarthy PJ, Grose RH, Cummins AG. The role of small intestinal bacterial overgrowth, intestinal permeability, endotoxaemia, and tumor necrosis factor alpha in the pathogenesis of non-alcoholic steatohepatitis. *Gut* 2001; 48(2): 206–211.

34. Sookoian S, Pirola CJ. Meta-analysis if the influence of I148M variant of patatin-like phospholipase domain containing 3 gene (PNPLA3) on the susceptibility and histological severity of nonalcoholic fatty liver disease. *Hepatology* 2011; 53: 1883–1894.

35. Chalasani N, Younossi Z, Lavine J, Diehl AM, Brunt EM, Cusi K, Charlton M, Sanyal AJ. The diagnosis and management of nonalcoholic fatty liver disease: Practice guideline by the American Gastroenterological Association, American Association for the Study of Liver Diseases, and American College of Gastroenterology. *Gastroenterology* 2012; 142: 1592–1609.

36. Festi D, Schiumerini R, Marzi L, Biase ARD, Mandolesi D, Montrone L, Scaioli E, Bonato G. Review article: The diagnosis of non-alcoholic fatty liver disease—availability and accuracy of non-invasive methods. *Aliment Pharmacol Ther* 2013; 37: 392–400.

37. Angulo P, Hui JM, Marchesini G, Bugianesi E, George J, Farrell GC, Enders F, Saksena S, Burt AD, Bida JP, Lindor K, Sanderson SO, Lenzi M, Adams LA, Kench J, Therneau TM, Day CP. The NAFLD fibrosis score: A noninvasive system that identifies liver fibrosis in patients with NAFLD. *Hepatology* 2007; 45: 846–854.

38. Machado MV, Cortez-Pinto H. Non-invasive diagnosis of non-alcoholic fatty liver disease. A critical appraisal. *J Hepatol* 2013; 58: 1007–1019.

39. Paredes AH, Torres DM, Harrison SA. Nonalcoholic fatty liver disease. *Clin Liver Dis* 2012; 16: 397–419.

40. Francque SMA, Verrijken AN, Mertens I, Hubens G, Marck EV, Pelckmans P, Michielsen P, Gaal LV. Noninvasive assessment of nonalcoholic fatty liver disease in obese or overweight patients. *Clin Gastroenterol Hepatol* 2012; 10: 1162–1168.

41. Castera L, Foucher J, Bernard PH, Carvalho F, Allaix D, Merrouche W, Couzigou P, de Ledinghen V. Pitfalls of liver stiffness measurement: A 5-year prospective study of 13,369 examinations. *Hepatology* 2010; 51: 828–835.

42. Myers RP, Pomier-Layrargues G, Kisch R, Pollett A, Beaton M, Levstik M, Duarte-Rojo A, Wong D, Crotty P, Elkashab M. Discordance in fibrosis staging between liver biopsy and transient elastography using the FibroScan XL probe. *J Hepatol* 2012; 56(3): 564–570.

43. Brunt EM, Janney CG, Di Bisceglie AM, Neuschwander-Tetri BA, Bacon BR. Nonalcoholic steatohepatitis: A proposal for grading and staging the histological lesions. *Am J Gastroenterol* 1999; 94(9): 2467–2474.

44. Noureddin M, Loomba R. Nonalcoholic fatty liver disease: Indications for liver biopsy and noninvasive biomarkers. *Clin Liver Dis* 2012; 1(4): 104–107.

45. Adams LA, Feldstein AE. Non-invasive diagnosis of nonalcoholic fatty liver and nonalcoholic steatohepatitis. *J Dig Dis* 2011; 12: 10–16.

46. Kim CH, Younossi ZM. Nonalcoholic fatty liver disease: A manifestation of the metabolic syndrome. *Cleve Clin J M* 2008; 75(10): 721–728.

47. Starley BQ, Calcagno CJ, Harrison SA. Nonalcoholic fatty liver disease and hepatocellular carcinoma: A weighty connection. *Hepatology* 2010; 51: 1820–1832.

48. O'Leary JG, Landaverde C, Jennings L, Goldstein RM, Davis GL. Patients with NASH and cryptogenic cirrhosis are less likely than those with hepatitis C to receive liver transplants. *Clin Gastroenterol Hepatol* 2011; 9(8): 700–704.

49. Patil DT, Yerian LM. Evolution of nonalcoholic fatty liver disease recurrence after liver transplantation. *Liver Transpl* 2012; 18: 1147–1153.

50. Promrat K, Kleiner DE, Niemeier HM, Jackvony E, Kearns M, Wands JR, Fava JL, Wing RR. Randomized controlled trial testing the effects of weight loss on nonalcoholic steatohepatitis. *Hepatology* 2010; 51(1): 121–129.

51. Kirk E, Reeds DN, Finck BN, Mayurranjan SM, Patterson BW, Klein S. Dietary fat and carbohydrates differentially alter insulin sensitivity during caloric restriction. *Gastroenterology* 2009; 136(5): 1552–1560.

52. Zivkovic AM, German JB, Sanyal AJ. Comparative review of diets for the metabolic syndrome: Implications for nonalcoholic fatty liver disease. *Am J Clin Nutr* 2007; 86: 285–300.

53. Molloy JW, Calcagno CJ, Williams CD, Jones FJ, Torres DM, Harrison SA. Association of coffee and caffeine consumption with fatty liver disease, nonalcoholic steatohepatitis, and degree of hepatic fibrosis. *Hepatology* 2012; 55(2): 429–436.

54. Harrison SA, Fecht W, Brunt EM, Neuschwander-Tetri BA. Orlistat for overweight subjects with nonalcoholic steatohepatitis: A randomized, prospective trial. *Hepatology* 2009; 49(1): 80–86.

55. Bradley D, Magkos F, Klein S. Effects of bariatric surgery on glucose homeostasis and type 2 diabetes. *Gastroenterology* 2012; 143: 897–912.

56. Mathurin P, Hollebecque A, Arnalsteen L, Buob D, Leteurtre E, Caiazzo R, Pigeyre M, Verkindt H, Dharancy S, Louvet A, Romon M, Pattou F. Prospective study of the long-term effects of bariatric surgery on liver injury in patients without advanced disease. *Gastroenterology* 2009; 137(2): 532–540.

57. Chavez-Tapia NC, Tellez-Avila FI, Barrientos-Gutierrez T, Mendez-Sanchez N, Lizardi-Cervera J, Uribe M. Bariatric surgery for non-alcoholic steatohepatitis in obese patients. *Cochrane Database Syst Rev* 2010; 20(1): CD007340.

58. Bugianesi E, Gentilcore E, Manini R, Natale S, Vanni E, Villanova N, David E, Rizzetto M, Marchesini G. A randomized controlled trial of metformin versus vitamin E or prescriptive diet in nonalcoholic fatty liver disease. *Am J Gastroenterology* 2005; 100: 1082–1090.

59. Loomba R, Lutchman G, Kleiner DE, Ricks M, Feld JJ, Borg BB, Modi A, Nagabhyru P, Sumner AE, Liang TJ, Hoofnagle JH. Clinical trial: Pilot study of metformin for the treatment of non-alcoholic steatohepatitis. *Aliment Pharmacol Ther* 2009; 29(2): 172–182.

60. Shields WW, Thompson KE, Grice SA, Harrison SA, Coyle WJ. The effect of metformin and standard therapy versus standard therapy alone in nondiabetic patients with insulin resistance and nonalcoholic steatohepatitis (NASH): A pilot trial. *Therap Adv Gastroenterol* 2009; 2(3): 157–163.

61. Belfort R, Harrison SA, Brown K, Darland C, Finch J, Hardies J, Balas B, Gastaldelli A, Tio F, Pulcini J, Berria R, Ma JZ, Dwivedi S, Havranek R, Fincke C, DeFronzo R, Bannayan GA, Schenker S, Cusi K. A placebo-controlled trial of pioglitazone in subjects with nonalcoholic steatohepatitis. *N Engl J Med* 2006; 355: 2297–2307.

62. Aithal GP, Thomas JA, Kaye PV, Lawson A, Ryder SD, Spendlove I, Austin AS, Freeman JG, Morgan L, Webber J. Randomized, placebo-controlled trial of pioglitazone in nondiabetic subjects with nonalcoholic steatohepatitis. *Gastroenterology* 2008; 135: 1176–1184.

63. Lutchman G, Apurva M, Kleiner DE, Promrat K, Heller T, Ghany M, Borg B, Loomba R, Liang TJ, Premkumar A, Hoofnagle JH. The effects of discontinuing pioglitazone in patients with nonalcoholic steatohepatitis. *Hepatology* 2007; 46: 424–429.

64. Kenny PR, Brady DE, Torres DM, Ragozzino L, Chalasani N, Harrison SA. Exenatide in the treatment of diabetic patients with non-alcoholic steatohepatitis: A case series. *Am J Gastroenterol* 2010; 105: 2707–2709.

65. Boettcher E, Csako G, Pucino F, Wesley R, Loomba R. Meta-analysis: Pioglitazone improves liver histology and fibrosis in patients with non-alcoholic steatohepatitis. *Aliment Pharmacol Ther* 2012; 35(1): 66–75.

66. Sanyal AJ, Chalasani N, Kowdley KV, McCullough A, Diehl AM, Bass NM, Neuschwander-Tetri BA, Lavine JE, Tonascia J, Unalp A, Van Natta M, Clark J, Brunt EM, Kleiner DE, Hoofnagle JH, Robuck PR. Pioglitazone, vitamin E, or placebo for nonalcoholic steatohepatitis. *N Engl J Med* 2010; 362: 1675–1685.

67. Lavine JE, Schwimmer JB, Van Natta ML, Molleston JP, Murray KF, Rosenthal P, Abrams SH, Scheimann AO, Sanyal AJ, Chalasani N, Tonascia J, Unalp A, Clark JM, Brunt EM, Kleiner DE, Hoofnagle JH, Robuck PR. Effect of vitamin E or metformin for treatment of nonalcoholic fatty liver disease in children and adolescents. The TONIC randomized controlled trial. *JAMA* 2011; 305(16): 1659–1668.

68. Abdelmalek MF, Sanderson SO, Angulo P, Soldevila-Pico C, Liu C, Peter J, Keach J, Cave M, Chen T, McClain CJ, Lindor KD. Betaine for nonalcoholic fatty liver disease: Results of a randomized placebo-controlled trial. *Hepatology* 2009; 50(6): 1818–1826.

69. Zein CO, Yerian LM, Gogate P, Lopez R, Kirwan JP, Feldstein AE, McCullough AJ. Pentoxifylline improves nonalcoholic steatohepatitis: A randomized placebo-controlled trial. *Hepatology* 2011; 54(5): 1610–1619.

6 Insulin, the Glycemic Index, and Carcinogenesis

*Livia S.A. Augustin, Cyril W.C. Kendall, Arash Mirrahimi,
Stephanie Nishi, and David J.A. Jenkins*

CONTENTS

INTRODUCTION

Cancer is the second leading cause of death after heart disease in developed countries and the third in developing countries accounting for 7.6 million deaths or 20% of all deaths globally from noncommunicable diseases [1]. Considerable evidence suggests an involvement of environmental causes including diet in the etiology of cancer. A 20-fold variation in cancer rates has been observed across geographic regions for several cancer types, and migrant studies have shown an increase in the risk for cancer in migrants from low-risk areas that approximates that of the host population [2–4]. McKeown-Eyssen [5] and Giovannucci [6] independently suggested that hyperglycemia and hyperinsulinemia may be important factors in promoting malignant transformation and tumor growth. Clinical conditions related to impaired glucose tolerance and insulin resistance including type 2 diabetes, obesity, the metabolic syndrome, and polycystic ovarian syndrome have been associated with greater risk of cancer at various sites. These conditions share similar metabolic risk factors including hyperglycemia, hyperinsulinemia, higher inflammatory markers, and unfavorable adipokine profiles, which may also be shared by cancer [7–9]. Metformin, a diabetic medication that reduces hyperglycemia and improves insulin resistance, significantly reduced total cancer incidence and mortality by 33% in people with type 2 diabetes [8] and cancer-related mortality in people with concomitant type 2 diabetes and cancer [10]. Carbohydrates are the dietary factors that primarily raise blood glucose and insulin levels, and they have been implicated in the etiology of cancer at various sites [6,11]. However, evidence suggests that different carbohydrates may impact cancer development differently, and hence, it has been proposed that the nature of the carbohydrates consumed, i.e., the glycemic index (GI), by virtue of differences in glycemic raising potential, may affect carcinogenesis differently [12].

CANCER

The word *cancer*, derived from the Latin for crab due to its crab-like growth in tissues, was first described in the books by Hippocrates (400 BC). Cancer is a complex disease of cells involving initially an accumulation of DNA mutations in critical genes of normal cells. Many cancer types arise

133

as a consequence of mutations, methylation/demethylation, in cellular proto-oncogenes and tumor-suppressor genes. The ability of DNA to change is central to its capacity to evolve and adapt to environmental pressures. For this reason, some believe that cancer is the price to pay for the long-term adaptability of the human species. Cancer concerns cells that are replicating, and hence, tissues that are more prone to develop cancer are those with higher replication rates such as those that interact more directly with the environment (skin, lungs, digestive tract), those that secrete hormones (breast, liver, and pancreas), and those involved in reproduction (endometrium, ovary, prostate). Bones and muscle cells have low replication rates in adults and higher in children, and hence, cancer in these tissues tends to be less frequent in adults compared to children. In youth, however, cancers tend to be mostly of genetic etiology due to the low environmental exposures. Experimentally, carcinogenesis is divided in at least three phases: initiation, promotion, and progression. The initiation phase is characterized by an acute damage to the genome. When this damage escapes the endogenous (e.g., body's own defenses) and exogenous or environmental protective mechanisms, DNA adducts then accumulate over time and a neoplasm may form. Of all the environmental mechanisms, diet has been proposed to be a large contributor. In 1914 Rous first observed that food restriction in mice reduced tumor metastasis [13], in the 1920's some observations suggested that obesity was associated with greater cancer mortality and in the 1930's high plant food consumption was suggested to reduce the chance of developing cancer [14]. In the 1980s, Doll and Peto [15] attempted to quantify the cancer risk attributable to various environmental causes and estimated that approximately 35% of cancer deaths could be avoided by dietary modifications alone [15]. This seems to still hold true today [16,17]. Dietary factors may affect cancer in both protecting and promoting growth and may have direct effects on initiation and/or promotion of cancers. The luminal effects of food components in the gastrointestinal tract may have direct or indirect effects by affecting systemic nutrient surges and altering hormonal and inflammatory pathways that alter risk for cancers of the breast, prostate, pancreas, liver, and endometrium. Red meat and food-derived heterocyclic amines found in processed meat are linked to increased cancer rates, particularly colon cancer, and to total cancer mortality [17–20]. Free radicals generated from dietary metabolic processes are known to result in DNA damage and produce genetic mutations [21]. Of the cancer protective dietary factors, vegetables, particularly of the brassica family, fruit, particularly citrus fruits, and whole grains have shown the strongest protective effects [18].

INSULIN

Insulin is a hormone produced by the beta cells in the islets of Langerhans, a region representing approximately 2% of the pancreas. Insulin release is stimulated by glucose and amino acid levels in the blood and by gut hormones produced by gastrointestinal cells during the ingestion of dietary carbohydrates and proteins. Preproinsulin is first produced in the beta cells and then converted into proinsulin, which in turn is converted into insulin releasing a carboxyl-peptide called C-peptide, which can be detected in the blood circulation and is considered a able marker of overall insulin release. Insulin is responsible for the uptake of glucose from the circulation to various tissues (muscle, adipose tissue, liver, heart) by binding to the insulin receptor, which produces a cascade of phosphorylation reactions. These reactions ultimately are responsible for the translocation of glucose transporters (e.g., GLUT-4 present in muscle and adipose tissue) from the inner cell to the cell surface, where it fuses with the plasma membrane allowing glucose to enter the cell and be used for energy production (ATP synthesis). In insulin resistance, the insulin receptors are often underfunctioning, and hence, more insulin is released by the pancreas to maintain normal blood glucose levels. This state is called compensatory hyperinsulinemia. When insulin resistance worsens or the pancreas produces less insulin than required to maintain normal blood glucose levels, impaired fasting or impaired postprandial hyperglycemia results. These conditions generally precede type 2 diabetes by a long time. Insulin is a growth hormone and may directly stimulate cancer promotion and progression, as suggested by in vitro and animal studies [22,23], or indirectly by enhancing the activity of other proteins and hormones with proliferating activity such as insulin-like growth factor-I (IGF-I) [24] and estrogen [25]. In turn, IGF-I may stimulate estrogen activity [26], and both IGF-I and estrogen may be cancer promoters and cancer risk factors [27–29]. Most cancer cells express both insulin receptors and IGF-I receptors.

GLYCEMIC INDEX AND CANCER

Dietary carbohydrates have been implicated in the etiology of cancer, however evidence suggests that the impact of carbohydrates on cancer risk may differ with different carbohydrate sources, hence, it has been proposed that the glycemic-raising nature of the carbohydrates consumed, i.e., the GI, may play a role in carcinogenesis [12]. The hypothesis is that high GI foods by virtue of their higher postprandial blood glucose responses may, in the long term, adversely affect cancer initiation, promotion, and/or progression. The dietary GI is a classification of carbohydrate foods based on postprandial blood glucose responses, where the low GI foods result in lower rises of blood glucose and insulin mainly due to the slower rate of carbohydrate absorption, whereas the high GI foods result in higher peaks and larger fluctuations for the same amount of carbohydrate ingested [30]. The GI methodology is recognized and described by the International Standards Organization (ISO 26642:2010) and by the World Health Organization [31]. The GI concept has been accepted by a number of health organizations worldwide, such as the World Health Organization, the International Diabetes Federation, the Canadian Diabetes Association, the European Association for the Study of Diabetes, and Dietary Guidelines for Healthy Living in India [31–35]. Whether a carbohydrate food may be high or low GI depends on many factors, which are characteristics of the carbohydrate food and not of the subject consuming it. Those factors that result in a low GI include type and amount of dietary fiber (higher viscous fiber), type of starch (higher amylose-to-amylopectin ratio), particle size of the grains (larger particles, whole kernels), food processing (cooling after cooking, cooking starch less, as in pasta al dente), macronutrients (higher protein and fat), and presence of organic acids such as vinegar [36]. Therefore, the GIs of different foods consumed in equicarbohydrate amounts vary and are summarized in the international GI tables [37]. A related topic is the glycemic load (GL), which has been developed for epidemiological studies to give an overall measure of the glycemic and insulinemic potential of the diet; hence, in this context, it is calculated as the daily average GI of a person's diet multiplied by the grams of total available carbohydrate consumed [38].

Many clinical trials indicate that consuming low GI diets instead of high GI diets has metabolic advantages including improvements in blood glucose, insulin, cholesterol, antioxidant defenses, and inflammatory markers [39–46]. Epidemiological studies suggest that low GI and GL diets are linked to lower risk of type 2 diabetes, coronary heart disease, and cancer [47–49]. Specifically investigating the dietary GI in cancer risk, the initial studies on colorectal and breast cancer suggested a protective effect of low GI diets compared to higher GI diets in populations with high carbohydrate intakes [50,51] and in others [52]. More recently, a meta-analysis and a subsequent case-control study on a large cancer database have confirmed some of the original findings with mild associations mainly for cancers of the breast [47,53], colorectum [53,54], and possibly prostate [54]. Furthermore, when investigating the association with cancer risk of two carbohydrate foods at the opposite end of the GI spectrum—pasta (low GI) and white bread (high GI)—it was found that bread increased breast and colorectal cancer risk, and pasta showed no association [55]. In the colorectal study, after stratifying by sex, no significant associations were seen in men with either bread or pasta while women were at two-fold increased risk of developing colorectal cancer when consuming higher intakes of white bread (odds ratio [OR]: 2.02, confidence interval [CI]: 1.46–2.80, P for trend = 0.0002), while pasta was of borderline statistical significance (OR: 1.37, CI: 1.00–1.88, P for trend < 0.164), regardless of their menopausal status or body mass index (BMI). In the breast cancer study, white bread but not pasta increased breast cancer risk in women albeit only in post-menopausal women and in those with high BMI (>25 kg/m^2) [55].

Possible mechanisms for the potential link between dietary GI and cancer risk may involve the IGF axis, and indeed low GI foods have been found to favorably increase the major binding protein IGFBP-3, which binds IGF-I, thus reducing its bioavailability [56]. Furthermore, free radical-dependent DNA damage is considered a major contributor to cancer initiation [57,58], and a link between postprandial glycemia and oxidative stress has been proposed through glucose-dependent mitochondrial free radical generation [59]. Several studies by Brownlee [59] and Ceriello et al. [60], independently, have documented the acute effects of an oral glucose load on increased oxidative stress measures that may be improved by taking antioxidants. Furthermore, large glycemic fluctuations may induce oxidative stress to a greater extent than in steady hyperglycemia [61]. These studies suggest that a high dietary GI by virtue of greater glucose fluctuations may be a source of oxidative stress and deplete antioxidant defenses. Botero et al. have shown that 1-week consumption of a low GI diet, compared to a high GI control diet, resulted in significantly greater total antioxidant economy in 12 young overweight and obese men [62]. Interestingly, slowing carbohydrate absorption and hence mimicking a low GI diet by use of the diabetes drug acarbose, an alpha-glucosidase inhibitor, significantly lowered oxidative stress [63]. Similarly, metformin, which improves insulin resistance/hyperglycemia and is associated with lower cancer incidence and mortality, has also been shown to reduce markers of oxidative stress [64].

Other mechanisms have been proposed for the metabolic benefits and disease risk reduction associated with low GI diets. High BMI is a risk factor for many cancers, and several clinical trials have shown body weight reductions with the consumption of low GI diets [43,65] and also in studies where weight loss was not the aim [41,42]. Fibrinolytic activity, which is generally linked to thrombosis, may also be linked to carcinogenesis [66] and was improved on low GI compared to high GI diets with reductions in plasminogen activator inhibitor-1 of up to 50% in people with type 2 diabetes [67,68]. Inflammation may play a stimulating role in cancer progression, and clinical trial evidence suggests a reduction in inflammatory markers (C-reactive protein) of up to 30% of baseline levels with low GI diets [39,46,69].

CONCLUSIONS

Overall, evidence suggests that alterations in the nature of dietary carbohydrates and hence in the rate of carbohydrate absorption may have important physiological and pathological consequences by, for example, modifying free radical generation. Some of the mechanisms by which low GI foods may confer protection in diabetes and cardiovascular disease development and complications, such as reducing insulin levels, may also play a role in carcinogenesis. However, more studies, particularly clinical trials, are required to test the hypothesis of a possible protective role of low GI diets in carcinogenesis by virtue of their lower glucose- and insulin-raising potential.

REFERENCES

1. World Health Organization (WHO). *Global Status Report on Noncommunicable Diseases 2010—Description of the Global Burden of NCDs, Their Risk Factors and Determinants.* Geneva, Switzerland: WHO, 2011. Available from: http://whqlibdoc.who.int/publications/2011/9789240686458_eng .pdf, Accessed December 2013.
2. King H, Li JY, Locke FB, Pollack ES, Tu JT. Patterns of site-specific displacement in cancer mortality among migrants: The Chinese in the United States. *Am J Public Health.* 1985;75(3):237–42.
3. Rastogi T, Devesa S, Mangtani P et al. Cancer incidence rates among South Asians in four geographic regions: India, Singapore, UK and US. *Int J Epidemiol.* 2008;37(1):147–60.
4. Ziegler RG, Hoover RN, Pike MC et al. Migration patterns and breast cancer risk in Asian-American women. *J Natl Cancer Inst.* 1993;85(22):1819–27.
5. McKeown-Eyssen G. Epidemiology of colorectal cancer revisited: Are serum triglycerides and/or plasma glucose associated with risk? *Cancer Epidemiol Biomarkers Prev.* 1994;3(8):687–95.
6. Giovannucci E. Insulin and colon cancer. *Cancer Causes Control.* 1995;6(2):164–79.

7. Giovannucci E, Harlan DM, Archer MC et al. Diabetes and cancer: A consensus report. *Diabetes Care.* 2010;33(7):1674–85.
8. Noto H, Goto A, Tsujimoto T, Noda M. Cancer risk in diabetic patients treated with metformin: A systematic review and meta-analysis. *PLoS One.* 2012;7(3):e33411.
9. Stattin P, Bjor O, Ferrari P et al. Prospective study of hyperglycemia and cancer risk. *Diabetes Care.* 2007;30(3):561–7.
10. Yin M, Zhou J, Gorak EJ, Quddus F. Metformin is associated with survival benefit in cancer patients with concurrent type 2 diabetes: A systematic review and meta-analysis. *Oncologist.* 2013;18(12):1248–55.
11. Franceschi S, Favero A, La Vecchia C et al. Food groups and risk of colorectal cancer in Italy. *Int J Cancer.* 1997;72(1):56–61.
12. Augustin LS, Franceschi S, Jenkins DJ, Kendall CW, La Vecchia C. Glycemic index in chronic disease: A review. *Eur J Clin Nutr.* 2002;56(11):1049–71.
13. Rous P. The influence of diet on transplanted and spontaneous mouse tumors. *J Exp Med.* 1914;20(5):433–51.
14. Stock P, Karn MN. A co-operative study of the habits, home life, dietary and family histories of 450 cancer patients and of an equal number of control patients. *Ann Eugen Human Genet.* 1933;5:30–3.
15. Doll R, Peto R. The causes of cancer: Quantitative estimates of avoidable risks of cancer in the United States today. *J Natl Cancer Inst.* 1981;66(6):1191–308.
16. McCullough ML, Giovannucci EL. Diet and cancer prevention. *Oncogene.* 2004;23(38):6349–64.
17. Willett WC. Diet, nutrition, and avoidable cancer. *Environ Health Perspect.* 1995;103 Suppl 8:165–70.
18. Kushi LH, Doyle C, McCullough M et al. American Cancer Society guidelines on nutrition and physical activity for cancer prevention: Reducing the risk of cancer with healthy food choices and physical activity. *CA Cancer J Clin.* 2012;62(1):30–67.
19. Pan A, Sun Q, Bernstein AM et al. Red meat consumption and mortality: Results from 2 prospective cohort studies. *Arch Intern Med.* 2012;172(7):555–63.
20. Santarelli RL, Pierre F, Corpet DE. Processed meat and colorectal cancer: A review of epidemiologic and experimental evidence. *Nutr Cancer.* 2008;60(2):131–44.
21. Ames BN, Gold LS. Endogenous mutagens and the causes of aging and cancer. *Mutat Res.* 1991;250(1–2):3–16.
22. Bjork J, Nilsson J, Hultcrantz R, Johansson C. Growth-regulatory effects of sensory neuropeptides, epidermal growth factor, insulin, and somatostatin on the non-transformed intestinal epithelial cell line IEC-6 and the colon cancer cell line HT 29. *Scand J Gastroenterol.* 1993;28(10):879–84.
23. Tran TT, Medline A, Bruce WR. Insulin promotion of colon tumors in rats. *Cancer Epidemiol Biomarkers Prev.* 1996;5(12):1013–15.
24. Ullrich A, Gray A, Tam AW et al. Insulin-like growth factor I receptor primary structure: Comparison with insulin receptor suggests structural determinants that define functional specificity. *EMBO J.* 1986;5(10):2503–12.
25. Nestler JE, Powers LP, Matt DW et al. A direct effect of hyperinsulinemia on serum sex hormone-binding globulin levels in obese women with the polycystic ovary syndrome. *J Clin Endocrinol Metab.* 1991;72(1):83–9.
26. Plymate SR, Hoop RC, Jones RE, Matej LA. Regulation of sex hormone-binding globulin production by growth factors. *Metabolism.* 1990;39(9):967–70.
27. Giovannucci E. Nutrition, insulin, insulin-like growth factors and cancer. *Horm Metab Res.* 2003;35(11–12):694–704.
28. Kaaks R, Lukanova A. Energy balance and cancer: The role of insulin and insulin-like growth factor-I. *Proc Nutr Soc.* 2001;60(1):91–106.
29. Parazzini F, La Vecchia C, Bocciolone L, Franceschi S. The epidemiology of endometrial cancer. *Gynecol Oncol.* 1991;41(1):1–16.
30. Jenkins DJ, Wolever TM, Taylor RH et al. Glycemic index of foods: A physiological basis for carbohydrate exchange. *Am J Clin Nutr.* 1981;34(3):362–6.
31. WHO. Carbohydrates in human nutrition. Report of a joint FAO/WHO expert consultation. *FAO Food Nutr Pap.* 1998;66:1–140.
32. Ceriello A, Colagiuri S. International Diabetes Federation guideline for management of postmeal glucose: A review of recommendations. *Diabet Med.* 2008;25(10):1151–6.
33. Mann JI, De Leeuw I, Hermansen K et al. Evidence-based nutritional approaches to the treatment and prevention of diabetes mellitus. *Nutr Metab Cardiovasc Dis.* 2004;14(6):373–94.
34. Misra A, Sharma R, Gulati S et al. Consensus dietary guidelines for healthy living and prevention of obesity, the metabolic syndrome, diabetes, and related disorders in Asian Indians. *Diabetes Technol Ther.* 2011;13(6):683–94.

35. Sievenpiper JL, Dworatzek PD. Food and dietary pattern-based recommendations: An emerging approach to clinical practice guidelines for nutrition therapy in diabetes. *Can J Diabetes*. 2013;37(1):51–7.
36. Jenkins DJ, Kendall CW, Augustin LS et al. Glycemic index: Overview of implications in health and disease. *Am J Clin Nutr*. 2002;76(1):266S–73S.
37. Atkinson FS, Foster-Powell K, Brand-Miller JC. International tables of glycemic index and glycemic load values: 2008. *Diabetes Care*. 2008;31(12):2281–3.
38. Salmeron J, Manson JE, Stampfer MJ, Colditz GA, Wing AL, Willett WC. Dietary fiber, glycemic load, and risk of non-insulin-dependent diabetes mellitus in women. *JAMA*. 1997;277(6):472–7.
39. Brand-Miller J, Hayne S, Petocz P, Colagiuri S. Low-glycemic index diets in the management of diabetes: A meta-analysis of randomized controlled trials. *Diabetes Care*. 2003;26(8):2261–7.
40. Goff LM, Cowland DE, Hooper L, Frost GS. Low glycaemic index diets and blood lipids: A systematic review and meta-analysis of randomised controlled trials. *Nutr Metab Cardiovasc Dis*. 2013;23(1):1–10.
41. Jenkins DJ, Kendall CW, Augustin LS et al. Effect of legumes as part of a low glycemic index diet on glycemic control and cardiovascular risk factors in type 2 diabetes mellitus: A randomized controlled trial. *Arch Intern Med*. 2012;172(21):1653–60.
42. Jenkins DJ, Kendall CW, McKeown-Eyssen G et al. Effect of a low-glycemic index or a high-cereal fiber diet on type 2 diabetes: A randomized trial. *JAMA*. 2008;300(23):2742–53.
43. Larsen TM, Dalskov SM, van Baak M et al. Diets with high or low protein content and glycemic index for weight-loss maintenance. *N Engl J Med*. 2010;363(22):2102–13.
44. McMillan-Price J, Petocz P, Atkinson F et al. Comparison of 4 diets of varying glycemic load on weight loss and cardiovascular risk reduction in overweight and obese young adults: A randomized controlled trial. *Arch Intern Med*. 2006;166(14):1466–75.
45. Rizkalla SW, Taghrid L, Laromiguiere M et al. Improved plasma glucose control, whole-body glucose utilization, and lipid profile on a low-glycemic index diet in type 2 diabetic men: A randomized controlled trial. *Diabetes Care*. 2004;27(8):1866–72.
46. Wolever TM, Gibbs AL, Mehling C et al. The Canadian trial of carbohydrates in diabetes (CCD), a 1-y controlled trial of low-glycemic-index dietary carbohydrate in type 2 diabetes: No effect on glycated hemoglobin but reduction in C-reactive protein. *Am J Clin Nutr*. 2008;87(1):114–25.
47. Barclay AW, Petocz P, McMillan-Price J et al. Glycemic index, glycemic load, and chronic disease risk—A meta-analysis of observational studies. *Am J Clin Nutr*. 2008;87(3):627–37.
48. Ma XY, Liu JP, Song ZY. Glycemic load, glycemic index and risk of cardiovascular diseases: Meta-analyses of prospective studies. *Atherosclerosis*. 2012;223(2):491–6.
49. Mirrahimi A, de Souza RJ, Chiavaroli L et al. Associations of glycemic index and load with coronary heart disease events: A systematic review and meta-analysis of prospective cohorts. *J Am Heart Assoc*. 2012;1(5):e000752.
50. Augustin LS, Dal Maso L, La Vecchia C et al. Dietary glycemic index and glycemic load, and breast cancer risk: A case-control study. *Ann Oncol*. 2001;12(11):1533–8.
51. Franceschi S, Dal Maso L, Augustin L et al. Dietary glycemic load and colorectal cancer risk. *Ann Oncol*. 2001;12(2):173–8.
52. Higginbotham S, Zhang ZF, Lee IM et al. Dietary glycemic load and risk of colorectal cancer in the women's health study. *J Natl Cancer Inst*. 2004;96(3):229–33.
53. Choi Y, Giovannucci E, Lee JE. Glycaemic index and glycaemic load in relation to risk of diabetes-related cancers: A meta-analysis. *Br J Nutr*. 2012;108(11):1934–47.
54. Hu J, La Vecchia C, Augustin LS et al. Glycemic index, glycemic load and cancer risk. *Ann Oncol*. 2013;24(1):245–51.
55. Augustin LS, Malerba S, Lugo A et al. Associations of bread and pasta with the risk of cancer of the breast and colorectum. *Ann Oncol*. 2013;24(12):3094–9.
56. Brand-Miller JC, Liu V, Petocz P, Baxter RC. The glycemic index of foods influences postprandial insulin-like growth factor-binding protein responses in lean young subjects. *Am J Clin Nutr*. 2005;82(2):350–4.
57. Beckman KB, Ames BN. Oxidative decay of DNA. *J Biol Chem*. 1997;272(32):19633–6.
58. Halliwell B. Oxidative stress and cancer: Have we moved forward? *Biochem J*. 2007;401(1):1–11.
59. Brownlee M. The pathobiology of diabetic complications: A unifying mechanism. *Diabetes*. 2005;54(6):1615–25.
60. Ceriello A, Bortolotti N, Motz E et al. Meal-induced oxidative stress and low-density lipoprotein oxidation in diabetes: The possible role of hyperglycemia. *Metabolism*. 1999;48(12):1503–8.
61. Monnier L, Mas E, Ginet C et al. Activation of oxidative stress by acute glucose fluctuations compared with sustained chronic hyperglycemia in patients with type 2 diabetes. *JAMA*. 2006;295(14):1681–7.

62. Botero D, Ebbeling CB, Blumberg JB et al. Acute effects of dietary glycemic index on antioxidant capacity in a nutrient-controlled feeding study. *Obesity (Silver Spring)*. 2009;17(9):1664–70.
63. Inoue I, Shinoda Y, Nakano T et al. Acarbose ameliorates atherogenecity of low-density lipoprotein in patients with impaired glucose tolerance. *Metabolism*. 2006;55(7):946–52.
64. Tessier D, Maheux P, Khalil A, Fulop T. Effects of gliclazide versus metformin on the clinical profile and lipid peroxidation markers in type 2 diabetes. *Metabolism*. 1999;48(7):897–903.
65. Ebbeling CB, Leidig MM, Sinclair KB, Seger-Shippee LG, Feldman HA, Ludwig DS. Effects of an ad libitum low-glycemic load diet on cardiovascular disease risk factors in obese young adults. *Am J Clin Nutr*. 2005;81(5):976–82.
66. Rakic JM, Maillard C, Jost M et al. Role of plasminogen activator-plasmin system in tumor angiogenesis. *Cell Mol Life Sci*. 2003;60(3):463–73.
67. Jarvi AE, Karlstrom BE, Granfeldt YE, Bjorck IE, Asp NG, Vessby BO. Improved glycemic control and lipid profile and normalized fibrinolytic activity on a low-glycemic index diet in type 2 diabetic patients. *Diabetes Care*. 1999;22(1):10–18.
68. Jensen L, Sloth B, Krog-Mikkelsen I et al. A low-glycemic-index diet reduces plasma plasminogen activator inhibitor-1 activity, but not tissue inhibitor of proteinases-1 or plasminogen activator inhibitor-1 protein, in overweight women. *Am J Clin Nutr*. 2008;87(1):97–105.
69. Gogebakan O, Kohl A, Osterhoff MA et al. Effects of weight loss and long-term weight maintenance with diets varying in protein and glycemic index on cardiovascular risk factors: The diet, obesity, and genes (DiOGenes) study: A randomized, controlled trial. *Circulation*. 2011;124(25):2829–38.

7 Nutrition and Cardiovascular Disease

Miguel A. Martinez-Gonzalez and Maira Bes-Rastrollo

CONTENTS

INTRODUCTION: CARDIOVASCULAR PREVENTION IN THE TWENTY-FIRST CENTURY

Cardiovascular disease (CVD) is the leading component of noncommunicable diseases (NCDs). Atherosclerotic and hypertensive diseases, mainly ischemic heart disease and stroke together with heart failure, whether resulting from ischemic heart disease or other causes, are the major CVD entities and represent the most important threats for population health in the twenty-first century. Ischemic heart disease and stroke have been projected for the year 2020 to rank first and second in frequency among causes of death, first and third among causes of years of life lost, and first and fourth among causes of disability-adjusted years of life lost, respectively [1]. In summary, CVD still remains the leading cause of death worldwide and a major cause of disability [1]. Furthermore, the projections of mortality from CVD for 2030 are somber and cumbersome [2].

Therefore, CVD constitutes a global health crisis and has a ubiquitous occurrence [3]. In addition to the well-known burden of mortality and disability caused by CVD in high-income countries, the important high-level Meeting of the United Nations General Assembly on NCDs held in September 2011 denounced that CVD will exert a devastating impact specifically on the working-age populations (ages 35–64 years) of low- and middle-income countries by the year 2030 [4].

In this dramatic context, the available evidence to support that most of the burden of CVD is preventable through diet and lifestyle is huge [2,5]. For no other chronic condition is there such a large body of scientific evidence on the effectiveness of preventive approaches. This body of evidence is mainly based on good-quality prospective observational cohorts and also on a few large randomized trials. Therefore, the prevention of CVD through diet and lifestyle, without any doubt, represents an absolute priority for public health. Diet is especially relevant in cardiovascular prevention, and consequently, the assessment of the *diet-heart hypothesis* has been one of the most active research areas in nutritional epidemiology during the last 50 years [6,7]. The identification and targeting of dietary factors with the greatest potential for preventing CVD are of major scientific and public health importance.

Substantial advances in understanding the role of specific nutritional factors as determinants of CVD have accrued during the last two decades. The priority of overall food patterns over single foods or individual nutrients, the importance of carbohydrate quality rather than quantity, and the specific roles of each fat subtype, some foods or their combination, sodium intake, and total energy balance represent several key findings of interest. In the present chapter, we summarize the current understanding of dietary factors as determinants of the occurrence of CVD.

HARD CLINICAL END POINTS

Many studies of nutritional epidemiology conducted to assess the diet-heart hypothesis have used as end point intermediate biomarkers of cardiovascular risk (reductions in blood pressure [BP], changes in lipids, inflammatory molecules, or other biomarkers) as a proxy for the risk of ischemic heart disease or stroke.

This approach could be flawed for several reasons [8]. In the first place, the existence of multiple pathways leading from diet to heart disease speaks against the simplistic approach of giving a high value to changes in any single biomarker. Second, the induction period can be variable for the different pathways in which diverse biomarkers are involved, and this fact severely limits the possibility of assessing at any time point any multiple combinations of biomarkers. Third, probably there are other pathways that are still less well known and can account for a substantial proportion of clinical events.

Therefore, the most sensible approach to investigate the diet-heart hypothesis is the use of hard clinical events as the end point. In the present review, we will specially highlight the results of studies assessing hard clinical events.

FOOD PATTERNS

In nutritional epidemiology, food pattern analysis is a methodological approach that captures different combinations of food intake and better reflects the complexity of the diet and its relationships with disease risk. Food pattern analysis has mostly replaced the traditional single-nutrient analysis in relation to chronic diseases, because that traditional approach has been challenged by several conceptual and methodological limitations. When an outcome is likely to be caused by a single nutrient, an exclusive focus on that nutrient may be the optimal approach; however, CVD has been associated with many dietary factors, and the food pattern approach may be the most useful option because it goes beyond nutrients or foods and examines the effects of the overall diet [9]. The focus on isolated nutrients or single foods makes it difficult to take into account any interaction between them. Many foods are consumed together, and there can be a wide range of potential interactions between different nutrients and foods. Food patterns adequately capture between-food synergies. In this context, for the assessment of the association between dietary factors and CVD, to shift the focus to overall dietary patterns is more useful than the reductionist and overly optimistic approach of attributing all the effects to a single nutrient or food. It is very unlikely that the intake of a single nutrient or food could exert a sufficiently strong effect as to substantially change the incidence rates of CVD. Conversely, the additive effect of small changes in many nutrients is more likely to show an effect.

In summary, the current paradigm in nutritional epidemiology is to use food pattern analysis instead of other classical analytical approaches focused on single nutrients. In addition, dietary patterns overcome problems of confounding by other aspects of the diet.

In the next paragraphs, we review the key components of food patterns that have been consistently shown to behave as determinants of CVD risk in high-quality longitudinal observational studies and large clinical trials.

VEGETABLES AND FRUITS

Food patterns that emphasize the consumption of fruits and vegetables have been associated with substantial improvements in several vascular risk factors, including lipid levels, BP, insulin resistance, inflammatory biomarkers, endothelial function, and weight control [10–14]. These benefits might be derived from several sources: (a) the wide variety of phytochemicals, micronutrients, and fiber present in fruits and vegetables; (b) the potentially improved bioavailability of these nutrients in their natural state when fruits and vegetables are consumed as fresh foods instead of cooked; and (c) the replacement of less healthful foods in the diet by fruit and vegetables. In prospective cohorts, greater fruit and vegetable consumption is associated with lower incidence of coronary heart disease (CHD) and stroke. A meta-analysis conducted by Dauchet et al. [15] found stronger inverse associations with CHD for the consumption of fruit than for vegetable consumption. The meta-analysis by He et al. [16] showed an inverse dose–response trend between both fruit and vegetables consumption and the risk of CHD. A narrative review by Ness and Powles [17] and two meta-analyses support the inverse association of fruit or vegetable consumption with stroke risk [18,19]. The meta-analysis by Dauchet et al. [18] showed that stroke risk was reduced by 11% for each additional serving per day of fruit and by a nonsignificant 3% for each additional serving per day of vegetables. The estimates of relative risk (RR) in the meta-analysis by He et al. [19] were 0.72 (95% CI: 0.66, 0.79) for fruit and 0.81 (95% CI: 0.72, 0.90) for vegetables for the comparison between the highest (≥5 servings/day) and the lowest (<3 servings/day) categories of consumption.

Potential differences in health effects contributed by specific types of fruits, vegetables, or their juices require further investigation.

DIETARY FIBER AND WHOLE GRAIN CONSUMPTION

A pooled analysis of 11 cohort studies conducted by Pereira et al. [20] found that dietary fiber intake was inversely associated with the incidence of CHD events and also with CHD mortality. Each 10-g/day increment of energy-adjusted and measurement error-corrected total dietary fiber was associated with a 14% (RR of 0.86; 95% CI: 0.78–0.96) lower risk of all coronary events and a 27% (RR of 0.73; 95% CI: 0.61–0.87) relative reduction in the risk of coronary death.

Not only the fiber content but also the degree of cereals processing (i.e., refined versus whole grains) is apparently important regarding their ability to provide an effective prevention against CVD. The American Heart Association (AHA) developed a pragmatic definition of whole grains based on the fiber content of whole wheat, that is, ≥1.1 g of naturally occurring dietary fiber per 10 g of carbohydrate in the grain product (e.g., bread or cracker) [21], but there is no universally accepted definition of whole grains. The term "whole grains" usually includes bran, germ, and endosperm from the natural cereal. Whole grain products (e.g., whole wheat breads, oats, barley, brown rice, brown pasta) are also known as "lente" carbohydrates because they have a slower (*lentus* in Latin) gastrointestinal absorption and generally produce slower glycemic and insulinemic responses than highly processed refined grains [22]. Bran is rich in dietary fiber, B vitamins, minerals, flavonoids, and tocopherols; germ contains numerous fatty acids, antioxidants, and phytochemicals. Endosperm essentially provides starch (carbohydrate polysaccharides) and storage proteins [23]. The degree of processing appears to act as an effect modifier of the effects of grain and carbohydrate consumption on the risk of CVD.

In large and well-conducted longitudinal epidemiologic studies, whole grain consumption has been consistently associated with lower incidence of CHD and possibly stroke. A meta-analysis on whole grains and CVD reported in its pooled estimate a significant 21% lower risk (95% CI: 15–27%) of CVD events associated with the consumption of 2.5 servings/day vs. 0.2 serving/day of whole grains [24]. The higher dietary fiber in whole grains apparently contributes to these benefits. But also other additional characteristics of whole grains, including slower digestion (lower glycemic responses) and higher content of minerals, phytochemicals, and fatty acids, are likely to play a key role in explaining these inverse associations [25,26]. Thus, similar to fruits and vegetables, health effects of whole grains may result from the interaction of synergistic effects of multiple elements that are unlikely to be matched by supplemental fiber alone, added bran, or isolated micronutrients. Another explanation of the beneficial effect of whole grains comes from dietary substitution for more highly refined/processed carbohydrates and starches that may themselves induce adverse cardiometabolic effects.

The removal of bran and germ that occurs in the refining process reduces dietary fiber, and this implies that important benefits are lost, including potential reductions in blood cholesterol levels and BP [27,28]. On the other hand, the refining process increases bioavailability and accelerates the digestion of starch in the remaining endosperm, which increases short-term and rapid glycemic responses [29].

Weight losses and improvements in glucose and insulin homeostasis, in endothelial function, and in inflammatory biomarkers have been reported in small randomized trials of whole grains [22,24,30]. These physiological benefits are consistent with the observed benefits in large epidemiologic studies using clinical end points as outcomes.

Fish and Omega-3 Fatty Acids

The finding that populations with a high fish consumption such as Alaskan Native Americans, Greenland Eskimos, or Japanese living in fishing villages had low rates of CVD helped to generate the hypothesis that fish consumption may protect against atherosclerosis. Kromhout et al. [31] found in the Dutch arm of the Seven Countries study that men who consumed 30 g/day of fish had 50% lower CHD mortality than those who rarely ate fish.

Subsequently, a wide collection of large cohort studies integrated in several meta-analyses and systematic reviews [32–42] have also found moderate inverse relationships between fish consumption and CVD [43].

In a recent dose–response meta-analysis including 18 studies, an increment of two servings a week of any fish was associated with a 4% (95% confidence interval [CI]: 1–7%) reduced risk of cerebrovascular disease [32].

A previous review by He et al. [40] reported a 7% lower risk of CHD mortality for each 20-g/day increase in fish intake.

Also randomized clinical trials (RCTs) (mostly conducted in secondary prevention) have assessed the effect of fish consumption or fish oil supplementation on CVD outcomes (mainly reinfarctions). The pioneering Diet and Reinfarction Trial (DART) [44] demonstrated that participants who increased their fish consumption to twice a week had a significant 29% reduction in total mortality after 2 years. The GISSI-Prevenzione trial [45] found that daily supplementation with n-3 fatty acids led to a 10% to 15% reduction in the main end points (death, nonfatal MI, and stroke). The Japan Eicosapentaenoic Acid Lipid Intervention Study (JELIS) [46] found that supplementation with eicosapentaenoic acid (EPA) (1800 mg/day) significantly reduced coronary events among patients receiving low-dose statin therapy after 4.6 years of follow-up. Fish and fish oil are among only a handful of dietary factors for which both long-term observational studies and RCTs of CVD outcomes have been successfully conducted.

The available evidence tends to suggest that greater cardiovascular benefits can be obtained with fish consumption and omega-3 fatty acids in secondary prevention than in primary prevention and in populations consuming low amounts of omega-3 fatty acids at baseline than among those with a higher baseline consumption of fish or omega-3 fatty acids [35]. Fish and other seafood are good sources of long-chain omega-3 polyunsaturated fatty acids (PUFAs), which include docosahexaenoic acid (DHA) and EPA, which are only synthesized from their plant-derived precursor, alpha-linolenic acid, in low amounts (<5%) in humans. Average EPA plus DHA contents of different seafood species vary by >10-fold. Fatty (oily) fish such as salmon, sardines, trout, white tuna, anchovies, and herring have the highest concentrations [43].

Small randomized trials have found that long-chain omega-3 fatty acids reduced triglyceride levels [47], systolic and diastolic BP [48], and resting heart rate [49]. RCT and observational studies also suggest that these oils may also improve endothelial function, reduce inflammation, normalize heart rate variability, improve myocardial relaxation and efficiency, and, at high doses, limit platelet aggregation [50]. These findings for physiological benefits are in agreement with the inverse association between fish consumption and the incidence of CHD and ischemic stroke, and especially risk of cardiac death.

However, some large trials using supplements of omega-3 fatty acids instead of the consumption of whole fish have found no effect on stroke [32].

Therefore, it is possible that the potential benefit of fish consumption on CVD could be attributed not simply to long-chain omega-3 fatty acids but also to a wider array of nutrients (and their interactions) that are abundant in fish. For example, fish are also rich in vitamin D and in multiple B vitamins, which have been inversely associated with the risk of CVD. Also essential amino acids and trace elements present in fish (e.g., arginine, calcium, magnesium, potassium, iodine, and selenium) may contribute to explain their reported favorable vascular effects. Another important issue to explain the cardiovascular protection by fish against CVD is that fish usually tend to replace in meals red or processed meats, which are less healthy foods.

Probably the benefits of eating fish can be superior to those provided by fish oil supplements, although definitive evidence on this comparison is not yet available. Potential adverse cardiovascular effects of methylmercury found in a few fish species are limited and conflicting; if present, the available evidence suggests that cardiovascular benefits of fish consumption are not counterbalanced for this potential adverse effect [51,52].

NUTS, LEGUMES, AND SOY

Nuts are a good source of unsaturated fatty acids, fiber, minerals (potassium, calcium, and magnesium), vitamins (folate and tocopherols), and other bioactive compounds, such as phytosterols and polyphenols [53,54]. In large prospective cohort studies, the consumption of tree nuts has been reported to be associated with lower CHD incidence [55,56]. Overall, cardiovascular benefits of modest nut consumption (≥2 servings/week versus never or almost never consumption) are supported by both effects on risk factors in short-term trials and the magnitude and consistency of reduced CVD risk observed in prospective cohort studies.

An important pooled analysis of primary data from 25 nut consumption trials including in total 583 participants showed impressive benefits of nut consumption on blood lipids, with reductions in total blood cholesterol concentrations of 10.9 mg/dL (5.1% change) and in low-density lipoprotein (LDL) cholesterol concentration (LDL-C) of 10.2 mg/dL (7.4% change). Reductions in triglyceride levels by 20.6 mg/dL (10.2%) were obtained only in subjects with blood triglyceride levels of at least 150 mg/dL but not in those with lower levels [57].

Beyond these short-term trials and beyond observational studies, the large *Prevención con Dieta Mediterránea* (PREDIMED) primary prevention randomized trial with 7447 participants reported a 30% relative reduction in major cardiovascular events (stroke, myocardial infarction [MI], or cardiovascular death) versus a control diet after a 4.8-year intervention with Mediterranean diet (MeDiet) supplemented with mixed nuts (mainly walnuts, but also almonds and hazel nuts) totaling a consumption of 30 g/day of mixed nuts. This finding, consistent with previous observational studies and small randomized trials on intermediate outcomes, provides first-line evidence to support the benefits of mixed nuts in cardiovascular prevention [58].

Epidemiological evidence for cardiovascular benefits from legumes (e.g., peas, beans, lentils, and chickpeas) is weaker than for nuts, although they may also provide beneficial effects taking into account the overall package of micronutrients, phytochemicals, and fiber provided by them. In a meta-analysis of RCTs, consumption of soy-containing foods showed an apparent beneficial effect lowering diastolic and systolic BP, even though the effects did not achieve statistical significance. Isolated soy protein or isoflavones (phytoestrogens) seem to have smaller effects, producing only modest reductions in LDL cholesterol and diastolic BP [59,60]. More investigation of the effects of legumes on CVD with well-conducted prospective cohorts and RCTs is required.

Dairy Products

Dairy products are a good source of potentially beneficial nutrients, such as magnesium, potassium, calcium, and bioactive peptides. On the other hand, the main type of fat in dairy products is saturated fat, specifically palmitic acid with adverse effects on blood lipids. Based on the lower content of calories, saturated fatty acids (SFA), and cholesterol of low-fat or nonfat dairy products, together with the scarce nutritional advantage of whole-fat dairy, the majority of dietary guidelines and scientific organizations recommend low-fat or nonfat dairy consumption [51].

Furthermore, different studies have suggested that dairy products might be associated with lower BP and reduced risk of hypertension. The consumption of low-fat dairy (but not of whole-fat diary) has been inversely associated with BP and with the risk of hypertension [61–63]. Potentially varying health effects of specific dairy foods (e.g., milk, yogurt, cheese, and butter) require further study.

Meats and Processed Meats

Food patterns associated with lower CVD risk such as the MeDiet [58,64,65], the Prudent dietary pattern [66], the dietary approaches to stop hypertension (DASH) diet [67], or the vegetarian diets [68] have a common denominator: they include a lower consumption of overall meats and specially of red and processed meats because diverse components of meats, such as SFA, cholesterol, heme iron, and others could increase cardiometabolic risk. In addition, in processed meats, high levels of salt and other preservatives might be detrimental for cardiovascular health. Available meta-analyses of prospective cohort studies evaluating the role of meat consumption on the risk of CHD have found that total red meat consumption was associated with overall higher risk of CHD, although the association was not statistically significant [55,69]. Consumption of processed meats but not unprocessed red meats was associated with higher incidence of CHD [69]. The adverse effects of preservatives (e.g., sodium, phosphates, and nitrites) specially present in processed meats and/or their methods of cooking preparation (e.g., high temperature commercial cooking/frying) could influence their health effects [69].

Sugar-Sweetened Beverages

Evidence from RCT, prospective cohorts, and ecological comparisons support positive associations between sugar-sweetened beverage (SSB) consumption and adiposity in children and adults [70]. This direct association between SSB and obesity or weight gain is most consistent among large prospective cohort studies with long follow-up and without undue adjustment for total energy intake, because total energy intake is an intermediate link between exposure and outcome, and therefore, it should not be treated as a confounder. The detrimental effect of SSB on adiposity is nowadays considered a resolved issue [71].

In the United States, the proportion of total dietary calories from SSBs increased to 222 calories/day per person in the period from 1965 to 2002, the same period that overweight/obesity was increasing rapidly [72]. On average, an American teenage boy drinks approximately 300 kcal/day of SSB and a teenage girl approximately 200 kcal [73]. Most SSB intake by children occurs at home, not at school [74].

Results from limited short-term trials suggested that calories in liquid form may be less satiating and thereby increase the total amount of daily calories consumed [75,76]. SSB intake can also displace more healthful beverages, such as milk [77].

Reduced SSB consumption improved weight loss or reduced weight gain in both children and adults [78]. In one multicomponent lifestyle intervention, the reduction of each 1 serving/day of SSB was associated with 0.65-kg greater weight loss [79].

A meta-analysis by Mattes et al. [80] including six RCTs reported that adding SSBs to the diets of participants significantly increased body weight in a dose-dependent manner. This finding has been confirmed by the most recent meta-analysis on this issue conducted by Malik et al. [70].

In another meta-analysis of prospective cohorts, higher SSB intake was associated with higher incidence of diabetes mellitus (DM) and metabolic syndrome [81].

A direct positive association between SSB intake and the incidence of CHD was observed in the Nurses' Health Study (including 88,520 women observed for up to 24 years). This study reported that the detrimental association persisted even after accounting for potential confounding factors. Among women who consumed two or more servings of SSBs per day, a 35% higher risk of developing CHD was found in comparison with those who consumed less than 1 serving per month (relative risk = 1.35; 95% CI, 1.07 to 1.69; P for trend < 0.001) [82]. The combination of highly refined carbohydrate calories, a liquid form that may minimize satiety, absence of other beneficial nutrients/constituents, displacement of more healthful beverages, and very high intake in many population subgroups renders reduction in SSB a key dietary target for improving individual and population cardiometabolic health [83].

ALCOHOLIC BEVERAGES

Light to moderate alcohol consumption (1 drink or less daily for women and 2 drinks or less daily for men) is associated with a reduced risk of CVD, whereas increasingly excessive consumption results in a detrimental effect. This is a very consistent finding of many observational epidemiologic studies. However, there are no trials, and therefore, there is no experimental evidence on alcohol consumption and hard cardiovascular end points. Alcohol consumption confers cardiovascular protection predominately through improvements in insulin sensitivity, reduced coagulation factors, and, especially, increased high-density lipoprotein (HDL) cholesterol [84]. On the other hand, habitual heavy alcohol intake is cardiotoxic, causing a large proportion of dilated cardiomyopathies of non-ischemic causes worldwide [85]. The ensuing ventricular dysfunction is often irreversible, even when alcohol consumption is stopped; continued drinking in such patients is associated with increased mortality. Both acute binges and higher habitual intake of alcohol have also been associated with higher risk of atrial fibrillation [86]. Conversely, in randomized trials and in the absence of weight gain, modest alcohol use reduces systemic inflammation and improves HDL cholesterol levels and insulin resistance [87–89]. Consistent with these effects, individuals who drink alcohol moderately (up to 2 drinks/day for men and 1 drink/day for women) experience a lower incidence of CHD and DM compared with nondrinkers [55,90].

In these observational studies, benefits of moderate alcohol intake could be overestimated, because the nonexposed group (nondrinkers) frequently includes former drinkers, those who have received a medical advice to quit drinking because of some chronic disease and other individuals who avoid alcohol because of poor health [91], and because heavy alcohol consumers are generally underrepresented in large longitudinal epidemiologic studies. Some nonalcohol components, including resveratrol and other polyphenols present in wine, more than in beer, and in beer more than in liquors, could have potential benefits. In this line of thought, greater benefits from moderate consumption of wine can be expected than from beer consumption and greater benefits from beer than from liquors. However, most available evidence supports the direct effects of alcohol itself irrespective of the type of beverage [87–89,92] because moderate intake of alcohol, regardless of whether it comes from wine, beer, or liquors, has been found to be associated with reduced rates of CHD in different populations [93]. Further research on this issue is needed.

A growing interest in the drinking pattern has received confirmation by epidemiological findings, because lowest cardiovascular risk has been observed among individuals who drink moderately on several days of the week, rather than among those who concentrate the same amount of alcohol in 1 or 2 drinking occasions during the week (i.e., binge drinkers) [94].

Other different adverse effects of alcohol, even in moderate doses, also need to be taken into account. Interestingly, increased alcohol intake leads to higher weight gain because an average serving of alcohol contributes approximately 120 to 200 kcal that, as discussed previously, may be less satiating than calories from solid foods [95]. Alcohol-related accidents, homicides, suicides, and social problems explain why alcohol use has an overall net adverse effect on population mortality [96]. Thus, alcohol use, especially among younger adults, is not advisable at all as a population-based strategy to reduce CVD risk. For adults who already drink alcohol, no more than moderate use can be encouraged.

An alcohol drinking pattern that is likely to be especially healthy can be denominated the "Mediterranean Alcohol Drinking Pattern Score" (MADP). This pattern reflects the traditional way of consuming alcohol in Mediterranean countries, and it is based on the idea of including in the pattern several dimensions of the drinking habits, in an analogy to the food pattern approach that is currently accepted as the most sensible method in nutritional epidemiology. Beyond the total amount of alcohol consumed, it seems interesting to capture other aspects of the conformity to a traditional MADP. We used data from the prospective cohort study of the SUN Project [97] to define a MADP that positively scored moderate alcohol intake, alcohol intake spread out over the week, low spirits consumption, wine preference, wine consumed during meals, and avoidance of binge drinking. Each 2-point increment in the MADP was associated with lower risk of cardiovascular mortality [HR (95% CI): 0.49 (0.31–0.79)]. Better adherence to the MADP was associated with reduced cardiovascular mortality as compared with abstention or departure from this pattern, throughout categories of ethanol intake. This reduction went beyond the inverse association usually observed for moderate alcohol drinking (Figure 7.1).

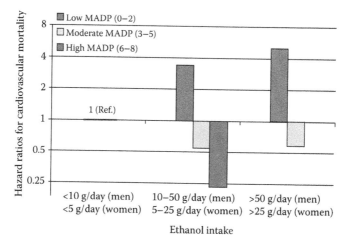

FIGURE 7.1 Hazard ratios of total mortality according to total alcohol intake and adherence to the mediterranean alcohol drinking pattern (MADP).

Phytochemicals

The beneficial effects of the incredibly rich combination of natural phytochemicals present in fruit and vegetables are probably superior to those of every thinkable polypill containing any mixture of artificial elements. There are more than 8000 phytochemicals present in whole foods. These compounds differ in solubility, molecular size, and polarity, characteristics that may affect their bioavailability and their biological properties in cells, organs, and tissues. A supplement given as a pill simply cannot mimic this balanced natural combination of bioactive compounds present in fruit, vegetables, extra-virgin olive oil, or red wine. Phytochemicals are naturally occurring compounds in plant foods. They include plant sterols, flavonoids, and sulfur-containing compounds [98]. For example, over 4000 different classes of flavonoids have been described. Their major dietary sources are tea, broccoli, kale, celery, onions, garlic, apples, and red wine.

A meta-analysis of seven cohort studies found that participants in the highest tertile of flavonol intake had a 20% (95% CI: 7–31%) lower risk of fatal CHD than those in the lowest tertile [99]. In a meta-analysis of RCTs, flavonoids-rich foods such as cocoa and soy decreased cardiovascular risk factors [59]. In particular, dark chocolate reduced systolic and diastolic BP.

Plant sterols occur naturally in fruits, vegetables, vegetables oils, nuts, and grains. Over 40 plant sterols (phytoesterols) have been identified. Except for the methyl groups in the side chain, sterols are structurally similar to dietary cholesterol. They inhibit cholesterol absorption in human intestines. Plant sterols lower blood cholesterol [100]. One major concern is that plant sterols modestly lower blood concentrations of carotenoids and some fat-soluble vitamins. Therefore, the long-term effects of food enriched with these phytochemicals need to be assessed.

The Mediterranean Diet

The available scientific evidence demonstrates that overall dietary patterns can improve health and prevent CVD in a greater extent than isolated food or nutrients [58,101]. Using different research approaches, several healthful dietary patterns have been identified. They share several key common characteristics, including an emphasis on fruits, vegetables, other plant foods such as legumes and nuts, and (in many patterns) whole grains and fish; with limited or occasional dairy products (mainly low-fat dairy); and often with very limited amounts of red meats or processed meats and fewer sugared beverages, refined carbohydrates, and other processed foods. These dietary patterns are each generally consistent with food-based priorities for CVD health ideal metrics.

In this context, the MeDiet is defined as the traditional dietary pattern found in Greece, Southern Italy, Spain, and other olive-growing countries of the Mediterranean basin in the early 1960s [102]. It consists in an abundant use of olive oil as the major culinary fat; a high consumption of plant-based foods (fruits, vegetables, legumes, nuts and seeds, and whole grain cereals); frequent but moderate intake of wine (especially red wine), usually with meals; consumption of fresh fish and seafood; moderate consumption of dairy products (especially yogurt and cheese), poultry, and eggs; and low consumption of sweet desserts and red and processed meat.

Randomized trials of dietary intervention constitute hallmarks in the acquisition of knowledge in this field. The availability of a randomized trial (the Lyon Diet Heart Study) showing a protective effect on CVD hard clinical end points was a strong point to support the causal effect of the MeDiet [55,103]. The Lyon trial was a secondary prevention trial because it only included survivors of a previous MI, and the number of observed events was modest. Surprisingly, the Lyon trial gave no special consideration to olive oil, which is traditionally accepted as the hallmark of the MeDiet and the major source of fat in Mediterranean countries. However, results of the Lyon trial were subsequently confirmed also for primary prevention by the recent PREDIMED trial conducted in 7447 initially healthy participants, without any previous history of CVD [58,104]. Participants in the PREDIMED trial were men and women from 55 to 80 years at high cardiovascular risk because they were diabetics or had at least three major vascular risk factors. They were randomly allocated to one of three diets: a MeDiet rich in nuts, a MeDiet rich in extra-virgin olive oil, and a control group receiving advice to reduce the intake of fat. A significant reduction in the risk of a combined cardiovascular end point (MI, stroke, or cardiovascular death) was observed for both groups allocated to MeDiet. The trial was stopped after a median follow-up of 4.8 years because of early evidence of benefit. The hazard ratio for a combined end point of MI, stroke, or cardiovascular death was 0.70 (95% CI: 0.54–0.92) for the MeDiet with extra-virgin olive oil and 0.72 (95% CI: 0.54–0.96) for the MeDiet with nuts.

We conducted a random effect meta-analysis to combine these two trials and found a relative 38% reduction in the risk of CVD after intervention with a MeDiet with pooled risk ratio of 0.62 (95% CI: 0.45–0.85) [105]. There was no evidence of heterogeneity, and we repeated the meta-analysis also using a fixed-effects model (Figure 7.1). We did not include another published trial (the Indo-Mediterranean Diet Heart Study) because its validity has been seriously questioned [106].

Together with the evidence from randomized trials, examining the evidence from observational studies is also important given that even RCTs are not completely free of limitations (i.e., subject compliance, disease latency, duration of exposure, or lifestyle changes) [55].

A meta-analysis published by Sofi et al. in 2010 [107] found a growing accrual of evidence supporting a substantial beneficial effect of the MeDiet on CVD clinical end points. After that meta-analysis, other seven new prospective observational studies were published [108–114] up to August 2013. Two of these studies [108,109] provided separated estimates for men and women. We repeated the meta-analysis adding these nine new estimates to those already included in the meta-analysis by Sofi et al.

The Northern Manhattan Study (n: 2568) [110] reported that a dietary pattern resembling the MeDiet was inversely associated with a composite outcome of CVD (ischemic stroke, MI, or vascular death). Nevertheless, the estimate for 1-point increase was not statistically significant. The Greek European Prospective Investigation into Cancer and Nutrition (EPIC) cohort, which had previously assessed only fatal coronary events [64], reported the updated results for 636 cases of CHD including both fatal and nonfatal cases [108]. Better adherence to the MeDiet was associated with a nonsignificant lower CHD incidence and a statistically significant reduction in mortality from CHD. Other results from this same cohort reported a significant inverse association with cerebrovascular disease [111]. The Dutch cohort of the EPIC study also found that higher adherence to a MeDiet was associated with lower risk of a combined CVD end point (fatal CVD, nonfatal MI, and nonfatal stroke) [112]. Among more than 77,000 adults living in the Subartic region (North Sweden), the Västerboten Intervention Program [109] showed that higher adherence to a MeDiet was associated with a significant reduction in cardiovascular mortality among women, but not among men. The authors concluded that the benefits of the MeDiet go beyond the Mediterranean geographical area and can be borrowed by other populations.

Two Italian rural male cohorts of the Seven Countries Study (n: 1139) [113] estimated a significant 26% relative reduction in CHD mortality for each 2.7-point increment in the Mediterranean Adequacy Index (MAI) (HR: 0.74; 95% CI: 0.55–0.99) after 20 years of follow-up. Since the authors used an index that ranges from 0 to over 100, when we converted the estimates to a 2-point increment within a 0 to 9 scale, the magnitude of the association was unusually strong.

The Danish MONICA cohort [114] assessed 1849 men and women and found a significant 8% relative reduction in the risk of CVD for each 1-unit increase in adherence to an 8-point scale.

The MORGEN study conducted in the Netherlands [115] included 8128 men and 9759 women aged 20–65 years and assessed a MeDiet operationalized according to 8 of the 9 items of the MDS proposed by Trichopoulou et al. [64] (moderate alcohol consumption was excluded). They found a nonsignificant inverse association with a combined CVD end point (fatal CVD, nonfatal MI, and stroke). We did not include these results in our meta-analysis because they were partly included in the EPIC-NL study [112].

Two cohort studies conducted in Spain [116,117] consistently showed a very similar inverse association, though the EPIC-Spain cohort [116] had narrower confidence intervals. They were

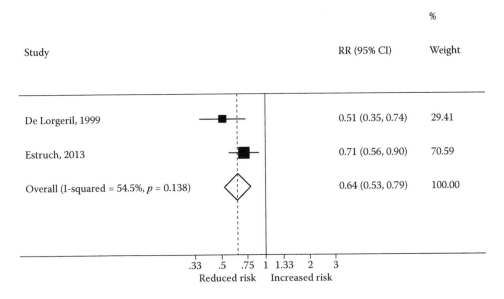

FIGURE 7.2 Meta-analysis of experimental studies (randomized trials) of Mediterranean diets for the prevention of cardiovascular clinical end-points. (From Martinez-Gonzalez MA, Bes-Rastrollo M. *Curr Opin Lipidol.* 2014;25:20–6.)

published ahead of print almost simultaneously and shortly before the meta-analysis by Sofi et al. [107]. They were already included in that previous meta-analysis.

We included nine estimates from seven new prospective cohort studies in our meta-analysis together with seven of the eight previous estimates included in the meta-analysis by Sofi et al. [107]. The initial report from the Greek EPIC cohort on CHD mortality [64] was excluded because it was subsequently updated [108]. Our new random-effect meta-analysis with 16 estimates showed that each 2-point increment in a 0 to 9 MDS was associated with a 10% relative reduction in the risk of CVD (risk ratio: 0.90; 95% CI: 0.86–0.94) (Figure 7.2). These results were highly consistent with the previous pooled estimate reported by Sofi et al. [107]. Therefore, our updated meta-analysis supported an inverse linear association between MeDiet and CVD. However, there was evidence of statistical heterogeneity ($I^2 = 77.5\%$; $p < 0.001$). After removing from the meta-analysis those studies with end points that only included fatal CVD [109,113,118], we observed not only a slightly stronger inverse association (risk ratio: 0.87; 95% CI: 0.85–0.90) but also that evidence of heterogeneity was not present any more ($I^2 = 19.8\%$, $p = 0.26$). A possible explanation for the heterogeneity due to studies that only included fatal CVD cases as outcome might be explained by the fact that mortality from CVD is related not only to incidence but also to the quality and timeliness of medical care. Another potential explanation may be related to differences in the methods used for case ascertainment (Figure 7.3).

Visual inspection of the funnel plots and the Egger's test ($p = 0.001$) suggested a potential possibility of publication bias. However, when we excluded the three studies based only on CVD fatal cases, the potential for publication bias disappeared ($p = 0.69$ in the Egger's test).

DISAPPOINTING RESULTS OF LOW-FAT DIETS

The MeDiet is relatively high in total fat. But as reviewed above, a wide body of consistent evidence supports the benefits of the MeDiet in cardiovascular prevention. In contrast, it is important to highlight the disappointing results found after using low-fat diets as a paradigm of a healthy diet to prevent CVD [119–121]. In sharp contrast with the MeDiet, the long-term compliance and sustainability of low-fat diets seem suboptimal. In any case, nutritional quality should be a higher priority than reducing fat intake [121]. In addition, to have a higher potential for long-term adherence than low-fat diets, the MeDiet has passed the tests of long-term sustainability, effectiveness, and nutritional quality [122,123]. The MeDiet represents a considerably more palatable alternative than the usual low-fat approaches for promoting healthy eating. Also, it has a strong background of a millenary tradition without any evidence of harm. A traditional MeDiet is a relatively low-cost nonpharmaceutical means of preventing CVD. It can be easily adopted by large sectors of the population. The promotion of this dietary pattern seems a feasible tool for the prevention of CVD in Public Health Nutrition.

DASH Diet

The food pattern known as DASH emphasizes the consumption of fruits, vegetables, and low-fat dairy products; including whole grains, poultry, fish, and nuts; and it is low in red meat, saturated fat, sweets, and SSBs [13,124]. The original DASH diet was low in total fat (27% energy) and higher (55% energy) in carbohydrates; additional modifications to build new DASH-type dietary patterns have been evaluated with an exchange of approximately 10% energy of carbohydrate for vegetable sources of monounsaturated fat or protein [124]. In controlled feeding trials, each of these DASH diets significantly lowered BP and improved blood lipids in comparison with usual Western diets [13,125]. This finding highlights the greater importance of specific food choices rather than macronutrient composition for maximization of CVD benefits. BP reduction was greatest when DASH diets were combined with reduced sodium intake [13]. In several observational studies, a better adherence to a DASH-type dietary pattern was associated with lower risk of CVD [51]. Currently, very few US adults, even those with elevated BP, follow a DASH dietary pattern [126].

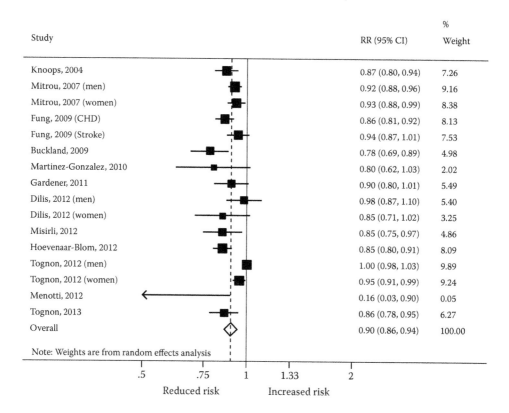

FIGURE 7.3 Meta-analysis of observational studies of adherence to the Mediterranean diet (for each +2 points in 0 to 9 score) and cardiovascular disease. (From Martinez-Gonzalez MA, Bes-Rastrollo M. *Curr Opin Lipidol.* 2014;25:20–6.)

Vegetarian Diets

A vegetarian dietary pattern includes several types of vegetarian diets: pesco-vegetarians (who consume fish); lacto-ovo-vegetarians (who consume milk and eggs); and strict vegans (who consume no animal products). Potentially different cardiometabolic effects of these different vegetarian diets are not established. Few RCTs of vegetarian diets have been conducted. Two small trials demonstrated that vegetarian diets versus typical Western diets reduced BP [127,128]. However, three other trials found no differences between lacto-vegetarian or vegan dietary pattern and conventional dietary recommendations for improving weight loss, BP, blood lipids, or insulin resistance [129–134]. In several observational studies, vegetarians versus nonvegetarians improved health outcomes [51,135–140]. Several characteristics of vegetarian diets could explain these relationships, including high consumption of plant-based foods and low consumption of meats, processed meats, and other processed and fast foods [137].

Because vegetarians are often generally more health conscious, other lifestyle characteristics, in addition to diet, may play a role as potential confounders on the observed lower rates of CVD. Overall, vegetarian diets have been studied less extensively than Mediterranean or DASH patterns, and although the foods that are not consumed (animal products) are their strictly defining feature, the more salient features for CVD benefits may be the foods that are typically consumed, in particular, more fruits, vegetables, legumes, nuts, and vegetable oils [83].

In a collaborative reanalysis of five prospective studies, mortality from CHD was reported to be significantly lower by 24% among vegetarians compared to nonvegetarians [135]. Subsequently, a meta-analysis of seven cohort studies confirmed a lower cardiovascular mortality in vegetarians, but inconsistent results for the association between vegetarian diets and death from any cause were found [140]. More recently, a 5-year follow-up of the Adventist Health Study-2 cohort showed an overall association of vegetarian dietary patterns with lower mortality [139]. Most available comparisons between vegetarians and nonvegetarians relied on a single measurement of diet at baseline, but dietary patterns may change over time and the length of exposure to vegetarianism may account for heterogeneity in results from different cohorts. When vegetarians were separated according to the length of their exposure to vegetarianism, the cardiovascular benefit was present only among those who have been vegetarian for at least 5 years [135].

The team of the PREDIMED trial evaluated a moderate pro-vegetarian diet. Since a pure vegetarian diet might not easily be embraced by many individuals, consuming preferentially plant-derived foods instead of animal-derived foods (i.e., a pro-vegetarian food pattern) would be a more easily understood message for health promotion. A pro-vegetarian food pattern was found to be related with a reduction in mortality from any cause, and especially in cardiovascular mortality [138].

Okinawa Diet

One of the regions with lowest rates of CHD in the world is the Japanese region Okinawa. Therefore, Japanese diets have been proposed as another healthful dietary pattern [141]. This traditional dietary pattern is characterized by soybean products, fish, seaweeds, fruits, vegetables, and green tea and low meat consumption [142]. However, Japanese diets often contain high sodium because of soy sauce and added salt at home, likely contributing to the relatively high incidence of stroke and some cancers. Very low-fat Japanese diets have also been associated with higher stroke risk, specially hemorrhagic stroke [143]. Food staples of traditional Okinawan diets are rich in antioxidant and relative low in calories. They include orange-yellow root vegetables and green leafy vegetables; wide varieties of seaweeds; tofu; and herbaceous plants [144]. Due to the appropriate energy balance, age-related weight gain is avoided. This is also an important advantage of the Okinawan food pattern [141]. Japanese dietary patterns seem another good option for CHD prevention, although the reason for relatively high rates of some cancer and stroke requires further investigation. Scientific evidence for benefits of these dietary patterns remains more limited than evidence supporting the MeDiet or the DASH diet.

QUALITY OF CARBOHYDRATES

The importance of carbohydrate quality, rather than quantity, has been one of the most important new insights related to diet and cardiometabolic health. Although carbohydrates have traditionally been classified as simple (e.g., monosaccharides and disaccharides) versus complex (e.g., starch and glycogen), several additional characteristics are relevant in determining cardiometabolic effects [83]. These include dietary fiber content; bran and germ content; food structure (e.g., intact, minimally processed, refined, or liquid); and potentially glycemic responses or induction of hepatic de novo lipogenesis following ingestion. The concept of the glycemic index (GI) defines the different glycemic responses to various carbohydrate-containing foods. The GI is measured as the 2-h area under the curve for blood glucose levels after ingesting a test food compared with a standard weight (50 g) of reference carbohydrate (glucose or white bread). In order to take into account the quantity of carbohydrates consumed for each food, the glycemic load (GL) was developed, derived from the product of the GI value of a food and its carbohydrate content. In the Nurses' Health Study, a higher dietary GL was associated with higher risk of CHD [145].

Our group of research has developed a score called Carbohydrate Quality Index (CQI) to evaluate the quality of carbohydrates. The criteria for a maximum CQI were as follows: higher dietary fiber, higher ratio whole grains/total grains, higher ratio solid carbohydrates/total carbohydrates, and lower GI. Based on the position of each subject according to the quintiles of each criterion, the score ranges from 4 points (lowest quality) to 20 points (highest quality). We observed that those subjects with the highest score (in the fifth quintile) exhibited a very low prevalence of inadequate nutrient intake (adjusted odds ratio: 0.03; 95% CI: 0.01–0.08 vs. the first quintile) in the elderly subjects at high CVD risk of the PREDIMED trial. Similar results were observed in the young Mediterranean cohort of the SUN Project [146].

QUALITY OF FATS

Earlier results from epidemiologic studies on the "diet-heart" hypothesis were based on ecological data relating dietary intake of saturated fat and cholesterol to rates of CHD in different countries. In the pioneering Seven Countries Study conducted by Keys [147], there was a strong correlation between intake of saturated fat as a percentage of calories and coronary death rates across 16 defined populations in seven countries ($r = 0.84$). Noteworthy, the correlation between energy from total fat and CHD incidence was modest ($r = 0.39$). Interestingly, the regions with the lowest (Crete) and the highest (Finland) CHD rates in the Seven Countries study had the same amount of total fat intake (approximately 40% of energy), which was the highest fat intake among the 16 populations of this pioneering ecological study.

Results from migration studies also suggested that changes in diet (especially increased saturated fat intake) and lifestyle rather than genetic factors were responsible for the differences in CHD rates among three Japanese populations living in Japan, Hawaii, and San Francisco [148]. However, concurrent changes in multiple aspects make it difficult to identify specific causal factors.

Beyond international comparisons or migration studies, several prospective cohort studies have directly addressed the specific associations between subtypes of dietary fat and the risk of CHD. Hu et al. [149] conducted a detailed prospective analysis among 80,082 women aged 34 to 59 years in the Nurses' Health Study. This large cohort study, with good control of confounding, showed that the type of fat was more important than the quantity of fat. Higher intake of saturated and trans fatty acids was associated with higher CHD risks, whereas greater intake of polyunsaturated and monounsaturated fats was associated with lower risk.

In a meta-analysis of four prospective cohort studies involving nearly 140,000 individuals, Mozaffarian et al. [150] estimated that each 2% increase in energy intake from trans fatty acids was associated with a 23% increase risk for CHD (pooled relative risk of 1.23; 95% CI: 1.11–1.37; $p <$ 0.001). Trans fatty acids raise LDL cholesterol and lower HDL cholesterol in comparison to natural cis-unsaturated fatty acids [151].

Two traditional trials conducted with the objective of replacing saturated by polyunsaturated fat, one conducted among institutionalized patients in a Los Angeles Veterans hospital [152] and another in a Finnish mental hospital [153], found statistically significant reductions in serum cholesterol and in nonfatal MI and coronary deaths associated with this change in fat subtypes. Total fat intake was not reduced. By contrast, prevention trials that lowered total fat did not find any significant reduction in serum cholesterol or in the rate of CHD events. In the Medical Research Council low-fat trial [154], there was no effect on the rate of reinfarction. Similarly, in the Women's Health Initiative Randomized Controlled Dietary Modification Trial previously cited [119], reduction in total fat intake did not significantly reduce the risk of CHD, stroke, or total CVD in postmenopausal women.

Recently, a controversy has emerged supporting that saturated fat intake is not the major risk factor for CVD [155]. Indeed, the results of a meta-analysis that included several prospective cohort studies did not support any significant association between saturated fat intake and CVD risk [156]. The key issue here might be the substitution. If saturated fat is substituted for refined carbohydrates, the effect will be essentially null because both are very likely associated with moderate adverse effects.

In any case, all these results suggest that overall dietary patterns play a more important role than total amount of macronutrients as nutritional determinants of CHD.

SALT INTAKE

There is compelling evidence that higher intake of sodium chloride (salt) is associated with elevated levels of BP [157]. Through its effects on BP, a reduction in salt intake will reduce stroke and CHD, as a meta-analysis of prospective observational studies has supported [158–161]. Long-term follow-up of salt-reduction trials is also consistent with lower CVD event rates after salt reduction [162,163].

Foods consumed in restaurants, pre-prepared, or packaged foods account for more than 50% of sodium intake in Western countries. The rest is derived from naturally occurring sources or added at home [162]. In Asian countries, most sodium is from soy sauce or is added at home [162]. Structural or policy-level approaches are very well suited for reducing population average levels of salt intake. Projected benefits are enormous. A national effort that reduced US salt intake by 3 g/day (<1.2 g/day less sodium) could annually prevent between 60,000 and 120,000 CHD events and 32,000 to 66,000 strokes, saving 194,000 to 392,000 quality-adjusted life-years and $10 to $24 billion in health care costs [164,165]. The best approach to reduce BP is that of using sodium reduction in combination with the DASH diet.

NUTRITIONAL INTERVENTIONS

Targeted goals to the individuals are more effective than any generic advice [166,167]. Clinical providers can help patients to accomplish targeted changes in the healthful dietary patterns and implement simple office-based assessments to inquire about and help them to set dietary goals. Clinic-based strategies are facilitated by health care systems changes, including scheduled visits for individual/group education and sustained in-person, telephone, or electronic feedback.

In the context of a Mediterranean dietary pattern, in order to have a feasible, reliable, and fast tool to evaluate adherence to the MeDiet, the PREDIMED trial intervention team developed and validated an instrument for rapid estimation of adherence to the MeDiet [168]. This tool has been demonstrated to be very useful in clinical practice. The score proposed was an adaptation of a previously validated 9-item index selecting the best cutoff points to discriminate between cases of MI and controls [169]. This 14-point screener was designed to assess adherence to the MeDiet and to allow for immediate feedback to participants. This 14-point score includes 14 questions as given in Table 7.1.

TABLE 7.1

PREDIMED 14-item Screener of Adherence to Mediterranean Diet (1 Point is Obtained for each Affirmative Answer)

	Frequency[a]
1. Do you use olive oil as the principal source of fat for cooking?	Yes
2. How much olive oil do you consume per day (including that used in frying, salads, meals eaten away from home, etc.)?	≥ 4 tablespoons[b]
3. How many servings of vegetables do you consume per day? Count garnish and side servings as 1/2 point; a full serving is 200 g.	≥ 2
4. How many pieces of fruit (including fresh-squeezed juice) do you consume per day?	≥ 3
5. How many servings of red meat, hamburger, or sausages do you consume per day? A full serving is 100–150 g.	<1
6. How many servings (12 g) of butter, margarine, or cream do you consume per day?	<1
7. How many carbonated and/or sugar-sweetened beverages do you consume per day?	<1
8. Do you drink wine? How much do you consume per week?	≥ 7 cups[c]
9. How many servings (150 g) of pulses do you consume per week?	≥ 3
10. How many servings of fish/seafood do you consume per week?	≥ 3
11. How many times do you consume commercial (not homemade) pastry such as cookies or cake per week?	<2
12. How many times do you consume nuts per week? (1 serving = 30 g)	≥ 3
13. Do you prefer to eat chicken, turkey, or rabbit instead of beef, pork, hamburgers, or sausages?	Yes
14. How many times per week do you consume boiled vegetables, pasta, rice, or other dishes with "sofrito" (a sauce of tomato, garlic, onion, and leeks sautéed in olive oil?	≥ 2

Note: Questionnaire from reference [168].
[a] Criterion to score 1 point. Otherwise, 0 recorded.
[b] 1 tablespoon = 13.5 g.
[c] 1 cup = 100 ml.

The 14-score PREDIMED screener showed a reasonable absolute agreement with the information gathered from the full-length food-frequency questionnaire, and it has shown strong inverse associations with metabolic syndrome and its components [170], cardiovascular risk factors [171], cardiovascular clinical end points [172], or obesity indexes such as body mass index, waist circumference, and waist-to-height ratio [173].

SUMMARY

During the last two decades, the body of knowledge on nutritional determinants of CVD has considerably increased. Although there is still a long road to cover the gaps in knowledge, a vast amount of high-quality studies are available to support the beneficial cardiovascular role of plant-based food patterns, tree nuts, virgin olive oil, whole grains, fish consumption, and moderate consumption of alcohol. These studies also support the detrimental role of processed foods, high salt intake, trans-fats, SSB, and processed meats.

The evidence knowledge can be summarized in the following dietary goals to reduce CVD:

- Consume more fruits.
- Consume more vegetables.
- Consume more whole grains. Increase your intake of fiber.
- Consume more legumes.
- Consume more fish.

- Consume more nuts.
- Consume low-fat dairy instead of whole-fat dairy.
- Use virgin olive oil.
- For hydration: drink water.
- If you consume alcohol: max. 2 daily servings for men, 1 daily serving for women. Otherwise, no alcohol consumption is recommended.
- Reduce your portion sizes.
- Do not forget physical activity (min. 150 min/week moderate activity).
- Consume less precooked and fried foods.
- Consume less meats and processed meats.
- Consume less refined sugars and partially hydrogenated vegetable oils.
- Do not put on weight. If you are overweight/obese try to lose weight.

REFERENCES

1. Mathers CD, Lopez AD, Murray CJL. The burden of disease and mortality by condition: Data, methods, and results for 2001. In: Lopez AD, Mathers CD, Ezzati M, Jamison DT, Murray CJL, eds. *Global Burden of Disease and Risk Factors*. Washington, DC: International Bank for Reconstruction and Development/ World Bank; 2006:45–240.
2. Mathers CD, Longcars D. Projections of global mortality and burden of disease from 2002 to 2030. *PLoS Med* 2006;3:e442.
3. Labarthe DR, Dunbar SB. Global cardiovascular health promotion and disease prevention: 2011 and beyond. *Circulation* 2012;125:2667–76.
4. United Nations General Assembly. *Political Declaration of the High-Level Meeting of the General Assembly on the Prevention and Control of Non-Communicable Diseases*. New York: United Nations; September 16, 2011. A/66/L.
5. US Burden of Disease Collaborators. The state of US health, 1990–2010: Burden of diseases, injuries, and risk factors. *JAMA* 2013;310:591–608.
6. Mozaffarian D, Ludwig DS. Dietary guidelines in the 21st century: A time for food. *JAMA* 2010;304:681–2.
7. Kris-Etherton PM, Etherton TD, Carlson J, Gardner C. Recent discoveries in inclusive food-based approaches and dietary patterns for reduction in risk for cardiovascular disease. *Curr Opin Lipidol* 2002;13:397–407.
8. Hu FB, Willett WC. Optimal diets for prevention of coronary heart disease. *JAMA* 2002;288:2569–78.
9. Martinez-Gonzalez MA, Martin-Calvo N. The major European dietary patterns and metabolic syndrome. *Rev Endocr Metab Disord* 2013;14:265–71.
10. Estruch R, Martínez-González MA, Corella D et al. PREDIMED Study Investigators. Effects of a Mediterranean-style diet on cardiovascular risk factors: A randomized trial. *Ann Intern Med* 2006;145:1–11.
11. Esposito K, Marfella R, Ciotola M, Di Palo C, Giugliano F, Giugliano G, D'Armiento M, D'Andrea F, Giugliano D. Effect of a Mediterranean-style diet on endothelial dysfunction and markers of vascular inflammation in the metabolic syndrome: A randomized trial. *JAMA* 2004;292:1440–6.
12. Elmer PJ, Obarzanek E, Vollmer WM, Simons-Morton D, Stevens VJ, Young DR, Lin PH, Champagne C, Harsha DW, Svetkey LP, Ard J, Brantley PJ, Proschan MA, Erlinger TP, Appel LJ. Effects of comprehensive lifestyle modification on diet, weight, physical fitness, and blood pressure control: 18-month results of a randomized trial. *Ann Intern Med* 2006;144:485–95.
13. Miller ER 3rd, Erlinger TP, Appel LJ. The effects of macronutrients on blood pressure and lipids: An overview of the DASH and OmniHeart trials. *Curr Atheroscler Rep* 2006;8:460–5.
14. Svendsen M, Blomhoff R, Holme I, Tonstad S. The effect of an increased intake of vegetables and fruit on weight loss, blood pressure and antioxidant defense in subjects with sleep related breathing disorders. *Eur J Clin Nutr* 2007;61:1301–11.
15. Dauchet L, Amouyel P, Hercberg S, Dallongeville J. Fruit and vegetable consumption and risk of coronary heart disease: A meta-analysis of cohort studies. *J Nutr* 2006;136:2588–93.
16. He FJ, Nowson CA, Lucas M, MacGregor GA. Increased consumption of fruit and vegetables is related to a reduced risk of coronary heart disease: Meta-analysis of cohort studies. *J Hum Hypertens* 2007;21:717–28.
17. Ness AR, Powles JW. Fruit and vegetables, and cardiovascular disease: A review. *Int J Epidemiol* 1997;26:1–13.

18. Dauchet L, Amouyel P, Dallongeville J. Fruit and vegetable consumption and risk of stroke: A meta-analysis of cohort studies. *Neurology* 2005;65:1193–7.

19. He FJ, Nowson CA, MacGregor GA. Fruit and vegetable consumption and stroke: Meta-analysis of cohort studies. *Lancet* 2006;367:320–6.

20. Pereira MA, O'Reilly E, Augustsson K, Fraser GE, Goldbourt U, Heitmann BL, Hallmans G, Knekt P, Liu S, Pietinen P, Spiegelman D, Stevens J, Virtamo J, Willett WC, Ascherio A. Dietary fiber and risk of coronary heart disease: A pooled analysis of cohort studies. *Arch Intern Med* 2004;164:370–6.

21. Lichtenstein AH, Appel LJ, Brands M, Carnethon M, Daniels S, Franch HA, Franklin B, Kris-Eterton P, Harris WS, Howard B, Karanja N, Lefevre M, Rudel L, Sacks F, Van Horn L, Winston M, Wylie-Rosett J. Diet and lifestyle recommendations revision 2006: A scientific statement from the American Heart Association Nutrition Committee. *Circulation* 2006;114:82–96.

22. De Munter JS, Hu FB, Spiegelman D, Franz M, van Dam RM. Whole grain, bran, and germ intake and risk of type 2 diabetes: A prospective cohort study and systematic review. *PLoS Med* 2007;4:e261.

23. Sabelli PA, Larikins BA. The development of endosperm in grasses. *Plant Physiol* 2009;149:14–26.

24. Mellen PB, Walsh TF, Herrington DM. Whole grain intake and cardiovascular disease: A meta-analysis. *Nutr Metab Cardiovasc Dis* 2008;18:283–90.

25. Jacobs DR Jr, Steffen LM. Nutrients, foods, and dietary patterns as exposures in research: A framework for food synergy. *Am J Clin Nutr* 2003;78:508S–13S.

26. Jacobs DR Jr, Tapsell LC. Food, not nutrients, is the fundamental unit in nutrition. *Nutr Rev* 2007;65:439–50.

27. Anderson JW, Randles KM, Kendall CW, Jenkins DJ. Carbohydrate and fiber recommendations for individuals with diabetes: A quantitative assessment and meta-analysis of the evidence. *J Am Coll Nutr* 2004;23:5–17.

28. Whelton SP, Hyre AD, Pedersen B, Yi Y, Whelton PK, He J. Effect of dietary fiber intake on blood pressure: A meta-analysis of randomized, controlled clinical trials. *J Hypertens* 2005;23:475–81.

29. Ludwig DS. The glycemic index: Physiological mechanisms relating to obesity, diabetes, and cardiovascular disease. *JAMA* 2002;287:2414–23.

30. Katcher HI, Legro RS, Kunselman AR, Gillies PJ, Demers LM, Bagshaw DM, Kris-Etherton PM. The effects of a whole grain-enriched hypocaloric diet on cardiovascular disease risk factors in men and women with metabolic syndrome. *Am J Clin Nutr* 2008;87:79–90.

31. Kromhout D, Bosschieter EB, de Lezenne Coulander C. The inverse relation between fish consumption and 20-year mortality from coronary heart disease. *N Engl J Med* 1985;312:1205–9.

32. Chowdhury R, Stevens S, Gorman D, Pan A, Warnakula S, Chowdhury S, Ward H, Johnson L, Crowe F, Hu FB, Franco OH. Association between fish consumption, long chain omega 3 fatty acids, and risk of cerebrovascular disease: Systematic review and meta-analysis. *BMJ* 2012;345:e6698.

33. Xun P, Qin B, Song Y, Nakamura Y, Kurth T, Yaemsiri S, Djousse L, He K. Fish consumption and risk of stroke and its subtypes: Accumulative evidence from a meta-analysis of prospective cohort studies. *Eur J Clin Nutr* 2012;66:1199–207.

34. Larsson SC, Orsini N. Fish consumption and the risk of stroke: A dose-response meta-analysis. *Stroke* 2011;42:3621–3.

35. Jacobson TA. Beyond lipids: the role of omega-3 fatty acids from fish oil in the prevention of coronary heart disease. *Curr Atheroscler Rep* 2007;9:145–53.

36. Wang C, Harris WS, Chung M, Lichtenstein AH, Balk EM, Kupelnick B, Jordan HS, Lau J. n-3 Fatty acids from fish or fish-oil supplements, but not alpha-linolenic acid, benefit cardiovascular disease outcomes in primary- and secondary-prevention studies: A systematic review. *Am J Clin Nutr* 2006;84(1):5–17.

37. Bouzan C, Cohen JT, Connor WE, Kris-Etherton PM, Gray GM, König A, Lawrence RS, Savitz DA, Teutsch SM. A quantitative analysis of fish consumption and stroke risk. *Am J Prev Med* 2005;29:347–52.

38. König A, Bouzan C, Cohen JT, Connor WE, Kris-Etherton PM, Gray GM, Lawrence RS, Savitz DA, Teutsch SM. A quantitative analysis of fish consumption and coronary heart disease mortality. *Am J Prev Med* 2005;29:335–46.

39. Yzebe D, Lievre M. Fish oils in the care of coronary heart disease patients: A meta-analysis of randomized controlled trials. *Fundam Clin Pharmacol* 2004;18(5):581–92.

40. He K, Song Y, Daviglus ML, Liu K, Van Horn L, Dyer AR, Greenland P. Accumulated evidence on fish consumption and coronary heart disease mortality: A meta-analysis of cohort studies. *Circulation* 2004;109:2705–11.

41. He K, Song Y, Daviglus ML, Liu K, Van Horn L, Dyer AR, Goldbourt U, Greenland P. Fish consumption and incidence of stroke: A meta-analysis of cohort studies. *Stroke* 2004;35:1538–42.

42. Whelton SP, He J, Whelton PK, Muntner P. Meta-analysis of observational studies on fish intake and coronary heart disease. *Am J Cardiol* 2004;93:1119–23.
43. Mozaffarian D, Rimm EB. Fish intake, contaminants, and human health: Evaluating the risks and the benefits. *JAMA* 2006;296:1885–99.
44. Burr ML, Fehily AM, Gilbert JF, Rogers S, Holliday RM, Sweetnam PM, Elwood PC, Deadman NM. Effects of changes in fat, fish, and fibre intakes on death and myocardial reinfarction: Diet and reinfarction trial (DART). *Lancet* 1989;2:757–61.
45. GISSI Prevenzione Investigators. Dietary supplementation with n-3 polyunsaturated fatty acids and vitamin E after myocardial infarction: Results of the GISSI-Prevenzione trial. Gruppo Italiano per lo Studio della Sopravvivenza nell'Infarto miocardio. *Lancet* 1999;354:447–55.
46. Yokoyama M, Origasa H, Matsuzaki M, Matsuzawa Y, Saito Y, Ishikawa Y, Oikawa S, Sasaki J, Hishida H, Itakura H, Kita T, Kitabatake A, Nakaya N, Sakata T, Shimada K, Shirato K; Japan EPA Lipid Intervention Study (JELIS) Investigators. Effects of eicosapentaenoic acid on major coronary events in hypercholesterolaemic patients (JELIS): A randomised open-label, blinded endpoint analysis. *Lancet* 2007;369:1090–8.
47. Eslick GD, Howe PR, Smith C, Priest R, Bensoussan A. Benefits of fish oil supplementation in hyperlipidemia: A systematic review and meta-analysis. *Int J Cardiol* 2009;136:4–16.
48. Geleijnse JM, Giltay EJ, Grobbee DE, Donders AR, Kok FJ. Blood pressure response to fish oil supplementation: Metaregression analysis of randomized trials. *J Hypertens* 2002;20:1493–9.
49. Mozaffarian D, Geelen A, Brouwer IA, Geleijnse JM, Zock PL, Katan MB. Effect of fish oil on heart rate in humans: A meta-analysis of randomized controlled trials. *Circulation* 2005;112:1945–52.
50. Mozaffarian D, Wu JHY. Omega-3 fatty acids and cardiovascular disease-effects on risk factors, molecular pathways, and clinical events. *J Am Coll Cardiol* 2011;58:2047–67.
51. Dietary Guidelines Advisory Committee. Report of the Dietary Guidelines Advisory Committee on the Dietary Guidelines for Americans. US Department of Agriculture, Agricultural Research Service, 2010. Available at http://www.cnpp.usda.gov/DGAs2010-DGACReport.htm (accessed October 23, 2013).
52. Mozaffarian D, Shi P, Morris JS, Spiegelman D, Grandjean P, Siscovick DS, Willet WC, Rim EB. Mercury exposure and risk of cardiovascular disease in two US cohort. *New Engl J Med* 2011;364:1116–25.
53. Ros E, Mataix J. Fatty acid composition of nuts—implications for cardiovascular health. *Br J Nutr* 2006;11:S29–35.
54. Ros E, Tapsell LC, Sabate J. Nuts and berries for heart health. *Curr Atheroscler Rep* 2010;11:397–406.
55. Mente A, de Koning L, Shannon HS, Anand SS. A systematic revie of the evidence supporting a causal link between dietary factors and coronary heart disease. *Arch Intern Med* 2009;169:659–69.
56. Bao Y, Han J, Hu FB, Giovannucci EL, Stampfer MJ, Willett WC, Fuchs CS. Association of nut consumption with total and cause-specific mortality. *N Engl J Med* 2013;369:2001–11.
57. Sabate J, Oda K, Ros E. Nut consumption and blood lipid levels: A pooled analysis of 25 intervention trials. *Arch Intern Med* 2010;170:821–7.
58. Estruch R, Ros E, Salas-Salvadó J, Covas MI, Corella D, Arós F, Gómez-Gracia E, Ruiz-Gutiérrez V, Fiol M, Lapetra J, Lamuela-Raventos RM, Serra-Majem L, Pintó X, Basora J, Muñoz MA, Sorlí JV, Martínez JA, Martínez-González MA; PREDIMED Study Investigators. Primary prevention of cardiovascular disease with a Mediterranean diet. *N Engl J Med* 2013;368:1279–90.
59. Hooper L, Kroon PA, Rimm EB, Cohn JS, Harvey I, Le Cornu KA, Ryder JJ, Hall WL, Cassidy A. Flavonoids, flavonoid-rich foods, and cardiovascular risk: A meta-analysis of randomized controlled trials. *Am J Clin Nutr* 2008;88:38–50.
60. Sacks FM, Lichtenstein A, Van Horn L, Harris W, Kris-Etherton P, Winston M. Soy protein, isoflavones, and cardiovascular health: An American Heart Association Science Advisory for professionals from the Nutrition Committee. *Circulation* 2006;113:1034–44.
61. McGrane MM, Essery E, Obbagy J, Lyon J, Macneil P, Spahn J, Van Horn L. Dairy consumption, blood pressure, and risk of hypertension: An evidence-based review of recent literature. *Curr Cardiovasc Risk Rep* 2011;5:287–98.
62. Alonso A, Beunza JJ, Delgado-Rodríguez M, Martínez JA, Martínez-González MA. Low-fat dairy consumption and reduced risk of hypertension: The Seguimiento Universidad de Navarra (SUN) cohort. *Am J Clin Nutr* 2005;82:972–9.
63. Toledo E, Alonso A, Martinez-Gonzalez MA. Differential association of low-fat and whole-fat dairy products with blood pressure and incidence of hypertension. *Curr Nutr Rep* 2012;1:197–204.
64. Trichopoulou A, Costacou T, Bamia C, Trichopulos D. Adherence to a Mediterranean diet and survival in a Greek population. *N Engl J Med* 2003;26:2599–608.

65. Martinez-Gonzalez MA, Gea A. Mediterranean diet: The whole is more than the sum of its parts. *Br J Nutr* 2012;108:577–8.

66. Fung TT, Willett WC, Stampfer MJ, Manson JE, Hu FB. Dietary patterns and the risk of coronary heart disease in women. *Arch Intern Med* 2001;161:1857–6.

67. Fung TT, Chiuve SE, McCullough ML, Rexrode KM, Logroscino G, Hu FB. Adherence to a DASH-style diet and risk of coronary heart disease and stroke in women. *Arch Intern Med* 2008;168:713–20.

68. Dominique Ashen M. Vegetarian diets in cardiovascular prevention. *Curr Treat Options Cardiovasc Med* 2013;15(6):735–45.

69. Micha R, Wallace S, Mozaffarian D. Red and processed meat consumption and risk of incident coronary heart disease, stroke, and diabetes: A systematic review and meta-analysis. *Circulation* 2010;121:2271–83.

70. Malik VS, Pan A, Willett WC, Hu FB. Sugar-sweetened beverages and weight gain in children and adults: A systematic review and meta-analysis. *Am J Clin Nutr* 2013;98:1084–102.

71. Hu FB. Resolved: There is sufficient scientific evidence that decreasing sugar-sweetened beverage consumption will reduce the prevalence of obesity and obesity-related diseases. *Obes Rev* 2013;14:606–19.

72. Duffey KJ, Popkin BM. Shifts in patterns and consumption beverages between 1965 and 2002. *Obesity (Silver Spring)* 2007;15:2739–47.

73. Lloyd-Jones D, Adams R, Carnethon M, De Simone G, Ferguson TB, Flegal K, Ford E, Furie K, Go A, Greenlund K, Haase N, Hailpern S, Ho M, Howard V, Kissela B, Kittner S, Lackland D, Lisabeth L, Marelli A, McDermott M, Meigs J, Mozaffarian D, Nichol G, O'Donnell C, Roger V, Rosamond W, Sacco R, Sorlie P, Stafford R, Steinberger J, Thom T, Wasserthiel-Smoller S, Wong N, Wylie-Rosett J, Hong Y; American Heart Association Statistics Committee and Stroke Statistics Subcommittee. Heart disease and stroke statistics—2009 update: A report from the American Heart Association Statistics Committee and Stroke Statistics Subcommittee. *Circulation* 2009;119:e21–181.

74. Wang YC, Bleich SN, Gortmaker SL. Increasing caloric contribution from sugar-sweetened beverages and 100% fruit juices among US children and adolescents, 1988–2004. *Pediatrics* 2008;121:e1604–14.

75. Stull AJ, Apolzan JW, Thalacker-Mercer AE, Iglay HB, Campbell WW. Liquid and solid meal replacement products differentially affect postprandial appetite and food intake in older adults. *J Am Diet Assoc* 2008;108:1226–30.

76. Zijlstra N, Mars M, de Wijk RA, Westerterp-Plantenga MS, de Graaaf C. The effect of viscosity on ad libitum food intake. *Int J Obes (Lond)* 2008;32:676–83.

77. Keller KL, Kirzner J, Pietrobelli A, St-Onge MP, Faith MS. Increased sweetened beverage intake is associated with reduced milk and calcium intake in 3-to 7-year-old children at multi-item laboratory lunches. *J Am Diet Assoc* 2009;109:497–501.

78. Wolff E, Sansinger ML. Soft drinks and weight gain: How strong is the link? *Medscape J Med* 2008;10:189.

79. Chen L, Appel LJ, Loria C, Lin PH, Champagne CM, Elmer PJ, Ard JD, Mitchell D, Batch BC, Svetkey LP, Caballero B. Reduction in consumption of sugar-sweetened beverages is associated with weight loss: The PREMIER trial. *Am J Clin Nutr* 2009;89:1299–306.

80. Mattes RD, Shikany JM, Kaiser KA, Allison DB. Nutritively sweetened beverage consumption and body weight: A systematic review and meta-analysis of randomized experiments. *Obes Rev* 2011;12:346–65.

81. Malik VS, Popkin BM, Bray GA, Despres JP, Willett WC, Hu FB. Sugar-sweetened beverages and risk of metabolic syndrome and type 2 diabetes: A meta-analysis. *Diabetes Care* 2010;33:2477–83.

82. Fung TT, Malik V, Rexrode KM, Manson JE, Willett WC, Hu FB. Sweetened beverage consumption and risk of coronary heart disease in women. *Am J Clin Nutr* 2009;89:1037–42.

83. Mozaffarian D, Appel LJ, Van Horn L. Components of a cardioprotective diet: New insights. *Circulation* 2011;123:2870–91.

84. Brien SE, Ronksley PE, Turner BJ, Mukamal KJ, Ghali WA. Effect of alcohol consumption on biological markers associated with risk of coronary heart disease: Systematic review and meta-analysis of interventional studies. *BMJ* 2011;342:d636.

85. Laonigro I, Correale M, Di Biase M, Altomare E. Alcohol abuse and heart failure. *Eur J Heart Fail* 2009;11:453–62.

86. Conen D, Tedrow UB, Cook NR, Moorthy MV, Buring JE, Albert CM. Alcohol consumption and risk of incident atrial fibrillation in women. *JAMA* 2008;300:2489–96.

87. Rim EB, Williams P, Fosher K, Criqui M, Stampfer MJ. Moderate alcohol intake and lower risk of coronary heart disease: Meta-analysis of effects on lipids and haemostatic factors. *BMJ* 1999;319:1523–8.

88. Shai I, Wainstein J, Harman-Boehm I, Raz I, Fraser D, Rudich A, Stampfer MJ. Glycemic effects of moderate alcohol intake among patients with type 2 diabetes: A multicenter, randomized, clinical intervention trial. *Diabetes Care* 2007;30:3011–16.

89. Joosten MM, Beulens JW, Kersten S, Hendriks HF. Moderate alcohol consumption increases insulin sensitivity and ADIPOQ expression in postmenopausal women: A randomized, crossover trial. *Diabetologia* 2008;51:1375–81.

90. Koppes LL, Dekker JM, Hendriks HF, Bouter LM, Heine RJ. Moderate alcohol consumption lowers the risk of type 2 diabetes: A meta-analysis of prospective observational studies. *Diabetes Care* 2005;28:719–25.

91. Fillmore KM, Stockwell T, Chikritzhs T, Bostrom A, Kerr W. Moderate alcohol use and reduced mortality risk: Systematic error in prospective studies and new hypotheses. *Ann Epidemiol* 2007;17:S16–23.

92. Mukamal KJ, Rim EB. Alcohol consumption: Risks and benefits. *Curr Atheroscler Rep* 2008;10:536–43.

93. Rimm EB, Klatsky A, Grobbee D, Stampfer MJ. Review of moderate alcohol consumption and reduced risk of coronary heart disease: Is the effect due to beer, wine, or spirits? *BMJ* 1996;312:731–6.

94. Mukamal KJ, Jensen MK, Gronbaek M, Stampfer MJ, Manson JE, Pischon T, Rimm EB. Drinking frequency, mediating biomarkers, and risk of myocardial infarction in women and men. *Circulation* 2005;112:1406–13.

95. Sayon-Orea C, Martinez-Gonzalez MA, Bes-Rastrollo M. Alcohol consumption and body weight: A systematic review. *Nutr Rev* 2011;69:419–31.

96. Danaei G, Ding EL, Mozaffarian D, Taylor B, Rehm J, Murray CJ, Ezzati M. The preventable cause of death in the United States: Comparative risk assessment of dietary, lifestyle, and metabolic risk factors. *PLoS Med* 2009;6:e1000058.

97. Gea A, Bes-Rastrollo M, Toledo E, Garcia-Lopez M, Beunza JJ, Estruch R, Martinez-Gonzalez MA. Mediterranean alcohol-drinking pattern and mortality in the SUN (Seguimiento Universidad de Navarra) Project: A prospective cohort study. *Br J Nutr* 2014;111(10):1871-80.

98. Rajaram S. The effect of vegetarian diet, plant foods, and phytochemicals on hemostasis and thrombosis. *Am J Clin Nutr* 2003;78:552S–8S.

99. Huxley RR, Neil HA. The relation between dietary flavonol intake and coronary heart disease mortality: A meta-analysis of prospective cohort studies. *Eur J Clin Nutr* 2003;57:904–8.

100. Law M. Plant sterol and stanol margarines and health. *BMJ* 2000;320:861–4.

101. Appel LJ. Dietary patterns and longevity: Expanding the blue zones. *Circulation* 2008;118:214–15.

102. Willett WC, Sacks F, Trichopoulou A, Drescher G, Ferro-Luzzi A, Helsing E, Trichopoulos D. Mediterranean diet pyramid: A cultural model for healthy eating. *Am J Clin Nutr* 1995;61 Suppl 6:S1402–6.

103. De Lorgeril M, Salen P, Martin JL, Monajud I, Delaye J, Mamelle N. Mediterranean diet, traditional risk factors, and the rate of cardiovascular complications after myocardial infarction: Final report of the Lyon Diet Heart Study. *Circulation* 1999;99:779–85.

104. Martinez-Gonzalez MA, Corella D, Salas-Salvado J, Ros E, Covas MI, Fiol M, Wärnberg J, Arós F, Ruíz-Gutiérrez V, Lamuela-Raventós RM, Lapetra J, Muñoz MÁ, Martínez JA, Sáez G, Serra-Majem L, Pintó X, Mitjavila MT, Tur JA, Portillo MP, Estruch R; PREDIMED Study Investigators. Cohort profile: Design and methods of the PREDIMED study. *Int J Epidemiol* 2012;41:377–85.

105. Martinez-Gonzalez MA, Bes-Rastrollo M. Dietary patterns, Mediterranean diet, and cardiovascular disease. *Curr Opin Lipidol* 2014;25(1):20–6.

106. Horton R. Expression of concern: Indo-Mediterranean Diet Heart Study. *Lancet* 2005;366:354–6.

107. Sofi F, Abbate R, Gensini GF, Casini A. Accruing evidence on benefits of adherence to the Mediterranean diet on health: An updated systematic review and meta-analysis. *Am J Clin Nutr* 2010;92:1189–92.

108. Dilis V, Katsoulis M, Lagiou P, Trichopoulos D, Naska A, Trichopoulou A. Mediterranean diet and CHD: The Greek European prospective investigation into cancer and nutrition cohort. *Br J Nutr* 2012;108:699–709.

109. Tognon G, Nilsson LM, Lissner L, Johansson I, Hallmans G, Lindahl B, Winkvist A. The Mediterranean diet score and mortality are inversely associated in adults living in the Subartic region. *J Nutr* 2012;142:1547–53.

110. Gardener H, Wright CB, Gu Y, Demmer RT, Boden-Albala B, Elkind MS, Sacco RL, Scarmeas N. Mediterranean diet and risk of ischemic stroke, myocardial infarction, and vascular death: The Northern Manhattan Study. *Am J Clin Nutr* 2011;94:1458–64.

111. Misirli G, Benetou V, Lagiou P, Bamia C, Trichopoulos D, Trichopoulou A. Relation of the traditional Mediterranean diet to cerebrovascular disease in a Mediterranean population. *Am J Epidemiol* 2012;176:1185–92.

112. Hoevenaar-Blom M, Nooyens ACJ, Kromhout D, Spijkerman AM, Beulens JW, van der Schouw YT, Bueno-de-Mesquita B, Verschuren WM. Mediterranean style diet and 12-year incidence of cardiovascular diseases: The EPIC-NL cohort study. *Plos ONE* 2012;7:e45458.

113. Menotti A, Alberti-Fidanza A, Fidanza F. The association of the Mediterranean Adequacy Index with fatal coronary events in an Italian middle-aged male population followed for 40 years. *Nutr Metab Cardiovasc Dis* 2012;22:369–75.

114. Tognon G, Lissner L, Sæbye D, Walker KZ, Heitmann BL. The Mediterranean diet in relation to mortality and CVD: A Danish cohort study. *Br J Nutr* 2014;111(1):151–9.

115. Hoevenaar-Blom MP, Spijkerman AM, Kromhout D, Verschuren WM. Insufficient sleep duration contributes to lower cardiovascular disease risk in addition to four traditional lifestyle factors: The MORGEN study. *Eur J Prev Cardiol* 2013, doi: 10.1177/2047487313493057.

116. Buckland G, González CA, Agudo A, Vilardell M, Berenguer A, Amiano P, Ardanaz E, Arriola L, Barricarte A, Basterretxea M, Chirlaque MD, Cirera L, Dorronsoro M, Egües N, Huerta JM, Larrañaga N, Marin P, Martínez C, Molina E, Navarro C, Quirós JR, Rodriguez L, Sanchez MJ, Tormo MJ, Moreno-Iribas C. Adherence to the Mediterranean diet and risk of coronary heart disease in the Spanish EPIC Cohort Study. *Am J Epidemiol* 2009;170:1518–29.

117. Martinez-Gonzalez MA, Garcia-Lopez M, Bes-Rastrollo M, Toledo E, Martínez-Lapiscina EH, Delgado-Rodriguez M, Vazquez Z, Benito S, Beunza JJ. Mediterranean diet and the incidence of cardiovascular disease: A Spanish cohort. *Nutr Metab Cardiovasc Dis* 2011;21:237–44.

118. Mitrou PN, Kipnis V, Thiébaut AC, Reedy J, Subar AF, Wirfält E, Flood A, Mouw T, Hollenbeck AR, Leitzmann MF, Schatzkin A. Mediterranean dietary pattern and prediction of all-cause mortality in a US population: Results from the NIH-AARP Diet and Health Study. *Arch Intern Med* 2007;167:2461–8.

119. Howard BV, Van Horn L, Hsia J, Manson JE, Stefanick ML, Wassertheil-Smoller S, Kuller LH, LaCroix AZ, Langer RD, Lasser NL, Lewis CE, Limacher MC, Margolis KL, Mysiw WJ, Ockene JK, Parker LM, Perri MG, Phillips L, Prentice RL, Robbins J, Rossouw JE, Sarto GE, Schatz IJ, Snetselaar LG, Stevens VJ, Tinker LF, Trevisan M, Vitolins MZ, Anderson GL, Assaf AR, Bassford T, Beresford SA, Black HR, Brunner RL, Brzyski RG, Caan B, Chlebowski RT, Gass M, Granek I, Greenland P, Hays J, Heber D, Heiss G, Hendrix SL, Hubbell FA, Johnson KC, Kotchen JM. Low-fat dietary pattern and risk of cardiovascular disease: The Women's Health Initiative Randomized Controlled Dietary Modification Trial. *JAMA* 2006;295:655–66.

120. Look AHEAD Research Group, Wing RR, Bolin P, Brancati FL, Bray GA, Clark JM, Coday M, Crow RS, Curtis JM, Egan CM, Espeland MA, Evans M, Foreyt JP, Ghazarian S, Gregg EW, Harrison B, Hazuda HP, Hill JO, Horton ES, Hubbard VS, Jakicic JM, Jeffery RW, Johnson KC, Kahn SE, Kitabchi AE, Knowler WC, Lewis CE, Maschak-Carey BJ, Montez MG, Murillo A, Nathan DM, Patricio J, Peters A, Pi-Sunyer X, Pownall H, Reboussin D, Regensteiner JG, Rickman AD, Ryan DH, Safford M, Wadden TA, Wagenknecht LE, West DS, Williamson DF, Yanovski SZ. Cardiovascular effects of intensive lifestyle intervention in type 2 diabetes. *N Engl J Med* 2013;369:145–54.

121. Despres JP, Poirier P. Looking back at Look AHEAD-giving lifestyle a chance. *Nat Rev Cardiol* 2013;10:184–6.

122. Serra-Majem L, Bes-Rastrollo M, Román-Viñas B, Pfrimer K, Sánchez-Villegas A, Martínez-González MA. Dietary patterns and nutritional adequacy in a Mediterranean country. *Br J Nutr* 2009;101 Suppl 2:S21–8.

123. Martínez-González MA, Salas-Salvado J, Estruch R. Intensive lifestyle intervention in type 2 diabetes. *N Engl J Med* 2013;369:2357.

124. Swain JF, McCarron PB, Hamilton EF, Sacks FM, Appel LJ. Characteristics of the diet patterns tested in the Optimal Macronutrient Intake Trial to Prevent Heart Disease (OmniHeart): Options for heart-healthy diet. *J Am Diet Assoc* 2008;108:257–65.

125. Appel LJ, Sacks FM, Carey VJ, Obarzanek E, Swain JF, Miller ER 3rd, Conlin PR, Erlinger TP, Rosner BA, Laranjo NM, Charleston J, McCarron P, Bishop LM; OmniHeart Collaborative Research Group. Effects of protein, monounsaturated fat, and carbohydrate intake on blood pressure and serum lipids: Results of the OmniHeart randomized trial. *JAMA* 2005;294:2455–64.

126. Mellen PB, Gao SK, Vitolins MZ, Goff DC Jr. Deteriorating dietary habits among adults with hypertension: DASH dietary accordance, NHANES 1988–1994 and 1999–2004. *Arch Intern Med* 2008;168:308–14.

127. Margetts BM, Beilin LJ, Vandongen R, Armstrong BK. Vegetarian diet in mild hypertension: A randomised controlled trial. *BMJ (Clin Res Ed)* 1986;293:1468–71.

128. Sciarrone SE, Strahan MT, Beilin LJ, Burke V, Rogers P, Rouse IR. Ambulatory blood pressure and heart rate responses to vegetarian meals. *J Hypertens* 1993;11:277–85.

129. Hakala P, Karvetti RL. Weight reduction on lactovegetarian and mixed diets: Changes in weight, nutrient intake, skinfold thicknesses and blood pressure. *Eur J Clin Nutr* 1989;43:421–30.

130. Barnard ND, Cohen J, Jenkings DJ, Turner-McCrievy G, Gloede L, Green A, Ferdowsian H. A low-fat vegan diet and a conventional diabetes diet in the treatment of type 2 diabetes: A randomized, controlled, 74-wk clinical trial. *Am J Clin Nutr* 2009;89:1588S–96S.

131. Burke LE, Styn MA, Steenkiste AR, Music E, Warziski M, Choo J. A randomized clinical trial testing treatment preference and two dietary options in behavioral weight management: Preliminary results of the impact of diet at 6 months: PREFER study. *Obesity (Silver Spring)* 2006;14:2007–17.

132. Burke LE, Hudson AG, Warziski MT, Styn MA, Music E, Elci OU, Sereika SM. Effects of a vegetarian diet and treatment preference on biochemical and dietary variables in overweight and obese adults: A randomized clinical trial. *Am J Clin Nutr* 2007;86:588–96.

133. Fung TT, Rexrode KM, Mantzoros CS, Manson JE, Willet WC, Hu FB. Mediterranean diet and incidence of and mortality from coronary heart disease and stroke in women. *Circulation* 2009;119:1093–100.

134. Nunez-Cordoba JM, Valencia-Serrano F, Toledo E, Alonso A, Martinez-Gonzalez MA. The Mediterranean diet and incidence of hypertension: The Seguimiento Universidad de Navarra (SUN) Study. *Am J Epidemiol* 2009;169:339–46.

135. Key TJ, Fraser GE, Thorogood M, Appleby PN, Beral V, Reeves G, Burr ML, Chang-Claude J, Frentzel-Beyme R, Kuzma JW, Mann J, McPherson K. Mortality in vegetarians and non-vegetarians: A collaborative analysis of 8300 deaths among 76,000 men and women in five prospective studies. *Public Health Nutr* 1998;1:33–41.

136. Fraser GE. Associations between diet and cancer, ischemic heart disease, and all-cause mortality in non-Hispanic white California Seventh-day Adventists. *Am J Clin Nutr* 1999;70:532S–8S.

137. Craig WJ, Mangels AR. Position of the American Dietetic Association: Vegetarian diets. *J Am Diet Assoc* 2009;109:1266–82.

138. Martínez-Gonzalez MA, Sanchez-Tainta A, Corella D, Salas-Salvadó J, Ros E, Arós F, Gómez-Gracia E, Fiol M, Lamuela-Raventós RM, Schröder H, Lapetra J, Serra-Majem L, Pinto X, Ruiz-Gutierrez V, Estruch R; for the PREDIMED Group. A provegetarian food pattern and reduction in total mortality in the Prevención con Dieta Mediterránea (PREDIMED) study. *Am J Clin Nutr.* May 28, 2014. pii: ajcn.071431. [Epub ahead of print].

139. Orlich MJ, Singh PN, Sabaté J, Jaceldo-Siegl K, Fan J, Knutsen S, Beeson WL, Fraser GE. Vegetarian dietary patterns and mortality in Adventist Health Study 2. *JAMA Intern Med* 2013;173:1230–8.

140. Huang T, Yang B, Zheng J, Li G, Wahlqvist ML, Li D. Cardiovascular disease mortality and cancer incidence in vegetarians: A meta-analysis and systematic review. *Ann Nutr Metab* 2012;60:233–40.

141. Wilcox BJ, Willcox DC, Todoriki H, Fujiyoshi A, Yano K, He Q, Curb JD, Suzuki M. Caloric restriction, the traditional Okinawan diet, and healthy aging: The diet of the world's longest-lived people and its potential impact on morbidity and life span. *Ann N Y Acad Sci* 2007;1114:434–55.

142. Shimazu T, Kuriyama S, Hozawa A, Ohmori K, Sato Y, Nakaya N, Nishino Y, Tsubono Y, Tsuji I. Dietary patterns and cardiovascular disease mortality in Japan: A prospective cohort study. *Int J Epidemiol* 2007;36:600–9.

143. Ding EL, Mozaffarian D. Optimal dietary habits for the prevention of stroke. *Semin Neurol* 2006;26:11–23.

144. Willcox DC, Willcox BJ, Todoriki H, Suzuki M. The Okinawan diet: Health implications of a low-calorie, nutrient-dense, antioxidant-rich dietary pattern low in glycemic load. *J Am Coll Nutr* 2009;28:500S–16S.

145. Liu S, Willett WC, Stampfer MJ, Hu FB, Franz M, Sampson L, Hennekens CH, Manson JE. A prospective study of dietary glycemic load, carbohydrate intake, and risk of coronory heart disease in US women. *Am J Clin Nutr* 2000;71:1455–61.

146. Sanchez-Tainta A, Zazpe I, Bes-Rastrollo M et al. Nutritional adequacy according to carbohydrates and fat quality in the PREDIMED trial (submitted).

147. Keys A. *Seven Countries: A Multivariate Analysis of Death and Coronary Heart Disease.* Cambridge, MA: Harvard University Press; 1980.

148. Kato H, Tillotson J, Nichaman MZ, Rhoads GG, Hamilton HB. Epidemiologic studies of coronary heart disease and stroke in Japanese men living in Japan, Hawaii and California. *Am J Epidemiol* 1973;97:372–85.

149. Hu FB, Stampfer MJ, Manson JE, Rimm E, Colditz GA, Rosner BA, Hennekens CH, Willett WC. Dietary fat intake and the risk of coronary heart disease in women. *N Engl J Med* 1997;337:1491–9.

150. Mozaffarian D, Katan MB, Ascherio A, Stampfer MJ, Willett WC. Trans fatty acid and cardiovascular disease. *N Engl J Med* 2006;354:1601–13.

151. Hu FB. Diet and lifestyle influences on risk of coronary heart disease. *Curr Atheroscler Rep* 2009;11:257–63.

152. Dayton S, Pearce ML, Hashimoto S, Dixon WJ, Tomiyasu U. A controlled clinical trial of a diet high in unsaturated fat in preventing complications of atherosclerosis. *Circulation* 1969;40:1S–63S.

153. Turpeinen O, Karvonen MJ, Pekkarienn M, Miettinen M, Elosuo R, Paavilainen E. Dietary prevention of coronary heart disease: The Finnish Mental Hospital Study. *Int J Epidemiol* 1979;8:99–118.

154. Morris JN, Ball KP, Antonis A et al. Controlled trial of soya-bean oil in myocardial infarction. *Lancet* 1968;2:693–9.

155. Malhotra A. Saturated fat is not the major issue. *BMJ* 2013;347:f6340.

156. Siri-Tarino PW, Sun Q, Hu FB, Krauss RM. Meta-analysis of prospective cohort studies evaluating the association of saturated fat with cardiovascular disease. *Am J Clin Nutr* 2010;91:535–46.

157. He FJ, MacCregor GA. A comprehensive review on salt and health and current experience of worldwide salt reduction programmes. *J Hum Hypertens* 2009;23:363–84.

158. Strazzulo P, D'Elia L, Kandala NB, Cappuccio FP. Salt intake, stroke, and cardiovascular disease: Meta-analysis of prospective studies. *BMJ* 2009;339:b4567.

159. Cook NR, Ctuler JA, Obarzanek E, Buring JE, Rexrode KM, Kumanyika SK, Appel LJ, Whelton PK. Long term effects of dietary sodium reduction on cardiovascular disease outcomes: Observational follow-up of the Trials of Hypertension Prevention (TOHP). *BMJ* 2007;334:885–8.

160. Appel LJ. At the tipping point: Accomplishing population-wide sodium reduction in the United States. *J Clin Hypertens (Greenwich)* 2008;10:7–11.

161. Ikehara S, Iso H, Date C, Kikuchi S, Watanabe Y, Inaba Y, Tamakoshi A. JACC Study Group. Salt preference and mortality from stroke and coronary heart disease for Japanese men and women: The JACC study. *Prev Med* 2012;54:32–7.

162. Brown IJ, Tzoulaki I, Candeias V, Elliott P. Salt intakes around the world: Implications for public health. *Int J Epidemiol* 2009;38:791–813.

163. Risk Factor Monitoring and Methods Branch Web Site. Applied Research Program, National Cancer Institute. Sources of sodium among the US population, 2005–06. Available at http://riskfactor.cancer.gov/diet/foodsources/sodium/ (accessed October 23, 2013).

164. Bibbins-Domingo K, Chjertow GM, Coxson PG, Moran A, Lightwood JM, Pletcher MJ, Goldman L. Projected effect of dietary salt reductions on future cardiovascular disease. *N Engl J Med* 2010;362:590–9.

165. Smith-Spangler CM, Juusola JL, Enns EA, Owens DK, Garber AM. Population strategies to decrease sodium intake and the burden of cardiovascular disease: A cost-effectiveness analysis. *Ann Intern Med* 2010;152:481–7.

166. World Health Organization. *Intervention on Diet and Physical Activity: What Works.* Geneva, Switzerland: WHO Press; 2009.

167. Artinian NT, Fletcher GF, Mozaffarian D, Kris-Etherton P, Van Horn L, Lichtenstein AH, Kumanyika S, Kraus WE, Fleg JL, Redeker NS, Meininger JC, Banks J, Stuart-Shor EM, Fletcher BJ, Miller TD, Hughes S, Braun LT, Kopin LA, Berra K, Hayman LL, Ewing LJ, Ades PA, Durstine JL, Houston-Miller N, Burke LE; American Heart Association Prevention Committee of the Council on Cardiovascular Nursing. Intervention to promote physical activity and dietary lifestyle changes for cardiovascular risk factor reduction in adults: A scientific statement from the American Heart Association. *Circulation* 2010;122:406–41.

168. Schroder H, Fito M, Estruch R, Martinez-Gonzalez MA, Corella D, Salas-Salvado J, Lamuela-Raventós R, Ros E, Salaverría I, Fiol M, Lapetra J, Vinyoles E, Gómez-Gracia E, Lahoz C, Serra-Majem L, Pintó X, Ruiz-Gutierrez V, Covas MI. A short screener is valid for assessing Mediterranean diet adherence among older Spanish men and women. *J Nutr* 2011;141:1140–5.

169. Martinez-Gonzalez MA, Fernandez-Jarne E, Serrano-Martinez M, Wright M, Gomez-Gracia E. Development of a short dietary intake questionnaire for the quantitative estimation of adherence to a cardioprotective Mediterranean diet. *Eur J Clin Nutr* 2004;58:1550–2.

170. Babio N, Bullo M, Basora J, Martinez-Gonzalez MA, Fernandez-Ballart J, Marquez-Sandoval F, Molina C, Salas-Salvadó J; Nureta-PREDIMED Investigators. Adherence to the Mediterranean diet and risk of metabolic syndrome and its components. *Nutr Metab Cardiovasc Dis* 2009;19:563–70.

171. Sanchez-Tainta A, Estruch R, Bullo M, Corella D, Gomez-Gracia E, Fiol M, Algorta J, Covas MI, Lapetra J, Zazpe I, Ruiz-Gutiérrez V, Ros E, Martínez-González MA; PREDIMED Group. Adherence to a Mediterranean-type diet and reduced prevalence of clustered cardiovascular risk factors in a cohort of 3, 204 high-risk patients. *Eur J Cardiovasc Rehabil* 2008;15:589–93.

172. Schröder H, Martinez-Gonzalez MA, Fito M, Fito M, Corella D, Estruch R, Ros E. Baseline adherence to the Mediterranean diet and major cardiovascular events in the PREDIMED trial JAMA Intern Med (in press).

173. Martinez-Gonzalez MA, Garcia-Arellano A, Toledo E, Salas-Salvado J, Buil-Cosiales P, Corella D, Covas MI, Schröder H, Arós F, Gómez-Gracia E, Fiol M, Ruiz-Gutiérrez V, Lapetra J, Lamuela-Raventos RM, Serra-Majem L, Pintó X, Muñoz MA, Wärnberg J, Ros E, Estruch R; for the PREDIMED Study Investigators. A 14-item Mediterranean diet assessment tool and obesity indexes among high-risk subjects: The PREDIMED trial. *PLOS One* 2012;7:e43134.

8 Risk Relationship between Insulin Resistance, Diabetes, and Atherosclerotic Cardiovascular Disease

Serena Del Turco, Rosa Sicari, and Amalia Gastaldelli

CONTENTS

INTRODUCTION

In recent years, there has been great interest in the concept of a clustering of risk factors for cardiovascular disease (CVD) occurring in a given individual to a greater degree than expected by chance. This clustering, commonly referred to as the "metabolic syndrome," has clinical manifestations frequently observed in obesity and is believed to be associated with underlying insulin resistance (IR) in the majority, of individuals. In its original conception, "syndrome X" [1] or the "insulin resistance syndrome" [2] provided a framework to understand the relationship or association between IR, multiple metabolic abnormalities, and the development of type 2 diabetes mellitus (T2DM). This "metabolic" clustering of risk factors (obesity, elevated triglycerides [TG] and low high-density lipoprotein [HDL] cholesterol, hypertension, IR, abnormal fasting or 2-h plasma glucose levels, and others) is used primarily to CVD risk profiling in an individual subject.

Early studies from UK Prospective Diabetes Study (UKPDS) showed that an increase in HbA1c of up to 10% was associated with a hazard ratio (HR) for CVD of 2.2 for myocardial infarction and of 1.8 for the development of stroke when compared to control subjects with HbA1c of 5% [3]. Not only T2DM and obesity *per se* are states of IR but also hypertriglyceridemia, hypertension, and coronary artery disease (CAD) [4]. So it is not surprising to find that over half of patients referred to cardiologists have metabolic syndrome [5–7]. In the presence of IR, the amount of secreted insulin is increased since more insulin is required to promote glucose disposal [8]. As a consequence, higher circulating insulin levels are needed to overcome IR and promote glucose disposal. This has relevant pathophysiologic and clinical consequences. The insulin-resistant state is associated with dyslipidemia, hyper-aggregation, and antifibrinolysis that may create a prothrombotic milieu favoring the occurrence of cardiovascular (CV) complications. The association between IR and cardiometabolic risk and, in particular, the role of insulin will be reviewed in the following sections.

FROM IR TO TYPE 2 DIABETES

IR is mainly due to a defect in insulin receptors. The insulin receptor is a transmembrane receptor tyrosine kinase that includes the insulin-like growth factor receptor (IGFR) and the insulin receptor-related receptor (IRR). These receptors are composed of two alpha and two beta subunits linked by disulfide bonds able to form homodimers or heterodimers that function as allosteric enzymes in which the alpha subunit inhibits the tyrosine kinase activity of the beta subunit. Insulin binds with high affinity to the alpha-subunit of the insulin receptor leading to subsequent autophosphorylation via beta subunits. As shown in Figure 8.1, activation of the insulin receptor leads to tyrosine phosphorylation of insulin receptor substrate 1 (IRS1), thereby initiating signal transduction. When IRS1 is alternatively phosphorylated on serine 307, its downstream signaling ability is diminished. Defects in IRS1 phosphorylation have, as a consequence, alterations in glucose and lipid metabolism. In particular, the two most critical signaling branches activated downstream from insulin receptors are the phosphatidylinositol 3-kinase (PI3K) pathway in vascular endothelium, skeletal

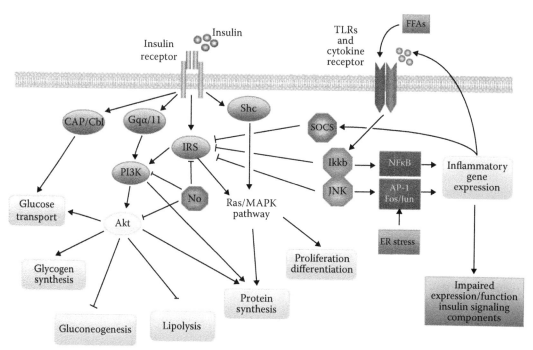

FIGURE 8.1 **(See color insert.)** Direct interaction of insulin signaling and inflammatory pathways. The insulin signaling cascade branches into two main pathways. The PI3K/AKT pathway mediates insulin action on nutrient metabolism including glucose uptake. The Ras/MAPK pathway mediates insulin's effect on gene expression but also interacts with the PI3K-AKT pathway to control cell growth and differentiation. Activation of the insulin receptor leads to tyrosine phosphorylation of IRS1, thereby initiating signal transduction. Stimulation of the NF-κB and AP-1 Fos/Jun inflammatory pathways results in the activation of the serine kinases, Ikkb and JNK1, which reduce the signaling ability of IRS1. Additional inflammation-related negative regulators of IRS proteins include the Socs proteins and NO, which are induced in inflammation and promote IRS degradation. NO also reduces PI3K/Akt activity by s-nitrosylation of Akt. (Reprinted from *FEBS Letters*, 582[1], De Luca C and Olefsky JM, Inflammation and insulin resistance, 97–105, Copyright 2008, with permission from Elsevier.)

muscle, and adipose tissue (for the control of vasodilator and metabolic actions of insulin), and the Ras/mitogen activated protein kinase (MAPK) pathway in various tissues (for mitogenic and growth effects of insulin) (Figure 8.1). The PI3K pathway is a key component of the metabolic effect of insulin on rapid stimulation of glucose uptake via the glucose transporter protein GLUT4 into its target metabolic tissues, i.e., skeletal muscle and fat [9,10].

In the natural history of T2DM, individuals progress from normal glucose tolerance (NGT) to impaired glucose tolerance (IGT) to overt T2DM, and this progression has been demonstrated in populations of diverse ethnic background [11]. The development of hyperglycemia, particularly in postprandial state, is due to an imbalance between IR and insulin secretion [8]. It is widely recognized that both IR and beta-cell dysfunction are important in the pathogenesis of glucose intolerance. In populations with a high prevalence of T2DM, IR is well established long before the development of any impairment in glucose homeostasis, particularly in subjects with ectopic fat accumulation. Although the relative contributions of IR and beta-cell function to the development of type 2 diabetes may differ among ethnic groups, the onset and pace of beta-cell failure determine the rate of progression of hyperglycemia [12]. The decline in insulin-secretion-to-insulin-resistance ratio starts already in NGT subjects with a 2-h plasma glucose concentration (PG) greater than 5.6 mmol/L [13]. We have shown that subjects with IGT (i.e., subjects with 2-h oral glucose tolerance test [OGTT] glucose between 140 and 200 mg/dL) have already lost a great part of their beta-cell function, i.e., their capacity to respond to the hyperglycemic stimulus by secreting more insulin [13].

IR is usually present at the level of different organs: in the muscle showing reduced glucose uptake, in the adipose tissue mainly as impaired suppression of lipolysis, in the liver with the result of increased glucose production, mainly as gluconeogenesis, and as impaired suppression of very low density lipoprotein (VLDL) secretion (Figure 8.2). Although the major insulin target tissues are liver, adipose tissue, and skeletal muscle, insulin receptors have also been found in the brain, heart, kidney, pulmonary alveoli, pancreatic acini, placenta vascular endothelium, monocytes, granulocytes, erythrocytes, and fibroblasts [14]. This dynamic interaction between insulin secretion and IR is essential to the maintenance of NGT, and interruption of this cross-talk between the beta-cell and peripheral tissues results in the progressive deterioration of glucose homeostasis (Figure 8.2).

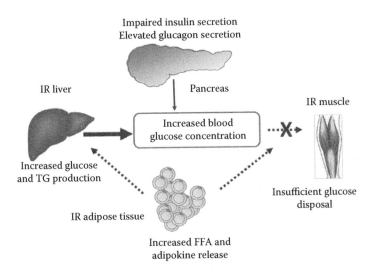

FIGURE 8.2 **(See color insert.)** Increased glucose concentration is due to IR at the level of different tissues. In the muscle, IR determines insufficient glucose disposal. In the liver, IR determines increased glucose production. In the presence of IR, the pancreas is required to secrete more insulin, but because of beta-cell dysfunction, the amount of secreted insulin is not sufficient to overcome IR and the subject develops hyperglycemia. IR at the level of adipose tissue is seen as impaired suppression of lipolysis, with excess FFA release and organ lipotoxicity.

Subjects with IR require more insulin to promote glucose uptake by peripheral tissues, and genetically predisposed individuals may lack the necessary beta-cell secretory capacity [8]. The resulting insulin deficiency disrupts the regulation of glucose production in the liver, glucose uptake in muscle, and the release of fatty acid from adipose tissue. The outcome is postprandial and later fasting hyperglycemia [15].

As long as the beta cell is able to secrete sufficient amounts of insulin to offset the severity of IR, glucose tolerance remains within normal ranges. However, postprandial glucose tends to be above normal levels long before fasting plasma glucose (diagnosis of diabetes requires a 2-h PG above 200 mg/dL). Thus, in the great majority of patients with T2DM, the diagnosis is often delayed since it is usually performed on the basis of fasting glycemia > 126 mg/dL. Although the relative contributions of IR and beta-cell function to the development of type 2 diabetes may differ in different ethnic groups, the onset and pace of beta-cell failure determine the rate of progression of hyperglycemia [12]. In addition, a reduced insulin-secretion-to-insulin-resistance ratio, which is an index of beta-cell dysfunction, is one of the strongest predictors of type 2 diabetes in subjects with IGT [16].

The major problem of a delayed diagnosis of diabetes is the silent but relentless progression of diabetes complications and, particularly among them, of CVDs [17]. Diabetic patients are known to have CV death rates that are three- to fourfold higher than those of subjects without T2DM in the presence of similar traditional factors such as elevated blood pressure, dyslipidemia, and smoking [18]. It has been observed that ~50% of diabetics already have some manifestations of CVD at the time of diagnosis [19], and this is possibly related to delayed diagnosis. Although the highest CVD risk belonged to patients with diabetes, it has been shown in a 20-year prospective study that the risk of CVD was 2.8-fold higher in subjects with a normal fasting plasma glucose at baseline that developed T2DM during follow-up compared to the control group that never developed T2DM [20].

CV burden can be assessed by advanced imaging techniques, such as carotid intima-media thickness (C-IMT) or arterial wall calcification. It has been shown that C-IMT is often increased in otherwise "asymptomatic" patients with T2DM [21], and it is a significant predictor of CVD [22], even in asymptomatic type 2 diabetic patients without a history of CVD [23]. We have recently shown that the "preclinical" C-IMT increase is associated independently of age with altered postprandial glucose profile, increased peripheral and hepatic IR, and decreased beta-cell function in subjects without T2DM [24].

IR, HYPERLIPIDEMIA, AND LIPOTOXICITY

Hyperlipidemia is a characteristic feature of subjects with IR. A high level of TG and cholesterol is the result not only of obesity and excess caloric intake but also of IR. Subjects with IR often display obesity and ectopic fat accumulation in liver, muscle, heart, pancreas, as well as epicardial and visceral fat [8]. Excess adiposity, in particular abdominal and ectopic fat accumulation, is believed to be the driving force behind the development of early CVD and increased overall mortality observed in obese individuals in population-based studies [25–37].

Abdominal obesity is associated with a greater risk of developing T2DM [38]. The Paris Prospective Study was the first large prospective study to confirm the close relationship between adipose tissue IR (i.e., elevated plasma free fatty acid [FFA] concentration) and the deterioration of glucose tolerance over time [39]. Visceral fat is believed to be more prone to lipolysis in response to counter-regulatory hormones and more resistant to the antilipolytic effect of insulin [40,41]. Moreover, it has been speculated that because it drains directly into the portal vein, FFA derived from the visceral bed would have a more direct impact on liver metabolism than fat from peripheral (subcutaneous) lipolysis [42]. In any case, the role of visceral fat and its relation to overall CV risk remain unsettled [41,43–45]. In a recent cross-sectional study across 21 research centers in Europe, simultaneously measuring insulin sensitivity (by euglycemic insulin clamp technique) and the cluster of risk factors associated with the metabolic syndrome, it was not possible to isolate different measures of adiposity (BMI, fat mass, or fat distribution) as more prominent than the others such as causative factors for IR or related CV risk factors [45]. We have found a closer correlation between visceral and liver fat accumulation than with BMI or subcutaneous fat [42,46]. However, while the "portal hypothesis" is appealing to the development of hepatic IR by visceral adipose tissue, the finding that in healthy obese individuals the contribution of visceral fat to the overall FFA pool increases only modestly (from ~10% to only ~25% compared to lean subjects) [47] suggests that expansion of subcutaneous fat adipose tissue also plays an important role in the development of hepatic IR. Moreover, the amount of FFA released from visceral fat, relative to whole body lipolysis, is minimum, i.e., ~5% or less [47], thus indicating that its contribution to peripheral (muscle) IR is marginal. However, visceral fat releases a number of adipocytokines (e.g., tumor necrosis factor-α [TNF-α], leptin, interleukins, etc.) implicated in the development of IR [48,49], thus explaining how a rather modest amount of adipose tissue (less than 15% of total body fat) could impair hepatic and peripheral (muscle) insulin action.

When subcutaneous adipose tissue becomes dysfunctional it is more likely that visceral and ectopic fat accumulate. A recent study showed that overfeeding determines different patterns of fat accumulation: in particular, only subjects that showed defective expression in the subcutaneous fat of lipid storage-related genes (DGAT2, SREBP1c, and CIDEA) exhibit the largest accumulation in visceral depot [50]. The incapacity of subcutaneous adipose tissue to metabolize circulating fatty acids determines ectopic fat accumulation in other organs such as liver, muscle, and pancreas, as well as heart [51]. Fat deposition occurs in the intrathoracic region as epicardial and mediastinal fat and inside cardiomyocytes. All of the cardiac fat depots have been shown to be markers of cardiac lipotoxicity, mitochondrial dysfunction, inflammation, local and systemic IR, atherosclerosis, and cardiac dysfunction [51]. Ectopic fat occurs concomitantly in several organs. Subjects with fatty liver also display epicardial fat accumulation (EPA) and reduced myocardial energy [52]. EPA thickness was correlated with endothelial dysfunction, as measured by reduced flow mediated vasodilation in patients with metabolic syndrome (MS) [53]. Pericardial fat was an independent risk factor for coronary artery stenosis in the Korean Atherosclerosis Study 2, although the odds ratio was small when adjusted for age gender and BMI (OR: 1.01, $p < 0.03$) [54]. In the Framingham Heart Study, it has been shown that both visceral and epicardial fat accumulations are associated with increased risk of coronary heart disease (CHD) myocardial infarction, and stroke [55]. However, although cardiac fat is associated with impairment in heart metabolism and cardiac dysfunction, the interplay between cardiac fat accumulation, IR, and cardiac dysfunction remains to be fully established.

IR AND ENDOTHELIAL DYSFUNCTION

Genetic predisposition and environmental factors contribute to the development of both IR and endothelial dysfunction. The molecular and cellular mechanisms that mediate IR and endothelial dysfunction are multiple (e.g., hyperinsulinemia, lipotoxicity, glucotoxicity, inflammation) and may also explain the relationship between metabolic disorders and CVD [56,57]. Reduced NO availability appears to be associated with endothelial exposure to high circulating levels of FFAs [58] and glucose [59] with subsequent vascular damage that amplifies both endothelial dysfunction and IR states [60]. Likewise, endothelial dysfunction may contribute to impaired insulin action, altering the transcapillary passage of insulin and its delivery to target tissues.

In vascular endothelium, insulin stimulates the production of nitric oxide (NO) by a similar signaling pathway as for glucose uptake in liver, adipose tissue, and skeletal muscle [61,62]. Endothelial-derived NO diffuses into adjacent vascular smooth muscle cells (VSMCs) where it activates guanylate cyclase, the enzyme that converts GTP to GMPc. Increased levels of cGMP lowers intracellular free calcium, promotes vasodilation, inhibits VSMC proliferation, and regulates angiogenesis [63]. Moreover, the insulin-mediated NO production in endothelial cells promotes anti-inflammatory and antithrombotic phenotype, decreasing the release of proinflammatory cytokines, the expression of adhesion molecules (CAMs), intercellular adhesion molecule-1 (ICAM-1), vascular adhesion molecule 1 (VCAM-1), and E-Selectin [64].

Activation of insulin receptors mediates a cascade of phosphorylation/dephosphorylation events, guanine nucleotide exchange events, and spatial positioning of adapter molecules that activate a complex network of signaling inputs whose balancing provides the specific cell response to insulin signaling. Of particular importance is the MAPK pathway that controls the production of endothelin-1 (ET-1), a potent vasoconstrictor involved in increased vascular permeability, the endothelial release of interleukin-6 (IL-6), and VSMC proliferation and is implicated in processes that characterize the early step of atherogenesis. The modification of insulin vasoconstrictor and vasodilator properties might also be involved in vascular pathophysiology of IR [56]. Insulin-mediated MAPK signaling pathway activation may lead to increased expression of plasminogen activator inhibitor 1 (PAI-1), the main inhibitor of fibrinolysis, VCAM-1, and E-Selectin and to platelet aggregation [65,66]. Interestingly, inhibition of PI3K or Akt branch amplifies the MAPK, suggesting that this signaling pathway may counteract proatherogenic effects mediated by the MAPK-dependent branch of insulin-signaling pathway, both increasing NO levels and inhibiting adhesion molecule expression.

IR, INFLAMMATION, AND ATHEROSCLEROSIS

Low-grade inflammation is one link between IR, type 2 diabetes, and CVD [67]. Increased plasma levels of inflammatory markers, as IL-6, TNF-α, and C-reactive protein (CRP) are associated with increased risk for several chronic diseases including IR, CAD, and T2DM [68]. The origins of the heightened inflammatory activity are diverse, although visceral obesity and ectopic fat are thought to play a central role in this process (Figure 8.3). Obesity indeed is associated with subclinical inflammation, as a consequence of nutrient overload, and with IR, dysmetabolism, and hypertension, each one an independent CV risk factor [69]. Moreover, the insulin-resistant state of obesity frequently involves high circulating levels of nonesterified fatty acids (FFAs), which cause ectopic fat accumulation and lipotoxicity, and therefore further oxidative stress and atherogenesis [51,70].

Potential molecular mechanisms that link insulin-resistant/obesity and inflammation involve inflammatory mediators such as TNF-α. The presence of TNF-α in obese compared with lean

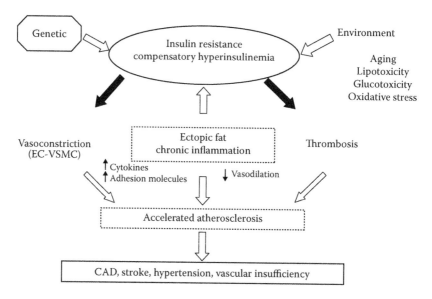

FIGURE 8.3 Ectopic fat accumulation and chronic inflammation are central in the development of IR and accelerated atherosclerosis. Genetic and environmental factors worsen the situation.

adipose tissue [71,72], its positive correlation with adiposity and IR [73], and the amelioration of insulin sensitivity after neutralization of TNF-α [74] supported the involvement of inflammation and its complications in obesity. TNF-α may activate serine kinase pathways, such as c-Jun NH2-terminal kinase (JNK) and IκB kinase (IKK), which phosphorylate serine residues of IRS-1 and impair insulin signaling [75–77]. Both JNK and IKK, which are members of two major proinflammatory cascades, are likely activated in insulin-resistant states and thus provide potential connections between inflammation and IR [76,77]. Increasing adiposity activates both JNK and IKKβ [78]. Besides serine phosphorylation of IRS-1, IKK-β can also influence insulin function through phosphorylation of the NF-κB inhibitor (IκB), leading to activation of NF-κB, a ubiquitous transcription factor that regulates the expression of many genes involved in inflammatory response, thus maintaining and potentiating inflammatory activation. JNK and IKKβ/NF-κB pathways are also activated by pattern recognition receptors, the toll-like receptors (TLRs) that recognize foreign substances, and the receptor for advanced glycation end products (RAGE) that bind advanced glycation end products, adducts formed between glucose and targeted proteins in hyperglycemia conditions [79]. Endogenous lipids or lipid conjugates might also activate one or more of the TLRs in obesity, a possibility supported by experiments showing that saturated fatty acids bind and activate toll-like receptor 4 (TLR-4) [80]. FFA can also bind TLR-4 on the surface of adipocyte and macrophages, constituting an important trigger of innate immunity through recognition of pathogen-associated molecular patterns [81]. The binding of FFA to TLR-4 activates NF-κB and MAP kinase pathways initiating a potent inflammatory response [82].

Systemic markers of oxidative stress were also found in adipose tissue. Intracellular reactive oxygen species (ROS) and ER stress play a pivotal role in JNK and IKKβ/NF-κB pathways increasing the expression of inflammatory cytokines and contributing to the development of obesity-induced IR [83]. Adipose tissue is an important endocrine tissue that secretes many biologically active proteins, as adipokines and inflammatory cytokines, whose circulating levels are increased during obesity [84]. A variety of biologically active derivatives are generated from adipose cells, including ROS, proinflammatory molecules (IL-1β, IL-6, TNF-α), angiogenetic factors (vascular endothelial growth factor, VEGF), hemostasis-modulating compounds (PAI-1), acute-phase reaction proteins (serum amyloid A [SAA] proteins, CRP), monocyte chemoattractant protein-1 (MCP-1), and hormones such as leptin, resistin, adiponectin, visfatin, and angiotensinogen (AGT). While leptin and adiponectin are true adipokines that appear to be produced exclusively by adipocytes, TNF-α, IL-6, MCP-1, visfatin, and PAI-1 are expressed as well at high levels in activated macrophages and/or other cells [85]. These cytokines and chemokines activate intracellular pathways that promote the development of IR and endothelial dysfunction, an initial step of atherogenesis [84].

Endothelial cells may increase the expression of one or more of the adhesion proteins ICAM-1, VCAM-1, E-selectin, or P-selectin in response to increased adiposity, playing an important role in adipose tissue inflammation. In both animal and human studies of genetic and diet-induced obesity, macrophages in adipose tissue contribute to release of inflammatory mediators, promoting obesity-induced IR [86,87]. When monocytes accumulate in adipose tissue, two distinct subsets of macrophages originate: resident activated macrophages (M2), characterized by the production of nitric oxide synthase 2 and IL-6, and infiltrative activated macrophages (M1) that express the chemokine (C-C motif) receptor 2 (CCR2) specific for MCP-1 and release IL-6 that favor lipid accumulation in macrophages [88]. M2 macrophages are recruited in visceral adipose tissues by MCP-1, released by adipocytes themselves, mimicking the chemotaxis of monocytes in the atheroma. In addition to cytokine and protease release, the actions of macrophages in inflammation include antigen presentation and T cell activation. Increasing adiposity leads to the recruitment of immune cells to adipose tissue, such as T cells [89], mast cells [90], and natural killer T (NKT) cells [91] in adipose tissue inflammation, but their role is not fully understood. Interferon-gamma (IFNγ), a typical T-helper 1 cytokine, likely regulates local expression of MCP-1, TNF-α, and other inflammatory mediators in adipocytes and macrophages, suggesting a role for adaptive immunity in obesity pathophysiology [92]. The cross-talk involving adipocytes, macrophages, and endothelial cells leads to production of mediators that act both in a paracrine and autocrine fashion generating local and systemic effects, respectively. In fact, the release of IL-6 by M1 macrophages into the circulation can also promote important systemic effects [93] such as increased production of liver-derived acute-phase inflammatory mediators and coagulation-related factors, correlated with atherothrombosis.

In addition to adipose tissue, also the liver can play a pivotal role in systemic inflammation and metabolic derangements in obesity [42,94]. Nonalcoholic fatty liver disease (NAFLD), from simple steatosis to steatohepatitis, advanced fibrosis, and cirrhosis, is often associated with abdominal obesity and inflammation. The liver contains a resident population of macrophage-like cells, the Kupffer cells, which can secrete inflammatory mediators upon activation, and other immune cells, including T and B lymphocytes, NK cells, hepatic stellate cells, and liver sinusoidal endothelial cells, which may also play roles in inflammation-induced IR [95]. The Kupffer cells can be activated by proinflammatory cytokines and FFAs, produced either by hepatocytes in response to steatosis or by abdominal fat tissue. Unlike adipose tissue, the liver does not accumulate macrophages or other immune cells in the context of obesity.

Cytokines accelerate the atherosclerotic process acting both directly on endothelial cell and indirectly on the liver, causing increased production of CRP, fibrinogen, PAI-1, and related factors, which, in turn, leads to endothelial dysfunction [42,51,96]. CRP induces endothelial dysfunction by impairing eNOS-dependent vasodilation and uncoupling of eNOS [97], by increasing endothelial cell adhesion molecule, MCP-1 and PAI-1 expression [98]. Similarly, there is evidence that SAA, an acute-phase inflammatory protein, may be a mediator of atherosclerosis. HDL particles containing SAA, rather than apolipoprotein (apo) A1, show adherence to vascular proteoglycans via the tethering region of SAA, suggesting the existence of "inflammatory HDL" [99].

IR, COAGULATION, AND PROTHROMBOTIC STATE

Subjects with type 2 diabetes often show alterations in hemostatic and fibrinolytic factors, including fibrinogen, factor VII, von Willebrand factor (vWF), tissue plasminogen activator (t-PA), and PAI-1, thus increasing hyper-aggregability, hypercoagulability, and hypofibrinolysis. These phenomena are the consequence of increased adipokine and insulin secretion that exerts important actions on vessel, platelet, coagulation, and fibrinolysis and contributes to a prothrombotic and systemic inflammatory state. Since these factors play an important role in the risk of developing CVD, their role in IR state is of great importance (Figure 8.4).

Increased fibrinogen levels appear to be initiated by an inflammatory profile and to be positively associated with IR. The basis for increased levels of fibrinogen is not clear, but it may be related to the presence of obesity. It has also been demonstrated that IR is associated with activation of the coagulation system. Factor VII activity has been shown to increase during postprandial hyperlipidemia, suggesting a risk for acute CAD events after consumption of a high-fat meal [100]. Moreover, in patients with CAD, a positive correlation was found between increased FVII activity levels and IR, BMI, and waist circumference [101].

A pathogenic role of hypofibrinolysis or increased PAI-1 levels is thought to play a role in the development of vascular disease in subjects with type 2 diabetes or IR.

Various studies have shown elevated levels of PAI-1, a fibrinolytic inhibitor, in obese individuals [102] as well as in patients with IR, type 2 diabetes, and CVDs [103,104]. PAI-1 is an adipocytokine secreted from a variety of cells including hepatocytes, vascular endothelial cells, SMCs, preadipocytes, and platelets [105,106]. It prevents fibrinolysis and promotes thrombosis, inactivating urokinase-type plasminogen activator (uPA) and t-PA, and so inhibiting plasminogen activation in vivo [107]. The link between elevated PAI-1 and IR has been studied extensively in animal and in vitro models. In a high-fat/high-carbohydrate diet model of obesity, PAI-1-deficient mice do not develop obesity and IR, suggesting that PAI-1 has also a direct role on the IR [108]. Hepatic cells respond to increased levels of insulin, VLDL, and FFAs by synthesizing and secreting PAI-1.

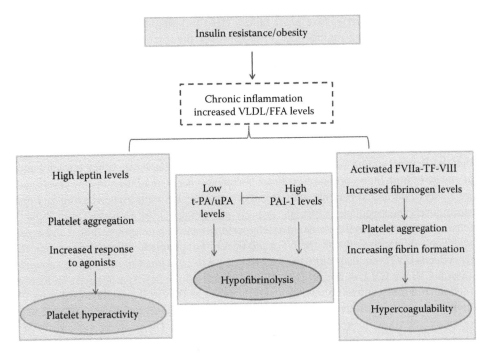

FIGURE 8.4 Increased IR and inflammation are related to platelet hyperactivity, hypercoagulability, and hypofibrinolysis. This altered coagulation profile presupposes a prothrombotic state.

Plasma PAI-1 levels are more closely related to fat accumulation and PAI-1 expression in the liver than in adipose tissue, suggesting that the liver is an important source of PAI-1 in insulin-resistant subjects [109]. Macrophages can synthesize PAI-1 [110] and induce its synthesis in adipose tissue through release of TNF-α [111]. Incubation of endothelial cells with VLDL also increases PAI-1 synthesis and secretion; a putative VLDL response element, recently identified in the gene for PAI-1, may be responsible for this induction [112]. Furthermore, adipose tissue appears to be the main source of PAI-1 in obese patients [113]. Studies of human adipocytes and adipose tissue explants have reported that insulin induces PAI-1 production in adipocytes [114].

Circulating levels of t-PA, an activator of clot dissolution, and vWF, a mediator of platelet adhesion and aggregation, both associated with the risk of developing CVD, are increased in subjects with MS and correlated with the HOMA-IR measure of insulin sensitivity [115]. vWF is produced almost exclusively by endothelial cells activated by proinflammatory cytokines [116] and contributes to thrombogenesis through platelet adhesion and aggregation [117]. High levels of vWF were found in the setting of atherosclerotic CVD and associated with risk of CVD in people with T2DM or IR [118]. Given that t-PA and vWF are mainly released by endothelium, their increased levels are indexes of endothelial dysfunction in subjects with IR and metabolic syndrome. Insulin infusion has been also shown to stimulate regional vasodilation and PAI-1 and t-PA expression in the forearm vascular beds of healthy subjects, suggesting that this alteration can lead to hypofibrinolysis and to development of atherosclerotic complications in patients with IR [119]. t-PA and PAI-1 levels are strongly associated and their increase reflects also a response to an inflammatory burst. Since t-PA forms complexes with PAI-1, its major inhibitor, circulating t-PA levels may reflect not only endothelial synthesis and release but also raised PAI-1 levels in IR and diabetes [120].

Obesity is also related to hypercoagulability. Hyperleptinemia, which is common in obesity, has been associated with acute thrombotic events in obesity since by binding on the platelet surface, leptin promotes platelet aggregation [121]. Leptin is also associated with obesity-related hypertension and chronic congestive heart failure (HF) in humans, and vascular endothelial and myocardial dysfunction in animal models [122]. However, the role of leptin and leptin resistance in the pathogenesis of hypertension and HF in obesity remains controversial.

IR AND HYPERTENSION

Many studies suggest an association between IR, compensatory hyperinsulinemia, and hypertension [123,124]. Hypertension is a major independent risk factor for the development of CVD [125], and the risk increases progressively with incremental rise in blood pressure [70]. Evidence suggests that the changes in glucose and insulin metabolism may play a role in the etiology and/or the clinical course of high blood pressure. A direct correlation between plasma insulin levels and blood pressure exists in untreated patients with essential hypertension with higher fasting and postprandial insulin levels independently of weight or body mass index [126]. However, only about 50% of hypertensive subjects are insulin-resistant and hyperinsulinemic. Numerous clinical and experimental studies have demonstrated that the blockade of renin angiotensin aldosterone system (RAAS) not only reduces CVD but also improves insulin sensitivity and glucose intolerance in nondiabetic patients with CVD or CV risk factors [127–129]. A systematic review synthesized results of several large randomized clinical trials showing a significant reduction in the incidence of type 2 diabetes in hypertensive patients treated with either angiotensin-converting enzyme inhibitors (ACEs) or angiotensin receptor blockers (ARBs) for 3–6 years [130]. These metabolic effects of ARBs have been explained by hemodynamic effects, such as improved delivery of insulin and glucose to the peripheral skeletal muscle, and nonhemodynamic effects, including direct effects on glucose transport and insulin signaling pathways, all of which decrease IR. However, the link between IR, hyperinsulinemia, and hypertension is still controversial. The Insulin Resistance Atherosclerosis Study (IRAS) performed in triethnic large population demonstrated a weak association between IR, but not hyperinsulinemia, and hypertension/high blood pressure in subjects without diabetes. This association was not confirmed in patients with type 2 diabetes [131]. A possible link is the accumulation of visceral and ectopic fat that occurs not only in liver and muscle but also in the heart and around the vessels [70] (see Figure 8.5). We have demonstrated a direct relationship between blood pressure and visceral and cardiac fat, and an inverse relationship with cardiac contractility as recently reviewed in ref [70]. In patients with visceral obesity, the systemic circulating RAAS is dysregulated [132]. Moreover, it has been shown that the adipose tissue expresses all components of the renin–angiotensin system necessary to generate angiotensin (Ang) peptides for local function [133]. The angiotensin type 1 (AT_1) and type 2 (AT_2) receptors mediate the effect of Ang II, and recent studies have shown that both receptors may modulate fat mass expansion through upregulation of adipose tissue lipogenesis (AT_2) and downregulation of lipolysis (AT_1). Thus, both receptors may have synergistic and additive effects to promote the storage of lipid in adipose tissue in response to the nutrient environment. The production of angiotensinogen (AGT) by adipose tissue in rodents also contributes to one third of the circulating AGT levels. Increased adipose tissue AGT production in the obese state may be responsible in part for the metabolic and inflammatory disorders associated with obesity. This supports the notion that besides the traditional role of Ang II produced by the liver in the control of blood pressure, Ang II produced by the adipose tissue may more accurately reflect the role of this hormone in the regulation of fat mass and associated disorders [134]. Other long-term effects of Ang II on CV structure include the promotion of inception and progression of vascular diseases through hemodynamic effects and direct effects on blood vessels and, indirectly, through the stimulation of aldosterone [135]. Biological actions of Ang II are transduced through the activation of angiotensin receptors. The AT_1 receptor, the best characterized, is responsible for mediating vasoconstriction, endothelial activation increased myocardial contractility, cell proliferation, and hypertrophy, all of which may contribute to progression of CVD [136]. Upregulation of the RAAS has been found in subjects with type 2 diabetes and obesity (Figure 8.5), where the chronic activation of inflammation leads to IR [137].

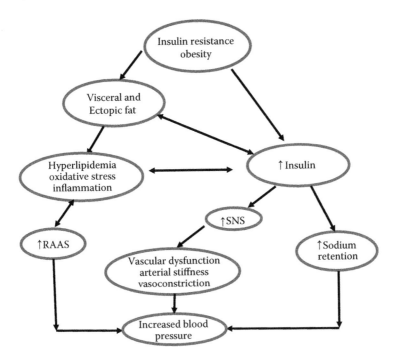

FIGURE 8.5   Proposed mechanisms linking obesity and IR to hypertension. (From Sironi AM et al., *Curr Pharm Des* 2011, 17[28]:3074–3080.)

The relationship between IR and hypertension can be explained also by abnormalities in vasodilation and blood flow. There is a direct cross-talk between insulin and Ang II signaling pathways in metabolic and CV tissues. Ang II negatively modulates insulin signaling. Insulin given intravenously causes vasodilation in normal subjects, and this response is deficient in obese, insulin-resistant subjects and in patients with T2DM. Ang II, via AT_1 receptors, counteracts Ins-PI3K-Akt signaling pathway in both vascular and skeletal tissues, resulting in inhibition of mechanisms involved in the vasodilator and glucose transport properties [138,139]. Ang II impairs endothelial-dependent relaxation, through AT1R, increasing generation of ROS in the vasculature that reacts with bioavailable NO to generate peroxinitrite [140,141]. In addition to generation of ROS, Ang II stimulates RhoA/ROK pathway signaling in VSMCs, inhibiting actions mediated by Ins signaling [142], such as activation of endothelial NO synthase activity, Na^+ pump activation, and Ca^{2+}-myosin light chain (MLC) desensitization.

There is also evidence that hypertension is associated to glucose intolerance [143]. The co-presence of glucose intolerance and hyperinsulinemia underlines a defect in insulin-stimulated glucose uptake in some patients with IR [123,144]. Studies in both human subjects and animals have provided contradictory results on the efficacy of lowering blood pressure to improve insulin sensitivity.

Blood flow influences the regulation of glucose uptake by tissue beds, and it seems possible that vasoconstriction may induce IR by decreasing insulin-mediated delivery of glucose to peripheral tissues leading to the development of prediabetes and type 2 diabetes.

The uptake of glucose is regulated by a specific glucose transporter, the GLUT-4, that mediates the transport of glucose in adipose tissue, skeletal muscle, and heart tissues that specifically express this protein [145]. Accumulating data indicate that Ang II and IR conditions are associated with impaired translocation and incorporation into plasma membrane of GLUT-4 [146,147], an abnormality corrected by AT_1 receptor blockade [146]. In particular, Ang II, acting via the AT_1 receptor, can reduce GLUT-4 translocation at multiple steps, both enhancing ROS generation [148–150] and inhibiting Ins-mediated PI3K-Akt signaling [151]. This mechanism explains glucose intolerance associated with hypertension in subjects with IR and T2DM.

The presence of defects in insulin-mediated glucose uptake by muscle and insulin inhibition of adipose tissue lipolysis does not imply that all tissues are equally insulin resistant [70]. In fact, hyperinsulinemia can increase reabsorption of sodium and water by kidney tubular cells [152], and this can be associated with a volume-dependent hypertension, explaining why insulin-resistant hyperinsulinemic, nondiabetic individuals are at increased risk to retain salt and water. Many evidences suggest that the sympathetic nervous system (SNS) is overactive in obese subjects [153]. This is in part due to IR since insulin per se causes an SNS shift of autonomic balance [154]. Sympathetic system activation is detected in insulin-resistant subjects as increased heart rate and blood pressure, baroreceptor dysfunction, enhanced lipolysis in visceral fat, as well as sodium retention [155].

CONCLUSIONS

The interplay between IR CV risk factors and development of clinically symptomatic CAD is complex. The evidence collected so far suggests a major role for IR in preintrusive and preclinical CAD, targeting a wide range of functions in endothelium, heart, liver, and adipose tissue that would link risk to disease development. Early strategies to counteract detrimental effects of IR should be developed in order to interrupt this vicious cycle.

REFERENCES

1. Reaven G: Role of insulin resistance in human disease. *Diabetes* 1988, **37**:1595–1607.
2. DeFronzo RA, Ferrannini E: Insulin resistance. A multifaceted syndrome responsible for NIDDM, obesity, hypertension, dyslipidemia, and atherosclerotic cardiovascular disease. *Diabetes Care* 1991, **14**(3):173–194.
3. Stratton IM, Adler AI, Neil HA, Matthews DR, Manley SE, Cull CA, Hadden D, Turner RC, Holman RR: Association of glycaemia with macrovascular and microvascular complications of type 2 diabetes (UKPDS 35): Prospective observational study. *BMJ* 2000, **321**(7258):405–412.
4. Bressler P, Bailey SR, Matsuda M, DeFronzo RA: Insulin resistance and coronary artery disease. *Diabetologia* 1996, **39**(11):1345–1350.
5. Chung EH, Curran PJ, Sivasankaran S, Chauhan MS, Gossman DE, Pyne CT, Piemonte TC, Waters J, Bilazarian S, Riskala N, Shoraki A, Nesto RW: Prevalence of metabolic syndrome in patients < or = 45 years of age with acute myocardial infarction having percutaneous coronary intervention. *Am J Cardiol* 2007, **100**(7):1052–1055.
6. Milani RV, Lavie CJ: Prevalence and profile of metabolic syndrome in patients following acute coronary events and effects of therapeutic lifestyle change with cardiac rehabilitation. *Am J Cardiol* 2003, **92**(1):50–54.
7. Savage PD, Banzer JA, Balady GJ, Ades PA: Prevalence of metabolic syndrome in cardiac rehabilitation/secondary prevention programs. *Am Heart J* 2005, **149**(4):627–631.
8. Gastaldelli A: Role of beta-cell dysfunction, ectopic fat accumulation and insulin resistance in the pathogenesis of type 2 diabetes mellitus. *Diabetes Res Clin Pract* 2011, **93** Suppl 1:S60–S65.
9. Cheatham B, Vlahos CJ, Cheatham L, Wang L, Blenis J, Kahn CR: Phosphatidylinositol 3-kinase activation is required for insulin stimulation of pp70 S6 kinase, DNA synthesis, and glucose transporter translocation. *Mol Cell Biol* 1994, **14**(7):4902–4911.
10. Le Marchand-Brustel Y, Gautier N, Cormont M, Van Obberghen E: Wortmannin inhibits the action of insulin but not that of okadaic acid in skeletal muscle: Comparison with fat cells. *Endocrinology* 1995, **136**(8):3564–3570.
11. Defronzo RA: Banting lecture. From the triumvirate to the ominous octet: A new paradigm for the treatment of type 2 diabetes mellitus. *Diabetes* 2009, **58**(4):773–795.
12. Ferrannini E, Gastaldelli A, Matsuda M, Miyazaki Y, Pettiti M, Glass L, DeFronzo RA: Influence of ethnicity and familial diabetes on glucose tolerance and insulin action: A physiological analysis. *J Clin Endocrinol Metab* 2003, **88**(7):3251–3257.
13. Gastaldelli A, Ferrannini E, Miyazaki Y, Matsuda M, DeFronzo RA: Beta-cell dysfunction and glucose intolerance: Results from the San Antonio metabolism (SAM) study. *Diabetologia* 2004, **47**(1):31–39.

14. Belfiore A, Frasca F, Pandini G, Sciacca L, Vigneri R: Insulin receptor isoforms and insulin receptor/insulin-like growth factor receptor hybrids in physiology and disease. *Endocr Rev* 2009, **30**(6):586–623.
15. Lebovitz HE: Type 2 diabetes: An overview. *Clin Chem* 1999, **45**(8 Pt 2):1339–1345.
16. Defronzo RA, Tripathy D, Schwenke DC, Banerji M, Bray GA, Buchanan TA, Clement SC, Henry RR, Kitabchi AE, Mudaliar S, Ratner RE, Stentz FB, Musi N, Reaven PD, Gastaldelli A: ACT NOW Study: Prediction of diabetes based on baseline metabolic characteristics in individuals at high risk. *Diabetes Care* 2013, **36**(11):3607–3612.
17. Cusi K: Cardiovascular risk management in type 2 diabetes: From clinical trials to clinical practice. *Endocrinologist* 2001, **11**(6):474–490.
18. Stamler J, Vaccaro O, Neaton JD, Wentworth D: Diabetes, other risk factors, and the 12-year cardiovascular mortality for men screened in the multiple risk factor intervention trial. *Diabetes Care* 1993, **16**:434–444.
19. Turner R, Cull C, Holman R: United Kingdom Prospective Diabetes Study 17: The effect of improved metabolic control on complications of NIDDM. *Ann Intern Med* 1996, **124**:136–145.
20. Hu FB, Stampfer M, Haffner SM, Solomon CG, Willett WC, Manson JE: Elevated risk of cardiovascular disease prior to clinical diagnosis of type 2 diabetes. *Diabetes Care* 2002, **25**:1129–1134.
21. Djaberi R, Schuijf JD, Jukema JW, Rabelink TJ, Stokkel MP, Smit JW, de Koning EJ, Bax JJ: Increased carotid intima-media thickness as a predictor of the presence and extent of abnormal myocardial perfusion in type 2 diabetes. *Diabetes Care* 2010, **33**(2):372–374.
22. Burke GL, Evans GW, Riley WA, Sharrett AR, Howard G, Barnes RW, Rosamond W, Crow RS, Rautaharju PM, Heiss G: Arterial wall thickness is associated with prevalent cardiovascular disease in middle-aged adults. The Atherosclerosis Risk in Communities (ARIC) Study. *Stroke* 1995, **26**(3):386–391.
23. Yoshida M, Mita T, Yamamoto R, Shimizu T, Ikeda F, Ohmura C, Kanazawa A, Hirose T, Kawamori R, Watada H: Combination of the Framingham risk score and carotid intima-media thickness improves the prediction of cardiovascular events in patients with type 2 diabetes. *Diabetes Care* 2012, **35**(1):178–180.
24. Andreozzi F, Gastaldelli A, Mannino GC, Sciacqua A, Succurro E, Arturi F, Folli F, Perticone F: Increased carotid intima-media thickness in the physiologic range is associated with impaired postprandial glucose metabolism, insulin resistance and beta cell dysfunction. *Atherosclerosis* 2013, **229**(2):277–281.
25. Peeters A, Barendregt JJ, Willekens F, Mackenbach JP, Al Mamun A, Bonneux L, NEDCOM, the Netherlands Epidemiology and Demography Compression of Morbidity Research Group: Obesity in adulthood and its consequences for life expectancy: A life-table analysis. *Ann Intern Med* 2003, **138**:1138–1145.
26. van Dam RM, Willett WC, Manson JE, Hu FB: The relationship between overweight in adolescence and premature death in women. *Ann Intern Med* 2006, **145**:91–97.
27. Abbasi F, Brown B, Lamendola C, McLaughlin T, Reaven G: Relationship between obesity, insulin sensitivity and coronary artery disease risk. *J Am Coll Cardiol* 2002, **40**:37–43.
28. National Institutes of Health Consensus Development Conference Statement: Health implications of obesity. *Ann Intern Med* 1985, **103**:1073–1077.
29. Pi-Sunyer F: Medical hazards of obesity. *Ann Intern Med* 1993, **119**(7):655–660.
30. Poirier P, Giles T, Bray G, Hong Y, Stern J: Obesity and cardiovascular disease: Pathophysiology, evaluation, and effect of weight loss. *Arterioscler Thromb Vasc Biol* 2006, **26**:968–976.
31. Wyatt SB, Winters KP, Dubbert PM: Overweight and obesity: Prevalence, consequences, and causes of a growing public health problem. *Am J Med Sci* 2006, **331**(4):166–174.
32. Bray G, Bellanger T: Epidemiology, trends, and morbidities of obesity and the metabolic syndrome. *Endocrine* 2006, **29**:109–117.
33. Gunnell D, Frankel S, Nanchahal K, Peters T, Davey Smith G: Childhood obesity and adult cardiovascular mortality. *Am J Clin Nutr* 1998, **67**:1111–1118.
34. World Health Organization: Obesity. Preventing and managing the global epidemic. Report of WHO consultation on obesity. World Health Organization, Geneva, June 3–5, 1997.
35. Hamilton M, Hamilton D, Zderic T: Role of low energy expenditure and sitting in obesity, metabolic syndrome, type 2 diabetes, and cardiovascular disease. *Diabetes* 2007, **45**:2655–2667.
36. Flegal K, Graubard B, Williamson D, Gail M: Cause-specific excess deaths associated with underweight, overweight, and obesity. *JAMA* 2007, **298**:2028–2037.
37. Despres JP, Cartier A, Cote M, Arsenault BJ: The concept of cardiometabolic risk: Bridging the fields of diabetology and cardiology. *Ann Med* 2008, **40**(7):514–523.
38. Cassano P, Rosner B, Vokonas P, Weiss S: Obesity and body fat distribution in relation to the incidence of non-insulin-dependent diabetes mellitus. *Am J Epidemiol* 1992, **136**:1474–1486.

39. Charles M, Eschwege E, Thibult N, Claude J-R, Warnet J-M, Rosselin G, Girard J, Balkau B: The role of non-esterified fatty acids in the deterioration of glucose tolerance in Caucasian subjects: Results of the Paris Prospective Study. *Diabetologia* 1997, **40**:1101–1106.
40. Ostman J, Arner P, Engfeldt P, Kager L: Regional differences in the control of lipolysis in human adipose tissue. *Metabolism* 1979, **29**:1198–1205.
41. Despres J: Cardiovascular disease under the influence of excess visceral fat. *Crit Pathw Cardiol* 2007, **6**:51–59.
42. Gaggini M, Morelli M, Buzzigoli E, DeFronzo RA, Bugianesi E, Gastaldelli A: Non-alcoholic fatty liver disease (NAFLD) and its connection with insulin resistance, dyslipidemia, atherosclerosis and coronary heart disease. *Nutrients* 2013, **5**(5):1544–1560.
43. Klein S: The case of visceral fat: Argument for the defense. *J Clin Invest* 2004, **113**:1530–1532.
44. Miles J, Jensen M: Visceral adiposity is not causally related to insulin resistance. *Diabetes Care* 2005, **28**:2326–2327.
45. Ferrannini E, Balkau B, Coppack S, Dekker J, Mari A, Nolan J, Walker M, Natali A, Beck-Nielsen H, and the RISC Investigators: Insulin resistance, insulin response, and obesity as indicators of metabolic risk. *J Clin Endocrinol Metab* 2007, **92**:2885–2892.
46. Gastaldelli A, Cusi K, Pettiti M, Hardies J, Miyazaki Y, Berria R, Buzzigoli E, Sironi AM, Cersosimo E, Ferrannini E, Defronzo RA: Relationship between hepatic/visceral fat and hepatic insulin resistance in nondiabetic and type 2 diabetic subjects. *Gastroenterology* 2007, **133**:496–506.
47. Nielsen S, Guo Z, Johnson C, Hensrud D, Jensen M: Splanchnic lipolysis in human obesity. *J Clin Invest* 2004, **113**:1582–1588.
48. Shoelson S, Lee J, Goldfine A: Inflammation and insulin resistance. *J Clin Invest* 2006, **116**:1793–1801.
49. Fontana L, Eagon J, Trujillo M, Scherer P, Klein S: Visceral fat adipokine secretion is associated with systemic inflammation in obese humans. *Diabetes* 2007, **56**:1010–1013.
50. Alligier M, Gabert L, Meugnier E, Lambert-Porcheron S, Chanseaume E, Pilleul F, Debard C, Sauvinet V, Morio B, Vidal-Puig A, Vidal H, Laville M: Visceral fat accumulation during lipid overfeeding is related to subcutaneous adipose tissue characteristics in healthy men. *J Clin Endocrinol Metab* 2013, **98**(2):802–810.
51. Morelli M, Gaggini M, Daniele G, Marraccini P, Sicari R, Gastaldelli A: Ectopic fat: The true culprit linking obesity and cardiovascular disease? *Thromb Haemost* 2013, **110**(4):651–660.
52. Perseghin G, Lattuada G, De Cobelli F, Esposito A, Belloni E, Ntali G, Ragogna F, Canu T, Scifo P, Del Maschio A, Luzi L: Increased mediastinal fat and impaired left ventricular energy metabolism in young men with newly found fatty liver. *Hepatology* 2008, **47**(1):51–58.
53. Aydin H, Toprak A, Deyneli O, Yazici D, Tarcin O, Sancak S, Yavuz D, Akalin S: Epicardial fat tissue thickness correlates with endothelial dysfunction and other cardiovascular risk factors in patients with metabolic syndrome. *Metab Syndr Relat Disord* 2010, **8**(3):229–234.
54. Kim TH, Yu SH, Choi SH, Yoon JW, Kang SM, Chun EJ, Choi SI, Shin H, Lee HK, Park KS, Jang HC, Lim S: Pericardial fat amount is an independent risk factor of coronary artery stenosis assessed by multidetector-row computed tomography: The Korean Atherosclerosis Study 2. *Obesity (Silver Spring)* 2011, **19**(5):1028–1034.
55. Mahabadi AA, Massaro JM, Rosito GA, Levy D, Murabito JM, Wolf PA, O'Donnell CJ, Fox CS, Hoffmann U: Association of pericardial fat, intrathoracic fat, and visceral abdominal fat with cardiovascular disease burden: The Framingham Heart Study. *Eur Heart J* 2009, **30**(7):850–856.
56. Kim JA, Montagnani M, Koh KK, Quon MJ: Reciprocal relationships between insulin resistance and endothelial dysfunction: Molecular and pathophysiological mechanisms. *Circulation* 2006, **113**(15):1888–1904.
57. Del Turco S, Gaggini M, Daniele G, Basta G, Folli F, Sicari R, Gastaldelli A: Insulin resistance and endothelial dysfunction: A mutual relationship in cardiometabolic risk. *Curr Pharm Des* 2013, **19**(13):2420–2431.
58. Potdar S, Kavdia M: NO/peroxynitrite dynamics of high glucose-exposed HUVECs: Chemiluminescent measurement and computational model. *Microvasc Res* 2009, **78**(2):191–198.
59. Steinberg HO, Tarshoby M, Monestel R, Hook G, Cronin J, Johnson A, Bayazeed B, Baron AD: Elevated circulating free fatty acid levels impair endothelium-dependent vasodilation. *J Clin Invest* 1997, **100**(5):1230–1239.
60. Cersosimo E, DeFronzo RA: Insulin resistance and endothelial dysfunction: The road map to cardiovascular diseases. *Diabetes Metab Res Rev* 2006, **22**(6):423–436.
61. Zeng G, Quon MJ: Insulin-stimulated production of nitric oxide is inhibited by wortmannin. Direct measurement in vascular endothelial cells. *J Clin Invest* 1996, **98**(4):894–898.

62. Zeng G, Nystrom FH, Ravichandran LV, Cong LN, Kirby M, Mostowski H, Quon MJ: Roles for insulin receptor, PI3-kinase, and Akt in insulin-signaling pathways related to production of nitric oxide in human vascular endothelial cells. *Circulation* 2000, **101**(13):1539–1545.

63. Garg UC, Hassid A: Nitric oxide-generating vasodilators and 8-bromo-cyclic guanosine monophosphate inhibit mitogenesis and proliferation of cultured rat vascular smooth muscle cells. *J Clin Invest* 1989, **83**(5):1774–1777.

64. Sudano I, Spieker LE, Hermann F, Flammer A, Corti R, Noll G, Luscher TF: Protection of endothelial function: Targets for nutritional and pharmacological interventions. *J Cardiovasc Pharmacol* 2006, **47** Suppl 2:S136–S150; discussion S172–S176.

65. Montagnani M, Golovchenko I, Kim I, Koh GY, Goalstone ML, Mundhekar AN, Johansen M, Kucik DF, Quon MJ, Draznin B: Inhibition of phosphatidylinositol 3-kinase enhances mitogenic actions of insulin in endothelial cells. *J Biol Chem* 2002, **277**(3):1794–1799.

66. Mukai Y, Wang CY, Rikitake Y, Liao JK: Phosphatidylinositol 3-kinase/protein kinase Akt negatively regulates plasminogen activator inhibitor type 1 expression in vascular endothelial cells. *Am J Physiol Heart Circ Physiol* 2007, **292**(4):H1937–H1942.

67. Van Gaal LF, Mertens IL, De Block CE: Mechanisms linking obesity with cardiovascular disease. *Nature* 2006, **444**(7121):875–880.

68. de Luca C, Olefsky JM: Inflammation and insulin resistance. *FEBS Lett* 2008, **582**(1):97–105.

69. Berg AH, Scherer PE: Adipose tissue, inflammation, and cardiovascular disease. *Circ Res* 2005, **96**(9):939–949.

70. Sironi AM, Sicari R, Folli F, Gastaldelli A: Ectopic fat storage, insulin resistance, and hypertension. *Curr Pharm Des* 2011, **17**(28):3074–3080.

71. Greenberg AS, Obin MS: Obesity and the role of adipose tissue in inflammation and metabolism. *Am J Clin Nutr* 2006, **83**(2):461S–465S.

72. Hotamisligil GS, Shargill NS, Spiegelman BM: Adipose expression of tumor necrosis factor-alpha: Direct role in obesity-linked insulin resistance. *Science* 1993, **259**(5091):87–91.

73. Fernandez-Real JM, Ricart W: Insulin resistance and chronic cardiovascular inflammatory syndrome. *Endocr Rev* 2003, **24**(3):278–301.

74. Cheung AT, Ree D, Kolls JK, Fuselier J, Coy DH, Bryer-Ash M: An in vivo model for elucidation of the mechanism of tumor necrosis factor-alpha (TNF-alpha)-induced insulin resistance: Evidence for differential regulation of insulin signaling by TNF-alpha. *Endocrinology* 1998, **139**(12):4928–4935.

75. Hotamisligil GS, Peraldi P, Budavari A, Ellis R, White MF, Spiegelman BM: IRS-1-mediated inhibition of insulin receptor tyrosine kinase activity in TNF-alpha- and obesity-induced insulin resistance. *Science* 1996, **271**(5249):665–668.

76. Hirosumi J, Tuncman G, Chang L, Gorgun CZ, Uysal KT, Maeda K, Karin M, Hotamisligil GS: A central role for JNK in obesity and insulin resistance. *Nature* 2002, **420**(6913):333–336.

77. Shoelson SE, Lee J, Yuan M: Inflammation and the IKK beta/I kappa B/NF-kappa B axis in obesity- and diet-induced insulin resistance. *Int J Obes Relat Metab Disord* 2003, **27** Suppl 3:S49–S52.

78. Tsatsanis C, Androulidaki A, Dermitzaki E, Charalampopoulos I, Spiess J, Gravanis A, Margioris AN: Urocortin 1 and Urocortin 2 induce macrophage apoptosis via CRFR2. *FEBS Lett* 2005, **579**(20):4259–4264.

79. Akira S, Uematsu S, Takeuchi O: Pathogen recognition and innate immunity. *Cell* 2006, **124**(4):783–801.

80. Lee JY, Sohn KH, Rhee SH, Hwang D: Saturated fatty acids, but not unsaturated fatty acids, induce the expression of cyclooxygenase-2 mediated through Toll-like receptor 4. *J Biol Chem* 2001, **276**(20):16683–16689.

81. Shi H, Kokoeva MV, Inouye K, Tzameli I, Yin H, Flier JS: TLR4 links innate immunity and fatty acid-induced insulin resistance. *J Clin Invest* 2006, **116**(11):3015–3025.

82. Janeway CA, Jr., Medzhitov R: Innate immune recognition. *Annu Rev Immunol* 2002, **20**:197–216.

83. Keaney JF, Jr., Larson MG, Vasan RS, Wilson PW, Lipinska I, Corey D, Massaro JM, Sutherland P, Vita JA, Benjamin EJ: Obesity and systemic oxidative stress: Clinical correlates of oxidative stress in the Framingham Study. *Arterioscler Thromb Vasc Biol* 2003, **23**(3):434–439.

84. Lau DC, Dhillon B, Yan H, Szmitko PE, Verma S: Adipokines: Molecular links between obesity and atherosclerosis. *Am J Physiol Heart Circ Physiol* 2005, **288**(5):H2031–H2041.

85. Fain O, Stirnemann J: Macrophage activation syndrome. *Rev Prat* 2004, **54**(9):935–939.

86. Xu H, Barnes GT, Yang Q, Tan G, Yang D, Chou CJ, Sole J, Nichols A, Ross JS, Tartaglia LA, Chen H: Chronic inflammation in fat plays a crucial role in the development of obesity-related insulin resistance. *J Clin Invest* 2003, **112**(12):1821–1830.

87. Weisberg SP, McCann D, Desai M, Rosenbaum M, Leibel RL, Ferrante AW, Jr.: Obesity is associated with macrophage accumulation in adipose tissue. *J Clin Invest* 2003, **112**(12):1796–1808.

88. Lumeng CN, Bodzin JL, Saltiel AR: Obesity induces a phenotypic switch in adipose tissue macrophage polarization. *J Clin Invest* 2007, **117**(1):175–184.

89. Nishimura S, Manabe I, Nagai R: Adipose tissue inflammation in obesity and metabolic syndrome. *Discov Med* 2009, **8**(41):55–60.

90. Liu H, Dear AE, Knudsen LB, Simpson RW: A long-acting glucagon-like peptide-1 analogue attenuates induction of plasminogen activator inhibitor type-1 and vascular adhesion molecules. *J Endocrinol* 2009, **201**(1):59–66.

91. Ohmura K, Ishimori N, Ohmura Y, Tokuhara S, Nozawa A, Horii S, Andoh Y, Fujii S, Iwabuchi K, Onoé K, Tsutsui H: Natural killer T cells are involved in adipose tissues inflammation and glucose intolerance in diet-induced obese mice. *Arterioscler Thromb Vasc Biol* 2010, **30**(2):193–199.

92. Karlsson EA, Beck MA: The burden of obesity on infectious disease. *Exp Biol Med (Maywood)* 2010, **235**(12):1412–1424.

93. Rocha VZ, Libby P: The multiple facets of the fat tissue. *Thyroid* 2008, **18**(2):175–183.

94. Gregor MF, Hotamisligil GS: Inflammatory mechanisms in obesity. *Annu Rev Immunol* 2011, **29**:415–445.

95. Racanelli V, Rehermann B: The liver as an immunological organ. *Hepatology* 2006, **43**(2 Suppl 1):S54–S62.

96. Bloomgarden ZT: Inflammation, atherosclerosis, and aspects of insulin action. *Diabetes Care* 2005, **28**(9):2312–2319.

97. Hein TW, Singh U, Vasquez-Vivar J, Devaraj S, Kuo L, Jialal I: Human C-reactive protein induces endothelial dysfunction and uncoupling of eNOS in vivo. *Atherosclerosis* 2009, **206**(1):61–68.

98. Paffen E, DeMaat MP: C-reactive protein in atherosclerosis: A causal factor? *Cardiovasc Res* 2006, **71**(1):30–39.

99. Lewis KE, Kirk EA, McDonald TO, Wang S, Wight TN, O'Brien KD, Chait A: Increase in serum amyloid a evoked by dietary cholesterol is associated with increased atherosclerosis in mice. *Circulation* 2004, **110**(5):540–545.

100. Miller GJ: Lipoproteins and thrombosis: Effects of lipid lowering. *Curr Opin Lipidol* 1995, **6**(1):38–42.

101. Karatela RA, Sainani GS: Interrelationships of factor VII activity and plasma leptin with insulin resistance in coronary heart disease. *Atherosclerosis* 2009, **209**(1):235–240.

102. Skurk T, Hauner H: Obesity and impaired fibrinolysis: Role of adipose production of plasminogen activator inhibitor-1. *Int J Obes Relat Metab Disord* 2004, **28**(11):1357–1364.

103. Takazoe K, Ogawa H, Yasue H, Sakamoto T, Soejima H, Miyao Y, Kawano H, Moriyama Y, Misumi K, Suefuji H, Kugiyama K, Yoshimura M: Increased plasminogen activator inhibitor activity and diabetes predict subsequent coronary events in patients with angina pectoris. *Ann Med* 2001, **33**(3):206–212.

104. Lyon CJ, Hsueh WA: Effect of plasminogen activator inhibitor-1 in diabetes mellitus and cardiovascular disease. *Am J Med* 2003, **115** Suppl 8A:62S–68S.

105. Bastelica D, Mavri A, Verdierl M, Berthet B, Juhan-Vague I, Alessi MC: Relationships between fibrinolytic and inflammatory parameters in human adipose tissue: Strong contribution of TNFalpha receptors to PAI-1 levels. *Thromb Haemost* 2002, **88**(3):481–487.

106. Dimova EY, Kietzmann T: Metabolic, hormonal and environmental regulation of plasminogen activator inhibitor-1 (PAI-1) expression: Lessons from the liver. *Thromb Haemost* 2008, **100**(6):992–1006.

107. Iwaki T, Urano T, Umemura K: PAI-1, progress in understanding the clinical problem and its aetiology. *Br J Haematol* 2012, **157**(3):291–298.

108. Ma LJ, Mao SL, Taylor KL, Kanjanabuch T, Guan Y, Zhang Y, Brown NJ, Swift LL, McGuinness OP, Wasserman DH, Vaughan DE, Fogo AB: Prevention of obesity and insulin resistance in mice lacking plasminogen activator inhibitor 1. *Diabetes* 2004, **53**(2):336–346.

109. Alessi MC, Bastelica D, Mavri A, Morange P, Berthet B, Grino M, Juhan-Vague I: Plasma PAI-1 levels are more strongly related to liver steatosis than to adipose tissue accumulation. *Arterioscler Thromb Vasc Biol* 2003, **23**(7):1262–1268.

110. Kishore P, Li W, Tonelli J, Lee DE, Koppaka S, Zhang K, Lin Y, Kehlenbrink S, Scherer PE, Hawkins M: Adipocyte-derived factors potentiate nutrient-induced production of plasminogen activator inhibitor-1 by macrophages. *Sci Transl Med* 2010, **2**(20):20ra15.

111. Pandey M, Loskutoff DJ, Samad F: Molecular mechanisms of tumor necrosis factor-alpha-mediated plasminogen activator inhibitor-1 expression in adipocytes. *FASEB J* 2005, **19**(10):1317–1319.

112. Eriksson P, Nilsson L, Karpe F, Hamsten A: Very-low-density lipoprotein response element in the promoter region of the human plasminogen activator inhibitor-1 gene implicated in the impaired fibrinolysis of hypertriglyceridemia. *Arterioscler Thromb Vasc Biol* 1998, **18**(1):20–26.

113. Shimomura I, Funahashi T, Takahashi M, Maeda K, Kotani K, Nakamura T, Yamashita S, Miura M, Fukuda Y, Takemura K, Tokunaga K, Matsuzawa Y: Enhanced expression of PAI-1 in visceral fat: Possible contributor to vascular disease in obesity. *Nat Med* 1996, **2**(7):800–803.

114. Fain JN, Madan AK: Insulin enhances vascular endothelial growth factor, interleukin-8, and plasminogen activator inhibitor 1 but not interleukin-6 release by human adipocytes. *Metabolism* 2005, **54**(2):220–226.

115. Ragab A, Abousamra NK, Higazy A, Saleh O: Relationship between insulin resistance and some coagulation and fibrinolytic parameters in patients with metabolic syndrome. *Lab Hematol* 2008, **14**(1):1–6.

116. Blann A: Von Willebrand factor and the endothelium in vascular disease. *Br J Biomed Sci* 1993, **50**(2):125–134.

117. Spiel AO, Gilbert JC, Jilma B: Von Willebrand factor in cardiovascular disease: Focus on acute coronary syndromes. *Circulation* 2008, **117**(11):1449–1459.

118. Frankel DS, Meigs JB, Massaro JM, Wilson PW, O'Donnell CJ, D'Agostino RB, Tofler GH: Von Willebrand factor, type 2 diabetes mellitus, and risk of cardiovascular disease: The Framingham Offspring Study. *Circulation* 2008, **118**(24):2533–2539.

119. Carmassi F, Morale M, Ferrini L, Dell'Omo G, Ferdeghini M, Pedrinelli R, De Negri F: Local insulin infusion stimulates expression of plasminogen activator inhibitor-1 and tissue-type plasminogen activator in normal subjects. *Am J Med* 1999, **107**(4):344–350.

120. Lowe GD, Danesh J, Lewington S, Walker M, Lennon L, Thomson A, Rumley A, Whincup PH: Tissue plasminogen activator antigen and coronary heart disease. Prospective study and meta-analysis. *Eur Heart J* 2004, **25**(3):252–259.

121. Konstantinides S, Schafer K, Koschnick S, Loskutoff DJ: Leptin-dependent platelet aggregation and arterial thrombosis suggests a mechanism for atherothrombotic disease in obesity. *J Clin Invest* 2001, **108**(10):1533–1540.

122. Yang R, Barouch LA: Leptin signaling and obesity: Cardiovascular consequences. *Circ Res* 2007, **101**(6):545–559.

123. Swislocki AL, Hoffman BB, Reaven GM: Insulin resistance, glucose intolerance and hyperinsulinemia in patients with hypertension. *Am J Hypertens* 1989, **2**(6 Pt 1):419–423.

124. Ferrannini E, Natali A, Capaldo B, Lehtovirta M, Jacob S, Yki-Jarvinen H: Insulin resistance, hyperinsulinemia, and blood pressure: Role of age and obesity. European Group for the Study of Insulin Resistance (EGIR). *Hypertension* 1997, **30**(5):1144–1149.

125. Lawes CM, Vander Hoorn S, Rodgers A: Global burden of blood-pressure-related disease, 2001. *Lancet* 2008, **371**(9623):1513–1518.

126. Sechi LA, Melis A, Tedde R: Insulin hypersecretion: A distinctive feature between essential and secondary hypertension. *Metabolism* 1992, **41**(11):1261–1266.

127. Perlstein TS, Henry RR, Mather KJ, Rickels MR, Abate NI, Grundy SM, Mai Y, Albu JB, Marks JB, Pool JL, Creager MA: Effect of angiotensin receptor blockade on insulin sensitivity and endothelial function in abdominally obese hypertensive patients with impaired fasting glucose. *Clin Sci (Lond)* 2012, **122**(4):193–202.

128. Rizos CV, Milionis HJ, Kostapanos MS, Florentin M, Kostara CE, Elisaf MS, Liberopoulos EN: Effects of rosuvastatin combined with olmesartan, irbesartan, or telmisartan on indices of glucose metabolism in Greek adults with impaired fasting glucose, hypertension, and mixed hyperlipidemia: A 24-week, randomized, open-label, prospective study. *Clin Ther* 2010, **32**(3):492–505.

129. Steinberger J, Daniels SR: Obesity, insulin resistance, diabetes, and cardiovascular risk in children: An American Heart Association scientific statement from the Atherosclerosis, Hypertension, and Obesity in the Young Committee (Council on Cardiovascular Disease in the Young) and the Diabetes Committee (Council on Nutrition, Physical Activity, and Metabolism). *Circulation* 2003, **107**(10):1448–1453.

130. Elliott WJ, Meyer PM: Incident diabetes in clinical trials of antihypertensive drugs: A network meta-analysis. *Lancet* 2007, **369**(9557):201–207.

131. Saad MF, Rewers M, Selby J, Howard G, Jinagouda S, Fahmi S, Zaccaro D, Bergman RN, Savage PJ, Haffner SM: Insulin resistance and hypertension: The insulin resistance atherosclerosis study. *Hypertension* 2004, **43**(6):1324–1331.

132. Aneja A, El-Atat F, McFarlane SI, Sowers JR: Hypertension and obesity. *Recent Prog Horm Res* 2004, **59**:169–205.

133. Engeli S, Negrel R, Sharma AM: Physiology and pathophysiology of the adipose tissue renin-angiotensin system. *Hypertension* 2000, **35**(6):1270–1277.

134. Yvan-Charvet L, Quignard-Boulange A: Role of adipose tissue renin-angiotensin system in metabolic and inflammatory diseases associated with obesity. *Kidney Int* 2011, **79**(2):162–168.

135. Mehta PK, Griendling KK: Angiotensin II cell signaling: Physiological and pathological effects in the cardiovascular system. *Am J Physiol Cell Physiol* 2007, **292**(1):C82–C97.

136. Hunyady L, Catt KJ: Pleiotropic AT1 receptor signaling pathways mediating physiological and pathogenic actions of angiotensin II. *Mol Endocrinol* 2006, **20**(5):953–970.

137. Dzau V: The cardiovascular continuum and renin-angiotensin-aldosterone system blockade. *J Hypertens Suppl* 2005, **23**(1):S9–S17.

138. Andreozzi F, Laratta E, Sciacqua A, Perticone F, Sesti G: Angiotensin II impairs the insulin signaling pathway promoting production of nitric oxide by inducing phosphorylation of insulin receptor substrate-1 on Ser312 and Ser616 in human umbilical vein endothelial cells. *Circ Res* 2004, **94**(9):1211–1218.

139. Wei Y, Sowers JR, Clark SE, Li W, Ferrario CM, Stump CS: Angiotensin II-induced skeletal muscle insulin resistance mediated by NF-kappaB activation via NADPH oxidase. *Am J Physiol Endocrinol Metab* 2008, **294**(2):E345–E351.

140. Pueyo ME, Arnal JF, Rami J, Michel JB: Angiotensin II stimulates the production of NO and peroxynitrite in endothelial cells. *Am J Physiol* 1998, **274**(1 Pt 1):C214–C220.

141. Berry C, Hamilton CA, Brosnan MJ, Magill FG, Berg GA, McMurray JJ, Dominiczak AF: Investigation into the sources of superoxide in human blood vessels: Angiotensin II increases superoxide production in human internal mammary arteries. *Circulation* 2000, **101**(18):2206–2212.

142. Sloniger JA, Saengsirisuwan V, Diehl CJ, Dokken BB, Lailerd N, Lemieux AM, Kim JS, Henriksen EJ: Defective insulin signaling in skeletal muscle of the hypertensive TG(mREN2)27 rat. *Am J Physiol Endocrinol Metab* 2005, **288**(6):E1074–E1081.

143. Shen DC, Shieh SM, Fuh MM, Wu DA, Chen YD, Reaven GM: Resistance to insulin-stimulated-glucose uptake in patients with hypertension. *J Clin Endocrinol Metab* 1988, **66**(3):580–583.

144. Pollare T, Lithell H, Berne C: Insulin resistance is a characteristic feature of primary hypertension independent of obesity. *Metabolism* 1990, **39**(2):167–174.

145. Carvalho E, Kotani K, Peroni OD, Kahn BB: Adipose-specific overexpression of GLUT4 reverses insulin resistance and diabetes in mice lacking GLUT4 selectively in muscle. *Am J Physiol Endocrinol Metab* 2005, **289**(4):E551–E561.

146. Henriksen EJ, Jacob S, Kinnick TR, Teachey MK, Krekler M: Selective angiotensin II receptor antagonism reduces insulin resistance in obese Zucker rats. *Hypertension* 2001, **38**(4):884–890.

147. Leguisamo NM, Lehnen AM, Machado UF, Okamoto MM, Markoski MM, Pinto GH, Schaan BD: GLUT4 content decreases along with insulin resistance and high levels of inflammatory markers in rats with metabolic syndrome. *Cardiovasc Diabetol* 2012, **11**:100.

148. Rudich A, Tirosh A, Potashnik R, Hemi R, Kanety H, Bashan N: Prolonged oxidative stress impairs insulin-induced GLUT4 translocation in 3T3-L1 adipocytes. *Diabetes* 1998, **47**(10):1562–1569.

149. Blendea MC, Jacobs D, Stump CS, McFarlane SI, Ogrin C, Bahtyiar G, Stas S, Kumar P, Sha Q, Ferrario CM, Sowers JR: Abrogation of oxidative stress improves insulin sensitivity in the Ren-2 rat model of tissue angiotensin II overexpression. *Am J Physiol Endocrinol Metab* 2005, **288**(2):E353–E359.

150. Wei Y, Sowers JR, Nistala R, Gong H, Uptergrove GM, Clark SE, Morris EM, Szary N, Manrique C, Stump CS: Angiotensin II-induced NADPH oxidase activation impairs insulin signaling in skeletal muscle cells. *J Biol Chem* 2006, **281**(46):35137–35146.

151. Csibi A, Communi D, Muller N, Bottari SP: Angiotensin II inhibits insulin-stimulated GLUT4 translocation and Akt activation through tyrosine nitration-dependent mechanisms. *PloS One* 2010, **5**(4):e10070.

152. DeFronzo RA, Cooke CR, Andres R, Faloona GR, Davis PJ: The effect of insulin on renal handling of sodium, potassium, calcium, and phosphate in man. *J Clin Invest* 1975, **55**(4):845–855.

153. Kotsis V, Stabouli S, Papakatsika S, Rizos Z, Parati G: Mechanisms of obesity-induced hypertension. *Hypertens Res* 2010, **33**(5):386–393.

154. Muscelli E, Emdin M, Natali A, Pratali L, Camastra S, Gastaldelli A, Baldi S, Carpeggiani C, Ferrannini E: Autonomic and hemodynamic responses to insulin in lean and obese humans. *J Clin Endocrinol Metab* 1998, **83**(6):2084–2090.

155. Reaven GM, Chen YD: Insulin resistance, its consequences, and coronary heart disease. Must we choose one culprit? *Circulation* 1996, **93**(10):1780–1783.

9 Strategies for the Prevention of Type 2 Diabetes

Harry G. Preuss and Jeffrey M. Preuss

CONTENTS

IMPORTANCE OF THE ISSUE

It is generally accepted that the recently recognized "diabetes epidemic" provides a significant health and socioeconomic problem for the citizens of the United States as well as populations throughout the world [1,2]. The health perturbations manifested in diabetics and the monetary costs thrust upon the general public bring all sorts of undesired misery. To provide a clear example of the problem, the International Diabetic Association estimates that 5–10% of the total health care budgets in many countries are devoted to various aspects of diabetic care [1]. Accordingly, much effort over the last few years has gone into seeking means to prevent or at least to delay onset and lessen manifestations of this detrimental chronic disorder. Up to this point, results from investigations examining preventive measures show some promise, especially when natural lifestyle measures that cause fat loss and/or enhance insulin sensitivity like proper diet and exercise are included in the various regimens.

After a proper discussion of background material, this review eventually focuses on the consideration that too much consumption of sugar and refined carbohydrates is a major factor in the diabetes epidemic through at least two mechanisms: first, by indirectly disturbing glucose–insulin metabolism and other hormonal systems secondary to increased fat accumulation from excess caloric intake, and second, by directly perturbing the glucose–insulin system. A hypothesis is put forth that changing this situation can play a significant role in prevention or at least delay and lessen deleterious manifestations.

OVERVIEW OF DIABETES MELLITUS

Frederick Banting with colleagues Best, Macleod, and Collip discovered and isolated insulin in the early 1920s [3–6]. Knowing full well the important role that insulin plays in the regulation of glucose homeostasis, most scholars initially believed that lack of insulin production and/or release was responsible for all known diabetes mellitus and that definitive treatment was finally at hand. Unfortunately, it became apparent shortly after this discovery that another even more ubiquitous form of diabetes exists where the level of circulating insulin is adequate or even more than adequate, at least initially. In this case, a poor response of the peripheral tissue to insulin early on, commonly referred to as insulin resistance (IR), is the primary basis for the diabetes [7,8]. Because of differences in the two pathogeneses, the original form of diabetes ascribed to a lack of insulin production/release occurring generally in younger individuals and requiring treatment with insulin (insulin dependent) was categorized as type 1 [9]. The other form, largely initiated by poor response to insulin by the peripheral tissues such as muscle and fat (IR), was categorized as type 2 (non-insulin dependent) [9].

Type 2 diabetes mellitus (T2D) rather than type 1 is the form this review concentrates upon, because it is by far the most prevalent form of diabetes mellitus (85–95%) and the form responsible for the current so-called "epidemic" [10–15]. In most cases, T2D is a chronic disorder with gradual deterioration of glucose–insulin homeostasis. As a result, diabetic patients endure a variety of microvascular (nephropathy, retinopathy, and peripheral neuropathy) and macrovascular (atherosclerosis, coronary vascular disease) complications that are associated with increased morbidity, mortality, and early signs of aging. A common scenario in the usually long-term course of T2D is development of IR, followed by a compensatory rise in circulating insulin concentrations—an attempt to adapt to this situation. Eventually, an inability of augmented insulin production to compensate for the IR develops leading to hyperglycemia, hyperinsulinemia, and further complications.

A milder level of IR at early onset may not augment circulating concentrations of glucose to levels required to diagnose clinical diabetes [16–20]. Although appearing nonalarming, nevertheless, this stage is still harmful and plays an important role in the eventual development of many chronic medical perturbations—especially those related to the cardiovascular system [21]. It is also in this stage that many physicians feel the timing is best for instituting prevention/treatment. This early stage is characteristically referred to as "prediabetic."

Consequently, appreciating the early pathology behind diabetes, such as in the prediabetic stage, is important [21]. While IR is a major component in the development of T2D, it has also been linked to many disorders that make up the ubiquitous metabolic syndrome [16–20]. The major features of this syndrome besides IR/T2D include central obesity, hypertension, and dyslipidemias—especially hypertriglyceridemia and low levels of HDL cholesterol [22]. In addition to participating in the development of many facets of the metabolic syndrome, the factors involved in diabetes also play a strong role in the aging process by promoting inflammation, endothelial dysfunction, production of advanced glycation end products (AGE), and oxidative stress [23,24].

T2D is a significant, long-term health problem associated with many chronic debilitating disorders that need to be prevented or, at least, ameliorated early on in order to obtain the best future health outcome. What is the present situation?

DIABETES EPIDEMIC: SUMMING UP THE PROBLEM

The estimated prevalence of diabetes in the United States released January 26, 2011 presents a reason for some alarm [12,13]. The best approximation is that there are 18.8 million diagnosed diabetics in the United States with another 7 million undiagnosed cases. As mentioned earlier, the majority of emerging diabetes is by far type 2. In addition to those already possessing T2D, a larger pool of potential victims lies out there; as it is believed that the prediabetic population may reach in the neighborhood of 79 million. Genetic differences may exist based upon the relative frequency of diabetes mellitus in various ethnic groups in the United States: 7.1% non-Hispanic whites, 8.4% Asian Americans, 12.6% non-Hispanic blacks, and 11.8% Hispanics [12,13]. The steadily growing numbers are unfortunate, because diabetes is already a leading cause of death in the United States—ranking fifth in the year 2000 [14].

Over the last 40 years, the occurrence of T2D has also escalated at an alarming rate throughout the world bringing with it all sorts of coinciding medical problems. A report by King et al. [10] supports the concept of the epidemic nature of diabetes in the world during the first part of the twenty-first century. This group predicted a rise in incidence to 5.4% of the world population by 2025, whereas Wild et al. [11] forecast a slightly lower but still alarming rise to 4.4% by the year 2030. Suffice it to say, whatever the correct prediction, all calculations indicate a sharp rise in occurrence. In the next 10–15 years, the incidence of T2D will escalate even more with India, China, and the United States predicted to have the most cases in that order [12].

Why such an alarming current upsurge in the number of diabetic patients? A concomitant increase in obesity may provide a clue [25]. Many experts believe that changes in modern lifestyle like a generally increased caloric intake coupled with insufficient exercise have contributed significantly not only to the worldwide epidemic of obesity but to diabetes as well. Recently, a new medical term burst upon the scene—"diabesity," because it is widely recognized that the incidence of T2D and obesity is increasing in parallel throughout the United States as well as throughout the world [10–15].

The diabetic epidemic is real, and there are available clues after examining certain aspects of the pathogenesis to suggest that diabetes can be prevented, onset delayed, and/or harmful manifestations at least ameliorated by natural lifestyle changes. This includes natural means to avoid or at least lessen body fat accumulation (especially in the visceral area).

Relationship of T2D to Overweight/Obesity

As emphasized above, the close proximity of the dual epidemics of diabetes and obesity in regard to time and locations may not just be coincidental—rather linkage is a strong possibility. In support, the fact that excess fat accumulation (overweight and obesity) increases the chance for developing diabetes and vice versa is well established [26–33]. More than 80% of type 2 diabetics are obese, whereas 10% of obese patients are diabetic [34]. Obesity, particularly the accumulation of mesenteric (abdominal) fat, like diabetes has long been associated with IR and many chronic disturbances of aging such as many cardiovascular maladies including hypertension, joint problems, and even some forms of cancer [26,31]. An excellent review describing the pathophysiology behind diabesity has been written [26].

Data from a representative sample of adults with diabetes participating in the NHANES between 1999 and 2006 have been assessed [35]. The prevalence of diabetes and levels of fasting glucose, insulin, c-peptide, and HbA1c were examined across different weight classes. The prevalence of diabetes was increased in the heavier weight classes. Consequently, it is not surprising that losing weight is an important way to prevent, delay, and ameliorate the development of diabetes [33].

As a first approximation, we recently examined data from 107 females, age 28 to 82 years, who were recruited for a "weight loss study" [36]. The group average BMI was 28.7 kg/m^2 ± 1.1 standard error of mean (SEM). When the various assessments of overweight/obesity (scale weight, BMI, and fat mass) were correlated with data assessing glucose–insulin function (fasting blood glucose, HbA1c, and circulating insulin levels), all correlations were statistically significantly positive over a wide age range ($p < 0.01$) (Table 9.1). Rising levels of circulating glucose, HbA1c, and insulin levels coinciding with increasing levels of various estimates of increasing fat mass strengthen the correlation.

It follows that behavioral changes leading to increased body weight are major contributing factors, directly or indirectly, in the rising incidence of diabetes. In addition, other associations with diabetes such as older age, urbanization, lack of exercise, and increased refined carbohydrate consumption may work, at least in part, via visceral fat accumulation secondary to poor dietary and

TABLE 9.1

Correlation of Body Composition with Fasting Blood Sugar (FBS), HbA1c, and Circulating Insulin Concentrations in 107 Female Subjects

	Scale Weight
FBS	$r = 0.25$
HbA1c	$r = 0.31$
Insulin	$r = 0.50$
	BMI
FBS	$r = 0.29$
HbA1c	$r = 0.39$
Insulin	$r = 0.57$
	Fat Mass
FBS	$r = 0.26$
HbA1c	$r = 0.31$
Insulin	$r = 0.50$

Source: Preuss HG, Kaats GR, *Original Internist*, 18:92–95, 2011.
Note: All values $p < 0.01$.

exercise habits [32]. The role of sugar consumption in the epidemic of obesity is still under some scrutiny [37], but the weight of evidence suggests that it is a major factor [38].

It seems reasonable in any regimen designed to prevent T2D to include weight reduction by lessening caloric intake when overweight or obesity is present. However, some have contended that there are "special calories"—those coming from refined carbohydrates like sugars that particularly need to be avoided [23]. Two reasons exist for this. First, when available, we tend to eat excess calories via sweets causing fat accumulation and the bad associations that come with this. Some even believe these foods are addictive to further the problem [39]. Second, sweet refined carbohydrates have the potential to further cause/worsen IR directly [23,24]. With the above in mind, a discussion on carbohydrates is in order.

BASIC INFORMATION ON CARBOHYDRATES

Carbohydrates, traditionally defined as compounds having a 1:2:1 molar ratio of carbon, hydrogen, and oxygen, are found mainly in fruits, grains, vegetables, and dairy products and serve as the principal source of energy throughout the globe [40]. The major classes of carbohydrates include monosaccharides (one monosaccharide unit) and disaccharides (two units)—both commonly referred to as sugars, oligosaccharides (3–9 units), and polysaccharides (>10 units). Starches are polymers of glucose units bound covalently either by alpha-(1,4) or alpha-(1,6) linkages.

To be absorbed, carbohydrates are eventually broken down into monosaccharides: first by alpha-amylase that splits starches into monosaccharide, disaccharide, trisaccharide, and oligosaccharide units, and then by alpha-glucosidases bound in the brush border of the small intestines that complete the breakdown of larger units into monosaccharides [40]. Drugs such as acarbose and natural supplements such as l-arabinose inhibit alpha-glucosidases like sucrase, whereas other natural products like bean and hibiscus extracts can block alpha-amylase. Thus, there are means to essentially slow absorption of carbohydrates and ameliorate the harmful effects of foods with high glycemic indices [41].

Sucrose, commonly referred to as "table sugar," is a disaccharide composed of glucose and fructose bound together. The historical origins of sucrose obtained from sugar cane and beets are intriguing [42]. After sucrose is broken down into individual monosaccharides by an alpha-glucosidase referred to as sucrase, glucose and fructose are then absorbed by different transport mechanisms [40]. Just recently, sucrose consumption by the general public has diminished, replaced by a commodity called high fructose corn syrup (HFCS), a stable product cheaper than sucrose. Two major forms of HFCS exist, such that the ratio of glucose to fructose is not 50:50 as in sucrose, but rather 45:55 or 55:45. Suffice it to say, the consumer still receives a goodly supply of each monosaccharide in the switch from table sugar to HFCS.

Diverse carbohydrates are absorbed at different rates—some relatively quickly (high glycemic index) and those more slowly absorbed (low glycemic index) [43,44]. Many dietary factors influence the rate of absorption, for example, the concomitant ingestion of viscous, soluble fibers lowers the glycemic index of a carbohydrate such as sucrose. This is important because the final rate with consideration of the amount taken in (load) can affect the insulin system greatly—rapidly absorbed carbohydrates are the ones associated with IR and many chronic health disturbances [43,44]. Carbohydrates not absorbed in the small intestines but swept distally are generally referred to as "resistant starches." When fermented distally in the large intestines, their breakdown products potentially offer many health benefits [41,44].

Worth repeating, many believe that excess ingestion of sugars and refined carbohydrate calories has a special role in the pathology behind the epidemic of T2D [45,46]. However, not everyone has found such an association [47]. Much of our information incriminating the role of excess sugar consumption derives from animal studies. Since the late 1970s, our laboratory has added sucrose to regular rodent feed to bring out various aspects of the metabolic syndrome such as IR and hypertension associated with perturbations in the renin–angiotensin and nitric oxide systems [48–51].

Most findings originating from earlier animal studies have been confirmed in clinical investigations. For example, 30 years later, the assumption derived from rat studies that heavy ingestion of sucrose, glucose, and fructose elevates blood pressure has been born out recently in clinical studies [52]. In animal models, however, body weight increases have not been a key factor in the development of these disorders, including IR [48–51]. Accordingly, this speaks to an additional mechanism behind sugar-induced IR other than obesity and fat accumulation—probably hormonal disturbances not directly linked to accumulation of fat mass.

Another piece of information is that T2D is more common in urban areas and in aging individuals. In both of these latter two population demographics, diabetes is increasing significantly. Finally, as indicated earlier, lack of exercise can also contribute to IR, a major perturbation in prediabetics and in T2D [53,54]. Suffice it to say, all the above associations may be interrelated by some means with perturbations in glucose and insulin metabolism.

When taken in excess, table sugar (sucrose) and HFCS are believed to be bad foods as far as wellbeing is concerned. These sugars are rapidly absorbed and make up a large portion of the daily caloric intake (high glycemic load), and contain fructose, considered by many to be a particularly bad sugar as far as health concerns. The question has been raised whether sugar is toxic [55]. What does history reveal?

SUGARS AND OTHER REFINED CARBOHYDRATES PLAY A MAJOR ROLE IN THE ESCALATING DIABETES EPIDEMIC

Early History

During World War 1, the incidence of arteriosclerotic heart disease dramatically fell in all countries where the food supply was inadequate from shortages brought on by war. Based upon available data, Paton [56] proposed that the incidence of obesity, arteriosclerosis, and diabetes declined from a lack of dietary sugar. In turn, such reasoning could explain the reverse—namely, the reason behind increases in these chronic disorders prior to the war when a remarkable boost in sugar intake had taken place. However, total agreement over this theory was lacking. Others, like Aschoff [57], favored an alternative hypothesis. He believed that low fat intake rather than low sugar intake during the war was the primary reason behind diminution of cardiovascular perturbations. Further support for the latter possibility came from Himsworth [58] who also noted a reduced incidence of diabetes mellitus among the general population during World War 1 and also associated it with the low-fat diets prevalent at the time.

While scientists took sides—sugars or fats—Yudkin [59] added to the confusion somewhat by pointing out that changes in intakes of sugars and fats were closely and positively correlated with each other during the war. Data from World War 2 also failed to solve the debate whether sugars or fats were more important in the genesis of atherosclerotic heart disease and diabetes mellitus; because once again, both low sugar and fat intakes occurred in the wake of decreased occurrence of diabetes mellitus [60].

Later History

Following World War 2 from 1957 on, a series of papers by John Yudkin continued to champion the theory that consumption of sugars and refined sweeteners were largely responsible for the increasing incidence of T2D and coronary heart disease [16,61–63]. To strengthen his contentions, he emphasized that the findings were clear that higher consumption of sucrose raises blood pressure and circulating triglycerides and insulin levels. Accordingly, Yudkin advocated a low carbohydrate diet for optimal health, a concept popularized later by Atkins and others with their ketogenic diets [64].

In 1974, roughly four decades ago, Ahrens [60] reported in his historical perspective on sucrose, hypertension, and heart disease that "the most striking recent dietary change has been the sevenfold increase in consumption of sucrose" in the Western diet. He was assessing an increased incidence of hypertension in the Western world. For the most part, his concepts were based on data provided earlier by Yudkin [59].

While Yudkin received modest backing for his "sugar hypothesis," the theory that fats are even more responsible for the increased prevalence of cardiovascular diseases received more support from both the academic world and the general public. Ancel Keys was largely responsible for such support. Keys published epidemiologic findings discussing the role of fats in cardiovascular diseases—the so-called seven country study that supported the concept that "fat causes heart disease" [65–67].

Roughly 10 years later, another nail was driven into the coffin of the sugar hypothesis. Bierman [68], Walker [69], and Nuttall and Gannon [42] reported that little evidence existed to point to sugar consumption as a cause of any health hazard except dental caries. They believed from the available evidence that high sucrose consumption does not contribute significantly to the prevalence of cardiovascular diseases, T2D, obesity, or micronutrient deficiencies.

Despite much opposition, Yudkin continued to favor sucrose over fats as the major nutritional promoter of many chronic disorders, especially cardiovascular perturbations and diabetes mellitus. In the 1970s and 1980s, Yudkin wrote that several factors may produce ischemic heart disease—smoking, physical inactivity, stress, and diet [16,61–63]. "We cannot therefore expect that any one isolated factor will show an exact association with the disease," since many biological variations are involved. Yudkin continued to emphasize to the scientific community that excess sucrose ingestion in animals and humans elevates circulating triglycerides and insulin and results in a diminished glucose tolerance in man and rat [16,61–63].

By 1973, as reported by Taubes and Kearns Couzens [70], the links between sugar, diabetes, and heart disease were troubling and prompted Senator George McGovern to convene a hearing of his Select Committee on Nutrition and Human Needs to address the issue. The question raised was whether excess intake by the public of dietary sugars and refined carbohydrates was largely responsible for the fact that the obesity rates had more than doubled since 1970, coinciding with the incidence of diabetes that had more than tripled [11–13]. Variations in sugar consumption were a very compelling explanation for differences in diabetic rates among populations. In 1983, Israel et al. [71]

reported that sensitive individuals may be adversely affected by high levels of sucrose present in the Westernized diet. They found in 24 carbohydrate-sensitive individuals consuming 5%, 18%, or 33% w/w sucrose in a crossover design that circulating uric acid and inorganic phosphorus levels as well as diastolic blood pressure increased with rising sucrose content. Consequently, more evidence was amassed to support Ahren's contention that dietary sucrose plays a major role in the ever-increasing incidence of hypertension [60,71–73]. A case is even made for the role of excess sugar ingestion with IR in the aging process [23,74].

Current History

In support of Yudkin's original concept, Lustig et al. [75] have more recently labeled sugar as a toxic compound. The majority of calories emanating from added sugars in a given day come from processed foods that include obvious sources like breads, cakes, jams, and ice cream [76]. However, goodly amounts of sugar calories are also present in abundance in tomato sauces, salad dressings, and cereals. Sodas and sugar-containing drinks are under the most careful scrutiny, because they supply roughly one third of calories from added sugars. Since 1970, it is estimated that the daily consumption of calories from sugary drinks has at least doubled. Two unfortunate results of this excess are a decreased intake of micronutrients [77,78] and increased body weight [79]. While the dietary Guidelines for Americans 2010 recommends that no more than 5% to 15% of calories should come from solid fats and sugars combined, approximately 13% of adult total calories come from added sugar alone between 2005 and 2010 [80]. It has been reported that children and adolescents derive roughly 16% of their calories from added sugars [81].

Excess intake of sugars and other refined carbohydrates, especially those rapidly absorbed and containing fructose, has long been considered deleterious to overall health. Evidence of this has only become stronger over time. It seems reasonable to apply all the means available to lessen intake and slow absorption of these ingredients. Concerning caloric intake from carbohydrates, sugar-sweetened beverages (SSBs) have come under increasing scrutiny.

SUGAR-SWEETENED BEVERAGES

Considering the overall intake of high glycemic carbohydrates, SSBs like soft drinks and fruit juices are significant sources of added sugars in the American diet [82,83]. These drinks not only supply scores of calories leading to bodily fat accumulation with subsequent IR but also make available rapidly absorbed sugars (sucrose or high-fructose corn syrup) in large amounts that directly encourage IR and the development of T2D [84]. During the latter part of the twentieth century, a number of studies performed in various settings showed in both adults and children that the rising level of obesity and T2D paralleled a concomitant rise in the consumption of SSBs [85–87]. Three supporting examples are given below.

In 51,603 females from the Nurses' Health Care Study, higher consumption of SSBs corresponded with a greater degree of weight gain and an enhanced risk for the development of diabetes [88]. The authors hypothesized that augmented weight gain from excess calories and the large amount of absorbable sugars was mainly responsible despite the fact that other factors could also be involved. Women with the higher intakes of sugar-sweetened drinks tended to be less physically active, smoke more, and consume less protein, alcohol, magnesium, and cereal fiber.

This brings up an intriguing question. How do liquid sources of sugars differ from solid sources? The investigators offered the suggestion that sugar-sweetened soft drinks and fruit punches display low satiety and do relatively little to lessen caloric intake from solid foods [89–91]. Consumption of fruit juice without added sugars and diet soda were not linked to an augmented risk of diabetes. A previous report indicated that increased consumption of diet soda in children had not been linked to obesity either [92].

In another study involving 43,960 African-American women, the investigators analyzed those individuals who gave a complete dietary history and weight information and were diabetes-free at baseline [93]. Concerning the main outcome measure, that is, the incidence of T2D, 2713 fresh cases of diabetes occurred over time. The onset of diabetes was more prevalent in those with the higher intake of both sugar-sweetened soft drinks and fruit drinks. The former association was almost entirely mediated through an increase in body mass index (BMI). Interestingly, in this particular study, sugar-sweetened fruit drinks were consumed at a greater rate than sugar-sweetened soft drinks. This observation was consistent with the finding that the proportion of energy derived from fruit drinks doubled from 1977 to 2001. Based on this, the authors make a cogent argument that the public should be aware that sweetened fruit drinks may not be a healthy alternative to soft drinks for avoiding T2D. Similar to the above study performed on nurses [88], this one reported that the consumption of "straight" orange and grapefruit juices and diet soda did not increase diabetic risk like the sweetened products.

In a recent study, Duffey et al. [94] examined data obtained from 2774 adults in the Coronary Risk Development in Young Adults (CARDIA) study over 7 years and found that SSB consumption was associated with increased cardiometabolic risk—higher waist circumference, low-density lipoprotein (LDL) cholesterol and triglycerides, and blood pressure [94].

The ingestion of sugar-added sodas and fruit juices has become more prevalent over recent years. This intake corresponds with a rise in the increased incidence of obesity and diabetes. SSBs provide rapidly absorbed sugar calories, many of which may come from fructose. Also, it has been questioned whether calories in beverages influence satiety to a proper degree. Since many believe these events are linked to T2D, at least to some extent, it seems wise to limit consumption.

ARTIFICIALLY SWEETENED BEVERAGES

Comparing results from various clinical studies frequently leads to confusion. Understanding the participation of artificially sweetened beverages (ASBs) in the diabetes epidemic is no exception. In the studies described in Sugar-Sweetened Beverages, three of the studies reported that, unlike SSB intake, ASB-drinking was not associated with T2D or obesity [88,92,93]. These results might be expected because ASBs obviously do not have high glycemic indices nor contain fructose—two major factors involved in perturbations associated with sugars. However, as depicted in Table 9.2 dealing with ASB studies, such findings are not universal. Table 9.2 lists seven studies performed over the last 10 to 11 years reporting the effects of ASBs on many metabolic events such as T2D and other manifestations of the metabolic syndrome [95–101].

Six of those studies listed in the table include data from SSB groups in their findings. With a single exception [98], all corroborated the deleterious effects from SSB consumption. In contrast, findings in the ASB groups were not as consistent. In the first listed two investigations [95,96], ASB ingestion decreased fat accumulation and T2D similar to the three studies mentioned above [86,90,91]. However, the last five studies presented data suggesting that ASB consumption was associated with harmful chronic effects [97–101].

A recent report by Fagherazzi et al. [101] tackled the issue of ASBs and their potential harm. Since less was known about ASB, 66,118 women were followed for roughly 20 years and 1369 developed T2D. Women in the highest quartile for both SSBs and ASBs showed increased risk, and there were strong positive trends in T2D risk across quartiles with ASBs as well as SSBs. While the investigators corroborated that SSBs are associated with increased risk of T2D. No association was found with 100% fruit juice. The final conclusion reached was that more randomized trials are necessary to determine conclusively the role of ASBs in the diabetes and obesity epidemics.

Sometimes well-controlled animal studies can contribute significantly to a final conclusion. They do not produce the compliance issues that are very common in clinical trials. Swithers and Davidson [102] found that reducing the correlation between sweet taste and caloric content (glucose vs. saccharin) resulted in increased caloric intake, increased body weight, and increased adiposity in rats. As other surmised in humans [88–90], it was hypothesized that rats are less able to judge caloric

TABLE 9.2

Recent Studies Examining ASB, SSB, and FJ on Type 2 Diabetes and Cardiometabolic Risk Factors

Source	Beverage	Comments
Raben et al. [95]	ASB– SSB+	Overweight subjects, 10-week study, consume sucrose or artificial sweetener $N = 21$, SSB, BW, and fat mass increased 1.6 and 1.3 kg, SBP increased 3.8 mm Hg $N = 20$, ASB, BW, and fat mass decreased 1.0 and 0.3 kg, SBP down 3.1 mm Hg
Yoshida et al. [96]	ASB– SSB+ FJ–	Estimates of insulin resistance assessed, SSB not ASB, nor FJ associated with increased risk
Dhingra et al. [97]	ASB+ SSB+	6039 observations on middle-aged individuals, Framingham Heart Study Regular and diet sodas associated with higher prevalence and incidence of multiple metabolic risk factors
Lutsey et al. [98]	ASB+ SSB–	9514 participants (45–64 years), ARIC study, food frequency questionnaires ASB but not SSB associated with incidence of metabolic syndrome
Nettleton et al. [99]	ASB+	Daily diet soda intake linked to greater risk Met syndrome (36%) & T2D (67%) Estimated by food frequency questionnaire over 3-year follow-up
De Koning et al. [100]	ASB+/– SSB+	SSB and ASB, average intakes estimated by food-frequency questionnaires Analysis of ASB data by different means resulted in conflicting results $N = 40,389$ healthy men
Fagherazzi et al. [101]	ASB+ SSB+ FJ (100%)–	Examined 66,118 women over 14 years, self-reported consumption 1369 incidences T2D, both SSB and ASB associated with increased T2D risk No association with 100% FJ consumption

Note: +, after beverage indicates positive association; –, indicates no association; ASB, artificially sweetened beverages; BW, body weight; FJ, fruit juice; SBP, systolic BP; SSB, sugar sweetened beverages; T2D, type 2 diabetes.

intake (satiety) in liquid form. de Matos Feijo et al. [103] reported that consumption of ASB such as saccharin and aspartame compared to sucrose increased weight gain in Wistar rats. The weight gain occurred despite no significant increase in calories consumed, and so, the investigators speculated that the weight gain was due either to decreased energy expenditure and/or fluid retention.

Replacement of SSBs with ASBs may not provide the answer to limiting the diabesity epidemic. Recent reports on the benefits of ASBs to help prevent diabesity have only created more confusion [104–109]. More data are needed to make a final determination.

FRUCTOSE

Over a span covering many years, several different research groups have consistently reported that consumption of sucrose compared to starch perturbs glucose tolerance [110–113]. These differences have been attributed, at least in part, to fructose release and subsequent metabolism following sucrose digestion [114]. In 1978, a review paper by Yudkin [115] published in the *Journal of the Royal Society of Medicine* stated clearly his reasons behind the different responses between sucrose and starch, "Present evidence suggests that most of the effects of sucrose are due in small part to its ease of digestion and absorption compared with starch, also in small part to its being a disaccharide, but chiefly to the fructose released when sucrose is digested." Accordingly, Yudkin proposed over 30 years ago two important pathophysiological principles favored even today—the harm from caloric sweeteners such as sucrose and HFCS lies both in their high glycemic indices (rapid absorption) and the presence of fructose [114,115].

Many findings have suggested that fructose presents a health problem. Hepatic metabolism of fructose favors de novo lipogenesis. Subsequent hepatic steatosis in the liver has been connected with many aspects of IR and the metabolic syndrome [87,116–119]. Other data suggest that high sugar consumption can play a role in heart failure [120,121], and the latter has been ascribed to the fructose moiety [122]. In addition, the unique ability of fructose to induce increased uric acid levels has been proposed as a major mechanism by which fructose can cause cardiorenal disease [123,124] and elevated blood pressure [123,125]. Sucrose ingestion is associated with retinal capillary damage [126–128], and the fructose moiety appears to be the culprit [129–131]. Fructose has been linked to obesity. It has been reported that beverages high in fructose produce smaller increases in satiety hormones and feeling of satiety than drinks sweetened with comparable amounts of glucose [132]. To add insult to injury, fructose consumption may exacerbate the various abnormalities already present in obese subjects [132].

Despite the potential harm attributed to fructose, the consumption of this monosaccharide is obviously increasing, because consumption of sucrose/HFCS has increased significantly from 1970 to 1997 [116]. Much of this is the result of increased consumption of soft drinks as well as breakfast cereals, deserts, and baked goods sweetened with sucrose and HFCS [133]. Important to note, countries with the highest availability of HFCS have a higher prevalence of T2D independent of obesity [82,134]. As a generality, HFCS, developed in early 1970s, is replacing sucrose in foods because of a longer shelf life and lower costs. Unfortunately, individuals obtain even more fructose (about 10%) on an average from HFCS containing 55% fructose than from sucrose [134].

Following the lead of Yudkin, Lustig et al. [75] also believe sugar is toxic mainly because of the fructose moiety present in sucrose. A popular theory is that consumption of HFCS in beverages may play a significant role in the epidemic of obesity [82]. Various aspects of fructose metabolism may be involved in obesity [116]. Suffice it to say, fructose consumption makes up a significant proportion of energy intake in the American diet, and the upsurge corresponds with increased prevalence of obesity.

What is known concerning fructose metabolism? Fructose does not stimulate insulin secretion nor enhanced leptin production—key afferent signals in regulating food intake and body weight. With fructose ingestion, there is less insulin response compared to glucose intake [116]. Because insulin response to meals has a significant role in leptin production, circulating leptin levels are decreased in turn [116,119,123]. Such may have deleterious long-term effects on the regulation of energy intake and body adiposity that depend on these two hormones to quell appetite. Additionally, fructose interferes with normal transport of and signaling by leptin. Leptin produces satiety and reduces dopamine signaling decreasing pleasure derived from food [75]. Another point to consider in the pathogenesis of obesity is that sugar consumption dampens suppression of the hormone ghrelin, which signals hunger [75]. Although fructose alone does not augment circulating insulin concentrations early on, the subsequent development of IR will eventually result in hyperinsulinemia.

Sources of fructose such as sucrose and HFCS are linked to numerous chronic conditions in addition to obesity [123]. In rodents, fructose consumption induces elevated systolic blood pressure, IR, impaired glucose tolerance (IGT), hyperinsulinemia, and hypertriglyceridemia [135–139]. In monkeys, fructose rapidly caused liver damage that relates to the duration of fructose consumption and total calories consumed [140]. Similar data obtained from humans are not readily available.

However, the implication that fructose is significantly involved in the pathogenesis of "sugar-induced chronic diseases" is not unanimously accepted. Sievenpiper [141] commented on a series of his studies where fructose substituted for other carbohydrates to maintain calories at a given level and did not find that fructose caused perturbations, that is, substitution of fructose for other sources of carbohydrates did not increase body weight, circulating lipids, blood pressure, uric acid, and even improved glycemic control. More precisely, this group did not find evidence that supports the view that fructose is harmful at typical intakes. "High levels of exposure and excess energy appear to be the dominant considerations for harm." These investigators did mention that larger, longer, and higher-quality studies are needed.

Among the popular sweeteners, fructose seems to be the most harmful. Accordingly, the most common dietary sources such as sucrose and HFCS should be limited in daily consumption. What is the evidence that such a strategy would be successful?

ROLE OF LOW CARBOHYDRATE DIETS IN PREVENTING AND TREATING DIABETES

Concerning the possibility that excess dietary loads of rapidly absorbed carbohydrates play a significant role in the increasing prevalence of glucose–insulin perturbations through augmenting fat accumulation (weight gain) and/or having a direct effect on insulin sensitivity [16,70], some clinical studies examining the effects of "low carbohydrate diets" have been carried out recently to determine such [142,143]. However, clinical studies, especially those investigating obesity, have their shortcomings including use of scale weight loss rather than changes in fat mass and nonrecognition of poor compliance by participants [144]. Suffice it to say, substantial differences among clinical investigations often exist. We will briefly describe a few below.

In 2003, 132 severely obese subjects (mean BMI 43) with a high prevalence of diabetes (39%) were assigned to receive either a carbohydrate-restricted diet (Low-Carb) or a calorie- and fat-restricted diet (Low-Fat) [145]. At the end of 6 months, the former group compared to the latter lost significantly more weight; mean −5.8 kg vs. −1.9 kg ($p = 0.002$). More improvements in insulin sensitivity and circulating triglyceride levels, even after adjustment for weight loss, were found in the Low-Carb group. Another report on the same study followed in 2004 that was based on results after 1 year [146]. Mean decrease in body weight did not prove to be statistically significantly different this time, mean −5.1 kg vs. −3.1 kg. However, triglyceride levels decreased more, and hemoglobin A1C levels improved more in the Low-Carb group even after adjustment for weight loss. Noting that the dropout rate was high (34%), it is not surprising that the investigators reported suboptimal dietary adherence of the enrolled persons.

In 2005, 96 insulin-resistant women with BMI exceeding 27 kg/m^2 were assigned to one of three dietary interventions: a high-carbohydrate, high-fiber (HC) diet, a high-fat (HF) Atkins diet, or a high-protein (HP) Zone diet [147]. Body weight, waist circumference, triglycerides, and insulin levels decreased with all diets, but with the exception of circulating insulin levels, the changes were significantly greater in the HF and HP groups compared to the HC group.

Nordmann et al. [142] examined data from five trials composed of 447 individuals with BMI exceeding 25 kg/m^2 in order to compare effects of low-carbohydrate diets without caloric restriction vs. low-fat, caloric-restricted diets. By 6 months, those individuals consuming the low-carbohydrate diets lost significantly more scale weight than subjects following the low-fat, caloric-restricted regimens (weighted mean difference was −3.3 kg). However, the difference did not reach statistical significance after 12 months (weighted mean difference −1.0 kg). In addition, triglyceride and HDL changed more favorably in the low-carbohydrate group, whereas LDL levels were more favorable in the low-fat group.

Six randomized control trials involving 202 participants were studied to determine the effects of low glycemic index or load diets on weight loss in overweight/obese individuals [143]. Compared to diets with a higher glycemic load, overweight/obese subjects lost more weight and total fat mass and had more improvement in their lipid profile. Another systematic review focused on data from randomized controlled trials of low-carbohydrate diets compared with low-fat/low-calorie ones [148]. These reviewers arrive at results similar to others: low-carbohydrate/high-protein diets are more effective at 6 months and are as effective as low-fat diets in reducing weight and cardiovascular disease up to 1 year.

Sacks et al. [149] examined the possible advantages with respect to weight loss from diets that featured different proportional macronutrient content: proteins, fats, or carbohydrates. Eight hundred eleven overweight adults were assigned to one of four diets containing different levels of the macronutrients. All the reduced calorie diets resulted in significant weight loss—it did not matter which macronutrient was emphasized in the diet.

The objective of a recently reported study by Krebs et al. [150] was to assess the value of a low-carbohydrate diet in obese patients with T2D. The principal end points were insulin sensitivity, glycemic control, and risk factors for cardiovascular disease. Measurements in 14 obese patients were made at baseline, 12 weeks, and 24 weeks. The diet was well tolerated, and the subjects achieved weight loss over 24 weeks. The weight loss was associated with a significant reduction in calorie intake. Glycemic control, measured by various means, improved significantly.

Although results may vary among clinical studies, the general trend with low carbohydrate diets is to show weight loss and improvement in glucose–insulin parameters. Could drugs help to achieve these goals even better?

DRUGS IN THE ROLE OF PREVENTATIVES

The idea that drugs developed to treat T2D would be examined very early on for their potential to prevent the onset of diabetes or as a minimum favorably influence the course is readily apparent [151]. Currently, a variety of oral medications are widely available for therapeutic application with many other potential agents coming on the scene [152]. The main classes of oral agents not only differ in their modes of action but their safety profiles and tolerability as well. The major, commonly used classes at present include insulin production and release stimulators (sulfonylureas, and meglitinides), reducers of hepatic glucose production (biguanides), and those that improve insulin action peripherally such as thiazolidinediones and biguanides.

The first generally used oral diabetic medications, sulfonylureas, were developed in 1955 with a second generation appearing in 1984. Sulfonylureas, the cornerstone of therapy for many years, work primarily by increasing endogenous insulin production and secretion. Accordingly, viable pancreatic beta cells to make insulin are needed in order for them to become effective. Unfortunately, hypoglycemia (2–4% incidence per year), weight gain, and dermatologic, hematologic, and gastrointestinal disturbances not infrequently appear with their use [152]. Of the sulfonylureas, glyburide causes more hypoglycemia than others but is not associated with cardiovascular problems or weight gain [153]. When a retrospective review of medical records for 150 consecutive patients with T2D in mid-1997 was performed, it was found that the use of this class of agents was often a poor choice. The investigators looked for duration of disease, accompaniment of other medical conditions, medical history, occurrence of contraindications, and presence of complications. Of 45 patients using glibenclamide, 40 (89%) had one or more risk factors for hypoglycemia, that is, age over 65 years, renal impairment or cognitive function, and living alone [154].

When using antidiabetic medicines such as sulfonylureas, clinicians not too infrequently consider whether medications of this type confer excess cardiovascular risks compared to other oral drug options. The relation between use of sulfonylureas to treat T2D and the risk of cardiovascular events has been vigorously debated, especially after results from the University Group Diabetes Project (UGDP) came to the surface [155–159]. The investigators observed a dose-response relation between sulfonylurea exposure and the risk of death—based upon observations collected over 30 years. In 2002, the relationship between use of metformin and sulfonylurea and mortality in new users of these agents was examined in 12,272 patients [159]. Metformin therapy alone or in combination with sulfonylurea was associated with reduced all-cause and cardiovascular mortality compared with sulfonylurea therapy alone. Despite this uncertainty, sulfonylureas for over 50 years have been a mainstay of therapy for diabetics.

Metformin, introduced in 1995, succeeded the earlier used biguanide—phenformin [160,161]. While phenformin was popular early on after its release, an unacceptably high incidence of lactic acidosis hastened its disuse and the development of a safer biguanide—metformin [160]. Metformin, like phenformin, is associated with lactic acidosis but to a much lesser extent [161]. Benefits far outweigh adverse side effects. Yet, because of this association, use of metformin is contraindicated in renal failure, hepatic dysfunction, congestive heart failure, and binge drinkers [152]. In addition, cautious use is recommended in the elderly and in anyone prior to radiography. While metformin carries the risk of lactic acidosis, one study reported that 66 of 70 metformin patients who subsequently developed lactic acidosis had at least one contraindication prior to use [154]. Some had two or three. For example, more than 20% had renal function below the well-published exclusion criteria.

Metformin decreases hepatic glucose production, lessens glucose absorption, and amplifies cellular glucose uptake [162]. Further, it results in elevated circulating levels of HDL and lowers triglycerides and LDL concentrations. It is not characteristically associated with hypoglycemia as monotherapy [152]; however, gastrointestinal disturbances (20%) are common [162].

Thiazolidinediones, released in 1999, are agonists of PPAR gamma [163], and stimulation of PPAR gamma is associated with enhanced insulin sensitivity [164]. Accordingly, thiazolidinediones enhance insulin sensitivity and lower hepatic gluconeogenesis but can cause hypoglycemia. However, the occurrence and extent of hypoglycemia can be ameliorated if the agent is used modestly [152]. An early thiazolidinedione, troglitazone was linked to hepatic toxicity and removed from the market. Because of this example, some still worry about liver damage and recommend frequent liver testing when using thiazolidinediones [152]. In reality, liver safety is no longer a major issue with the present thiazolidinediones according to a recent review [163]. Although this same review also reported no differences between rosiglitazone and pioglitazone in fluid retention, weight gain, and bone fractures, pioglitazone was judged cardioprotective, while rosiglitazone was judged cardiotoxic [162,163].

The majority of patients with T2D are overweight or obese, and obesity is associated with coronary heart disease. It is generally accepted that weight loss, in most instances, can improve diabetes and the cardiovascular situation. Ironically, improvement of glycemic control with insulin secretagogues such as sulfonylureas has been associated with weight gain. Insulin has been linked to weight gain. In contrast, biguanides, such as metformin, usually cause weight loss [165]. Alpha-glucosidase inhibitors are neutral. Thiazolidinediones are typically associated with weight gain and increased risk of edema [166–168].

Since postprandial hyperglycemia may contribute to the development of T2D in addition to development and/or worsening of many chronic diabetic-associated conditions, the addition of so-called carbohydrate blockers, in this case inhibitors of alpha-glucosidase enzymes, is of interest [41,169]. Alpha-glucosidase enzymes, located in the villus wall of the gastrointestinal tract, hasten the breakdown of disaccharides such as sucrose into monosaccharides like glucose and fructose—allowing absorption of the formed monosaccharides. In this way, they slow/prevent carbohydrate absorption and can produce benefits from this action [170]. Recently, a review of 19 trials carried out to evaluate the clinical efficacy and safety profile of acarbose, the most common pharmaceutical blocker, used alone and combined with other antidiabetic drugs was published [171]. The overall picture indicated that acarbose given as monotherapy or added to other antidiabetics was effective. It lowered HbA1c levels, seemed to improve lipid profiles, and reversed IGT toward normal response. Even though good acute responses were noted, it was the opinion of the investigators that long-term studies were needed to determine actual utility. Regarding adverse events, use is associated with a high incidence of gastrointestinal disturbances such as flatulence and diarrhea, which remits somewhat with time [172,173].

As a general rule, antidiabetic drugs have provided over the years their share of adversities. Aside from hypoglycemia, chronic use of many has been associated with various cardiovascular abnormalities. Weight gain with the development of edema has also been a problem. Unfortunately, the ability to prevent diabetes during treatment does not seem to last with discontinuance of the regimen making it likely that an attempt to overcome diabetes would have to result in lifetime continuance.

This would be fine in the case of lifestyle changes; but based upon past experiences, long-term drug usage could result in unhealthful adverse side effects.

CLINICAL STUDIES EXAMINING PREVENTION OF T2D

To date, interventions aimed at preventing diabetes and overcoming the diabetes epidemic have included lifestyle changes such as modification of diet and exercise as well as using many drugs developed for the treatment of the metabolic disorder [174,175]. A brief description of results from some planned research investigations follows.

Among 47- to 49-year-old males in the early 1990s, 41 subjects with early-stage T2D and 181 subjects with IGT were tested to determine if long-term, lifestyle changes could prevent diabetes [176]. With the lifestyle changes in play, body weights were reduced over time by 2.3–3.7%, and 50% of patients experienced signs of diabetic remission in a follow-up after 6 years. Blood pressure, lipids, and hyperinsulinemia were significantly reduced. Improvement in glucose tolerance correlated with weight reduction. The investigators concluded that long-term intervention with proper diet and exercise was effective even after several years—strengthening the concept that one might prevent or postpone manifestations of diabetes after choosing the right regimen.

In 1997, results from the Da Qing IGT and diabetes study were published [177]. Data had been gathered in 1986 from 33 health care clinics in the city of Da Qing. The 577 subjects with IGT had been divided into four groups: control and three treatment groups. The treatment groups included a diet-only group, an exercise-only group, and a diet-plus-exercise group. The investigators found that all three treatments compared to control led to a statistically significant greater decrease in the incidence of diabetes over a 6-year period: 68% in control, 44% in diet only, 41% in exercise only, and 46% in diet plus exercise. The authors concluded that among individuals with IGT, diet and exercise led to a significant decrease in the incidence of diabetes over a 6-year period that ended in 1992.

The question subsequently arose as to how long these benefits could last beyond the period of active intervention [178]. In 2006, 14 years after the intervention, the participants were reevaluated to determine the lasting effects of the earlier intervention. The average annual incidence of diabetes was 7% for the intervention group and 11% for the control. Participants in the intervention group went an average of 3.6 fewer years without diabetes compared to control. Whether a reduction in cardiovascular diseases occurred could not be determined.

This 2001 study performed by Tuomilehto et al. [179] randomly assigned 172 male and 350 female subjects with a mean age of 55 years, a mean BMI of 31, and IGT to either an intervention or control group]. Over the 3.2-year duration of follow up, an oral glucose tolerance test was performed annually. The weight loss after 1 and 2 years was 4.2% and 3.5% in the intervention group as compared to 0.8% and 0.8%, respectively, in the control group ($p < 0.001$ for both periods). The incidence of diabetes averaged 11% in the intervention group and 23% in control at the end of the study ($p < 0.001$). A safe conclusion is that some portion of T2D can be favorably influenced by lifestyle changes that are associated with weight loss in overweight individuals.

A follow-up of the above study was designed to determine if risk reduction from lifestyle changes remained after discontinuation of active counseling [180]. After 4 years of study, the participants who were free of diabetes were followed another 3 years for a total study time of 7 years. The incidence of T2D was 4.3% and 7.4%, respectively, in the intervention and control groups. Sustained good lifestyle practices with reduction in disease incidence remained after active counseling was discontinued.

In the ensuing years, drugs were included in regimens to prevent or delay onset of T2D. Chiasson et al. [181] randomly assigned patients with IGT to receive 100 mg acarbose ($n = 714$) or placebo ($n = 715$) three times daily. Acarbose, an antidiabetic agent in common use, decreases the absorption of carbohydrates in the small intestines. Two hundred twenty-one (32%) of patients receiving acarbose and 285 (42%) in the placebo group eventually developed diabetes. The most frequent side effects were flatulence and diarrhea. The authors concluded that acarbose could delay T2D in those with IGT.

Buchanan et al. [182] randomized women with gestational diabetes to placebo ($n = 133$) or the insulin sensitizer troglitazone (400 mg/day; $n = 133$) in the so-called TRIPOD study (Troglitazone in Prevention of Diabetes). During a medium follow-up of 30 months, the average incidence rate for T2D was 12.1% in the placebo group and 5.4% in the troglitazone treatment group ($p < 0.01$). Accordingly, treatment of women with troglitazone was deemed to delay and perhaps prevent onset of T2D. Women who completed the TRIPOD study were offered participation in the PIPOD study (Pioglitazone in the Prevention of Diabetes) [183]. The risk of diabetes found at 4.6% per year in PIPOD was similar to that found in those taking troglitazone in TRIPOD. The conclusion from both studies was that thiazolidinedione drugs could favorably delay the onset of diabetes in Hispanic women with prior gestational diabetes.

At the inception of the Diabetes Prevention Program (DPP) study reported in 2002 [184], it was postulated that a lifestyle intervention program that included lowering elevated glucose levels, reducing overweight, living a more active lifestyle, or taking the antidiabetic drug, metformin, would ameliorate severity of, delay development of, and/or prevent diabetes. Nondiabetic subjects (3234) with elevated fasting blood glucose, mean age 51 years, and mean BMI 34.0 were assigned to three groups: a placebo group, a metformin group (850 mg twice daily), or a lifestyle modification program that had a 7% weight loss goal and at least 150 min of physical activity per week as goals. After an average 2.8 years of follow-up, the incidence of diabetes was 11.0%, 7.8%, and 4.8%, respectively. Results from the DPP indicate that individuals at risk for developing diabetes can prevent or delay onset of diabetes by reducing through diet and exercise modest amounts of excess weight. The group participants in the lifestyle intervention decreased risk of developing diabetes by 58%. The lifestyle intervention regimen proved significantly more effective than metformin usage, which in itself proved effective, compared to placebo. Of interest, while the lifestyle intervention proved effective for all age groups, metformin therapy became less effective with age—being no better than placebo in patients over the age of 60. Also, based on a list of 34 T2D-associated genes to form a gene-risk score (GRS), those with the greatest risk, that is, the highest GRS score, still showed improvement with a lifestyle regimen, but those receiving metformin had virtually no improvement compared to placebo.

In the DPP study described above, troglitazone was used initially in a separate grouping but was discontinued later when the drug was associated with severe liver injury [184]. A publication in 2005 compared both the short-term results during the course of trial and the longer-term results after troglitazone use was discontinued with the other trial groups [185]. The troglitazone group ended activity after a mean of 0.9 years, and at that time, the diabetes incident rate was 3.0 cases per 100 patient years compared to 12.0 (placebo), 6.7 (metformin), and 5.1 (intensive lifestyle intervention) cases per 100 person-years in the other three groups. However, for the 3 years after troglitazone withdrawal, the incidence rate for diabetes was similar to the placebo group suggesting that troglitazone was effective only during its limited period of actual use.

After completion of the DPP study, 88% of the enrolled patients entered a 10-year follow-up period [186]. However, all three groups (placebo, lifestyle intervention, and metformin) were now offered lifestyle intervention. After a few years, diabetes incidence rates were similar between the groups—5.9/100 person-years for the original lifestyle group, 4.9 for the metformin group, and 5.6 for the placebo group. The investigators interpreted the findings to mean that prevention or delay of diabetes with lifestyle intervention can persist for at least 10 years.

Torgerson et al. [187] postulated that based on the fact that T2D is closely linked to overweight and obesity, addition of a weight-losing drug (Orlistat) to a lifestyle regimen change would be even more effective than a lifestyle regimen change alone. In a 4-year double-blind prospective study, 3305 subjects were assigned to lifestyle change plus either Orlistat 120 mg or placebo three times daily. All subjects had a BMI exceeding 30 kg/m² with normal (79%) or impaired (21%) glucose tolerance. The dropout numbers were large—only 52% of the Orlistat-treated group compared with

34% of the placebo group finishing the 4-year study. The cumulative incidence of diabetes was 9.0% with placebo and 6.2% with Orlistat. Of note, only subjects in the IGT group showed the improvement relative to placebo. Average weight loss in the treated group, comparable in the impaired and normal glucose tolerance subgroups, exceeded that of the placebo group—5.8 vs. 3.0 kg ($p < 0.001$). The investigators concluded that Orlistat did contribute to diabetes prevention in a setting of lifestyle change. However, the fact that those with normal glucose tolerance did not share in this benefit despite losing as much weight as in the IGT group is unexplained.

Kosaka et al. [188] examined whether an intensive lifestyle intervention designed to achieve and maintain ideal body weight was beneficial in subjects with IGT. A control group was composed of 356 individuals, whereas the intensive intervention group contained 102 individuals. Control subjects were urged to maintain a BMI < 24.0 kg/m^2 and the intervention group <22.0 kg/m^2. The cumulative 4-year incidence of diabetes in the control group was 9.3% vs. 3.0% in the intervention group ($p < 0.001$). This was associated with body weight decrease of 0.39 kg in control compared to 2.18 kg in the intervention group ($p < 0.001$). This study indicates that lifestyle intervention aimed at achieving ideal body weight in men with IGT can be successful.

In 2006, Gerstein et al. [189] designed a study to determine the ability of rosiglitazone to prevent T2D in individuals at high risk of developing the condition. The subjects were aged 30 years or more and had impaired fasting glucose or IGT or both. The subjects, who up to the initiation of the study were without evidence of cardiovascular disease, were assigned to receive rosiglitazone (8 mg daily) or placebo for a median of 3 years. Development of diabetes or death was the end point. Subjects (11.6%) receiving rosiglitazone in contrast to 26.0% given placebo developed diabetes; 50.5% of treated subjects and 30.3% receiving placebo became normoglycemic ($p < 0.001$). Cardiovascular event rates were the same in both groups, although congestive heart failure (0.5% compared to 0.1%) was greater in the rosiglitazone group. Under the conditions of study, rosiglitazone was effective in preventing T2D.

High-risk Japanese patients eating standard diets, taking regular exercise, and possessing IGT were randomly assigned to placebo ($n = 883$) or oral voglibose, a so-called carbohydrate inhibitor like acarbose, 0.2 mg three times a day ($n = 897$) [190]. Subjects in the alpha-glucosidase group had a lower risk to progress to diabetes compared to placebo (50 vs. 106; $p < 0.0014$). The conclusion was that voglibose can help to prevent diabetes.

In a recent study, 602 patients with frequent follow-up received pioglitazone or placebo for a medium follow-up of 2.4 years [168]. As compared to placebo, pioglitazone reduced the risk of conversion of IGT to T2D by 72%. Other benefits included a reduced rate of carotid intima thickening, a lowered diastolic blood pressure, and an increase in the level of HDL. On the negative side, pioglitazone was associated with significant weight gain, increased plasma volume, and edema. In a letter to the editor that followed, McCowen and Fajtova noting the parallel rise in HbA1c between the placebo and pioglitazone groups once the drug was stopped suggested that the drug only had short-term effects [191]. In other words, evidence that prevention remained after stopping the drug was not strong.

The above studies, designed to examine means to prevent or at least ameliorate the ramifications of diabetes and thus end the diabetes epidemic, show promise. They include lifestyle changes such as modification of diet and exercise as well as use of antidiabetic drugs. The success in one study using Orlistat was attributed to weight loss. With the development of various classes of antidiabetic agents, it has commonly been hypothesized that each one could be used early on to prevent development of glucose–insulin perturbations. In the above studies, metformin, thiazolidinediones, and alpha-glucosidase inhibitors were all associated with favorable effects over the period of use, but whether their antidiabetic effects remain after discontinuance remains in doubt.

POTENTIAL OF DIETARY SUPPLEMENTS TO AID IN PREVENTION

As discussed above, drugs have been used along with lifestyle changes in various research protocols designed to examine diabetes prevention. While inclusion of drugs appears to have some merit, their removal, by and large, eventually causes loss of their favorable effects [166]. No doubt the major fear resulting in removal is the potential for eventual harm via adverse reactions [151–153]. Of note, natural dietary substances were not employed in the major clinical studies despite the fact that many of them have profound potential to overcome IR and have virtually no adverse reactions. As a general rule, natural dietary supplements compared to drugs have less active strength but also less harm as relates to adverse reactions. Unfortunately, little cogent clinical research has been performed on these natural products. The major reasons behind this are simple. The usual manufacturer of natural agents compared to the drug manufacturers has meager cash available to sponsor definitive research. Funding is even more difficult to obtain because of the complexity in patenting natural substances.

We previously classified the major antidiabetic drugs as insulin stimulators that increase production and release of insulin (sulfonylureas and meglitinides), block gastrointestinal absorption of carbohydrates (acarbose, voglibose), reduce hepatic glucose production (biguanides), and improve insulin action peripherally (thiazolidinediones and biguanides). As a first approximation, a similar classification of natural dietary supplements would look like this: stimulate insulin (*Gymnema sylvestre*, fenugreek, garlic [192,193]), block gastrointestinal absorption of carbohydrates (bean extract, hibiscus extract, l-arabinose [41,194,195]), reduce hepatic glucose production (biotin [196]), and improve insulin action peripherally (trivalent chromium [197], cinnamon [198,199], maitake mushroom SX fraction [200], and bitter melon [201]).

It would be interesting to test the ability of some of these natural constituents over many years to see how they influence the course of the diabetes epidemic.

REFERENCES

1. Smyth S, Heron A: Diabetes and obesity: The twin epidemics. *Nat Med* 12:75–80, 2005.
2. Emery N: The global diabetes epidemic brought to you by global development. *The Atlantic*, July 2, 2012. Available at www.theatlantic.com/health/.../07/...diabetes-epidemic.../259305/ (accessed March 5, 2013).
3. No Author Listed: Frederick Grant Banting (1891–1941), co discoverer of insulin. *JAMA* 198:660–661, 1966.
4. Rafuse J: Seventy-five years later, insulin remains Canada's major medical-research coup. *Canad Med Assoc J* 155:1306–1308, 1996.
5. Preuss HG: The insulin system in health and disease (Editorial). *J Am Coll Nutr* 16:393–394, 1997.
6. Rosenfeld L: Insulin: Discovery and controversy. *Clin Chem* 48:2270–2288, 2002.
7. Himsworth H: Diabetes mellitus: A differentiation into insulin-sensitive and insulin-insensitive types. *Lancet* 1:127–130, 1936.
8. Ginsberg H, Kimmerling G, Olefsky JM, Reaven GM: Further evidence that insulin resistance exists in patients with chemical diabetes. *Diabetes* 23:674–678, 1974.
9. Olefsky JM: Diabetes mellitus. In: *Cecil Textbook of Medicine* (19th ed). Wyngaarden JB, Smith LH Jr, Bennett JC (eds). WB Saunders Co., Philadelphia, PA, pp. 1291–1310, 1992.
10. King H, Aubert RE, Herman WH: Global burden of diabetes, 1995–2025: Prevalence, numerical estimates, and projections. *Diabetes Care* 22:1414–1431, 1998.
11. Wild S, Roglic G, Green A et al.: Global prevalence of diabetes: Estimates for the year 2000 and projections for 2030. *Diabetes Care* 27:1047–1053, 2004.
12. American Diabetic Association: Diabetes statistics, 2011. Available at http://www.diabetes.org/diabetes-basics/diabetes-statistics/.
13. National Diabetes Information Clearinghouse (NDIC): National diabetes statistics, 2011. Available at http://diabetes.niddk.nih.gov/pubs/statistics/#Estimated.
14. Winer N, Sowers JR: Epidemiology of diabetes. *J Clin Pharmacol* 44:397–405, 2004.
15. Yaturu S, Jain SK: Obesity and type 2 diabetes. In: *Obesity: Epidemiology, Pathophysiology, and Prevention* (2nd ed). Bagchi D, Preuss HG (eds). CRC Press, Boca Raton, FL, pp. 211–238, 2012.
16. Yudkin J: Sucrose, coronary heart disease, diabetes and obesity. Do hormones provide a link? *Am Heart J* 115:493–498, 1988.
17. Reaven GM: Role of insulin resistance in human disease (Banting Lecture 1988). *Diabetes* 37:1595–1607, 1988.
18. Broughton DL, Taylor RL: Review: Deterioration of glucose tolerance with age: The role of insulin resistance. *Age Aging* 20:221–225, 1991.

19. Sowers JR: Is hypertension an insulin resistant state? Metabolic changes associated with hypertension and antihypertensive therapy. *Am Heart J* 122:932–935, 1991.

20. DeFronzo RA, Ferrannini E: Insulin resistance. A multifaceted syndrome responsible for NIDDM, obesity, hypertension, dyslipidemia, and atherosclerotic cardiovascular disease. *Diabetes Care* 14:173–194, 1991.

21. Haffner SM, Stern MP, Hazuda HP et al.: Cardiovascular risk factors in confirmed diabetic individuals: Does the clock start ticking before the onset of clinical diabetes? *JAMA* 263:2893–2898, 1990.

22. Ford ES, Giles WH, Dietz WH: Prevalence of metabolic syndrome among US adults. *JAMA* 287:356–359, 2002.

23. Preuss HG, Bagchi D, Clouatre D: Insulin resistance: A factor of aging. In: *The Advanced Guide to Longevity Medicine*. Ghen MJ, Corso N, Joiner-Bey H, Klatz R, Dratz A (eds). IMPAKT Communications, Boulder, CO, pp. 239–250, 2001.

24. Preuss HG, Echard B, Bagchi D et al.: Anti-aging nutraceuticals. In: *Anti-Aging Therapeutics*. Klatz R, Goldman R (eds), American Academy of Anti-Aging Medicine, Boca Raton, FL, pp. 219–224, 2008.

25. Eckel RH, Kahn SE, Ferrannini E et al.: Obesity and type 2 diabetes: What can be unified and what needs to be individualized? *J Clin Endocrinol Metab* 96:1654–1663, 2011.

26. Beck-Nielsen H, Hother-Nielsen O: Obesity in non-insulin-dependent diabetes mellitus. In: *Diabetes Mellitus: A Fundamental and Clinical Text*. Lippincott-Raven Publishers, Philadelphia, PA, pp. 475–484, 1996.

27. Ohlson LO, Larsson B, Svardsudd K et al.: The influence of body fat distribution on the incidence of diabetes mellitus. 13.5 years of follow-up of the participants in the study of men born in 1913. *Diabetes* 34:1055–1058, 1985.

28. Lundgren H, Bengtsson C, Blohme G et al.: Adiposity and adipose tissue distribution in relation to the incidence of diabetes in women. Results from a prospective study in Gothenburg, Sweden. *Int J Obes* 13:413–423, 1989.

29. Colditz GA, Willett WC, Rotnitzky A, Manson JE: Weight gain as a risk factor for clinical diabetes mellitus in women. *Ann Intern Med* 122:481–486, 1995.

30. Resnick HE, Valsania P, Halter JB, Lin X: Relation of weight gain and weight loss on subsequent diabetes risk in overweight adult. *J Epidemiol Community Health* 54:596–602, 2000.

31. Mokdad AH, Ford ES, Bowman BA et al.: Prevalence of obesity, diabetes, and obesity-related health risk factors, 2001. *JAMA* 289:76–79, 2003.

32. Snijder MB, Dekker JM, Visser M et al.: Associations of hip and thigh circumferences independent of waist circumference with the incidence of type 2 diabetes. The Hoorn Study. *Am J Clin Nutr* 77:1192–1197, 2003.

33. Aucott LS: Influences of weight loss on long-term diabetes outcome. *Proc Nutr Soc* 67:54–59, 2008.

34. Harris MI, Hadden WC, Knowler WC, Bennett PH: Prevalence of diabetes and impaired glucose tolerance and plasma glucose levels in US population aged 20–74 yr. *Diabetes* 36:523–534, 1987.

35. Nguyen NT, Nguyen XM, Lane J, Wang P: Relationship between obesity and diabetes in a US adult population: Findings from the National Health and Nutrition Examination Survey, 1999–2006. *Obes Surg* 21:351–355, 2011.

36. Preuss HG, Kaats GR: Examining possible causes for age-related blood pressure elevations in 107 female volunteering for a weight loss study. *Orig Internist* 18:92–95, 2011.

37. Van Baak MA, Astrup A: Consumption of sugars and body weight. *Obes Rev* 10(Suppl 1):9–23, 2009.

38. Te Morenga L, Mallard S, Mann J: Dietary sugars and body weight: Systemic review and meta-analysis of randomized controlled trials and cohort studies. *BMJ* 346:e7492, 2012.

39. Ifland JR, Sheppard K, Preuss HG et al.: Refined food addiction: A classic substance use disorder. *Med Hypotheses* 72:518–526, 2009.

40. Sanders LM, Lupton JR: Carbohydrates. In: *Present Knowledge in Nutrition* (10th ed). Erdman JW Jr, Macdonald IA, Zeisel SH (eds). Wiley-Blackwell, Ames, IA, pp. 83–96, 2012.

41. Preuss HG: Bean amylase inhibitor and other carbohydrate absorption blockers: Effects on diabesity and general health. *J Am Coll Nutr* 28:266–276, 2009.

42. Nuttall FQ, Gannon MC: Sucrose and disease. *Diabetes Care* 4:305–310, 1981.

43. Jenkins DJA, Srichaikul K, Mirrahimi A et al.: Glycemic index. In: *Obesity: Epidemiology, Pathophysiology, and Prevention* (2nd ed). Bagchi D, Preuss HG (eds). CRC Press, Boca Raton, FL, pp. 495–500, 2012.

44. Erik E, Aller JG, Abete I et al.: Starches, sugars, and obesity. *Nutrients* 3:341–369, 2011.

45. Basu S, Stuckler D, McKee M, Galea G: Nutritional determinants of worldwide diabetes: An econometric study of food markets and diabetes prevalence in 173 countries. *Public Health Nutr* 16:179–186, 2013.

46. Basu S, Yoffe P, Hills N, Lustig RH: The relationship of sugar to population-level diabetes prevalence: An economic analysis of a repeated cross-sectioned data. *PLoS* 8(2):ie57873, 2013.
47. Laville M, Nazare JA: Diabetes, insulin resistance and sugars. *Obes Rev* 10(Suppl 1):24–33, 2009.
48. Preuss MB, Preuss HG: Effects of sucrose on the blood pressure of various strains of Wistar rats. *Lab Invest* 43:101–107, 1980.
49. Fournier RD, Chiueh CC, Kopin IJ et al.: The interrelationship between excess CHO ingestion, blood pressure and catecholamine excretion in SHR and WKY. *Am J Physiol* 250:E381–E385, 1986.
50. Preuss HG, Echard B, Bagchi D, Perricone NV: Maitake mushroom extracts ameliorate progressive hypertension and other chronic metabolic perturbations in aging female rats. *Int J Med Sci* 7:169–180, 2010.
51. Preuss HG, Echard MT, Bagchi D, Perricone NV: Effects of astaxanthin on blood pressure and insulin sensitivity are not directly interdependent. *Int J Med Sci* 8:126–138, 2011.
52. Chen L, Caballero B, Mitchell DC et al.: Reducing consumption of sugar-sweetened beverages is associated with reduced blood pressure: A prospective study among US adults. *Circulation* 121:2398–2406, 2010.
53. DiLoreto C, Fanelli C, Lucidi P et al.: Make your diabetic patient well: Long-term impact of different amounts of physical activity on type 2 diabetes. *Diabetes Care* 28:1295–1302, 2005.
54. Preuss HG, Bagchi D, Kaats GR: Role of exercise in weight management and other health benefits: Emphasis on pedometer-based program. In: *Obesity: Epidemiology, Pathophysiology, Prevention* (2nd ed). Bagchi D, Preuss HG (eds). Taylor and Francis Group, Boca Raton, FL, pp. 409–415, 2012.
55. Taubes G: Is sugar toxic? *NY Times*, April 17, 2011. Available at http://www.nytimes.com/2011/04/17/magazine/mag-17Sugar-t.html?pagewanted=all&_r=0.
56. Paton JHP: Relation of excessive carbohydrate ingestion to catarrhs and other diseases. *Brit Med J* 1:738, 1933.
57. Aschoff L: Observations concerning the relationship between cholesterol metabolism and vascular disease. *Brit Med J* 2:1131–1134, 1932.
58. Himsworth HP: Diet and the incidence of diabetes mellitus. *Clin Sci* 2:117–148, 1935.
59. Yudkin J: Patterns and trends in carbohydrate consumption and their relation to disease. *Proc Nutr Soc* 23:149–162, 1964.
60. Ahrens RA: Sucrose, hypertension, and heart disease: An historical perspective. *Am J Clin Nutr* 27:403–422, 1974.
61. Yudkin J: Sucrose and cardiovascular disease. *Proc Nutr Soc* 31:331–337, 1972.
62. Yudkin J, Morland J: Sugar and myocardial infarction. *Am J Clin Nutr* 20:503–506, 1964.
63. Yudkin J, Szanto SS: Hyperinsulinism and atherogenesis. *Br Med J* 1:349, 1971.
64. Atkins R: *Dr Atkins' New Diet Revolution* (Revised ed). Evans, HarperCollins, New York, 2001.
65. Keys A, Aravanis C, Blackburn HW et al.: Epidemiologic studies related to coronary heart disease: Characteristics of men aged 40–59 in seven countries. *Acta Med Scand* 460(Suppl):1–392, 1967.
66. Keys A: Coronary heart disease in seven countries. *Nutrition* 13:250-252, 1997.
67. Keys A, Aravanis C, Blackburn H et al.: *Seven Countries. Multivariate Analysis of Death and Coronary Heart Disease.* Harvard University Press, Cambridge, MA and London, 1980.
68. Bierman EL: Carbohydrate, sucrose and human disease. *Am J Clin Nutr* 32:2712–2722, 1979.
69. Walker ARP: Sucrose, hypertension, and heart disease. (Letter to Editor). *Am J Clin Nutr* 28:195–202, 1975.
70. Taubes G, Kearns Couzens K: Big sugar's sweet little lies. *Mother Jones*, November/December 2012.
71. Israel KD, Michelis OE 4th, Reiser S, Keeney M: Serum uric acid, inorganic phosphorus, and glutamic-oxalacetic transaminase and blood pressure in carbohydrates-sensitive adults consuming three different levels of sucrose. *Ann Nutr Metab* 27:425–435, 1983.
72. Preuss HG, Fournier RD: Effects of sucrose ingestion on blood pressure. *Life Sci* 30:879–886, 1982.
73. Preuss HG, Gondal JA, Lieberman SL: Association of macronutrients and energy intake with hypertension. *J Am Coll Nutr* 15:21–35, 1996.
74. Preuss HG: Effects of glucose/insulin perturbations on aging and chronic disorders of aging: The evidence. *J Am Coll Nutr* 16:397–403, 1997.
75. Lustig RH, Schmidt LA, Brindis CD: The toxic truth about sugar. *Nature* 482:27–29, 2012.
76. Ervin RB, Ogden CL: *Consumption of Added Sugars among US Adults, 2005–2010.* NCHS Data Brief, no. 122. National Center for Health Statistics, Hyattsville, MD, May 2013.
77. Marriott BP, Olsho L, Hadden L, Conner P: Intake of added sugars and selected nutrients in the United States, National Health and Nutrition Examination Survey (NHANES) 2003–2006. *Crit Rev Food Sci Nutr* 50:228–258, 2010.
78. Bowman SA: Diets of individuals based on energy intakes from added sugars. *Fam Econ Nutr Rev* 12:31–38, 1999.

79. Vartanian LR, Schwartz MB, Brownell KD: Effects of soft drink consumption on nutrition and health. A systematic review and meta-analysis. *Am J Public Health* 97:667–675, 2007.
80. US Department of Agriculture and US Department of Health and Human Services: *Dietary Guidelines for Americans, 2010* (7th ed). US Government Printing Office, Washington, DC, 2010.
81. Ervin RB, Kit BK, Carroll MD, Ogden CL: *Consumption of Added Sugars among US Children and Adolescents, 2005–2008*. NCHS Data Brief, no. 87. National Center for Health Statistics, Hyattsville, MD, May 2013.
82. Bray GA, Nielsen SJ, Popkin BM: Consumption of high-fructose corn syrup in beverages may play a role in the epidemic of obesity. *Am J Clin Nutr* 79:537–543, 2004.
83. Johnson RK, Appel LJ, Brands M et al.: Dietary sugars intake and cardiovascular health: A scientific statement from the American Heart Association. *Circulation* 120:1011–1020, 2009.
84. Akgun S, Ertel NH: The effects of sucrose, fructose, and high-fructose corn syrup meals on plasma glucose and insulin in non-insulin-dependent diabetic subjects. *Diabetes Care* 88:279–283, 1985.
85. Putnam JJ, Allshouse JE: *Food Consumption, Prices, and Expenditures 1970–97*. Statistical Bulletin No. 965. Food and Rural Economics Division, Economic Research Service. US Dept of Agriculture, Washington, DC, 1999.
86. French SA, Lin BH, Guthrie JF: National trends in soft drink consumption among children and adolescents age 6 to 17 years: Prevalence, amounts, and sources, 1977/1978 to 1994/1998. *J Am Diet Assoc* 103:1326–1331, 2003.
87. Malik VS, Popkin BM, Bray GA et al.: Sugar-sweetened beverages, obesity, type 2 diabetes mellitus, and cardiovascular disease risk. *Circulation* 121:1356–1364, 2010.
88. Schulze MB, Manson JE, Ludwig DS et al.: Sugar-sweetened beverages, weight gain, and incidence of type 2 diabetes in young and middle-aged women. *JAMA* 292:927–934, 2004.
89. Mattes RD: Dietary compensation by humans for supplemental energy provided as ethanol or carbohydrates in fluids. *Physiol Behav* 59:179–187, 1996.
90. DiMeglio DP, Mattes RD: Liquid versus solid carbohydrates: Effects on food intake and body weight. *Int J Obes Relat Metab Disord* 24:794–800, 2000.
91. DeCastro JM: The effects of the spontaneous ingestion of particular foods or beverages on the meal pattern and overall nutrient intake of humans. *Physiol Behav* 53:1133–1144, 1993.
92. Ludwig DS, Peterson KE, Gortmaker S: Relation between consumption of sugar-sweetened drinks and childhood obesity: A prospective observational analysis. *Lancet* 357:505–508, 2001.
93. Palmer JR, Boggs DA, Krishnan S et al.: Sugar-sweetened beverages and incidence of type 2 diabetes mellitus in African American women. *Arch Intern Med* 168:1487–1492, 2008.
94. Duffey KJ, Gordon-Larsen P, Steffen LM et al.: Drinking caloric beverages increases the risk of adverse cardiometabolic outcomes in the Coronary Risk Development in Young Adults (CARDIA) Study. *Am J Clin Nutr* 92:954–959, 2010.
95. Raben A, Vasilaras TH, Moller AC, Astrup A: Sucrose compared with artificial sweeteners: Different effects on ad libitum food intake and body weight after 10 wk of supplementation in overweight subjects. *Am J Clin Nutr* 76:721–729, 2002.
96. Yoshida M, McKeown NM, Rogers G et al.: Surrogate markers of insulin resistance are associated with consumption of sugar-sweetened drinks and fruit juice in middle and older-aged adults. *J Nutr* 137:2121–2127, 2007.
97. Dhingra R, Sullivan L, Jaques PF et al.: Soft drink consumption and risk of developing cardiometabolic risk factors and the metabolic syndrome in middle-aged adults in the community. *Circulation* 116:480–488, 2007.
98. Lutsey PL, Steffan LM, Stevens J: Dietary intake and the development of the metabolic syndrome: The Atherosclerotic Risk in Communities Study. *Circulation* 117:754–761, 2008.
99. Nettleton JA, Lutsey PL, Wang Y et al.: Diet soda intake and risk of incident metabolic syndrome and type 2 diabetes in the Multi-Ethnic Study of Atherosclerosis (MESA). *Diabetes Care* 32:688–694, 2009.
100. de Koning L, Malik VS, Rimm EB et al.: Sugar-sweetened and artificially sweetened beverage consumption and risk of type 2 diabetes in men. *Am J Clin Nutr* 93:1321–1327, 2011.
101. Fagherazzi G, Vilier A, Sartorelli DS et al.: Consumption of artificially and sugar-sweetened beverages and incident type 2 diabetes in the Etude Epidemiologique aupres des femmes del la Mutuelle Generale de L'Education Nationale-European Prospective investigation into cancer and nutrition cohort. *Am J Clin Nutr* 97:517–523, 2013. doi:103945/ajcn112.050997.
102. Swithers SE, Davidson TL: A role for sweet taste: Calorie predictive relations in energy regulation by rats. *Behav Neurosci* 122:161–173, 2008.

103. de Matos Feijo F, Ballard CR, Faletto KC et al.: Saccharin and aspartame, compared with sucrose, induce greater weight gain in Adult Wistar rats, at similar total caloric intake levels. *Appetite* 60:203–207, 2012.
104. Mattes RD, Popkin BM: Nonnutritive sweetener consumption in humans: Effects on appetite and food intake and their putative mechanisms. *Am J Clin Nutr* 89:1–14, 2009.
105. Brown RJ, de Banate MA, Rother KI: Artificial sweeteners: A systematic review of metabolic effects in youth. *Int J Pediatr Obes* 5:305–312, 2010.
106. Wiebe N, Padwal R, Field C et al.: A systemic review on the effect of sweeteners on glycemic response and clinically relevant outcomes. *BMC Med* 9:123–141, 2011.
107. Pepino MY, Bourne C: Non-nutritive sweeteners, energy balance, and glucose homeostasis. *Curr Opin Clin Nutr Metab Care* 14:391–395, 2012.
108. Raben A, Richelsen B: Artificial sweeteners: A place in the field of functional foods? Focus on obesity and related metabolic disorders. *Curr Opin Clin Nutr Metab Care* 15:597–604, 2012.
109. Swithers SE: Artificial sweeteners produce the counterintuitive effect of inducing metabolic derangements. *Trends Endocrinol Metab* 24:431–441, 2013.
110. Uram JA, Friedman L, Kline OL: Influence of diets on glucose tolerance. *Am J Physiol* 192:521–524, 1958.
111. Cohen AM, Teitelbaum A: Effects of dietary sucrose and starch on oral glucose tolerance and insulin-like activity. *Am J Physiol* 206:105–108, 1964.
112. Cohen AM, Teitelbaum A, Balogh M, Groen JJ: Effect of interchanging bread and sucrose as main source of carbohydrate in a low fat diet on the glucose tolerance curve of healthy volunteer subjects. *Am J Clin Nutr* 19:59–62, 1966.
113. Hallfrisch J, Lazar D, Jorgensen C, Reiser S: Insulin and glucose responses in rats fed sucrose or starch. *Am J Clin Nutr* 32:787–793, 1979.
114. Bruckdorfer KR, Khan IH, Yudkin J: Fatty acid synthetase activity in the liver and adipose tissue of rats fed with various carbohydrates. *Biochem J* 129:439–446, 1972.
115. Yudkin J: Carbohydrate confusion. *J Royal Soc Med* 71:551–556, 1978.
116. Elliott SS, Keim NL, Stern JS et al.: Fructose, weight gain, and the insulin resistance syndrome. *Am J Clin Nutr* 76:911–922, 2002.
117. Havel PJ: Control of energy homeostasis and insulin action by adipocyte hormones: Leptin acylation stimulating protein, and adiponectin. *Curr Opin Lipidol* 13:51–59, 2002.
118. Havel PJ: Dietary fructose: Implications for dysregulation of energy homeostasis and lipid/carbohydrate metabolism. *Nutr Rev* 63:133–157, 2005.
119. Tappy L, Le KA, Tran C, Paquot N: Fructose and metabolic diseases: New findings, new questions. *Nutr* 26:1044–1049, 2010.
120. Sen S, Kundu BK, Wu HC-J et al.: Glucose regulation of load-induced mTor signaling and ER stress in mammalian heart. *J Am Heart Assoc* 17:2(3):e004796, 2013.
121. Wiernsperger N, Geloen A, Rapin J-R: Fructose and cardiometabolic disorders: The controversy will, and must, continue. *Clinics* 65:729–738, 2010.
122. Teff KL, Grudziak J, Townsend RR et al.: Endocrine and metabolic effects of consuming fructose- and glucose-sweetened beverages with meals in obese men and women: Influence of insulin resistance on plasma triglyceride responses. *J Clin Endocrinol Metab* 94:1562–1569, 2009.
123. Johnson RJ, Segal MS, Sautin Y et al.: Potential role of sugar (fructose) in the epidemic of hypertension, obesity, and the metabolic syndrome, diabetes, kidney disease, and cardiovascular disease. *Am J Clin Nutr* 86:899–906, 2007.
124. Cox L, Stanhope KL, Schwarz JM et al.: Consumption of fructose- but not glucose-sweetened beverages for 10 weeks increases circulating concentrations of uric acid, retinol binding protein-4, and gamma-glutamyl transferase activity in overweight/obese humans. *Nutr Metab* 9(1):68, 2012.
125. Jalal DL, Smits G: Increased fructose associates with elevated blood pressure. *J Am Soc Nephrol* 21:1543–1549, 2010.
126. Cohen AM, Michaelson IC, Yanko L: Retinopathy in rats with disturbed carbohydrate metabolism following a high sucrose diet. *Am J Opthalmol* 73:863–869, 1972.
127. Papachristodoulou D, Heath H: Ultrastructural alterations during the development of retinopathy in sucrose-fed and streptozotocin-diabetic rats. *Exp Eye Res* 25:371–384, 1977.
128. Thornber JM, Eckhert CD: Protection against sucrose-induced retinal capillary damage in the Wistar rat. *J Nutr* 114:1070–1075, 1984.
129. Boot-Handford R, Hezath H: Identification of fructose as the retinopathic agent associated with the ingestion of sucrose-rich diets in the rat. *Metabolism* 29:1247–1252, 1980.

130. More NS, Rao NA, Preuss HG: Early sucrose-induced retinal vascular lesions in SHR and WKY rats. *Ann Lab Clin Sci* 16:419–426, 1986.
131. Preuss HG, Fournier RD, Chieuh CC et al.: Refined carbohydrates affect blood pressure and retinal vasculature in SHR and WKY. *J Hypertens* 4:S459–S462, 1986.
132. Page KA, Chan O, Arora J et al.: Effects of fructose vs glucose on regional cerebral blood flow in brain regions involved with appetite and reward pathways. *JAMA* 309:63–70, 2013.
133. Drewnowski A, Rehm CD: Energy intakes of US children and adults by food purchase location and by specific food sources. *Nutr J* 12:59, 2013.
134. Goran MI, Ulijaszek SJ, Ventura EE: High fructose corn syrup and diabetes prevalence: A global perspective. *Glob Public Health* 8:55–64, 2013.
135. Tobey TA, Nondon CE, Zavaroni I, Reaven GM: Mechanism of insulin resistance in fructose-fed rats. *Metabolism* 31:608–612, 1982.
136. Reaven GM: Effects of fructose on lipid metabolism. *Am J Clin Nutr* 35:627, 1982.
137. Yeh TC, Liu CP, Cheng WH et al.: Caffeine intake improves fructose-induced hypertension and insulin resistance by enhancing central insulin signaling. *Hypertension* 63:535–541, 2014.
138. Preuss HG, Fournier RD, Preuss J et al.: Effects of different refined carbohydrates on the blood pressure of SH and WKY Rats. *J Clin Biochem Nutr* 5:9–20, 1988.
139. Reaven GM, Ho H, Hoffman BB: Effects of a fructose-enriched diet on plasma insulin and triglyceride concentration in SHR and WKY rats. *Horm Metab Res* 22:363–365, 1990.
140. Kavanagh K, Wylie AT, Tucker KL et al.: Dietary fructose induces endotoxemia and hepatic injury in calorically controlled primates. *Am J Clin Nutr* 98:349–357, 2013. doi: 10.3945/ajcn.112.057331.
141. Sievenpiper JL: Fructose: Where does the truth lie? *J Am Coll Nutr* 31:149–151, 2012.
142. Nordmann AJ, Nordmann A, Briel M et al.: Effects of low-carbohydrate vs. low-fat diets on weight loss and cardiovascular risk factors: A meta-analysis of randomized controlled trials. *Arch Intern Med* 166:285–293, 2006.
143. Thomas DE, Elliott EJ, Baur L: Low glycaemic index or low glycaemic load diets for overweight and obesity. *Cochrane Database Syst Rev* 18(3):CD005105, 2007.
144. Kaats GR, Preuss HG: Challenges to the conduct and interpretation of weight loss research. In: *Obesity: Epidemiology, Pathophysiology, Prevention* (2nd ed). Bagchi D, Preuss HG (eds). Taylor and Francis Group, Boca Raton, FL, pp. 833–852, 2012.
145. Samaha FF, Iqbal N, Seshadri P et al.: A low-carbohydrate as compared with a low-fat diet in severe obesity. *N Eng J Med* 348:2074–2081, 2003.
146. Stern L, Iqbal N, Seshadri P et al.: The effects of low-carbohydrate versus conventional weight loss diets in severely obese adults: One-year follow-up of a randomized trial. *Ann Int Med* 18:778–785, 2004.
147. McAuley KA, Hopkins CM, Smith KJ et al.: Comparison of high-fat and high-protein diets with a high-carbohydrate diet in insulin-resistant obese women. *Diabetologia* 48:8–16, 2005.
148. Hession M, Rolland C, Kulkarni U et al.: Systematic review of randomized controlled trials of low-carbohydrate vs. low-fat/low-calorie diets in the management of obesity and its comorbidities. *Obes Rev* 10:36–50, 2009.
149. Sacks FM, Bray GA, Carey VJ et al.: Comparison of weight-loss diets with different compositions of fat, protein, and carbohydrates. *N Engl J Med* 360:859–873, 2009.
150. Krebs JD, Bell D, Hall R et al.: Improvements in glucose metabolism and insulin sensitivity with a low-carbohydrate diet in obese patients with type 2 diabetes. *J Am Coll Nutr* 32:11–17, 2013.
151. Krentz AJ, Bailey CJ: Oral antidiabetic agents: Current role in type 2 diabetes mellitus. *Drugs* 65:385–411, 2005.
152. Ketz J: Review of oral antidiabetic agents. 2001. Available at https://www.clevelandclinicmeded.com/medicalpubs/pharmacy/MayJune2001/oral_antidiabetic.htm (accessed January 24, 2013).
153. Gangji AS, Cukierman T, Gerstein HC et al.: A systematic review and meta-analysis of hypoglycemia and cardiovascular events: A comparison of glyburide with other secretagogues and with insulin. *Diabetes Care* 30:389–394, 2007.
154. Yap WS, Peterson GM, Vial JH et al.: Review of management of type 2 diabetes mellitus. *J Clin Pharm Therapeut* 23:457–465, 1998.
155. Cornfield J: The University Diabetes Program. A further statistical analysis of mortality findings. *JAMA* 217:1676–1687, 1971.
156. Schwartz TB, Meinert CL: The UGDP controversy: Thirty-four years of contentious ambiguity laid to rest. *Prospect Biol Med* 47:564–574, 2004.
157. Simpson SH, Majumdar SR, Tsuyuki RT et al.: Dose-response relation between sulfonylurea drugs and mortality in type 2 diabetes mellitus: A population-based cohort study. *CMAJ* 174:169–174, 2006.

158. Eurich DT, McAlister FA, Blackburn DF et al.: Benefits and harm of antidiabetic agents in patients with diabetes and heart failure: Systematic review. *BMJ* 335:497–506, 2007.
159. Johnson JA, Majumdar SR, Simpson SH, Toth EL: Decreased mortality associated with the use of metformin compared with sulfonylurea monotherapy in type 2 diabetes. *Diabetes Care* 25:2244–2248, 2002.
160. Ching CK, Laic K, Poon NT et al.: Hazards posed by a banned drug—phenformin is still hanging around. *Hong Kong Med J* 14:50–54, 2008.
161. McGuiness ME, Talbert RL: Phenformin-induced lactic acidosis: A forgotten adverse drug reaction. *Ann Pharmacother* 27:1183–1187, 1993.
162. Stein SA, Lamos EM, Davis SN: A review of the efficacy and safety of oral antidiabetic drugs. *Expert Opin Drug Saf* 12:153–175, 2013.
163. Tolman KG: The safety of thiazolidinediones. *Expert Opin Drug Saf* 10:419–428, 2011.
164. Bortolini M, Wright MB, Bopst M, Balas B: Examining the safety of PPAR agonists—current trends and future prospects. *Expert Opin Drug Saf* 12:65–79, 2013.
165. Cheng V, Kashyep SR: Weight considerations in pharmacotherapy for type 2 diabetes. *J Obes* 9:207–212, 2011.
166. Fonseca V: Effect of thiazolidinediones on body weight in patients with diabetes mellitus. *Am J Med* 115(Suppl 8A):425–485, 2003.
167. Wilding J: Thiazolidinediones, insulin resistance, and obesity: Finding a balance. *Int J Clin Prac* 60:1272–1280, 2006.
168. DeFronzo RA, Tripathy D, Schwenke DC et al.: (Act now Study): Pioglitazone for diabetes prevention in impaired glucose tolerance. *N Eng J Med* 364:1104–1115, 2011.
169. Scheen AJ: Clinical efficacy of acarbose in diabetes mellitus: A critical review of controlled trials. *Diabetes Metab* 24:311–320, 1998.
170. Barrett ML, Uldani JK: A proprietary alpha-amylase inhibitor from white bean (*Phaseolus vulgaris*): A review of clinical studies on weight loss and glycemic control. *Nutr J* 10:24, 2011.
171. Derosa G, Maffioli P: Efficacy and safety profile evaluation of acarbose alone and in association with other antidiabetic drugs: A systematic review. *Clin Therapeut* 6:1221–1236, 2012.
172. Hoffman J, Spengler M: Efficacy of 24-week monotherapy with acarbose, metformin, or placebo in dietary-treated NIDDM patients: The Essen-II study. *Am J Med* 103:483–490, 1997.
173. Hotta N, Kakuta H, Sano T et al.: Long-term effect of acarbose on glycaemic control in non-insulin-dependent diabetes mellitus: A placebo-controlled double-blind study. *Diabet Med* 10:134–138, 1993.
174. Shin J-A, Lee J-H, Kim H-S et al.: Prevention of diabetes: A strategic approach for individual patients. *Diabetes Metab Res Rev* 28:79–84, 2012.
175. American Diabetes Association: Diabetes mellitus and exercise. *Diabetes Care* 25:S64–S70, 2002.
176. Eriksson K-F, Lindgarde F: Prevention of type 2 (non-insulin-dependent) diabetes mellitus by diet and physical exercise. The 6-year Malmo feasibility study. *Diabetologia* 34:891–898, 1991.
177. Pan XR, Li GW, Hu YH et al.: Effects of diet and exercise in preventing NIDDM in people with impaired glucose tolerance. The Da Qing IGT and diabetes study. *Diabetes Care* 20:537–544, 1997.
178. Li G, Zhang P, Wang J et al.: The long-term effect of lifestyle interventions to prevent diabetes in the China Da Qing Diabetes Prevention Study: A 20-year follow-up study. *Lancet* 371:1783–1789, 2008.
179. Tuomilehto J, Lindstrom J, Eriksson JG et al.: Prevention of type 2 diabetes mellitus by changes in lifestyle among subjects with impaired glucose tolerance. *N Engl J Med* 344:1343–1350, 2001.
180. Lindstrom J, Ilanne-Parikka P, Peltonen M et al.: Sustained reduction in the incidence of type 2 diabetes by lifestyle intervention: Follow-up of the Finnish Diabetes Prevention Program. *Lancet* 368:1673–1679, 2006.
181. Chiasson JL, Josse RG, Gornis R et al.: Acarbose for prevention of type 2 diabetes mellitus: The STOP-NIDDM randomized trial. *Lancet* 359:2072–2077, 2002.
182. Buchanan TA, Xiang AH, Peters RK et al.: Preservation of pancreatic beta-cell function and prevention of type 2 diabetes by pharmacological treatment of insulin resistance in high-risk Hispanic women. *Diabetes* 51:2796–2803, 2002.
183. Xiang AH, Peters RK, Kios SL et al.: Effect of pioglitazone on pancreatic beta-cell function and diabetes risk in Hispanic women with prior gestational diabetes. *Diabetes* 55:517–522, 2006.
184. Knowler WC, Barrett-Connor E, Fowler SB et al.: Reduction in the incidence of type 2 diabetes with lifestyle intervention or metformin. *New Engl J Med* 346:393–403, 2002.
185. Knowler WC, Hamman RF, Edelstein SL et al.: Prevention of type 2 diabetes with troglitazone in the Diabetes Prevention Program. *Diabetes* 54:1150–1156, 2005.

186. Knowler WC, Fowler SE, Hamman RF et al.: 10-year follow-up of diabetes incidence and weight loss in the Diabetes Prevention Program outcomes study. *Lancet* 374:1677–1686, 2009.

187. Torgerson JS, Hauptman J, Boldrin MN, Sjostrom L: Xenical in the prevention of diabetes in obese subjects (XENDOS) study: A randomized study of orlistat as an adjunct to lifestyle changes for the prevention of type 2 diabetes in obese patients. *Diabetes Care* 27:155–161, 2004.

188. Kosaka K, Noda M, Kuzuya T: Prevention of type 2 diabetes by lifestyle intervention. A Japanese trial in IGT males. *Diabetes Res Clin Pract* 67:152–162, 2005.

189. Gerstein HC, Yusuf S, Bosch J et al.: Effect of rosiglitazone on the frequency of diabetes in patients with impaired glucose tolerance or impaired fasting glucose: A randomised controlled study. *Lancet* 368:1096–1105, 2006.

190. Kawamori R, Tajima N, Iwamoto Y et al.: Voglibose for prevention of type 2 diabetes mellitus: A randomized, double-blind trial in Japanese individuals with impaired glucose tolerance. *Lancet* 373:1607–1614, 2009.

191. McCowen KC, Fajtova VT: Pioglitazone for diabetes prevention. *N Eng J Med* 365:182–183, 2011.

192. Al-Romaiyan A, King AJ, Persaud SJ, Jones PM: A novel extract of *Gymnema sylvestre* improves glucose tolerance in vivo and stimulates insulin secretion and synthesis *in vitro*. *Phytother Res* 27:1006–1011, 2013.

193. Rizvi SI, Mishra N: Traditional Indian medicines used for the management of diabetes mellitus. *J Diabetes Res* 2013:712092, 2013.

194. Preuss HG, Echard B, Talpur N et al.: Inhibition of starch and sucrose gastrointestinal absorption in rats by various dietary supplements alone and combined. Acute studies. *Int J Med Sci* 4:196–202, 2007.

195. Preuss HG, Bagchi D, Echard B et al.: Inhibition of starch and sucrose gastrointestinal absorption in rats by various dietary supplements alone and combined. Subchronic studies. *Int J Med Sci* 4:209–215, 2007.

196. McCarty MF: High-dose biotin, an inducer of glucokinase expression, may synergize with chromium picolinate to enable a definitive nutritional therapy for type II diabetes. *Med Hypotheses* 52:401–406, 1999.

197. Anderson RA, Cheng N, Bryden N et al.: Elevated intakes of supplemental chromium improve glucose and insulin variables in individuals with type 2 diabetes. *Diabetes* 46:1786–1791, 1997.

198. Qin B, Panickar KS, Anderson RA: Cinnamon: Potential role in the prevention of insulin resistance, metabolic syndrome, and type 2 diabetes. *J Diabetes Sci Technol* 4:685–693, 2010.

199. Preuss HG, Echard B, Polansky MM, Anderson R: Whole cinnamon and aqueous extracts ameliorate sucrose-induced blood pressure elevations in spontaneously hypertensive rats. *J Am Coll Nutr* 25:144–150, 2006.

200. Preuss HG, Echard B, Bagchi D et al.: Enhanced insulin-hypoglycemic activity in rats consuming a specific glycoprotein extracted from maitake mushroom. *Mol Cell Biochem* 306:105–113, 2007.

201. Clouatre D, Echard B, Preuss HG: Effects of bitter melon extracts in diabetic and normal rats on blood glucose and blood pressure regulation. *J Med Foods* 14:1496–1504, 2011.

10 Bariatric Surgery for Type 2 Diabetes Mellitus Resolution

Geltrude Mingrone and Marco Castagneto

CONTENTS

INTRODUCTION

The term "bariatric" derives from the Greek word "barus," which means heavy, and it is, therefore, used in relation to obesity and to surgical operations that have the aim of reducing the volume of food intake or the amount of calories absorbed by the intestine.

Although the first attempt to the clinical application of this type of surgery dates back to the early 1950s, it was not until the late 1970s and the 1980s that bariatric surgery became a suitable treatment option for the so-called "morbid" obesity (body mass index [BMI] > 40 kg/m^2). Increased body mass increases the likelihood and risk of associated diseases particularly type 2 diabetes mellitus (T2DM), hypertension and cardiovascular complications, obstructive sleep apnea, certain types of cancer, and osteoarthritis [1].

Among the very first clinical applications of bariatric surgery in the early 1960 there was the early clinical application of the ileal bypass, which was aimed at the treatment of metabolic diseases such as hyperlipidemias and related cardiovascular risk [2].

Until the 1990s, bariatric surgery was regarded with some disfavor because of metabolic and surgical complications and also because obesity itself was not perceived as a real disease. However, in the last decades, the "obesity epidemics" with its health, social, and economic burden have become progressively manifest. The World Health Organization statistics show that worldwide obesity has more than doubled since 1980, which means that in 2008, a half billion adults were obese (BMI ≥ 30 kg/m^2) [3]. This has led overweight and obesity to become the fifth greater risk for death. Obesity has been found to contribute to diabetes (44%), coronary heart disease (3%), and certain types of cancer. The link between obesity and diabetes (about 60% of diabetic people are obese) has been well known for a long time, including its association with environmental and behavioral factors as well as having a definite genetic background. It has been estimated that the present world population of diabetic patients is about 366 million and is projected to be 552 million by 2030 [4]. In the

United States, in 2010, diabetic subjects were estimated to number 20.9 million, being a threefold increase from 1980 [5].

In addition, it should be emphasized that this epidemiologic situation is not confined to the Western more affluent countries, but it is rapidly spreading to the Middle East and Asian areas as well as to lower income populations. The actual threat of the "diabesity" epidemic resides in the fact that current therapeutic management of obesity with or without type 2 diabetes, excluding prevention, is far from satisfactory and long lasting [6]. This consideration together with the undeniable effectiveness of weight loss surgery and the progressive development and safe use of the laparoscopic approach has stimulated great interest in this therapeutic modality.

The value of this surgical modality of therapy applies not only to obesity itself but also to the treatment of T2DM, since weight loss through diet and exercise is traditionally a prerequisite to a successful glycemic control. Incidental diabetes improvement after gastrointestinal surgery for other diseases has long been observed. At present, the extensive experience and application of bariatric surgery documented by patient observation, systematic review, and clinical trials have consistently demonstrated that there is a high rate of improvement or resolution of T2DM after surgery. Moreover, the early improvement or reversal of carbohydrate metabolic abnormalities before significant BMI reduction, as well as the different responses to different operations, suggest that weight loss may not be the only determinant of this remarkable phenomenon.

The purpose of this article is to present the available data on the effects of different bariatric operations on T2DM pathophysiology and to discuss features and possible mechanisms of its resolution.

BARIATRIC SURGICAL PROCEDURES

Although description of all of the available bariatric operations is beyond the scope of this review, it is useful to make reference to the main procedures that have been developed over the last 50 years and that, thanks to the laparoscopic approach, have now become the standard surgical armamentarium of bariatric surgery.

Weight losing operations on the gastrointestinal tract are usually classified as restrictive or malabsorptive depending on whether they are effective by reducing caloric intake or by limiting caloric absorption. In the first instance, early satiety is obtained with reduction of the gastric volume; in the second case, food absorption is incomplete because part of the intestine is bypassed and therefore is excluded from food transit and also from early mixing with biliopancreatic juices, which enhance substrate digestion. However, very few procedures are purely either restrictive or malabsorptive, but most are a combination of these two modalities. The next four sections are the outline of the four procedures that are commonly performed and that have now accounted for the 344,221 operations done worldwide in 2008, 220,000 of which were done in the United States and Canada alone [7].

GASTRIC BANDING

Laparoscopic adjustable gastric banding (LAGB) is a purely restrictive operation that consists of the placement of an inflatable cuff slightly below the esophagogastric junction. This creates a small upper pouch with an outlet whose diameter can be finely adjusted by inflating the silicon chamber. LAGB was the prevailing procedure performed in 2008 with a frequency of 42.3%, although its use has been declining in recent years particularly in Europe [8].

Various reports and meta-analysis indicate that 46% excess weight loss (EWL) at 2 years has been maintained at and beyond 10 years, according to a longitudinal Australian study [9]. However, this benefit has required a price of significant revisional procedures [9]. However, other authors have reported less satisfactory results in the long term [10,11]. Overall, this operation displays a lower weight loss but also a lower mortality (around 0.5%) compared to the other procedures [12].

SLEEVE GASTRECTOMY

Sleeve gastrectomy (SG) consists of the resection of the stomach along the greater curvature preserving the pylorus, and therefore fashioning a gastric tube of about 200 mL. This procedure was originally conceived by Marceau et al. [13] as part of a variant of biliopancreatic diversion (BPD) called a "duodenal switch" (DS), where the gastric remnant was anastomosed below the pylorus to the loop of the gut called the biliary limb. Later, Regan et al. [14] applied this technique to high-risk super obese patients (BMI > 60 kg/m²) as a two-stage operation, where the gastric resection is performed first. It soon became apparent that quite a few patients needed the second stage because very remarkable weight loss was achieved in this way. Therefore, SG has become an independent operation that lately has gained increasing popularity with an employment rate of about 15% of all bariatric operations. EWL is 50% to 60% with a recorded surgical mortality of 0.4%. However, morbidity at 1 year has been 10.8% [15].

ROUX-EN-Y GASTRIC BYPASS

Roux-en-Y gastric bypass (RYGB) (Figure 10.1), carried out just below the esophagogastric junction, consists of the divisions of the stomach into two parts or pouches: the upper one, whose volume is about 25 mL, is then anastomosed to the distal end of the jejunum, which is sectioned at about 50 cm from the duodenal-jejunal junction becoming the so called alimentary tract. The distal larger gastric pouch with the duodenum and part of the jejunum are therefore excluded from food transit and carry the biliopancreatic juice through an anastomosis of the proximal jejunal end to the side of the alimentary tract. RYGB is considered the gold standard of bariatric surgery, and, in fact, it now

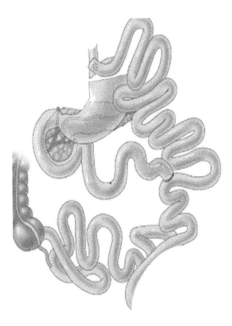

FIGURE 10.1   RYGB: it consists of the division, with a surgical stapler, of the stomach leaving a small upper pouch (20–30 mL) and a large distal gastric remnant. The jejunum is then divided at about 0.5 m from the duodenal–jejunal junction (ligament of Treitz): its distal end is then connected to the upper gastric pouch (alimentary limb) while the proximal end, carrying the biliopancreatic juice (biliopancreatic limb), is reattached to the gastrointestinal tract about 1–1.5 m from the gastrojejunal anastomosis.

accounts for nearly half of all such operations. The reported excessive weight loss is 60%, and the mortality range is 0.5–1%. Morbidity at 1 year is 14.9% [12,15].

BILIOPANCREATIC DIVERSION

BPD (Figure 10.2) is primarily a malabsorptive operation, where, in its original design, the stomach is resected in its midportion leaving a residual volume of about 400 mL, and the duodenal stump is then closed just below the pylorus [16]. The ileum is transected 2.5 m from the ileocecal valve, and its distal end is anastomosed to the stomach. Finally, the proximal end of the ileum, carrying the biliopancreatic juices, is connected in an end-to-side fashion to the small bowel, 50 cm proximal to the ileocecal valve. As mentioned before, Marceau et al. [13] conceived a variant of this operation, called duodenal switch (DS), in which the stomach is resected along the greater curvature, like in the SG, which derives from this procedure. The duodenum is then divided just distal to the pylorus and is anastomosed to the ileum 2.5–3 m from the ileocecal valve. The distal duodenal stump is closed, and the proximal end of the divided small bowel is connected with the ileum 50 cm from the ileocecal valve.

The essentially malabsorptive nature of this operation is due to the fact that most of the small bowel is excluded from food transit and that the absorption process takes place in the terminal 2.5 m of intestine and, in particular, in the last 50 cm where the biliopancreatic juices are mixed with the chime.

BPD, initially performed as an open procedure and then laparoscopically, is a very effective long-term weight losing procedure with some inherent risk of protein–calorie and micronutrient malnutrition. Experience with this more demanding type of surgery has been concentrated in a few centers, and, for this reason, its use has been more limited than the other bariatric operations. Excessive weight loss at 5 years is 75% and perioperative mortality is 0.75–1% [15,16].

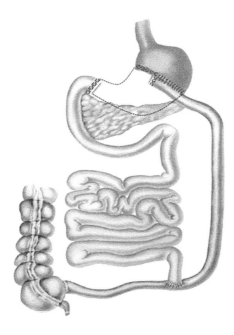

FIGURE 10.2 BPD: in its original design, BPD includes a partial gastric resection leaving a pouch of about 400 mL with duodenal stump closure. The ileum is then transected 2.5 m from the ileocecal junction: the distal end is connected to the gastric pouch (alimentary limb) while the proximal end, carrying the biliopancreatic juice (biliary limb), is reattached to the small bowel 50 cm proximal to the ileocecal valve (common limb).

BARIATRIC SURGERY AND RESOLUTION OF T2DM

The beneficial effect of gastrointestinal surgery on the diabetic state has long been observed. The expanded acceptance and employment of bariatric surgery has made these observations more specific and has been increasingly supported by clinical and investigative evidence. The well-known Swedish Obese Subjects study (SOS) [17] of over 4000 obese subjects followed for up to 20 years, half of them having undergone various types of bariatric surgery and the other half being matched controls, shows that at 2 years, 72% of the operated diabetic patients were in remission compared to 21% in the traditional treatment group. At 10 years, 36% of the SOS patients were still diabetes free. As a corollary to these findings, since T2DM is closely linked to the cardiovascular risk, in the surgical group, the SOS study reported a statistically significant 29% reduction of mortality and a 37% reduction of cardiovascular events. Moreover, recent data from the same study show that in the glucose-tolerant subjects at baseline who were followed up for 15 years, diabetes developed in 110 out of 1658 patients in the surgically treated group compared to 392 out of 1771 patients in the control group, with an incidence of 6.8 and 28.4 per million persons per year, respectively [18].

Besides this large, long-term prospective study, there are numerous case series, as well as several carefully planned clinical investigations, all supporting the above findings and defining the different effects by bariatric procedure. These studies also provide information on the reversal of carbohydrate metabolism abnormalities [19].

In 2004, Buchwald et al. [20] published their well-known systematic review of the literature and their meta-analysis and showed that the diabetes remission rate was higher for BPD (95%), intermediate for RYGB (80%), and lower for LAGB (57%). These results were maintained at and beyond 2 years and were matched by the rate of EWL and also by improvement of the other obesity-related comorbidities. A subsequent analysis of the literature using only the more recent contributions found equivalent diabetes reversal rates for LAGB and RYGB [21].

On the other hand, sleeve gastrectomy, which as noted has gained increased popularity, displays a very favorable immediate glycemic control profile, comparable to the other procedures, although long-term follow-ups are not yet available [22]. A systematic review on this topic shows that diabetes resolved in 66.2% and improved in 26.9%, whereas a prospective study with an 18-month follow-up resulted in an 80% diabetes reversal, together with a significant improvement of comorbidities compared to none in the normally treated diabetic group [23,24]. All these reports are further supported by observational studies comparing surgery with conventional antidiabetic therapy [25,26]. Among them, in a retrospective case-matched study in T2DM obese patients, the group of the University of Minnesota found, at 1 year, an incidence of diabetes remission of only 3.4% in the medically treated group compared to that in the surgical groups: 81% in DS, 58% in RYGB, and 20% in LAGB [27,28].

It must be underlined that the different rates of diabetes remission among these studies are related to multiple variables like diabetes duration and duration of follow-up, but above all, it depends on the criteria used for definition of diabetes reversal. While most of the earlier reports mainly used clinical assessment and discontinuation of antidiabetic therapy for T2DM remission, the more recent studies rely also on biochemical parameters such as fasting blood glucose (<126 mg/dL) and more specifically on glycated hemoglobin.

Recently, the American Diabetes Association has endorsed new and stricter standards for diabetes remission, requiring a fasting glucose of less than 100 mg/dL and an HbA1c below 6% without hypoglycemic medications for 1 year after surgery [29]. Based on these criteria, diabetes remission rates are, as expected, lower than those previously reported, as shown in the analysis of Pournaras et al. [30].

The favorable effect of surgery in T2DM patients with BMI > 35 kg/m^2 has stimulated interest also regarding the use of surgery in subjects with BMI less than 35, or even in lean diabetic patients in whom it was difficult to maintain satisfactory metabolic control. On this topic, single case reports have been previously described in the 1990s. Mingrone et al. [31] published their experience of two teenage normal-weight sisters with hereditary hyperchylomicronemia and intractable diabetes mellitus in spite of massive insulin infusion. These young women underwent the high lipid malabsorptive BPD operation with complete resolution of the highly insulin-resistant diabetic state, which has now persisted some 20 years later and without appreciable weight loss.

Generally, it can be stated that bariatric surgery in the under 35 BMI subjects displays a similar beneficial effect on T2DM improvement, as found in the more obese patients. Clinical experience with this cohort is well summarized in a recent systematic review and observational studies [32]. The high effectiveness of RYGB is further validated, whereas SG shows a remission rate superior to what has been reported for patients with >35 BMI obesity [33,34]. On the contrary, in the same category of subjects, BPD achieves inferior results, which can be explained by the small numbers of cases analyzed or, possibly, by the different metabolic characteristics of the lower BMI diabetics [35]. Another more recent systematic review found an overall remission rate of 80% without antidiabetic medication, with no mortality [36]. In a long-term retrospective study in RYGB patients with BMI 30–35 kg/m^2 and a long-standing T2DM, Cohen et al. [37] showed a remission rate of 88% with a median follow-up of 5 years. Finally, Lee et al. [38] in a randomized study in diabetic patients with BMI < 35 compared RYGB with SG and again found at 1 year a higher remission rate after the former procedure compared to the latter one (93% vs. 47%). It is worth noting that even in the thinner patients, there are no reports of body weight dropping out of the normal ranges with any type of operations so far examined. Although all the evidences accumulated from individual studies on the positive effect of bariatric surgery on T2DM are consistently in agreement, we recognize that randomized prospective studies comparing different surgical operations with medical therapy are necessary for validation. At the present time, four randomized prospective studies [39–42], most of them recently published, are available for analysis. These studies compare traditional or intensive medical therapy with the most common bariatric operations. They confirm the previously reported nonrandomized studies on the superior performance of the surgical options. The first of these randomized studies was carried out in Australia by Dixon et al. [39] in 2008. The surgical procedure that they tested was LAGB, and a follow-up of 2 years was reached by the majority of patients with diabetes of short duration. Remission, defined as fasting glycemia of <126 mg/dL and HbA1c < 6.2% without antidiabetic medications, occurred in 73% of the surgical group in contrast to 13% in the conventional therapy group. Also the T2DM improvement was matched by weight reduction. Recently, paired prospective randomized studies, published in the *New England Journal of Medicine*, provide validation of the beneficial effect of the surgical option in T2DM obese patients [40,41].

One of these studies performed by our group [40] showed at 2 years a statistically significant T2DM remission rate of 95% for BPD versus 75% for RYGB, with respect to 0% for the medical group. Although both surgical procedures produced similar EWL, the diabetes reversal was much prompter with BPD. It is worth noting that the patient's initial weight was not predictive of a successful metabolic outcome. Also the patients' time course of weight loss after surgery did not correlate with the normalization of glycemia.

Schauer et al. [41] compared RYGB and SG with intensive antidiabetic therapy. The primary end point in this study was the attainment of a glycated hemoglobin of 6% or lower at 1 year, which was reached by 42% of RYGB, 37% of SG versus 12% in the medically treated patients.

Finally, a recent randomized clinical trial [42] studied the effect of lifestyle-intensive medical management with or without RYGB on comorbid risk factors in 120 diabetic patients with BMI < 35 kg/m^2, recruited in US and Taiwan centers. At 1 year, the composite end point, HbA1c < 7.0%, LDL cholesterol < 100 mg/dl, and systolic blood pressure < 130 mm Hg, was achieved in 49% of RYGB and in 19% of the medical management group.

Data gathered so far provide solid and conclusive support to the guidelines set forth by the National Institutes of Health (NIH) consensus conference on bariatric surgery for obese subjects with BMI > 35, done some 20 years ago [43]. Concerning T2DM in patients with BMI < 35, the available data indicate a similar beneficial effect of surgery [42]. However, it might be possible, especially in the low BMI range, that there may be subgroups of subjects that have different patho-physiologic features and therefore may have a different response to the various surgical operations.

Although we have so far provided the evidence supporting the substantial, long-term remission of T2DM after bariatric surgery, unfortunately, this disease may relapse overtime. The SOS study [17] reports 36% of relapse rate at 10 years among subjects who initially had diabetes reversal. However, it should be pointed out that these data are not stratified by type of operation, which, as previously reported, appear to have quite different impacts on glycemic control. In fact, Arterburn et al. [44] in a retrospective multisite study recently analyzed T2DM long-term remission and relapse rates after RYGB. While they found a 68.2% complete remission within 5 years after surgery, however, one third of their patients suffered a relapse in the next 5 years, with an overall median duration of remission of 8.3 years.

On the other hand, in a retrospective study of 312 diabetic patients undergoing BPD, Scopinaro et al. [45] found only 12 failures at 10 years. In addition, these authors found that in slightly obese or non-obese individuals, the effect of BPD on glycemic control improvement was less conspicuous. These data suggest that the various operations may have different effects depending also on the individual pathophysiologic characteristics of T2DM.

Certainly, there are features that are predictive of a lower response to surgery: diabetes of long duration (>5 years), older age, multiple drug antidiabetic therapy, and low C-peptide levels are independently associated with a less favorable long-term outcome [38,46].

Although the main aim of bariatric surgery in T2DM patients is weight loss, its temporal decrease does not always correlate with the improvement of glucose metabolism. In the four previously quoted prospective randomized studies [39–42], normalization of blood glucose was found to correlate with weight loss only after LAGB but not with RYGB, SG, or BPD operated subjects. These data suggest that other factors should be taken into consideration in order to explain this phenomenon [46]. Quite a few reports have shown that bariatric surgery, besides producing weight loss, also improves other obesity-related comorbidities like hypertension, dyslipidemia, and cardiovascular risk factors. The corollary of these results is a reduced mortality with respect to usual medical therapy. These results are even more remarkable in diabetics. A recent systematic review has lent further support to these observations showing regression of left ventricular hypertrophy and improvement of diastolic function in this category of subjects [47].

MECHANISMS OF T2DM REVERSAL AFTER BARIATRIC SURGERY

Losing weight has been for a long time, and still is, the main goal of treatment in T2DM with reduction of obesity primarily because of its well-known clinical effectiveness. The scientific basis for this strategy is the demonstration that even a moderate diet-induced weight loss is able to produce a marked improvement of insulin resistance, which is also the goal of type 2 diabetes therapy [48].

Nevertheless, as noted earlier, a large body of data has been collected indicating that weight loss alone cannot account for the improvement in carbohydrate metabolism after the various bariatric operations, which also produce additional different features. Moreover, acute calorie restriction, although able to improve peripheral insulin resistance, does not appear to permanently reduce the intake regimen of bariatric surgery patients in the long term. It stems from these considerations that there is now special interest on the mechanisms of T2DM reversal after weight-reducing surgery, with the aim of gaining further insight in the pathophysiology of this disease.

INSULIN RESISTANCE

Even though all bariatric operations so far examined bring about an improvement of glycemic control, their impact on its determinants, i.e., insulin resistance and insulin secretion, is different. Keeping in mind that insulin resistance determined by the homeostatic model assessment for insulin resistance (HOMA-IR) is a measure of its hepatic component only, in LAGB HOMA-IR significantly improves only 6 months after surgery and progressively decreases to 15% of baseline levels at 18 months together with a relevant weight loss. Dixon et al. [39], in their already quoted randomized prospective study on LAGB, reached the conclusion that weight loss seems to be the main determinant of T2DM improvement. This contention is very much in line with the purely restrictive nature of the operation, which does not appear to substantially interfere with the basic physiology of the gastrointestinal tract.

On the contrary, different characteristics are displayed by both SG and RYGB, which, in the systematic review of Rao et al. [49] and in Schauer et al.'s [41] prospective randomized study, show a progressive improvement of HOMA-IR, which has been maintained up to 2 years follow-up. Peterli et al. [50] in addition demonstrated, for both SG and RYGB, an augmented insulin response to a test meal 1 week and 3 months after operation, which is synchronous with the elevation of the intestinal glucagon-like peptide 1 (GLP-1). However, it should be noted that insulin levels are not equivalent to insulin secretion, the former representing the balance between production and clearance. The best methods to measure insulin secretion are based on circulating C-peptide levels, which contrary to insulin is not cleared by the liver.

Studies in rodents confirm weight-independent improvement of glucose and of lipid metabolism after both operations, which is mediated by an increase in GLP-1 response to mixed meals. There is very good evidence that RYGB, as well as SG, achieves better glycemic control through increased insulin secretion and restoration of the first phase of insulin response. However, there are conflicting results concerning the cause of the early insulin resistance improvement, which generally occurs before a substantial weight loss is achieved with these two operations [51–54]. Thus, an enhanced secretory response after RYGB might account, at least partially, for the development of postprandial hyperinsulinemic hypoglycemia.

Obviously, besides GLP-1, there are other hormones and mediators that should be taken into consideration [55] and that will be dealt with in more detail in another Chapter 11. Circulating levels of ghrelin, for instance, which is produced by the gastric fundus, are also reduced, especially after SG, and so is its diabetogenic effect through lipolysis induction without changes in GH, cortisol, and epinephrine secretion [56].

Quite different metabolic and neurohormonal features are displayed by BPD and its DS variant, which, as previously reported, have been proven to be the most effective procedures in the surgical therapy of T2DM in both the short and long terms. Insulin sensitivity, measured by the more accurate euglycemic hyperinsulinemic clamp technique, normalizes very early after surgery when weight loss is still negligible [57,58]. This feature, in turn, generates a drastically reduced need of insulin, whose secretion postsurgery drops to normal values. The different pathophysiologic effects of BPD and RYGB are further substantiated by a recent prospective randomized study [40], which shows that time to diabetes remission was 4 months for BPD and 10 months for RYGB despite comparable weight loss.

Concerning gastrointestinal hormones, we found with BPD a consistent increased GLP-1 and a decreased gastrointestinal polypeptide (GIP) after meals. These results are in line with an enhancement of insulin sensitivity.

On a more pathophysiological point, these data, as well as many other experimental and clinical studies, indicate that, in addition to weight loss and calorie restriction, the antidiabetic effect of surgery resides on the release of enteric hormones and incretins. Depending on the section of the gastrointestinal tract involved, two pathophysiological theories, respectively called the "foregut and hindgut hypotheses," which are discussed in Chapter 11, have been proposed [59]. However, other factors such as bile flow alteration, modification of delivery, and absorption of nutrients and autonomic nerve modulation may also play a role in T2DM remission.

We have recently found [60] that the duodenum and jejunum of diabetic mice, as well as in insulin-resistant humans, secrete circulating protein factor/s that in vitro impair insulin signaling in the myocytes by stimulating the mammalian target of rapamycin complex 2 (mTORC2). This feature, in turn, promotes Akt phosphorylation at Ser473 while reducing the Akt phosphorylation at

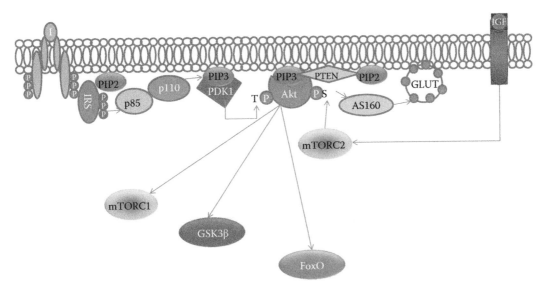

FIGURE 10.3 Putative mechanism of action of the protein factor/s secreted by the duodenum/jejunum on skeletal muscle cells. We hypothesize that this factor (jejunum) binds the insulin growth factor (IGF)-receptor activating the enzymatic mTORC2 with subsequent phosphorylation of a key enzyme in cellular glucose uptake and utilization, Akt, on its serine473 residue (S). Binding to its receptor, insulin activates the enzyme pyruvate dehydrogenase kinase 1 (PDK1), which activates the Akt by phosphorylating its threonine308 (T) residue. The excessive phosphorylation of Akt on serine473 reduces the activity of this enzyme with consequent reduction of the glucose transporter GLUT4 transduction on the muscle cell membranes. The insulin receptor, composed by 4 subunits, is schematically represented on the left.

Thr308 with proteolysis of glycogen synthase kinase (GSKβ) and enhanced activity of this enzyme, which acts by inactivating the glycogen synthase and thus reduces the glycogen production induced by insulin. Activation of PI 3-kinase and Akt is known to be critical in the mechanism of insulin action on glucose transporter GLUT-4 translocation and glucose interiorization. In addition, mTORC2 negatively feeds back to the insulin receptor substrate (IRS-1), thus promoting insulin resistance due to mTORC2-mediated degradation of IRS-1. A reduced strength of insulin signaling via the IRS-1/PI 3-kinase pathway also results in a diminished glucose uptake and utilization in insulin target tissues. This pathway is depicted in Figure 10.3.

CONCLUSION

Remission of T2DM following bariatric surgery is a well-established phenomenon, which pertains not only to frank obesity but also to mild obesity and even to normal weight subjects [20,61]. This result translates to long-term reduction of mortality and morbidity for all cases. In particular, it results to a 37% decrease of deleterious cardiovascular events in diabetics compared to 16% in nondiabetic patients [17]. In addition, at 10–15 years follow-up, bariatric surgery was found to be markedly more effective in preventing the onset of new cases of type 2 diabetes [18]. Presently, from the clinical point of view, the criteria set forth by the NIH consensus conference of 1991 [43] substantially still apply, even though the International Diabetes Federation position statement strongly supports the surgical option at an earlier stage of the disease before complications have been established.

As it is well known, BMI > 35 is taken as the discriminant indicator for bariatric surgery in poorly controlled T2DM patients. On the other hand, recent data show that initial weight is not a reliable predictor of T2DM reversal after surgery, and, therefore, other criteria, as already mentioned, should be employed instead [61]. Moreover, it appears that diabetic disease with distinct pathophysiological features responds differently to the various bariatric operations, which may have somewhat different mechanisms of action. In this regard, prospective randomized studies comparing specific surgical procedures in well-defined subgroups of patients are, indeed, needed in order to make the specific surgical treatment of diabetes a timely and evidence-based choice.

Of course, there are many more targets at stake: first of all is a more complete understanding of the role of the gastrointestinal tract and its mediators and neurohormones in the onset and reversal of T2DM. If carefully done with biochemical and endocrine mediator effects characterized, this could lead to the development of new agents and/or new procedures capable of reproducing the same effect as surgery. Another important question regards beta-cell physiology and the possibility of preserving or recovering its beneficial function.

In conclusion, diabetes is such a worldwide epidemic that it can only be dealt with by more basic and broadly available means. At present, bariatric or rather metabolic surgery represents a very important clinical and investigative tool to assist us to acquire new knowledge of this disease.

ACKNOWLEDGMENT

We would like to express our deep gratitude to our long-time friend and colleague John H. Siegel MD, the late Emeritus Professor of New Jersey Medical School, University of Medicine and Dentistry of New Jersey: his generous support, suggestions, and assistance have been a special award to us.

REFERENCES

1. Baker MT. The history and evolution of bariatric surgical procedures. *Surg Clin North Am*. 2011, 91: 1181–201.
2. Buchwald H, Varco RL. Ileal bypass in patients with hypercholesterolemia and atherosclerosis. Preliminary report on therapeutic potential. *JAMA*. 1966, 196: 627–30.
3. World Health Organization. Obesity and overweight: Fact sheet, May 2012. Available at http://www.who.int.
4. Wild S, Roglic G, Green A, Sicree R, King H. Global prevalence of diabetes: Estimates for the year 2000 and projections for 2030. *Diabetes Care*. 2004, 27: 1047–53.
5. Centers for Disease Control and Prevention. National diabetes fact sheet, 2011. Available at http://www.cdc.gov.
6. Anjum Q. Diabesity—a future pandemic. *J Pak Med Assoc*. 2011, 61: 321.
7. Buchwald H, Oien DM. Metabolic/bariatric surgery worldwide 2011. *Obes Surg*. 2013. 23: 427–36.
8. Mathus-Vliegen EM, de Wit LT. Health-related quality of life after gastric banding. *Br J Surg*. 2007, 94: 457–65.
9. O'Brien PE, MacDonald L, Anderson M, Brennan L, Brown WA. Long-term outcomes after bariatric surgery: Fifteen-year follow-up of adjustable gastric banding and a systematic review of the bariatric surgical literature. *Ann Surg*. 2013, 257: 87–94.
10. Worni M, Ostbye T, Shah A, Carvalho E, Schudel IM, Shin JH, Pietrobon R, Guller U. High risks for adverse outcomes after gastric bypass surgery following ailed gastric banding: A population-based trend analysis of the United States. *Ann Surg*. 2013, 257: 279–86.
11. Chakravarty PD, McLaughlin E, Whittaker D, Byrne E, Cowan E, Xu K, Bruce DM, Ford JA. Comparison of laparoscopic adjustable gastric banding (LAGB) with other bariatric procedures: A systematic review of the randomised controlled trials. *Surgeon*. 2012, 10: 172–82.
12. Dixon JB, le Roux CW, Rubino F, Zimmet P. Bariatric surgery for type 2 diabetes. *Lancet*. 2012, 379: 2300–11.
13. Marceau P, Biron S, St Georges R, Duclos M, Potvin M, Bourque RA. Biliopancreatic diversion with gastrectomy as surgical treatment of morbid obesity. *Obes Surg*. 1991, 1: 381–7.
14. Regan JP, Inabnet WB, Gagner M, Pomp A. Early experience with two-stage laparoscopic Roux-en-Y gastric bypass as an alternative in the super-super obese patient. *Obes Surg*. 2003, 13: 861–4.
15. DeMaria EJ, Pate V, Warthen M, Winegar DA. Baseline data from American Society for Metabolic and Bariatric Surgery-designated Bariatric Surgery Centers of Excellence using the Bariatric Outcomes Longitudinal Database. *Surg Obes Relat Dis*. 2010, 6: 347–55.

16. Scopinaro N, Adami GF, Marinari GM, Gianetta E, Traverso E, Friedman D, Camerini G, Baschieri G, Simonelli A. Biliopancreatic diversion. *World J Surg*. 1998, 22: 936–46.
17. Sjöström L, Lindroos AK, Peltonen M, Torgerson J, Bouchard C, Carlsson B, Dahlgren S, Larsson B, Narbro K, Sjöström CD, Sullivan M, Wedel H. Swedish Obese Subjects Study Scientific Group. Lifestyle, diabetes, and cardiovascular risk factors 10 years after bariatric surgery. *N Engl J Med*. 2004, 351: 2683–93.
18. Carlsson LM, Peltonen M, Ahlin S, Anveden Å, Bouchard C, Carlsson B, Jacobson Lönroth H, Maglio C, Näslund I, Pirazzi C, Romeo S, Sjöholm K, Sjöström E, Wedel H, Svensson PA, Sjöström L. Bariatric surgery and prevention of type 2 diabetes in Swedish obese subjects. *N Engl J Med*. 2012, 36: 695–704.
19. Muscelli E, Mingrone G, Camastra S, Manco M, Pereira JA, Pareja JC, Ferrannini E. Differential effect of weight loss on insulin resistance in surgically treated obese patients. *Am J Med*. 2005, 118: 51–7.
20. Buchwald H, Avidor Y, Braunwald E, Jensen MD, Pories W, Fahrbach K, Schoelles K. Bariatric surgery: A systematic review and meta-analysis. *JAMA*. 2004, 292: 1724–37.
21. Meijer RI, van Wagensveld BA, Siegert CE, Eringa EC, Serné EH, Smulders YM. Bariatric surgery as a novel treatment for type 2 diabetes mellitus: A systematic review. *Arch Surg*. 2011, 146: 744–50.
22. Shi X, Karmali S, Sharma AM, Birch DW. A review of laparoscopic sleeve gastrectomy for morbid obesity. *Obes Surg*. 2010, 20: 1171–7.
23. Gill RS, Birch DW, Shi X, Sharma AM, Karmali S. Sleeve gastrectomy and type 2 diabetes mellitus: A systematic review. *Surg Obes Relat Dis*. 2010, 6: 707–13.
24. Leonetti F, Capoccia D, Coccia F, Casella G, Baglio G, Paradiso F, Abbatini F, Iossa A, Soricelli E, Basso N. Obesity, type 2 diabetes mellitus, and other comorbidities: A prospective cohort study of laparoscopic sleeve gastrectomy vs medical treatment. *Arch Surg*. 2012, 147: 694–700.
25. Inge TH, Miyano G, Bean J, Helmrath M, Courcoulas A, Harmon CM, Chen MK, Wilson K, Daniels SR, Garcia VF, Brandt ML, Dolan LM. Reversal of type 2 diabetes mellitus and improvements in cardiovascular risk factors after surgical weight loss in adolescents. *Pediatrics*. 2009, 123: 214–22.
26. Hofsø D, Nordstrand N, Johnson LK, Karlsen TI, Hager H, Jenssen T, Bollerslev J, Godang K, Sandbu R, Røislien J, Hjelmesaeth J. Obesity-related cardiovascular risk factors after weight loss: A clinical trial comparing gastric bypass surgery and intensive lifestyle intervention. *Eur J Endocrinol*. 2010, 163: 735–45.
27. Dorman RB, Serrot FJ, Miller CJ, Slusarek BM, Sampson BK, Buchwald H, Leslie DB, Bantle JP, Ikramuddin S. Case-matched outcomes in bariatric surgery for treatment of type 2 diabetes in the morbidly obese patient. *Ann Surg*. 2012, 255: 287–93.
28. Leslie DB, Dorman RB, Serrot FJ, Swan TW, Kellogg TA, Torres-Villalobos G, Buchwald H, Slusarek BM, Sampson BK, Bantle JP, Ikramuddin S. Efficacy of the Roux-en-Y gastric bypass compared to medically managed controls in meeting the American Diabetes Association composite end point goals for management of type 2 diabetes mellitus. *Obes Surg*. 2012, 22: 367–74.
29. Buse JB, Caprio S, Cefalu WT, Ceriello A, Del Prato S, Inzucchi SE, McLaughlin S, Phillips GL 2nd, Robertson RP, Rubino F, Kahn R, Kirkman MS. How do we define cure of diabetes? *Diabetes Care*. 2009, 32: 2133–5.
30. Pournaras DJ, Aasheim ET, Søvik TT, Andrews R, Mahon D, Welbourn R, Olbers T, le Roux CW. Effect of the definition of type II diabetes remission in the evaluation of bariatric surgery for metabolic disorders. *Br J Surg*. 2012, 99: 100–3.
31. Mingrone G, Henriksen FL, Greco AV, Krogh LN, Capristo E, Gastaldelli A, Castagneto M, Ferrannini E, Gasbarrini G, Beck-Nielsen H. Triglyceride-induced diabetes associated with familial lipoprotein lipase deficiency. *Diabetes*. 1999, 48: 1258–63.
32. Maggard-Gibbons M, Maglione M, Livhits M, Ewing B, Maher AR, Hu J, Li Z, Shekelle PG. Bariatric surgery for weight loss and glycemic control in nonmorbidly obese adults with diabetes: A systematic review. *JAMA*. 2013, 309: 2250–61.
33. Abbatini F, Capoccia D, Casella G, Coccia F, Leonetti F, Basso N. Type 2 diabetes in obese patients with body mass index of 30–35 kg/m^2: Sleeve gastrectomy versus medical treatment. *Surg Obes Relat Dis*. 2012, 8: 20–4.
34. Serrot FJ, Dorman RB, Miller CJ, Slusarek B, Sampson B, Sick BT, Leslie DB, Buchwald H, Ikramuddin S. Comparative effectiveness of bariatric surgery and nonsurgical therapy in adults with type 2 diabetes mellitus and body mass index <35 kg/m^2. *Surgery*. 2011, 150: 684–91.
35. Scopinaro N, Adami GF, Papadia FS, Camerini G, Carlini F, Fried M, Briatore L, D'Alessandro G, Andraghetti G, Cordera R. Effects of biliopancreatic diversion on type 2 diabetes in patients with BMI 25 to 35. *Ann Surg*. 2011, 253: 699–703.

36. Li Q, Chen L, Yang Z, Ye Z, Huang Y, He M, Zhang S, Feng X, Gong W, Zhang Z, Zhao W, Liu C, Qu S, Hu R. Metabolic effects of bariatric surgery in type 2 diabetic patients with body mass index < 35 kg/m². *Diabetes Obes Metab.* 2012, 14: 262–70.

37. Cohen RV, Pinheiro JC, Schiavon CA, Salles JE, Wajchenberg BL, Cummings DE. Effects of gastric bypass surgery in patients with type 2 diabetes and only mild obesity. *Diabetes Care.* 2012, 35: 1420–8.

38. Lee WJ, Chong K, Ser KH, Lee YC, Chen SC, Chen JC, Tsai MH, Chuang LM. Gastric bypass vs sleeve gastrectomy for type 2 diabetes mellitus: A randomized controlled trial. *Arch Surg.* 2011, 146: 143–8.

39. Dixon JB, O'Brien PE, Playfair J, Chapman L, Schachter LM, Skinner S, Proietto J, Bailey M, Anderson M. Adjustable gastric banding and conventional therapy for type 2 diabetes: A randomized controlled trial. *JAMA.* 2008, 299: 316–23.

40. Mingrone G, Panunzi S, De Gaetano A, Guidone C, Iaconelli A, Leccesi L, Nanni G, Pomp A, Castagneto M, Ghirlanda G, Rubino F. Bariatric surgery versus conventional medical therapy for type 2 diabetes. *N Engl J Med.* 2012, 366: 1577–85.

41. Schauer PR, Kashyap SR, Wolski K, Brethauer SA, Kirwan JP, Pothier CE, Thomas S, Abood B, Nissen SE, Bhatt DL. Bariatric surgery versus intensive medical therapy in obese patients with diabetes. *N Engl J Med.* 2012, 366: 1567–76.

42. Ikramuddin S, Korner J, Lee WJ, Connett JE, Inabnet WB, Billington CJ, Thomas AJ, Leslie DB, Chong K, Jeffery RW, Ahmed L, Vella A, Chuang LM, Bessler M, Sarr MG, Swain JM, Laqua P, Jensen MD, Bantle JP. Roux-en-Y gastric bypass vs intensive medical management for the control of type 2 diabetes, hypertension, and hyperlipidemia: The Diabetes Surgery Study randomized clinical trial. *JAMA.* 309: 2240–9.

43. NIH Conference. Gastrointestinal surgery for severe obesity. Consensus Development Conference Panel. *Ann Intern Med.* 1991, 115: 956–61.

44. Arterburn DE, Bogart A, Sherwood NE, Sidney S, Coleman KJ, Haneuse S, O'Connor PJ, Theis MK, Campos GM, McCulloch D, Selby J. A multisite study of long-term remission and relapse of type 2 diabetes mellitus following gastric bypass. *Obes Surg.* 2013, 23: 93–102.

45. Scopinaro N, Marinari GM, Camerini GB, Papadia FS, Adami GF. Specific effects of biliopancreatic diversion on the major components of metabolic syndrome: A long-term follow-up study. *Diabetes Care.* 2005, 28(10): 2406–11.

46. Tice JA. Bariatric surgery for the treatment of type 2 diabetes mellitus. CTAF 2012, California Technology Assessment Forum. Report June 20, 2012. Available at http://www.ctaf.org.

47. Vest AR, Heneghan HM, Agarwal S, Schauer PR, Young JB. Bariatric surgery and cardiovascular outcomes: A systematic review. *Heart.* 2012, 98: 1763–77.

48. Bogardus C, Lillioja S, Mott DM, Hollenbeck C, Reaven G. Relationship between degree of obesity and in vivo insulin action in man. *Am J Physiol.* 1985, 248: 286–91.

49. Rao RS, Yanagisawa R, Kini S. Insulin resistance and bariatric surgery. *Obes Rev.* 2012, 13: 316–28.

50. Peterli R, Steinert RE, Woelnerhanssen B, Peters T, Christoffel-Courtin C, Gass M, Kern B, von Fluee M, Beglinger C. Metabolic and hormonal changes after laparoscopic Roux-en-Y gastric bypass and sleeve gastrectomy: A randomized, prospective trial. *Obes Surg.* 2012, 22: 740–8.

51. Chambers AP, Jessen L, Ryan KK, Sisley S, Wilson-Pérez HE, Stefater MA, Gaitonde SG, Sorrell JE, Toure M, Berger J, D'Alessio DA, Woods SC, Seeley RJ, Sandoval DA. Weight-independent changes in blood glucose homeostasis after gastric bypass or vertical sleeve gastrectomy in rats. *Gastroenterology.* 2011, 141: 950–8.

52. Salinari S, Bertuzzi A, Guidone C, Previti E, Rubino F, Mingrone G. Insulin sensitivity and secretion changes after gastric bypass in normotolerant and diabetic obese subjects. *Ann Surg.* 2013, 257: 462–8.

53. Campos GM, Rabl C, Peeva S, Ciovica R, Rao M, Schwarz JM, Havel P, Schambelan M, Mulligan K. Improvement in peripheral glucose uptake after gastric bypass surgery is observed only after substantial weight loss has occurred and correlates with the magnitude of weight lost. *J Gastrointest Surg.* 2010, 14: 15–23.

54. Nannipieri M, Mari A, Anselmino M, Baldi S, Barsotti E, Guarino D, Camastra S, Bellini R, Berta RD, Ferrannini E. The role of beta-cell function and insulin sensitivity in the remission of type 2 diabetes after gastric bypass surgery. *J Clin Endocrinol Metab.* 2011, 96: 1372–9.

55. Laferrère B. Diabetes remission after bariatric surgery: Is it just the incretins? *Int J Obes (Lond).* 2011, 35: S22–5.

56. Vestergaard ET, Gormsen LC, Jessen N, Lund S, Hansen TK, Moller N, Jorgensen JO. Ghrelin infusion in humans induces acute insulin resistance and lipolysis independent of growth hormone signaling. *Diabetes.* 2008, 57: 3205–10.

57. Guidone C, Manco M, Valera-Mora E, Iaconelli A, Gniuli D, Mari A, Nanni G, Castagneto M, Calvani M, Mingrone G. Mechanisms of recovery from type 2 diabetes after malabsorptive bariatric surgery. *Diabetes*. 2006, 55: 2025–31.
58. Castagneto M, Mingrone G. The effect of gastrointestinal surgery on insulin resistance and insulin secretion. *Curr Atheroscler Rep*. 2012, 14: 624–30.
59. Rubino F, Schauer PR, Kaplan LM, Cummings DE. Metabolic surgery to treat type 2 diabetes: Clinical outcomes and mechanisms of action. *Annu Rev Med*. 2010, 61: 393–411.
60. Salinari S, Debard C, Bertuzzi A, Durand C, Zimmet P, Vidal H, Mingrone G. Jejunal proteins secreted by db/db mice or insulin-resistant humans impair the insulin signaling and determine insulin resistance. *PLoS One*. 2013, 8:e562585.
61. Cummings DE. Metabolic surgery for type 2 diabetes. *Nat Med*. 2012, 18: 656–8.

11 Incretin Response after Bariatric Surgery

Roxanne Dutia and Blandine Laferrère

CONTENTS

INTRODUCTION

Certain types of bariatric surgery increase incretin levels, including glucagon-like peptide-1 (GLP-1) and gastric inhibitory peptide (GIP). These hormones, which are predominantly secreted from the gut, are responsible for 50–60% of insulin secretion [1], and the *incretin effect* has been shown to be impaired in those with type 2 diabetes [2]. It has been hypothesized that manipulation of the gastrointestinal anatomy via certain types of bariatric surgeries leads to changes in incretin levels that impact metabolism and glucose homeostasis. This chapter will briefly review physiology of incretins, provide a thorough review of the impact of different types of bariatric surgeries on incretin levels and associated improvements in metabolism and glucose homeostasis, present possible mechanisms for the changes in incretin levels and favorable metabolic effects after bariatric surgery, as well as discuss the significance of the incretins in the context of energy balance and glucose metabolism.

INCRETINS: BRIEF OVERVIEW

GLP-1

GLP-1 is primarily secreted by L-cells of the small intestine; however, a small amount is also produced in the brain [3]. Proglucagon is synthesized and cleaved by the prohormone convertase (PC) 1/3 in L-cells of the gut to yield GLP-1 [4,5]. GLP-1 is expressed throughout the small intestine; however, expression density increases distally [6,7]. Active forms include GLP-$1_{7\text{-}36}$ and GLP-$1_{7\text{-}37}$, with the former amidated form comprising the majority (~80%) [8]. GLP-$1_{7\text{-}36}$ is degraded within minutes by dipeptidyl peptidase (DPP)-4 to the inactive GLP$_{9\text{-}36}$ form [9]. GLP-1 is secreted in response to various nutrients including carbohydrate, fat, and protein [10] and binds to the G-protein–coupled GLP-1 receptor in the β-cells of the pancreas, leading to enhanced insulin secretion [11]. GLP-1 may also reduce food intake by mediating effects via GLP-1 receptors in the brain [12,13]. GLP-1 receptor knockout (KO) mice have severely impaired glucose tolerance [14], and GLP-1 has been shown to enhance β-cell glucose sensing [15]. Other potential actions of GLP-1 include inhibition of gastrointestinal motility, gastric acid, and exocrine pancreatic and glucagon secretion, decreased appetite, increased postprandial glucose-dependent insulin secretion, and improved insulin sensitivity [16].

GIP

Pro-GIP is synthesized and cleaved by PC1/3 [17] in the K-cells of the gut to yield GIP, which is expressed in the duodenum and jejunum [18]. GIP is secreted in response to nutrients including glucose and fat [19,20]. GIP binds to the G-protein-coupled GIP receptor [21] expressed in various tissues including the brain, gut, and adipose tissue; however, its incretin effects are likely due to its expression in the β-cells of the pancreas [21]. Disruption of GIP receptor signaling deteriorates glucose tolerance [22]. GIP-$1_{1\text{-}42}$ is degraded by DPP-4 to the inactive form GLP-$1_{3\text{-}42}$ [23].

Evidence *in vitro* and in rodent models suggests an antiapoptotic effect of GIP [24] and GLP-1 [25] on pancreatic β-cells.

EFFECTS OF BARIATRIC SURGERY ON INCRETIN LEVELS AND RELATED METABOLIC AND GLUCOREGULATORY EFFECTS

ROUX-EN-Y GASTRIC BYPASS

In rodent models, Roux-en-Y gastric bypass (RYGBP) surgery has been shown to reduce body weight and adiposity as well as improve glucose metabolism [26–28]. This metabolic improvement is accompanied by increased postprandial GLP-1 levels [26–28] and pancreatic GLP-1 receptor expression [28]; however, postprandial GIP levels are generally reported as unchanged [26,27].

Similar effects of RYGBP have been reported in humans. RYGBP leads to a sustainable reduction in body weight and remission of diabetes in 40–80% of cases [29,30]. Numerous human studies have shown that nutrient-stimulated GLP-1 levels are markedly elevated after RYGBP in both subjects with and without diabetes [31–49]. This postprandial elevation in GLP-1 has been shown to be independent of reductions in body weight [32,41,42,44,50]. Elevations in postprandial GLP-1 are observed as quickly as 2, 7, and 14 days [34,38,39,49] after surgery, and persist in subjects greater than 10 years after RYGBP [40]. However, the variance in GLP-1 response increases with years after surgery [51]. Levels of fasting GLP-1 are usually unchanged [33–35,39,45,47,50,52] after RYGBP surgery; however, isolated studies have observed an increase [33] or decrease [34]. Similar to rodents, the effects of RYGBP on GIP levels are less consistent. Postprandial levels have been reported as unchanged or transiently increased or decreased [31,33,37,39,47]. Fasting levels are generally reported as unchanged [33,39], but a reduction has been reported [35].

Although countless studies have shown an improvement in diabetes after RYGBP, the role of GLP-1 in this improvement has been highlighted by antagonism with Exendin 9-39, a GLP-1 receptor antagonist.

Exendin 9-39 treatment significantly attenuated the enhanced insulin secretion rates in subjects post-RYGBP [53], and worsened glucose tolerance in post-RYGBP subjects with a history of diabetes [54]. However, non-incretin–mediated mechanisms including intestinal gluconeogenesis [55] and increased uptake of glucose by the intestine [56] have also been suggested to contribute to improvements in diabetes. Several case studies have highlighted the importance of the altered nutrient route to improvements in glucose metabolism after surgery. Direct feeding into the gastric remnant of a subject post-RYGBP leads to higher glucose, lower insulin, and a severely diminished postprandial GLP-1 response, compared to oral feeding in this subject [57]. Another case study showed that administration of nutrients via a gastrostomy tube into the gastric remnant improved hypoglycemia and dampened hypersecretion of GLP-1 and insulin in a post-RYGBP subject with neuroglycopenia [58].

DUODENAL–JEJUNAL BYPASS

Most studies investigating the effects of duodenal–jejunal bypass (DJB) on metabolic and glucoregulatory end points and incretin hormones have been performed in rodents. In rodents, DJB surgery [59–66] improves glucose tolerance without any significant reduction in body weight [59–66]. Improvements in β-cell area and islet fibrosis [61], as well as suppressed hepatic glucose production and improved glucose disposal rate [60], were observed after DJB. Postprandial GLP-1 levels [59–61,63–69] are also elevated after DJB and are further enhanced if the DJB procedure is combined with vertical sleeve gastrectomy (VSG) [70]. The improvement in glucose tolerance after DJB is suggested to be GLP-1-dependent as this effect is abolished by GLP-1 receptor antagonism [66]. An increase in GLP-1 expression in selective sections of the intestine including the duodenum [62], gastrojejunum [62], mid-jejunum [66,71], and ileum [66] has also been observed after DJB. Effects of DJB on GIP are mixed; however, some studies have reported enhancement in postprandial GIP release [61] or an increase in intestinal GIP expression in the jejunum (without any change in plasma levels) [60].

Few studies have investigated the effects of DJB in humans, and most studies have investigated this procedure in subjects with a lower BMI range (<30 kg/m^2) [72–75]. In humans, DJB improves glycemia, with or without concomitant weight loss, and this has been reported between 3 and 12 months post-surgery [72–75]. DJB has also been shown to significantly increase postprandial GLP-1 [75,76] without any change in GIP [75].

BILIOPANCREATIC DIVERSION

In rats, biliopancreatic diversion (BPD) has been shown to decrease food intake and body weight, improve glucose tolerance, and increase postprandial GLP-1 levels [77,78]. In humans, BPD has been shown to improve glucose metabolism and β-cell function [79–82] as early as 1 week after surgery. Although evidence suggests that the effects on glucose metabolism may be due to weight loss [80], the rapidity in improvement suggests otherwise [82]. Studies also show a consistent enhancement in postprandial GLP-1 secretion [79–82] and a significant reduction in GIP [81,82] after BPD in humans.

ILEAL TRANSPOSITION

Ileal transposition (IT) has been performed in rodent models. IT in various diabetes rat models has been shown to improve glucose tolerance and insulin sensitivity, often in the absence of weight loss [83–85]. However, a reduction in weight [69,77,86] and adiposity [85] has been observed. IT also consistently enhances postprandial GLP-1 secretion [66,77,83–86], and postprandial GIP is either increased [84] or unchanged [85]. Additionally, IT has been shown to increase gene expression of *proglucagon* [83–86] and *proconvertase 1/3* [83] in the transposed ileum. A comparison of IT compared with sub-IT (transposed ileum is transplanted more distally down the small intestine) showed a greater improvement in glucose tolerance and enhanced GLP-1 release, highlighting the importance of quick nutrient delivery to the ileum [65]. Furthermore, a rodent study aimed at parsing out the importance of the hindgut and foregut to the improvement in glucose homeostasis after bariatric surgery compared DJB, DJB+IT, and IT to sham-operated rats and observed a slight but significant synergistic effect of DJB+IT on glucose tolerance and insulin secretion, compared to either surgery alone [65]; however, no greater postprandial GLP-1 response was observed [65]. In two different comparison studies between DJB/modified JB versus IT, both procedures equally improved glucose tolerance; however, hypersecretion of postprandial GLP-1 was significantly greater after IT [69,77].

VERTICAL SLEEVE GASTRECTOMY

The effect of VSG on incretins bears similarity to RYGBP. VSG also decreases weight and adiposity and improves glucose metabolism [87,88]. In rats, most studies have observed an increase in postprandial GLP-1 levels after VSG that are comparable to post-RYGBP levels and independent of weight loss [87,88]; however, one study observed no increase [67]. Fasting GLP-1 levels were unchanged after VSG in rats, similar to what has been observed after RYGBP [89]. Increases in postprandial GLP-1 after RYGBP and VSG were also accompanied by improved glucose tolerance and enhanced insulin secretion, and these effects were blunted by GLP-1 receptor antagonism, demonstrating GLP-1's role in glucose metabolism after these procedures [87,88].

In humans, postprandial GLP-1 levels are consistently reported to be elevated after VSG in subjects with or without diabetes [49,52,90–92]. Increases are reported as early as 3–7 days [49,52,90], sustained 1–2 years after VSG [92,93], and are independent of weight loss [94]. Studies have reported a comparable increase in postprandial GLP-1 after VSG versus RYGBP, from 1 week to 2 years after surgery [49,93,95], although some have observed a greater effect after RYGBP [52,96]. Similar to RYGBP, most studies show no change in fasting GLP-1 after VSG [52,91,94,95], although an increase and decrease have been reported [90,96]. One study observed that postprandial GIP levels were comparably increased after VSG and RYGBP [95]. VSG has also been coupled to intestinal surgeries including enterectomy [97] and ileal interposition [98] to either the duodenum or jejunum; these surgeries have been reported to increase postprandial GLP-1 levels, and the latter has been shown to increase GIP as well.

GASTRIC BANDING

Although gastric banding is a common procedure that can lead to substantial weight loss and improvement in comorbidities, it does not stimulate GLP-1 release [50,99]. Thus, the effects of GB on improvements in weight gain and glucose metabolism are likely exclusively due to caloric restriction.

ENDOLUMINAL SLEEVE

Placement of an endoluminal sleeve in rats has been shown to reduce body weight independently of food intake, improve glucose metabolism and insulin sensitivity, and enhance postprandial GLP-1 secretion independently of weight loss [100]. Although a significant lowering of glucose levels was obtained when only the pylorus was covered, greater duodenal exclusion led to enhanced glycemic control [100]. In humans, this sleeve appears effective for weight loss and improvement in glucose homeostasis [101,102]; however, effects on incretins are yet to be reported [103].

POTENTIAL MECHANISMS FOR INCREASED INCRETIN LEVELS AFTER BARIATRIC SURGERY

FOREGUT AND HINDGUT HYPOTHESES

The *foregut hypothesis* and *hindgut hypothesis* are two theories, heavily debated in the literature, that aim to explain the favorable improvements in weight loss and glucose metabolism after

RYGBP and other bariatric surgeries that alter the nutrient route. The foregut hypothesis purports that nutrient exclusion from the proximal small intestine is key to improving glucose metabolism. This theory is supported by animal and human studies using various forms of bariatric surgery including intestinal bypass and intestinal sleeves. For example, in rats, gastrojejunal bypass and duodenal–jejunal or endoluminal sleeves increase GLP-1 levels and improve glucose metabolism independently of weight loss [59,100,104]. Studies in humans using endoluminal sleeves likewise report similar effects on glucose homeostasis [101,102]. Furthermore, comparison of glucose delivery via a gastrostomy tube in RYGBP patients showed blunted plasma insulin and GLP-1 responses versus delivery via the oral route [105]. However, recent studies in both rodents and humans using VSG, which does not have an intestinal bypass component, also show an improvement in glucose metabolism, independent of weight loss [49,87,96]. Some studies report that GLP-1 levels after VSG are similar to post-RYGBP [49,87,93,95,96], although others report somewhat lower levels [52,96]. VSG, a procedure that does not exclude nutrients from contact with the proximal small intestine, but does increase gastric emptying and nutrient transit time [106], suggests that other mechanisms may also be important.

The hindgut hypothesis purports that the accelerated delivery of nutrients to the distal small intestine stimulates L-cell secretion of GLP-1 and other hormones, and leads to weight-independent improvements in glucose metabolism [66,85,86,107]. Furthermore, transposing the ileum to more proximal sections of the intestine (i.e., IT) improves glucose tolerance and increases GLP-1 to levels observed after duodenal–jejunal bypass [66,69]. Gastric emptying, which is accelerated after liquid consumption in RYGBP patients [48,108,109], also supports the hindgut hypothesis.

BILE ACIDS

There is evidence that both fasting and postprandial circulating bile acids are increased after certain types of bariatric surgery. In humans, an increase in fasting bile acid levels has been observed after RYGBP, from 3 months up to several years after surgery [110–112]. However, bile acid levels are not increased after gastric banding, even after equivalent weight loss compared to RYGBP. RYGBP may also impact the metabolism of specific classes or types of bile acids [113,114]. For example, postprandial conjugated bile acid response, diminished in the obese, can be restored approximately 1 year after RYGBP, with no change in unconjugated bile acids [115]. Furthermore, RYGBP subjects in diabetes remission have higher levels of the bile acids cholic acid, deoxycholic acid, and chenodeoxycholic acid than subjects with diabetes that did not undergo remission after RYGBP [116].

The change in bile acid metabolism after RYGBP may contribute to increased GLP-1 and subsequent metabolic improvements observed after surgery. Administration of bile acids in humans has been shown to improve glucose control and concomitantly stimulate insulin, peptide YY (PYY), and GLP-1 release [117–120]. *In vitro*, individual bile acids have also been reported to stimulate GLP-1 release [121]. Additionally after RYGBP, a positive correlation between fasting total bile acids and postprandial GLP-1, and a negative correlation between total bile acids and postprandial glucose, have been observed [110].

Data from rodent models supports the human data. IT and VSG in rats increase fasting plasma bile acids and improve glycemia, independent of weight loss [122,123]. Furthermore, direct delivery of bile acids to the mid-jejunum (via a catheter from the common bile duct) in rats increased plasma total bile acids and tauroursodeoxycholic acid levels, improved glucose metabolism, increased GLP-1 levels, promoted weight loss, and reduced adiposity and liver steatosis [124]. In rodents, inhibition of the bile acid transporter, responsible for bile acid reabsorption in intestine, increases fecal bile acid excretion, improves glycemic control, and increases circulating GLP-1 and insulin levels [125]. In human clinical trials, bile acid sequestrants, which bind to bile acids, increase bile acid excretion and lower cholesterol via increased bile acid synthesis; they also improve glycemic control and some stimulate GLP-1 release [126–128].

Evidence suggests that bile acids may mediate glycemic effects via the cell surface TGR-5 receptor [129]. In mice, TGR-5 receptor activation improves glucose homeostasis and stimulates GLP-1 release [130]. Furthermore, bile acid sequestrant-induced improvements in glycemic control were partly dependent upon TGR-5 receptor activation and subsequent GLP-1 release [131]. These rodent studies are corroborated by *in vitro* data showing that bile acid activation of the TGR-5 receptor (which, like GLP-1, is expressed in intestinal L-cells) stimulates GLP-1 release [121,130,132]. Certain bile acids are better ligands for the TGR-5 receptor; both free and conjugated bile acids lithocholic acid, deoxycholic acid, chenodeoxycholic acid, and cholic acid (in order of decreased potency) activate TGR-5 [129].

MICROBIOTA

Recent evidence suggests that RYGBP leads to changes in the composition of microbiota in the gut, potentially producing beneficial colonic fermentation that can impact incretin levels and subsequent glucose metabolism and energy balance.

Differences in gut microbiota populations have been observed in obese versus lean individuals, as well as after weight loss. The gut of mice and humans are predominantly populated with *Firmicutes* and *Bacteroidetes* microbiota, and both obese mice and humans have a significant reduction in *Bacteroidetes* and a compensatory increase in *Firmicutes* compared to lean controls [133,134]. Furthermore, high-fat-diet feeding in rodents has been shown to increase *Firmicutes* and decrease *Bacteroidetes* populations—an effect that can be rapidly reversed by changing the diet [135]. *Bacteroidetes* populations are also increased after diet therapy in humans [134], and the increase in this population was significantly correlated with weight loss [134].

RYGBP has also been shown to alter gut microbial populations. After RYGBP, there is an increase in the bacterial richness and diversity in the gut [136]. Cross-sectional data showed that post-RYGBP subjects have an even lower proportion of *Firmicutes* compared to both lean and obese controls [137], and a longitudinal study found that the *Bacteroidetes* proportion was significantly increased 3 months after RYGBP [138]. In rats, an increase in *Bacteroidetes* along the anastomosed jejunum, through the ileum, and in the colon and an increase in *Bifidobacterium* along the proximal jejunum, through the ileum, cecum, and colon, were observed [139]. Recently, *Akkermansia muciniphila* has garnered some attention as it found to be reduced in mice with obesity and/or type 2 diabetes, and administration of this bacteria can reverse the metabolic effects of high-fat feeding in mice [140]. Furthermore, *Akkermansia* levels were found to be increased after RYGBP in mice, independent of changes in body weight and food intake [141]. Altering the gut microbial populations after RYGBP with probiotic supplementation may provide an additional benefit, in addition to the endogenous changes in microbiota post-RYGBP. For example, administration of *Lactobacillus* to post-RYGBP subjects led to a reduction in bacterial overgrowth and a greater excess weight loss early after surgery [142].

Changes in the gut microflora post-RYGBP may contribute to the increase in GLP-1 observed. Prebiotic use (indigestible carbohydrates including oligofructose, inulin, etc.) leads to changes in bacterial populations that are reminiscent to those observed after weight loss and RYGBP. For example, prebiotics selectively increase *Bifidobacteria* [143–147], decrease *Firmicutes*, and increase *Bacteroidetes* populations [148]. Furthermore prebiotic use leads to increases in short-chain fatty acid (SCFA; acetate, butyrate, and propionate) content in the colon and plasma [149–151], a concomitant increase in *proglucagon* mRNA (colonic) and plasma GLP-1 [149–153], and a reduction in GIP [150]. Similarly, prebiotics have also been shown to stimulate L-cell proliferation in the colon and increase intestinal *proglucagon* mRNA expression and circulating GLP-1 levels [148,154]. These increased GLP-1 levels may be partly responsible for the beneficial metabolic effects of prebiotic use including reductions in weight gain and adiposity (which may be independent of caloric intake) and improvement in insulin secretion and glucose tolerance [148–150,152,153,155–162].

OTHER POTENTIAL MECHANISMS

There are also other, less explored mechanisms by which incretin levels may be increased after bariatric surgery for which further study is warranted.

Malabsorption after Gastric Bypass

Although significant carbohydrate malabsorption in the small intestine does not appear to occur after RYGBP [108,163], it is possible that carbohydrates are fermented to SCFA in the colon, leading to increased GLP-1 levels. For example, α-glucosidase inhibitors, which inhibit carbohydrate digestion leading to increased carbohydrate metabolism by colonic bacteria, improve glucose tolerance and increase GLP-1 levels [164]. Additionally, a strong inverse correlation between colonic fermentation and glucose tolerance, and positive correlation between colonic fermentation and satiety, have been reported [162]. Furthermore, *in vitro*, SCFAs stimulate *proglucagon* mRNA and GLP-1 release from the colon, and mRNA expression is further increased by reducing the pH to mimic the fermentation environment of the large intestine [153]. This effect of SCFAs on *proglucagon* transcription is likely via the SCFA receptors, free fatty acid receptor (FFAR)-2 and/or FFAR-3, localized to L-cells in the intestine [152,165,166]. In fact, prebiotics stimulate L-cell differentiation and upregulate expression of FFAR-2 [152,165,166]. It has been shown that the FFAR-2 is critical for SCFA-induced GLP-1 and insulin release and improvements in glucose tolerance [165], whereas FFAR-3 receptor is not [145,165]. Additionally, GLP-1 has been shown to be essential for the beneficial effects of prebiotics on glucose tolerance and hepatic insulin sensitivity [167].

Change in Meal Pattern and Duration

After RYGBP, the rate of food intake is decreased [168] and meal duration is increased [169], which could potentially impact the release of satiety hormones, including GLP-1. For example, it has been shown that meal duration modulates the release of satiety hormones in healthy, lean persons, with 30 min inducing greater satiety hormone release than either 5- or 120-min meals [170,171]. After RYGBP, a decrease in meal size as well as an increase in meal frequency are also observed in both humans and rats [168,172]; however, the impact of meal size and frequency to incretin hormone levels and satiety is inconsistent [173–179].

Alterations in Post-Translational Processing of GLP-1

RYGBP surgery could also modulate post-translational modification of GLP-1. Plasma levels of DPP-4, the enzyme responsible for degradation of GLP-1, are lower after RYGBP, but not after matched caloric restriction, suggesting that RYGBP can alter DPP-4 activity independent of body weight changes [180]. This is corroborated by rodent data, which observed a reduction in DPP-4 activity in the serum and the anastomosed jejunum area (but not distal jejunum or ileum) of rats after RYGBP [139]. It is plausible that RYGBP can lead to alterations in other enzymes responsible for GLP-1 production including PC-1; however, this has yet to be studied.

Trophic Effects

RYGBP has been shown to lead to gut hypertrophy and an increase in L-cells, potentially via a GLP-2-mediated mechanism [181,182]. GLP-2, although not an incretin *per se*, is a trophic factor derived from *proglucagon* that is also increased after RYGBP [39,95,182]. Increased L-cell numbers could contribute to increased GLP-1 levels after RYGBP.

CONCLUSIONS AND SIGNIFICANCE OF INCRETIN CHANGES AFTER BARIATRIC SURGERY

Diet and lifestyle interventions are often unsuccessful, partly because compensatory systems are engaged to favor the storage of calories for survival. However, bariatric surgery appears to evade

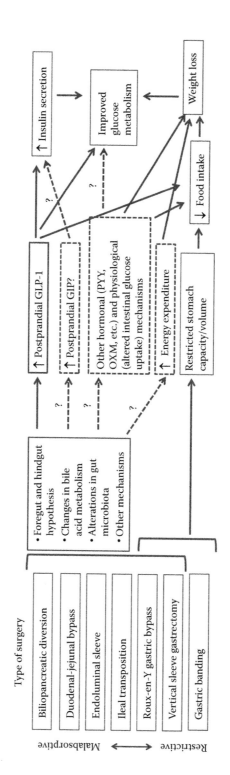

FIGURE 11.1 Potential mechanisms underlying changes in incretin hormones, and subsequent changes in energy and glucose metabolism. GLP-1, glucagon-like peptide-1; OXM, oxyntomodulin; PYY, peptide YY.

this evolutionary obstacle and offer remarkably sustainable weight loss and improvement in comorbidities. All bariatric surgeries are not created equal, and different types of surgeries lead to differing degrees of weight loss and diabetes resolution, due to varied physical changes and activated hormonal systems after the surgery. Bariatric surgery is no longer a one-size-fits-all intervention for the obese, but rather a promising tool for weight loss and resolution of comorbidities that should be tailored to the physiological needs of the patient, based on not just body mass but also existing comorbidities. In the future, as our understanding of the mechanisms of weight loss and improvement in comorbidities after bariatric surgery expands, invasive bariatric surgery techniques may be utilized less frequently. It is possible that the same benefits of invasive surgeries may be achieved by less invasive techniques or by targeting the physical and hormonal systems perturbed after surgery.

This idea has been explored with the incretins. The strong evidence linking GLP-1 with weight loss and improved glucose metabolism has led to the development of numerous pharmaceutical and nutraceutical agents to target this system. For example, the pharmaceutical industry has generated long-lasting GLP-1 receptor agonists as well as inhibitors of the GLP-1 degrading enzyme, DPP-4. Other therapies to enhance endogenous GLP-1 production, including functional foods such as prebiotics or those that could accelerate gastric emptying, also have the potential to work via this system. Although these therapies are effective, they cannot recapitulate the dramatic weight loss and improvement in comorbidities observed after bariatric surgery, demonstrating that incretins are significant but do not act autonomously. Other gut hormones, including ghrelin, oxyntomodulin, and PYY, may work in concert with the incretins, and thus, future therapies will require a combination approach to mimic the powerful effect of this surgery. It is possible that surgery provides a buffer for counterregulatory mechanisms that are usually activated with traditional weight loss techniques. Future research on the incretin systems and other altered systems after bariatric surgery will move the field forward and potentially offer patients alternative therapies that provide the same metabolic benefits after surgery (Figure 11.1).

REFERENCES

1. Nauck MA, Homberger E, Siegel EG, Allen RC, Eaton RP, Ebert R, Creutzfeldt W. 1986. Incretin effects of increasing glucose loads in man calculated from venous insulin and C-peptide responses. *The Journal of Clinical Endocrinology and Metabolism* 63:492–498.
2. Nauck M, Stockmann F, Ebert R, Creutzfeldt W. 1986. Reduced incretin effect in type 2 (non-insulin-dependent) diabetes. *Diabetologia* 29:46–52.
3. Phillips LK, Prins JB. 2011. Update on incretin hormones. *Annals of the New York Academy of Sciences* 1243:E55–E74.
4. Bell GI, Santerre RF, Mullenbach GT. 1983. Hamster preproglucagon contains the sequence of glucagon and two related peptides. *Nature* 302:716–718.
5. Zhu X, Zhou A, Dey A, Norrbom C, Carroll R, Zhang C, Laurent V, Lindberg I, Ugleholdt R, Holst JJ, Steiner DF. 2002. Disruption of PC1/3 expression in mice causes dwarfism and multiple neuroendocrine peptide processing defects. *Proceedings of the National Academy of Sciences of the United States of America* 99:10293–10298.
6. Eissele R, Goke R, Willemer S, Harthus HP, Vermeer H, Arnold R, Goke B. 1992. Glucagon-like peptide-1 cells in the gastrointestinal tract and pancreas of rat, pig and man. *European Journal of Clinical Investigation* 22:283–291.
7. Theodorakis MJ, Carlson O, Michopoulos S, Doyle ME, Juhaszova M, Petraki K, Egan JM. 2006. Human duodenal enteroendocrine cells: Source of both incretin peptides, GLP-1 and GIP. *American Journal of Physiology Endocrinology and Metabolism* 290:E550–E559.
8. Orskov C, Rabenhoj L, Wettergren A, Kofod H, Holst JJ. 1994. Tissue and plasma concentrations of amidated and glycine-extended glucagon-like peptide I in humans. *Diabetes* 43:535–539.
9. Deacon CF, Johnsen AH, Holst JJ. 1995. Degradation of glucagon-like peptide-1 by human plasma in vitro yields an N-terminally truncated peptide that is a major endogenous metabolite in vivo. *The Journal of Clinical Endocrinology and Metabolism* 80:952–957.
10. Mansour A, Hosseini S, Larijani B, Pajouhi M, Mohajeri-Tehrani MR. 2013. Nutrients related to GLP1 secretory responses. *Nutrition* 29:813–820.

11. Doyle ME, Egan JM. 2007. Mechanisms of action of glucagon-like peptide 1 in the pancreas. *Pharmacology & Therapeutics* 113:546–593.

12. Kanoski SE, Fortin SM, Arnold M, Grill HJ, Hayes MR. 2011. Peripheral and central GLP-1 receptor populations mediate the anorectic effects of peripherally administered GLP-1 receptor agonists, liraglutide and exendin-4. *Endocrinology* 152:3103–3112.

13. Turton MD, O'Shea D, Gunn I, Beak SA, Edwards CM, Meeran K, Choi SJ, Taylor GM, Heath MM, Lambert PD, Wilding JP, Smith DM, Ghatei MA, Herbert J, Bloom SR. 1996. A role for glucagon-like peptide-1 in the central regulation of feeding. *Nature* 379:69–72.

14. Scrocchi LA, Brown TJ, MaClusky N, Brubaker PL, Auerbach AB, Joyner AL, Drucker DJ. 1996. Glucose intolerance but normal satiety in mice with a null mutation in the glucagon-like peptide 1 receptor gene. *Nature Medicine* 2:1254–1258.

15. Holz GGT, Kuhtreiber WM, Habener JF. 1993. Pancreatic beta-cells are rendered glucose-competent by the insulinotropic hormone glucagon-like peptide-1(7-37). *Nature* 361:362–365.

16. Holst JJ. 2004. On the physiology of GIP and GLP-1. *Hormone and Metabolic Research* 36:747–754.

17. Ugleholdt R, Poulsen ML, Holst PJ, Irminger JC, Orskov C, Pedersen J, Rosenkilde MM, Zhu X, Steiner DF, Holst JJ. 2006. Prohormone convertase 1/3 is essential for processing of the glucose-dependent insulinotropic polypeptide precursor. *The Journal of Biological Chemistry* 281:11050–11057.

18. Polak JM, Bloom SR, Kuzio M, Brown JC, Pearse AG. 1973. Cellular localization of gastric inhibitory polypeptide in the duodenum and jejunum. *Gut* 14:284–288.

19. Tseng CC, Jarboe LA, Wolfe MM. 1994. Regulation of glucose-dependent insulinotropic peptide gene expression by a glucose meal. *The American Journal of Physiology* 266:G887–G891.

20. Lardinois CK, Starich GH, Mazzaferri EL. 1988. The postprandial response of gastric inhibitory polypeptide to various dietary fats in man. *Journal of the American College of Nutrition* 7:241–247.

21. Usdin TB, Mezey E, Button DC, Brownstein MJ, Bonner TI. 1993. Gastric inhibitory polypeptide receptor, a member of the secretin-vasoactive intestinal peptide receptor family, is widely distributed in peripheral organs and the brain. *Endocrinology* 133:2861–2870.

22. Miyawaki K, Yamada Y, Yano H, Niwa H, Ban N, Ihara Y, Kubota A, Fujimoto S, Kajikawa M, Kuroe A, Tsuda K, Hashimoto H, Yamashita T, Jomori T, Tashiro F, Miyazaki J, Seino Y. 1999. Glucose intolerance caused by a defect in the entero-insular axis: A study in gastric inhibitory polypeptide receptor knockout mice. *Proceedings of the National Academy of Sciences of the United States of America* 96:14843–14847.

23. Kieffer TJ, McIntosh CH, Pederson RA. 1995. Degradation of glucose-dependent insulinotropic polypeptide and truncated glucagon-like peptide 1 in vitro and in vivo by dipeptidyl peptidase IV. *Endocrinology* 136:3585–3596.

24. Kim SJ, Winter K, Nian C, Tsuneoka M, Koda Y, McIntosh CH. 2005. Glucose-dependent insulinotropic polypeptide (GIP) stimulation of pancreatic beta-cell survival is dependent upon phosphatidylinositol 3-kinase (PI3K)/protein kinase B (PKB) signaling, inactivation of the forkhead transcription factor Foxo1, and down-regulation of bax expression. *The Journal of Biological Chemistry* 280:22297–22307.

25. Farilla L, Hui H, Bertolotto C, Kang E, Bulotta A, Di Mario U, Perfetti R. 2002. Glucagon-like peptide-1 promotes islet cell growth and inhibits apoptosis in Zucker diabetic rats. *Endocrinology* 143:4397–4408.

26. Shin AC, Zheng H, Townsend RL, Sigalet DL, Berthoud HR. 2010. Meal-induced hormone responses in a rat model of Roux-en-Y gastric bypass surgery. *Endocrinology* 151:1588–1597.

27. Meirelles K, Ahmed T, Culnan DM, Lynch CJ, Lang CH, Cooney RN. 2009. Mechanisms of glucose homeostasis after Roux-en-Y gastric bypass surgery in the obese, insulin-resistant Zucker rat. *Annals of Surgery* 249:277–285.

28. Liu Y, Zhou Y, Wang Y, Geng D, Liu J. 2011. Roux-en-Y gastric bypass-induced improvement of glucose tolerance and insulin resistance in type 2 diabetic rats are mediated by glucagon-like peptide-1. *Obesity Surgery* 21:1424–1431.

29. Buchwald H, Estok R, Fahrbach K, Banel D, Jensen MD, Pories WJ, Bantle JP, Sledge I. 2009. Weight and type 2 diabetes after bariatric surgery: Systematic review and meta-analysis. *The American Journal of Medicine* 122:248–256.

30. Schauer PR, Kashyap SR, Wolski K, Brethauer SA, Kirwan JP, Pothier CE, Thomas S, Abood B, Nissen SE, Bhatt DL. 2012. Bariatric surgery versus intensive medical therapy in obese patients with diabetes. *The New England Journal of Medicine* 366:1567–1576.

31. Laferrère B, Heshka S, Wang K, Khan Y, McGinty J, Teixeira J, Hart AB, Olivan B. 2007. Incretin levels and effect are markedly enhanced 1 month after Roux-en-Y gastric bypass surgery in obese patients with type 2 diabetes. *Diabetes Care* 30:1709–1716.

32. Laferrère B, Teixeira J, McGinty J, Tran H, Egger JR, Colarusso A, Kovack B, Bawa B, Koshy N, Lee H, Yapp K, Olivan B. 2008. Effect of weight loss by gastric bypass surgery versus hypocaloric diet on glucose and incretin levels in patients with type 2 diabetes. *The Journal of Clinical Endocrinology and Metabolism* 93:2479–2485.

33. Jorgensen NB, Jacobsen SH, Dirksen C, Bojsen-Moller KN, Naver L, Hvolris L, Clausen TR, Wulff BS, Worm D, Lindqvist Hansen D, Madsbad S, Holst JJ. 2012. Acute and long-term effects of Roux-en-Y gastric bypass on glucose metabolism in subjects with Type 2 diabetes and normal glucose tolerance. *American Journal of Physiology Endocrinology and Metabolism* 303:E122–E131.

34. Umeda LM, Silva EA, Carneiro G, Arasaki CH, Geloneze B, Zanella MT. 2011. Early improvement in glycemic control after bariatric surgery and its relationships with insulin, GLP-1, and glucagon secretion in type 2 diabetic patients. *Obesity Surgery* 21:896–901.

35. Falken Y, Hellstrom PM, Holst JJ, Naslund E. 2011. Changes in glucose homeostasis after Roux-en-Y gastric bypass surgery for obesity at day three, two months, and one year after surgery: Role of gut peptides. *The Journal of Clinical Endocrinology and Metabolism* 96:2227–2235.

36. Promintzer-Schifferl M, Prager G, Anderwald C, Mandl M, Esterbauer H, Shakeri-Leidenmuhler S, Pacini G, Stadler M, Bischof MG, Ludvik B, Luger A, Krebs M. 2011. Effects of gastric bypass surgery on insulin resistance and insulin secretion in nondiabetic obese patients. *Obesity* 19:1420–1426.

37. Bose M, Teixeira J, Olivan B, Bawa B, Arias S, Machineni S, Pi-Sunyer FX, Scherer PE, Laferrère B. 2010. Weight loss and incretin responsiveness improve glucose control independently after gastric bypass surgery. *Journal of Diabetes* 2:47–55.

38. Pournaras DJ, Osborne A, Hawkins SC, Vincent RP, Mahon D, Ewings P, Ghatei MA, Bloom SR, Welbourn R, le Roux CW. 2010. Remission of type 2 diabetes after gastric bypass and banding: Mechanisms and 2 year outcomes. *Annals of Surgery* 252:966–971.

39. Jacobsen SH, Olesen SC, Dirksen C, Jorgensen NB, Bojsen-Moller KN, Kielgast U, Worm D, Almdal T, Naver LS, Hvolris LE, Rehfeld JF, Wulff BS, Clausen TR, Hansen DL, Holst JJ, Madsbad S. 2012. Changes in gastrointestinal hormone responses, insulin sensitivity, and beta-cell function within 2 weeks after gastric bypass in non-diabetic subjects. *Obesity Surgery* 22:1084–1096.

40. Dar MS, Chapman WH, 3rd, Pender JR, Drake AJ, 3rd, O'Brien K, Tanenberg RJ, Dohm GL, Pories WJ. 2012. GLP-1 response to a mixed meal: What happens 10 years after Roux-en-Y gastric bypass (RYGB)? *Obesity Surgery* 22:1077–1083.

41. Bradley D, Conte C, Mittendorfer B, Eagon JC, Varela JE, Fabbrini E, Gastaldelli A, Chambers KT, Su X, Okunade A, Patterson BW, Klein S. 2012. Gastric bypass and banding equally improve insulin sensitivity and beta cell function. *The Journal of Clinical Investigation* 122:4667–4674.

42. Isbell JM, Tamboli RA, Hansen EN, Saliba J, Dunn JP, Phillips SE, Marks-Shulman PA, Abumrad NN. 2010. The importance of caloric restriction in the early improvements in insulin sensitivity after Roux-en-Y gastric bypass surgery. *Diabetes Care* 33:1438–1442.

43. Kashyap SR, Daud S, Kelly KR, Gastaldelli A, Win H, Brethauer S, Kirwan JP, Schauer PR. 2010. Acute effects of gastric bypass versus gastric restrictive surgery on beta-cell function and insulinotropic hormones in severely obese patients with type 2 diabetes. *International Journal of Obesity* 34:462–471.

44. Campos GM, Rabl C, Peeva S, Ciovica R, Rao M, Schwarz JM, Havel P, Schambelan M, Mulligan K. 2010. Improvement in peripheral glucose uptake after gastric bypass surgery is observed only after substantial weight loss has occurred and correlates with the magnitude of weight lost. *Journal of Gastrointestinal Surgery: Official Journal of the Society for Surgery of the Alimentary Tract* 14: 15–23.

45. Korner J, Inabnet W, Febres G, Conwell IM, McMahon DJ, Salas R, Taveras C, Schrope B, Bessler M. 2009. Prospective study of gut hormone and metabolic changes after adjustable gastric banding and Roux-en-Y gastric bypass. *International Journal of Obesity* 33:786–795.

46. Vidal J, Nicolau J, Romero F, Casamitjana R, Momblan D, Conget I, Morinigo R, Lacy AM. 2009. Long-term effects of Roux-en-Y gastric bypass surgery on plasma glucagon-like peptide-1 and islet function in morbidly obese subjects. *The Journal of Clinical Endocrinology and Metabolism* 94:884–891.

47. Korner J, Bessler M, Inabnet W, Taveras C, Holst JJ. 2007. Exaggerated glucagon-like peptide-1 and blunted glucose-dependent insulinotropic peptide secretion are associated with Roux-en-Y gastric bypass but not adjustable gastric banding. *Surgery for Obesity and Related Diseases: Official Journal of the American Society for Bariatric Surgery* 3:597–601.

48. Morinigo R, Moize V, Musri M, Lacy AM, Navarro S, Marin JL, Delgado S, Casamitjana R, Vidal J. 2006. Glucagon-like peptide-1, peptide YY, hunger, and satiety after gastric bypass surgery in morbidly obese subjects. *The Journal of Clinical Endocrinology and Metabolism* 91:1735–1740.

49. Peterli R, Steinert RE, Woelnerhanssen B, Peters T, Christoffel-Courtin C, Gass M, Kern B, von Fluee M, Beglinger C. 2012. Metabolic and hormonal changes after laparoscopic Roux-en-Y gastric bypass and sleeve gastrectomy: A randomized, prospective trial. *Obesity Surgery* 22:740–748.

50. Bose M, Machineni S, Olivan B, Teixeira J, McGinty JJ, Bawa B, Koshy N, Colarusso A, Laferrère B. 2010. Superior appetite hormone profile after equivalent weight loss by gastric bypass compared to gastric banding. *Obesity* 18:1085–1091.

51. Van der Schueren BJ, Homel P, Alam M, Agenor K, Wang G, Reilly D, Laferrère B. 2012. Magnitude and variability of the glucagon-like peptide-1 response in patients with type 2 diabetes up to 2 years following gastric bypass surgery. *Diabetes Care* 35:42–46.

52. Peterli R, Wolnerhanssen B, Peters T, Devaux N, Kern B, Christoffel-Courtin C, Drewe J, von Flue M, Beglinger C. 2009. Improvement in glucose metabolism after bariatric surgery: Comparison of laparoscopic Roux-en-Y gastric bypass and laparoscopic sleeve gastrectomy: A prospective randomized trial. *Annals of Surgery* 250:234–241.

53. Salehi M, Prigeon RL, D'Alessio DA. 2011. Gastric bypass surgery enhances glucagon-like peptide 1-stimulated postprandial insulin secretion in humans. *Diabetes* 60:2308–2314.

54. Jorgensen NB, Dirksen C, Bojsen-Moller KN, Jacobsen SH, Worm D, Hansen DL, Kristiansen VB, Naver L, Madsbad S, Holst JJ. 2013. The exaggerated glucagon-like peptide-1 response is important for the improved beta-cell function and glucose tolerance after Roux-en-Y gastric bypass in patients with type 2 diabetes. *Diabetes* 62:3044–3052.

55. Mithieux G, Andreelli F, Magnan C. 2009. Intestinal gluconeogenesis: Key signal of central control of energy and glucose homeostasis. *Current Opinion in Clinical Nutrition and Metabolic Care* 12:419–423.

56. Saeidi N, Meoli L, Nestoridi E, Gupta NK, Kvas S, Kucharczyk J, Bonab AA, Fischman AJ, Yarmush ML, Stylopoulos N. 2013. Reprogramming of intestinal glucose metabolism and glycemic control in rats after gastric bypass. *Science* 341:406–410.

57. Dirksen C, Hansen DL, Madsbad S, Hvolris LE, Naver LS, Holst JJ, Worm D. 2010. Postprandial diabetic glucose tolerance is normalized by gastric bypass feeding as opposed to gastric feeding and is associated with exaggerated GLP-1 secretion: A case report. *Diabetes Care* 33:375–377.

58. McLaughlin T, Peck M, Holst J, Deacon C. 2010. Reversible hyperinsulinemic hypoglycemia after gastric bypass: A consequence of altered nutrient delivery. *The Journal of Clinical Endocrinology and Metabolism* 95:1851–1855.

59. Pacheco D, de Luis DA, Romero A, Gonzalez Sagrado M, Conde R, Izaola O, Aller R, Delgado A. 2007. The effects of duodenal-jejunal exclusion on hormonal regulation of glucose metabolism in Goto-Kakizaki rats. *American Journal of Surgery* 194:221–224.

60. Jiao J, Bae EJ, Bandyopadhyay G, Oliver J, Marathe C, Chen M, Hsu JY, Chen Y, Tian H, Olefsky JM, Saberi M. 2013. Restoration of euglycemia after duodenal bypass surgery is reliant on central and peripheral inputs in Zucker fa/fa rats. *Diabetes* 62:1074–1083.

61. Speck M, Cho YM, Asadi A, Rubino F, Kieffer TJ. 2011. Duodenal-jejunal bypass protects GK rats from {beta}-cell loss and aggravation of hyperglycemia and increases enteroendocrine cells coexpressing GIP and GLP-1. *American Journal of Physiology Endocrinology and Metabolism* 300:E923–E932.

62. Woods M, Lan Z, Li J, Wheeler MB, Wang H, Wang R. 2011. Antidiabetic effects of duodenojejunal bypass in an experimental model of diabetes induced by a high-fat diet. *The British Journal of Surgery* 98:686–696.

63. Liu SZ, Sun D, Zhang GY, Wang L, Liu T, Sun Y, Li MX, Hu SY. 2012. A high-fat diet reverses improvement in glucose tolerance induced by duodenal-jejunal bypass in type 2 diabetic rats. *Chinese Medical Journal* 125:912–919.

64. de Luis D, Domingo M, Romero A, Gonzalez Sagrado M, Pacheco D, Primo D, Conde R. 2012. Effects of duodenal-jejunal exclusion on beta cell function and hormonal regulation in Goto-Kakizaki rats. *American Journal of Surgery* 204:242–247.

65. Liu S, Zhang G, Wang L, Sun D, Chen W, Yan Z, Sun Y, Hu S. 2012. The entire small intestine mediates the changes in glucose homeostasis after intestinal surgery in Goto-Kakizaki rats. *Annals of Surgery* 256:1049–1058.

66. Kindel TL, Yoder SM, Seeley RJ, D'Alessio DA, Tso P. 2009. Duodenal-jejunal exclusion improves glucose tolerance in the diabetic, Goto-Kakizaki rat by a GLP-1 receptor-mediated mechanism. *Journal of Gastrointestinal Surgery: Official Journal of the Society for Surgery of the Alimentary Tract* 13: 1762–1772.

67. Li F, Zhang G, Liang J, Ding X, Cheng Z, Hu S. 2009. Sleeve gastrectomy provides a better control of diabetes by decreasing ghrelin in the diabetic Goto-Kakizaki rats. *Journal of Gastrointestinal Surgery: Official Journal of the Society for Surgery of the Alimentary Tract* 13:2302–2308.

68. Yan L, Zhu Z, Wu D, Zhou Q, Wu Y. 2011. Effects of sleeve gastrectomy surgery with modified jejunoileal bypass on body weight, food intake and metabolic hormone levels of rats. *Journal of Huazhong University of Science and Technology Medical Sciences* 31:784–788.

69. Wang TT, Hu SY, Gao HD, Zhang GY, Liu CZ, Feng JB, Frezza EE. 2008. Ileal transposition controls diabetes as well as modified duodenal jejunal bypass with better lipid lowering in a nonobese rat model of type II diabetes by increasing GLP-1. *Annals of Surgery* 247:968–975.

70. Sun D, Liu S, Zhang G, Chen W, Yan Z, Hu S. 2012. Type 2 diabetes control in a nonobese rat model using sleeve gastrectomy with duodenal-jejunal bypass (SGDJB). *Obesity Surgery* 22:1865–1873.

71. Kindel TL, Yoder SM, D'Alessio DA, Tso P. 2010. The effect of duodenal-jejunal bypass on glucose-dependent insulinotropic polypeptide secretion in Wistar rats. *Obesity Surgery* 20:768–775.

72. Cohen RV, Rubino F, Schiavon C, Cummings DE. 2012. Diabetes remission without weight loss after duodenal bypass surgery. *Surgery for Obesity and Related Diseases: Official Journal of the American Society for Bariatric Surgery* 8:e66–e68.

73. Ramos AC, Galvao Neto MP, de Souza YM, Galvao M, Murakami AH, Silva AC, Canseco EG, Santamaria R, Zambrano TA. 2009. Laparoscopic duodenal-jejunal exclusion in the treatment of type 2 diabetes mellitus in patients with BMI < 30 kg/m2 (LBMI). *Obesity Surgery* 19:307–312.

74. Ferzli GS, Dominique E, Ciaglia M, Bluth MH, Gonzalez A, Fingerhut A. 2009. Clinical improvement after duodenojejunal bypass for nonobese type 2 diabetes despite minimal improvement in glycemic homeostasis. *World Journal of Surgery* 33:972–979.

75. Lee HC, Kim MK, Kwon HS, Kim E, Song KH. 2010. Early changes in incretin secretion after laparoscopic duodenal-jejunal bypass surgery in type 2 diabetic patients. *Obesity Surgery* 20:1530–1535.

76. Naslund E, Gryback P, Hellstrom PM, Jacobsson H, Holst JJ, Theodorsson E, Backman L. 1997. Gastrointestinal hormones and gastric emptying 20 years after jejunoileal bypass for massive obesity. *International Journal of Obesity and Related Metabolic Disorders: Journal of the International Association for the Study of Obesity* 21:387–392.

77. Zhang GY, Wang TT, Cheng ZQ, Feng JB, Hu SY. 2011. Resolution of diabetes mellitus by ileal transposition compared with biliopancreatic diversion in a nonobese animal model of type 2 diabetes. *Canadian Journal of Surgery* 54:243–251.

78. Borg CM, le Roux CW, Ghatei MA, Bloom SR, Patel AG. 2007. Biliopancreatic diversion in rats is associated with intestinal hypertrophy and with increased GLP-1, GLP-2 and PYY levels. *Obesity Surgery* 17:1193–1198.

79. Valverde I, Puente J, Martin-Duce A, Molina L, Lozano O, Sancho V, Malaisse WJ, Villanueva-Penacarrillo ML. 2005. Changes in glucagon-like peptide-1 (GLP-1) secretion after biliopancreatic diversion or vertical banded gastroplasty in obese subjects. *Obesity Surgery* 15:387–397.

80. Marfella R, Barbieri M, Ruggiero R, Rizzo MR, Grella R, Mozzillo AL, Docimo L, Paolisso G. 2010. Bariatric surgery reduces oxidative stress by blunting 24-h acute glucose fluctuations in type 2 diabetic obese patients. *Diabetes Care* 33:287–289.

81. Salinari S, Bertuzzi A, Asnaghi S, Guidone C, Manco M, Mingrone G. 2009. First-phase insulin secretion restoration and differential response to glucose load depending on the route of administration in type 2 diabetic subjects after bariatric surgery. *Diabetes Care* 32:375–380.

82. Guidone C, Manco M, Valera-Mora E, Iaconelli A, Gniuli D, Mari A, Nanni G, Castagneto M, Calvani M, Mingrone G. 2006. Mechanisms of recovery from type 2 diabetes after malabsorptive bariatric surgery. *Diabetes* 55:2025–2031.

83. Patriti A, Aisa MC, Annetti C, Sidoni A, Galli F, Ferri I, Gulla N, Donini A. 2007. How the hindgut can cure type 2 diabetes. Ileal transposition improves glucose metabolism and beta-cell function in Goto-kakizaki rats through an enhanced Proglucagon gene expression and L-cell number. *Surgery* 142:74–85.

84. Strader AD, Clausen TR, Goodin SZ, Wendt D. 2009. Ileal interposition improves glucose tolerance in low dose streptozotocin-treated diabetic and euglycemic rats. *Obesity Surgery* 19:96–104.

85. Cummings BP, Strader AD, Stanhope KL, Graham JL, Lee J, Raybould HE, Baskin DG, Havel PJ. 2010. Ileal interposition surgery improves glucose and lipid metabolism and delays diabetes onset in the UCD-T2DM rat. *Gastroenterology* 138:2437–2446.

86. Strader AD, Vahl TP, Jandacek RJ, Woods SC, D'Alessio DA, Seeley RJ. 2005. Weight loss through ileal transposition is accompanied by increased ileal hormone secretion and synthesis in rats. *American Journal of Physiology Endocrinology and Metabolism* 288:E447–E453.

87. Chambers AP, Jessen L, Ryan KK, Sisley S, Wilson-Perez HE, Stefater MA, Gaitonde SG, Sorrell JE, Toure M, Berger J, D'Alessio DA, Woods SC, Seeley RJ, Sandoval DA. 2011. Weight-independent changes in blood glucose homeostasis after gastric bypass or vertical sleeve gastrectomy in rats. *Gastroenterology* 141:950–958.

88. Chambers AP, Stefater MA, Wilson-Perez HE, Jessen L, Sisley S, Ryan KK, Gaitonde S, Sorrell JE, Toure M, Berger J, D'Alessio DA, Sandoval DA, Seeley RJ, Woods SC. 2011. Similar effects of Roux-en-Y gastric bypass and vertical sleeve gastrectomy on glucose regulation in rats. *Physiology & Behavior* 105:120–123.

89. Wang Y, Yan L, Jin Z, Xin X. 2011. Effects of sleeve gastrectomy in neonatally streptozotocin-induced diabetic rats. *PloS One* 6:e16383.

90. Basso N, Capoccia D, Rizzello M, Abbatini F, Mariani P, Maglio C, Coccia F, Borgonuovo G, De Luca ML, Asprino R, Alessandri G, Casella G, Leonetti F. 2011. First-phase insulin secretion, insulin sensitivity, ghrelin, GLP-1, and PYY changes 72 h after sleeve gastrectomy in obese diabetic patients: The gastric hypothesis. *Surgical Endoscopy* 25:3540–3550.

91. Papamargaritis D, le Roux CW, Sioka E, Koukoulis G, Tzovaras G, Zacharoulis D. 2012. Changes in gut hormone profile and glucose homeostasis after laparoscopic sleeve gastrectomy. *Surgery for Obesity and Related Diseases: Official Journal of the American Society for Bariatric Surgery* 9:192–201.

92. Dimitriadis E, Daskalakis M, Kampa M, Peppe A, Papadakis JA, Melissas J. 2013. Alterations in gut hormones after laparoscopic sleeve gastrectomy: Prospective Clinical and Laboratory Investigational Study. *Annals of Surgery* 257:647–654.

93. Lee WJ, Chen CY, Chong K, Lee YC, Chen SC, Lee SD. 2011. Changes in postprandial gut hormones after metabolic surgery: a comparison of gastric bypass and sleeve gastrectomy. *Surgery for Obesity and Related Diseases: Official Journal of the American Society for Bariatric Surgery* 7:683–690.

94. Valderas JP, Irribarra V, Rubio L, Boza C, Escalona M, Liberona Y, Matamala A, Maiz A. 2011. Effects of sleeve gastrectomy and medical treatment for obesity on glucagon-like peptide 1 levels and glucose homeostasis in non-diabetic subjects. *Obesity Surgery* 21:902–909.

95. Romero F, Nicolau J, Flores L, Casamitjana R, Ibarzabal A, Lacy A, Vidal J. 2012. Comparable early changes in gastrointestinal hormones after sleeve gastrectomy and Roux-en-Y gastric bypass surgery for morbidly obese type 2 diabetic subjects. *Surgical Endoscopy* 26:2231–2239.

96. Ramon JM, Salvans S, Crous X, Puig S, Goday A, Benaiges D, Trillo L, Pera M, Grande L. 2012. Effect of Roux-en-Y gastric bypass vs sleeve gastrectomy on glucose and gut hormones: A prospective randomised trial. *Journal of Gastrointestinal Surgery: Official Journal of the Society for Surgery of the Alimentary Tract* 16:1116–1122.

97. Santoro S, Malzoni CE, Velhote MC, Milleo FQ, Santo MA, Klajner S, Damiani D, Maksoud JG. 2006. Digestive adaptation with intestinal reserve: A neuroendocrine-based operation for morbid obesity. *Obesity Surgery* 16:1371–1379.

98. DePaula AL, Macedo AL, Schraibman V, Mota BR, Vencio S. 2009. Hormonal evaluation following laparoscopic treatment of type 2 diabetes mellitus patients with BMI 20–34. *Surgical Endoscopy* 23: 1724–1732.

99. Rodieux F, Giusti V, D'Alessio DA, Suter M, Tappy L. 2008. Effects of gastric bypass and gastric banding on glucose kinetics and gut hormone release. *Obesity* 16:298–305.

100. Munoz R, Carmody JS, Stylopoulos N, Davis P, Kaplan LM. 2012. Isolated duodenal exclusion increases energy expenditure and improves glucose homeostasis in diet-induced obese rats. *American Journal of Physiology Regulatory, Integrative and Comparative Physiology* 303:R985–R993.

101. Rodriguez-Grunert L, Galvao Neto MP, Alamo M, Ramos AC, Baez PB, Tarnoff M. 2008. First human experience with endoscopically delivered and retrieved duodenal-jejunal bypass sleeve. *Surgery for Obesity and Related Diseases: Official Journal of the American Society for Bariatric Surgery* 4:55–59.

102. Escalona A, Pimentel F, Sharp A, Becerra P, Slako M, Turiel D, Munoz R, Bambs C, Guzman S, Ibanez L, Gersin K. 2012. Weight loss and metabolic improvement in morbidly obese subjects implanted for 1 year with an endoscopic duodenal-jejunal bypass liner. *Annals of Surgery* 255:1080–1085.

103. Gersin KS, Rothstein RI, Rosenthal RJ, Stefanidis D, Deal SE, Kuwada TS, Laycock W, Adrales G, Vassiliou M, Szomstein S, Heller S, Joyce AM, Heiss F, Nepomnayshy D. 2010. Open-label, sham-controlled trial of an endoscopic duodenojejunal bypass liner for preoperative weight loss in bariatric surgery candidates. *Gastrointestinal Endoscopy* 71:976–982.

104. Rubino F, Marescaux J. 2004. Effect of duodenal-jejunal exclusion in a non-obese animal model of type 2 diabetes: A new perspective for an old disease. *Annals of Surgery* 239:1–11.

105. Pournaras DJ, Aasheim ET, Bueter M, Ahmed AR, Welbourn R, Olbers T, le Roux CW. 2012. Effect of bypassing the proximal gut on gut hormones involved with glycemic control and weight loss. *Surgery for Obesity and Related Diseases: Official Journal of the American Society for Bariatric Surgery* 8:371–374.

106. Melissas J, Leventi A, Klinaki I, Perisinakis K, Koukouraki S, de Bree E, Karkavitsas N. 2013. Alterations of global gastrointestinal motility after sleeve gastrectomy: A prospective study. *Annals of Surgery* 258(6): 976–982.

107. Patriti A, Facchiano E, Annetti C, Aisa MC, Galli F, Fanelli C, Donini A. 2005. Early improvement of glucose tolerance after ileal transposition in a non-obese type 2 diabetes rat model. *Obesity Surgery* 15:1258–1264.

108. Wang G, Agenor K, Pizot J, Kotler DP, Harel Y, Van Der Schueren BJ, Quercia I, McGinty J, Laferrère B. 2012. Accelerated gastric emptying but no carbohydrate malabsorption 1 year after gastric bypass surgery (GBP). *Obesity Surgery* 22:1263–1267.

109. Horowitz M, Collins PJ, Harding PE, Shearman DJ. 1986. Gastric emptying after gastric bypass. *International Journal of Obesity* 10:117–121.

110. Patti ME, Houten SM, Bianco AC, Bernier R, Larsen PR, Holst JJ, Badman MK, Maratos-Flier E, Mun EC, Pihlajamaki J, Auwerx J, Goldfine AB. 2009. Serum bile acids are higher in humans with prior gastric bypass: Potential contribution to improved glucose and lipid metabolism. *Obesity* 17:1671–1677.

111. Simonen M, Dali-Youcef N, Kaminska D, Venesmaa S, Kakela P, Paakkonen M, Hallikainen M, Kolehmainen M, Uusitupa M, Moilanen L, Laakso M, Gylling H, Patti ME, Auwerx J, Pihlajamaki J. 2012. Conjugated bile acids associate with altered rates of glucose and lipid oxidation after Roux-en-Y gastric bypass. *Obesity Surgery* 22:1473–1480.

112. Jansen PL, van Werven J, Aarts E, Berends F, Janssen I, Stoker J, Schaap FG. 2011. Alterations of hormonally active fibroblast growth factors after Roux-en-Y gastric bypass surgery. *Digestive Diseases* 29:48–51.

113. Pournaras DJ, Glicksman C, Vincent RP, Kuganolipava S, Alaghband-Zadeh J, Mahon D, Bekker JH, Ghatei MA, Bloom SR, Walters JR, Welbourn R, le Roux CW. 2012. The role of bile after Roux-en-Y gastric bypass in promoting weight loss and improving glycaemic control. *Endocrinology* 153:3613–3619.

114. Kohli R, Bradley D, Setchell KD, Eagon JC, Abumrad N, Klein S. 2013. Weight loss induced by Roux-en-Y gastric bypass but not laparoscopic adjustable gastric banding increases circulating bile acids. *The Journal of Clinical Endocrinology and Metabolism* 98:E708–E712.

115. Ahmad NN, Pfalzer A, Kaplan LM. 2013. Roux-en-Y gastric bypass normalizes the blunted postprandial bile acid excursion associated with obesity. *International Journal of Obesity* 37:1553–1559.

116. Gerhard GS, Styer AM, Wood GC, Roesch SL, Petrick AT, Gabrielsen J, Strodel WE, Still CD, Argyropoulos G. 2013. A role for fibroblast growth factor 19 and bile acids in diabetes remission after Roux-en-Y gastric bypass. *Diabetes Care* 36:1859–1864.

117. Adrian TE, Gariballa S, Parekh KA, Thomas SA, Saadi H, Al Kaabi J, Nagelkerke N, Gedulin B, Young AA. 2012. Rectal taurocholate increases L cell and insulin secretion, and decreases blood glucose and food intake in obese type 2 diabetic volunteers. *Diabetologia* 55:2343–2347.

118. Wu T, Bound MJ, Standfield SD, Gedulin B, Jones KL, Horowitz M, Rayner CK. 2012. Effects of rectal administration of taurocholic acid on glucagon-like peptide-1 and peptide YY secretion in healthy humans. *Diabetes, Obesity & Metabolism* 15:474–477.

119. Izukura M, Hashimoto T, Gomez G, Uchida T, Greeley GH, Jr., Thompson JC. 1991. Intracolonic infusion of bile salt stimulates release of peptide YY and inhibits cholecystokinin-stimulated pancreatic exocrine secretion in conscious dogs. *Pancreas* 6:427–432.

120. Adrian TE, Ballantyne GH, Longo WE, Bilchik AJ, Graham S, Basson MD, Tierney RP, Modlin IM. 1993. Deoxycholate is an important releaser of peptide YY and enteroglucagon from the human colon. *Gut* 34:1219–1224.

121. Parker HE, Wallis K, le Roux CW, Wong KY, Reimann F, Gribble FM. 2012. Molecular mechanisms underlying bile acid-stimulated glucagon-like peptide-1 secretion. *British Journal of Pharmacology* 165:414–423.

122. Kohli R, Kirby M, Setchell KD, Jha P, Klustaitis K, Woollett LA, Pfluger PT, Balistreri WF, Tso P, Jandacek RJ, Woods SC, Heubi JE, Tschoep MH, D'Alessio DA, Shroyer NF, Seeley RJ. 2010. Intestinal adaptation after ileal interposition surgery increases bile acid recycling and protects against obesity-related comorbidities. *American Journal of Physiology Gastrointestinal and Liver Physiology* 299:G652–G660.

123. Cummings BP, Bettaieb A, Graham JL, Stanhope KL, Kowala M, Haj FG, Chouinard ML, Havel PJ. 2012. Vertical sleeve gastrectomy improves glucose and lipid metabolism and delays diabetes onset in UCD-T2DM rats. *Endocrinology* 153:3620–3632.

124. Kohli R, Setchell KD, Kirby M, Myronovych A, Ryan KK, Ibrahim SH, Berger J, Smith K, Toure M, Woods SC, Seeley RJ. 2013. A surgical model in male obese rats uncovers protective effects of bile acids post-bariatric surgery. *Endocrinology* 154:2341–2351.

125. Chen L, Yao X, Young A, McNulty J, Anderson D, Liu Y, Nystrom C, Croom D, Ross S, Collins J, Rajpal D, Hamlet K, Smith C, Gedulin B. 2012. Inhibition of apical sodium-dependent bile acid transporter as a novel treatment for diabetes. *American Journal of Physiology Endocrinology and Metabolism* 302:E68–E76.

126. Shang Q, Saumoy M, Holst JJ, Salen G, Xu G. 2010. Colesevelam improves insulin resistance in a diet-induced obesity (F-DIO) rat model by increasing the release of GLP-1. *American Journal of Physiology Gastrointestinal and Liver Physiology* 298:G419–G424.

127. Suzuki T, Oba K, Igari Y, Matsumura N, Watanabe K, Futami-Suda S, Yasuoka H, Ouchi M, Suzuki K, Kigawa Y, Nakano H. 2007. Colestimide lowers plasma glucose levels and increases plasma glucagon-like PEPTIDE-1 (7-36) levels in patients with type 2 diabetes mellitus complicated by hypercholesterol-emia. *Journal of Nippon Medical School* 74:338–343.

128. Smushkin G, Sathananthan M, Piccinini F, Man CD, Law JH, Cobelli C, Zinsmeister AR, Rizza RA, Vella A. 2012. The effect of a bile acid sequestrant on glucose metabolism in subjects with type 2 diabetes. *Diabetes* 62:1094–1101.

129. Kawamata Y, Fujii R, Hosoya M, Harada M, Yoshida H, Miwa M, Fukusumi S, Habata Y, Itoh T, Shintani Y, Hinuma S, Fujisawa Y, Fujino M. 2003. A G protein-coupled receptor responsive to bile acids. *The Journal of Biological Chemistry* 278:9435–9440.

130. Thomas C, Gioiello A, Noriega L, Strehle A, Oury J, Rizzo G, Macchiarulo A, Yamamoto H, Mataki C, Pruzanski M, Pellicciari R, Auwerx J, Schoonjans K. 2009. TGR5-mediated bile acid sensing controls glucose homeostasis. *Cell Metabolism* 10:167–177.

131. Potthoff MJ, Potts A, He T, Duarte JA, Taussig R, Mangelsdorf DJ, Kliewer SA, Burgess SC. 2012. Colesevelam suppresses hepatic glycogenolysis by TGR5-mediated Induction of GLP-1 action in DIO mice. *American Journal of Physiology Gastrointestinal and Liver Physiology* 304:G371–G380.

132. Reimann F, Habib AM, Tolhurst G, Parker HE, Rogers GJ, Gribble FM. 2008. Glucose sensing in L cells: A primary cell study. *Cell Metabolism* 8:532–539.

133. Ley RE, Backhed F, Turnbaugh P, Lozupone CA, Knight RD, Gordon JI. 2005. Obesity alters gut microbial ecology. *Proceedings of the National Academy of Sciences of the United States of America* 102:11070–11075.

134. Ley RE, Turnbaugh PJ, Klein S, Gordon JI. 2006. Microbial ecology: Human gut microbes associated with obesity. *Nature* 444:1022–1023.

135. Turnbaugh PJ, Backhed F, Fulton L, Gordon JI. 2008. Diet-induced obesity is linked to marked but reversible alterations in the mouse distal gut microbiome. *Cell Host & Microbe* 3:213–223.

136. Kong LC, Tap J, Aron-Wisnewsky J, Pelloux V, Basdevant A, Bouillot JL, Zucker JD, Dore J, Clement K. 2013. Gut microbiota after gastric bypass in human obesity: Increased richness and associations of bacterial genera with adipose tissue genes. *The American Journal of Clinical Nutrition* 98:16–24.

137. Zhang H, DiBaise JK, Zuccolo A, Kudrna D, Braidotti M, Yu Y, Parameswaran P, Crowell MD, Wing R, Rittmann BE, Krajmalnik-Brown R. 2009. Human gut microbiota in obesity and after gastric bypass. *Proceedings of the National Academy of Sciences of the United States of America* 106:2365–2370.

138. Furet JP, Kong LC, Tap J, Poitou C, Basdevant A, Bouillot JL, Mariat D, Corthier G, Dore J, Henegar C, Rizkalla S, Clement K. 2010. Differential adaptation of human gut microbiota to bariatric surgery-induced weight loss: Links with metabolic and low-grade inflammation markers. *Diabetes* 59:3049–3057.

139. Osto M, Abegg K, Bueter M, le Roux CW, Cani PD, Lutz TA. 2013. Roux-en-Y gastric bypass surgery in rats alters gut microbiota profile along the intestine. *Physiology & Behavior* 119:92–96.

140. Everard A, Belzer C, Geurts L, Ouwerkerk JP, Druart C, Bindels LB, Guiot Y, Derrien M, Muccioli GG, Delzenne NM, de Vos WM, Cani PD. 2013. Cross-talk between *Akkermansia muciniphila* and intestinal epithelium controls diet-induced obesity. *Proceedings of the National Academy of Sciences of the United States of America* 110:9066–9071.

141. Liou AP, Paziuk M, Luevano JM, Jr., Machineni S, Turnbaugh PJ, Kaplan LM. 2013. Conserved shifts in the gut microbiota due to gastric bypass reduce host weight and adiposity. *Science Translational Medicine* 5:178ra141.

142. Woodard GA, Encarnacion B, Downey JR, Peraza J, Chong K, Hernandez-Boussard T, Morton JM. 2009. Probiotics improve outcomes after Roux-en-Y gastric bypass surgery: a prospective randomized trial. *Journal of Gastrointestinal Surgery: Official Journal of the Society for Surgery of the Alimentary Tract* 13:1198–1204.

143. Menne E, Guggenbuhl N, Roberfroid M. 2000. Fn-type chicory inulin hydrolysate has a prebiotic effect in humans. *The Journal of Nutrition* 130:1197–1199.

144. Gibson GR, Beatty ER, Wang X, Cummings JH. 1995. Selective stimulation of bifidobacteria in the human colon by oligofructose and inulin. *Gastroenterology* 108:975–982.

145. 1991. NIH conference. Gastrointestinal surgery for severe obesity. Consensus Development Conference Panel. *Annals of Internal Medicine* 115:956–961.

146. Sghir A, Chow JM, Mackie RI. 1998. Continuous culture selection of bifidobacteria and lactobacilli from human faecal samples using fructooligosaccharide as selective substrate. *Journal of Applied Microbiology* 85:769–777.

147. Tuohy KM, Rouzaud GC, Bruck WM, Gibson GR. 2005. Modulation of the human gut microflora towards improved health using prebiotics—assessment of efficacy. *Current Pharmaceutical Design* 11:75–90.
148. Everard A, Lazarevic V, Derrien M, Girard M, Muccioli GG, Neyrinck AM, Possemiers S, Van Holle A, Francois P, de Vos WM, Delzenne NM, Schrenzel J, Cani PD. 2011. Responses of gut microbiota and glucose and lipid metabolism to prebiotics in genetic obese and diet-induced leptin-resistant mice. *Diabetes* 60:2775–2786.
149. Reimer RA, McBurney MI. 1996. Dietary fiber modulates intestinal proglucagon messenger ribonucleic acid and postprandial secretion of glucagon-like peptide-1 and insulin in rats. *Endocrinology* 137:3948–3956.
150. Belobrajdic DP, King RA, Christophersen CT, Bird AR. 2012. Dietary resistant starch dose-dependently reduces adiposity in obesity-prone and obesity-resistant male rats. *Nutrition & Metabolism* 9:93.
151. Keenan MJ, Zhou J, McCutcheon KL, Raggio AM, Bateman HG, Todd E, Jones CK, Tulley RT, Melton S, Martin RJ, Hegsted M. 2006. Effects of resistant starch, a non-digestible fermentable fiber, on reducing body fat. *Obesity* 14:1523–1534.
152. Cani PD, Hoste S, Guiot Y, Delzenne NM. 2007. Dietary non-digestible carbohydrates promote L-cell differentiation in the proximal colon of rats. *The British Journal of Nutrition* 98:32–37.
153. Zhou J, Martin RJ, Tulley RT, Raggio AM, McCutcheon KL, Shen L, Danna SC, Tripathy S, Hegsted M, Keenan MJ. 2008. Dietary resistant starch upregulates total GLP-1 and PYY in a sustained day-long manner through fermentation in rodents. *American Journal of Physiology Endocrinology and Metabolism* 295:E1160–E1166.
154. Parnell JA, Reimer RA. 2012. Prebiotic fibres dose-dependently increase satiety hormones and alter Bacteroidetes and Firmicutes in lean and obese JCR:LA-cp rats. *The British Journal of Nutrition* 107:601–613.
155. Cani PD, Neyrinck AM, Fava F, Knauf C, Burcelin RG, Tuohy KM, Gibson GR, Delzenne NM. 2007. Selective increases of bifidobacteria in gut microflora improve high-fat-diet-induced diabetes in mice through a mechanism associated with endotoxaemia. *Diabetologia* 50:2374–2383.
156. Piche T, des Varannes SB, Sacher-Huvelin S, Holst JJ, Cuber JC, Galmiche JP. 2003. Colonic fermentation influences lower esophageal sphincter function in gastroesophageal reflux disease. *Gastroenterology* 124:894–902.
157. Freeland KR, Wilson C, Wolever TM. 2010. Adaptation of colonic fermentation and glucagon-like peptide-1 secretion with increased wheat fibre intake for 1 year in hyperinsulinaemic human subjects. *The British Journal of Nutrition* 103:82–90.
158. Cani PD, Lecourt E, Dewulf EM, Sohet FM, Pachikian BD, Naslain D, De Backer F, Neyrinck AM, Delzenne NM. 2009. Gut microbiota fermentation of prebiotics increases satietogenic and incretin gut peptide production with consequences for appetite sensation and glucose response after a meal. *The American Journal of Clinical Nutrition* 90:1236–1243.
159. Tarini J, Wolever TM. 2010. The fermentable fibre inulin increases postprandial serum short-chain fatty acids and reduces free-fatty acids and ghrelin in healthy subjects. *Applied Physiology, Nutrition, and Metabolism* 35:9–16.
160. Verhoef SP, Meyer D, Westerterp KR. 2011. Effects of oligofructose on appetite profile, glucagon-like peptide 1 and peptide YY3-36 concentrations and energy intake. *The British Journal of Nutrition* 106:1757–1762.
161. Parnell JA, Reimer RA. 2009. Weight loss during oligofructose supplementation is associated with decreased ghrelin and increased peptide YY in overweight and obese adults. *The American Journal of Clinical Nutrition* 89:1751–1759.
162. Nilsson AC, Ostman EM, Holst JJ, Bjorck IM. 2008. Including indigestible carbohydrates in the evening meal of healthy subjects improves glucose tolerance, lowers inflammatory markers, and increases satiety after a subsequent standardized breakfast. *The Journal of Nutrition* 138:732–739.
163. Odstrcil EA, Martinez JG, Santa Ana CA, Xue B, Schneider RE, Steffer KJ, Porter JL, Asplin J, Kuhn JA, Fordtran JS. 2010. The contribution of malabsorption to the reduction in net energy absorption after long-limb Roux-en-Y gastric bypass. *The American Journal of Clinical Nutrition* 92:704–713.
164. Arakawa M, Ebato C, Mita T, Fujitani Y, Shimizu T, Watada H, Kawamori R, Hirose T. 2008. Miglitol suppresses the postprandial increase in interleukin 6 and enhances active glucagon-like peptide 1 secretion in viscerally obese subjects. *Metabolism: Clinical and Experimental* 57:1299–1306.
165. Tolhurst G, Heffron H, Lam YS, Parker HE, Habib AM, Diakogiannaki E, Cameron J, Grosse J, Reimann F, Gribble FM. 2012. Short-chain fatty acids stimulate glucagon-like peptide-1 secretion via the G-protein-coupled receptor FFAR2. *Diabetes* 61:364–371.

166. Kaji I, Karaki S, Tanaka R, Kuwahara A. 2011. Density distribution of free fatty acid receptor 2 (FFA2)-expressing and GLP-1-producing enteroendocrine L cells in human and rat lower intestine, and increased cell numbers after ingestion of fructo-oligosaccharide. *Journal of Molecular Histology* 42:27–38.
167. Cani PD, Knauf C, Iglesias MA, Drucker DJ, Delzenne NM, Burcelin R. 2006. Improvement of glucose tolerance and hepatic insulin sensitivity by oligofructose requires a functional glucagon-like peptide 1 receptor. *Diabetes* 55:1484–1490.
168. Laurenius A, Larsson I, Bueter M, Melanson KJ, Bosaeus I, Forslund HB, Lonroth H, Fandriks L, Olbers T. 2012. Changes in eating behaviour and meal pattern following Roux-en-Y gastric bypass. *International Journal of Obesity* 36:348–355.
169. Laferrère B. 2012. Gut feelings about diabetes. *Endocrinologia y Nutricion: Organo de la Sociedad Espanola de Endocrinologia y Nutricion* 59:254–260.
170. Kokkinos A, le Roux CW, Alexiadou K, Tentolouris N, Vincent RP, Kyriaki D, Perrea D, Ghatei MA, Bloom SR, Katsilambros N. 2010. Eating slowly increases the postprandial response of the anorexigenic gut hormones, peptide YY and glucagon-like peptide-1. *The Journal of Clinical Endocrinology and Metabolism* 95:333–337.
171. Lemmens SG, Martens EA, Born JM, Martens MJ, Westerterp-Plantenga MS. 2011. Staggered meal consumption facilitates appetite control without affecting postprandial energy intake. *The Journal of Nutrition* 141:482–488.
172. Zheng H, Shin AC, Lenard NR, Townsend RL, Patterson LM, Sigalet DL, Berthoud HR. 2009. Meal patterns, satiety, and food choice in a rat model of Roux-en-Y gastric bypass surgery. *American Journal of Physiology Regulatory, Integrative and Comparative Physiology* 297:R1273–R1282.
173. Jackson SJ, Leahy FE, Jebb SA, Prentice AM, Coward WA, Bluck LJ. 2007. Frequent feeding delays the gastric emptying of a subsequent meal. *Appetite* 48:199–205.
174. Leidy HJ, Armstrong CL, Tang M, Mattes RD, Campbell WW. 2010. The influence of higher protein intake and greater eating frequency on appetite control in overweight and obese men. *Obesity* 18:1725–1732.
175. Speechly DP, Buffenstein R. 1999. Greater appetite control associated with an increased frequency of eating in lean males. *Appetite* 33:285–297.
176. Speechly DP, Rogers GG, Buffenstein R. 1999. Acute appetite reduction associated with an increased frequency of eating in obese males. *International Journal of Obesity and Related Metabolic Disorders: Journal of the International Association for the Study of Obesity* 23:1151–1159.
177. Taylor MA, Garrow JS. 2001. Compared with nibbling, neither gorging nor a morning fast affect short-term energy balance in obese patients in a chamber calorimeter. *International Journal of Obesity and Related Metabolic Disorders: Journal of the International Association for the Study of Obesity* 25:519–528.
178. Munsters MJ, Saris WH. 2012. Effects of meal frequency on metabolic profiles and substrate partitioning in lean healthy males. *PloS One* 7:e38632.
179. Smeets AJ, Westerterp-Plantenga MS. 2008. Acute effects on metabolism and appetite profile of one meal difference in the lower range of meal frequency. *The British Journal of Nutrition* 99:1316–1321.
180. Alam ML, Van der Schueren BJ, Ahren B, Wang GC, Swerdlow NJ, Arias S, Bose M, Gorroochurn P, Teixeira J, McGinty J, Laferrère B. 2011. Gastric bypass surgery, but not caloric restriction, decreases dipeptidyl peptidase-4 activity in obese patients with type 2 diabetes. *Diabetes, Obesity & Metabolism* 13:378–381.
181. Hansen CF, Bueter M, Theis N, Lutz T, Paulsen S, Dalboge LS, Vrang N, Jelsing J. 2013. Hypertrophy dependent doubling of L-cells in Roux-en-Y gastric bypass operated rats. *PloS One* 8:e65696.
182. le Roux CW, Borg C, Wallis K, Vincent RP, Bueter M, Goodlad R, Ghatei MA, Patel A, Bloom SR, Aylwin SJ. 2010. Gut hypertrophy after gastric bypass is associated with increased glucagon-like peptide 2 and intestinal crypt cell proliferation. *Annals of Surgery* 252:50–56.

12 Medical Obesity Management

Lisa Marie DeRosimo

According to the National Health and Nutrition Examination Survey (NHANES 2009–2010), about a third of United States adults are classified as obese [1]. These individuals have a body mass index (BMI) ≥ 30. The goal of this chapter is to review the current medical interventions for obesity management. Numerous books have been published on this topic alone. This brief chapter seeks to offer esoteric strategies for the clinician who is evaluating and treating patients with obesity. First, dietary interventions will be reviewed, followed by a discussion of the role of physical activity in weight management. Then, adjunct therapies including behavior modification and pharmacological interventions will be discussed. Finally, a summary of how to apply these therapies in a clinical setting will be provided.

The benefits of mild weight loss (5–10% of initial weight) have been found to improve numerous disease processes, although few longitudinal studies have been completed [2]. However, a study by Dr. Foster and colleagues [3] shows that obese subjects have unrealistic expectations for their goal weight. When asked about their desired weight loss goal, 38% was the amount needed for subjects to reach their dream weight, while weight loss of 17% would be a disappointment for them. Thus, there is a gap between medically significant and personally significant weight loss. In order to minimize this discrepancy, it is helpful to remember and remind the patient of the three goals of weight management. These goals are to prevent further weight gain, to lower body weight by at least 5%, and then to maintain the lower body weight for the rest of their lives.

The traditional understanding of obesity is that more energy is taken in than is expended over a long period of time [4]. The excess calories that are consumed lead to an accumulation of body fat. In general, ingesting 3500 calories more than expended will lead to a gain of approximately 1 pound of fat. However, obesity is a disease with diverse etiologies for this energy mismatch [5]. There is an influence of both genetic and environmental factors. Prenatal influences can include genetics, race, ethnicity, and in utero environment. After birth, environmental issues like socioeconomic level, infant feeding history, education level, food sensitivities, sedentary lifestyle, hormonal imbalances, sleep disorders, medication-induced weight gain, eating disorders, and an obesity-prone environment contribute to the problem of excess weight gain.

In terms of genetics, if one parent is obese, there is a 50% chance of a child being obese. If both parents are obese, the probability rises to 80% [6]. In one overfeeding study, weight gain varied greatly among 12 monozygotic twin pairs who were chronically overfed 1000 kcal/day [7]. However, weight gain was very similar between each member of a twin pair. Though less common, there are also genetic mutations that cause obesity [8].

It is important to do a thorough medical evaluation, in order to discern the etiology of the obesity and to tailor the therapy to the patient. An appropriate medical history for evaluation of the obese patient should include the following: history of weight gain, previous weight loss attempts, anorectic use, psychiatric history, dietary history, exercise history, past medical history, family history, social history, and obesity-related review of systems. The physical examination of the obese patient should include vital signs; obesity parameters (weight, height, neck and waist circumference, and percentage of body fat); as well as a comprehensive physical exam. A thorough laboratory exam should also be done, which may include complete blood count (CBC); comprehensive metabolic panel; thyroid panel (TSH, free T3, free T4); lipids (cholesterol, triglycerides, LDL, HDL); fasting insulin; 2 h postprandial glucose; urinalysis; and 25-hydroxy vitamin D level. An electrocardiogram should be performed, if coronary or metabolic risk factors are present. Further screening may also include a sleep study or resting metabolic rate evaluation [9–12].

After the comprehensive evaluation is completed, therapy can be created that best suits the patient's profile. First, an appropriate eating plan should be prescribed. The role of dietary intervention is to provide a diet that will reduce the amount of energy consumed. In theory, this will tip the energy balance equation in favor of weight loss. The ideal diet for long-term weight management is unknown. Given the plethora of studies, it may be reasonable to recognize that the best diet is the one that is most effective and sustainable for the patient.

When it comes to prescribing a diet for the patient, there are a few points to keep in mind. Diet is the most important part of a weight management program. Patients will need to make food choices for the rest of their lives. Education on basic nutritional principles can be beneficial for long-term relapse prevention, which is reviewed later in this chapter. The 2010 United States Dietary Goals (USDG) [13] recommend consuming a diet with 45–65% calories from carbohydrate, 10–35% calories from protein, and 20–35% calories from fat. Foods have different energy contents based on their macronutrient composition [14]. A customized nutritional plan can be created, based upon individual eating patterns, food likes, and food dislikes noted in the medical history.

Weight loss diets can be classified into several categories: starvation diet (0–200 kcal/day), very-low-calorie diet (VLCD)/protein-sparing modified fast, low-calorie diet (800–1500 kcal/day), balanced deficit diet (reduction of 500 or more kcal/day), and self-directed and fad diets. Starvation diets are never prescribed in the current medical community. Often, patients will admit to fasting for 1 or more days, in their previous weight loss attempts. The terms *VLCD* and *protein-sparing modified fast* may be used interchangeably. VLCDs contain less than 800 kcal/day from either a liquid source or lean protein sources [4]. There are many commercial formulas available, or store-bought foods can be used with proper planning. The results are excellent for quick weight loss needs. VLCDs have been found to be safe, in an appropriate medical setting with adequate patient monitoring [15].

The best candidates for VLCD have obesity in the presence of immediate and urgent health problems that may be lessened by weight loss. The patient should be obese (BMI > 30) and ideally needs to lose 30 or more pounds. Being overweight (BMI ≥ 27) is an acceptable criterion, if comorbidities are present. Often, a VLCD is used before surgery, in order to achieve quick weight loss. A screening electrocardiogram (EKG) is recommended before use of a VLCD (Table 12.1).

TABLE 12.1
Contraindications for the Use of VLCD

Absolute Contraindications for VLCD

Type 1 diabetes	High-risk job
Epilepsy	Arrhythmias
Recent infarction	Psychosis
Substance abuse	Pregnancy/lactation
Unstable medical disease	Age over 70 years
BMI under 30	

Relative Contraindications for VLCD

Congestive heart failure	Transient ischemic attack
DVT	NSAID use
Severe psychiatric illness	Lithium use
Age under 16 years	

Note: DVT, deep venous thrombosis; NSAID, non-steroidal anti-inflammatory drug.

The typical composition of a VLCD is 400–800 kcal/day with 75–105 g/day protein (1.5 g/kg ideal body weight [IBW] men, 1.2 g/kg IBW women); 50–100 g/day carbohydrate; and 10–20 g/day fat. Vitamin and mineral supplementation is usually necessary. Recommended levels are as follows: potassium, 25 mEq/day; calcium, 200–1000 mg/day; sodium, 2–3 g/day; water/fluid, >2 L/day; and a multivitamin with at least 100% of the recommended daily allowance. Serious health complications can range from constitutional symptoms to gastrointestinal (gall stones, malaise) and electrolyte imbalance; essential fatty acid deficiency; skin, hair, and nail changes; amenorrhea; and gout. Psychological issues can also develop. These diets are for short-term use, typically less than 24 weeks and with diligent medical supervision.

Monitoring during the use of VLCDs is mandatory. An initial history; physical; labs (CBC, comprehensive metabolic panel, lipids, TSH); and EKG should be performed. Weekly office visits are advised. Frequent electrolyte checks should be performed as well as a CBC every 3 months. A rhythm strip is recommended with each 30 pounds of weight loss. Weight-sensitive medications (i.e., Coumadin, insulin, hyperglycemic agents, digoxin, antidepressants, lithium) should be closely monitored and adjusted as needed.

A low-calorie diet provides caloric restriction typically to the amount between 1000 and 1200 kcal/day for women and 1200–1600 kcal/day for men. Types of low-calorie diets include calorie-reduced/balanced diets (counting calories or points), portion-controlled diets (use of some pre-packaged foods), low-fat diets (counting fat grams), and low-carbohydrate diets (carbohydrates restricted). In contrast, balanced deficit diets, provide less restriction than low-calorie diets. Calories typically are reduced by 500–1000 calories daily. Macronutrients are generally 15% protein, 55% carbohydrate, 30% fat, based on US dietary goals [4].

There are also a wide variety of other diets that have been studied for weight loss. Mediterranean, ketogenic, dietary approaches to stop hypertension (DASH), and low glycemic index are a few examples. The dilemma is that no single diet has been found that provides superior long-term weight control [16]. A study was done to compare weight loss on Atkins, Ornish, Zone, and Weight Watchers diets. Adherence was best when initial weight loss was quickest. However, long-term results and drop-out were similar between the four groups.

In practice, setting a reasonable goal provides the most benefit for the patient. The focus should be on 5–10% weight loss. When that goal is achieved, a new goal of 5–10% weight loss can be set. Simple plans are easier to implement and maintain. Food diaries are a wonderful tool to help with tracking caloric intake, and they will be discussed further in the section on behavior modification. Nutrition education can give patients autonomy to make food choices, after their weight loss phase is completed.

After implementing an appropriate diet, physical activity should be considered for the weight management plan. In regard to the role of physical activity in long-term weight management, the data are mixed. It seems reasonable that activity would benefit the energy balance equation by increasing energy expenditure. However, numerous studies have been conducted, and the results are often confusing and frustrating for the person seeking to lose weight [17]. The 2007 American Heart Association Position Statement on Physical Activity and Public Health provides a summary of the role of physical activity in weight loss. "Despite the intuitive appeal of the idea that physical activity helps in losing weight, it appears to produce only modest increments of weight loss beyond those achieved by dietary measures and its effects no doubt vary among people" [18].

Physical activity can be described as exercise and nonexercise activities [19]. Exercise is defined as physical activity that is planned or structured. Repetitive movements are orchestrated to improve physical fitness. Nonexercise activity is physical activity involving nonvolitional exercise. These movements lead to nonexercise activity thermogenesis (NEAT). NEAT has been explored for weight management, as it provides a means of calorie expenditure without the restraints of a regular exercise routine. NEAT is also referred to as lifestyle activity. It is helpful to implement NEAT in a patient's treatment plan, as NEAT can be an important source of total energy expenditure. Individual variation in NEAT varies as much as tenfold [20] (Table 12.2).

TABLE 12.2

Examples of NEAT

Park car further away

Use stairs instead of elevator

Avoid moving platforms

Fidget or pace while talking on phone

House cleaning

Initiating a physical activity intervention has associated risks. However, prevention of musculo-skeletal injury, arrhythmia, and sudden cardiac death (induced by vigorous physical activity) can be reduced by proper screening and appropriate activity prescription. Stress testing is recommended, prior to starting a vigorous-intensity plan in asymptomatic males over 45 years old and asymptomatic females over 55 years old. Asymptomatic persons with diabetes or metabolic syndrome should also be considered for additional screening [18].

A physical activity prescription should consider several points. First, assess the current level of activity (which activity, frequency, duration) as well as past activity level (i.e., college sports) and favorite activities of the patient. Barriers to exercise (medical, physical, social, family) may be present, and the patient may be reluctant to begin a program. Identifying and offering realistic alternatives is essential for incorporating activity into the weight management plan.

The perfect activity regimen is unknown. The best time for exercise is the most convenient time for the patient. It is more important to exercise regularly than be concerned about whether morning or evening is more effective [18,21]. The patient should decide what exercise, what time, and what location work best, while the clinician documents specifics for accountability. Use of a specific exercise prescription noting the frequency, time, and duration may improve compliance. Combining some aerobic (cardiovascular fitness) and anaerobic (basal metabolic rate) activities are most beneficial [20]. A physical activity prescription should include the type of activity, time, frequency, intensity, and enjoyment level. Writing the prescription or setting up an activity contract with the patient can improve compliance.

The question arises as to how much activity is enough. According to the United States Department of Health and Human Services (USDHHS), general health will benefit from moderate aerobic exercise (150 min/week) and strength training. Prevention of weight gain and acute weight loss requires 150–300 min/week of aerobic activity, and prevention of weight regain in the maintenance phase requires 200–420 min/week [22,23]. These numbers can be daunting to an obese sedentary patient, and it is important to recognize this barrier to success. When prescribing a physical activity plan, it is prudent to start slow and increase the time and frequency incrementally. Low- or no-impact activities such as aqua classes or water walking are helpful for beginners. Recumbent bikes or chair exercises can also provide a safe and easy starting point. Balance training and strength training with light weights or bands can also provide success that will encourage the patient to pursue more challenging activities as they lose weight, gain strength, and improve endurance.

According to the National Weight Control Registry (NWCR) [24,25], activity is an integral part of long-term weight management. Setting the right activity behaviors early in the treatment plan can facilitate and improve transition to the maintenance phase. A physical activity plan that is most realistic for your patient will be the most sustainable in the long term.

An adjunct to the foundation of a proper eating plan and activity prescription is pharmacotherapy. The ideal pharmaceutical agent would be specific for weight loss and have no abuse potential. It would decrease hunger or increase satiety and increase thermogenesis. There would be no significant side effects, and it could be used for the long term. The drug would also be affordable. To date, this medication has yet to be discovered. The goal of this section is to review the pharmacologic options available for the clinician today. Medications that are not available in the United States will be briefly mentioned, but they have no significant role currently in the choice of a pharmacologic therapy. However, it is beneficial to be aware of these agents, as many patients may have used them in the past.

When considering the use of medications, it is important to understand the risks and benefits. It is also important to discuss these risks and benefits with the patient and assure their understanding. Risks may be minimized when the medications are used properly with close medical supervision. It is prudent to use a consent form, which is signed by the patient. This consent form would illustrate the patients' awareness of the risks and their decision to pursue pharmacotherapy [9].

At present, there are no universally acceptable criteria for prescribing antiobesity medications. Etiology of the obesity and comorbidities varies extensively. It is the clinician's duty to determine the best pharmacologic choice. Prescribing guidelines established by the American Society of Bariatric Physicians (ASBP) [9] suggest the following parameters for deciding to use an anorectic agent. BMI should be ≥30 in a healthy patient. BMI can be ≥27, when comorbidities are present. Other indications for use include body weight > 120% of well-documented long-standing healthy weight after the age of 18 years, body fat > 30% for females, body fat > 25% in males, waist or waist/hip ratio presenting increased cardiovascular risks, or comorbid condition aggravated by the patient's excess adiposity. These guidelines also suggest that anorectic agents may be used to prevent weight regain after successful weight loss or as a prevention of weight gain in patients with a familial predisposition to obesity and its comorbidities.

The first class of antiobesity drugs that will be reviewed are those that decrease energy intake. This class of medications acts in the central nervous system. Their mechanism of action is to alter release and reuptake of neurotransmitters involved in appetite (norepinephrine, serotonin, and dopamine) [26]. Currently available appetite suppressants in this class are phentermine, diethylpropion, benzphetamine, and phendimetrazine. These anorectic agents are approved by the Food and Drug Administration (FDA) for short-term use in combination with lifestyle changes in adults with a BMI > 30 or BMI > 27 with comorbidities. They decrease food intake and increase resting energy expenditure. Phentermine and diethylpropion are chemically related to amphetamines [27]. Phentermine and diethylpropion are Drug Enforcement Administration (DEA) schedule IV controlled substances, indicating a relatively low potential for abuse [28]. Phendimetrazine and benzphetamine are class III of the DEA schedule, suggesting a greater risk for addiction potential. Mazindol and phenylpropanolamine are other agents in this class that are not currently available in the United States. Absolute contraindications to use of these sympathicomimetic agents are advanced arteriosclerosis, coronary artery disease, moderate/severe hypertension, hyperthyroidism, glaucoma, agitation, drug abuse, and pregnancy. Adverse effects of use may include headache, dry mouth, constipation or diarrhea, insomnia, restlessness and euphoria, palpitations, tachycardia, hypertension and cardiac arrhythmias, dizziness, blurred vision or ocular irritation, and impotence or decreased libido. In practice, these medications have been found to be safe in the treatment of obesity. There is little or no risk of abuse [9], and this class is the oldest class of antiobesity agents available today.

Serotonin-based appetite suppressants include fluoxetine, chlorphentermine, fenfluramine, and dexfenfluramine. None of these drugs are currently FDA approved for weight loss. Dopaminergic agents include amphetamines like methylphenidate and dextroamphetamine. These are DEA schedule II controlled substances. They exert their action by inhibiting dopamine reuptake. Adverse effects may include agitation, insomnia, tachycardia, and hypertension. These agents have abuse potential, and they are not recommended or approved for obesity management. Sibutramine is a medication that inhibits both norepinephrine and serotonin reuptake. Individuals on sibutramine with a higher risk for cardiovascular disease were found to have a greater incidence of cardiovascular events than those individuals on placebo medication [29]. It was voluntarily withdrawn from use in 2010.

Bupropion [30] is an antidepressant that inhibits both norepinephrine and dopamine reuptake. It is structurally similar to the appetite suppressant diethylpropion. Bupropion is currently FDA approved in the treatment of depression, attention deficit/hyperactivity disorder (ADHD), and smoking cessation. Bupropion is not approved as a primary antiobesity agent, though it may be a useful adjunct for patients with a dual diagnosis of depression, ADHD, or tobacco use. Side effects include allergic reaction, anxiety, confusion, seizure, dry mouth, nausea, headache, and dizziness. As this drug may lower the seizure threshold, it should not be used in patients with bulimia. Bupropion may also worsen symptoms of anxiety in some individuals.

Two new drugs have recently been approved by the FDA for obesity therapy. Lorcaserin is a selective 5-HT2C receptor agonist that inhibits feeding behavior primarily by central nervous system action [31]. Side effects include headache, nausea, and dizziness. The FDA approved lorcaserin in June 2012 to treat adults with BMI ≥ 30 or ≥ 27 in the presence of at least one comorbidity. Although lorcaserin use was not associated with valvular diseases in its placebo-controlled trials, it was recommended to be used with caution in patients with congestive heart failure. If the patient does not lose ≥5% of baseline body weight after 12 weeks, locaserin should be discontinued.

The second new antiobesity medication, Qsymia, is a combination of two medications available today (topiramate and phentermine) [32]. In July 2012, the FDA approved phentermine plus extended-release topiramate in combination with diet and physical activity for treatment of obesity among adults with BMI ≥ 30 or ≥ 27 and at least one obesity-related comorbidity. Topiramate is an FDA-approved anticonvulsant medication with a side effect of weight loss. Topiramate is also currently approved for migraine prophylaxis. Topiramate is not approved as a monotherapy in obesity. It acts centrally to enhance GABA-evoked current. Topiramate also blockades sodium and calcium ion channels in the periphery. Its mechanism of action for weight loss is unknown. Common adverse events include paresthesias, short-term memory loss, taste impairment, and sedation. Metabolic acidosis and glaucoma are rare but real potential side effects. Bicarbonate levels should be monitored regularly, during the use of topiramate [33].

When low-dose, controlled-release phentermine was combined with topiramate in large randomized controlled trials, the subjects lost significantly more weight than those on a placebo over a 56-week period [34]. The most common adverse events were dry mouth, paresthesias, constipation, insomnia, dizziness, tachycardia, hypertension, and dysgeusia. Qsymia carries a warning of potential congenital abnormalities during the first trimester of gestation. A risk evaluation and mitigation strategy (REMS) is in place that restricts prescribing to trained clinicians. Documentation of effective contraception and monthly pregnancy tests for reproductive-age women is required. It is currently available only by mail-order pharmacy. The company is also required to carry out a long-term cardiovascular outcomes trial.

There are also antiobesity medications that affect digestion. Orlistat was approved by the FDA in 2003, and it may be prescribed for up to 4 years for weight loss or maintenance in adults. It is the only antiobesity agent approved for use in obese adolescents [35]. Orlistat acts by inhibiting gastric and pancreatic lipases. It reduces the absorption of approximately 30% of ingested dietary fat within 2 h of a meal. Orlistat needs to be used in accordance with a low-fat, calorie-controlled diet. Supplementation with a daily multivitamin is critical because orlistat leads to decreased absorption of fat-soluble vitamins [36]. The vitamin should be taken at least 2 h prior to the use of orlistat.

The most common adverse events with orlistat are oily stool, oily spotting, oily evacuation, abdominal pain, and fecal urgency. Elevated liver enzymes and vitamin malabsorption are potential adverse effects. Orlistat should not be prescribed to patients with cholestasis, liver disease, or chronic malabsorption. The withdrawal rate is as high as 35% in clinical trials, secondary to undesirable side effects. A lower dose of orlistat was approved as an over-the-counter medication for obese adults in 2007. The recommended dosing on a three-times-a-day regimen is a significant limitation to the wide use of this agent. A similar-acting medication, cetilistat, is currently in clinical trials (Table 12.3).

Acarbose is an agent that competitively and reversibly inhibits pancreatic α-amylase and intestinal α-glucosidase in the intestinal brush border [37]. This delays carbohydrate absorption, leading to lower postprandial insulin and glucose levels. Acarbose is approved for diabetes treatment, and it produces small weight losses in some studies. Acarbose is not approved for monotherapy for obesity. Side effects include abdominal pain, diarrhea, and flatulence.

TABLE 12.3
FDA Approved Obesity Agents and Their Dosages

	Method of Action	Dosage
Phentermine	Decrease energy intake	15–37.5 mg po qd
Diethylpropion	Decrease energy intake	25–75 mg po qd
Benzphetamine	Decrease energy intake	25–50 mg po tid prn
Phendimetrazine	Decrease energy intake	35–105 mg po qd
Qsymia	Decrease energy intake	3.75/23–15/92 mg po qd
Locaserin	Decrease energy intake	10 mg po q 12 h
Orlistat	Lipase inhibitor	60–120 mg po TID prn

There are several other agents available for the treatment of diabetes that also have weight loss efficacy. None are available as monotherapy for the treatment of obesity. They are all useful adjuncts for obese patients with the comorbidity of diabetes. Metformin is a biguanide that inhibits intestinal glucose absorption, reduces hepatic glucose production, and increases insulin sensitivity in peripheral insulin-targeted tissues [38]. Metformin induces modest weight loss and improves fertility in polycystic ovary syndrome. Metformin is approved for the treatment of type 2 diabetes in adults and children over the age of 10 years. It may have an effect in diabetes prevention and is recommended for use in metabolic syndrome. The main adverse effects of metformin are diarrhea, nausea, vomiting, and flatulence. Metformin is contraindicated in renal failure, secondary to the risk of metabolic acidosis. Metformin should be withheld in critically ill patients and when imaging contrast agents are administered.

Amylin is a pancreatic β-cell hormone that reduces food intake, slows gastric emptying, and reduces postprandial glucagon secretion. Pramlintide, a synthetic analog of amylin, is approved for the treatment of both type 1 and type 2 diabetes. It produces small weight losses in obese and diabetic adults [39]. Adverse effects are nausea and abdominal discomfort. This medication is not approved for monotherapy for obesity; however, it may be a useful agent in obese patients with diabetes.

Incretin hormones such as glucagon-like peptide-1 (GLP-1) agonists simulate glucoregulatory actions of mammalian glucagon-like peptide 1. This includes enhanced glucose-dependent insulin release, suppression of inappropriate glucagon release, delayed gastric emptying, and reduction in food intake through direct central action on receptors in the hypothalamus and area postrema [40,41]. Exenatide and liraglutide, GLP-1 analogs, are approved by the FDA for adjunct treatment of type 2 diabetes mellitus in adults. Weight loss is a side effect of the therapy; however, they are not approved for use in obesity therapy alone. Side effects include nausea, vomiting, diarrhea, dyspepsia, headache, and hypoglycemia. They are contraindicated in severe renal impairment or patients with a history of pancreatitis or gastroparesis.

There are currently no medications augmenting energy expenditure that are approved for clinical use in the treatment of obesity. Thermogenic agents are appealing in theory, as they would increase metabolic rate by adrenergic mechanisms [42]. Thyroid hormones can increase energy expenditure but only when given in doses that cause hyperthyroidism. Thus, thyroid hormone treatments are not recommended or approved for weight loss. Ephedrine, a drug that increases release of norepinephrine, exerts an effect on beta 3 noradrenergic receptors. The thermogenic effects of ephedrine can be increased when methylxanthines such as caffeine (which inhibit phosphodiesterases) are used in combination with ephedrine. Side effects include tremor, nervousness, insomnia, and increased blood pressure and pulse. Ephedrine was banned by the FDA in 2004.

Pharmacologic agents that may be available in the future include tesofensine, a triple monoamine reuptake inhibitor, cannabinoid (CB) receptor inhibitors, and gut-derived hormones (ghrelin).

Combination therapies also show promise for efficacy in the long-term management of obesity. Naltrexone and bupropion or zonisamide and bupropion are some combinations being tested clinical trials at present.

In summary, numerous studies have been done in search of the ideal anorectic agent. This agent has not yet been identified. There are several agents that are useful for the clinician, as part of a comprehensive weight management program. The success of weight loss agents, independent of diet, activity, and behavior interventions, is too small to recommend their use exclusively. Tailoring the pharmacotherapy to the patient's comorbidities can be a very useful addition for the overall weight management plan. Many agents have been banned secondary to concerns of long-term adverse consequences. It is prudent to thoroughly review the risk/benefit profile with each patient before beginning therapy. A comprehensive informed-consent form is recommended for each patient prescribed an antiobesity agent. The clinician should be familiar with the DEA regulations, state medical board regulations, and the ASBP standards of care for prescribing appetite suppressants. Standards of care vary by state. Antiobesity agents can be a useful adjunct to modification of diet, activity, and lifestyle. However, these agents must be prescribed cautiously and carefully monitored for efficacy and side effects.

The last component of a comprehensive medical weight loss program that will be discussed is behavior therapy. The goal of behavior therapy is to identify areas of difficulty through self-monitoring. Techniques to replace maladaptive behaviors with behaviors that promote weight control are taught to the patient. A behavioral or lifestyle assessment can investigate the nutritional patterns, work schedule, family situation, social connections, and exercise habits of the patient. The tools used to complete a behavior assessment include the following: intake questionnaires, food diaries, exercise logs, and depression and anxiety scales. Lifestyle assessment may also assess onset of obesity (rapid or gradual); time frame (childhood, puberty, pregnancy, menopause); and major life changes. It is often beneficial to directly ask the patient: "Why do you think you gained weight?"

When evaluating the patient initially, common mental disorders should be assessed. A mental status exam can illuminate potential barriers to treatment such as undiagnosed psychiatric illness or difficulties with judgment or impulse control. Untreated psychiatric illnesses that will impair successful weight control include eating disorders, personality disorders, mood disorders, and anxiety and attention deficit disorders. There are numerous screening forms (i.e., Beck Depression Inventory) available for the clinician to detect mental illness.

Binge eating disorder is one mental illness that is very common. Thirty percent of weight control participants meet the criteria for diagnosis, and 50% of severely obese patients meet the criteria for diagnosis [43]. It is imperative for the clinician to distinguish between binge eating behaviors and overeating. Overeating occurs at social functions, and there is an abundance of food that is readily available. The mood is usually relaxed or positive, and other people are also overeating. In contrast, binge eating disorder is classified as occurring at least two times per week for at least 6 months, without purging or compensatory behavior. There is usually marked distress, guilt, or depressive feelings. The patient may also hide food or eat in secret. There is a sensation of being out of control. The patient may not be physically hungry throughout the day; thus, food deprivation and dieting are common triggers to binge [44]. A patient with an undiagnosed psychiatric illness will be less likely to respond to behavior therapy and change.

A person's decision to change a behavior is influenced by both the conscious and the subconscious mind [45]. The conscious mind holds wishes, desires, and aspirations (free will), while the subconscious mind is simply a stimulus–response reflex (habits, tendencies). Prochaska et al. [46] describe the stages of change, which progress from precontemplation, contemplation, preparation, and action through the maintenance phase. Patients exhibit signs of readiness to change when their conversation moves toward desires, reasons, needs, and steps to begin change. It is important to determine how ready, willing, and able a patient is to change. Signs of readiness include change talk, a resolve to succeed, questions about change, and envisioning and experimenting with change. Patients are resistant to change when they argue, interrupt, or ignore or negate the clinician's suggestions.

If the patient is in the early stage or precontemplation, the most important tools are to support the patient and provide information on the risks of obesity. When the patient is in the contemplation stage, giving more information on change and the benefits of weight loss can be helpful. Preparation and action are the phases when the patient is most ready to implement a plan of change. Setting small realistic goals, developing a plan of action, and rewarding success are key for long-term success. Behavior techniques are best utilized in the preparation and action phases. Maintenance is after weight loss has occurred, and patients are continuing their new habits into their lifestyle. Positive reinforcement of the new behaviors and continued accountability are useful in this stage as well as provides a contingency plan for any relapses to old habits.

It is beneficial to ascertain the motivators for weight management at the time of the physician/patient interview. For example, a patient may go to the clinician's office because his/her spouse forced them. The clinician's plan will be markedly different than that for a patient who wants to lose 30 pounds for his/her high school reunion in a month. A clinician needs to listen to the patient, discern his/her motivation, and formulate an appropriate plan of therapy. It is impossible to provide effective individualized treatment without understanding patients and their motivation.

A useful tool to implement behavioral change is motivational interviewing. Motivational interviewing emphasizes the patient's personal choices and control of the decision of what to do [43,47]. There is a partnership between the patient and clinician. The patient provides the reasons to change rather than the clinician. The goal of the clinician is to discover what motivates change in behavior and to find areas in the resistance to change that can be exploited. Four guiding principles of motivational interviewing are to resist the righting influence, to understand patient motivation, to listen to the patient, and to empower the patient. The righting influence is the desire to impose one's medical beliefs on the patient. This is not successful for long-term change. When the clinician listens to patients and strives to understand their motivations, then tools to empower change can be successfully implemented.

Behavioral therapies in obesity management derive from learning theory. The essence is to identify difficulties for the patient and target a treatment intervention to substitute adaptive responses that facilitate weight management. Components of the therapy include self-monitoring, goal setting, problem solving, contingency management, stimulus control, stress management, social support, cognitive restructuring, relapse prevention, and rewards [48].

After doing an initial assessment, the clinician should target problem areas for the patient. The treatment plan will include dietary changes, activity changes, possible medication changes, and behavior changes. It is most effective to target one area for success at a time. Set realistic goals for the patient and review them routinely. If patients feel overwhelmed, they are more likely to stop the program. Rewarding goal achievement and changed behavior can keep the patient motivated. It is important to realize that changing behavior is a process, and it will take effort on the patient's behalf. Close follow-up initially can enhance success.

The core of behavior therapy enables the patient to effectively solve problems, control tempting stimuli, restructure their thought processes, and utilize a contingency plan. The lifestyle exercise attitudes relationships nutrition (LEARN) program for weight management is one version of behavioral therapy available for clinicians [49]. As the clinician guides patients in behavior change, patients are better able to prevent relapsing to their former habits. Long-term stress management and a good social support network have also been found to be helpful in lifestyle change. The clinician is the conductor of this process. The goal is to identify areas of change, to offer methods that are helpful for the patient, and to keep the patient accountable. When new methods are used repeatedly, the method can become a habit. The goal is for the patient to replace maladaptive behavior with new ones that support weight loss and maintenance over the long term. Changing a habit takes time, and the amount of time to change is different for each person [50].

Behavioral therapies are most important for long-term relapse prevention. Sadly, 65% of successful "losers" regain some or all of the weight lost initially. Risk factors for weight regain include recent weight loss (within the last 2 years), larger weight losses (>30% maximum weight), depression, dietary disinhibition, binge eating disorder, decreased energy expenditure, increased calorie intake from fat, decreased eating restraint, and increased hunger [51]. Successful weight maintenance has been defined in several ways. Basically, weight maintenance is when at least 5% or more of initial weight is lost and maintained within 5–10 pounds for at least a year.

The NWCR, established in 1994, follows a large cohort of individuals prospectively who have achieved this weight loss success. The NWCR prospectively follows people who have successfully maintained at least a 30-pound weight loss for a year or longer. Their observations show that successful "losers" maintain a low-calorie, low-fat diet and a lifestyle with a high level of physical activity. Seventy-five percent of these individuals weigh weekly, and 90% exercise an hour a day [52]. Ninety-eight percent of these people utilize some form of portion control, and 78% eat breakfast daily. Physical activity is reported to be a significant component for weight loss, maintenance, and loss of any regained weight for these individuals. Strategies for success in these cohorts include monitoring systems and a weight buffer zone (no gain over 3 pounds). These individuals also have a plan of action for any weight regain. These individuals utilize techniques to manage stress effectively, and their overall attitude is positive.

In summary, behavioral therapies are integral to developing lifestyle changes that patients can use for long-term weight maintenance. Realistic goals and self-monitoring techniques are essential. Long-term accountability (small groups, weight checks, e-mails, phone calls) can facilitate long-term relapse prevention [51]. Documenting the patient's goals and tailoring the treatment to the individual patient enhances compliance. Food diaries and exercise logs are simple inexpensive methods to keep the patient accountable. Partial meal replacements may also facilitate long-term success. Controlling culprit stimuli (traveling, eating in restaurants, late night eating) and stress management techniques can also prevent relapse [53]. Changing the way patients think about themselves and the environment can be helpful. It is also prudent to create a contingency plan. Contracts and good social support are also tools for eliciting long-term lifestyle changes. Physical activity is essential for long-term weight management [52]. Weight management is a process, and lifestyle modification is the key to success.

Obesity is a complex mix of family, community, and societal issues. It is not solely an issue of personal responsibility. It is difficult to make good decisions in an environment where healthy options are not always available. Simple techniques to set patients up for success are multiple. Weight maintenance is often more challenging than weight loss. Sustainable lifestyle changes are required for long-term success. Prior maladaptive habits will not succeed, after a lower weight is reached. Eventually, the weight will be regained. Encouraging free enrollment with the NWCR is a simple way to maintain accountability for the patient. Periodic questionnaires are sent to patients, in order to assess their progress on a prospective basis.

The medical weight management program that is most sustainable is most likely to succeed. Good nutrition and physical activity are powerful therapies for long-term weight maintenance. Pharmacological intervention may enhance the efficacy of dietary, activity, and behavioral interventions. Frequent personal contact attenuates regain. Each patient is unique, so a "one-size-fits-all" treatment plan will not succeed in the long term. Listening to the patient can provide nearly all the information needed for a successful plan of therapy. In conclusion, the medical management of obesity is both an art and a science. There is no one perfect plan, and the relapse rate is high. However, listening to patients, holding them accountable to an individualized weight management plan, and encouraging their success can facilitate long-term change and improve their quality of life.

REFERENCES

1. CDC/NCHS. National health and nutrition examination survey, 2009–2010. Available at http://www.cdc.gov.nchs.data.
2. Bischoff SC, Damms-Machado A, Betz C, Herpertz S, Legenbauer T, Löw T, Wechsler JG, Bischoff G, Austel A, Ellrott T. Multicenter evaluation of an interdisciplinary 52-week weight loss program for obesity with regard to body weight, comorbidities and quality of life—a prospective study. *Int J Obes.* 2012;36(4):614–24.

3. Foster GD, Wadden TA, Vogt RA, Brewer G. What is a reasonable weight loss? Patient's expectations and evaluations of obesity treatment outcomes. *J Consult Clin Psychol.* 1997;65:79–85.

4. Bray G, Bouchard C. *Handbook of Obesity: Clinical Applications*, 3rd Edition. New York: Informa Healthcare and CRC Press New York, 2008.

5. National Institutes of Health. Available at http://nhlbi.nih.gov/health/health-topics/topics/obes/causes.html.

6. Whitaker RC, Wright JA, Pepe MS, Seidel KD, Dietz WH. Predicting obesity in young adulthood from childhood and parental obesity. *N Engl J Med.* 1997;337(13):869–73.

7. Bouchard C, Tremblay A, Despres JP, Nadeau A, Lupien PJ, Theriault G, Dussault J, Moorjani S, Pinault S, Fournier G. The response to long-term overfeeding in identical twins. *N Engl J Med.* 1990;322:1477–82.

8. Farooqi IS, O'Rahilly S. Monogenic obesity in humans. *Am Rev Med.* 2005;56:443–58.

9. American Society of Bariatric Physicians. Overweight and obesity evaluation and management, 2010. Available at http://www.asbp.org.

10. Bray GA. Classification and treatment of the obese patient. In: Bray GA, Bouchard C, eds. *Handbook of Obesity Evaluation and Treatment Essentials.* New York: Informa Healthcare, 2010:177–95.

11. Cooper JT. Evaluation of the obese patient. In: Steelman GM, Westman EC, eds. *Obesity: Evaluation and Treatment Essentials.* New York: Informa Healthcare, 2010:35–42.

12. Kushner RF, Aronne LJ. Obesity and the primary care physician. In: Bray G, Bouchard C, eds. *Handbook of Obesity: Clinical Applications*, 3rd Edition. New York: Informa Healthcare, 2008:117–29.

13. United States Dietary Goals, 2010. Available at http://fnic.nal.usda.gov/dietary-guides.

14. Mahan KL, Escott-Stump SE. *Krause's Food and Nutrition Therapy*, 12th Edition. Philadelphia, PA: WB Saunders, 2008.

15. Tsai AG, Wadden TA. The evolution of very-low-calorie diets: An update and meta-analysis. *Obesity* 2006;14:1283–93.

16. Dansinger ML, Gleason JA, Griffith JL, Selker HP, Schaefer EJ. Comparison of the Atkins, Ornish, Weight Watchers, and Zone diets for weight loss and heart disease risk reduction. *JAMA.* 2005;293(1):43–53.

17. Church T. Exercise and weight management. In: Bray G, Bouchard C, eds. *Handbook of Obesity: Clinical Applications*, 3rd Edition. New York: Informa Healthcare and CRC Press New York, 2008:291–302.

18. Thompson PD, Franklin BA, Balady GJ, Blair SN, Corrado D, Estes NA 3rd, Fulton JE, Gordon NF, Hassel WL, Link MS, Maron BJ, Mittleman MA, Peliccia A, Wenger NK, Willich SN, Costa F. Exercise and acute cardiovascular events: placing the risks into perspective: A scientific statement from the American Heart Association Council on nutrition, physical activity and metabolism and the council on clinical cardiology. *Circulation.* 2007;115:2358–68.

19. US Department of Health and Human Services. Physical activity and health: a report of the surgeon general. Atlanta. US Department of Health and Human Services Center for chronic disease prevention and health promotion, 1996. Available at http://www.cdc.gov/ncdphp/dnpa/physical/terms/index.htm.

20. Anderson RE, Wadden TA, Bartlett SJ, Zemel B, Verde TJ, Franckiowiak SC. Effects of lifestyle activity verses structured aerobic exercise in obese women. *JAMA.* 1999;281:335–40.

21. Meriweather RA, Lee JA. Physical activity counseling. *Am Fam Phys.* 2008;77:1129–36.

22. US Department of Health and Human Services. Physical activity guidelines for Americans, 2008. Available at http://www.health.gov/paguidelines/default.aspx.

23. Donnelly JE, Blair SN, Jakicic JM, Manore MM, Rankin JW, Smith BK. American College of Sports Medicine Position Stand. Appropriate physical activity intervention strategies for weight loss and prevention of weight regain for adults. *Med Sci Sports Exerc.* 2009;41(2):459–71.

24. Klem ML, Wing RR, McGuire MT, Seagle HM, Hill JO. A descriptive study of individuals successful at long term maintenance of substantial weight loss. *Am J Clin Nutr.* 1997;66(2):239–46.

25. Hill JO, Thompson H, Wyatt H. Weight maintenance: What's missing? *J Am Diet Assoc.* 2005;105(5 Suppl 1):S63–6.

26. Samanin R, Garattini S. Neurochemical mechanism of action of anorectic drugs. *Pharmacol Toxicol.* 1993;73:63–8.

27. Kaplan LM. Pharmacologic therapies for obesity. *Gastroenterol Clin North Am.* 2010;39:69–79.

28. Drug Enforcement Administration, Office of Diversion Control. List of scheduling actions controlled substances regulated chemicals, US Department of Justice 2014. Available at http://www.deadiversion.usdoj.gov/schedules.index.html.

29. James WP, Caterson ID, Coutinho W, Finer N, Van Gaal LF, Maggioni AP, Torp-Pedersen C, Sharma AM, Shepherd GM, Rode RA, Renz CL. Effect of sibutramine on cardiovascular outcomes in overweight and obese subjects. *N Eng J Med.* 2010;363:905–17.

30. Anderson JW, Greenway FL, Fujioka K, Gadde KM, McKenney J, O'Neil PM. Bupropion SR enhances weight loss: A 48-week double blind, placebo-controlled trial. *Obes Res.* 2002;10:633–41.

31. Martin CK, Redman LM, Zhang J, Sanchez M, Anderson CM, Smith SR, Ravussin E. Locaserin, a 5-HT(2c) receptor agonist, reduces body weight by decreasing energy intake without influencing energy expenditure. *J Clin Endocrinol Metab.* 2011;96:837–45.

32. Phentermine/Topiramate ER (prescribing information). Mountain View, CA: VIVUS Inc., July 2012. Available at http://www.qsymia.com.

33. Astrup A, Toubro S. Topimate. A new potential pharmacological treatment for obesity. *Obes Res.* 2004;12(Suppl):167s–73s.

34. Gadde KM, Allison DB, Ryan DH, Peterson CA, Troupin B, Schwiers ML, Day WW. Effects of low-dose, controlled release, phentermine plus topiramate combination on weight and associated comorbidities in overweight and obese adults (CONQUER): A randomized, placebo-controlled phase 3 extension study. *Lancet* 2011;377:1341–52.

35. Chanoine JP, Hampl S, Jensen G. Effect of orlistat on weight and body composition in obese adolescents. *JAMA.* 2005;293:2873–83.

36. McDuffe JR, Calis KA, Booth SL, Uwaifo GI, Yanovski JA. Effects of orlistat on fat-soluble vitamins in adolescents. *Phamacotherapy.* 2002;22:814–22.

37. Salvatore T, Giugliano D. Pharmacokinetic-pharmacodynamic relationships of Acarbose. *Clin Pharmacokinet.* 1996;30:94–106.

38. Mehnert H. Metformin, the rebirth of a biguanide: Mechanism of action and place in the prevention and treatment of insulin resistance. *Exp Clin Endocrinol Diabetes.* 2001;109(Suppl 2):S259–64.

39. Singh-Franco D, Perez A, Harrington C. The effect of pramlintide acetate on glycemic control and weight in patients with type 2 diabetes mellitus and in obese patients without diabetes: A systematic review and meta-analysis. *Diabetes Obes Metab.* 2011;13:169–80.

40. DeFronzo RA, Ratner RE, Han J, Kim DD, Fineman MS, Baron AD. Effects of exenatide (exendin-4) on glycemic control and weight over 30 weeks in metformin treated patients with type 2 diabetes. *Diabetes Care.* 2005;28(5):1092–100.

41. Amori RE, Lau J, Pittas AG. Efficacy and safety of incretin therapy in type 2 diabetes. *JAMA.* 2007;298:184–206.

42. Astrup A, Toubro S. Drugs with thermogenic properties. In: Bray G, Bouchard C, eds. *Handbook of Obesity: Clinical Applications*, 3rd Edition. New York: Informa Healthcare and CRC Press New York, 2008:405–16.

43. Rollick S, Miller WR, Butler CC. *Motivational Interviewing in Health Care: Helping Patients Change Behavior.* New York: The Guilford Press, 2008.

44. Sim LA, McAlpine DE, Grothe KB, Clark MM. Identification and treatment of eating disorders in the primary care setting. *Mayo Clin Proc.* 2010;85(8):746–51.

45. Lipton BH. *The Biology of Belief: Unleashing the Power of Consciousness, Matter and Miracles.* Carlsbad, CA: Hay House, 2008.

46. Prochaska JO, Velicer WF, Rossi JS, Goldstein MG, Marcus BH, Rakowski W, Fiore C, Harlow LL, Redding CA, Rosenbloom D, Rossi SR. Stages of change and decisional balance for 12 problem behaviors. *Health Psychol.* 1994;13(1):39–46.

47. Miller WR, Rollick S. *Motivational Interviewing. Preparing People for Change.* 2nd Edition. New York: The Guilford Press, 2002.

48. Foster GD, Makris AP, Baile BA. Behavioral treatment of obesity 1234. *AJCN.* 2005;82:230s–35s.

49. Brownell KD. *The LEARN Program for Weight Management.* Dallas, TX: American Health Publishers Co., 2000.

50. Lally P, Van Jaarsveld C, Potts HW, Wardle J. How are habits formed: Modeling habit formation in the real world. *Eur J Soc Psych.* 2010;40:998–1009.

51. Wadden TA, Butryn ML, Byrne KJ. Efficacy of lifestyle modification for long term weight control. *Obes Res.* 2004;12:151S–61S.

52. The National Weight Control Registry. Research findings. 2014. Available at http://www.nwcr.ws.research.default.htm.

53. Foreyt JP. Weight loss: Counseling and long term management. Medscape Diabetes and Endocrinology, 2004. Available at http://www.medscape.org/viewarticle/493028.

13 Peripheral Endocrine Response to Weight Loss

Priya Sumithran and Joseph Proietto

CONTENTS

INTRODUCTION

Long-term maintenance of weight loss is one of the most challenging aspects of obesity management. Of 228 overweight United States residents randomly surveyed, only 20.6% reported having intentionally lost at least 10% of their initial weight and kept it off for at least 1 year (Wing and Hill 2001), and a meta-analysis concluded that 4.5 years after completing a structured weight loss program involving a hypocaloric diet with or without exercise, the average weight loss maintained was 3.2% (Anderson et al. 2001). Why is it so difficult to maintain weight loss in the long term? A possible explanation is that physiological changes that accompany diet-induced weight loss may encourage regain of lost weight.

BODY WEIGHT REGULATION

Despite considerable variation in food intake from day to day, most adults maintain a fairly stable body weight over time. Although large weight changes may occur in humans and animals following sustained dietary restriction or overfeeding, when *ad libitum* feeding is resumed, weight and adiposity generally return to baseline levels (Bernstein et al. 1975; Pasquet and Apfelbaum 1994). This homeostatic regulation of body weight is controlled primarily by the hypothalamus, where peripheral signals conveying information about short-term food intake and long-term energy balance are integrated to affect appetite and energy expenditure.

HOMEOSTATIC REGULATION

The primary brain region involved in the homeostatic control of food intake, the arcuate nucleus (ARC) of the hypothalamus, contains two interconnected groups of neurons with opposing effects on energy balance. Food intake is stimulated by neurons that co-express neuropeptide Y (NPY) and agouti-related peptide (AgRP), and inhibited by neurons expressing pro-opiomelanocortin (POMC) and cocaine- and amphetamine-regulated transcript (CART). Projections from the ARC travel to other hypothalamic regions including the paraventricular nucleus, where the appetite-suppressing thyrotropin-releasing hormone (TRH), corticotrophin-releasing hormone (CRH), and oxytocin are produced, and the lateral hypothalamus, which is the source of appetite-stimulating melanin-concentrating hormone (MCH) and orexins.

Signals from the periphery, reflecting short- and long-term energy balance, influence the relative activity of the two circuits. Insulin and the adipocyte hormone leptin are signals of long-term energy balance. Hormones from the gastrointestinal tract and pancreas, such as ghrelin, cholecystokinin (CCK), glucagon-like peptide 1 (GLP-1), amylin, pancreatic polypeptide (PP), and peptide YY (PYY), along with several others (Table 13.1), relay information related to meals via the bloodstream and the vagus nerve to the hypothalamus and hindbrain, including the area postrema and the nucleus of the solitary tract. Reciprocal projections between these areas allow integration of signals to influence food intake and energy expenditure (Figure 13.1).

HEDONIC PATHWAYS

In addition to its nutritional value, food also has rewarding properties. The cortex and reward circuits in the limbic system ("hedonic" pathways) transmit information to the hypothalamus related to

TABLE 13.1
Peptides and Hormones Involved in Appetite Regulation

Location	Appetite-Suppressing	Appetite-Stimulating
	Central	
Hypothalamus	POMC (Krude et al. 2003)	Neuropeptide Y (Billington et al. 1991)
	Nesfatin-1 (Oh-I et al. 2006)	AgRP (Rossi et al. 1998)
	TRH (Vijayan and McCann 1977)	Orexins (Sakurai et al. 1998)
	CRH (Britton et al. 1982)	MCH (Shimada et al. 1998)
	Oxytocin (Arletti et al. 1989)	Endocannabinoids (Di Marzo et al. 2001)
	Serotonin (Blundell 1977)	Opioids (Jalowiec et al. 1981)
	Histamine (Sakata et al. 1988)	
	Urocortin (Spina et al. 1996)	
	Peripheral	
Gastrointestinal tract	Cholecystokinin (Muurahainen et al. 1988)	Ghrelin (Wren et al. 2001)
	GLP-1 (Flint et al. 1998)	
	Peptide YY (Batterham et al. 2002)	
	Oxyntomodulin (Cohen et al. 2003)	
	Enterostatin (Erlanson-Albertsson and York 1997)	
	Bombesin (Muurahainen et al. 1993)	
	Uroguanylin (Valentino et al. 2011)	
Pancreas	Amylin (Chapman et al. 2007)	
	Insulin (Porte and Woods 1981)	
	Pancreatic polypeptide (Batterham et al. 2003)	
Adipocytes	Leptin (Zhang et al. 1994)	

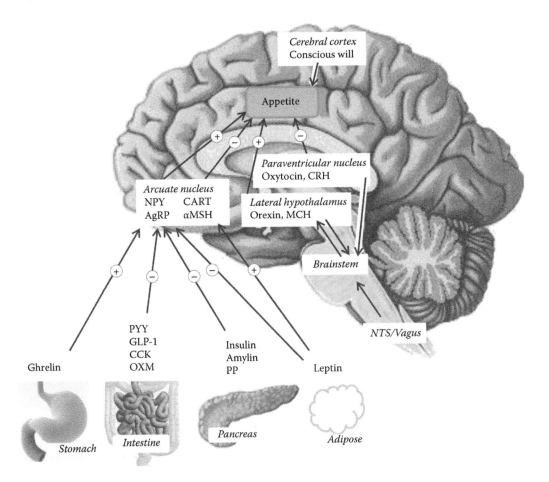

FIGURE 13.1 **(See color insert.)** Selected pathways involved in body weight regulation.

the sight, smell, and taste of food, along with emotional and social factors, which are all integrated to influence energy balance. In the short term, these hedonic pathways can override the homeostatic system, resulting in a desire to consume palatable food despite adequate energy stores and food availability.

There are interactions between these two systems of appetite regulation. For example, leptin affects taste and reward pathways (Fulton et al. 2000), ghrelin stimulates the mesolimbic dopaminergic pathway and increases consumption of sweet foods (Naleid et al. 2005; Disse et al. 2010), and stimulation of the cannabinoid 1 (CB1) receptor increases not only food intake but also a preference for palatable foods (Koch and Matthews 2001).

ADAPTATIONS TO WEIGHT LOSS

Diet-induced weight loss is accompanied by a multitude of physiological changes that collectively predispose to weight regain, many of which persist well beyond the period of initial weight reduction.

REDUCED ENERGY EXPENDITURE

In weight-stable adults, total energy expenditure (TEE) is comprised of approximately 60% resting energy expenditure (REE, involving processes such as maintaining transmembrane ion gradients and resting cardiopulmonary activity); 10% thermic effect of food (TEF, the energy required to digest, transport, and deposit nutrients); and 30% nonresting energy expenditure (NREE, largely as physical activity) (Leibel et al. 1995).

A 10% weight loss induced by dietary restriction leads to a reduction in TEE of 15% more than predicted by alterations in body mass and composition, in both normal-weight and obese persons (Leibel et al. 1995), which persists for more than 1 year in people who maintain a reduced body weight (Rosenbaum et al. 2008a). Most of this is accounted for by a reduction in NREE, due to increased efficiency of skeletal muscle at low workloads (Doucet et al. 2003; Rosenbaum et al. 2003). There is mixed evidence as to whether REE also declines more than predicted (Doucet et al. 2001; Schwartz et al. 2012).

ALTERATIONS IN AUTONOMIC NERVOUS SYSTEM

Obesity is associated with increased activity of the sympathetic nervous system (SNS) (Grassi et al. 2005). Chronic stimulation may blunt SNS responsiveness (Scheidegger et al. 1984) and thereby impair energy expenditure, postprandial thermogenesis, and fat oxidation (Julius et al. 2000; Greenfield and Campbell 2008). In the obese, diet-induced weight loss is accompanied by a reduction in sympathetic and an increase in cardiac parasympathetic activity (Arone et al. 1995; Rissanen et al. 2001). The increase in cardiac parasympathetic tone is not sustained following several months of weight loss maintenance (Laaksonen et al. 2003; Straznicky et al. 2011). In contrast, maintenance of weight loss has divergent effects on markers of sympathetic function, with a recent study showing a sustained reduction in whole-body noradrenaline spillover but a rebound in muscle sympathetic nerve activity during weight loss maintenance, indicating either a reduction in sympathetic outflow elsewhere or a mismatch between sympathetic nerve firing and noradrenaline overflow (Straznicky et al. 2011).

SUPPRESSION OF HYPOTHALAMIC–PITUITARY–THYROID AXIS

Thyroxine (T4) and triiodothyronine (T3) release from the thyroid gland is stimulated by thyroid-stimulating hormone (TSH) from the anterior pituitary, as a result of stimulation by TRH from the paraventricular nucleus of the hypothalamus. T4 is converted to the more biologically active T3 in peripheral target tissues. Dietary restriction results in impaired TSH response to TRH, reductions in circulating TSH and T3, and increased production of reverse T3 (rT3), an inactive molecule. Variable effects of energy restriction on total and free T4 have been demonstrated (O'Brian et al. 1980; Romijn et al. 1990; Rosenbaum 2005). There are conflicting reports regarding the extent to which these changes are sustained during prolonged weight loss maintenance (O'Brian et al. 1980; Näslund et al. 2000; Weinsier et al. 2000; Hukshorn et al. 2003; Rosenbaum et al. 2005). As well as being an important determinant of REE, thyroid hormones play a key role in adaptive thermogenesis and increase mitochondrial uncoupling in skeletal muscle (al-Adsani et al. 1997; Bianco et al. 2005). As such, suppression of the hypothalamic–pituitary–thyroid (HPT) axis, along with reduction in SNS activity, may be among the mechanisms by which skeletal muscle work efficiency is increased after weight loss (Rosenbaum et al. 2000; Bianco et al. 2005).

STIMULATION OF HYPOTHALAMIC–PITUITARY–ADRENAL AXIS

The production and release of cortisol from the adrenal cortex is stimulated by adrenocorticotropic hormone from the pituitary. This is, in turn, driven by CRH release from the paraventricular nucleus. In rodents, glucocorticoids are required for increases in hypothalamic NPY and AgRP and reduction in POMC messenger RNA (mRNA) to occur during fasting (Makimura et al. 2003) and have been shown to inhibit the suppression of food intake and body weight by leptin (Zakrzewska et al. 1997). Increased activation of the hypothalamic–pituitary–adrenal (HPA) axis has been demonstrated in obese humans, particularly in those with predominantly abdominal obesity (Marin et al. 1992; Pasquali et al. 1993), although the cause and physiological significance of this is not clear. In lean people, food restriction results in stimulation of the HPA axis (Fichter and Pirke 1986). Studies have yielded mixed results on the effects of dietary restriction on the HPA axis in the obese, but increased HPA activation, demonstrated by increased circulating cortisol and reduced dexamethasone suppression or diurnal variation of cortisol production, has often been reported, particularly with severe energy restriction (Galvao-Teles et al. 1976; Edelstein et al. 1983; Torgerson et al. 1999; Johnstone et al. 2004; Ho et al. 2007; Tomiyama et al. 2010). Following weight loss in obese participants, fasting plasma cortisol has been shown to correlate with appetite (Doucet et al. 2000).

ALTERATIONS IN HYPOTHALAMIC–PITUITARY–GONADAL AXIS

In adults, pulsatile release of gonadotropin-releasing hormone (GnRH) from the hypothalamus promotes the release of luteinizing hormone (LH) and follicle-stimulating hormone (FSH) from the anterior pituitary. In the ovaries, FSH and LH stimulate the production of steroid hormones including estradiol (E2) and progesterone and are instrumental in follicular development and ovulation. In the testes, FSH stimulates spermatogenesis, and LH stimulates testosterone production. Circulating testosterone is largely bound to proteins such as albumin and sex-hormone–binding globulin (SHBG). In most tissues, the fraction of testosterone that is not bound to SHBG is considered biologically active (Mah and Wittert 2009).

In centrally obese men and women, premenopausal and postmenopausal women, hyperinsulinemia mediates several changes in the hypothalamic–pituitary–gonadal (HPG) axis, including reduced SHBG and increased E2 due to aromatization of testosterone in adipose tissue and increased ovarian production of estrogen (Haffner 2000; Diamanti-Kandarakis and Bergiele 2001; Mah and Wittert 2009). In obese men, total and free testosterone are reduced, which may be due to reduced LH pulse amplitude, increased circulating estrogen resulting in negative feedback on GnRH and LH secretion, and a possible effect of leptin on androgen production (Mah and Wittert 2009). In contrast, in women, abdominal obesity and hyperinsulinemia are associated with excessive production of androgens, a key feature of polycystic ovary syndrome (PCOS). Insulin resistance and hyperandrogenism can disturb ovarian function in premenopausal women through mechanisms that are not clearly elucidated, resulting in anovulation (Diamanti-Kandarakis and Bergiele 2001). FSH and LH are not significantly different in obese women compared with lean women (Kopelman et al. 1981), although centrally obese women with PCOS have higher LH than comparably obese women without PCOS (Pasquali et al. 2000). Evidence for the involvement of leptin in the regulation of gonadal function and fertility is the reversal of hypogonadotrophic hypogonadism and delayed puberty in people with genetically-based leptin deficiency following leptin administration (Licinio et al. 2004).

The effect of weight loss on the HPG axis may be dependent on the degree of dietary restriction and the prevailing fat stores. In lean men and women, weight loss due to restriction of food intake or intensive exercise results in hypothalamic hypogonadism and subfertility, which is reversible following weight regain or cessation of dietary restriction/training (Frisch 1987; Roemmich and Sinning 1997; Karila et al. 2008). In overweight or obese men, complete fasting for 10 days leading to loss of 4% starting weight resulted in hypogonadotrophic hypogonadism (Klibanski et al. 1981), and a 14% weight loss induced by a 6-week very-low-energy diet (VLED) has also resulted in reductions in free testosterone and LH, which was partially attenuated by leptin replacement (Hukshorn et al. 2003). However, several other studies have shown improvements in HPG axis dysfunction following weight loss in the obese, such as increases in total and free testosterone and SHBG in men, with no change in total or free E2 (Pasquali et al. 1988; Strain et al. 1988). The changes in testosterone and SHBG may be proportional to the degree of weight loss and are partially attenuated after 12 months of weight loss maintenance (Niskanen et al. 2004). In overweight women, modest weight loss (in the order of 5 kg) reduces insulin and androgens, thereby improving menstrual disturbances, ovulation, and fertility in premenopausal women (Pasquali et al. 1989; Kiddy et al. 1992). A greater degree of weight loss (>10%) may be required before a reduction in estrogens is seen (O'Dea et al. 1979; Schapira et al. 1994; Campbell et al. 2012).

Since hypogonadism is associated with weight gain, central adiposity, and loss of lean body mass in both men and women (Donato et al. 2006; Haseen et al. 2010; Hamilton et al. 2011), it is conceivable that the suppression of the HPG axis seen following weight loss under some conditions may predispose to weight regain.

ALTERATIONS IN ADIPOCYTE AND GASTROINTESTINAL HORMONES

There is accumulating evidence that diet-induced weight loss results in changes in circulating concentrations of several peripheral hormones involved in appetite regulation, which collectively promote weight regain and restoration of energy balance.

Leptin reduces food intake and increases energy expenditure by inhibiting the hypothalamic expression of AgRP and NPY and stimulating that of POMC (Pelleymounter et al. 1995; Stephens et al. 1995; Schwartz et al. 1997). Leptin secretion is proportional to fat mass during energy balance at usual body weight (Considine et al. 1996) but is profoundly reduced by dietary restriction and is significantly lower during dynamic weight loss than during weight loss maintenance (Rosenbaum et al. 1997; Keim et al. 1998). During a dietary energy deficit, changes in leptin correlate inversely with self-reported appetite, and leptin administration reduces appetite (Keim et al. 1998; Westerterp-Plantenga et al. 2001). The importance of leptin as a signal of energy depletion is highlighted by the reversal of many weight loss–induced physiological responses (such as changes in thyroid hormones, the autonomic nervous system, energy expenditure, skeletal muscle efficiency, and regional brain activation) following administration of leptin in weight-reduced people to achieve pre–weight loss levels (Rosenbaum et al. 2005, 2008b).

Other hormonal changes that accompany diet-induced weight loss include increased circulating ghrelin (which promotes hunger) and gastric inhibitory polypeptide (GIP, which may stimulate energy storage) (Hauner et al. 1988; Wren et al. 2001). An increase in PP has also been reported, along with reductions in PYY, CCK, insulin, and amylin (Sumithran et al. 2011), with studies reporting varying effects of weight loss on GLP-1 secretion (Verdich et al. 2001; Adam et al. 2006; Sumithran et al. 2011). Since these hormones have all been shown to inhibit food intake (Porte and Woods 1981; Muurahainen et al. 1988; Flint et al. 1998; Batterham et al. 2002, 2003; Chapman et al. 2007), the majority of weight loss–induced alterations in their release should predispose weight-reduced people to weight regain, by increasing hunger, reducing satiety, and promoting energy storage.

The alterations in hormone release appear to persist beyond the period of negative energy balance. Our research group conducted a study involving 50 overweight or obese men and women who underwent a 10-week VLED-based weight loss program followed by a 12-month period of attempted weight loss maintenance (Sumithran et al. 2011). Participants were required to lose at least 10% of their starting weight, and in the 34 people who completed the study, peripheral appetite-mediating hormones were measured prior to weight loss, following the weight loss period, and again 12 months later. Initial weight loss of 13.5 ± 0.5 kg (mean ± SE; 14% of baseline weight) was accompanied by significant reductions in circulating leptin, PYY, CCK, insulin, and amylin, and increases in ghrelin, GIP, and PP (Sumithran et al. 2011). At the end of the 12-month follow-up period, during which participants regained a mean of 5.5 ± 1.0 kg, hormone levels remained significantly different from pre–weight loss values (Figure 13.2).

INCREASED APPETITE

Diet-induced weight loss brings about a sustained increase in subjective ratings of hunger (Doucet et al. 2000; Sumithran et al. 2011). In the study described prior, participants were asked to rate their appetite using a visual analog scale while fasting and for 4 h following a standardized meal.

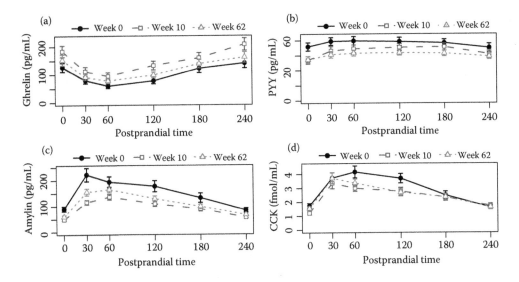

FIGURE 13.2 Peripheral appetite-mediating hormones before and after weight loss.

Ratings of hunger, urge and desire to eat, and prospective consumption increased after weight loss, and there was no attenuation of this effect 12 months later (Figure 13.3). Reported preoccupation with thoughts of food was higher, and fullness was lower at 12 months compared with pre-weight loss (Sumithran et al. 2011). Several studies have reported the appetite changes to be related to alterations in circulating leptin following weight loss (Keim et al. 1998; Heini et al. 1998; Doucet et al. 2000). Furthermore, weight-reduced adults may also experience an increase in the perceived rewarding properties of food and a preference for high-calorie foods (Drewnowski et al. 1985; Cameron et al. 2008).

In contrast to nonsurgical methods of weight loss, bariatric surgical procedures, such as laparoscopic adjustable gastric banding (LAGB) and Roux-en-Y gastric bypass (RYGB), reduce appetite and are more likely to bring about sustained reductions in body weight (Dixon et al. 2005; Borg et al. 2006). Gastrointestinal hormone changes following RYGB (such as lack of increase in ghrelin, and exaggerated postprandial release of GLP-1 and PYY) favor appetite suppression (Cummings et al. 2002; Korner et al. 2005; Morinigo et al. 2006) whereas LAGB and dietary restriction induce similarly anorexigenic changes in gastrointestinal and adipocyte hormones (Dixon et al. 2005), and the mechanism by which LAGB suppresses appetite remains to be elucidated (Burton and Brown 2011).

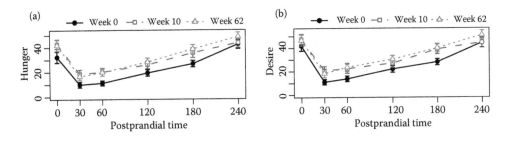

FIGURE 13.3 Reported appetite before and after weight loss.

ALTERATIONS IN REGIONAL BRAIN ACTIVATION

Alterations in brain activity patterns in response to food stimuli have been demonstrated using functional brain imaging techniques in obese people after diet-induced weight loss. For example, one study reported increased activity in the limbic (reward) system and areas involved in executive function and decision-making, along with reduced activity in the hypothalamus and areas involved in the emotional control of food intake, integrative cognitive control functions, and motor planning, compared to baseline in weight-reduced participants (Rosenbaum et al. 2008b), which may indicate a state of increased responsiveness to food reward with decreased control of food intake. Others have shown altered activation in several brain areas involved in the control of complex aspects of eating behavior including the insula, inferior visual cortex, posterior cingulate cortex, posterior hippocampus, and amygdala in response to food stimuli in weight-reduced individuals compared with obese and lean controls (DelParigi et al. 2004; Cornier et al. 2009). The insula is involved in mediating the desirability of food (Gordon et al. 2000), and activation in this area in response to images of high-calorie foods is stimulated by ghrelin (Malik et al. 2008) and attenuated by leptin administration in weight-reduced or congenitally leptin-deficient adults (Baicy et al. 2007; Rosenbaum et al. 2008b).

CONCLUSION

Diet-induced weight loss is accompanied by coordinated changes in several neuroendocrine and metabolic systems, which result in increased appetite, reduced energy expenditure, and predisposition to fat storage. These mechanisms would confer a survival advantage if food were scarce but facilitate weight regain in an environment in which energy-dense food is abundant and physical activity is nonessential.

REFERENCES

Adam, T. C. M., M. P. G. M. Lejeune, and M. S. Westerterp-Plantenga. 2006. Nutrient-stimulated glucagon-like peptide 1 release after body-weight loss and weight maintenance in human subjects. *The British Journal of Nutrition* 95 (1):160–7.

al-Adsani, H., L. J. Hoffer, and J. E. Silva. 1997. Resting energy expenditure is sensitive to small dose changes in patients on chronic thyroid hormone replacement. *The Journal of Clinical Endocrinology and Metabolism* 82 (4):1118–25.

Anderson, J. W., E. C. Konz, R. C. Frederich, and C. L. Wood. 2001. Long-term weight-loss maintenance: A meta-analysis of US studies. *The American Journal of Clinical Nutrition* 74 (5):579–84.

Arletti, R., A. Benelli, and A. Bertolini. 1989. Influence of oxytocin on feeding behavior in the rat. *Peptides* 10 (1):89–93.

Arone, L. J., R. Mackintosh, M. Rosenbaum, R. L. Leibel, and J. Hirsch. 1995. Autonomic nervous system activity in weight gain and weight loss. *The American Journal of Physiology* 269 (1 Pt 2):R222–5.

Baicy, K., E. D. London, J. Monterosso, M.-L. Wong, T. Delibasi, A. Sharma, and J. Licinio. 2007. Leptin replacement alters brain response to food cues in genetically leptin-deficient adults. *Proceedings of the National Academy of Sciences of the United States of America* 104 (46):18276–9.

Batterham, R. L., M. A. Cowley, C. J. Small, H. Herzog, M. A. Cohen, C. L. Dakin, A. M. Wren, A. E. Brynes, M. J. Low, M. A. Ghatei, R. D. Cone, and S. R. Bloom. 2002. Gut hormone PYY_{3-36} physiologically inhibits food intake. *Nature* 418 (6898):650–4.

Batterham, R. L., C. W. Le Roux, M. A. Cohen, A. J. Park, S. M. Ellis, M. Patterson, G. S. Frost, M. A. Ghatei, and S. R. Bloom. 2003. Pancreatic polypeptide reduces appetite and food intake in humans. *The Journal of Clinical Endocrinology and Metabolism* 88 (8):3989–92.

Bernstein, I. L., E. C. Lotter, P. J. Kulkosky, D. Porte, Jr., and S. C. Woods. 1975. Effect of force-feeding upon basal insulin levels of rats. *Proceedings of the Society for Experimental Biology and Medicine* 150 (2):546–8.

Bianco, A. C., A. L. Maia, W. S. da Silva, and M. A. Christoffolete. 2005. Adaptive activation of thyroid hormone and energy expenditure. *Bioscience Reports* 25 (3–4):191–208.

Billington, C. J., J. E. Briggs, M. Grace, and A. S. Levine. 1991. Effects of intracerebroventricular injection of neuropeptide Y on energy metabolism. *American Journal of Physiology* 260 (2 Pt 2):R321–7.

Blundell, J. E. 1977. Is there a role for serotonin (5-hydroxytryptamine) in feeding? *International Journal of Obesity* 1 (1):15–42.

Borg, C. M., C. W. Le Roux, M. A. Ghatei, S. R. Bloom, A. G. Patel, and S. J. B. Aylwin. 2006. Progressive rise in gut hormone levels after Roux-en-Y gastric bypass suggests gut adaptation and explains altered satiety. *The British Journal of Surgery* 93 (2):210–5.

Britton, D. R., G. F. Koob, J. Rivier, and W. Vale. 1982. Intraventricular corticotropin-releasing factor enhances behavioral effects of novelty. *Life Sciences* 31 (4):363–7.

Burton, P. R., and W. A. Brown. 2011. The mechanism of weight loss with laparoscopic adjustable gastric banding: Induction of satiety not restriction. *International Journal of Obesity* 35 Suppl 3:S26–30.

Cameron, J. D., G. S. Goldfield, M.-J. Cyr, and E. Doucet. 2008. The effects of prolonged caloric restriction leading to weight-loss on food hedonics and reinforcement. *Physiology and Behavior* 94 (3):474–80.

Campbell, K. L., K. E. Foster-Schubert, C. M. Alfano, C.-C. Wang, C.-Y. Wang, C. R. Duggan, C. Mason, I. Imayama, A. Kong, L. Xiao, C. E. Bain, G. L. Blackburn, F. Z. Stanczyk, and A. McTiernan. 2012. Reduced-calorie dietary weight loss, exercise, and sex hormones in postmenopausal women: Randomized controlled trial. *Journal of Clinical Oncology: Official Journal of the American Society of Clinical Oncology* 30 (19):2314–26.

Chapman, I., B. Parker, S. Doran, C. Feinle-Bisset, J. Wishart, C. W. Lush, K. Chen, C. Lacerte, C. Burns, R. McKay, C. Weyer, and M. Horowitz. 2007. Low-dose pramlintide reduced food intake and meal duration in healthy, normal-weight subjects. *Obesity (Silver Spring)* 15 (5):1179–86.

Cohen, M. A., S. M. Ellis, C. W. Le Roux, R. L. Batterham, A. J. Park, M. Patterson, G. S. Frost, M. A. Ghatei, and S. R. Bloom. 2003. Oxyntomodulin suppresses appetite and reduces food intake in humans. *The Journal of Clinical Endocrinology and Metabolism* 88 (10):4696–701.

Considine, R. V., M. K. Sinha, M. L. Heiman, A. Kriauciunas, T. W. Stephens, M. R. Nyce, J. P. Ohannesian, C. C. Marco, L. J. McKee, and T. L. Bauer. 1996. Serum immunoreactive-leptin concentrations in normal-weight and obese humans. *The New England Journal of Medicine* 334 (5):292–5.

Cornier, M.-A., A. K. Salzberg, D. C. Endly, D. H. Bessesen, D. C. Rojas, and J. R. Tregellas. 2009. The effects of overfeeding on the neuronal response to visual food cues in thin and reduced-obese individuals. *PLoS One* 4 (7):e6310.

Cummings, D. E., D. S. Weigle, R. S. Frayo, P. A. Breen, M. K. Ma, E. P. Dellinger, and J. Q. Purnell. 2002. Plasma ghrelin levels after diet-induced weight loss or gastric bypass surgery. *The New England Journal of Medicine* 346 (21):1623–30.

DelParigi, A., K. Chen, A. D. Salbe, J. O. Hill, R. R. Wing, E. M. Reiman, and P. A. Tataranni. 2004. Persistence of abnormal neural responses to a meal in postobese individuals. *International Journal of Obesity and Related Metabolic Disorders: Journal of the International Association for the Study of Obesity* 28 (3):370–7.

Di Marzo, V., S. K. Goparaju, L. Wang, J. Liu, S. Batkai, Z. Jarai, F. Fezza, G. I. Miura, R. D. Palmiter, T. Sugiura, and G. Kunos. 2001. Leptin-regulated endocannabinoids are involved in maintaining food intake. *Nature* 410 (6830):822–5.

Diamanti-Kandarakis, E., and A. Bergiele. 2001. The influence of obesity on hyperandrogenism and infertility in the female. *Obesity Reviews: An Official Journal of the International Association for the Study of Obesity* 2 (4):231–8.

Disse, E., A.-L. Bussier, C. Veyrat-Durebex, N. Deblon, P. T. Pfluger, M. H. Tschop, M. Laville, and F. Rohner-Jeanrenaud. 2010. Peripheral ghrelin enhances sweet taste food consumption and preference, regardless of its caloric content. *Physiology & Behavior* 101 (2):277–81.

Dixon, A. F. R., J. B. Dixon, and P. E. O'Brien. 2005. Laparoscopic adjustable gastric banding induces prolonged satiety: A randomized blind crossover study. *The Journal of Clinical Endocrinology and Metabolism* 90 (2):813–9.

Donato, G. B., S. C. Fuchs, K. Oppermann, C. Bastos, and P. M. Spritzer. 2006. Association between menopause status and central adiposity measured at different cutoffs of waist circumference and waist-to-hip ratio. *Menopause (New York)* 13 (2):280–5.

Doucet, E., P. Imbeault, S. St-Pierre, N. Almeras, P. Mauriege, J.-P. Despres, C. Bouchard, and A. Tremblay. 2003. Greater than predicted decrease in energy expenditure during exercise after body weight loss in obese men. *Clinical Science (London, England: 1979)* 105 (1):89–95.

Doucet, E., P. Imbeault, S. St-Pierre, N. Almeras, P. Mauriege, D. Richard, and A. Tremblay. 2000. Appetite after weight loss by energy restriction and a low-fat diet-exercise follow-up. *International Journal of Obesity and Related Metabolic Disorders: Journal of the International Association for the Study of Obesity* 24 (7):906–14.

Doucet, E., S. St-Pierre, N. Almeras, J. P. Despres, C. Bouchard, and A. Tremblay. 2001. Evidence for the existence of adaptive thermogenesis during weight loss. *The British Journal of Nutrition* 85 (6):715–23.

Drewnowski, A., J. D. Brunzell, K. Sande, P. H. Iverius, and M. R. Greenwood. 1985. Sweet tooth reconsidered: Taste responsiveness in human obesity. *Physiology and Behavior* 35 (4):617–22.

Edelstein, C. K., P. Roy-Byrne, F. I. Fawzy, and L. Dornfeld. 1983. Effects of weight loss on the dexamethasone suppression test. *The American Journal of Psychiatry* 140 (3):338–41.

Erlanson-Albertsson, C., and D. York. 1997. Enterostatin—a peptide regulating fat intake. *Obesity Research* 5 (4):360–72.

Fichter, M. M., and K. M. Pirke. 1986. Effect of experimental and pathological weight loss upon the hypothalamo–pituitary–adrenal axis. *Psychoneuroendocrinology* 11 (3):295–305.

Flint, A., A. Raben, A. Astrup, and J. J. Holst. 1998. Glucagon-like peptide 1 promotes satiety and suppresses energy intake in humans. *Journal of Clinical Investigation* 101 (3):515–20.

Frisch, R. E. 1987. Body fat, menarche, fitness and fertility. *Human Reproduction (Oxford, England)* 2 (6):521–33.

Fulton, S., B. Woodside, and P. Shizgal. 2000. Modulation of brain reward circuitry by leptin. *Science* 287 (5450):125–8.

Galvao-Teles, A., L. Graves, C. W. Burke, K. Fotherby, and R. Fraser. 1976. Free cortisol in obesity: Effect of fasting. *Acta Endocrinologica* 81 (2):321–9.

Gordon, C. M., D. D. Dougherty, S. L. Rauch, S. J. Emans, E. Grace, R. Lamm, N. M. Alpert, J. A. Majzoub, and A. J. Fischman. 2000. Neuroanatomy of human appetitive function: A positron emission tomography investigation. *The International Journal of Eating Disorders* 27 (2):163–71.

Grassi, G., R. Dell'Oro, F. Quarti-Trevano, F. Scopelliti, G. Seravalle, F. Paleari, P. L. Gamba, and G. Mancia. 2005. Neuroadrenergic and reflex abnormalities in patients with metabolic syndrome. *Diabetologia* 48 (7):1359–65.

Greenfield, J. R., and L. V. Campbell. 2008. Role of the autonomic nervous system and neuropeptides in the development of obesity in humans: Targets for therapy? *Current Pharmaceutical Design* 14 (18):1815–20.

Haffner, S. M. 2000. Sex hormones, obesity, fat distribution, type 2 diabetes and insulin resistance: Epidemiological and clinical correlation. *International Journal of Obesity and Related Metabolic Disorders: Journal of the International Association for the Study of Obesity* 24 Suppl 2:S56–8.

Hamilton, E. J., E. Gianatti, B. J. Strauss, J. Wentworth, D. Lim-Joon, D. Bolton, J. D. Zajac, and M. Grossmann. 2011. Increase in visceral and subcutaneous abdominal fat in men with prostate cancer treated with androgen deprivation therapy. *Clinical Endocrinology* 74 (3):377–83.

Haseen, F., L. J. Murray, C. R. Cardwell, J. M. O'Sullivan, and M. M. Cantwell. 2010. The effect of androgen deprivation therapy on body composition in men with prostate cancer: Systematic review and meta-analysis. *Journal of Cancer Survivorship: Research and Practice* 4 (2):128–39.

Hauner H., G. Glatting, D. Kaminska and E. Pfeiffer. 1988. Effects of gastric inhibitory polypeptide on glucose and lipid metabolism of isolated rat adipocytes. *Annals of Nutrition Metabolism* 32:282–8.

Heini, A. F., C. Lara-Castro, K. A. Kirk, R. V. Considine, J. F. Caro, and R. L. Weinsier. 1998. Association of leptin and hunger-satiety ratings in obese women. *International Journal of Obesity and Related Metabolic Disorders: Journal of the International Association for the Study of Obesity* 22 (11):1084–7.

Ho, J. T., J. B. Keogh, S. R. Bornstein, M. Ehrhart-Bornstein, J. G. Lewis, P. M. Clifton, and D. J. Torpy. 2007. Moderate weight loss reduces renin and aldosterone but does not influence basal or stimulated pituitary–adrenal axis function. *Hormone and Metabolic Research* 39 (9):694–9.

Hukshorn, C. J., P. P. C. A. Menheere, M. S. Westerterp-Plantenga, and W. H. M. Saris. 2003. The effect of pegylated human recombinant leptin (PEG-OB) on neuroendocrine adaptations to semi-starvation in overweight men. *European Journal of Endocrinology/European Federation of Endocrine Societies* 148 (6):649–55.

Jalowiec, J. E., J. Panksepp, A. J. Zolovick, N. Najam, and B. H. Herman. 1981. Opioid modulation of ingestive behavior. *Pharmacology, Biochemistry, and Behavior* 15 (3):477–84.

Johnstone, A. M., P. Faber, R. Andrew, E. R. Gibney, M. Elia, G. Lobley, R. J. Stubbs, and B. R. Walker. 2004. Influence of short-term dietary weight loss on cortisol secretion and metabolism in obese men. *European Journal of Endocrinology/European Federation of Endocrine Societies* 150 (2):185–94.

Julius, S., M. Valentini, and P. Palatini. 2000. Overweight and hypertension: A 2-way street? *Hypertension* 35 (3):807–13.

Karila, T. A. M., P. Sarkkinen, M. Marttinen, T. Seppala, A. Mero, and K. Tallroth. 2008. Rapid weight loss decreases serum testosterone. *International Journal of Sports Medicine* 29 (11):872–7.

Keim, N. L., J. S. Stern, and P. J. Havel. 1998. Relation between circulating leptin concentrations and appetite during a prolonged, moderate energy deficit in women. *The American Journal of Clinical Nutrition* 68 (4):794–801.

Kiddy, D. S., D. Hamilton-Fairley, A. Bush, F. Short, V. Anyaoku, M. J. Reed, and S. Franks. 1992. Improvement in endocrine and ovarian function during dietary treatment of obese women with polycystic ovary syndrome. *Clinical Endocrinology* 36 (1):105–11.

Klibanski, A., I. Z. Beitins, T. Badger, R. Little, and J. W. McArthur. 1981. Reproductive function during fasting in men. *The Journal of Clinical Endocrinology and Metabolism* 53 (2):258–63.

Koch, J. E., and S. M. Matthews. 2001. Delta9-tetrahydrocannabinol stimulates palatable food intake in Lewis rats: Effects of peripheral and central administration. *Nutritional Neuroscience* 4 (3):179–87.

Kopelman, P. G., N. White, T. R. Pilkington, and S. L. Jeffcoate. 1981. The effect of weight loss on sex steroid secretion and binding in massively obese women. *Clinical Endocrinology* 15 (2):113–6.

Korner, J., M. Bessler, L. J. Cirilo, I. M. Conwell, A. Daud, N. L. Restuccia, and S. L. Wardlaw. 2005. Effects of Roux-en-Y gastric bypass surgery on fasting and postprandial concentrations of plasma ghrelin, peptide YY, and insulin. *The Journal of Clinical Endocrinology and Metabolism* 90 (1):359–65.

Krude, H., H. Biebermann, and A. Gruters. 2003. Mutations in the human proopiomelanocortin gene. *Annals of the New York Academy of Sciences* 994:233–9.

Laaksonen, D. E., T. Laitinen, J. Schonberg, A. Rissanen, and L. K. Niskanen. 2003. Weight loss and weight maintenance, ambulatory blood pressure and cardiac autonomic tone in obese persons with the metabolic syndrome. *Journal of Hypertension* 21 (2):371–8.

Leibel, R. L., M. Rosenbaum, and J. Hirsch. 1995. Changes in energy expenditure resulting from altered body weight. *The New England Journal of Medicine* 332 (10):621–8.

Licinio, J., S. Caglayan, M. Ozata, B. O. Yildiz, P. B. de Miranda, F. O'Kirwan, R. Whitby, L. Liang, P. Cohen, S. Bhasin, R. M. Krauss, J. D. Veldhuis, A. J. Wagner, A. M. DePaoli, S. M. McCann, and M.-L. Wong. 2004. Phenotypic effects of leptin replacement on morbid obesity, diabetes mellitus, hypogonadism, and behavior in leptin-deficient adults. *Proceedings of the National Academy of Sciences of the United States of America* 101 (13):4531–6.

Mah, P. M., and G. A. Wittert. 2009. Obesity and testicular function. *Molecular and Cellular Endocrinology* 316 (2):180–6.

Makimura, H., T. M. Mizuno, F. Isoda, J. Beasley, J. H. Silverstein, and C. V. Mobbs. 2003. Role of glucocorticoids in mediating effects of fasting and diabetes on hypothalamic gene expression. *BMC Physiology* 3:5.

Malik, S., F. McGlone, D. Bedrossian, and A. Dagher. 2008. Ghrelin modulates brain activity in areas that control appetitive behavior. *Cell Metabolism* 7 (5):400–9.

Marin, P., N. Darin, T. Amemiya, B. Andersson, S. Jern, and P. Bjorntorp. 1992. Cortisol secretion in relation to body fat distribution in obese premenopausal women. *Metabolism: Clinical and Experimental* 41 (8):882–6.

Morinigo, R., V. Moize, M. Musri, A. M. Lacy, S. Navarro, J. L. Marin, S. Delgado, R. Casamitjana, and J. Vidal. 2006. Glucagon-like peptide-1, peptide YY, hunger, and satiety after gastric bypass surgery in morbidly obese subjects. *The Journal of Clinical Endocrinology and Metabolism* 91 (5):1735–40.

Muurahainen, N. E., H. R. Kissileff, and F. X. Pi-Sunyer. 1993. Intravenous infusion of bombesin reduces food intake in humans. *American Journal of Physiology* 264 (2 Pt 2):R350–4.

Muurahainen, N., H. R. Kissileff, A. J. Derogatis, and F. X. Pi-Sunyer. 1988. Effects of cholecystokinin-octapeptide (CCK-8) on food intake and gastric emptying in man. *Physiology and Behavior* 44 (4–5):645–9.

Näslund E., I. Anderson, M. Degerblad, P. Kogner, J. Kral, S. Rösner, and P. Hellström. 2000. Associations of leptin, insulin and resistance and thyroid function with long-term weight loss in dieting obese men. *Journal of Internal Medicine* 243:299–308.

Naleid, A. M., M. K. Grace, D. E. Cummings, and A. S. Levine. 2005. Ghrelin induces feeding in the mesolimbic reward pathway between the ventral tegmental area and the nucleus accumbens. *Peptides* 26 (11):2274–9.

Niskanen, L., D. E. Laaksonen, K. Punnonen, P. Mustajoki, J. Kaukua, and A. Rissanen. 2004. Changes in sex hormone-binding globulin and testosterone during weight loss and weight maintenance in abdominally obese men with the metabolic syndrome. *Diabetes, Obesity and Metabolism* 6 (3):208–15.

O'Brian, J. T., D. E. Bybee, K. D. Burman, R. C. Osburne, M. R. Ksiazek, L. Wartofsky, and L. P. Georges. 1980. Thyroid hormone homeostasis in states of relative caloric deprivation. *Metabolism: Clinical and Experimental* 29 (8):721–7.

O'Dea, J. P., R. G. Wieland, M. C. Hallberg, L. A. Llerena, E. M. Zorn, and S. M. Genuth. 1979. Effect of dietery weight loss on sex steroid binding sex steroids, and gonadotropins in obese postmenopausal women. *The Journal of Laboratory and Clinical Medicine* 93 (6):1004–8.

Oh-I, S., H. Shimizu, T. Satoh, S. Okada, S. Adachi, K. Inoue, H. Eguchi, M. Yamamoto, T. Imaki, K. Hashimoto, T. Tsuchiya, T. Monden, K. Horiguchi, M. Yamada, and M. Mori. 2006. Identification of nesfatin-1 as a satiety molecule in the hypothalamus. *Nature* 443 (7112):709–12.

Pasquali, R., D. Antenucci, F. Casimirri, S. Venturoli, R. Paradisi, R. Fabbri, V. Balestra, N. Melchionda, and L. Barbara. 1989. Clinical and hormonal characteristics of obese amenorrheic hyperandrogenic women before and after weight loss. *The Journal of Clinical Endocrinology and Metabolism* 68 (1):173–9.

Pasquali, R., S. Cantobelli, F. Casimirri, M. Capelli, L. Bortoluzzi, R. Flamia, A. M. Labate, and L. Barbara. 1993. The hypothalamic–pituitary–adrenal axis in obese women with different patterns of body fat distribution. *The Journal of Clinical Endocrinology and Metabolism* 77 (2):341–6.

Pasquali, R., F. Casimirri, N. Melchionda, R. Fabbri, M. Capelli, L. Plate, D. Patrono, V. Balestra, and L. Barbara. 1988. Weight loss and sex steroid metabolism in massively obese man. *Journal of Endocrinological Investigation* 11 (3):205–10.

Pasquali, R., A. Gambineri, D. Biscotti, V. Vicennati, L. Gagliardi, D. Colitta, S. Fiorini, G. E. Cognigni, M. Filicori, and A. M. Morselli-Labate. 2000. Effect of long-term treatment with metformin added to hypocaloric diet on body composition, fat distribution, and androgen and insulin levels in abdominally obese women with and without the polycystic ovary syndrome. *The Journal of Clinical Endocrinology and Metabolism* 85 (8):2767–74.

Pasquet, P., and M. Apfelbaum. 1994. Recovery of initial body weight and composition after long-term massive overfeeding in men. *The American Journal of Clinical Nutrition* 60 (6):861–3.

Pelleymounter, M. A., M. J. Cullen, M. B. Baker, R. Hecht, D. Winters, T. Boone, and F. Collins. 1995. Effects of the obese gene product on body weight regulation in ob/ob mice. *Science* 269 (5223):540–3.

Porte, D., Jr., and S. C. Woods. 1981. Regulation of food intake and body weight by insulin. *Diabetologia* 20 Suppl:274–80.

Rissanen, P., A. Franssila-Kallunki, and A. Rissanen. 2001. Cardiac parasympathetic activity is increased by weight loss in healthy obese women. *Obesity Research* 9 (10):637–43.

Roemmich, J. N., and W. E. Sinning. 1997. Weight loss and wrestling training: Effects on growth-related hormones. *Journal of Applied Physiology (Bethesda, Md.: 1985)* 82 (6):1760–4.

Romijn, J. A., R. Adriaanse, G. Brabant, K. Prank, E. Endert, and W. M. Wiersinga. 1990. Pulsatile secretion of thyrotropin during fasting: A decrease of thyrotropin pulse amplitude. *The Journal of Clinical Endocrinology and Metabolism* 70 (6):1631–6.

Rosenbaum, M., R. Goldsmith, D. Bloomfield, A. Magnano, L. Weimer, S. Heymsfield, D. Gallagher, L. Mayer, E. Murphy, and R. L. Leibel. 2005. Low-dose leptin reverses skeletal muscle, autonomic, and neuroendocrine adaptations to maintenance of reduced weight. *Journal of Clinical Investigation* 115 (12):3579–86.

Rosenbaum, M., J. Hirsch, D. A. Gallagher, and R. L. Leibel. 2008a. Long-term persistence of adaptive thermogenesis in subjects who have maintained a reduced body weight. *The American Journal of Clinical Nutrition* 88 (4):906–12.

Rosenbaum, M., J. Hirsch, E. Murphy, and R. L. Leibel. 2000. Effects of changes in body weight on carbohydrate metabolism, catecholamine excretion, and thyroid function. *The American Journal of Clinical Nutrition* 71 (6):1421–32.

Rosenbaum M., Nicolson M., Hirsch J., Murphy E., Chu F, and Leibel R. 1997. Effects of weight change on plasma leptin concentrations and energy expenditure. *The Journal of Clinical Endocrinology and Metabolism* 82:3647–54.

Rosenbaum, M., M. Sy, K. Pavlovich, R. L. Leibel, and J. Hirsch. 2008b. Leptin reverses weight loss-induced changes in regional neural activity responses to visual food stimuli. *Journal of Clinical Investigation* 118 (7):2583–91.

Rosenbaum, M., K. Vandenborne, R. Goldsmith, J.-A. Simoneau, S. Heymsfield, D. R. Joanisse, J. Hirsch, E. Murphy, D. Matthews, K. R. Segal, and R. L. Leibel. 2003. Effects of experimental weight perturbation on skeletal muscle work efficiency in human subjects. *American Journal of Physiology. Regulatory, Integrative and Comparative Physiology* 285 (1):R183–92.

Rossi, M., M. S. Kim, D. G. Morgan, C. J. Small, C. M. Edwards, D. Sunter, S. Abusnana, A. P. Goldstone, S. H. Russell, S. A. Stanley, D. M. Smith, K. Yagaloff, M. A. Ghatei, and S. R. Bloom. 1998. A C-terminal fragment of Agouti-related protein increases feeding and antagonizes the effect of alpha-melanocyte stimulating hormone in vivo. *Endocrinology* 139 (10):4428–31.

Sakata, T., K. Fukagawa, K. Ookuma, K. Fujimoto, H. Yoshimatsu, A. Yamatodani, and H. Wada. 1988. Modulation of neuronal histamine in control of food intake. *Physiology and Behavior* 44 (4–5):539–43.

Sakurai, T., A. Amemiya, M. Ishii, I. Matsuzaki, R. M. Chemelli, H. Tanaka, S. C. Williams, J. A. Richardson, G. P. Kozlowski, S. Wilson, J. R. Arch, R. E. Buckingham, A. C. Haynes, S. A. Carr, R. S. Annan, D. E. McNulty, W. S. Liu, J. A. Terrett, N. A. Elshourbagy, D. J. Bergsma, and M. Yanagisawa. 1998. Orexins and orexin receptors: A family of hypothalamic neuropeptides and G protein-coupled receptors that regulate feeding behavior. *Cell* 92 (4):573–85.

Schapira, D., P. Wolff, N. Kumar, J. Anderson, N. Aziz, G. Lyman, and M. Swanson. 1994. The effect of weight-loss on estimated breast-cancer risk and sex-hormone levels. *Oncology Reports* 1 (3):613–7.

Scheidegger, K., M. O'Connell, D. C. Robbins, and E. Danforth, Jr. 1984. Effects of chronic beta-receptor stimulation on sympathetic nervous system activity, energy expenditure, and thyroid hormones. *The Journal of Clinical Endocrinology and Metabolism* 58 (5):895–903.

Schwartz, A., J. L. Kuk, G. Lamothe, and E. Doucet. 2012. Greater than predicted decrease in resting energy expenditure and weight loss: Results from a systematic review. *Obesity (Silver Spring)* 20 (11):2307–10.

Schwartz, M. W., R. J. Seeley, S. C. Woods, D. S. Weigle, L. A. Campfield, P. Burn, and D. G. Baskin. 1997. Leptin increases hypothalamic pro-opiomelanocortin mRNA expression in the rostral arcuate nucleus. *Diabetes* 46 (12):2119–23.

Shimada, M., N. A. Tritos, B. B. Lowell, J. S. Flier, and E. Maratos-Flier. 1998. Mice lacking melanin-concentrating hormone are hypophagic and lean. *Nature* 396 (6712):670–4.

Spina, M., E. Merlo-Pich, R. K. Chan, A. M. Basso, J. Rivier, W. Vale, and G. F. Koob. 1996. Appetite-suppressing effects of urocortin, a CRF-related neuropeptide. *Science (New York)* 273 (5281):1561–4.

Stephens, T. W., M. Basinski, P. K. Bristow, J. M. Bue-Valleskey, S. G. Burgett, L. Craft, J. Hale, J. Hoffmann, H. M. Hsiung, A. Kriauciunas, W. Mackellar, P. Rasteck Jr., B. Schoner, D. Smith, F. Tinsley, X. Zhang and M. Heiman. 1995. The role of neuropeptide Y in the antiobesity action of the obese gene product. *Nature* 377 (6549):530–2.

Strain, G. W., B. Zumoff, L. K. Miller, W. Rosner, C. Levit, M. Kalin, R. J. Hershcopf, and R. S. Rosenfeld. 1988. Effect of massive weight loss on hypothalamic-pituitary-gonadal function in obese men. *The Journal of Clinical Endocrinology and Metabolism* 66 (5):1019–23.

Straznicky, N. E., M. T. Grima, N. Eikelis, P. J. Nestel, T. Dawood, M. P. Schlaich, R. Chopra, K. Masuo, M. D. Esler, C. I. Sari, G. W. Lambert, and E. A. Lambert. 2011. The effects of weight loss versus weight loss maintenance on sympathetic nervous system activity and metabolic syndrome components. *The Journal of Clinical Endocrinology and Metabolism* 96 (3):E503–8.

Sumithran, P., L. A. Prendergast, E. Delbridge, K. Purcell, A. Shulkes, A. Kriketos, and J. Proietto. 2011. Long-term persistence of hormonal adaptations to weight loss. *The New England Journal of Medicine* 365 (17):1597–604.

Tomiyama, A. J., T. Mann, D. Vinas, J. M. Hunger, J. Dejager, and S. E. Taylor. 2010. Low calorie dieting increases cortisol. *Psychosomatic Medicine* 72 (4):357–64.

Torgerson, J. S., B. Carlsson, K. Stenlof, L. M. Carlsson, E. Bringman, and L. Sjostrom. 1999. A low serum leptin level at baseline and a large early decline in leptin predict a large 1-year weight reduction in energy-restricted obese humans. *The Journal of Clinical Endocrinology and Metabolism* 84 (11):4197–203.

Valentino, M. A., J. E. Lin, A. E. Snook, P. Li, G. W. Kim, G. Marszalowicz, M. S. Magee, T. Hyslop, S. Schulz, and S. A. Waldman. 2011. A uroguanylin-GUCY2C endocrine axis regulates feeding in mice. *The Journal of Clinical Investigation* 121 (9):3578–88.

Verdich, C., S. Toubro, B. Buemann, J. L. Madsen, J. J. Holst, and A. Astrup. 2001. The role of postprandial releases of insulin and incretin hormones in meal-induced satiety—effect of obesity and weight reduction. *International Journal of Obesity and Related Metabolic Disorders: Journal of the International Association for the Study of Obesity* 25 (8):1206–14.

Vijayan, E., and S. M. McCann. 1977. Suppression of feeding and drinking activity in rats following intraventricular injection of thyrotropin releasing hormone (TRH). *Endocrinology* 100 (6):1727–30.

Weinsier, R. L., T. R. Nagy, G. R. Hunter, B. E. Darnell, D. D. Hensrud, and H. L. Weiss. 2000. Do adaptive changes in metabolic rate favor weight regain in weight-reduced individuals? An examination of the set-point theory. *The American Journal of Clinical Nutrition* 72 (5):1088–94.

Westerterp-Plantenga M., W. Saris, C. Hukshorn and L. Campfield. 2001. Effects of weekly administration of pegylated recombinant human OB protein on appetite profile and energy metabolism in obese men. *The American Journal of Clinical Nutrition* 74:426–34.

Wing, R. R., and J. O. Hill. 2001. Successful weight loss maintenance. *Annual Review of Nutrition* 21:323–41.

Wren, A. M., L. J. Seal, M. A. Cohen, A. E. Brynes, G. S. Frost, K. G. Murphy, W. S. Dhillo, M. A. Ghatei, and S. R. Bloom. 2001. Ghrelin enhances appetite and increases food intake in humans. *The Journal of Clinical Endocrinology and Metabolism* 86 (12):5992–5.

Zakrzewska, K. E., I. Cusin, A. Sainsbury, F. Rohner-Jeanrenaud, and B. Jeanrenaud. 1997. Glucocorticoids as counterregulatory hormones of leptin: Toward an understanding of leptin resistance. *Diabetes* 46 (4):717–9.

Zhang, Y., R. Proenca, M. Maffei, M. Barone, L. Leopold, and J. M. Friedman. 1994. Positional cloning of the mouse obese gene and its human homologue. *Nature* 372 (6505):425–32.

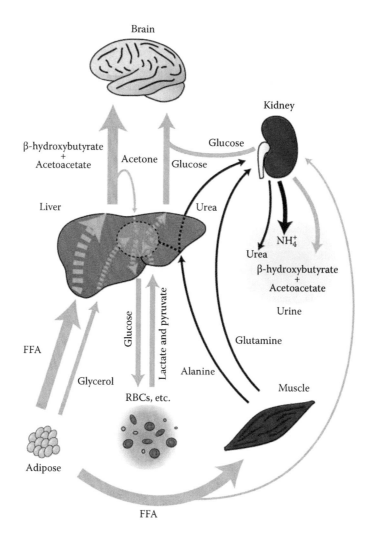

FIGURE 1.1 Overall scheme of starvation fuel metabolism.

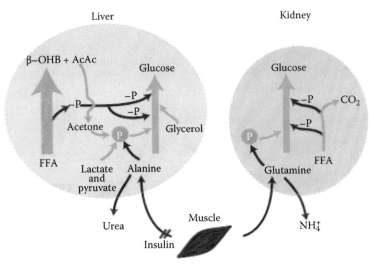

FIGURE 1.2 Glucogenesis in starvation in liver and kidney.

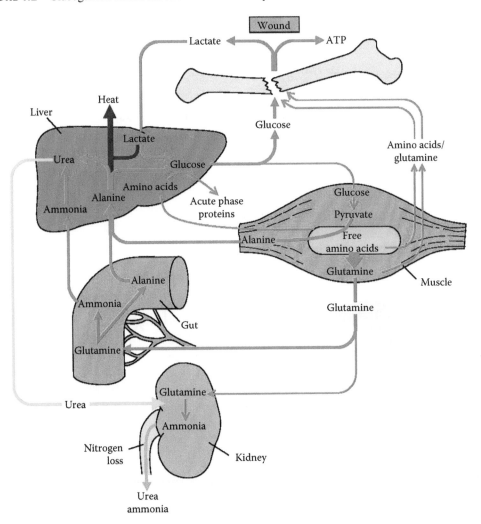

FIGURE 1.9 Metabolic response to critical illness.

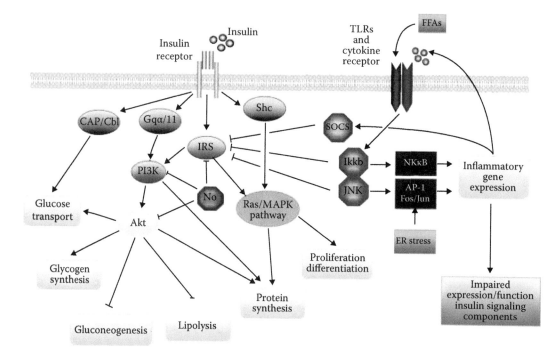

FIGURE 8.1 Direct interaction of insulin signaling and inflammatory pathways.

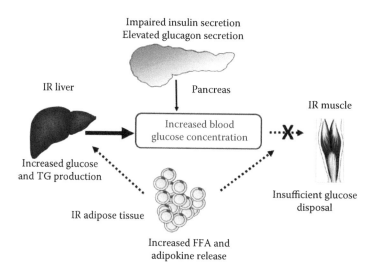

FIGURE 8.2 Increased glucose concentration is due to **IR** at the level of different tissues.

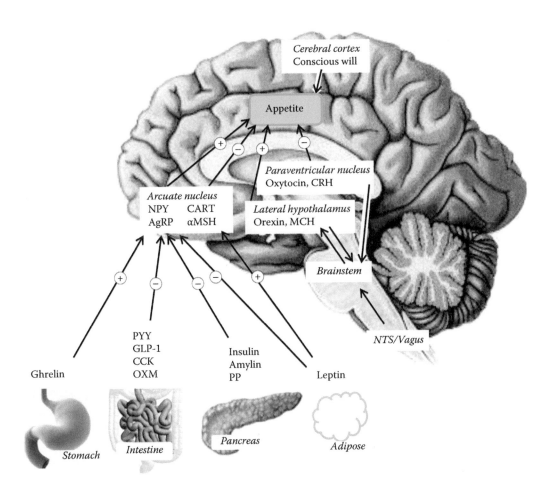

FIGURE 13.1 Selected pathways involved in body weight regulation.

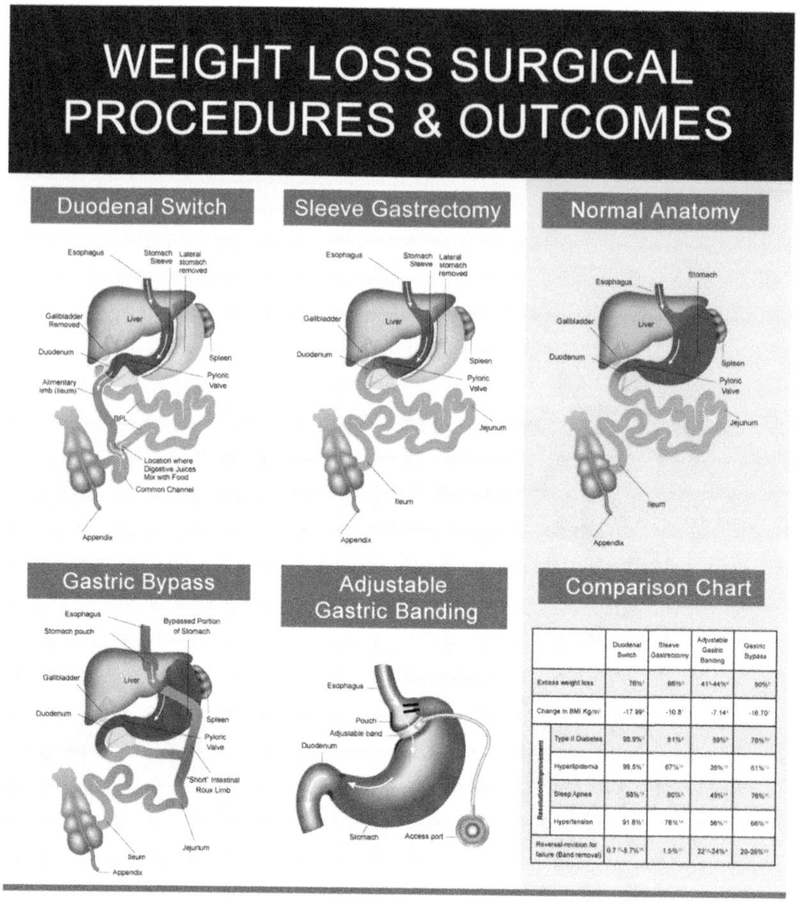

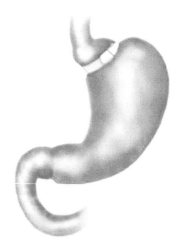

WEIGHT LOSS SURGICAL PROCEDURES & OUTCOMES

Duodenal Switch

Sleeve Gastrectomy

Normal Anatomy

Gastric Bypass

Adjustable Gastric Banding

Comparison Chart

	Duodenal Switch	Sleeve Gastrectomy	Adjustable Gastric Banding	Gastric Bypass
Excess weight loss	76%	66%	41–44%	50%
Change in BMI Kg/m²	-17.99	-10.8	-7.14	-16.70
Type II Diabetes	98.9%	81%	59%	78%
Hyperlipidemia	99.5%	67%	35%	61%
Sleep Apnea	58%	80%	45%	76%
Hypertension	91.8%	76%	56%	66%
Reversal-revision for failure (Band removal)	0.7–3.7%	1.5%	22–34%	20–25%

FIGURE 14.1   Weight loss surgical procedures and outcomes.

FIGURE 15.1   Adjustable gastric banding.

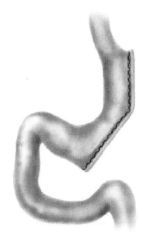

FIGURE 15.2   Sleeve gastrectomy.

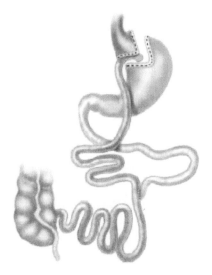

FIGURE 15.3   Roux-en-Y gastric bypass.

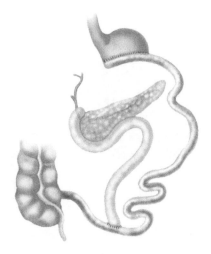

FIGURE 15.4   Biliopancreatic diversion.

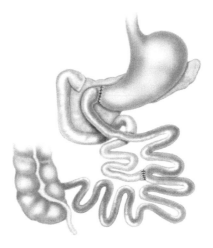

FIGURE 15.5 Duodenal–jejunal bypass.

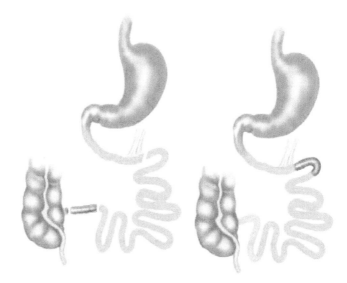

FIGURE 15.6 Ileal interposition.

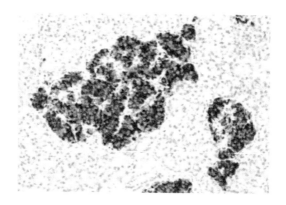

FIGURE 18.1 Middle of figure shows enlarged islet from patient with immunohistochemical staining for insulin.

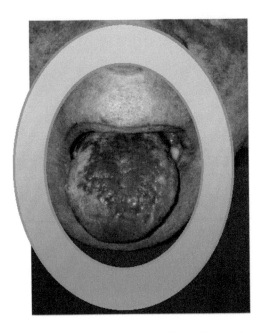

FIGURE 21.8 Atrophic glossitis and cheilitis in a patient with multiple B vitamin deficiencies.

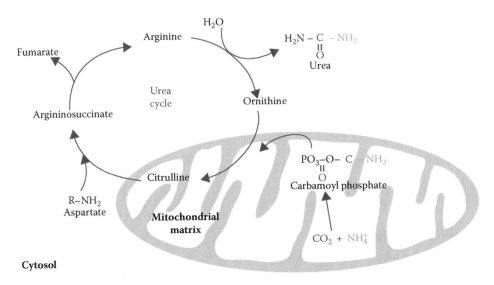

FIGURE 27.1 Simplified urea cycle depicting the key enzymes involved in the pathway.

14 An Overview of Surgical Weight Loss Options

Amrita G. Sawhney and Michael Fishman

CONTENTS

INTRODUCTION

The consequences of morbid obesity increase the risk for serious medical illness, impact health and quality of life, and reduce survival. A clinical imperative for effective, meaningful, and sustainable weight loss exists to prevent these diseases from manifesting and reversing those that have already occurred. The key to successful weight loss is a permanent alteration in eating behavior and caloric intake (i.e., food choices and portion sizes) combined with an increase in daily caloric expenditure. But, accomplishing these fundamental changes through lifestyle and pharmaceutical therapy has been a difficult process for patients and providers alike. Surgical approaches to weight loss must be considered when more conservative measures fail.

All bariatric procedures have the capacity to reduce food intake. Some have been shown to alter food selection choices. A metabolic effect has been observed after certain bariatric procedures that favorably alters hormonal balance within the gastrointestinal (GI) tract. This action may improve glucose metabolism and help resolve diabetes. But it also has a significant role in changing a patient's perception of hunger and satiety.

The metabolism can be increased naturally by exercise. It may also be possible to increase energy expenditure through the use of specific agents, such as herbal and pharmaceutical stimulants. But we are now beginning to recognize that some weight loss procedures may also result in an increased metabolic rate.

In this chapter, we will review the background of the three types of bariatric surgery and their practical use. We will explore guidelines for patient selection and discuss which surgery is best suited for which patient. We will discuss the mechanisms by which each procedure assists in weight loss and the associated risks of complications.

HISTORICAL OVERVIEW

Bariatric surgery has evolved over the past 60 years. The early attempts at surgical weight control provided invaluable experience and research outcomes but were associated with significant risks. The evolution of the methodologies over the past six decades has led to the application of procedures with improved outcomes and reduced rates of mortality and morbidity. Many types of weight loss surgeries were developed. These are often presented chronologically. They can also be categorized by the type of procedure: malabsorptive, restrictive, and combined (Table 14.1).

The restrictive procedures function purely to restrict the intake of oral consumption by creating a smaller stomach capacity (or reservoir) to eat into. Malabsorptive procedures impair caloric intake by causing an alteration of the GI capacity to absorb nutrients. Combination procedures restrict food intake and selection by the creation of a small reservoir but also add a component of GI malabsorption.

Among the restrictive procedures are vertical banded gastroplasty (VBG), laparoscopic adjustable gastric banding (LAGB), and the sleeve gastrectomy (SG). The malabsorptive procedures include the duodenal switch (DS; biliopancreatic diversion [BPD]) and two new devices, which are in the testing stage (duodenal sleeve and gastric aspirator). The combined procedures are essentially limited to the various forms of Roux-en-Y gastric bypass (RYGB).

The jejunoileal bypass (JIB), a malabsorptive procedure developed in the 1950s, was the earliest recognized form of weight loss surgery. The concept emerged from observation by surgeons that a shortened gut led to weight loss and resistance to weight regain despite increased caloric intake [1]. Several pioneering surgeons were independently involved in its genesis. Victor Henrickson in Gothenburg, Sweden, is recognized for performing intestinal resection for weight management in 1953. In the same year, Richard Varco of the University of Minnesota performed a JIB operation, although his results were not published [2]. In 1954, Dr. Arnold J. Kremer, also from the University of Minnesota, along with his colleagues Drs. Linder and Nelson, were among the first to perform JIB surgery [3].

The JIB procedure circumvented a large portion of the GI tract and created significant malabsorption. In the native GI tract, there are approximately 700 cm or 22 feet of small bowel. In the JIB, only 30–40 cm of the small bowel is retained in the absorptive stream [4]. The majority of the small bowel is bypassed, creating a severe form of surgical malabsorption, leading to approximately one-third of calories absorbed compared to an intact small bowel. This, therefore, is the principal mechanism of weight loss. Because the shortened length of the bowel results in rapid transit time from the stomach to the colon, frequent liquid stools result, particularly after ingestion of fats or refined carbohydrates [1]. Thus, the JIB also causes weight loss from a deterrent physiologic feedback effect on caloric intake.

In 1962, Payne and DeWind performed end-to-end jejunocolonic shunt in 10 patients. In addition to weight loss, they observed uncontrollable diarrhea, dehydration, and electrolyte imbalance in the patients. Subsequently, they advised against such jejunocolonic anastomoses and went on to

TABLE 14.1
Types of Weight Loss Operations

Malabsorptive	Restrictive	Combined
Jejunoileal bypass	Vertical banded gastroplasty	Loop gastric bypass
Jejunoileal bypass jejunocolonic shunt	Silastic ring vertical gastroplasty	Stapled gastric bypass
Jejunoileal bypass end-to-end anastomosis	Lap band	Transected gastric bypass
Jejunoileal bypass end-to-side anastomosis	Sleeve gastrectomy	Banded gastric bypass
Biliopancreatic diversion		Distal Roux-en-Y gastric bypass
Biliopancreatic diversion with a duodenal switch		

recommend an end-to-side jejunoileostomy instead [5]. Another JIB modification was developed by Scott with an end-to-end anastomosis [6]. The Payne modification was designed to decrease bacterial overgrowth by diminishing the amount of reflux from the colon into the small bowel. Scott claimed that his modification achieved superior weight loss by preventing reflux of nutrients into the bypassed segment.

Various forms of the JIB procedure were performed until the 1970s, when they fell out of favor [7]. This was due to the recognition of associated long-term complications. These could be quite severe, causing major organ damage, including liver failure (7%), renal failure (37%), severe fluid and electrolyte imbalances from diarrhea (29%), calcium oxalate nephrolithiasis (29%), vitamin deficiencies, malnutrition, and death [8].

Halverson et al. [9] performed a review of 101 carefully screened obese patients who underwent JIB and were followed for a mean of 32 months. They reported that 3% died postoperatively of liver failure and/or its complications. Another death was attributed to pulmonary embolism and another from severe diarrhea and cachexia. Reversal was required in 19% due to liver failure or electrolyte disturbances. Overall, 58% had major complications [9]. Thus, while the JIB did result in long-term weight loss, its complications were thought to be so considerable that its replacement became inevitable. Although the procedure was abandoned, there are still patients with JIB procedures who may present for treatment, and metabolic physicians must be prepared to participate in their care (Table 14.2) [10].

In 1967, Mason and Ito [11] developed the first series of gastric bypass (GBP) operations for obese patients. They had observed that postoperative females who underwent partial gastrectomy for peptic ulcer disease remained underweight and found weight regain a challenge. The GBP was designed as a combined restrictive and malabsorptive operation. A small stomach pouch was created in congruity to the esophagus. Most of the stomach, the duodenum, and 2 feet of the proximal jejunum were excluded from the nutrient stream.

Many modifications of this procedure have occurred since its development, including the first stapled GBP by Alden in 1977 [12]. The GBP proved to be a safe and effective surgical alternative to the JIB, resulting in a 50% loss of excess body weight (EBW). However, it is not without its own risk of complications, including nausea, vomiting, dumping syndrome, marginal ulcers, bile reflux, gastritis, gastric dilation, gastric blowout, and nutritional deficiencies (i.e., iron; calcium; vitamins A, D, E, and B_{12}; and thiamine).

In 1978, Wilkinson and Peloso [13] developed a purely restrictive weight loss procedure by placing a nonadjustable band around the upper part of the stomach. This consisted of a 2 cm Marlex mesh wrapped around the upper part of the stomach. However, the nonadjustable band, and other

TABLE 14.2
Complications of Jejunoileal Bypass

Problem	Mechanism
Steatohepatitis Possible cirrhosis	Amino acid deficiency
Renal oxalosis	Excess oxalate absorption; oxalate not bound by calcium
Fat-soluble vitamin deficiency	Malabsorption; steatorrhea
Gallstones	Bile acid loss; mobilization of cholesterol
Enteritis	Bacterial overgrowth
Arthritis	Bacterial toxin; autoimmune
Fatigue syndrome	Vitamin deficiency; multifactorial
Bypass encephalopathy	Possible deficiency; possible D-lactic acid deficiency
Bypass dermatitis	Possible antigen–antibody complex (enteric bacteria)

Source: Singh D., *World J. Gastroenterol.*, 1518, 2009.

forms that followed in the 1980s had high failure rates due to inability to control the stomal diameter, pouch dilation, and erosion. Therefore, they were eventually abandoned.

In 1979, Scopinaro in Italy developed a new form of malabsorptive procedure, the BPD [14]. This operation differed from the JIB since no small bowel was rendered surgically nonfunctional and a 200–250 cm^2 gastric pouch was formed. By allowing flow of pancreatic juices and bile in the two small bowel limbs, bypass enteritis was minimized, and decreases in the rate of hepatic failure were seen. The operation improved the frequency and extent of diarrhea. However, nutrient deficiencies, including protein malnutrition, limited its appeal [15].

In 1982, several restrictive gastroplasty operations were undertaken, including the VBG by Edward Mason [16]. A variant of this procedure was the silastic ring vertical gastroplasty (SRVG) [17]. Both the VBG and SRVG involved stapling the stomach, thereby leaving a 10–30 cm^2 pouch. The small bowel was not rerouted, and the procedures were fairly simple to perform. This made VBG a popular surgical weight loss option. In the 1990s, such procedures accounted for nearly 90% of bariatric operations performed in the United States [1].

In 1986, Lubomyr Kuzmak reported the first clinical use of an adjustable gastric band in weight loss surgery. Other surgeons using the adjustable band technique included Knut Kolle [18] and Molina [19]. The advantage of the band was that it preserved the natural anatomy of the GI tract, without requiring any anastomosis or stapling of the stomach. Furthermore, the size of the stomal diameter could be varied based on the patient's requirements. This latter function was enabled through the use of an implanted port, which instilled saline into the bladder of the adjustable band.

In 1988, Hess [20] developed a variation of the BPD by performing a duodenal switch (BPD-DS). This operation preserved the pyloric sphincter, which prevented dumping syndrome and decreased the rate of marginal ulcer development. Stomach volume was decreased with an SG. The duodenum is divided, and a 250 cm Roux limb is created. A duodenobiliopancreatc limb was also created, which is anastomosed to the Roux limb 50 cm from the ileocecal junction. As with the BPD, patients must be closely monitored for nutritional deficiencies. They may experience malodorous stools, body odor, and flatus if their diet is not carefully controlled. This procedure is primarily considered to be malabsorptive but does add a component of restriction by means of the creation of a gastric sleeve.

In 1993, a significant step toward what we know as modern bariatric surgery was taken by Dr. Alan Wittgrove [21] when he performed the first laparoscopic gastric bypass (LGB) operation in San Diego, California. The advantages over the open procedure were evident. Banka et al. [22] have published a retrospective cohort study of 41,094 open cases and 115,177 laparoscopic cases. Their work shows that more open cases had complications, higher mortality, longer length of stay, and higher total hospital charges [22].

Also in 1993, one of the earliest vertical sleeve gastrectomies (VSGs) was performed by Dr. Jamieson in Australia [23]. This was followed by Dr. Johnston in England in 1996 and Dr. Michelle Gagner in New York in 2001. The VSG was seen as an alternative to GBP because of decreased rates of nutritional deficiencies, marginal ulcer development, dumping syndrome, and intestinal obstruction [24,25]. The VSG is thought of as a mainly restrictive procedure.

CURRENT COMMON WEIGHT LOSS PROCEDURES

Currently, there are three weight loss procedure types in use at most bariatric surgery centers: the gastric band, SG, and RYGB. In addition, because of the strong data on diabetes resolution, there has been a recent increase in the use of the DS. The metabolic consequences of these procedures are discussed in detail elsewhere in this text. Figure 14.1, reproduced with permission from Dr. Ara Keshishian [26], illustrates these procedures and provides a comparison of outcomes for these procedures.

Most surgeons perform these procedures laparoscopically, with an option to open the abdomen if necessary. Figure 14.2 shows the percentage change in performed open gastric bypass (OGB), LGB, laparoscopic SG (LSG), and LAGB between 2008 and 2012 [27]. Of particular note are the

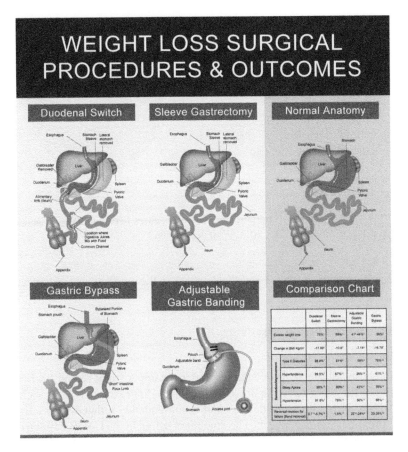

FIGURE 14.1 **(See color insert.)** Weight loss surgical procedures and outcomes. Notes: [1]Biertho L et al. Is biliopancreatic diversion with duodenal switch indicated for patients with body mass index <50 kg/m²? *SOARD* 2010;6:508–515. [2]Shi X, Karmali S, Sharma AM et al. A review of laparoscopic sleeve gastrectomy for morbid obesity. *Obes Surg.* 2010;20:1171–1177. [3]Phillips E, Ponce J, Cunneen SA et al. Safety and effectiveness of REALIZE adjustable gastric band: 3-year prospective study in the United States. *Surg Obes Relat Dis.* 2009;5:588–597. [4]van Nieuwenhove Y et al. Long-term results of a prospective study of laparoscopic adjustable gastric banding for morbid obesity. *Obes Surg.* 2001;21:582–587. [5]O'Brian P et al. Systematic review of medium-term weight loss after bariatric surgery. *Obes Surg.* 2006;16:1301–1040. [6]Buchwald H. Bariatric surgery, a systematic review and meta-analysis. *JAMA* 2004;292:1724–1738. [7]Uglioni B et al. Midterm results of primary vs. secondary laparoscopic sleeve gastrectomy (LSG) as an isolated operation. *Obes Surg.* 2009;19(4):401–406. [8]Cottam et al. Laparoscopic sleeve gastrectomy and an initial weight loss procedure for high risk patients with morbid obesity. *Surg Endosc.* 2006;20:859–863. [9]Tice JA, Karliner L, Walsh J et al. Gastric banding or bypass? A systematic review comparing the two most popular procedures. *Am J Med.* 2008;121:885–893. [10]Tice et al. Gastric banding or bypass? A systematic review comparing the two popular procedures. *Am J Med.* 2008;121:885–893. [11]Benaiges et al. Laparoscopic sleeve gastrectomy and laparoscopic gastric bypass are equally effective for reduction of the cardiovascular risk in severely obese patients at one year follow up. *Surg Obes.* 2011 (in press). [12]Post-approval statistical analysis of clinical trial data. *Ethicon Endo Surgery.* [13]Cottam et al. A case-controlled match-paired cohort study of lap. RNY gastric bypass and lap band patient in a single US center with three year follow up. *Obes Surg.* 2006;16:534–540. [14]Biertho L et al. Is biliopancreatic diversion with duodenal switch indicated for patients with body mass index <50 kg/m²? *SOARD* 2010;6:508–515. [15]Marcaeu et al. Duodenal switch: Long term results. *Obes Surg.* 2007;17;1421–1430. [16]Anthone et al. The duodenal switch operation for the treatment of morbid obesity. *Ann Surg.* 2003;238:618–628. [17]Dapri et al. Lap seromyotomy for long stenosis after sleeve gastrectomy with or without duodenal switch. *Obes Surg.* 2009;19:495–499. [18]Ray J et al. Safety, efficacy and durability of laparoscopic adjustable gastric banding in a single surgeon US community hospital. *SOARD* 7;2011:140–144. [19]Christou et al. Weight gain after short and long gastric bypass in patients followed for longer than 10 years. *Ann Surg.* 2006;244:734–740. (From Keshishian, A., http://www.dssurgery.com/weight-loss-surgery-poster.php. With permission.)

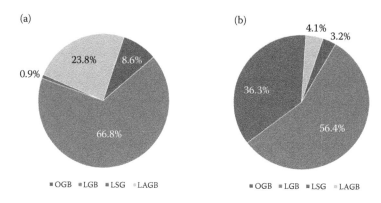

FIGURE 14.2 Percent distribution of bariatric surgery procedures between 2008 (a) and 2012 (b). (From Nguyen NT et al., *J. Am. Coll. Surg.*, 216, 2013. With permission.)

increase in the performance of the SG and the decrease in the performance of the gastric band during this period.

RESTRICTIVE WEIGHT LOSS PROCEDURES

Gastric Banding

The gastric band is an adjustable device that encircles the upper stomach and restricts food intake. The surgeon places the band under laparoscopic guidance approximately 1 cm below the gastro-esophageal junction. The balloon inside the band is subsequently inflated with saline and thereby creates a small proximal stomach pouch. The amount of saline in the LAGB balloon determines the diameter of the surgically created canal between the small proximal stomach pouch and the rest of the stomach. The degree of narrowing of the canal corresponds to the rate at which food and liquid leave the small proximal stomach pouch and hence affects satiety and calories consumed. This volume of saline "fill" can be increased as needed to achieve weight loss goals or decreased if patients develop issues with tolerance such as acid reflux and vomiting.

There are several different band types available in the market. Each has slightly different characteristics, which may have particular advantages or disadvantages for the individual patient. The Lap-Band AP system made by Allergan is one device option (Figure 14.3). The band is designed to create a closed high-pressure system. This high-pressure system allows for an easily achieved restriction on intake while also limiting the ability of patients to overeat. Another advantage of this high-pressure system is higher restriction with less volume adjustments. This allows for less fluid to be added to the band to achieve optimal restriction.

As a downside of this high-pressure system, patients who eat past the point of satiety will often have high incidences of emesis and food becoming "stuck" in the band. This may necessitate multiple return trips to the surgeon's office or hospital for removal of fluid from the band. Also, because of significant pressure changes with minimal fluid adjustments, the band can become overtightened. As a result, some have advocated that adjustments be made under fluoroscopic guidance.

A second device option is the REALIZE Adjustable Gastric Band by Ethicon. The design is similar to the Lap-Band; however, unlike its competitor, the REALIZE band functions in a low-pressure system. The low pressure has the advantage of leading to less frequent episodes of emesis. This is because the lower pressure allows the balloon to give slightly, which often allows passage of an impacted food bolus.

The final device option, although not available in the United States but used in Europe and elsewhere, is the Cousin Bioring, a new-generation adjustable gastric band. Much like the REALIZE

(a)   (b)

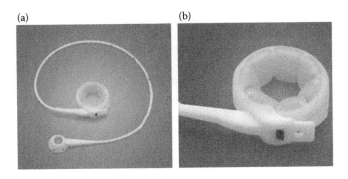

FIGURE 14.3   The Lap-Band. (Permission from : Apollo Endosurgery.)

band, the Cousin Bioring is a low-pressure system. It differs from the REALIZE band in size and the configuration of the port [28].

Regardless of specific device chosen, the insertion of the gastric band leads to an early and prolonged satiety. In this way, the band leads to smaller portion sizes. Patients who tend to eat large portions of food at one sitting often have excellent weight loss after a gastric banding because it limits their portions. Burton and Borwon [29] studied the mechanism of gastric band weight loss utilizing video manometry and nuclear studies of gastric emptying. His group found that the food bolus leaves the stomach pouch only 1–2 min after the intake stops, caused by esophageal peristaltic contractions that lead to periodic forward flow and reflux. This activity in the lower esophagus is thought to be linked to the early satiety appreciated by the patient.

The bands are adjusted utilizing a port that is anchored to the abdominal wall musculature and hidden under the patient's skin. This port is then connected to the balloon in the band with tubing that crosses the abdominal fascia and enters the peritoneal cavity. The port is accessed utilizing a noncoring needle similar to that used for intravenous infusion port devices. The port itself contains a silicone block, which is self-sealing, reducing the risk of a leak at the port site.

The first adjustment is usually scheduled for 4–6 weeks after surgery. These adjustments can be done in an office setting or in a fluoroscopy suite if fluoroscopy is utilized for adjustments. If fluoroscopy is not used, most surgeons utilize a method of injecting a measured volume of saline with each adjustment and order an oral liquid trial following the adjustment to ensure that the band is not overly tightened. This protocol can be specific to each surgeon and is usually based on practice experience as well as guidelines from the manufacturer [30].

Some surgeons begin with 1 mL of fluid at the time of the first fill and then continue to closely monitor the patient for adjustments [31]. The advantage of this approach is that it can be done in the office, making it easier for patients to undergo adjustments. The downside is that there is some margin for error because the anatomy and rate of gastric emptying is not observed with the newly tightened band. By utilizing fluoroscopy, the surgeon can visualize the opening in the band after the patient takes barium by mouth and adjust it accordingly. The other advantage of the fluoroscopic technique is that the esophagus, stomach, and band are visualized and inspected for early or late physiologic or structural changes due to the banding.

In general, patients are evaluated on an ongoing basis to determine whether they need additional fill volume. The goal of a an ideally filled band is to create a sensation of prolonged postmeal satiety, steady and progressive weight loss planned over 18 months to 3 years, and avoidance of negative restrictive symptoms. Table 14.3, modified from Favretti et al. [31], shows the indications for band adjustments.

Along with a new eating behavior, it is crucial that band patients exercise as well. The band itself does not increase metabolism, so to be successful with weight loss after banding, the patient must exercise [32].

TABLE 14.3

LAGB Adjustment Indications

Fluid May Be Added		No Adjustment	Fluid May Be Removed	
(+) Fluoroscopy	**(−) Fluoroscopy**		**(+) Fluoroscopy**	**(−) Fluoroscopy**
Stenosis of the gastric outlet with compensatory consumption of high-calorie liquids or very soft foods	Inadequate weight loss	Adequate weight loss	Wide outlet (>8 mm)	Vomiting, heartburn, reflux
Esophageal dilation (>2×)	Inadequate post meal satiety	Tolerating adequate variety of food	Immediate passage of barium swallow (1 peristaltic wave)	Coughing, wheezing at night
Esophageal atony	Tolerating increased meal volume	No negative symptoms	Inadequate range of tolerated food	Inadequate range of tolerated food
Esophageal emptying after more than 4–5 peristaltic waves	Between-meal hunger		Overly tight band causing patient to consume high-calorie liquid or very soft foods	Overly tight band causing patient to consume high-calorie liquid or very soft foods
Reflux				
Pouch dilation and insufficient emptying				

Source: Favretti F et al., *Am. J. Surg.*, 184, 2002.

Weight loss with the adjustable gastric band is variable. In an optimal scenario, a patient would lose 10–15 pounds the first month and then 1–2 pounds per week after. This weight loss is still less efficient then in the GBP or SG, which we will discuss later. Although there has been shown to be some improvement in weight-related comorbidities after gastric banding, the impact appears to be less favorable then a bypass or sleeve [33,34].

Although the gastric band is the least invasive surgical option, it does carry its own risks and associated morbidity. These include migration of implant (band erosion, band slippage, port displacement); tubing-related complications (port disconnection, tubing); band leak; esophageal spasm; gastroesophageal reflux disease (GERD); inflammation of the esophagus or stomach, and port-site infection [35]. Of these complications, some require further surgical intervention. Tubing-related complications are typically minor in their effect on patients and are usually easily corrected with minor surgery. However, migration of the implant and band leaks require removal of the band and, sometimes, additional procedures. Specifically, band erosions require not only removal of the band but also repair of the eroded portion of the stomach. In terms of GERD and inflammation of the stomach and esophagus, these are often relieved with removal of fluid from the band, thereby allowing food boluses to empty with less exposure to mucosal lining of the esophagus and stomach.

In patients with gastric bands, prolonged vomiting or exposure of caustic food boluses to the esophagus from the band being too tight can lead to chronic changes in the esophagus. These include but are not limited to esophageal dysmotility and Barrett's esophagus. For these reasons, it is very important to carefully follow band patients and intervene when symptoms arise or worsen. Utilizing fluoroscopy for adjustments allows the surgeon to intervene early should any of the afore-mentioned conditions be noted.

SG

The SG achieves weight loss by restricting the amount of food consumed without malabsorption. No foreign body is used. Initially, some surgeons adopted it as part of a staged operation for morbidly obese patients to allow them to lose weight and reduce comorbidities and return to the operating room as better surgical candidates (reduced surgical risk) for the second-stage procedures, which were more complicated and carried greater risk [36]. Chu et al. [37] published the first report of the SG used as the initial stage in super-obese patients who then underwent laparoscopic BPD with DS (LBPD-DS). Later, the SG came into its own as a single-step procedure as reports of its use were published in the literature.

One such report by Moon Han et al. in 2005 [38] reported a series of 130 patients who underwent SG. The authors reported a 75% resolution of dyslipidemia, 100% resolution of diabetes, 93% resolution of hypertension, and 100% resolution of joint pain in 1 year. In a study that included super-morbid and morbidly obese subjects, Langer et al. [39] reported that patients who underwent LSG achieved a mean excess weight loss of 46% at 6 months and 56% at 12 months postoperatively. They concluded that the SG as a single-step procedure was adequate for many patients.

Frezza [40] lists the advantages of SG as decreased stomach size without loss of function, pyloric preservation that prevents dumping, avoidance of malabsorption symptoms, 1-day postoperative hospitalization, the ability to perform SG laparoscopically even in patients weighing over 500 lbs, and the ability to use SG in patients with anemia or Crohn's disease who cannot undergo bypass. This has led other surgeons to utilize SG as a single-step procedure reserved not only for the super-morbidly obese but also for those with a body mass index (BMI) < 50 kg/m^2 [41,42].

An important consideration in the eventual success of the SG is the sleeve volume. Weiner et al. [43] studied this issue in a prospective trial of 120 patients who underwent LSG. Three groups were studied. In the first, LSG was performed without the use of a calibration tube; in the second, a 44-French-diameter calibration tube was used; and in the third, a 32-French-diameter calibration tube was used. They reported that the percentage of excess BMI loss was significantly higher for patients who underwent LSG with tube calibrations and that LSG with large sleeve volume was associated with a slight weight gain during 5 years of observation.

Stomach distensibility after SG and final stomach volume are also important factors in the success of this operation. Yehoshua et al. [44] studied 17 patients who underwent LSG utilizing volume and pressure in the entire pre-op stomach, in the removed gastric fundus, and finally, in the newly formed "sleeve" stomach after LSG. They demonstrated that the distensibility of the total stomach and excised portion were similar to each other. The distensiblity of the sleeve portion was 10 times less than that of the removed portion, and it represented 10% of the original volume of the total stomach. They conclude that the relatively high intraluminal pressure achieved in the sleeve accounts for early satiety experienced by patients and state that the size of the sleeve is important to prevent long-term dilation. A smaller sleeve ensures complete removal of the gastric fundus, which has the greatest potential for postoperative dilation.

After SG, stomach emptying is altered. This may be due to disruption of the nervous synctium of the stomach, which occurs along with resection of the greater curvature [45]. Furthermore, the procedure generally results in removal of the stomach's natural pacemaker. Although the specific effects of the SG on gastric emptying are still unclear, most authors believe that it actually accelerates nutrient flow into the duodenum [45]. The increase in transit of undigested nutrients may be the explanation for the altered incretin secretion by intestinal L cells after a sleeve procedure.

The SG is believed to exert a favorable effect on the GI endocrine system. Evidence suggests that the sleeve can act to decrease the release of gastric-secreted ghrelin, while increasing the release of intestinal glucagon-like peptide-1 (GLP-1) [46]. Therefore, the SG seems optimally suited to result in a decrease in hunger and an increase in satiety.

The combination of the diminished ghrelin-induced hunger, restrictive smaller stomach, altered gastric emptying, and increased incretin-related satiety leads to rapid, effective weight loss. Several studies have shown a comparable result of the SG to the RYGB in terms of weight loss and diabetes resolution. Because there is no alteration of intestinal anatomy, the SG has no malabsorptive component and, therefore, less risk of metabolic derangements.

Like all surgical procedures, the SG is also associated with certain risks and complications specific to the procedure. Insertion of the bougie tube may stretch the gastroesophageal junction. This has been associated with esophageal perforation in rare instances. The procedure is performed by utilizing a stapling device that staples and separates the stomach. Because of this, there exists a risk of a leak from this staple line.

Frezza et al. [47] report that the SG is a generally safe operation with some negatives, which include lack of reversibility and stapling complications. They retrospectively reviewed 53 cases of LSG between 2005 and 2008 and found that five patients (9.4%) developed complications [47]. These included three patients who developed postoperative staple line hemorrhage or bleeding and two patients who developed staple line leaks. In the same paper, they reviewed 17 published papers, which included 810 patients who underwent LSG. Table 14.4, adapted from Frezza et al. shows their findings. Other studies have shown a 1–7% occurrence rate of staple line leaks after LSG [48].

Gastroesophageal reflux disease (GERD) is another notable complication of SG. In a group of 176 patients, Carter et al. [49] report that 36.6% had GERD symptoms preoperatively, and this increased to 49% immediately after surgery and persisted at 47.2% over a month after LSG. They concluded that GERD was not relieved with LSG and those patients without GERD preoperatively were at an increased risk for it after.

Himpens et al. [50] reported a biphasic increase in GERD to 6 months postoperatively and then another increase in reflux from 3 to 6 years after LSG [50]. Braghetto et al. [51] also found GERD problematic after SG. They evaluated the lower esophageal sphincter (LES) using manometry before and after SG and demonstrated that the operation leads to a decrease in LES pressure. They

---

TABLE 14.4
Sleeve Gastrectomy Complications

Complication	Number	Percentage
Reoperations	29	3.6
Leak	7	0.8
Prolonged ventilator requirements	5	0.6
Strictures	6	0.7
Renal insufficiency	4	0.5
Postoperative hemorrhage	3	0.4
Atelectasis	2	0.2
Pulmonary embolus	2	0.2
Delayed gastric emptying	2	0.2
Gastric dilation	1	0.1
Prolonged vomiting	1	0.1
Subphrenic abscess	2	0.2
Trocar site infection	1	0.1
Urinary tract infection	1	0.1
Splenic injury	1	0.1
Trocar site hernia	1	0.1
Death	4	0.5

Source: Frezza EE et al., *Obes. Surg.*, 19, 2009.

stated that this may result in reflux symptoms and esophagitis due to a partial resection of the sling fibers during the gastrectomy.

Although the SG is not a malabsorptive procedure, it can result in the disturbances in calcium, vitamin D, and parathyroid hormone (PTH), which can leave some patients vulnerable to osteoporosis [52]. Patients with GERD may be even more at risk. The use of H2 blockers can impede the breakdown of calcium salts, and the use of proton pump inhibitors can lead to decreased osteoclast formation [48].

COMBINED RESTRICTIVE AND MALABSORPTIVE WEIGHT LOSS PROCEDURES

RYGB

Although the recent trend has been to increase the performance of SG procedures, the RYGB has remained the most commonly performed procedure for weight loss in the United States, with an estimated 140,000 cases performed per year [53]. At many centers, the RYGB is still considered the "gold standard" of weight loss surgery.

The RYGB produces weight loss through a confluence of mechanisms. This can be illustrated by considering the operation as a complex that includes several subprocedures. Each of these components can have different effects on weight loss and metabolism.

The first component of the RYGB is the creation of a small gastric pouch. This entails isolating the gastric cardia and separating it from the rest of the stomach. The remainder of the stomach, which is still connected to the pylorus and duodenum, is referred to as the gastric remnant. The gastric pouch has a volume of <100 mL. This greatly restricts gastric capacity and reduces mealtime food consumption. The rate of consumption is also altered by this component of the procedure.

Patients who eat too much food or eat too quickly after an RYGB will discover that food "backs up" into the esophagus. This overflow of food into the esophagus produces an unpleasant feeling of lower chest fullness. It also may result in a hypersalivation response and may eventually cause vomiting. Patients tell us that they quickly learn to avoid these unpleasant experiences by eating smaller meals, chewing more thoroughly, and eating more slowly.

The creation of the gastric pouch is also believed to suppress gastric production of the hormone ghrelin. This hormone plays an important role in stimulating hunger and regulating blood glucose. Therefore, the absence of this hormone reduces the desire to eat and may also contribute to the diabetes resolution seen after GBP.

The bypassed portion of the stomach, or remnant, remains in continuity with the rest of the GI tract. This may be thought of as a second component of the GBP. The gastric remnant is no longer within the path of nutrient flow. This appears to have an impact on food selection and taste preferences. Patients who have had a GBP report a preference for foods that are less sweet than before their surgery.

In their study, Bueter et al. [54] evaluated sucrose taste perception in humans after RYGB. They found that these patients were able to detect lower concentrations of sucrose compared to controls. Tichansky et al. [55] report that 82% of RYBG patients had a change in taste in food and beverages. Among these patients, 92% reported the change as a decrease in the intensity of taste, 68% of patients reported the development of aversion to certain foods, and 83% agreed that the loss of taste led to better weight loss. Scruggs et al. [56] reported that postoperative taste preference alteration was not accounted for by common mediators of taste such as zinc levels, glycemic status, liver and kidney function, or age. Furthermore, studies using functional magnetic resonance imaging (MRI) have shown that GBP surgery patients report a shift in food preference away from high-calorie foods, which may explain why they tend to seek out fewer "fast food" options after surgery [57].

In addition to bypassing the remnant stomach, the entire duodenum has been bypassed. This can be considered the third component of the RYGB. Bypassing the duodenum has the obvious effect of reducing nutrient absorption, since the duodenum is our most important nutrient absorptive surface. In addition, bypassing the duodenum appears to have an effect on the metabolic rate [58]. Studies have shown that diet-induced thermogenesis (DIT) is increased through this maneuver. The DIT is also referred to as the specific dynamic action (SDA) or the thermic effect of food (TEF) [59].

A fourth component of the RYGB is the creation of a conduit between the gastric pouch and the jejunum. The segment connecting the pouch to the small intestine is called the Roux limb. The Roux limb begins at a narrow opening at the anastomosis between the pouch and the small bowel. Therefore, this "stoma" contributes to the restriction of nutrient flow. As chewed and swallowed (but undigested) food leaves the pouch, it enters the intestine at the level of the jejunum. The presence of undigested food in the jejunum appears to be a potent stimulator of the L cells.

Foods that contain refined carbohydrates exert an osmotic effect at this level and produce a rapid fluid shift. This distends the bowel and leads to a "dumping syndrome." Here, again, patients learn to avoid these types of foods to prevent the unpleasant symptoms. Therefore, caloric intake is altered.

A fifth component of the RYGB is the maldigestion created by the bypassed intestinal segment. The complex process of digestion requires emulsification by bile and enzymatic breakdown from pancreatic and luminal enzymes. The bypassed GI segment containing the remnant stomach, duodenum, biliary, and pancreatic secretions is called the biliopancreatic limb. Although this limb of the GI tract will eventually meet the Roux limb, the distance between the food bolus and the digestive secretions will lead to an uncoordinated digestion. Therefore, some degree of maldigestion and malabsorption will occur.

While this malabsorption may be beneficial in terms of weight loss, its negative effect is that the essential vitamins and minerals will also be incompletely absorbed. This is precisely why patients who have had GBP require close, lifelong supervision by a metabolic physician.

The sixth component of the RYGB relates to the change in enteroendocrine secretion from the L cells of the distal intestine. Although this subject is covered in much greater detail elsewhere in this text, it should be included here as part of a description of the surgery. The release of hormones such as GLP-1 has powerful effects on glucose metabolism. This is certainly a significant component in the reversal of diabetes seen after GBP [53]. However, additional enteroendocrine hormones such as Peptide YY (PYY) are also secreted. Together, these may play further roles in reducing food intake through an induction of satiety.

Much like the previously described procedures, the RYGB also has associated risks. Surgical risks include anastomotic leak, stricture at the gastrojejunostomy, and internal hernias. Along with these technical risks, there are also metabolic risks associated with the malabsorptive component of the surgery as well as dumping syndrome.

Benotti et al. [60] evaluated clinical outcome data among 185,315 patients in the Bariatric Outcome Longitudinal Database to determine the major risk factors associated with mortality in a 30-day period following RYGB surgery. While the overall mortality rate was low at 0.1%, there were several factors associated with higher risk. These were increasing BMI, increasing age, male gender, pulmonary hypertension, congestive heart failure, and liver disease.

Melinek et al. [61] from the Departments of Pathology and Laboratory Medicine and General Surgery, UCLA School of Medicine, performed a series of autopsies on RYGB patients to shed some light on postoperative mortality. Autopsies were performed on 10 patients between 1994 and 2000. During the same time frame, at UCLA, 1067 patients underwent a GBP procedure (December 1993 to July 2000). The rate of major complications was 5.8%, and the mortality rate was 1.3%. Of the 10 patients in the group studied by Melinek et al., five deaths were attributable to technical complications, which included anastomotic leak, wound infection, jejunal necrosis, intestinal obstruction, hepatic artery ligation, wound dehiscence, and mesenteric vein thrombosis. Five of the deaths were attributed to underlying comorbid conditions. They also noted that 8 of 10 patients showed microscopic evidence of pulmonary emboli, despite provision of deep vein thrombosis prophylaxis. Also notable was the prevalence of steatohepatitis (80%) and fibrosis (70%).

The potential metabolic risks after RYGB require lifelong surveillance by physicians trained to monitor these patients. Metabolic risks are due to a multitude of factors. These include decreased intake, altered GI anatomy, use of antiacid agents, and possibly bacterial overgrowth.

Anemia is a significant concern. In a prospective study by Brolin et al. [62], iron deficiency was observed in 47% approximately 4 years after RYGB, with females affected more than twice as much as males. Dalcanale et al. [63] reviewed nutritional deficits 5 years after RYGB surgery. They found the following deficiencies in the 75 patients they studied: magnesium (32.1%), iron (29.8%), ferritin (36.0%), zinc (40.5%), vitamin B_{12} (61.8%), vitamin D_3 (60.5%), and β-carotene (56.8%).

MALABSORPTIVE WEIGHT LOSS PROCEDURES

The DS

As discussed previously, the BPD originated in Genoa, Italy, with Dr. Scopinaro. The DS was a US adaptation originally presented by Hess in 1988. The BPD and DS are more complex procedures than other weight loss operations and have been utilized infrequently in the US. However, based on the strength of recent data, there has been a renewed interest in the DS.

Recent studies are showing that DS may be more effective in achieving weight loss goals when compared to RYGB. One such study at two medical centers in Norway and Sweden compared patients with a BMI of 50–60 mg/m^2 who were randomized to undergo either GBP or DS. The DS patients lost more weight and had a greater reduction in total and LDL cholesterol and body fat percentage. However, the DS patients did experience more adverse events [64].

Even more compelling is the postoperative effect of the DS on glucose metabolism. In their meta-analysis, Buchwald et al. [41] showed that diabetes resolution was best for DS when compared to the other procedures: 98.9% for BPD or DS, 83.7% for GBP, 71.6% for gastroplasty, and 47.9% for gastric banding. Mingrone et al. [65] studied the effect of weight loss surgery in a randomized control trial of 60 patients. Patients had a BMI > 35 kg/m^2, were diagnosed with diabetes for at least 5 years, had a glycated hemoglobin level of 7.0% or more, and were between the ages of 30 and 60 years. The patients were randomized to receive medical therapy, GBP, or BPD. At 2 years, diabetes resolution was 0% in the medical therapy group, 75% in the GBP group, and 95% in the BPD group. Glycated hemoglobin levels decreased in all groups, with the greatest decrease observed in the two surgery groups. Their research also demonstrated that "age, sex, baseline BMI, duration of diabetes, and weight changes were not significant predictors of diabetes remission at 2 years or of improvement in glycemia at 1 and 3 months" [65].

Roslin et al. [66] report that hyperinsulinemic hypoglycemia is common after RYGB and may result in weight regain. In this small study, 45 patients (38 available for analysis) were randomized to receive RYGB, SG, or DS. Postoperative RYGB patients undergoing glucose challenge were more likely to experience larger rises in blood sugar, higher 1-hour insulin levels, and a greater reduction in blood glucose compared to DS patients.

Risks of the DS include surgical and metabolic factors. Hess et al. [67] reported on a series of 1404 BPD/DS. Amongst the first 1300 patients, major complications included gastric leaks (0.7%), mortality (0.57%), revisions (3.7%), and reversals (0.61%). The eight reversals were due to diarrhea, low protein, malnutrition, excess weight loss, protein loss, cirrhosis, and ovarian malignancy.

Aasheim et al. [68] compared vitamin deficiencies between DS and RYGB. They found a greater risk of vitamin A and vitamin D deficiency in the first year postoperatively and a greater risk of thiamine deficiency in the first few months postoperatively. Anemia was noted to increase after DS. Marceau et al. [69] reported an increase in moderate anemia from 5.7% to 14% postoperatively, and severe anemia increased from 0.2% to 0.8% postoperatively. They also reported a decrease in calcium with an associated rise in PTH independent of vitamin D status. Serum calcium was below normal in 20% of patients studied. Because of this, they recommended calcium supplementation as a routine measure for DS patients.

Malabsorptive Weight Loss Devices

Two new malabsorptive techniques have been recently been developed as weight loss procedures—the endoluminal sleeve and gastric aspirator. The endoluminal sleeve is an endoscopically deployed device that lines the GI tract from the pylorus to the jejunum with a plastic covering. In this way, it provides a conduit for the food bolus to pass through the GI tract without exposing it to the duodenal mucosa. The result is a significant decline in digestion and absorption of ingested food. The endoluminal sleeve has been shown to result in weight loss and improvement in glycemic control in moderately obese subjects with type 2 diabetes mellitus (T2DM). This device is undergoing clinical trials but is not available in the United States [70,35].

The gastric aspirator is another malabsorptive device that is currently available outside the United States. This device is implanted in the stomach, essentially the same way as a percutaneous gastrostomy (PEG) tube. Unlike a PEG tube, however, this tube anchors to a device that allows patients to "aspirate" part of their ingested food contents, thereby decreasing the amount "consumed." In this way, it allows patients to eat whatever amount of food they want and then correct for overeating by evacuating their stomach. Further clinical investigation is underway to determine whether this device can serve a meaningful role in surgical weight loss [70].

SELECTION CRITERIA

In 1991, the National Institutes of Health (NIH) published the first set of selection criteria for weight loss surgery. This was based on a consensus conference for GI surgery in morbidly obese patients [71]. However, it is important to note that the 1991 statement refers to the VBG and the GBP, which were the two most prevalent procedures being performed at the time. A summary of the 1991 selection criteria is shown in Table 14.5 [72].

In 2004, the American Society for Bariatric Surgery (ASBS) convened a consensus conference to update the 1991 NIH consensus statement [73]. The ASBS was motivated by certain factors in the ensuing 13 years following the publication of the 1991 NIH guidelines. These included an expanded list of surgical options, the introduction of laparoscopic minimally invasive techniques, evidence that delaying weight loss surgery can affect chances for the full reversal of diabetes, evidence that weight loss surgery can improve life expectancy, and evidence that weight loss surgery can be cost effective within 4 years compared to the expenditure for morbidly obese patients without surgery [73].

Table 14.6 shows the findings and conclusions of the 2004 consensus panel.

After patients meet these requirements, they can be considered candidates for surgical weight loss. However, a final determination should depend upon a multidisciplinary evaluation that includes input from primary health care providers, metabolic physicians, surgeons, dieticians, and psychologists. This team approach ensures that the selection process is objective and likely to optimally prepare the patient for surgery.

Our practice is to obtain further input from cardiology and gastroenterology specialists for any patient anticipating weight loss surgery. This will generally include cardiac stress testing and the option of additional testing such as an echocardiogram or coronary artery catheterization. It is not

---

TABLE 14.5

Selection Criteria for Weight Loss Surgery (NIH 1991 Guidelines)

BMI ≥ 40 kg/m^2 or BMI ≥ kg/m^2 with significant obesity-related comorbidities

Age between 16 and 65 years

Acceptable operative risk

Documented failure at nonsurgical approaches to long-term weight loss

Psychologically stable patient with realistic expectations

Commitment to long-term follow-up

Resolution of alcohol or substance abuse

Absence of active schizophrenia and untreated severe depression

Source: Schneider BE, *Diabetes Care*, 28, 2005.

TABLE 14.6

ASBS 2004 Patient Selection Criteria (An Update of the NIH 1991 Consensus Statement)

Surgery candidates should have attempted weight loss by nonoperative means. These include self-directed dieting, nutritional counseling, and commercial and hospital-based weight loss programs. Patients should not be required to complete formal nonoperative obesity therapy as a prerequisite for surgery.

The patient is best evaluated by a multidisciplinary team.

Patients should have a comprehensive medical examination prior to surgery.

Patients with class I obesity (BMI 30–40 kg/m^2) with a comorbid condition that may be cured or markedly improved by weight loss may become candidates for surgery after evaluating additional data and long-term risk-and-benefit analysis.

Bariatric surgery can be considered in adolescents at experienced centers.

Source: Buchwald H, *J. Am. Coll. Surg.*, 200, 2005.

uncommon to identify patients with significant subclinical coronary disease who may require revascularization before any consideration for weight loss surgery.

An upper endoscopy is also advised. This will help to identify any esophageal, gastric, or duodenal pathology, which may alter the decision for surgery. A further consideration is the fact that after a procedure such as the RYGB, access to the remnant stomach, duodenum, and biliopancreatic region will be impossible via endoscopic means. Therefore, it is important to be certain that there is no underlying pathology in these regions.

We have had the experience of identifying esophageal and gastric tumors during these evaluations, which were asymptomatic at the time. These patients were then referred for oncologic treatment rather than bariatric surgery.

If the patient has any pulmonary issues, especially sleep apnea, input from a pulmonology specialist is warranted. The patient may develop pulmonary complications after surgery and anesthesia. Furthermore, there is a high likelihood that continuous positive airway pressure and other respiratory therapies can be decreased as the patient loses weight postoperatively. Expert guidance in this process is advised.

The role of the metabolic physician in the preoperative evaluation has several components. Firstly, it is the metabolic physician who should direct the attempts at nonsurgical weight loss and affirm that the patients require surgical intervention to achieve their weight loss goal. Secondly, the metabolic physician should obtain nutritional data to confirm that the patient is optimally suited to undergo surgery on the basis of macro and micronutrient parameters. The patient should be committed to ongoing monitoring of these parameters after surgery in order to prevent the risk of metabolic complications.

A third function for the metabolic physician in the preoperative setting involves patients with diabetes. The patient should be appropriately counseled on adjustment of diabetic medications, particularly insulin. Patients must also be prepared for the necessary monitoring and medication adjustments to their diabetes care after surgery.

The final step in preparing the patient for weight loss surgery is the selection of a specific weight loss procedure. The goal is to select the procedure that will optimize the patient's weight loss efforts and obtain the metabolic benefits while minimizing the risk. We have proposed a methodology for surgical procedure selection based on certain patient characteristics. In this evaluation, we utilize the patient's BMI, eating patterns/behaviors, ability to exercise, prior surgeries, anticipated pregnancies, and diabetes history.

The first set of criteria can be based around the patient's BMI. In general, patients with supermorbid obesity, with a BMI greater than 50, should be considered for more aggressive approaches. Therefore, we generally do not recommend gastric banding for these individuals. Instead, the SG, GBP, or DS is usually considered.

The next criterion relates to the patient's eating patterns and behavior. We have found that patients who are excessive sweet eaters are not good candidates for gastric banding. This is because they often eat foods that melt or exit the small pouch quickly. Therefore, they never eat foods with sufficient volume to allow the band to create a sense of fullness. This type of eating pattern tends to nullify the utility of the band.

Similarly, patients who have behavioral or compulsive eating patterns are generally not good candidates for gastric banding. This is because they are unlikely to experience a change in eating desire and food preferences after simple gastric restriction. However, procedures that excise the ghrelin-secreting gastric cells, such as the gastric sleeve, GBP, and DS, alter food-seeking behavior. Furthermore, food preferences have been shown to be dramatically changed by these procedures. Therefore, patients with significant behavioral eating patterns tend to be recommended for weight loss procedures other than the gastric band.

Another important criterion has to do with the patient's ability to exercise. Patients who are physically able to exercise and prepared to commit to a rigorous program of physical activity may do better with a less aggressive procedure. These highly motivated patients are an important subset of those seeking weight loss surgery. They may have already made a vigorous attempt at nonsurgical weight loss only to be frustrated by the lack of progress. In our experience, gastric banding has served such patients well.

Patients who have undergone extensive prior abdominal surgery may be difficult candidates for the more aggressive forms of weight loss surgery, such as GBP and DS. Tissue adhesions from previous operations may make it difficult or impossible to liberate segments of bowel in order to perform the surgical anastomoses. Therefore, in such patients, we often suggest consideration of gastric-only procedures that focus on the upper abdomen.

An important subset of surgical weight loss candidates includes women of childbearing age. A pregnancy test must be performed prior to surgery since it would be inappropriate to undergo the weight loss procedure while the patient is pregnant. However, the issue of pregnancy after weight loss surgery is another significant consideration. Procedures that involve a degree of malabsorption, such as the GBP or DS may produce micronutrient deficiencies, which complicate normal fetal growth. For this reason, we generally prefer gastric restrictive procedures for patients who inform us of their desire to become pregnant in the foreseeable future. However, it should be stressed that all weight loss surgery patients are advised to use effective birth control methods within the first 2 years of surgery.

Another important criterion involves the patient's history of diabetes. Much has been discussed about the value of weight loss surgery and diabetes resolution. But it is clear that not all patients with diabetes will achieve this important goal. Furthermore, it is also clear that some procedures work better for certain patients. In the studies by Dixon [74] on the effects of gastric banding on diabetes resolution, patients with a relatively recent onset of diabetes achieved a high percentage of resolution after gastric banding. This is likely to be due to the fact that such patients still have preserved beta cell function and the capacity to secrete insulin. Therefore, we would recommend the use of gastric banding for patients who have had a history of diabetes of less than 2 years.

Beta cell function is known to deteriorate progressively in the course of diabetes. The capacity to maintain normal insulin secretion is lost as time progresses. A cutoff point is reached at which insulin secretion is significantly below normal, after which the patient generally requires insulin. This cutoff point is believed to occur at around 7.5 years into the diagnosis of type 2 diabetes mellitus.

The data by Schauer et al. [75] showed that both the gastric sleeve and GBP could resolve diabetes 12 months postoperatively. Patients had an average duration of type 2 diabetes of greater than 8 years. The diabetes resolution was 42% in the GBP group and 37% in the SG group. Guidone et al. [76] demonstrated diabetes resolution after GBP and BPD 24 months postoperatively. The patients had a history of type 2 diabetes for more than 5 years. Decreases in hemoglobin A1c were 25.18% in the GBP group and 43.01% in the BPD group.

Based on this information, we tend to recommend either the gastric sleeve or GBP for patients who have had type 2 diabetes for more than 2 years but less than 8 years. However, we tend to prefer either GBP or DS for patients with type 2 diabetes of more than 8 years' duration.

CONCLUSION

Weight loss surgery has evolved considerably over the last 60 years. During this time, certain procedures have fallen by the wayside, while others have come to the forefront. In this chapter, we have provided a historical review on the developments in the field. Experience has guided us to focus on procedures that can be performed safely and provide reliable, sustainable results. Most bariatric centers now offer three standard procedures: the adjustable gastric band, the SG, and the GBP. Because of the recent data regarding diabetes resolution, malabsorptive techniques such as the DS are gaining popularity.

In this chapter, we have attempted to review the major procedures in detail. Each procedure has its own unique role in the spectrum of weight loss surgery as well its own set of risks and benefits. As the field of bariatric surgery continues to develop, new procedures are likely to be developed. Furthermore, new approaches may provide as-yet unforeseen technological benefits.

REFERENCES

1. Fobi MAL. Surgical treatment of obesity: A review. *J Natl Med Assoc.* 2004;96:61–70.
2. Buchwald H, Buchwald JN. Evolution of operative procedures for the management of morbid obesity. *Obes Surg.* 2002;12:705–715.
3. Kremen AJ, Linner JH, Nelson CH. An experimental evaluation of the nutritional importance of proximal and distal small intestine. *Ann Surg.* 1954;140:439–448.
4. Griffen WO Jr, Young VL, Stevenson CC. A prospective comparison of gastric and jejunoileal bypass procedures for morbid obesity. *Ann Surg.* 1977;186:500–509.
5. Payne JH, DeWind LT. Surgical treatment of obesity. *Am J Surg.* 1969;118(2):141–146.
6. Scott HW, Sandstead HH, Brill AB. Experience with a new technique of intestinal bypass in the treatment of morbid obesity. *Ann Surg.* 1971;174:560–572.
7. Griffen WO Jr, Bivins BA, Bell RM. The decline and fall of the jejunoileal bypass. *Surg Gynecol Obstet.* 1983;157:301–308.
8. Requarth JA, Burchard KW, Colacchio TA, Stukel TA, Mott LA, Greenberg ER, Weismann RE. Long-term morbidity following jejunoileal bypass. The continuing potential need for surgical reversal. *Arch Surg.* 1995;130:318–325.
9. Halverson JD, Wise L, Wazna MF, Ballinger WF. Jejunoileal bypass for morbid obesity. A critical appraisal. *Am J Med.* 1978;64(3):461–475.
10. Singh D, Laya AS, Clarkston WK, Allen MA. Jejunoileal bypass: A surgery of the past and a review of its complications. *World J Gastroenterol.* 2009;15(18):2277–2279.
11. Mason ER, Ito C. Gastric bypass in obesity. *Surg Clinic North Am.* 1967;47:1345–1352.
12. Alden JF. Gastric and jejunoileal bypass a comparison in the treatment of morbid obesity. *Arch Surg.* 1977;112:799–806.
13. Wilkinson LH, Peloso OA. Gastric (reservoir) reduction for morbid obesity. *Arch Surg.* 1981;116(5):602–605.
14. Scopinaro N, Gianetta E, Civalleri D et al. Biliopancreatic bypass for obesity: II. Initial experience in man. *Br J Surg.* 1979;66:618–620.
15. Scopinaro N, Gianetta E, Adami GF et al. Biliopancreatic diversion for obesity at 18 years. *Surgery.* 1996;119:261–268.
16. Mason EE. Vertical banded gastroplasty for obesity. *Arch Surg.* 1982;117:701–706.
17. Laws HL. Standardized gastroplasty orifice. *Ann J Surg.* 1981;141:393.
18. Kolle K, Bo O. Gastric banding. Proceedings of the 7th Congress, Organization Mondiale de gastronterologie, Stockholm, Sweden, 1982;37.

19. Molina M. Gastric banding, an experience with more than 500 cases. Presented at Symposium on Surgical Treatment of Obesity, Los Angeles, 1984.

20. Hess DW. Biliopancreatic diversion with a duodenal switch procedure. Presentation at the Seventh Annual Symposium, Surgical Treatment of Obesity, Los Angeles, 1989.

21. Wittgrove AC, Clark GW, Tremblay LJ. Laparoscopy gastric bypass, Roux-en-Y: Preliminary report of five cases. *Obes Surg*. 1994;4:353–357.

22. Banka G, Woodard G, Hernandez-Boussard T, Morton JM. Laparoscopic vs open gastric bypass surgery: Differences in patient demographics, safety, and outcomes. *Arch Surg*. 2012;147(6):550–556.

23. Jamieson AC. Why the operation I prefer is the modified long verticle gastroplasty. *Obes Surg*. 1993;3(3):297–301.

24. Gehrer S, Kern B, Peters T, Christoffel-Courtin C, Peterli R. Fewer nutrient deficiencies after laparoscopic sleeve gastrectomy (LSG) than after laparoscopic Roux-Y-gastric bypass (LRYGB)—A prospective study. *Obes Surg*. 2010;20(4):447–453.

25. Giurgius M. *Overview of Bariatric Surgery*. University of Kentucky PPT, Lexington, KY.

26. Keshishian A. Available at http://www.dssurgery.com/weight-loss-surgery-poster.php.

27. Nguyen NT, Nguyen B, Gebhart A, Hohmann S. Changes in the makeup of bariatric surgery: A national increase in use of laparoscopic sleeve gastrectomy. *J Am Coll Surg*. 2013;216:252–257.

28. Niville E, Dams A, Reremoser S, Verhelst H. A mid-term experience with the Cousin Bioring—Adjustable gastric band. *Obes Surg*. 2012;22(1):152–157.

29. Burton PR, Borwon WA. The mechanism of weight loss with laparoscopic adjustable gastric banding: Induction of satiety not restriction. *Int J Obes (Lond)*. 2011;35(3):S26–S30.

30. The LAP-BAND® System. Surgical aid in the treatment of obesity: A decision guide for adults, 2011. Available at http://www.lapbandcentral.com.

31. Favretti F, O'Brien P, Dixon JB. Patient management after LAP-BAND placement. *Am J Surg*. 2002; 184:38S–41S.

32. Livhits M, Mercado C, Yermilov I, Parikh JA, Durson E, Mehran A, Ko CY, Gibbons M. Exercise following bariatric surgery: Systematic review. *Obes Surg*. 2010;20(5):657–665.

33. Belachew M, Belva PH, Desaive C. Long-term results of laparoscopic adjustable gastric banding for the treatment of morbid obesity. *Obes Surg*. 2002;12:564–568.

34. O'Brien PE, Dixon JB, Brown W et al. The laparoscopic adjustable gastric band. (Lap Band): A prospective study of medium-term effects on weight, health and quality of life. *Obes Surg* 2002;12:652–660.

35. Schouten R, Rijs CS, Bouvy ND et al. A multicenter, randomized efficacy study of the EndoBarrier Gastrointestinal Liner for presurgical weight loss prior to bariatric surgery. *Ann Surg*. 2010;251(2):236–243.

36. Regan JP, Inabnet WB, Gagner M et al. Early experience with two-stage laparoscopic Roux-en-Y gastric bypass as an alternative in the super-super obese patient. *Obes Surg*. 2003;13:861–864.

37. Chu CA, Gagner M, Quinn T et al. Two-stage laparoscopic biliopancreatic diversion with duodenal switch: An alternative approach to super super morbid obesity. *Surg Endosc*. 2003;16:S069 (abst).

38. Moon Han S, Kim WW, Oh JH. Results of laparoscopic sleeve gastrectomy (LSG) at 1 year in morbidly obese Korean patients. *Obes Surg*. 2005;15(10):1469–1475.

39. Langer FB, Bohdjalian A, Felbergbauer FX, Fleischmann E, Reza Hoda MA, Ludvik B. Does gastric dilatation limit the success of sleeve gastrectomy as a sole operation for morbid obesity? *Obes Surg*. 2006;16(2):166–171.

40. Frezza E. Laparoscopic vertical sleeve gastrectomy for morbid obesity. The future procedure of choice? *Surg Today*. 2007;37(4):275–281.

41. Buchwald H1, Estok R, Fahrbach K, Banel D, Jensen MD, Pories WJ, Bantle JP, Sledge I. Weight and type 2 diabetes after bariatric surgery: Systematic review and meta-analysis. *Am J Med*. 2009 Mar;122(3):248–265.e5.

42. Givon-Madhala O, Spector R, Wasserberg N et al. Technical aspects of laparoscopic sleeve gastrectomy in 25 morbidly obese patients. *Obes Surg*. 2007;17:722–727.

43. Weiner RA, Weiner S, Pomhoff I, Jacobi C, Makarewicz W, Weigand G. Laparoscopic sleeve gastrectomy—Influence of sleeve size and resected gastric volume. *Obes Surg*. 2007;17(10):1297–1305.

44. Yehoshua RT, Eidelman LA, Stein M, Fichman S, Mazor A, Chen J, Bernstine H, Singer P, Dickman R, Shikora SA, Rosenthal RJ, Rubin M. Laparoscopic sleeve gastrectomy—Volume and pressure assessment. *Obes Surg*. 2008;18:1083–1088.

45. Braghetto I, Davanzo C, Korn O, Csendes A, Valladares H, Herrera E, Gonzalez P, Papapietro K. Scintigraphic evaluation of gastric emptying in obese patients submitted to sleeve gastrectomy compared to normal subjects. *Obes Surg*. 2009;19(11):1515–1521.

46. Peterli R, Steinert RE, Woelnerhanssen B, Peters T, Christoffel-Courtin C, Gass M, Kern B, Von Fluee M, Beglinger C. Metabolic and hormonal changes after laparoscopic Roux-en-Y gastric bypass and sleeve gastrectomy: A randomized, prospective trial. *Obes Surg.* 2012;22(5):740–748.

47. Frezza EE, Reddy S, Gee LL, Wachtel MS. Complications after sleeve gastrectomy for morbid obesity. *Obes Surg.* 2009;19:684–687.

48. Deitel M, Gagner M, Erickson AL, Crosby RD. Third International Summit: Current status of sleeve gastrectomy. *Surg Obes Relat Dis.* 2011;7(6):749–759.

49. Carter PR, LeBlanc KA, Hausmann MG, Kleinpeter KP, deBarros SN, Jones SM. Association between gastroesophageal reflux disease and laparoscopic sleeve gastrectomy. *Surg Obes Relat Dis.* 2011;7(5):569–572.

50. Himpens J, Dobbeleir J, Peeters G. Long-term results of laparoscopic sleeve gastrectomy for obesity. *Ann Surg.* 2010;252:319–324.

51. Braghetto I, Lanzarini E, Korn O, Valladares H, Molina JC, Henriquez A. Manometric changes of the lower esophageal sphincter after sleeve gastrectomy in obese patients. *Obes Surg.* 2010;20:357–362.

52. Deitel M. Bariatric surgery, proton pump inhibitors, and possibility of osteoporosis. *Surg Obes Relat Dis.* 2010;6:461–462.

53. Story of Obesity Surgery—Gastric Bypass and Laparoscopic Bypass. American Society for Metabolic and Bariatric Surgery. Brief History and Summary of Bariatic Surgery Chapter 3. May 2005.

54. Bueter M, Miras, Chichger H, Fenske H, Ghatei MA, Bloom SR, Unwin RJ, Lutz TA, Spector AC, le Roux CW. Alterations of sucrose preference after Roux-en-Y gastric bypass. *Physiol Behav.* 2011;104(5):709–721.

55. Tichansky DS, Boughter JD Jr, Madan AK. Taste change after laparoscopic Roux-en-Y gastric bypass and laparoscopic adjustable gastric banding. *Surg Obes Relat Dis.* 2006;2:440–444.

56. Scruggs DM, Buffington C, Cowan GS Jr. Taste acuity of the morbidly obese before and after gastric bypass surgery. *Obes Surg.* 1994;4:24–28.

57. Scholtz S, Miras AD, Chhina N, Prechtl CG, Sleeth ML, Daud NM, Ismail NA, Durighel G, Ahmed AR, Olbers T, Vincent RP, Alaghband-Zadeh J, Ghatei MA, Waldman AD, Frost GS, Bell JD, le Roux CW, Goldstone AP. Obese patients after gastric bypass surgery have lower brain-hedonic responses to food than after gastric banding. *Gut.* 2014;63(6):891–902.

58. Faria SL, Faria OP, Buffington C, de Almeida Cardeal M, Rodrigues de Gouvêa H. Energy expenditure before and after Roux-en-Y gastric bypass. *Obes Surg.* 2012;22(9):1450–1455.

59. Wilms B, Ernst B, Schmid SM, Thurnheer M, Schultes B. Enhanced thermic effect of food after Roux-en-Y gastric bypass surgery. *J Clin Endocrinol Metab.* 2013;98(9):3776–3784.

60. Benotti P, Wood GC, Winegar DA, Petrick AT, Still CD, Argyropoulos G, Gerhard GS. Risk factors associated with mortality after Roux-en-Y gastric bypass surgery. *Ann Surg.* 2014;259(1):123–130.

61. Melinek J, Livingston E, Cortina G, Fishbein MC. Autopsy findings following gastric bypass surgery for morbid obesity. *Arch Pathol Lab Med.* 2002;126(9):1091–1095.

62. Brolin RE, Gorman JH, Gorman RC, et al. Are vitamin B12 and folate deficiency clinically important after Roux-en-Y gastric bypass? *J Gastrointest Surg.* 1998;2:436–442.

63. Dalcanale L, Oliveira C, Faintuch J, Nogueira MA, Rondo P, Lima V, Mendonca S, Pajecki D, Mancini M, Carrilho FJ. Long-term nutritional outcome after gastric bypass. *Obes Surg.* 2010;20(2):181–187.

64. Sovik TT. Duodenal switch bested gastric bypass for weight loss. *Ann Intern Med.* 2011;155:281–291.

65. Mingrone G, Panunzi S, De Gaetano A, Guidone C, Iaconelli A, Leccesi L, Nanni G, Pomp A, Castagneto M, Ghirlanda G, Francesco Rubino F. Bariatric surgery versus conventional medical therapy for type 2 diabetes. *N Engl J Med.* 2012;366:1577–1585.

66. Roslin MS, Dudiy Y, Brownlee A, Weiskopf J, Shah P. Response to glucose tolerance testing and solid high carbohydrate challenge: Comparison between Roux-en-Y gastric bypass, vertical sleeve gastrectomy, and duodenal switch. *Surg Endosc.* 2014;28(1):91–99.

67. Hess DS, Hess DW, Oakley RS. The biliopancreatic diversion with the duodenal switch: Results beyond 10 years. *Obes Surg.* 2005;15:408–416.

68. Aasheim ET, Bjorkman S, Sovik TT, Engstrom M, Hanvold SE, Mala T, Olbers T, Bohmer T. Vitamin status after bariatric surgery: A randomized study of gastric bypass and duodenal switch. *Am J Clin Nutr.* 2009;90:15–22.

69. Marceau P, Biron S, Hould FS, Lebel S, Marceau S, Lescelleur O, Biertho L, Simard S. Duodenal switch: Long-term results. *Obes Surg.* 2007;17:1421–1430.

70. ASPIRE BARIATRICS. Available at http://www.aspirebariatrics.com/clinical-results.html.

71. NIH Conference Consensus Development Conference Panel. Gastrointestinal surgery for severe obesity. *Ann Intern Med.* 1991;115:956–961.

72. Schneider BE, Min EC. Surgical management of morbid obesity. *Diabetes Care*. 2005;28:475–480.
73. Buchwald H. Consensus Conference Statement; Bariatric surgery for morbid obesity: Health implications for patients, health professionals, and third-party payers. *J Am Coll Surg*. 2005;200:593–604.
74. Dixon JB, O'Brien PE, Playfair J, Chapman L, Schachter LM, Skinner S, Proietto J, Bailey M, Anderson M. Adjustable gastric banding and conventional therapy for type 2 diabetes: A randomized controlled trial. *JAMA*. 2008;299(3):316–323.
75. Schauer PR, Kashyap SR, Wolski K, Brethauer SA, Kirwan JP, Pothier CE, Thomas S, Abood B, Nissen SE, Bhatt DL. Bariatric surgery versus intensive medical therapy in obese patients with diabetes. *N Engl J Med*. 2012;366(17):1567–1576.
76. Guidone C, Manco M, Valera-Mora E, Iaconelli A, Gniuli D, Mari A, Nanni G, Castagneto M, Calvani M, Mingrone G. Mechanisms of recovery from type 2 diabetes after malabsorptive bariatric surgery. *Diabetes*. 2006;55(7):2025–2031.

15 Diabetes Surgery

Alpana Shukla, Rajesh T. Patel, and Francesco Rubino

CONTENTS

INTRODUCTION

Type 2 diabetes mellitus (T2DM) is a major health priority globally due to the severe burden it places on health care systems. The estimated worldwide prevalence of T2DM among adults was 285 million in 2010, and this is projected to increase to 439 million by 2030 [1]. The management of diabetes has historically been solely a physician's domain and has revolved around lifestyle intervention combined with pharmacotherapy to address insulin resistance and/or defective beta-cell function, the core issues in the pathophysiology of this disease. While the pharmacological armamentarium to treat T2DM has expanded considerably, few patients are able to achieve and maintain optimal glycemic targets in the long term. Moreover, weight gain from insulin usage and the risk of hypoglycemia often preclude intensive medical management.

Several gastrointestinal (GI) procedures originally devised to produce significant and durable weight loss among the morbidly obese can also induce remission or dramatic improvement of T2DM and other obesity-related comorbidities. While improvement of diabetes and other metabolic disorders is an expected outcome of weight loss by any means, evidence from both experimental animal studies [2,3] and clinical investigations [4,5] suggests that these effects are partly independent of weight loss. This knowledge provided a rationale to the idea of a "diabetes surgery" intended as a surgical approach specifically aimed at the treatment of T2DM [6].

At the 2007 Rome *Diabetes Surgery Summit*, a group of leading international scholars first recommended consideration of GI surgery to intentionally treat type 2 diabetes. After that meeting, the concept of "metabolic surgery" has rapidly emerged to more broadly indicate a surgical approach aimed at the control of metabolic illnesses, not just excess weight. In view of the abundant data now available to attest to the efficacy and safety of bariatric surgery to treat T2DM in obese patients, the International Diabetes Federation (IDF) more recently issued a formal position statement [7], recommending the use of bariatric surgery in patients with diabetes and body mass index (BMI) > 35 kg/m² and as an alternative treatment option in patients with a BMI of 30–35 kg/m² inadequately controlled with optimal medical regimens.

ANATOMIC CHARACTERISTICS OF PROCEDURES AND INTERVENTIONS

CONVENTIONAL PROCEDURES

On the basis of previous theories about the mechanism of weight loss, the various surgical options for treating obesity were classified into restrictive, malabsorptive, or combined procedures. In light of the knowledge that GI operations engage endocrine and metabolic mechanisms of action, this classification has now become obsolete, but it is mentioned here as it is still found in many reports or books on bariatric surgery for practical reasons. In general, procedures involving a restriction/resection of gastric tissue are referred to as "restrictive," whereas procedures that involve intestinal bypass are considered "malabsorptive" or "mixed" (malabsorptive + restrictive). It must be noted that in this classification, the term *malabsorption* was used to indicate the putative mechanism of action and not a clinical syndrome and that, in fact, clinically relevant malabsorption is not a common outcome of all intestinal bypass procedures (i.e., with standard gastric bypass surgery, clinical malabsorption is rare).

Laparoscopic Adjustable Gastric Banding

Laparoscopic adjustable gastric banding (LAGB; Figure 15.1) is a surgical procedure in which a band is placed around the upper portion of the stomach, distal to the esophagogastric junction. The band divides the stomach into a small pouch above the band and large pouch below the band. Adjusting the size of the opening between the two parts of the stomach, by injecting or removing saline from the band (which is connected to a tube and port placed under the skin), controls how much food passes from the upper to the lower part of the stomach. The procedure is reversible, but of course, this requires a laparoscopic reoperation.

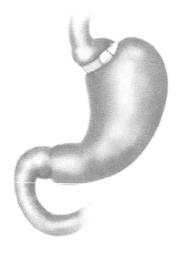

FIGURE 15.1   (**See color insert.**) Adjustable gastric banding.

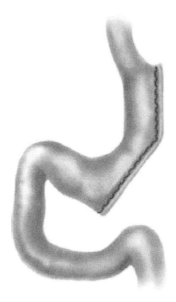

FIGURE 15.2 (See color insert.) Sleeve gastrectomy.

Sleeve Gastrectomy

Sleeve gastrectomy (SG; Figure 15.2) is a procedure in which a major portion of the stomach is surgically removed along a line roughly parallel to the greater curvature, reducing the gastric volume to about 25% of its original size. This results in a sleevelike or tubelike structure lacking the entire hormonally active gastric fundus. The procedure permanently reduces the stomach size and is irreversible.

Roux-en-Y Gastric Bypass

Roux-en-Y gastric bypass (RYGB; Figure 15.3) is currently the most commonly performed bariatric procedure worldwide. The procedure involves manipulation of both stomach and intestine by

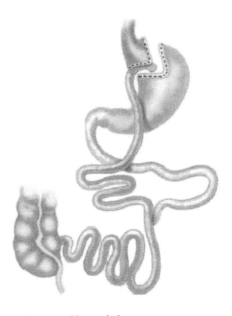

FIGURE 15.3 (See color insert.) Roux-en-Y gastric bypass.

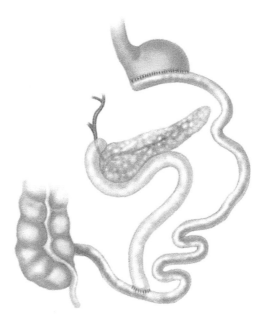

FIGURE 15.4 (See color insert.) Biliopancreatic diversion.

creating a small gastric pouch off the proximal stomach and connecting such pouch directly to the small intestine at the level of the mid jejunum, thereby excluding (bypassing) a large portion of the stomach, entire duodenum, and proximal jejunum (usually the first 50–100 cm of jejunum) from the transit of nutrients. The excluded small intestine (biliopancreatic limb) carries bile and pancreatic secretions and is reconnected to the distal small intestine via a second anastomosis. The segment of jejunum above the lower anastomosis and directly connected to the stomach is not exposed to bile or pancreatic juice and is called "alimentary limb." Bile and nutrients mix in the distal jejunum and can be absorbed through the remaining portion of the small bowel ("common limb").

Biliopancreatic Diversion

Biliopancreatic diversion (BPD; Figure 15.4) is a "malabsorptive" operation that combines a moderate restrictive component (reducing stomach size to 200–500 mL) with a very long intestinal bypass, which causes food to be poorly digested and absorbed. There are two variants of BPD: In the original technique (the classic Scopinaro procedure), the stomach is reduced by means of a horizontal resection that removes the entire antrum and the pylorus; in the BPD–duodenal switch (BPD/DS) variant, the gastric resection is vertical (similar to SG) and involves preservation of the lesser curvature, antrum, pylorus, and first 1 cm of duodenum (duodenal switch). Bile and nutrients mix only in a short 50–100 cm long "common limb," the terminal portion of the ileum proximal to the ileocecal valve. The common limb is where most nutrient absorption takes place after this procedure, thereby resulting in significant nutrient malabsorption that, in some cases, can result in clinically relevant complications.

NOVEL PROCEDURES

Duodenal–Jejunal Bypass

Duodenal–jejunal bypass (DJB; Figure 15.5) is an investigational operation, first described by Rubino and Marescaux [2] as an experimental procedure to investigate mechanisms of action of GI surgery. The procedure has also been used in clinical research studies for patients with type 2

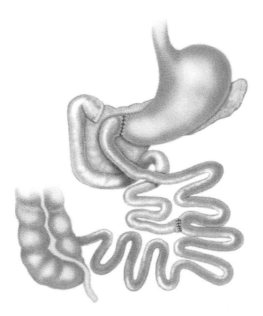

FIGURE 15.5   (**See color insert.**) Duodenal–jejunal bypass.

diabetes who are not obese [8]. The operation consists of a stomach-sparing bypass of a short portion of proximal small intestine (duodenum and proximal jejunum), comparable to the segment excluded in a standard RYGB. In a variant of this procedure, the DJB is performed in association with an SG (DJB/SG). DJB and DJB/SG have been reported to improve T2DM in overweight or nonobese patients, but the relative efficacy and safety of the procedure compared to standard operations has not been yet investigated in rigorous clinical trials. Recently, Cohen et al. [8] have reported 5-year follow-up data of a prospective series of DJB and DJB/SG. In addition to its yet limited clinical application, DJB has been utilized by several groups as an experimental procedure for research into the mechanisms of action of bariatric/metabolic surgery given its peculiar anatomic characteristics that allow for specific investigation of the role of intestinal bypass and exclusion of the proximal bowel for nutrient contact [9,10]. An endoluminal approach aimed at reproducing mechanisms and effects of DJB (endoluminal DJB or endoluminal sleeve—vide infra) has been also recently used in clinical studies for the treatment of diabetes and obesity.

Ileal Interposition

Ileal interposition (IT; Figure 15.6) is an investigational procedure in which a small segment of ileum (terminal part of the small intestine) with its vascular and nervous supplies is translocated to the proximal small intestine, accelerating its exposure to undigested nutrients. IT can also be performed in association with duodenal exclusion (ITDSG) or with SG (IT/SG). The concept of IT has been tested in rodents [11] and in humans [12].

Endoluminal Duodenojejunal Sleeve

Endoluminal duodenojejunal sleeve (ELS) is a flexible plastic sleeve that creates a barrier between ingested nutrients and the mucosa of the proximal small bowel (duodenum–jejunum) without causing actual anatomic interruption of GI continuity. This method was originally used in rodents to investigate the hypothesis that separation of ingested nutrients from other content of the intestinal lumen (bile/pancreatic juice) and from the intestinal mucosa could have direct antidiabetic effects, thus explaining, at least in part, the effect of RYGB or BPD on T2DM [13,14]. The method then has been studied in several clinical investigations, which showed it to result in substantial reduction of

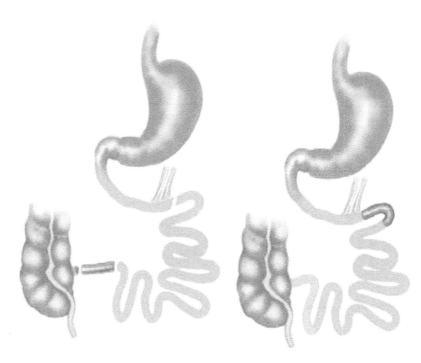

FIGURE 15.6 **(See color insert.)** Ileal interposition.

hemoglobin A1c (HbA1c) levels and changes in gut hormones [15–17]. A large, multicenter clinical trial to evaluate the safety and efficacy of an endoluminal duodenal sleeve is currently being performed in the United States.

MECHANISMS OF GLYCEMIC CONTROL FOLLOWING METABOLIC SURGERY

Weight loss by any means can diminish the metabolic abnormalities of obese type 2 diabetic subjects [18]. Numerous studies have proven that restriction of calories leads to a rapid improvement in glucose homeostasis in obese and diabetic subjects [19,20]. Because substantial reduction of caloric intake is difficult to sustain over the long term, weight regain is common with lifestyle modifications. Weight loss can also be achieved by medical therapy; however, it is usually minimal or moderate, and it is associated with side effects of drugs and weight regain. Subjects with T2DM who undergo bariatric surgery for morbid obesity, especially RYGB or BPD, experience sustained weight loss and substantial improvement in glucose metabolism and are frequently able to maintain glycemic control without insulin injections or medications [6,21]. Postoperative food deprivation followed by major weight loss after bariatric surgery is an intuitive, if somewhat simplistic, explanation for the glycemic improvements. Insulin sensitivity is increased markedly after bariatric surgery [21], accompanied by enhanced markers of insulin signaling in key target tissues, favorable changes in enzymes mediating fatty acid and glucose metabolism, elevated adiponectin levels, and decreases in intramuscular and intrahepatic lipids [5,14]. However, growing evidence indicates that the antidiabetic mechanisms of some of these operations cannot be explained by changes in caloric intake and body weight alone.

The following lines of evidence indicate that rearrangement of GI anatomy seems to confer additional antidiabetic effects independently of weight loss.

1. The first piece of experimental evidence in support of weight-independent mechanisms is derived from the animal investigations using the DJB model developed by Rubino and Marescaux [2] in rodents showing that the improvement of type 2 diabetes after duodenal

jejunal bypass is not only secondary to decreased food intake, weight loss, or the reduction in lipid and carbohydrate absorption [3]. These observations have led to the hypothesis that the exclusion of the proximal small intestine (duodenum and proximal jejunum) from the passage of food contributes to the resolution (or improvement) of diabetes after other diversionary procedures (i.e., RYGB, BPD) and that the proximal small intestine may be instrumental in the pathogenesis of the disease [2,22]. To further investigate the hypothesis that duodenal exclusion per se may activate direct antidiabetic effects, Francesco Rubino and his colleagues Stefano Sereno and Antonello Forgione, then at the European Institute of Telesurgery in Strasbourg, France, used an endoluminal duodenal tube (sleeve) that excludes the nutrients from contact with the duodenal mucosa and other intestinal content (bile, pancreatic juice) [13]. In these experiments, a flexible silicone tube was inserted in the duodenum–jejunum of Goto-Kakizaki rats, a nonobese model of type 2 diabetes. A control group of matched animals received the same type of endoluminal tube but with multiple openings to allow for nutrient contact with bile and intestinal mucosa. The intact endoluminal tube improved oral glucose tolerance in these animals, while fenestration of the tube sabotaged the effect [13]. Similar experiments comparing ELS and a sham operation in matched rodents [14] corroborated these results. The device theoretically mimics the "DJB," while neural connectivity is maintained and the distal small bowel receives less processed foodstuffs. Contrary to DJB, the duodenojejunal endoluminal sleeve is able to do this without disrupting bowel continuity or creating new anastomosis. This method has been shown to improve diabetes in lean rodents [13,14] as well as in clinical trials [16,17].

2. Rapidity of diabetes control after surgery. T2DM normally resolves rapidly following RYGB and BPD, long before substantial weight loss has occurred. In contrast, purely restrictive operations such as LAGB ameliorate diabetes only after substantial weight loss is achieved in spite of similar perioperative restriction in calorie intake in both procedures [23].

3. Interventions resulting in similar weight loss but different degrees of improvement in glucose homeostasis. RYGB achieves greater improvement of glucose tolerance and beta-cell function than an equivalent-magnitude weight loss achieved by purely gastric restrictive bariatric surgery such as LAGB [24], calorie restrictions [4], or SG [25]. Fatty diabetic Zucker rats undergoing gastric bypass also show better glucose tolerance and insulin sensitivity than sham-operated animals with equivalent dietary-induced weight loss [26].

4. Ileal interposition improves glucose homeostasis out of proportion to weight loss in rat models of obesity and diabetes [27,28]. Animals with IT show dramatic increase in glucagon-like peptide-1 (GLP-1), peptide YY (PYY), and enteroglucagon [28,29]. Enhanced GLP-1 is an obvious candidate to explain at least part of the glycemic effect of IT by inducing satiety and reduction in body weight, without malabsorption or gastric restriction.

The exact molecular mechanisms underlying improved glycemic control post–GI surgery or endoluminal sleeve devices remain unclear. In spite of anatomical and functional differences between procedures, glucose homeostasis is improved after all these types of operations [13]. This may be explained by partial overlap in the mechanism of action of the various procedures. However, given the specific physiological role of the stomach and of the various intestinal segments in regulating glucose homeostasis, it is also plausible that different GI surgeries may have distinct effects and mechanisms on of action.

It has been suggested that surgery may affect the "enteroinsular axis," which involves several key peptides believed to have a role in regulating insulin secretion, including incretin peptides, especially GLP-1. These factors are produced by intestinal enteroendocrine cells in response to ingestion of carbohydrates or fats, which in turn cause the release of insulin from the pancreas [30,31] and induce satiety/reduced appetite [32]; these changes after bariatric surgery could potentially explain the effects on obesity and diabetes.

The postprandial GLP-1 response to an oral glucose load or mixed test meal is consistently augmented following RYGB or BPD [4,33], while no change is observed after LAGB [5]. Increased PYY levels have been reported following RYGB and IT [5], an effect that may contribute to increased satiety and weight loss. Levels of ghrelin, an orexigenic hormone, do not show the expected physiological rise following weight loss after gastric bypass [34] and are substantially reduced after SG [9,33].

It has been suggested that the increase in GLP-1 and PYY after procedures that involve intestinal bypass (RYGB, BPD) results from the expedited presentation of relatively undigested nutrients to the distal small bowel rich in GLP-1/PYY-producing L cells ("hindgut theory"). However, SG also induces a similar and substantial rise in postprandial GLP-1 and PYY, despite the anatomy of this operation not including intestinal rerouting. In fact, a recent experimental study from our group suggests that increased postprandial levels of GLP-1 may be explained by modifications of gastric anatomy and physiology (emptying) rather than by the intestinal bypass per se, questioning the hindgut theory as a mechanism for the enhanced GLP-1 response after bariatric procedures [9]. Whatever the mechanisms responsible for the enhancement of GLP-1 (and PYY) response to nutrients, the exact role of increased incretin hormones in the surgical control of diabetes remains unclear; recent studies suggest that changes in gut hormones alone may not explain the entire story. In fact, blockage of GLP-1 action in animals [35] and humans [36] does not entirely prevent glycemic benefits of either SG or RYGB.

A number of well-conducted animal and human mechanistic investigations have recently expanded the number of weight-independent antidiabetic mechanisms that could explain the benefits of GI surgery. These mechanisms include changes in intestinal nutrient-sensing regulating insulin sensitivity [10], disruption of vagal afferent and efferent innervations [10], perturbations of bile acid metabolism [37], taste alterations [38], and enhancement of intestinal glucose uptake in the alimentary limb after diversionary procedures [39].

It has also been proposed that the exclusion of the proximal intestine from the nutrient flow may exert its direct antidiabetic effects by downregulating one or more yet unidentified "anti-incretin factors" [6,13]. Such factor(s) would have the physiologic role to prevent postprandial hypoglycemia and beta-cell proliferation (contrasting antiapoptosis effect of incretins), whereas an imbalance between incretins and anti-incretin may lead to insulin resistance and diabetes. Preliminary experimental evidence for the existence of intestinal signals that reduce insulin sensitivity in diabetic subjects has been recently reported [40,41].

Elucidating the fascinating mechanisms by which GI surgery can improve diabetes (and induce weight loss) has become the focus of intense research in recent years. Elucidating these mechanisms would provide an unprecedented opportunity to shed light on the elusive causes of diabetes and obesity and may also help find new targets for novel drugs and interventions that mimic the effects of bariatric and metabolic surgery.

CLINICAL EFFICACY OF BARIATRIC/METABOLIC SURGERY IN PATIENTS WITH TYPE 2 DIABETES

RESULTS OF METABOLIC/DIABETES SURGERY IN PATIENTS WITH A BMI > 35 KG/M²

The outcomes of metabolic surgery on diabetes and associated comorbidities in patients with a BMI > 35 kg/m² have been well documented over many years.

A meta-analysis by Buchwald et al. [42] including 22,094 patients with T2DM reported an overall 77% remission rate of T2DM (defined as persistent normoglycemia without diabetes medications after bariatric surgery). The mean procedure-specific resolution of T2DM was 48% for LAGB, 68% for vertical banded gastroplasty (VBG), 84% for RYGB, and 98% for BPD. A major limitation of this study was the retrospective nature of the majority of series included in the meta-analysis and the short duration of follow-up.

The multicenter Swedish Obese Subjects (SOS) study, a large prospective observational study, compared bariatric surgery (LAGB, $n = 156$; VBG, $n = 451$; RYGB, $n = 34$) versus conservative medical management in a group of well-matched obese patients. At 2 years, 72% of diabetic subjects in the surgical group achieved remission of T2DM, compared to 21% in the medically treated arm [43]. At 10 years, the relative risk of incident T2DM was three times lower and the rates of recovery from T2DM were three times greater for patients who underwent surgery compared to individ uals in the control group. The proportion of subjects in whom the remission was sustained at 10 years declined to 36% in the surgical group and 13% in the medical group. An important consideration in interpreting the long-term results of the SOS study is the fact that approximately 95% of patients underwent less effective gastric restrictive procedures rather than RYGB or BPD, therefore potentially underestimating the effects of surgery. On the other hand, it must be noted that an intention-to-treat analysis was applied in the analysis of this study; since many patients originally included in the control (conventional therapy) group have eventually undergone surgery over the years, this type of analysis may provide the false impression that long-term diabetes remission, albeit minimal, could also be obtained by the medical treatment in the study.

Two large case-series studies by Pories et al. (330 patients) [44] and Schauer et al. (191 patients) [45] focused principally on diabetes outcomes after RYGB. Mean fasting blood glucose (FBG) decreased from clearly diabetic values to near-normal levels (117 and 98 mg/dL in the two studies, respectively), and HbA1c fell to normal levels (6.6% and 5.6%) without diabetes medication in 89% and 82% of patients, respectively.

More recently, laparoscopic SG has garnered considerable interest as a low-morbidity surgical procedure that leads to effective weight loss and control of metabolic disease. A systematic review by Gill et al. [46] of 27 studies involving 673 patients (mean follow-up of 13.1 months) has reported a T2DM resolution rate of 66.2% in obese subjects and improved glycemic control in 26.9%. The mean decrease in blood glucose and HbA1c after SG was −88.2 mg/dL and −1.7%, respectively. SG therefore represents a very effective procedure in terms of both weight reduction and control of T2DM. However, it remains unclear whether the procedure provides similar efficacy compared to RYGB or BPD. While several short-term case-controlled studies suggest that there is no significant difference in the rates of diabetes remission between RYGB and SG [47], long-term (5 years and beyond) studies [48] and randomized clinical trials [49,50] show higher rates of diabetes remission, lower usage of diabetes medications, and better beta-cell function [25] after RYGB than after SG, in spite of equivalent weight loss.

More recently, several randomized controlled clinical trials comparing medical versus surgical management of T2DM have been reported. The STAMPEDE trial compared intensive medical therapy alone versus medical therapy plus RYGB or SG in 150 obese patients (BMI, 27–43 kg/m^2) with uncontrolled T2DM [50]. The primary end point was the proportion of patients with a glycated hemoglobin (HbA1c) level of 6.0% or less 12 months after treatment. The proportion of patients who reached the primary end point was 12% for the medical group, 42% in the RYGB group, and 37% in the SG group. Glycemic control was demonstrated to improve in all three groups, with a mean HbA1c level of 7.5 ± 1.8% in the medical therapy group, 6.4 ± 0.9% in the gastric bypass group, and 6.6 ± 1.0% in the SG group. All patients in the RYGB group who achieved the primary end point of the study (HbA1c < 6.0%) did so without the need for diabetes medications, unlike patients in the SG group; although the study was not powered to demonstrate differences between surgical procedures, these findings suggest a potential greater antidiabetic effect of RYGB. Secondary end points, including BMI, body weight, waist circumference, and the homeostasis model assessment of insulin resistance (HOMA-IR) improved more significantly in the surgical groups than the medical therapy group.

Another randomized controlled trial (RCT) from Italy [51] involving 60 patients (BMI ≥ 35 kg/m^2) with T2DM of at least 5 years' duration and an HbA1c level of 7.0% or more compared conventional medical therapy to RYGB and BPD. The primary end point was the rate of partial diabetes remission at 2 years (as defined by an expert panel of the American Diabetes Association, partial remission indicates a fasting glucose level < 100 mg/dL and an HbA1c level < 6.5% in the absence of pharmacological therapy). At 2 years' follow-up, diabetes remission had occurred in no patients in the medical therapy group versus 75% in the RYGB group and 95% in the BPD group. All patients in the surgical groups were able to discontinue their pharmacotherapy (oral hypoglycemic agents and insulin) within 15 days after the operation. At 2 years, the average baseline HbA1c levels (8.65 ± 1.45%) had decreased in all groups, but patients in the two surgical groups had the greatest degree of improvement (average HbA1c levels, 7.69 ± 0.57% in the medical therapy group, 6.35 ± 1.42% in the RYGB group, and 4.95 ± 0.49% in the BPD group). Similar results were also reported in two other randomized clinical trials where surgery was compared to medical therapy of diabetes in patients with a BMI of 30–40. In the Diabetes Surgery Study trial [52], 120 patients were randomized to receive intensive lifestyle and medical therapy with or without RYGB. The primary end point was a composite outcome including achievement of HbA1c < 7.0%, LDL cholesterol < 100 mg/dL, and systolic blood pressure < 130 mm Hg. After 12 months, 28 participants (49%; 95% confidence interval [CI], 36–63%) in the gastric bypass group and 11 (19%; 95% CI, 10–32%) in the lifestyle–medical management group achieved the primary end points (odds ratio [OR], 4.8; 95% CI, 1.9–11.7). Participants in the RYGB group also required 3.0 fewer medications than those receiving lifestyle–medical therapy alone. Twenty-two serious adverse events were reported in the RYGB group and 15 in the lifestyle–medical management group. In an earlier RCT, Dixon et al. [53] found greater reduction of HbA1c with LAGB compared with usual medical treatment in patients with recently diagnosed diabetes.

RESULTS OF BARIATRIC/METABOLIC SURGERY ON DIABETES IN PATIENTS WITH A BMI < 35 KG/M²

While bariatric surgery is widely recognized for its positive effects on comorbidities in morbidly obese patients, there is also now mounting evidence from observational studies and RCTs that less obese patients may obtain similar benefits following metabolic surgery. Cohen et al. [54] published results from a prospective study of 66 diabetic patients (BMI, 30–35 kg/m²) who elected to have the RYGB and were followed up for up to 6 years. Remission of diabetes occurred in 88% of patients (defined as an HbA1c < 6.5% without the use of hypoglycemic medication), while improvement of diabetes was seen in 11% of patients, which led to a decrease in the usage of pharmacotherapy and withdrawal of insulin.

Some of the recent prospective randomized controlled trials comparing surgery versus medical therapy have also included lower-BMI patients (<35 kg/m²). Dixon et al. [53] reported in 2008 an RCT comparing LAGB versus conventional therapy in 60 obese patients (BMI > 30 and < 40 kg/m²) with recently diagnosed (<2 years) T2DM. The primary outcome measure was the remission of T2DM (defined as fasting plasma glucose < 126 mg/dL and an HbA1c level < 6.2% while taking no glycemic therapy). After a 2-year follow-up, remission of T2DM was achieved in 73% in the surgical group and 13% in the conventional therapy-group; the main predictor of remission was weight loss. Secondary outcome measures, such as insulin sensitivity and levels of triglycerides and HDL were also improved in the surgical group.

Lee et al. [49] compared the efficacy of RYGB versus SG on T2DM resolution (remission defined as fasting plasma glucose < 126 mg/dL, HbA1c < 6.5%, without the use of oral hypoglycemics or insulin) in non–morbidly obese patients (BMI < 35 kg/m²) who, prior to surgery, had inadequately controlled T2DM. The resolution rate was 93% in the RYGB group compared with 47% in the SG group. The RYGB group also had a higher remission rate for metabolic syndrome than the SG group.

In the most recently published Diabetes Surgery Study (DSS) study, 120 participants who had an HbA1c level of 8.0% or higher, BMI between 30.0 and 39.9, C peptide level > 1.0 ng/mL, and type 2 diabetes for at least 6 months were randomized to lifestyle-intensive medical management or RYGB. After 12 months, the composite goal of HbA1c < 7.0%, LDL cholesterol < 100 mg/dL, and systolic blood pressure < 130 mm Hg was achieved in 49% in the gastric bypass group and 19% in the lifestyle-intensive medical management group. Regression analyses indicated that achieving the composite end point was primarily attributable to weight loss.

Despite evidence of efficacy of surgery in the control of diabetes in moderately obese and overweight patients deriving from several prospective series and even short-term results of randomized trials, defining the appropriate role of diabetes surgery in less obese or nonobese patients warrants further and long-term investigation. In particular, the impact of surgery on microvascular and macrovascular complications of diabetes needs to be assessed with long-term follow-up.

EFFECT OF SURGERY ON CARDIOVASCULAR MORBIDITY AND MORTALITY IN PATIENTS WITH T2DM

It is now evident that apart from its glycemic effects, bariatric surgery confers nonglycemic benefits, including improvement of cardiovascular risk factors such as dyslipidemia and hypertension. More importantly, bariatric/metabolic surgery seems to be associated with a reduction in overall mortality and diabetes-related mortality [55]. Adams et al. [56] conducted a retrospective cohort study including 7925 severely obese patients and 7925 similarly obese matched controls. After a mean follow-up of 8.4 years, it was demonstrated that surgery reduced overall mortality by 40%, cardiovascular mortality by 56%, cancer mortality by 60%, and diabetes-related mortality by 92% [59].

The meta-analysis by Buchwald et al. [42] showed a marked decrease in the levels of total cholesterol, LDL cholesterol, and triglycerides after GI surgery. An improvement in hyperlipidemia was shown in approximately 70% of patients, and hypertension was shown to improve or resolve in 79% of patients. Lee et al. [49] have demonstrated these beneficial effects of GI surgery in patients with a BMI < 35 kg/m^2. In another study, Cohen et al. [54] prospectively followed up patients with T2DM who had gastric bypass and demonstrated that the predicted 10-year risk of cardiovascular disease, calculated by the United Kingdom Prospective Diabetes Study (UKPDS) risk engine, fell substantially after surgery. There was a 71% decrease in the risk of coronary heart disease, 84% decrease in risk of fatal events, 50% decrease in the risk of stroke, and 57% decrease in the risk of fatal stroke [54].

A recent analysis of the SOS study looked at the effects of bariatric surgery on cardiovascular events with a mean follow-up of 13.3 years [57]. The results showed that bariatric surgery was associated with a reduction in the incidence of fatal and nonfatal cardiovascular events.

BARIATRIC, METABOLIC, AND DIABETES SURGERY: DEFINITIONS AND IMPLICATIONS FOR CLINICAL PRACTICE

Historically, the term *bariatric surgery* has been a synonym of *weight loss surgery*. The term *metabolic surgery* has emerged over the last decade from the recognition that benefits and mechanisms of action of bariatric surgery extend beyond weight loss. The terms *metabolic* and diabetes surgery indicate a surgical approach whose primary intent is the control of metabolic alterations/hyperglycemia, in contrast to *bariatric surgery*, conceived as a mere weight-reduction therapy. We recently showed that offering surgery to treat metabolic disease or diabetes rather than as a mere weight-reduction therapy can significantly influence patient selection, with important ramifications for clinical care. We analyzed data from a prospective database of 200 patients who underwent surgery at two distinct surgical programs within the same tertiary care center: the section of GI metabolic surgery, where surgery was offered and promoted as an approach primarily aimed at the treatment of diabetes or metabolic syndrome and the section of bariatric surgery, a traditional weight loss surgery program. The results of this analysis revealed distinct demographic and clinical characteristics of surgical candidates. Metabolic surgery patients were older (45.8 ± 13.4 vs. 41.8 ± 11.7, $P < .05$), had a lower body mass index (42.4 ± 7.1 vs. 48.6 ± 9.5 kg/m^2; $P < .01$), and had a higher prevalence of males (42% vs. 26%, $P < .05$). The prevalence of diabetes, hypertension, dyslipidemia, and cardiovascular disease was also significantly higher in patients operated on in the metabolic surgery program, as was the severity of diabetes (higher glycated hemoglobin levels, greater percentage of insulin use) [58]. An intuitive consequence of the change in goals of surgery and patient selection is the need to redefine the success and failure of surgical treatment. While excess weight loss has been a traditional measure of the efficacy of bariatric surgery, remission/improvement of metabolic disease (T2DM, hypertension, obstructive sleep apnea, and dyslipidemia) and cardiovascular disease risk reduction are more rational measures of outcomes in metabolic surgery. A recent position statement of the IDF recommends the use of diabetes-specific parameters as a measure of the efficacy of treatment when bariatric surgery is performed with the intent to treat diabetes. These recommendations include assessment of glycated hemoglobin levels, C peptide, fasting glycemia, insulin levels, and lipid profile and regular monitoring of blood pressure, among others.

The substantial difference between a weight-centric approach as in bariatric surgery and a disease-based approach as in metabolic/diabetes surgery has profound implications for the organization of centers offering metabolic and diabetes surgery. The model of care of metabolic surgery should be shaped around the goal of optimizing disease control and achieving a cure when possible; like in other fields of medicine (i.e., oncologic surgery, endocrine surgery, etc.), this entails the integration of surgical and medical therapies not as alternative strategies but as complementary treatments when indicated. The development of metabolic surgery requires availability of multidisciplinary expertise, use of rational and disease-based criteria for surgical indications, and the development of specific pathways of care, coherent with the intent to treat diabetes and metabolic illness.

REFERENCES

1. Shaw JE, Sicree RA, Zimmet PZ. Global estimates of the prevalence of diabetes for 2010 and 2030. *Diabetes Res Clin Pract.* 2010;87(1):4–14.
2. Rubino F, Marescaux J. Effect of duodenal–jejunal exclusion in a nonobese animal model of type 2 diabetes: A new perspective for an old disease. *Ann Surg.* 2004;239:1–11.
3. Rubino F, Forgione A, Cummings DE et al. The mechanism of diabetes control after gastrointestinal bypass surgery reveals a role of the proximal small intestine in the pathophysiology of type 2 diabetes. *Ann Surg.* 2006;244(5):741–9.
4. Laferrère B, Teixeira J, McGinty J et al. Effect of weight loss by gastric bypass surgery versus hypocaloric diet on glucose and incretin levels in patients with type 2 diabetes. *J Clin Endocrinol Metab.* 2008;93:2479–85.
5. Thaler JP, Cummings DE. Minireview: Hormonal and metabolic mechanisms of diabetes remission after gastrointestinal surgery. *Endocrinology.* 2009;150(6):2518–25.
6. Rubino F, Gagner M. Potential of surgery for curing type 2 diabetes mellitus. *Ann Surg.* 2002;236(5):554–9.
7. Zimmet P, Alberti KG, Rubino F et al. IDF's view of bariatric surgery in type 2 diabetes. *Lancet.* 2011;378(9786):108–10.
8. Cohen RV, Schiavon CA, Pinheiro JS, Correa JL, Rubino F. Duodenal–jejunal bypass for the treatment of type 2 diabetes in patients with body mass index of 22–34 kg/m². *Surg Obes Relat Dis.* 2007;3:195–7.
9. Patel RT, Shukla AP, Ahn SM, Moreira M, Rubino F. Surgical control of obesity and diabetes: The role of intestinal vs. gastric mechanisms in the regulation of body weight and glucose homeostasis. *Obesity (Silver Spring).* 2014;22(1):159–69.
10. Breen DM, Rasmussen BA, Kokorovic A, Wang R, Cheung GW, Lam TK. Jejunal nutrient sensing is required for duodenal–jejunal bypass surgery to rapidly lower glucose concentrations in uncontrolled diabetes. *Nat Med.* 2012;18(6):950–5.
11. Koopmans HS, Sclafani A, Fichtner C, Aravich PF. The effects of ileal transposition on food intake and body weight loss in VMH-obese rats. *Am J Clin Nutr.* 1982;35(2):284–93.
12. DePaula AL, Macedo AL, Prudente AS, Queiroz L, Schraibman V, Pinus J. Laparoscopic sleeve gastrectomy with ileal interposition ("neuroendocrine brake")—pilot study of a new operation. *Surg Obes Relat Dis.* 2006;2:464–6.
13. Rubino F, Schauer PR, Kaplan LM, Cummings DE. Metabolic surgery to treat type 2 diabetes: Clinical outcomes and mechanisms of action. *Annu Rev Med.* 2010;61:393–411.
14. Aguirre V, Stylopoulos N, Grinbaum R et al. An endoluminal sleeve induces substantial weight loss and normalizes glucose homeostasis in rats with diet-induced obesity. *Obesity (Silver Spring).* 2008;16:2585–92.

15. Schouten R, Rijs CS, Bouvy ND, Hameeteman W, Koek GH, Janssen IM, Greve JW. A multicenter, randomized efficacy study of the EndoBarrier gastrointestinal liner for presurgical weight loss prior to bariatric surgery. *Ann Surg*. 2010;251(2):236–43.

16. Tarnoff M, Rodriguez L, Escalona A, Ramos A, Neto M, Alamo M, Reyes E, Pimentel F, Ibanez L. Open label, prospective, randomized controlled trial of an endoscopic duodenal–jejunal bypass sleeve versus low calorie diet for pre-operative weight loss in bariatric surgery. *Surg Endosc*. 2009;23(3):650–6.

17. Sorli C, Rodriguez L, Reyes E et al. Pilot clinical study of an endoscopic, removable duodenal–jejunal bypass liner for the treatment of type 2 diabetes. *Diabetes Technol Therap*. 2009;11(11):725–32.

18. Pi-Sunyer FX. *Clinical Guidelines on the Identification, Evaluation, and Treatment of Overweight and Obesity in Adults: The Evidence Report*. NIH Publication No. 98-4083. Washington, DC: National Heart, Lung, and Blood Institute, The National Institute of Diabetes and Digestive and Kidney Diseases, 1998, pp. 39–41.

19. Goodpaster BH, Kelley DE, Wing RR, Meier A, Thaete FL. Effects of weight loss on regional fat distribution and insulin sensitivity in obesity. *Diabetes*. 1999;48:839–47.

20. Knowler WC, Barrett-Connor E, Fowler SE, Hamman RF, Lachin JM, Walker EA, Nathan DM. Reduction in the incidence of type 2 diabetes with lifestyle intervention or metformin. *N Engl J Med*. 2002;346:393–403.

21. Bradley D, Magkos F, Klein S. Effects of bariatric surgery on glucose homeostasis and type 2 diabetes. *Gastroenterology*. 2012;143(4):897–912.

22. Rubino F. Is type 2 diabetes an operable intestinal disease? A provocative yet reasonable hypothesis. *Diabetes Care*. 2008;31(Suppl 2):S290–6.

23. Pontiroli AE, Pizzocri P, Librenti MC, Vedani P, Marchi M, Cucchi E, Orena C, Paganelli M, Giacomelli M, Ferla G, Folli F. Laparoscopic adjustable gastric banding for the treatment of morbid (grade 3) obesity and its metabolic complications: A three-year study. *J Clin Endocrinol Metab*. 2002;87:3555–61.

24. Pattou F, Beraud G, Arnalsteen L et al. Restoration of beta cell function after bariatric surgeryin type 2 diabetic patients: A prospective controlled study comparing gastric banding and gastric bypass. *Obes Surg*. 2007;17:1041–3.

25. Kashyap SR, Bhatt DL, Wolski K et al. Metabolic effects of bariatric surgery in patients with moderate obesity and type 2 diabetes: Analysis of a randomized control trial comparing surgery with intensive medical treatment. *Diabetes Care*. 2013;36(8):2175–82.

26. Meirelles K, Ahmed T, Culnan DM, Lynch CJ, Lang CH, Cooney RN. Mechanisms of glucose homeostasis after Roux-en-Y gastric bypass surgery in the obese, insulin-resistant Zucker rat. *Ann Surg*. 2009;249:277–85.

27. Koopmans HS, Ferri GL, Sarson DL, Polak JM, Bloom SR. The effects of ileal transposition and jejunoileal bypass on food intake and GI hormone levels in rats. *Physiol Behav*. 1984;33:601–9.

28. Strader AD, Vahl TP, Jandacek RJ et al. Weight loss through ileal transposition is accompanied by increased ileal hormone secretion and synthesis in rats. *Am J Physiol Endocrinol Metab*. 2005;288:E447–53.

29. Mason EE. Ileal transposition and enteroglucagon/GLP-1 in obesity (and diabetic?) surgery. *Obes Surg*. 1999;9:223–8.

30. Carrel G, Egli L, Tran C, Schneiter P, Giusti V, D'Alessio D, Tappy L. Contributions of fat and protein to the incretin effect of a mixed meal. *Am J Clin Nutr*. 2011;94(4):997–1003.

31. Fujita Y, Wideman RD, Speck M, Asadi A, King DS, Webber TD, Haneda M, Kieffer TJ. Incretin release from gut is acutely enhanced by sugar but not by sweeteners in vivo. *Am J Physiol Endocrinol Metab*. 2009;296:E473–9.

32. Cho YM, Fujita Y, Kieffer TJ. Glucagon-like peptide-1: Glucose homeostasis and beyond. *Annu Rev Physiol*. 2014;76:535–59.

33. Shukla A, Rubino F. Secretion and function of gastrointestinal hormones after bariatric surgery: Their role in type 2 diabetes. *Can J Diabetes*. 2011;35(2):115–22.

34. Cummings DE. Gastric bypass and nesidioblastosis—too much of a good thing for islets? *N Engl J Med*. 2005;353:300–2.

35. Wilson-Pérez HE, Chambers AP, Ryan KK, Li B, Sandoval DA, Stoffers D, Drucker DJ, Pérez-Tilve D, Seeley RJ. Vertical sleeve gastrectomy is effective in two genetic mouse models of glucagon-like Peptide 1 receptor deficiency. *Diabetes*. 2013;62(7):2380–5.

36. Jiménez A, Casamitjana R, Viaplana-Masclans J, Lacy A, Vidal J. GLP-1 action and glucose tolerance in subjects with remission of type 2 diabetes after gastric bypass surgery. *Diabetes Care*. 2013;36(7):2062–9.

37. Patti ME, McMahon G, Mun EC, Bitton A, Holst JJ, Goldsmith J, Hanto DW, Callery M, Arky R, Nose V, Bonner-Weir S, Goldfine AB. Severe hypoglycaemia postgastric bypass requiring partial pancreatectomy: evidence for inappropriate insulin secretion and pancreatic islet hyperplasia. *Diabetologia*. 2005;48:2236–40.

38. Wilson-Pérez HE, Chambers AP, Sandoval DA, Stefater MA, Woods SC, Benoit SC, Seeley RJ. The effect of vertical sleeve gastrectomy on food choice in rats. *Int J Obes (Lond)*. 2013;37(2):288–95.
39. Saeidi N, Meoli L, Nestoridi E, Gupta NK, Kvas S, Kucharczyk J, Bonab AA, Fischman AJ, Yarmush ML, Stylopoulos N. Reprogramming of intestinal glucose metabolism and glycemic control in rats after gastric bypass. *Science*. 2013;341(6144):406–10.
40. Salinari S, le Roux CW, Bertuzzi A, Rubino F, Mingrone G. Duodenal–jejunal bypass and jejunectomy improve insulin sensitivity in Goto-Kakizaki diabetic rats without changes in incretins or insulin secretion. *Diabetes*. 2014;63(3):1069–78.
41. Salinari S, Debard C, Bertuzzi A, Durand C, Zimmet P, Vidal H, Mingrone G. Jejunal proteins secreted by db/db mice or insulin-resistant humans impair the insulin signaling and determine insulin resistance. *PLoS One*. 2013;8(2):e56258.
42. Buchwald H, Avidor Y, Braunwald E et al. Bariatric surgery: A systematic review and meta-analysis. *JAMA*. 2004;292(14):1724–37.
43. Sjöström L, Lindroos AK, Peltonen M et al. Swedish Obese Subjects Study Scientific Group. Lifestyle, diabetes and cardiovascular risk factors 10 years after bariatric surgery. *N Engl J Med*. 2004;351(26):2683–93.
44. Pories WJ, Swanson MS, MacDonald KG et al. Who would have thought it? An operation proves to be the most effective therapy for adult-onset diabetes mellitus. *Ann Surg*. 1995;222:339–50.
45. Schauer PR, Burguera B, Ikramuddin S et al. Effect of laparoscopic Roux-en Y gastric bypass on type 2 diabetes mellitus. *Ann Surg*. 2003;238(4):467–84.
46. Gill RS, Birch DW, Shi X et al. Sleeve gastrectomy and type 2 diabetes mellitus: A systematic review. *Surg Obes Relat Dis*. 2010;6(6):707–13.
47. Yaghoubian A, Tolan A, Stabile BE et al. Laparoscopic Roux-en-Y gastric bypass and sleeve gastrectomy achieve comparable weight loss at 1 year. *Am Surg*. 2012;78(12):1325–8.
48. Brethauer SA, Aminian A, Romero-Talamás H et al. Can diabetes be surgically cured? Long-term metabolic effects of bariatric surgery in obese patients with type 2 diabetes mellitus. *Ann Surg*. 2013;258(4):628–36.
49. Lee WJ, Chong K, Ser KH et al. Gastric bypass vs sleeve gastrectomy for type 2 diabetes mellitus: A randomized controlled trial. *Arch Surg*. 2011;146(2):143–8.
50. Schauer PR, Kashyap SR, Wolski K et al. Bariatric surgery versus intensive medical therapy in obese patients with diabetes. *N Engl J Med*. 2012;366(17):1567–76.
51. Mingrone G, Panunzi S, De Gaetano A et al. Bariatric surgery versus conventional medical therapy for type 2 diabetes. *N Engl J Med*. 2012;366(17):1577–85.
52. Ikramuddin S, Korner J, Lee WJ et al. Roux-en-Y gastric bypass vs intensive medical management for the control of type 2 diabetes, hypertension, and hyperlipidemia: The Diabetes Surgery Study randomized clinical trial. *JAMA*. 2013;309(21):2240–9.
53. Dixon JB, O'Brien PE, Playfair J et al. Adjustable gastric banding and conventional therapy for type 2 diabetes: A randomized controlled trial. *JAMA*. 2008;299(3):316–23.
54. Cohen RV, Pinheiro JC, Schiavon CA et al. Effects of gastric bypass surgery in patients with type 2 diabetes and only mild obesity. *Diabetes Care*. 2012;35(7):1420–8.
55. Sjöström L, Narbro K, Sjöström CD et al. Swedish Obese Subjects Study. Effects of bariatric surgery on mortality in Swedish obese subjects. *N Engl J Med*. 2007;357(8):741–52.
56. Adams TD, Gress RE, Smith SC et al. Long-term mortality after gastric bypass surgery. *N Engl J Med*. 2007;357(8):753–61.
57. Sjöström L, Peltonen M, Jacobson P et al. Bariatric surgery and long-term cardiovascular events. *JAMA*. 2012;307(1):56–65.
58. Rubino F, Shukla A, Pomp A et al. Bariatric, metabolic, and diabetes surgery: What's in a name? *Ann Surg*. 2014;259(1):117–22.

16 Metabolic Changes Post-Bariatric Surgery

Juliana S. Simonetti and Caroline Apovian

CONTENTS

INTRODUCTION

It has been well established that bariatric surgery has significant effects on obesity-related comorbidities such as type 2 diabetes, hypertension, lipid dysfunction, and other cardiovascular risk factors. Bariatric surgery is considered the most effective treatment of obesity due to its significant effects in decreasing obesity-related comorbidities [1]. Multiple studies have shown that it has a profound effect on the metabolic and nutritional status that goes beyond caloric restriction and malabsorption since significant changes on glycemic control and blood pressure, to list a few, are seen even prior to the weight loss being achieved [2]. The changes in the gastrointestinal hormones, which include glucagon-like peptide-1 (GLP-1), peptide tyrosine tyrosine (PYY), oxyntomodulin (OXM), glucose-dependent insulinotropic polypeptide (GIP), and ghrelin, are thought to play an important role in the metabolic changes post-bariatric surgery and in long-term maintenance of weight loss.

The gastrointestinal (GI) tract is the largest endocrine organ in the body, where more than 30 known peptide hormone genes are expressed, with more than 100 different hormonally active peptides produced [3]. The hormone changes post-bariatric surgery seem to play a very important role in weight loss. In this chapter, we will review some of the key hormones that have been found to affect appetite, energy balance, and glucose–insulin homeostasis in each type of bariatric surgical procedure.

BARIATRIC PROCEDURES

Bariatric surgery was initially conceived 50 years ago with the observation that patients who developed short bowel syndrome or underwent partial gastrectomy, performed for other diseases, had significant weight loss [4]. In its early stages, bariatric surgery was marked by questionable results with unacceptably high risks [5]. Much has changed over the last five decades, and today, minimally invasive surgery has become the most performed type of bariatric procedure in the United States, which has helped reduce complications and improve outcomes [5]; the US Agency for Healthcare Research and Quality (AHRQ) reported the risk of death from bariatric surgery to be about 0.1% and the overall likelihood of major complications to be about 4% [6]. In addition, several studies have demonstrated that bariatric surgery increases life expectancy by 89% [6] and decreases the risk of death from diabetes by 92%, from cancer by 60%, and from coronary artery disease by 56% [7], as compared to those obese persons who do not have surgery. Data published in 2011 showed a significant increase in bariatric surgeries in the United States, with the number reaching 220,000 in 2009 [6]. Given significant advancements in surgical techniques, bariatric surgery has become first-line treatment for those with severe obesity and related comorbidities.

TABLE 16.1
Summary of Bariatric Procedures

	Types of Operation	% Excess Weight Loss (%EWL)[a]	Description
Restrictive	Adjustable gastric band (AGB) (Figure 16.1)	50–60%	An adjustable silicone band is placed around the stomach laparoscopically, below the gastroesophageal junction, reducing gastric size to about 15 mL [4,5].
	Sleeve gastrectomy (SG) (Figure 16.2)	33–83%	Partial gastrectomy of the greater curvature of the stomach, creating a 100–150 mL tubular stomach [8].
	Vertical banded gastroplasty (VBG) (Figure 16.3)	63–70%	Horizontal gastric stapling is placed across the fundus, creating a gastric pouch using a naturally distensible portion of stomach, and then positioning a ring around the stomach from the lesser curvature to the initial gastrectomy [8].

(continued)

TABLE 16.1 (Continued)
Summary of Bariatric Procedures

Types of Operation		% Excess Weight Loss (%EWL)[a]	Description
Malabsorptive combined	Roux-en-Y gastric bypass (RYGB) (Figure 16.4)	70–80%	Creates a small stomach pouch of 15–30 mL and the Roux limb 75–150 cm in length that reroutes a portion of the alimentary tract to bypass the distal stomach and the proximal small bowel [8,9], rerouting nutrient flow from the stomach directly into the proximal jejunum through a gastrojejunal anastomosis [4].
	Biliopancreatic diversion (Figure 16.5)	77–88%	Distal gastrectomy with a long Roux-en-Y reconstruction where the enteroenterostomy is placed at a distal ileal level.

[a] %EWL, percentage of excess weight loss, is calculated from the following equation: (weight loss in kg/excess weight in kg) × 100, where excess weight = total body weight − ideal body weight. Information for %EWL was obtained from Lim, R.B. et al., *Curr. Probl. Surg.* 47, 2010.

Bariatric procedures are classified as either restrictive or malabsorptive, or a combination of both, with multiple techniques being used, leading to variable outcomes and weight loss (Table 16.1). In general, malabsorptive procedures lead to a greater percentage of weight loss, which may be attributed to its alteration of gut hormonal milieu and, somewhat, of macronutrient absorption [10]. Patients who have restrictive procedures tend to have more gradual weight loss. Restrictive bariatric operations limit the capacity of the stomach to accommodate food and constrict the flow of ingested nutrients, leading to weight loss. There are three restrictive procedures, the laparoscopic adjustable gastric band (LAGB), sleeve gastrectomy (SG), and vertical banded gastroplasty (VBG). LAGB, a purely restrictive procedure, is the second-most-performed bariatric procedure in the United States [5] (Figure 16.1). SG is a partial gastrectomy of the fundus and body of the stomach, which initially was considered a solely restrictive procedure (Figure 16.2), yet there is a growing consensus that this procedure involves neuroendocrine changes due to stomach resection and expedited delivery of nutrients into the small intestine, leading to weight loss and markedly improved glucose homeostasis [11]. VBG involves placing horizontal gastric staples across the fundus, creating a gastric pouch using a naturally distensible portion of the stomach, and then positioning a ring around the stomach from the lesser curvature to the initial gastrectomy [8] (Figure 16.3). VBG procedures have now fallen out of favor, and only very few of these procedures are performed due to numerous complications and the advent of the laparoscopic adjustable banding procedure [12].

Most of the malabsorptive procedures are combined with a form of restriction of the stomach volume with rearrangement of the intestine that causes nutrients to bypass the distal part of the stomach and the proximal small bowel [9]. The Roux-en-Y gastric bypass (RYGB) is the most common bariatric procedure in the United States and Canada [13]. In RYGB, the gastric volume is restricted by creating a 15–30 mL gastric pouch, while the nutrient flow is rerouted from the stomach directly into the proximal jejunum through a gastrojejunal anastomosis [14], connecting the Roux limb to the biliopancreatic limb to form a common channel (Figure 16.4). There are also variations in the procedure, with some leaving the remnant stomach and others resecting it. The differences in the procedure have been shown to have no difference in mortality or weight loss outcome [6]. Other combined malabsorptive and restrictive procedures include the biliopancreatic diversion (BPD), also called the Scopinaro procedure, where a partial gastrectomy of the distal stomach is performed along with a long RYGB, and the enteroenterostomy is placed on the distal ileal level (Figure 16.5). More frequently performed is the BDP with duodenal switch (BPD-DS) where an SG is performed and Roux limb is anastomosed to the duodenum instead of the stomach [4,15]. This procedure is not often performed in the United States due to rates of complications [4].

Initially, weight loss from these procedures was first described as a result of their restrictive and/ or malabsorptive mechanism; however, there is a growing body of evidence that the neuroendocrine effects of bariatric surgery play a key role in weight loss and glucose–insulin homeostasis, leading to improvement and resolution of obesity-related comorbidities [16].

THE GUT AS AN ENDOCRINE ORGAN

GHRELIN

Ghrelin is also known as the hunger hormone, an orexigenic neuropeptide that peaks preprandially and decreases after food intake. This amino acid peptide is secreted by cells in the stomach fundus

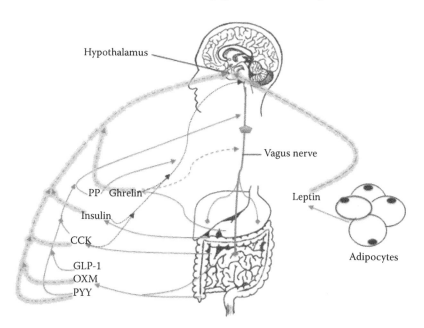

FIGURE 16.6   This figure reviews the brain-gut mechanism via Vagus nerve and gastro-intestinal hormones. The enteric nervous system transmits information about mechanical, chemical and neurohumoral stimuli to the CNS via the vagal and sympathetic nerves that control appetite. Ghrelin secreted by the stomach acts on vagus nerve, hypothalamus and hindbrain to stimulate appetite. The anorectic hormones, which include insulin, GLP-1, PYY, OXM, and Leptin act on vagus nerve and/or at the hypothalamus to induce satiety. PP and CCK are also anoretic hormones secreted by the pancreas and the small intestine. PP acts on vagus nerve and the hindbrain, while CCK acts on vagus nerve, hypothalamus, and hindbrain to decrease food intake and induce satiety. (Adapted from Mendieta-Zeron H, Lopez M, Dieguez C. Gastrointestinal peptides controlling body weight homeostasis. *Gen Comp Endocrinol*. 2008;155:481–495.)

(and in smaller amounts by the duodenum, jejunum, and ileum) [17]. Ghrelin is an appetite stimulant through action in the central nervous system (CNS) via neuropeptide Y (NPY) and agouti-related protein (AgRP) neurons in the hypothalamus (Figure 16.6), leading to enhanced appetite, gastric motility, and adipogenesis. However, ghrelin levels are decreased in those with obesity. A theory initially put forth was that lower levels of ghrelin were attenuated in those with obesity, leading to a delay in satiety. In addition, Tschop and colleagues [18] propose that decreased plasma ghrelin concentration observed in obesity represents a physiological adaptation to the positive energy balance, which may be a consequence of elevated insulin or leptin. Given the location of ghrelin-producing cells in the fundus of the stomach, bariatric surgery would reduce nutrients to ghrelin-producing cells and therefore further decrease ghrelin levels and induce satiety. The data from multiple studies investigating ghrelin levels post-op have been contradictory, some showing a decrease in the levels post-RYGB and others showing no changes [19]. The possible difficulty in identifying its direct connection with obesity is that ghrelin is activated when acylated, which may vary at different times of the day. There is no standard measure of ghrelin, that is, it can be measured as total, acylated, or deacylated [4]. The conflicting study results on ghrelin levels in obesity and post-bariatric surgery makes its role in energy balance and appetite and satiety regulation unclear.

L-CELL-DERIVED PEPTIDES: GLP-1, PYY, AND OXM

GLP-1

GLP-1 is an amino acid peptide released from the L-cells, which are located in distal gut, predominantly the ileum and colon, and in small numbers in the small bowel. Secretion of GLP-1 from L-cells in the intestine is triggered by ingestion of food, particularly glucose and monounsaturated fatty acids. GLP-1 plays a major role in glucose–insulin regulation and energy homeostasis via its incretin effect, enhancing glucose-stimulated insulin secretion from the β-cell [4,20]. In addition, it causes suppression of glucagon release from the pancreas and enhances growth and survival of β-cells. It is related to satiety by slowing gastric emptying and intestinal motility via the presence of nutrients in the distal gut. The peripheral GLP-1 is thought to cross the blood–brain barrier and bind to receptors in the CNS. Neurons in the nucleus of the solitary tract with projections to the paraventricular and arcuate nucleus of the hypothalamus also synthesize GLP-1 and are thought to be involved with the sensation of satiety and decrease in food intake. Postprandial GLP-1 secretion is attenuated in those with obesity [21]. Hyperinsulinemia is thought to be the culprit in the mechanism of decrease in GLP-1 in those with obesity and insulin resistance (IR). Insulin exerts a direct stimulatory effect on GLP-1 secretion from the intestinal L-cell, and IR in the L-cell impairs both homologous and heterologous secretagogue-induced GLP-1 secretion [22]. Pharmacological GLP-1 agonists have been available, such as exenatide, and their administration to obese humans reduces caloric intake by 15%, leading to weight loss [18].

Postprandial GLP-1 is found to increase after RYGB procedure as early as 2 days post-op, while it is unchanged in nonsurgical weight loss [23]. The plasma level-, meal-, or glucose-stimulated GLP-1 response increases fivefold to tenfold from presurgical levels [24]. In addition, plasma levels were found to be significantly higher in patients who had other intestinal rearrangement procedures besides RYGB, such as BPD and jejunoileal bypass (JIB). The increase of GLP-1 post-gastric bypass procedure is thought to be due to direct delivery of nutrients to the distal gut, resulting in higher GLP-1 secretion from the L-cells. This theory is also supported by the fact that GLP-1 increases post-SG; although this procedure does not involve intestinal rearrangement, it causes accelerated gastric emptying with rapid delivery of nutrient-rich chyme to the hindgut. The plasma levels of GLP-1 post-SG were less prominent than in RYGB. A few studies reported that GLP-1 level magnitude correlated with gastric emptying time and amount of weight loss post-op [25]. There is no increase in GLP-1 post-LAGB. This suggests that the higher percentage of weight loss post-rearrangement procedures and SG may be related to satiety effects of GLP-1 [25].

GLP-1 levels were also found to be higher post-RYGB in patients without diabetes than those with diabetes, although they had similar weight losses [26]. Research attempting to elucidate the mechanism for GLP-1 elevation post-op isolated dipeptidyl peptidase 4 (DDP-4) activity, which is significantly decreased post-op. DDP-4 is responsible for degrading GLP-1, so its inhibition leads to higher levels of GLP-1. Higher GLP-1 levels post-RYGB are also likely to be a cause for post-op hyperinsulinemia hypoglycemia and the resolution of type 2 diabetes mellitus (T2DM).

PYY

PYY is a 36-amino acid peptide cosecreted with GLP-1 by L-cells in the GI tract, mainly in the ileum and colon, and in the brain in response to meal stimulation and is degraded by Dipeptidyl peptidase-4 inhibitor (DPP-IV). PYY3-36, its active form, is a potent anorectic hormone, which inhibits food intake by binding to Y-2 neuronal receptors and inhibiting the release of NPY [27]. PYY produces satiety through its role in the "ileal break" which is caused by nutrients, especially triglycerides, reaching the ileum and a feedback mechanism via GLP-1 and PYY, leading to delay in gastric emptying and inhibition of acid secretion [28]. PYY levels are found to be lower in those with obesity and higher in normal-weight individuals [16]. Dysregulation of PYY is implicated in obesity, and its secretion in response to feeding may be blunted in obese individuals [24].

Postprandial plasma PYY is increased post-RYGB and other rearrangement procedures, similar to GLP-1. There are reports of PYY rising as early as 2 days after gastric bypass surgery [23] and increasing progressively to 6 months [29]. PYY was also found to be higher in post-SG patients when compared to other restrictive procedures and caloric restrictive weight loss. Higher levels of PYY post-gastric bypass has also being linked to better weight loss outcome [29]. The explanation for increase in PYY post-bariatric bypass surgery is similar to the increase in GLP-1, which is due to nutrient-rich chyme entering the distal jejunum directly from the stomach pouch and having direct contact with L-cells, leading to secretion of GLP-1 and PYY [24].

There is good evidence that attenuated appetite and increased weight loss after RYGB and other rearrangement procedures (BPD and JIB), as well as in laparoscopic sleeve gastrectomy (LSG), is associated with greater levels of GLP-1 and PYY [25]. This is not true for the purely restrictive procedure, such as LAGB. These findings suggest that the increase in GLP-1 and PYY have a strong association with weight loss post-bariatric surgery in the short and long term and may be key players in the mechanism of weight loss post-op. Further understanding of these hormones may also offer important targets for the medical treatment of obesity.

Oxyntomodulin (OXM)

OXM is a 37-amino acid peptide and is cosecreted with GLP-1 and PYY from the intestinal L-cells in response to food ingestion in proportion to meal calorie content [30]. Like GLP-1 and PYY, it is an anorectic hormone and is also degraded by DPP-IV. It also has an incretin effect (stimulates insulin released from the β-cells in response to ingestion of meals and inhibits glucagon), but OXM binds to GLP-1 or glucagon receptors with a lower affinity [4]. Similarly to GLP-1 and PYY, it inhibits gastric acid secretion and motility and has positive effects on glucose homeostasis [28]. Central injection of OXM into rodents' brains reduces food intake and weight gain, suggesting that OXM signals food ingestion to hypothalamic appetite-regulating circuits [30]. It was also found that OXM suppresses fasting plasma ghrelin (appetite stimulant), which may explain the mechanism by which OXM causes appetite suppression and decreases caloric intake, leading to weight loss. Studies looking at OXM post-RYGB surgery and other rearrangement surgeries have demonstrated that like GLP-1 and PPY, its levels increase in the post-op period [4]. One study looked at OXM plasma levels in response to OGTT that showed a twofold increase 1 month after gastric bypass procedure but not after an equivalent amount of weight was lost via diet [26]. Since OXM, GLP-1, and PYY are cosecreted from L-cells and have synergist effect on energy expenditure and appetite suppression [31], it becomes difficult to distinguish individual roles of each hormone post-bariatric surgery on weight loss. The prevailing hypothesis for weight loss post-gastric bypass surgery and sleeve gastrectomy is the combined supraphysiologic effect of all 3 hormones via local and systemic receptors throughout the gut, pancreas, and autonomic nervous system.

GLUCAGON-LIKE PEPTIDE-2

Glucagon-like peptide-2 (GLP-2) is a 33-amino acid hormone cosecreted by L-cells in the gut and the brain in response to food intake. Similarly to GLP-1, GLP-2 is cleaved from the larger proglucagon molecule. Contrary to other anorexic hormones secreted by L-cells, GLP-2 does not have a direct effect in food intake and satiety [4]. It does, however, play an important role in growth-promoting and cytoprotective effects in the GI tract by increasing crypt cell proliferation and increasing mucosal cell mass via inhibition of apoptosis [32]. Human studies looking at GLP-2 post-RYGB showed that postprandial GLP-2 plasma levels were increased in obese humans 1 month post-op and peaked at 6 months. This trophic effect may lead to increasing the number of cells producing GLP-1 and PYY and therefore contributes to long-term effect of weight loss post-bariatric surgery [26]. It is currently used as a therapeutic agent for the treatment of GI diseases involving malabsorption, inflammation, and/or mucosal damage [33].

GIP

GIP is a 42-amino acid peptide secreted from the intestinal K-cells located mainly in the duodenum and proximal jejunum in response to luminal nutrients especially lipids. GIP and GLP-1, both have a major role in glucose regulation via incretin effect, which stimulates insulin secretion in a glucose-dependent manner [34]. GIP also has a significant affect on fatty acid metabolism via activation of lipoprotein lipase, leading to lipogenesis and fat deposition [35]. GIP was found to have a direct link to obesity via subcutaneous adipose deposition. Human studies showed that GIP in combination with hyperinsulinemia and hyperglycemia leads to an increase in abdominal subcutaneous adipose tissue [36]. It has been suggested that GIP oversecretion with enhancement in receptor signaling may propagate the development of obesity, IR, and type 2 diabetes. This is supported by evidence from animal studies that looked at mice with a GIP receptor antagonist, which prevented diet-induced obesity and preserved insulin sensitivity when compared to high-fat-fed controls [37].

Given the location of the GIP-producing K-cells on the proximal part of the intestine and, it has been proposed that GIP levels decrease post-GBS since the K-cells are exposed to less nutrients, leading to less fat accumulation and long-term weight loss. However, there are contradicting study results, showing both a decrease and an increase or no change in GIP levels post-RYGB or duodenal–jejunal bypass surgery. Many of these discrepancies may be explained by differences in the surgical bypass limb length, time from the surgery, timing of test (fasting or postprandial), type of assay used, and changes in GIP receptor sensitivity [37].

CHOLECYSTOKININ

Cholecystokinin (CCK; pancreozymin) is a brain and gut peptide. In the gut, it is produced in I-cells of the small intestine, mainly in the duodenum. CCK is related to the release of pancreatic enzymes, contraction of the gallbladder, and inhibition of gastric emptying. In the brain, its role is unclear; however, CCK has been found to relate to food satiety in patients with bulimia nervosa, in whom it is decreased when compared to healthy controls. The hypothesis of its relation to satiety is that CCK inhibits gastric emptying and food intake; thus, in patients with bulimia nervosa its low levels contribute to impaired satiety, leading to binge behavior [38,39]. Study findings on CCK changes post-gastric bypass surgery have been inconclusive. A Swiss prospective, randomized 1-year trial of post-LRYGB and LSG found that CCK concentrations increased in both groups [40]. However, there are other studies that found no changes in fasting or postprandial CCK seen after RYGB or VBG, or JIB.

BILE ACIDS

Bile acids are important regulators of energy balance via activation of TGR5 and an increase in the resting energy expenditure [1]. Bile acids bind to TGR5, a plasma membrane–bound G protein receptor that is present in enteroendocrine cells, skeletal muscles, and brown adipose tissue, which leads to increase in GLP-1, improving insulin secretion and sensitivity [41]. Activation of the TGR5 receptor also mediates the conversion of T_4 to T_3 in the skeletal muscle and brown adipose tissue, which may facilitate weight loss by increasing resting energy expenditure [42]. In addition, bile acids can also increase insulin secretion through the activation of the farnesoid X receptor (FXR) in pancreatic β-cells. Activation of FXR triggers a cascade of controls in the fed-fasted state metabolism [43]. A small prospective study done by Kohli et al. [44] showed that plasma bile acid more than doubled after RYGB; however, it did not change or was found to be lower after LAGB. Another study by Steinert et al. [45] shows similar findings with lower basal concentrations of bile acid in obese patients in the presurgical period compared to healthy controls and an increase 1 year postsurgery. The exact mechanism of increased bile acids post-bariatric surgery is not well known, but it has been hypothesized that with malabsorptive procedures such as RYGB, there is an increase in the delivery of nutrients with bile to the distal intestine, leading to stimulation of L-cell secretion, with subsequent release of PYY, GLP-1, and OXM, hormones involved in satiety and decreased appetite [46].

LEPTIN

Leptin is a hormone secreted by adipocytes, which is involved in long-term energy balance by acting primarily in the hypothalamus to decrease food intake and increase energy expenditure [16]. Leptin is secreted in proportion to the amount of whole-body adipose tissue mass [47]. Leptin is a product of the obesity gene (*ob* gene), and it functions by binding to the leptin receptor [48]. Leptin increases with a decrease in body fat related to a reduction in food intake. However, leptin levels are increased in obese patients, suggesting that obesity is related to leptin resistance [49].

Several studies have demonstrated significantly lower fasting leptin concentrations in the post-RYGB patients compared to pre-RYGB, normal-weight, overweight, and obese subjects [16]. Leptin decreases after RYGB significantly correlate with changes in body mass index (BMI) and fat mass [2]. However, a study done by Beckman and colleagues [50] showed a decrease in leptin as soon as 2 weeks post-RYGB, before significant changes in absolute body weight were observed. There were similar findings in another study at 3 weeks post-RYGB [51]. The explanation for the fast changes prior to a significant change in the body weight is likely that a small percentage of leptin is also secreted by the stomach, which is significantly altered after RYGB, and this manipulation may cause the initial decrease, followed by even lower levels later due to a decrease in fat mass [52].

PANCREATIC POLYPEPTIDE

Pancreatic polypeptide (PP) is a gut hormone released from the pancreas in response to food intake. PP belongs to a family of peptides, NPY and PYY [53]. Plasma PP concentrations increase proportionally to caloric intake [54], and they are inversely proportional to adiposity, with high levels in anorexic subjects and reduced levels in obese subjects [55].

PP causes a negative energy balance by decreasing food intake and gastric emptying, and increasing energy expenditure via modification of feeding regulatory peptides and vagovagal activity [1].

PP is also found to reduce leptin in white adipose tissue. A small study looked at PP concentrations pre-RYGB and 6–9 months after surgery and found that PP levels pre-op and post-op were unchanged [56]. There were similar results in other small studies looking at PP levels post-gastric bypass, and most concluded that PP is not significantly altered by any of the bariatric procedures [1,57].

VAGAL NERVE

The GI tract is innervated by the autonomic nervous system, which includes a parasympathetic division (vagal and pelvic nerves) and a sympathetic division (splanchnic nerve). In addition to the autonomic nervous system, the GI track has its own enteric nervous system that is primarily involved in coordination of motility patterns and release of peptides from endocrine cells [58]. The enteric nervous system transmits information about mechanical, chemical, and neurohumoral stimuli to the CNS via the vagal and sympathetic nerves [55]. The vagus nerve plays a major role in regulating GI motility and secretion as well as hunger and satiety via nutrient signal and its afferent sensory nerve fibers. Vagal stimulation has been shown to reduce food intake and body weight in rats [59], while subdiaphragmatic vagotomy or abdominal afferent denervation completely blocks the inhibition of food intake following intestinal exposure to carbohydrates or fatty acids [60]. So it is believed that the vagus nerve and the neural connections between the intestine and the brain play an essential part in weight loss post-gastric bypass. During bariatric surgery, different surgical techiniques may affect the vagal innervation, leading to blockage of ghrelin—a peptide produced in the stomach that stimulates both feeding and growth hormone (GH) secretion [26,61]. There have been a few studies that investigated whether or not vagectomy might lead to additional weight loss; however, the results are varied. One study, which evaluated clinical outcomes of 40 patients with severe obesity post-laparoscopic RYGB with and without the preservation of the vagal nerve showed that there was no difference in postoperative weight loss, satiety, or plasma ghrelin between the two groups [62]. In contrast, a study done by Kral and colleagues [63] demonstrated that those patients who had truncal vagotomy with VBG compared to VBG alone had better weight loss at 1-year and at 5-years follow-up (51% of excess weight vs. 34% at 1 year and 61% vs. 28% at 5 years). The patients who had truncal vagotomy also reported less hunger and a decrease in frequency of band adjustment. In a small prospective study looking at the efficacy of laparoscopic truncal vagotomy alone in the treatment of severe obesity, preliminary results have shown subjects with variable excess weight loss; however, the intervention has generally been safe [64]. Other studies have related the change in weight post-GBS to vagal dysfunction, leading to transient fall of ghrelin and PP and increase in GLP-1 and PYY, suggesting that the hormones' action via the vagal pathway might mediate the weight loss [26,65].

GLUCOSE HOMEOSTASIS AND RESOLUTION OF T2DM

The improvement of T2DM post-bariatric surgery was initially thought to be due to weight loss and a decrease in fat mass; however, the improved insulin sensitivity was seen very early in the post-op phase, prior to patients losing any significant amount of weight. In addition, the degree of insulin sensitivity improvement post-RYGB exceeds that of an equivalent amount lost via diet and exercise [66]. Pories and colleagues [67] were the first to describe the antidiabetic effects of gastric bypass surgery in 1992. They showed that 82.9% of patients with T2DM were able to maintain normal levels of plasma glucose, glycosylated hemoglobin, and insulin at an average of 7.6 years post-op. This, in turn, has triggered several studies looking at hormonal changes related to gastric bypass surgery and the mechanism of diabetes remission.

The different types of bariatric procedures have different effects on insulin sensitivity and rate of T2DM remission. A meta-analysis of 136 studies done by Buchwald and colleagues [68] showed that the mean procedure resolution of T2DM was 48% for LAGB, 68% for VBG, 84% for RYGB, and 98% for BPD. Gastric banding and other purely restrictive procedures such as VBG seem to have less effect on T2DM resolution than procedures related to intestinal diversion (RYGB) where nutrients are directly delivered to the distal intestine and there are changes to the neuroendocrine connections of the gut [69]. The explanations for this weight-independent antidiabetic effect of RYGB are based on two theories: (1) The "hindgut" theory proposes that rapid delivery of nutrients to the distal bowel leads to increased secretion of incretins such as GLP-1, which causes improved glucose-dependent insulin secretion. (2) The "foregut" theory states that bypassing of the duodenum results in the exclusion from nutrient contact and subsequent release of a putative signal that is responsible for IR and/or abnormal glycemic control [69,70]. There is a growing number of studies that are investigating RYGB for treatment of diabetes in those with BMI < 35 kg/m². Lee and colleagues [71] reported the effect of gastric bypass for T2DM with BMI < 35 kg/m²—RYGB normalized hyperglycemia in 90% of those patients, with a mean HbA1c of 5.6% at 1 year [72]. Although much progress has been made in explaining the mechanism of diabetes resolution with bariatric surgery, many aspects regarding surgical treatment of T2DM are still questionable and unexplained, and further studies are warranted, especially in patients who are not obese.

CONCLUSION

As obesity becomes one of the most pressing and costly health problems of our generation, it is imperative to understand the role of the gut hormones and their association with hunger and satiety. Currently, bariatric surgery has been shown to be the only treatment of obesity to cause significant and long-lasting weight loss [73]. This, in turn, translates to improvement and resolution of comorbidities such as T2DM and hypertension hyperlipidemia, and improvement of mortality. In a large case–control study of nearly 16,000 patients followed for an average of 8 years, patients who were severely obese and had RYGB versus nonsurgical patients had reduced all-cause mortality by 40%, cardiovascular mortality by 56%, cancer mortality by 60%, and diabetes-related mortality by 92% [74].

Based on a strong body of evidence, it is clear that bariatric surgery leads to weight loss and glucose homeostasis not only via restrictive and malabsorptive mechanisms but also through anatomical rearrangement with rerouting of the intestine, changes in enteric nerve connections, and changes in gut hormones. Although some of the data had variable results, the majority of the studies showed that GLP-1, PYY, and OXM concentrations were higher and ghrelin levels were typically lower post-RYGB when compared to the concentrations of these hormones in individuals who were normal and overweight and those who lost weight by diet alone [16]. Other hormones such as CCK, PP, and leptin, in addition to bile acids, have also been shown to cause favorable changes post-bariatric surgery. Most of the hormone changes post-op can be attributed to the partial gastrectomy in combination with an increase in nutrient delivery to the distal intestine (Table 16.2). This, in turn, leads to stimulation of L-cells, resulting in synergistic action of GLP-1, PYY, and other L-cells products, combined with a decrease in GIP and ghrelin, the trophic role of GLP-2 (which causes a decrease in appetite), improved satiety, and consequently, weight loss [4]. In addition, modified neural signals from the enteric system and changes in the vagal nerve connectivity can influence hormone action on satiety. Bariatric surgery has the most striking effect on insulin sensitivity, often leading to resolution of T2DM. RYGB may become the treatment of choice not only for obese patients with T2DM but also for patients who are overweight. Even though much progress has been achieved in the understanding of gut hormones over the last 50 years since the first bariatric surgery was performed, more long-term studies are needed to fully comprehend their synchronized mechanisms and eventually develop less invasive treatments for obesity.

TABLE 16.2

Summary of Hormone Changes in Obesity and Post-Bariatric Surgery

Gut Hormones	Mechanism of Action	Changes in Obesity	Hormonal Changes Post-op[1]
Ghrelin	Appetite stimulant Secreted by cells in the stomach fundus, ↑ preprandial and ↓ w/ food intake ↑ gastric motility ↑ adipogenesis	↓ (Possible related to delay satiety)	↓ or no changes
GLP-1	Anoretic hormone Secreted by L-cells on distal gut ↑ glucose-stimulated insulin secretion from the β-cell [4,20] ↓ gastric emptying ↓ intestinal motility via the presence of nutrients in the distal gut → satiety	↓	↑ post-RYGB and SG No change post-LAGB
PYY	Anoretic hormone Cosecreted with GLP-1 by L-cells in the ileum and colon and brain by feedback mechanism via GLP-1 and PYY ↓ gastric emptying ↓ acid secretion [28]	↓	↑ post-RYGB and SG
OXM	Anoretic hormone Cosecreted with GLP-1 and PYY from the intestinal L-cells in response to food ingestion proportional to meal calorie content ↑ glucose-stimulated insulin secretion from the β-cell ↓ glucagon ↓ acid secretion and motility	↓	↑ post-RYGB and SG
CCK	Anoretic hormone Secreted by I-cells of the small intestine ↑ pancreatic enzymes, ↑contraction of gallbladder ↓ gastric emptying In the brain, may be related to food satiety	Questionable ↑ (↓ in BN → impaired satiety leading to binge behavior [38,39])	↑ or no changes post-RYGB, VBG, or JIB
PP	Anoretic hormone Released from the pancreas ↑ proportionally to caloric intake [54] and inversely proportional to adiposity ↓ food intake ↓ gastric emptying ↑ energy expenditure ↓ leptin in white adipose tissue	↓	No changes post-op
Bile acids	Binds to TGR5, a plasma membrane–bound G protein receptor, in enteroendocrine cells in skeletal muscles and brown adipose tissue ↑ GLP-1 ↑ insulin secretion and sensitivity [41] ↑ conversion of T_4 to T_3 in the skeletal muscle and brown adipose tissue ↑ resting energy expenditure [1] ↑ weight loss [42]	↓	↑↑ post-RYGB No changes post-LAGB

(continued)

TABLE 16.2 (Continued)

Summary of Hormone Changes in Obesity and Post-Bariatric Surgery

Gut Hormones	Mechanism of Action	Changes in Obesity	Hormonal Changes Post-op[1]
Leptin	Anoretic hormone	↑	↑ post-RYGB
	Secreted by adipocytes in proportion to the amount of whole-body adipose tissue mass [47], acts primarily in the hypothalamus	(Related to leptin resistance [48])	
	↓ food intake		
	↑ energy expenditure [16]		
	↓ body fat		
GIP	Secreted by the intestinal K-cells, mainly in the duodenum and proximal jejunum in response to luminal lipids	↑↑	↓ post-RYGB
	↑ insulin secretion in a glucose-dependent manner [34]		
	↑ lipoprotein lipase		
	↑ lipogenesis		
	↑ fat deposition [35]		

REFERENCES

1. Vincent RP, Le Roux CW. Changes in gut hormones after bariatric surgery. *Clin Endocrinol.* 2008;69(2): 173–179.
2. Korner J, Inabnet W, Conwell IM et al. Differential effects of gastric bypass and banding on circulating gut hormone and leptin levels. *Obesity (Silver Spring).* 2006;14(9):1553–1561.
3. Rehfeld JF. A centenary of gastrointestinal endocrinology. *Horm Metab Res.* 2004;36(11–12):735–741.
4. Ionut V, Burch M, Youdim A et al. Gastrointestinal hormones and bariatric surgery induced weight loss. *Obes Res J.* 2013;21(6):1093–1103.
5. Crookes PF. Surgical treatment of morbid obesity. *Annu Rev Med.* 2006;57:243–264.
6. Fact sheet. Metabolic & bariatric surgery. American Society for Metabolic and Bariatric surgery. Available at: http://s3.amazonaws.com/publicASMBS/MediaPressKit/MetabolicBariatricSurgeryOverviewJuly2011 .pdf. Updated on May 2011.
7. Sjostrom L, Narbro K, Sjostrom CD et al. Effects of bariatric surgery on mortality in Swedish obese subjects. *N Engl J Med.* 2007;357:741–752.
8. Lim RB, Blackburn G, Jones DB. Benchmarking best practices in weight loss surgery. *Curr Probl Surg.* 2010;47(2):79–174.
9. Blackburn GL, Hutter MM, Harvey AM et al. Expert panel on weight loss surgery: Executive report update. *Obesity (Silver Spring).* 2009;17(5):842–862.
10. Poirier P, Cornier MA, Mazzone T et al. Bariatric surgery and cardiovascular risk factors, A Scientific Statement from the American Heart Association. *Circulation.* 2011;123:1683–1701.
11. Melissas J, Koukouraki S, Askoxylakis J et al. Sleeve gastrectomy: A restrictive procedure? *Obes Surg.* 2007;17(1):57–62.
12. Zhao Y, Encinosa W. *Bariatric Surgery Utilization and Outcomes in 1998 and 2004: Statistical Brief #23. Healthcare Cost and Utilization Project (HCUP) Statistical Briefs [Internet].* Rockville (MD): Agency for Health Care Policy and Research (US), January 2006–2007.
13. Buchwald H, Oien DM. Metabolic/bariatric surgery worldwide 2008. *Obes Surg.* 2009;19:1605–1611.
14. Cummings D, Joost Overduin J, Foster-Schubert K. Gastric bypass for obesity: Mechanisms of weight loss and diabetes resolution. *J Clin Endocrinol Metab.* 2004;89(6):2608–2615.

15. Christou NV, Sampalis JS, Liberman M et al. Surgery decreases long-term mortality, morbidity, and health care use in morbidly obese patients. *Ann Surg*. 2004;240:416–423; discussion 423–424.

16. Beckman LM, Beckman TR, Earthman CP. Changes in gastrointestinal hormones and leptin after Roux-en-Y gastric bypass procedure: A review. *J Am Diet Assoc*. 2010;110(4):571–584.

17. Pujanek M, Bronisz A, Małecki P, Junik R. Pathomechanisms of the development of obesity in some endocrinopathies—An overview. *Endokrynol Pol*. 2013;64(2):150–155.

18. Tschop M, Weyer C, Tataranni PA et al. Circulating ghrelin levels are decreased in human obesity. *Diabetes*. 2001;50(4):707–709.

19. Cummings DE, Shannon MH. Ghrelin and gastric bypass: Is there a hormonal contribution to surgical weight loss? *J Clin Endocrinol Metab*. 2003;88(7):2999–3002.

20. Habib AM, Richards P, Cairns LS et al. Overlap of endocrine hormone expression in the mouse intestine revealed by transcriptional profiling and flow cytometry. *Endocrinology*. 2012;153(7):3054–3065.

21. Ranganath LR, Beety JM, Morgan LM et al. Attenuated GLP-1 secretion in obesity: Cause or consequence? *Gut*. 1996;38(6):916–919.

22. Lim GE, Huang GJ, Flora N et al. Insulin regulates glucagon-like peptide-1 secretion from the enteroendocrine L cell. *Endocrinology*. 2009;150:580–591.

23. Le Roux CW, Welbourn R, Werling M et al. Gut hormones as mediators of appetite and weight loss after Roux-en-Y gastric bypass. *Ann Surg*. 2007;246(5):780–785.

24. Scott WR, Batterham RL. Roux-en-Y gastric bypass and laparoscopic sleeve gastrectomy: Understanding weight loss and improvements in type 2 diabetes after bariatric surgery. *Am J Physiol Regul Integr Comp Physiol*. 2011;301(1):R15–27.

25. Morinigo R. Glucagon-like peptide-1, peptide YY, hunger, and satiety after gastric bypass surgery in morbidly obese subjects. *J Clin Endocrinol Metab*. 2006;91:1735–1740.

26. Ionut V, Bergman RN. Mechanisms responsible for excess weight loss after bariatric surgery. *J Diabetes Sci Technol*. 2011;5(5):1263–1282.

27. Ballantyne GH. Peptide YY(1-36) and peptide YY(3-36): Part I. Distribution, release and actions. *Obes Surg*. 2006;16(5):651–658.

28. Maljaars PW, Keszthelyi D, Masclee AA. An ileal brake-through? *Am J Clin Nutr*. 2010;92(3):467–468.

29. Morínigo R, Vidal J, Lacy AM et al. Circulating peptide YY, weight loss, and glucose homeostasis after gastric bypass surgery in morbidly obese subjects. *Ann Surg*. 2008;247(2):270–275.

30. Cohen MA, Ellis SM, Le Roux CW, Batterham RL. Oxyntomodulin suppresses appetite and reduces food intake in humans. *J Clin Endocrinol Metab*. 2003;88(10):4696–4701.

31. Wynne K, Park AJ, Small CJ, Meeran K, Ghatei MA, Frost GS, Bloom SR. Oxyntomodulin increases energy expenditure in addition to decreasing energy intake in overweight and obese humans: A randomised controlled trial. *Int J Obes (Lond)*. 2006;30(12):1729–1736.

32. Estall JL, Drucker DJ. Glucagon-like peptide-2. *Annu Rev Nutr*. 2006;26:391–411.

33. Le Roux CW, Borg C, Wallis K et al. Gut hypertrophy after gastric bypass is associated with increased glucagon-like peptide 2 and intestinal crypt cell proliferation. *Ann Surg*. 2010;252(1):50–56.

34. Edholm T, Degerblad M, Grybäck P. Differential incretin effects of GIP and GLP-1 on gastric emptying, appetite, and insulin-glucose homeostasis. *Neurogastroenterol Motil*. 2010;22(11):1191–1200.

35. McIntosh CH, Widenmaier S, Kim SJ. Glucose-dependent insulinotropic polypeptide (gastric inhibitory polypeptide; [GIP]). *Vitam Horm*. 2009;80:409–471.

36. Asmar M, Simonsen L, Madsbad S et al. Glucose-dependent insulinotropic polypeptide may enhance fatty acid re-esterification in subcutaneous abdominal adipose tissue in lean humans. *Diabetes*. 2010;59(9):2160–2163.

37. Kindel TL, Yoder SM, D'Alessio DA, Tso P. The effect of duodenal-jejunal bypass on glucose-dependent insulinotropic polypeptide secretion in Wistar rats. *Obes Surg*. 2010;20(6):768–775.

38. Gene ID: 885, CCK cholecystokinin (*Homo sapiens* [human]), updated on July 27, 2013.

39. Hannon-Engel S. Regulating satiety in bulimia nervosa: The role of cholecystokinin. *Perspect Psychiatr Care*. 2012;48(1):34–40.

40. Peterli R, Steinert RE, Woelnerhanssen B, Peters T et al. Metabolic and hormonal changes after laparoscopic Roux-en-Y gastric bypass and sleeve gastrectomy: A randomized, prospective trial. *Obes Surg*. 2012;22(5):740–748.

41. Chen X, Lou G, Meng Z, Huang W. TGR5: A novel target for weight maintenance and glucose metabolism. *Exp Diabetes Res*. 2011;2011:853501.

42. Pournaras DJ, Glicksman C, Vincent RP et al. The role of bile after Roux-en-Y gastric bypass in promoting weight loss and improving glycaemic control. *Endocrinology*. 2012;153(8):3613–3619.

43. Dufer M, Horth K, Wagner R et al. Bile acids acutely stimulate insulin secretion of mouse β-cells via farnesoid X receptor activation and K(ATP) channel inhibition. *Diabetes*. 2012;61:1479–1489.

44. Kohli R, Bradley D, Setchell K et al. Weight loss induced by Roux-en-Y gastric bypass but not laparoscopic adjustable gastric banding increases circulating bile acids. *JCEM*. 2013;98:E708–E712.

45. Steinert RE, Peterli R, Keller S et al. Bile acids and gut peptide secretion after bariatric surgery: A 1-year prospective randomized pilot trial. *Obesity*. 2013;21(12):E660–E668.

46. Katsuma S, Hirasawa A, Tsujimoto G. Bile acids promote glucagon-like peptide-1 secretion through TGR5 in a murine enteroendocrine cell line STC-1. *Biochem Biophys Res Commun*. 2005;329(1):386–390.

47. Friedman JM. Obesity in the new millennium. *Nature*. 2000;404:632–634.

48. Green ED, Maffei M, Braden VV et al. The human obese (OB) gene: RNA expression pattern and mapping on the physical, cytogenetic, and genetic maps of chromosome 7. *Genome Res*. 1995;5(1):5–12.

49. Meister B. Control of food intake via leptin receptors in the hypothalamus. *Vitam Horm*. 2000;59: 265–304.

50. Beckman LM, Beckman TR, Sibley SD, Earthman CP. Changes in gastrointestinal hormones and leptin after Roux-en-Y gastric bypass surgery. *JPEN J Parenter Enteral Nutr*. 2011;35:169–180.

51. Rubino F, Gagner M, Gentileschi P et al. The early effect of the Roux-en-Y gastric bypass on hormones involved in body weight regulation and glucose metabolism. *Ann Surg*. 2004;240:236–242.

52. Schubert ML. Gastric secretion. *Curr Opin Gastroenterol*. 2008;24:659–664.

53. Batterham RL, Le Roux CW, Cohen MA, Bloom SR. Pancreatic polypeptide reduces appetite and food intake in humans. *JCEM*. 2003;88:3989–3992.

54. Small CJ, Bloom SR. Gut hormones and the control of appetite. *Trends Endocrinol Metab*. 2004;15:259–263.

55. Mendieta-Zeron H, Lopez M, Dieguez C. Gastrointestinal peptides controlling body weight homeostasis. *Gen Comp Endocrinol*. 2008;155:481–495.

56. Meryn S, Stein D, Straus EW. Pancreatic polypeptide, pancreatic glucagon and enteroglucagon in morbid obesity and following gastric bypass operation. *Int J Obes*. 1986;10:37–42.

57. Le Roux CW, Aylwin SJ, Batterham RL et al. Gut hormone profiles following bariatric surgery favor an anorectic state, facilitate weight loss, and improve metabolic parameters. *Ann Surg*. 2006;243:108–114.

58. Naslund E, Hellstrom PM. Appetite signaling: From gut peptides and enteric nerves to brain. *Physiol Behav*. 2007;92:256–262.

59. Laskiewicz J, Krolczyk G, Zurowski G et al. Effects of vagal neuromodulation and vagotomy on control of food intake and body weight in rats. *J Physiol Pharmacol*. 2003;54:603–610.

60. Page A, Symonds E, Peiris M et al. Peripheral neural targets in obesity. *Br J Pharmacol*. 2012;166(5):1537–1558.

61. Date Y, Murakami N, Toshinai K et al. The role of the gastric afferent vagal nerve in ghrelin-induced feeding and growth hormone secretion in rats. *Gastroenterology*. 2002;123(4):1120–1128.

62. Perathoner A, Weiss H, Santner W et al. Vagal nerve dissection during pouch formation in laparoscopic Roux-Y-gastric bypass for technical simplification: Does it matter? *Obes Surg*. 2009;19(4):412–417.

63. Kral JG, Görtz L, Hermansson G, Wallin GS. Gastroplasty for obesity: Long-term weight loss improved by vagotomy. *World J Surg*. 1993;17(1):75–79.

64. Boss TJ, Peters J, Patti MG et al. *Laparoscopic Truncal Vagotomy for Weight-Loss: A Prospective, Dual-Center Safety and Efficacy Study*. Scientific Session of the Society of American Gastrointestinal and Endoscopic Surgeons (SAGES), Philadelphia, PA, April 9–12, 2008.

65. Sundbom M, Holdstock C, Engström BE, Karlsson FA. Early changes in ghrelin following Roux-en-Y gastric bypass: Influence of vagal nerve functionality? *Obes Surg*. 2007;17(3):304–310.

66. Thaler JP, Cummings DE. Minireview: Hormonal and metabolic mechanisms of diabetes remission after gastrointestinal surgery. *Endocrinology*. 2009;150(6):2518–2525.

67. Pories WJ, Swanson MS, MacDonald KG et al. Who would have thought it? An operation proves to be the most effective therapy for adult-onset diabetes mellitus. *Ann Surg*. 1995;222(3):339–350.

68. Buchwald H, Avidor Y, Braunwald E et al. Bariatric surgery: A systematic review and meta-analysis. *JAMA*. 2004;292:1724–1737.

69. Rubino F, Schauer PR, Kaplan LM, Cummings DE. Metabolic surgery to treat type 2 diabetes: Clinical outcomes and mechanisms of action. *Annu Rev Med*. 2010;61:393–411.

70. Cummings DE, Overduin J, Foster-Schubert KE. Gastric bypass for obesity: Mechanisms of weight loss and diabetes resolution. *JCEM*. 2004;89:2608–2615.

71. Lee WJ, Wang W, Lee YC et al. Effect of laparoscopic mini-gastric bypass for type 2 diabetes mellitus: Comparison of BMI > 35 and <35 kg/m². *J Gastrointest Surg.* 2008;12:945–952.
72. Spector D, Shikora S. Neuro-modulation and bariatric surgery for type 2 diabetes mellitus. *Int J Clin Pract Suppl.* 2010;166:53–58.
73. Sjostrom L, Lindroos AK, Peltonen M et al. Lifestyle, diabetes, and cardiovascular risk factors 10 years after bariatric surgery. *N Engl J Med.* 2004;351:2683–2693.
74. Adams TD, Gress RE, Smith SC et al. Long-term mortality after gastric bypass surgery. *N Engl J Med.* 2007;357:753–761.

17 Metabolic Monitoring of the Bariatric Surgery Patient

L.E. Sasha Stiles

CONTENTS

PROLOGUE

This chapter is designed as a primer for when to recommend weight loss surgery and how to care for metabolic surgery patients before and after surgery. The optimal evaluation of a metabolic surgery patient should result in a well-informed patient who is optimally prepared for his/her procedure and is committed to the necessary postoperative monitoring. The decision-making process for weight loss and metabolic surgery is explored. The components of immediate and long-term postoperative follow-up to prevent the avoidable metabolic complications of surgery are also reviewed. Finally, there is information on weight loss failure, weight regain after surgery, and the relationships between successful surgery and successful pregnancy.

PREOPERATIVE EVALUATION

How do we, patient and physician alike, decide that it is time for surgery? What tools do we use? How do we assess readiness, safety, and compelling need for surgery? When do we sway the hesitant patient that timely surgery is their best option? When would surgery be inappropriate or at least untimely? What type of surgery do we recommend for the patients?

As with any specialized medical endeavor, the metabolic evaluation requires certain specific tools and concepts that will be applied to the patient evaluation. Discussion on the bariatric evaluation begins by describing some of the structural components necessary to assist in answering these questions.

MEASUREMENTS

In general, the preoperative evaluation of a bariatric surgery patient begins with the body mass index (BMI). This measurement has been the recognized standard for determining the need for weight loss surgery. Unfortunately, it has also been used by the insurance industry to disallow candidates who do not meet criteria by this measurement. At the May 2013 National Institutes of Health (NIH) Conference on the Long-Term Outcomes of Bariatric Surgery, there was much discussion that focusing only on BMI is misguided. In a recent Swedish Obesity Study [1] and in current discussions with the author at NIH, it is clear that the true benefits of weight loss surgery are related far more to comorbidity than weight loss alone.

However, BMI has been utilized for decades and remains a gold standard for communication between patients and providers [2]. BMI is defined as one's weight in kilograms divided by height in meters squared. A complete description of this measure appears elsewhere. It is important for the metabolic physician to know the ranges for BMI in terms of the weight category. The following list can apply for all cultures except Asians [3]:

BMI < 18.5 = underweight
BMI 18.5–24.9 = normal weight
BMI 25–29.9 = overweight
BMI 30–34.9 = obesity I
BMI 35–39.5 = obesity II
BMI 40+ = obesity III

For reasons that are explained elsewhere, the burden of obesity is greater in Asian populations at a lower BMI, where obesity begins at BMI 23, obesity II at BMI 25, and obesity III at a BMI of 30 [4].

Another important derived parameter is the *ideal body weight* (IBW). This calculation began as a standard in the Metropolitan Life Insurance tables approximately 50 years ago. The tables present ranges of weight for height based on healthy young working men and women of the time [5]. Even though these tables are not directly applicable in today's society, they provide us with a concept of a gender-specific, stature-based weight, which assumes a normal percentage of body fat. The studies that produced the data showed that lean body mass (LBM) variations between individuals of the same gender and stature were relatively minor. Therefore, most of the difference in individual body weight was due to excess body fat.

The concept of *excess body weight* (EBW) delineates this weight difference from the IBW. EBW is calculated simply as the difference between IBW and actual body weight. Many bariatric surgery programs record post-op success based on the percentage of EBW loss (%EBWL).

In addition to height, weight, BMI, and EBW, a patient considering bariatric surgery should appreciate several anthropometric body measurements, including waist circumference (WC), neck circumference (NC), and body fat. *WC* is a sound and reproducible measurement that affords us some insight into the extent of central obesity. This should be measured at the interval between the top of the iliac crest laterally and the bottom of the lowest rib laterally, which is about 1–2 in. no matter ones' height. Another acceptable option is to measure at the umbilicus. The measurement should be taken at the end of a gentle (not forced) exhalation with a snug (but not tight) tape measure horizontally.

It is also useful to obtain a baseline measurement of the *NC*. NC can provide insight to the upper body fat distribution. It can also correlate with the risk of obstructive sleep apnea (OSA). OSA is generally considered if the neck circumference is >17 for men and >16 for women. NC is measured midway in the neck, just below the laryngeal prominence (Adam's apple).

Body fat measurement should be performed to establish a baseline of the quantity of EBW as adipose tissue. It can be obtained by the use of simple devices such as skin fold calipers, taken at standard regions on the body (triceps, biceps, shoulder blade, waist, hip, mid-thigh, etc.). A number of more technical approaches also exist. Bioelectrical impedance analysis (BIA) is performed as a bipolar (two limbs) or tetrapolar (four limbs) technique. The latter is considered more accurate and has the advantage of yielding some regional information on fat distribution. DEXA scanning is currently considered the most accurate means of obtaining body fat percentage but requires a small amount of radiation exposure at a significant additional cost.

In the discussion of a weight loss process, it is useful to provide objective information regarding the caloric intake and energy output. The American diet affords an extraordinary ability to intake large amounts of excess calories, often without the patient's awareness. Therefore, food logs are frequently found to be fraught with reporting inaccuracies. However, the use of apps for handheld devices that allow the patient to record their intake in real time is encouraging. Still, it remains to be seen if such methods will improve the accuracy of diet self-reporting.

Objective data on the resting energy expenditure (REE) or resting metabolic rate (RMR) can be obtained by *estimates of energy expenditure* such as the Harris–Benedict equation. REE/RMR is a component of the daily total energy expenditure (TEE). In general, REE represents approximately 75% of TEE. The remaining 25% is composed of the thermic effect of food (TEF) or specific dynamic action (SDA) and active energy expenditure (AEE). The TEF/SDA comprises approximately 5% and the AEE 20% of TEE. AEE is further composed of spontaneous physical activity (SPA) and nonexercise activity thermogenesis (NEAT). The latter includes activities such as sitting, fidgeting, and posture maintenance.

The REE/RMR can be measured by a technique known as *indirect calorimetry* (IC). IC is based on the knowledge that energy expenditure is closely related to oxygen consumption. Therefore, REE/RMR can be measured by measuring oxygen consumption in a patient at rest. There are a number of devices available to obtain the measurement. Our clinic utilizes an inexpensive handheld indirect calorimeter [7].

RMR is unique to each person and is affected by a number of factors as age, weight, body composition, medications, gender, hormones, and caffeine substances, to name a few. Assessing RMR (and thus caloric needs) is recommended to achieve a specific weight loss on all patients preferably early in their weight management career. Repeat assessments during times of weight gain or weight plateau are extremely helpful in defining the etiology of these roadblocks.

AEE can be estimated by several methods. Simple devices such as pedometers capture the number of strides taken. More complex digital accelerometers are now widely available.

The use of *metabolic equivalents* (MET) represents an easy tool for estimating calories expended during activity [6]. A MET is defined as the ratio of a metabolic rate (and therefore a rate of energy consumption) during a specific physical activity to a reference rate of the metabolic rate at rest.

Examples of MET Tables

0.9 ME = sleeping

1.0 ME = at rest

2.0 ME = walking or strolling at 2 mph

3.0 ME = bowling, golfing, slow dancing

4.0 ME = dancing fast, biking < 10 mph, climbing stairs

5.0 ME = brisk walking 4 mph, slow jogging

6.0 ME = hiking, brisk doubles tennis, biking > 10 mph

7.0 ME = usual weight loss surgery energy expenditure

8.0 ME = biking or running 7.5 mph

10.0 ME = 6-min mile running

11.0 ME = swimming butterfly

In order to calculate calories burned during exercise,

EX 1: to burn 150 calories sleeping, it takes 150 min at 1 met to burn 150 calories

EX 2: to burn 150 calories slow walking (2 met) = 2 mph = 150/2 met = 75 min slow walking to burn 150 calories

EX 3: to burn 150 calories brisk walking (5 met) = 4 mph = 150/5 = 30 min brisk walking to burn 150 calories

BARIATRIC HISTORY AND PHYSICAL [8–10]

Obesity HPI

It is often valuable to ask patients what they think has contributed to their weight gain. Some have good insight. They may report a change in jobs, a move from the city to the suburb, and a decrease in activity and exercise. Many recall a stressful period in their lives when food was used as a source of comfort. Some relate the weight gain to the use of specific medications such as antidepressants and psychotropics. Others simply do not know. Either way, many patients are completely overwhelmed by their condition and are confused by their failures to reverse it.

The metabolic physician has an opportunity to provide insight for the patient regarding the cause of his or her weight gain and the difficulty in managing its treatment. A scientific, stepwise approach should be used to evaluate and eliminate all possible causes (see Chapters 2 and 10). Scientific advancements have elucidated the complex changes of the weight-reduced state (see Chapter 11). Patients may benefit from recognition of these approaches so that they can gain clarity into their own condition.

The patient's weight milestones can add an understanding on the disease progression. Examples of these include weight after high school, weight at marriage, and pregnancy-related weight gain. Ask when the weight gain occurred and its trajectory. It is valuable to obtain the patient's prior weight set points. What were the stable weights in the patient's life? Was one of these weights an optimal weight for the patient? Can this weight act as a goal?

It is important for the metabolic physician and patient to agree on the goal weight for the bariatric process. The goal must be achievable and sustainable. In our clinic, the adjusted body weight (ABW) is used as a general target. The ABW is frequently considered the goal weight after bariatric surgery. It is calculated by utilizing the maximum body weight and the IBW. Subtracting the IBW from the maximum body weight yields the EBW. The ABW assumes that a percentage (25%) of the total EBW is not fat. Therefore, the formula for ABW is IBW + EBW/4.

The obesity history should include an objective evaluation of the patient's dietary intake. This should encompass both meal time (nutritive) eating and snacking (nonnutritive) food consumption.

The meal time dietary intake can be categorized into such groups as standard American diet, calorie counting, low fat, low carbohydrate, etc. Often the patient reports following any specific diet, which is labeled as uncontrolled. The percentage of the patient's meals outside of the home should be recorded. In particular, the frequency of fast food restaurant consumption should be noted.

In addition to the macronutrient components of the meals, eating patterns should be assessed. For example, does the patient choose large portions? Do they have second and third helpings? Do they drink sufficient amounts of water with their meals? Do they eat quickly? Do they eat past the point of fullness?

In the category of nonnutritive eating, patterns of snacking as well as emotional eating are included. Snacking is not initiated because of hunger. It does not conform to a structure of portion size or time constraints. Therefore, the quantity of calories consumed during snacking may be excessive. Similarly, emotional eating generally does not occur in the context of a meal and permits excessive caloric intake with limited control. It is important to identify the triggers that initiate patterns of emotional eating so that the patient can explore alternative coping mechanisms.

OTHER OBESITY HISTORICAL COMPONENTS

Be certain to review the *allergies* and *medications*. Ask the patient to bring in the meds they are taking, many of which may contribute to their weight gain. Document the *family history*, particularly for diabetes, all cardiovascular diseases, central obesity, cancer, depression, and lipid disorders. The family history may predict the possibility of metabolic syndrome for the patients as well as their offspring.

Document the *social history*, including employment, disability, alcohol, drugs, and smoking histories. Consider who lives in the patient's home. Review the patient's pattern of *exercise*. What is the patient physically able to do? What might they like? Are there issues with shortness of breath, pain in weight-bearing joints, cardiac limitations, and most importantly time management limitations? I have found that time management (putting everyone else first, having two or three jobs) is often the hardest hurdle to overcome for many of my patients [11,12].

Take a complete *surgical history*. Note any abdominal surgeries: gall bladder, appendicitis, abdominal hernia, weight-loss surgeries, and others. Detail any female surgery: cesarian sections, tubal ligations, ovarian surgeries, hysterectomy, and others. Be certain to review the previous *hospitalizations* for often this will turn up new history of old problems that are still relevant.

The *review of systems* (ROS) must be detailed. The history of many of the patients is voluminous, and doing a careful review of systems often turns up important information. In the cardiovascular ROS, ask about deep vein thrombosis (DVT), pulmonary embolism, Greenfield filter placement, use of blood thinners, heart attacks, hypertension, undiagnosed chest pain, angina, congestive heart failure, arrhythmias/palpitations, cardiac-related syncope, pulmonary artery hypertension, or other cardiac symptoms or conditions [13–15,16]. Note the results of cardiac studies especially stress tests, echocardiograms (with mention of ejection fraction), and lower extremity Dopplers, lung spiral CT, or other lung scans [16,17]. A history of significant edema and right heart failure usually suggests longstanding poorly controlled sleep apnea.

In the dermatologic ROS, it is important to recognize the presence of cellulitis, lymphedema, psoriasis, and easy bruising, among others. The ROS for endocrinology should include detail on diabetes, prediabetes, gestational diabetes, Cushing's, and other endocrinopathies [18]. To the list of etiologies for confusing overnight glucose elevations, add the stress of poor sleep quality afforded by insufficiently treated sleep apnea.

For the GI ROS, consider gall bladder issues, ulcerative colitis/Crohn's, diarrhea, nausea or vomiting, gastro-esophageal reflux disease (GERD), hiatal hernia, ulcers, *Helicobacter pylori*, endoscopy, hepatitis, diverticulosis, diverticulitis, fatty liver, cirrhosis, bowel obstruction, and colonoscopy [19].

In the ROS for heme/vascular/lymphatic, review anemias, iron deficiency, thalassemia trait, hemochromatosis, blood transfusions, venous insufficiency, clotting disorders, etc. In females, note the number of pregnancies and consequences. Ask about polycystic ovary syndrome (PCOS), irregular menses, heavy menses, hysterectomy, tubal ligation, birth control, and menopause. Review the latest cancer screens.

For the musculoskeletal ROS, focus on issues regarding the weight-bearing joints. However, upper body issues, such as carpal tunnel, can also be important. Note all issues of back pain, knee pain, foot pain, ankle pain, hip pain, and gout, with attention to the specifics of each [20,21]. Observe thigh girth and wide-based gaits, which contribute to lower extremity instability and injury.

In the pulmonary ROS, note any history of asthma, chronic obstructive pulmonary disease (COPD), sleep apnea, snoring, restless sleep, smoking history, pulmonary function tests, resting oxygen saturation, and peak flow [22,23]. For the neurology ROS, review the history of sciatica, disk disease with neurological compromise, seizures, fibromyalgia, multiple sclerosis, cerebrovascular accident (CVA), transient ischemic attack (TIA), neuropathy, pseudotumor cerebri, vertigo, syncope, unsteady balance, or gait.

In reviewing the urological/renal ROS, note any history of pyelonephritis, urinary frequency, kidney stones, renal insufficiency, incontinence, and prostatitis. Review the patient's history of inflammatory processes such as rheumatoid arthritis, SLE, and other autoimmune disorders [24].

The psychological ROS is of particular importance for a potential bariatric surgery patient. The patient should have undergone a thorough psychologist consultation, which should alert you to unstable DSMIII–IV diagnoses. Pay special attention to eating disorders including bulimia, recent suicide attempts, recent severe depression, and unstable bipolar and schizophrenic patients. Furthermore, since absorption of medications may vary with surgery, a patient on multiple psychiatric meds is at risk of destabilization after surgery [25,26].

OBESITY PHYSICAL EXAM

Vitals: Take the blood pressure with the patient seated. Measure the pulse rate and rhythm, and note any irregularity. Record the respiratory rate temperature. Measure the height, weight, waist, and neck circumference. Calculate the BMI.

HEENT: Note whether the head is normocephalic and atraumatic. Check the eyes for pupillary responses and scleral pigmentation. Check for oropharyngeal lesions. Look for moon facies, rounding with plethora (Cushing's), smooth tongue (low B vitamins), puffy nonpitting eyelids (low thyroid), and stained teeth (bulimia).

Skin: Examine the patient for the presence of acanthosis, hirsutism (Cushing's, PCOS), jaundice, coarse and dry hair, hair thinning (low thyroid), and skin thinning (Cushing's).

Neck: Note if there are any masses. Check for carotid bruits.

Chest: Note dorsocervical hump (Cushing's) and supraclavicular fat pad.

Lungs: Listen and report if clear, wheezes, rales, rhonchi, or diminished breath sounds.

COR: Note if regular or irregular, murmur, split S2 first intercostal space (cor Pulm), S3.

Abdomen: Describe central obesity, liver firmness, significant scars, hernias (inguinal, umbilical, ventral, or incisional), inguinal lymph nodes, and description of pannes.

Extremities: Note varicosities, nonhealing ulcers, taut, pitting edema, lymphedema, palpitation of digits for gout, bunion, ulcer, and other deformities.

Neuromuscular: Note if cranial nerves II–XII are intact. Note gait, balance, resting tremor (Parkinson's), intention tremor (cerebellar, multiple sclerosis), static tremor (hyperthyroid or benign essential tremor), proximal muscle weakness (Cushing's), any difficulty going from sitting to standing, and heel toe walk.

Psychological evaluation: Consider judgment and insight, orientation to time–place–person, mood and affect, memory and concentration, and significant eating issues.

Your initial *assessment* takes into consideration an extraordinary data collection, comorbidity evaluation, and treatments that can ensure safe elective surgery.

PREOPERATIVE TESTING

The history and physical as outlined above may provide clues for conditions that require preoperative evaluation. In addition, a number of studies are ordered routinely in preparation for bariatric surgery. In addition to the standard CXR, EKG, and lab tests, a full preoperative bariatric assessment should include tests that assess not only the risk for surgery but the postoperative weight loss process as well.

ADDITIONAL LAB TESTS TO CONSIDER PREOPERATIVELY

Nicotine levels: A value > 2 ng indicates continued tobacco use, which may complicate postoperative recovery. Smoking cessation can be verified after 2 months by obtaining a urine cotinine.

Pregnancy testing: It is imperative that bariatric surgery not take place if the patient is pregnant.

Glucose control: A HbA1C of less than 8 is encouraged.

Liver functions testing: Liver enzyme elevations should be investigated for the possibility of hepatitis, fatty liver, and cirrhosis. Ultrasound and other imaging studies may be necessary.

Uric acid: Gout and hyperuricemia are common in the obese and can be exacerbated during periods of dehydration or extreme weight loss.

Pre-albumin: This is a good indicator of the patient's general nutritional status meeting to surgery. Consider postponing surgery if the level is <20.

Iron studies: Since iron deficiency is a common problem after bariatric surgery, the preoperative evaluation provides an opportunity to correct preexisting deficiency. On the other hand, a high ferritin level may be seen in liver disease. A ferritin level > 500 should be investigated for the presence of hemochromatosis. A ferritin level < 20 should be explored. Women with heavy variable menstrual patterns are at risk of profound anemia after surgery and deserve extra counseling and treatment preoperatively.

Vitamin D: Vitamin D deficiency is very common. It is believed that it would be beneficial to normalize vitamin D status prior to surgery. The preoperative goal is a D25OH level of 30 or higher.

ADDITIONAL STUDIES TO CONSIDER PREOPERATIVELY

GI: An upper endoscopy is advisable before any bariatric procedure. This is useful to exclude GERD and peptic ulcer disease and to rule out esophageal and gastric abnormalities that may be difficult to treat after surgery. *H. pylori* testing is usually recommended.

Pulmonary: Pulmonary function tests (PFTs) with an arterial blood gas (ABG) is ordered for all patients with a BMI > 60, OSA, or a history of asthma. *Sleep studies* are recommended for patients with an enlarged neck circumference, habitual snoring, restless sleep, and daytime sleepiness. For those patients already on continuous positive airway pressure (CPAP), an assessment of *CPAP Compliance* is important. Many insurance carriers now require documented efficacy before allowing a patient to keep a CPAP machine. It is recommended that patients demonstrate compliance with CPAP for 70% over at least 4 h.

Cardiac: Patients with an abnormal EKG or a history of heart disease should be referred to a cardiologist for stress testing and echocardiogram prior to surgery. Our institution recommends one of several stress test modalities, which access echo wall motion on most patients with significant comorbidities and an exercise-induced ischemic EKG analysis on all patients.

Vascular: Venous Dopplers are generally obtained before surgery. Preoperative inferior vena cava (IVC) filters are recommended for patients with a BMI > 50.

PREOPERATIVE NUTRITION

Preoperative nutrition is not different from nutrition for the breadth of the American population, only perhaps more critical. Promote lean protein sources, whole grains, fruits and vegetables, and low fat dairy. If you can help patients change eating habits preoperatively, then these habits may hopefully remain long after surgery: Eat slowly, take 20 min for meals, sit down while eating, learn not to eat and drink at the same time, practice chewing 20 times, encourage snacks made of a combination of protein and fruit or vegetables, and, by meal planning, eliminate the common tendency for mindless snacking.

The difficulty is that people do just about anything to prove to you preoperatively that they are ready for surgery. The importance of a strong preoperative program is to create a rigorous preoperative review and create a strong physician–patient relationship that will continue years after surgery, for it is often much later in a patient's postoperative course that he or she stops exercising, stops his or her vitamins, and reverts to mindless eating. Everything you do up front should be done to foster a healthy long-term relationship.

The patient is generally asked to provide food logs at each preoperative visit, which are evidence of compliance with pre-op nutrition. Food logging skills hopefully mentor a postoperative habit for long-term success. Weight stabilization, weight loss, and A1C improvements can all help further assess nutritional compliance.

In the past, great attention was given to preoperative weight loss as a must for surgery [27]. It was seen initially as a way to evaluate motivation. But many also saw it as a way to block needy patients from surgery. Since then, it has been verified that by putting patients on a very low calorie diet (VLCD) ("liver shrinking") diet for 1–4 weeks before surgery, patients achieved a decrease in visceral fat and thus a safer surgery [28]. Weight gain stabilization has remained a key "hope" in the preoperative period. But the recognition of many metabolic processes involving gut hormones has shed new light on this population's ability to lose weight preoperatively. Limited mobility in this population also increases the difficulty in losing weight. Also, strenuous exercise preoperatively can further deteriorate the spine and weight-bearing joints. Unfortunately, the capacity to provide frequent, safe, and effective exercise for this population is beyond the financial means for most patients and programs alike.

An initial functional assessment by physical therapists is key to assessing exercise potentials and limitations. Exercise logs should be collected at each preoperative visit as evidence of compliance with exercise. Improvements in safely monitored 6-min walk tests provide information on compliance and cardiopulmonary fitness for surgery.

Preoperative vitamin supplementation is recommended for patients preparing for bariatric surgery, even if there is no evidence of preexisting deficiency. This includes multivitamins (2/day), calcium citrate 500 mg TID, vitamin D3 2000 IU/day, iron (30 µg elemental Fe), and B12 1000 µg/day.

MATCHING THE PATIENT TO THE BARIATRIC SURGERY TYPE

In this discussion, the scope will be limited to the three major existing procedures: gastric band, sleeve gastrectomy, and gastric bypass. These procedures are performed at our medical center, and our surgeons have good outcomes on each. To a certain extent, any of the procedures will produce the desired outcome: effective and sustained weight loss. However, some of the unique differences make one procedure better than the others for specific subsets of patients.

For example, each of the three has differing effects on the amount of weight loss, food intake control, energy expenditure, VAT reduction, microbiota alteration, glucose metabolism, and enteroendocrine stimulation. A detailed discussion on this topic is available elsewhere in this volume.

In general, patients who have a greater amount of weight to lose should select a more aggressive procedure. Patients are usually counseled to expect a 50% EBWL with the band, 60% from the sleeve, and 70% from the bypass. Similarly, the amount of visceral adipose tissue lost is less with the band than with the sleeve or the bypass. Suppression of food intake can occur with all procedures but seems to be more pronounced with the bypass, than with the sleeve or band.

Since the band does not appear to have effects on gut hormone production, it is less powerful than either the sleeve or the bypass in resolving diabetes. Nonetheless, there are good data on diabetes resolution after gastric banding in patients who have had diabetes for less than 2 years. Therefore, this option can be recommended for newly diagnosed diabetics. Patients who have had long-standing diabetes, particularly those who are on insulin, are strongly recommended to consider either a sleeve or bypass.

IMMEDIATE POSTOPERATIVE HOSPITAL FOLLOW-UP

There are three major reasons why a metabolic physician should make a post-op in-hospital visit. First, there is no better time to cement a strong postoperative relationship with your patient and their family. Next, the metabolic physician is usually the practitioner best suited to discuss postoperative medications. Third, if complications arise, the metabolic physician serves as a knowledgeable member of the medical team in assisting with resolution of the issues.

Because of the restrictions on pill size and absorption, many of the routine medications taken for hypertension, diabetes, gout, and lipids must be changed postoperatively. For example, *diuretics* are generally discontinued after bariatric surgery due to concerns of dehydration. Other *hypertension* medications must be lowered after bariatric surgery to prevent hypotension. In our experience, topical clonidine may provide a practical solution for bridging the patient over until he or she can resume his or her regular medications.

Allopurinol is discouraged directly after surgery as dehydration from the surgery can cause stone precipitation. *Colchicine* is recommended if the uric acid is >7.5 and/or symptoms of gout occur. Because of this, it is generally not recommended to proceed with weight loss surgery if the uric acid is >7.0.

In the category of diabetes management, many patients experience early type 2 diabetes resolution after bariatric surgery, even before discharge. This is particularly true if the patient is not requiring insulin. Certainly, *sulfonylureas* and *metformin* should be avoided due to the risk of complications from this therapy. Patients who continue to experience hyperglycemia (glucose over 150 mg/dL) may require some form of glucose controlling therapy upon discharge. Extensive use of DPP-IV inhibitors has been made for this situation. But some patients will require sliding scale coverage with *regular insulin*.

Even in this circumstance, it is frequently observed that the patient's diabetes does come under good control after several more weeks. Therefore, patients who are being discharged on hypoglycemic therapy after bariatric surgery are always instructed to contact us immediately if their blood sugar remains consistently below 125 mg/dL.

Lipid medications are generally not restarted until 1 month after surgery due to concerns re liver enzyme elevations during periods of possible ketosis and significant weight loss, as well as potential for nausea. Often, it is found that there is sufficient improvement in the lipid profile after 1 month that they can be discontinued completely. However, lipid levels are continuously evaluated, as they often revert to the presurgical baseline in susceptible patients 1 to 2 years after surgery.

Vitamin and nutrition education for the postoperative period is usually covered by the hospital dietitians. That said, be ready to discuss anything along these lines that comes up in your hospital visit. Arrange for a first office-based postoperative visit. Usually, this is coordinated with visits to the surgeon, bariatric dietitian, and psychologist.

In addition to modifying the patient's existing medications, it is generally recommended that patients are discharged on a proton pump inhibitor. It is also preferred to give the patient a prescription for an easily absorbed antiemetic to prevent severe vomiting. Patients who are at risk for thromboembolism (i.e., those with a personal or family history of DVT as well as patients with a BMI > 50) are given low-dose anticoagulation per 5 days postoperatively.

Finally, there are a few things you might emergently encounter during your hospital visit, which should alert you to serious GI, pulmonary, cardiac, renal, and vascular complications. Hypoxia or CO_2 retention, shortness of breath, significant hypertension, heart rate > 120, or any fever > 101 should alert you to a potential leak or wound infection. Decreased urine output or increased BUN/CR may be a sign of myocardial infarction (MI); however, this could also be a fluid issue or bleeding. Therefore, it is important for the metabolic physician to play the role of an astute hospitalist in caring for the bariatric patient.

POST-OP OUTPATIENT METABOLIC MONITORING

The stronger your relationship to the surgical program, the greater your ability to assist your patient's weight loss. The metabolic physician is often the first one the patient turns to with the daily concerns related to dehydration, pain, nausea, and vomiting. An early postoperative clinic visit is recommended to assess the following:

1. Weakness and fever, which could signify a surgical leak.
2. Tachycardia > 120, which could indicate a surgical leak or a pulmonary embolism. This can also be a sign of dehydration, along with dry mucus membranes and general fatigue. Always stress how the new diet is a full-time job. Suggest drinking a 5-mL pill cup of water every 5–10 min, or even set an alarm every 10 min to remind them to drink.
3. Check for calf tenderness as a harbinger for DVT.
4. Stress active mobility to prevent DVT and atelectasis. Patients who are inactive during the postoperative period are far more likely to develop a DVT or PE. On the other hand, it is important that the patient not overexert themselves during the first month after surgery. This is particularly true with regard to weight lifting, which may compromise their surgical incision integrity.
5. Medications need to be reviewed. Nothing bigger than a tic-tac® should be swallowed. Most meds can be crushed or spansules can be used. All extended release meds need to be changed to immediate release. The timing of medications, especially if there is significant post-op nausea, can be a challenge for weeks to months after surgery.
6. Renewed ankle swelling can occur, and diuretics carefully added back at a lower dose.
7. Blood pressure can be quite variable as you reintroduce or eliminate medications.
8. Review glucometer readings and food logs. Usually you will be rapidly decreasing any diabetic medications.
9. Anticoagulants, such as Coumadin, need special attention due to the composition of the postoperative diet.
10. There are many dietary changes. The bariatric dietitians are very capable of reviewing these with your patient should you have concern. Each surgical program has slightly different thoughts about protein drinks. Refer to other sections in this book for specifics. That said, make sure your patients are not eating too much or too fast, or alternatively not eating at all because they are not hungry.
11. Listen to the chest and make sure they are using their incentive spirometers.
12. Examine the wound. Slight oozing around the incision of a serosanguinous nature is normal. At times, the drainage can be copious as deep surgical fluids migrate to the lower abdominal wall. Hematomas are common. The extravasated heme migrates downward and outward with gravity, causing patient concerns. Reassure your patients, but be sure you assess for cellulitis.
13. Bleeding: Early bright red blood orally or per rectum can be normal due to an especially high number of staples from an uncomplicated surgery. Painless melena several days later can represent the same. Bleeding from marginal ulcers tends to occur much later and

is accompanied by significant pain. Be alert to when any drains have bright red blood accompanied by orthostatic vital signs, low urine output or vomiting blood, or systolic blood pressure < 100 or tachycardia > 120.

14. Celebrate with your patient! Become enthusiastic and curious about exercise goals and family reactions.

Postoperative Lab Review [29]

An important component of the postoperative metabolic physician visit is the review of routine bariatric laboratory data. Such testing is generally performed every 6 months within the first 2 years of the operation and annually thereafter. The laboratory analysis is quite extensive and generally includes a complete blood count (CBC), complete metabolic profile (CMP), serum phosphate, magnesium, international normalized ratio (INR), lipid profile, thyroid stimulating hormone (TSH), parathyroid hormone (PTH), and urinalysis. A vitamin panel should be obtained, including: vitamins A, D, K, E, B1, B6, B9 (folate), B12, and C. Iron studies, as well as zinc and copper levels, should be monitored.

As the patient progresses through postoperative period, it will be the metabolic physician seeing them for routine care. Knowing everything you can about the timing of and the meaning of these labs is critical. Margaret Furtado, who contributed to the American Society for Metabolic and Bariatric Surgery (ASMBS) nutritional guidelines, recently gave this author an enlightening list of metabolic monitoring pearls that I now pass on to you [28]:

1. Difficulty seeing at night might be the night blindness of vitamin A deficiency.
2. Numbness or tingling in hands or feet could be B1, B6, or B12 neuropathy.
3. Ask if your patient has burning in their feet, later progressing to their calves and knees. Thiamine deficiency can progress rapidly in just over an hour. Wernicke's encephalopathy is seen most commonly with post-op vomiting, but also can occur with poor preoperative nutrition and lack of vitamin intake postoperatively.
4. Has your patient become forgetful lately? Low B12 or B1 or hypoglycemia can cause this.
5. Is your patient experiencing brain fog or lethargy? This could be related to too little carbohydrate intake. Patients should be on at least 70 g of carbohydrates by 3 months and 100 g by 6 months post-op.
6. If their carbohydrates are too low, they may be too weak to exercise and thus promote metabolic bone disease.
7. Your patient may complain of foaming or a white discharge from their mouth after eating. This is a symptom of sialorrhea (commonly known to our surgical patients as sliming). You need to differentiate between "sliming" vs. true vomiting. Sliming occurs when one tends to eat rapidly and repeatedly gulp food too quickly. Eating slowly, not drinking with meals, and eating moist foods helps.
8. Has your patient ever been unsteady on their feet? These can be symptoms of thiamin, copper, or vitamin B12 deficiency.
9. If your patient is reaching for ice chips, they probably have pica from iron deficiency.
10. Dumping syndrome is the jejuna response to undigested carbohydrates. Enteroglucagon and other gut hormones cause an influx of fluids into the lumen. Patients may also complain of a runny nose, excessive salivation, nausea and vomiting, tremulousness and anxiety, tachycardia, presyncope, and diarrhea. Review medication for hidden sugar content and 24-h food logs for the same. Take special care to review liquid substances. Unfortunately, it is not enough to check for high sugary or fatty foods. Do they experience these symptoms frequently? Are they retesting their tolerance of these obvious trigger foods frequently? The more they test, the higher the risk of dietary indiscretions later.

11. Is extreme sustained hypoglycemia nesidioblastosis? Service's initial well-publicized assertion that gastric bypass creates an environment for nesidioblastosis has recently been disproved by examination of pathological series. Probably all hypoglycemic complaints can be handled by strict adherence to frequent complex carbohydrates and lean protein as directed by your bariatric dietitians [30].

WEIGHT LOSS CONCERNS AFTER WEIGHT LOSS SURGERY

How can we predict which patients are more vulnerable to weight loss failure after surgery? Christou et al. [31] and Reinhold [32] described the accepted excess weight loss (EWL) at 3, 6, and 12 months and further for RYGB. Acceptable norms range from 50% to 77% EWL by 24 months. Five- and ten-year data are less accurate due to significant loss of follow-up. Ritz et al. [33] has recently provided a simple and profound yardstick by which one can predict weight loss failure and hopefully do something about it before it becomes a reality. Weight loss failure in this study is defined as <25% weight loss at 2 years, and weight loss success is defined as >50% EWL at 2 years. These two groups showed very different weight loss time lines. Specifically the weight loss failure group's profile consistently showed that <30% weight loss at 6 months was far more likely. There are studies that assert that patients with BMI > 60 attain a lower % EBWL. In fact, those with BMI > 60 were more likely to regain weight after 1 year [34].

Poor weight loss is multifactorial. Some failure can be mechanical due to a dilated gastric pouch. This can be caused either by surgical technique or maladaptive eating behavior. A relapse of the patient's prior eating disorder can occur, especially after the honeymoon period of hunger reduction [35–37]. There is also a worrisome return to other addictions, such as alcohol, that can contribute to very early weight regain.

There is a risk that the patient will be unable to sustain the new eating behaviors and exercise requirements essential to continued weight loss. There are issues of weight bias, weight loss stigma, and time management, which deserve full attention on every visit. Life events in patients and their families can overwhelm the patients. The metabolic physician can play a vital role during these distressing times to help the patients save their weight loss before they give up hope.

How to best succeed in maintaining weight loss? Institute a full lifestyle change before surgery and engender full support from the patient's family, both preoperatively and postoperatively. Patients that continue to take their vitamins, that get their regular checkups, that continue to track their meals and their exercise, that weigh themselves regularly, that snack safely and not mindlessly, and who are able to get good support for their life issues are the ones who are more likely to succeed.

Considerable research has been done to discover which diabetic patients will succeed and which will enjoy the most complete remission of their diabetes. The recent SOS review shows that the earlier the diabetes at the time of surgery, the more likely the remission at 20 years while reviewing the long-term cardiovascular mortality trends [38].

WEIGHT REGAIN AFTER WEIGHT LOSS SURGERY

Obesity providers and society in general tend to assume that when the patients fail to lose enough weight or regain a significant amount of weight, maladaptive behavior is to blame. As a metabolic physician, it is critical to carefully evaluate at least three broad areas of concern: (1) anatomical or surgical issues, (2) behavioral issues, and (3) biological issues.

Weight loss averages 50% EWL after banding, 60% after the sleeve, 65% after RYGB, and 75% after biliopancreatic diversion (BPD)/duodenal switch. Ten years later, there is a sustained weight loss average of 35% across the board. It is important to realize that this 35% includes 20–30% weight regain, which was initially lost during the first 1–2 years after surgery [1].

Behavioral concerns, which contribute to poor diet and nutrition, include overeating, frequently processed grains, and poor fat choices. Often, these foods have limited nutrition and vitamin content as well as poor quality protein. Mindless eating, eating too fast, meal skipping, grazing, and restaurant eating, to name a few, contribute to poor eating habits which often recur after surgery. Weight regain is also attributed to a relapse into a sedentary lifestyle and a lack of physical activity.

Anatomical concerns specifically related to an enlarged pouch or demise of gastric band integrity or stretching of the sleeve have been implicated in weight regain. Revisional surgery of gastric bypass afforded a 37% increase in EWL and 53.7% EWL in converting a restrictive to a malabsorptive surgery [39,40]. Surgical revisional technology and the full range of surgical options are covered elsewhere. The reason for an enlarged pouch could be from maladaptive behavior; however, it could also be from specific tissue characteristics or the surgical structuring of the initial pouch.

Biologic/metabolic reasons for weight regain are less well known but possibly the most important. My colleague, Cynthia Buffington, has provided me with important insights into the biology of fat and its implication in weight loss and weight regain. Her analysis compels us to understand the adipocyte as a target organ.

Biological conditions can be set into play while the patient is initially becoming obese, which later resist weight loss and promote weight regain. Defects of a lifetime of aberrant food disposal are not corrected necessarily by weight loss. Rather these defects can promote other problems.

For example, the number of fat cells in an obese person can be as many as 10 times as numerous as in a lean individual. But obesity promotes adipose tissue growth both in fat cell number and size. More fatty acid (FA) is transported into fat cells, triglyceride synthesis is increased, and there is a reduction of triglyceride breakdown into its components of FAs and glycerol. Obesity causes an increased conversion of glucose into free FAs, resulting in increased lipogenesis. Obesity also causes a decreased ability of muscle to oxidize fat, possibly related to aberrant mitochondrial function and number [41].

All of the above changes in fat oxidation contribute to higher BMIs [42]. Further, the increase in triglyceride synthesis contributes to insulin resistance. As muscle is not able to oxidize this fat, it causes an increase in adipose tissue expansion. Thus, a greater number of calories will be stored as fat.

So does weight loss improve the defects in muscle oxidation? Weight loss surgery further reduces gene regulation of FA oxidation. Fat cell size does significantly decrease after weight loss surgery. Fat cell numbers remain elevated with the capacity to readily re-accumulate fat [43].

Obesity is known for increasing fat cell size and leptin hypersecretion [44]. As fat cell size falls, leptin secretion dramatically decreases, thus suggesting a weight regain potential in the postsurgical relationship of leptin to fat cells. The adipose tissue of formerly obese individuals has more vascularization and mesenchymal stem cells that are adipogenic. This suggests that obese fat cells are committed to an adipogenic lineage [45]. Weight loss causes an increased capacity for fat storage and decreased ability to utilize fat. Both of these impede weight loss success and long-term weight loss maintenance.

Weight loss is also associated with a greater decline in energy expenditure than can be explained by the reduction in calorie intake alone. This may be related to an increase in circulating organochlorines, which has been seen after BPD. Organochlorines are felt to contribute to a decline in energy expenditure via adverse actions on thyroid hormone function [46].

Leptin signals caloric sufficiency and prevents further weight gain by increasing EE and reducing appetite. However, leptin levels decrease with weight loss. A leptin threshold needed to cause satiety increases with weight gain. After weight loss, leptin levels decline, but the leptin threshold does not [47]. This gap between leptin levels and threshold may decrease the EE and signal increased food seeking.

Weight loss surgery can induce a decline in the omega-3 FAs, docosahexaenoic acid (DHA) and eicosapentaenoic acid (EPA), resulting in a 15% reduction of cerebral DHA. This decline has been implicated in increased stress and depression. It may play a role in increasing production of cortisol after weight loss surgery [48]. This is in addition to the fact that obesity is often accompanied by increases in cortisol through the stimulation of the hypothalamic–pituitary–adrenal axis.

Can we increase fat oxidation? Control insulin levels? Reduce the risk for adipose tissue re-expansion, and prevent declines in energy expenditure? Improve hormone profiles and nutrient status? What biological/metabolic tools are available to us? Said a different way, let us reframe the behavioral habits or long-term success into biological factors that fight adiposity and thus weight regain. The following general guidelines have been found to be of benefit to the patients.

Exercise

Exercise promotes FA oxidation and reduces fat synthesis from carbohydrates while increasing muscle mass. Exercise helps prevent the decline of energy expenditure that occurs postoperatively. Exercise reduces appetite and releases stress. Moderate regular exercise reduces fat-free mass. Maintaining fat-free mass is a known predictor of improved postsurgical weight loss [49].

Protein

Soy, fish, chicken, turkey, eggs, pork, milk, and cheese are examples of proteins that contain sufficient essential amino acids to stimulate protein synthesis and thus preserve muscle mass. Increased lean muscle mass prevents both the decline in EE and the decline in fat oxidation, which occur postsurgery. Quality protein also stabilizes insulin levels and increases satiety. Whey protein stimulates protein synthesis due to its highly digestible leucine (14%) greater than casein (10%), milk (10%), egg protein (8.5%), muscle protein (8%), soy protein isolate (8%), and wheat protein (7%).

Calcium

Low intake of calcium results in increased calcitriol. Calcitriol is known to promote obesity. Calcium increases the fecal fat content. Dietary calcium enhances fat breakdown and inhibits fat uptake [50].

(n-3)/(n-6) EFA Omega-3

Obese patients tend to have low n-3 EFA, at least in part due to the high level of n-6 in diets consisting of grain-fed animals and processed grains/foods. Fish oil supplements decrease fat mass in non-obese patients [51]. Foods rich in n-3 EFA are salmon, sardines, herring, mackerel, tuna, halibut, anchovies, avocado, kale, spinach, mustard greens, sesame seeds, pumpkin seeds, buffalo, deer and grass-fed animals, flax–hemp–walnut and wheat germ oils, and fish oil (linolenic acid, EPA, DHA).

Dietary Fiber

Fiber reduces the absorption of sugar and fat. High-fiber foods also have the highest antioxidant potential, thus decreasing inflammatory processes [52]. The per capita intake of fiber in the United States is among the lowest in the world (15 g vs. the recommended 30 g). Obese individuals are said to consume <10 g/day and in weight loss only <5 g/day. Significant fiber is found in fruits, vegetables, nuts, beans, and whole grains. Fiber increases satiety due to bulk and water absorption qualities. Soluble fiber reduces glucose absorption. Insulin levels and fat absorption are reduced. Fermentable fiber stimulates GLP-1 and PYY in the distal gut, as well as bifidobacterium [53].

Sleep

Less than 7 h of restorative sleep at night promotes obesity via a multitude of mechanisms [54].

The take home point: by understanding the mechanisms that sustain high adipose tissue in the form of poor weight loss and definite vulnerability for weight gain, the patients can be better served. Discussions on the behaviors of weight regain can now be fueled with the science of fat deposition and removal.

The following is a summary of the above discussion:

1. Increased capacity for adipose tissue re-expansion
   a. Reduced fat oxidation
   b. Reduced EE (fat oxidation, body composition, pollutants, leptin, ghrelin)
   c. Increased appetite (regulators)
   d. Fat-promoting hormones
   e. Micronutrient deficits
   f. Macronutrient aberrant composition (fat, processed grains)
2. Biological contributors to weight regain may be modified by lifestyle changes involving
   a. Exercise
   b. Energy expenditure
   c. The influence of high-quality protein and calcium
   d. Contributions of fish and n-3/n-6 FFAs
   e. The use of high fiber foods vs. processed foods
   f. Decrease in fat-promoting hormones as insulin and cortisol
   g. The need for at least 7 h of restorative sleep

PREGNANCY CONCERNS PREWEIGHT OR POSTWEIGHT LOSS SURGERY

"To begin the cure of obesity, we must provide excellence in health care of all women of child bearing age, especially the more disenfranchised."—John Kral MD, MPH.

Natural selection states that certain heritable traits that make an organism more likely to reproduce become more common in a population. These traits are stored in the DNA, i.e., our hard wiring. This genetic expression allows switching on and off of the software (enzymes, cofactors, immune modulators) as a response to environmental changes.

Epigenetics is the study of mitotically heritable alterations in gene-expression potential that are not caused by changes in DNA sequence. Nowhere is this more critical than in the epigenetic variability afforded to a woman of childbearing age and the developing fetus. Pre-pregnancy weight and nutrition do influence the future of the offspring. Post-pregnancy central obesity is implicated in midlife vulnerability to future adverse cardiovascular outcomes.

Below are the guidelines and implications for pregnancy after surgery:

- 71 g protein/day
- 500 mg folate
- Calcium 100 mg/day for breastfeeding or 1300 mg/day if <19 years old
- Iron 10 mg/day
- Regular meals and snacks
- 30 g of fiber: 9 g whole grains, fruits, and vegetables
- 8 cups of water and no alcohol
- One prenatal vitamin a day

These nutritional goals are achievable for most postoperative bariatric surgery patients. But there are obvious nutritional issues in the immediate postoperative period. Pregnancy tests prior to surgery are mandatory. Two forms of birth control after surgery are also recommended. However, should a woman become pregnant shortly after surgery, careful attention to the above details assures the health of the fetus and the mother.

If the pregnant postsurgical candidate is unable to maintain appropriate intake, both maternal and fetal well-being may be jeopardized. Immediate referral to a high-risk obstetrician should be initiated if this occurs. Certainly, the same is true if a bariatric patient becomes pregnant within

2 years of her surgery. Intrauterine growth evaluation should be evaluated by serial fetal ultrasound. If maternal weight loss is greater than 2 lbs. a week and it cannot be ameliorated, supplemental nutrition, including enteral, and even TPN, may be necessary.

CASE FOR A MOTHER'S HEALTH

As stated above, there is a relationship to pre-pregnancy weight, pregnancy weight gain, postpartum weight, and comorbidity in mothers. Therefore, following recommendations are made.
Weight gain guidelines for pregnancy:

- 25–35 lbs. for BMI 20–24
- 15–25 lbs. for BMI 25–29
- 15 lbs. for BMI > 30

Some 45% of women begin pregnancy overweight or obese [55], and 43% of pregnant women gain more weight than recommended [55]. Maternal overweight and obesity are associated with gestational diabetes, hypertension, and newborn macrosomia [56].

Women who are overweight or obese before they become pregnant tend to retain or gain more weight after pregnancy than non-overweight women [57]. Nulliparous overweight or obese women, especially age 19 or younger, are the most vulnerable for the largest sustained weight gain [58]. Black women and those with diabetes tend to gain more weight as well [59].

During pregnancy, fat is preferentially distributed abdominally, and the remaining postpartum adiposity often rests centrally. This weight gain pattern is predictive of cardiovascular disease, diabetes, and early mortality in women. Pre-pregnant and postpartum weight gains are modifiable risk factors that provide us with a unique vantage point for altering the course of obesity.

CASE FOR THE CHILD OBESITY RISK

"The Developmental Origins of Obesity: Programmed Adipogenesis" has been explored by Desai et al. [60]. Prenatal, in utero, and infant environmental exposures provide developmental programming for obese offspring. Low birth weight, catch-up growth, and high birth weight (often macrosomic) infants are most often the consequence of maternal obesity with or without gestational diabetes.

The fetus develops with maternal nutrition, hormones, and an individual metabolic environment. Changes in this uterine environment now are believed to alter everything from organ development, cellular composition, to gene expression of the epigenome. Therefore, maternal nutrition, oxygenation, and placental perfusion have profound effects on the fetus.

Obesity later in life is associated with a U-shaped infant birth weight curve. In this light, any deviation from normal birth weight potentially predisposes the infant to obesity and metabolic syndrome. Catch-up growth also deserves a warning. Infants that are born small and remain small exhibit less obesity and metabolic syndrome than those who start small and catch up to normal body weight [61,62]. The lack of LBM creates an environment suitable to weight regain in later life. Low birth weight infants and preterm infants are born with less lean body weight [63]. Normal birth weight newborns that have accelerated weight gain during the first 2 years exhibit this same phenomenon of higher body fat [64].

Adipogenesis primarily occurs during prenatal and postnatal development [65]. Epigenetic modifications of transcription factors and or histones are involved in this process (i.e., PPAR, C/EBP, SREBP1, PPARgamma) [66]. Lipogenic enzymes (FA synthase and lipoprotein lipase) are turned on to create increased fat uptake and synthesis promoting lipid accumulation within the adipocyte [67].

Desai examined LBW infants born to gestational diabetic and diabetic mothers. Collectively, his observation of these epigenetic alterations and related altered leptin expression indicates increased susceptibility to retain fat in adipocytes well as the ability of lipid accumulation to alter adipocyte endocrine function. For the infant born to a gestational or established diabetic mother, this may be the seat of insulin insensitivity and inflammation.

The U Laval Mother–Child Obesity Study in Quebec provided compelling, 20-year data on offspring born to a mother before or after weight loss surgery [68–70]. Children born to the same mother after her sustained EWL of 50% or greater from weight loss surgery had a 50% less risk for developing obesity even as an adult. The absolute risk declined from 35% to 11%. These data add credence to the epigenetic effects of obesity.

CONCLUSIONS

This chapter has provided the reader with information related to the care of bariatric surgery patients. The process of recommending weight loss surgery and how to care for metabolic surgery patients before and after surgery has been explored. The components of immediate and long-term postoperative follow-up necessary to prevent the avoidable metabolic complications of surgery have been reviewed. Weight loss failure, weight regain after surgery, and the relationships between successful surgery and successful pregnancy have also been discussed.

It is this author's hope that the information provided can assist in the careful planning and follow-up of a successful weight loss surgery patient. The metabolic physician can play a critical role in the proper preparation for surgery, the appropriate monitoring after surgery, and the achievement of significant, sustainable weight loss. Dedication to these patients can provide the structure that they need to get an optimal outcome from their weight loss procedure.

REFERENCES

1. Shiwaku K, Anuurad E, Enkhmaa B. Predictive values of anthropometric measurements for multiple metabolic disorders in Asian populations. *Diabetes Res Clin Pract* 2005;69(1):52–62.
2. Page KA, Kit H. Association of all-cause mortality with overweight and obesity using standard body mass index categories: A systematic review and meta-analysis. *JAMA* 2013;309(1):71–82.
3. Gallagher D, Heymsfield SB. Healthy percentage body fat ranges: An approach for developing guidelines based on body mass index. *Am J Clin Nutr* 2000;72:694–701.
4. NHLBI/NIDDK. Asian BMI Classification. 1998; Clinical Guidelines.
5. Sandowski SA. What is the ideal body weight? *Family Practice* 2000;17:348–51.
6. Ainsworth BE, Haskell WL, Leon AS. Compendium of physical activities: Classification of energy costs of human physical activities. *Med Sci Sports Exerc* 1993;25(1):71–80.
7. Hall KD, Heymsfield SB, Kemnitz JW. Energy balance and its components: Implications for bod weight regulation. *Am J Clin Nutr* 2012;95:989–94.
8. Leslie D, Kellogg TA, Ikramuddin S. Bariatric surgery primer for the internist: Keys to the surgical consultation. *Med Clin North Am* 2007;91(3):353–81.
9. Kuruba R, Koche LS, Murr MM. Preoperative assessment and perioperative care of patients undergoing bariatric surgery. *Med Clin North Am* 2007;91(3):339–51.
10. Catheline JM, Bihan H, Le Quang T. Preoperative cardiac and pulmonary assessment in bariatric surgery. *Obes Surg* 2000;18:271–7.
11. Sharma L, Lou C, Cahue S. The mechanism of the effect of obesity in knee osteoarthritis. The mediating role of malalignment. *Arth Rheum* 2000;43(3):568–75.
12. Van Gool CH, Penninx BW, Kempen GI. Effects of exercise adherence on physical function among overweight older adults with knee osteoarthritis. *Arth Rheum* 2005;53(1):24–32.
13. Torquati A, Wright K. Effects of gastric bypass operation on Framingham and actual risk of cardiovascular events in class II-III obesity. *Am Col Surg* 2007;204:771–6.
14. Flood C, Fleisher L. Preparation of the cardiac patient for the non-cardiac surgery. *Am Fam Phys* 2007;75:656–64.
15. Alpert M, Fraley MA. Management of obesity cardiomyopathy. *Expert Rev Cardiovasc Ther* 2005; 3:225–30.

16. Poirier P, Cornier MA, Mazzone T. Bariatric surgery and cardiovascular risk factors ASCI statement from the AHA. *Circulation* 2011;123(15):1983–701.
17. Fraley MA, Birchem N. Obesity and the electrocardiogram. *Obes Rev* 2005;6:275–81.
18. Mechsnick H, Garber AJ. American Assn Clin Endocrinologists position paper on obesity and obesity medicine. *End Pract* 2012;18:142–8.
19. Markel TA, Matter SG. Management of gastrointestinal disorders in the bariatric patient. *Med Clin North Am* 2007;91:443–50.
20. Felson DT, Lawrence RC, Hochberg MC. Osteoarthritis: New insights. Part 2: Treatment approaches. *Ann Int Med* 2009;133(9):726–50.
21. Messier SP, Getekunst DJ, Davis C. Weight loss reduces knee-joint loads in overweight and obese older adults with knee osteoarthritis. *Arth Rheum* 2005;53(7):2026–32.
22. Celli BR, Cote CG. The body mass index, airflow obstruction, dyspnea and exercise capacity index in COPD. *NEJM* 2004;350:1005–12.
23. Gupta PK, Gupta H, Kaushik M. Predictors of pulmonary complications after bariatric surgery. *SOARD* 2012;8:574–81.
24. Christou NV, Lieberman M, Sampaalis F. Bariatric surgery reduces cancer risk in morbidly obese patients. *SOARD* 2008;4:691–5.
25. Spitznagal MB, Garcia S, Miller LA. Cognitive function predicts weight loss after bariatric surgery. *SOARD* 2013;9:453–61.
26. Buffington CK. Alcohol use and the health risks: Survey results. *Bariatric Times* 2007;4:21–3.
27. Still CD, Benotti PWG, Gerhard GS. Outcomes of preoperative weight loss in high-risk patients undergoing gastric bypass surgery. *Arch Surg* 2007;142:994–8.
28. Lewis MC, Phillips ML, Slavotinek JP. Changes in liver size and fat content after treatment with Optifast VLCD. *Obes Surg* 2006;6:690–701.
29. Aills L, Blankenship J, Buffington C. ASMBS Allied Health nutritional guidelines for the surgical weight loss patient. *SOARD* 2008;4(5 suppl):s73–108.
30. Meier JJ, Butler AE, Galasso R. Hyperinsulinemic hypoglycemia after gastric bypass surgery is not accompanied by islet hypoplasia or increased Beta cell turnover. *Diabetes Care* 2006;7:154–9.
31. Christou NV, Look D, Maclean LD. Weight gain after short and long limb gastric bypass in patients followed for longer than 10 years. *Ann Surg* 2006;244:734–40.
32. Reinhold RB. Critical analysis of long term weight loss following gastric bypass. *Surg Gyn Obes* 1982;155:385–94.
33. Ritz P, Caiazzo R, Becouarn G. Early prediction of failure to lose weight after obesity surgery. *SOARD* 2013;9:118–22.
34. Ochner CN, Jochner MC, Caruso EA. Effect of preoperative body mass index on weight loss after obesity surgery. *SOARD* 2013;9:423–8.
35. Lutfi R, Torquati A, Sckhar N. Predictors of success after laparoscopic gastric bypass: A multivariate analysis of socioeconomic factors. *Surg Endosc* 2006;20:864–7.
36. Harvin G, DeLegge M, Garrow DA. The impact of race on weight loss after Roux-en-Y gastric bypass surgery. *Obes Surg* 2008;18:39–42.
37. Bond DS, Thomas JG, Unick JL. Self-reported and objectively measured sedentary behavior in bariatric surgery candidates. *SOARD* 2013;9:123–8.
38. Sjostrom L, Peltonen M, Jacobson P. Bariatric surgery and long-term cardiovascular events. *JAMA* 2012;307:56–65.
39. Shimazu H, Annaberdyev S, Motamarry I. Revisional bariatric surgery for unsuccessful weight loss and complications. *Obes Surg* 2013;23(11):1766–73.
40. Iannelli A, Schneck AS, Hebuterne X. Gastric pouch resizing for Roux-en-Y gastric bypass failure in patients with a dilated pouch. *SOARD* 2013;9:260–8.
41. Fabris R, Mingrone G, Milan M, Manco M, Granzotto M, Dalla Pozza A, Scarda A, Serra R, Greco AV, Federspil G, Vettor R. Further lowering of muscle lipid oxidative capacity in obese subjects after biliopancreatic diversion. *J Clin Endo Metab* 2004;89:1753–9.
42. Lofgren I, Herron K, Zern T. Waist circumference is a better predictor than BMI of coronary mortality disease risk in overweight menopausal women. *J Nutr* 2004;134(5):1071–6.
43. Hernández-Alvarez MI, Chiellini C, Manco M, Naon D, Liesa M, Palacín M, Mingrone G, Zorzano A. Genes involved in mitochondrial biogenesis function are induced in response to bilio-pancreatic disease in morbidly obese individuals with normal glucose tolerance but not in type 2 diabetic patients. *Diabetologia* 2009;52(8):1618–27.

44. Lofgren P, Andersson I, Adolfsson B. Long-term prospective controlled studies demonstrate adipose tissue hypercellularity and relative leptin deficiency with post obese state. *J Clinc Endo Metab* 2005;90(11):16207–13.

45. Baptista LS, da Silva KR, da Pedrosa CS. Adipose tissue of control and ex-obese patients exhibit differences in blood vessel content and resident mesenchymal stem cell population. *Obes Surg* 2009; 9:1304–12.

46. Hue O, Marcotte J, Berrigan F. Increased plasma levels of toxic pollutants accompanying weight loss induced by hypocaloric diet or by bariatric surgery. *Obes Surg* 2006;9:1145–54.

47. Rosenbaum M, Leibel RL. Adaptive thermogenesis in humans. *Int J Obes* 2010;34 suppl 1:547–55.

48. Myers MG Jr, Leibel RL, Seeley RJ. Obesity and leptin resistance: Distinguishing cause from effect. *Trends Endo Metab* 2010;11:643–51.

49. Metcalf B, Rabkin RA, Rabkin JM. Weight loss composition and the effects of exercise following obesity surgery as measured by bioelectrical impedance analysis. *Obesity* 2005;3:183–6.

50. Zemel MB. Calcitriol and energy metabolism. *Nutr Rev* 2008;66(10 suppl 2):5139–46.

51. Zemel MB, Sun X, Sobhan I. Oxidative and inflammatory stress in overweight and obese subjects. *Phys Sportsmet* 2009;37(2):29–39.

52. Friedman GD, Cutter GR, Donahue RP. Cardia: Study design, recruitment, and some characteristics of the examined subjects. *J Clin Epid* 1988;41(11):1105–16.

53. Delzenne NM. A place for dietary fiber in the management of the metabolic syndrome. *Clin Opin Clin Nutr Metab Care* 2005;8(6):636–40.

54. Knutson KL, Spiegel K, Penev P. Metabolic consequences of sleep deprivation. *Sleep Med Rev* 2007;11(3):163–78.

55. Reinold C, Dalenius K, Brindley P, Smith B, Grummer-Strawn L. *Pregnancy Nutrition Surveillance 2009 Report.* Atlanta: U.S. Department of Health and Human Services, Centers for Disease Control and Prevention; 2011.

56. Catalano PM. Increasing maternal obesity and weight gain during pregnancy: The obstetric problems of plentitude. *Obes Gyn* 2007;110:743–4.

57. Gunderson E. Childbearing and obesity in women: Weight before, during and after pregnancy. *Obst Gyn Clin North Am* 2009;36(2):327–32.

58. Chu SY, Callaghan WM, Bisch CL. Gestational weight gain by body mass index among US women delivering live births, 2004–5: Fueling future obesity. *Am J Obes Gyne* 2009;200:271.e1–7.

59. Britz SE, McDermott KC, Pierce CB. Changes in maternal weight 5–10 years after a first delivery. *Womens Health* 2012;8(5):513–9.

60. Desai M, Beall M, Ross MG. Developmental origins of obesity: Programmed adipogenesis. *Curr Diab Rep* 2013;13:27–33.

61. Monteiro PO, Victora CG. Rapid growth in infancy and childhood and obesity in later life—A systematic review. *Obes Res* 2005;62:143–54.

62. Baird J, Fisher D, Lucas P. Being big or growing fast: Systematic review of size and growth in infancy and later obesity. *BMJ* 2005;331(7522):929.

63. Finken MJ, Keijzer-Veen MG, Dekker FW. Preterm birth weight and postnatal growth in a population based longitudinal study from birth into adult life. *Diabetologia* 2006;493:478–85.

64. Ong KK, Ahmed ML, Emmett PM. Association between postnatal catch-up growth and obesity in childhood prospective cohort study. *BMJ* 2000;320(7240):967–71.

65. Wabitsch M. The acquisition of obesity: Insight from cellular and genetic research. *Proc Nutr Soc* 2000;592:325–30.

66. Janesick A, Bloomgerg B. Obesogens, stem cells and the developmental programming of obesity. *Int J Androl* 2012;353:437–48.

67. Boizar M, Le Liepvre X, Lernarchand P. Obesity-related overexpression of fatty-acid synthase gene in adipose tissue involves sterol regulatory element-binding protein transcription factors. *J Biol Chem* 1998;273(44):29164–7.

68. Smith J, Cianflone K, Biron S. Effects of maternal surgical weight loss in mothers on intergenerational transmission of obesity. *J Clin Endo Metab* 2009;94(11):4275–83.

69. Kral JG, Biron S, Simard S, Hould FS, Lebel S, Marceau S, Marceau P. Large maternal weight loss from obesity surgery prevents transmission of obesity to children who were followed for 2 to 18 years. *Pediatrics* 2006;118(6):e1644–9.

70. Kral JG, Biron S, Simard S. Large maternal weight loss from obesity surgery prevents of obesity to children who were followed for 2 to 18 years. *Pediatrics* 2006;118(6):e1644–9.

18 Hypoglycemia after Roux-en-Y Gastric Bypass Surgery

Shannon Roque, Sridhar Nambi, and Michael M. Rothkopf

CONTENTS

INTRODUCTION

Bariatric surgery, and in particular, the Roux-en-Y gastric bypass (RYGB), has unquestionable benefits in obese patients with diabetes mellitus. Resolution of diabetes has occurred in up to 85% of patients after this procedure. A substantial improvement in glucose control is noted, even in those in whom diabetes resolution does not occur.

However, these procedures are not without potential metabolic drawbacks, among the most disturbing of which is the development of reactive hypoglycemia. A mild, often asymptomatic form of hypoglycemia has been a well-known effect of gastric bypass (GB) surgery. This condition occurs as part of the dumping syndrome. However, a more severe form of hypoglycemia with neuroglycopenic symptoms has been described.

This condition appears to differ in significant ways from other forms of fasting or reactive hypoglycemia. These patients may face life-threatening hypoglycemic episodes, which are unresponsive to conservative therapy. GB reversal or even pancreatectomy has been suggested for these severe cases.

In this chapter, we will provide an overview of the issues related to hypoglycemia after RYGB based on our experience in the management of over 10,000 postoperative bariatric surgery patients. We will provide an overview of both fasting and postprandial hypoglycemia. We will review the literature on hypoglycemia after RYGB and outline current controversies as to the pathogenesis of this condition. Finally, we will present recommendations for the evaluation and management of these patients.

BIOCHEMISTRY OF HYPOGLYCEMIA

Glucose is the brain's preferred metabolic fuel. But since the brain can neither produce nor store glucose, it requires a continuous supply from the circulation [1]. The brain's GLUT1 transporter has a very low Km for glucose (Km = the substrate concentration at which the reaction rate is half of Vmax). This permits glucose to enter the cells freely via zero-order kinetics at physiologic levels (roughly 90 mg/dL or 5 mM/L) [2]. This means that glucose transport is normally independent of the plasma concentration.

Clinical hypoglycemia occurs when the plasma glucose concentration is less than 55 mg/dL (3 mM/L). At this level, glucose transport is approaching first-order kinetics, making it substrate-dependent and jeopardizing energy delivery to the brain [2]. To defend against this, cyclic AMP-mediated, hormonal counterregulatory mechanisms initiate hepatic glycogenolysis to quickly correct the hypoglycemia. Cyclic AMP also signals the hepatocyte nucleus to initiate gene expression for gluconeogenesis, thereby preparing for the provision of a long-term alternative supply of glucose [3].

If the hypoglycemia defense mechanisms fail, or if they are overwhelmed by the presence of excess insulin, symptomatic hypoglycemia can result. The initial symptoms of hypoglycemia are categorized as neurogenic. They are primarily due to the elevated levels of counterregulatory hormones such as epinephrine, glucagon, and cortisol. The neurogenic symptoms include sweating, shakiness, tachycardia, palpitations, and anxiety [1].

On the other hand, neuroglycopenic symptoms are more directly related to the reduced glucose transport to the brain and the failure of adenosine triphosphate (ATP) production via oxidative phosphorylation [4]. The neuroglycopenic symptoms include a sensation of hunger, weakness, tiredness, dizziness, inappropriate behavior (sometimes mistaken for inebriation), difficulty with concentration, confusion, and blurred vision. If hypoglycemia is not corrected from this point, sodium–potassium ion pumps will stall and neurologic membrane action potentials will be compromised. This may result in seizure, coma, or even death in extreme cases [1].

FASTING HYPOGLYCEMIA

One of the first steps in the diagnostic evaluation of a patient with hypoglycemia is to differentiate between fasting hypoglycemia and reactive hypoglycemia. Therefore, the timing of symptom onset relative to food ingestion is a crucial factor in the decision analysis [5].

Fasting hypoglycemia typically occurs in the morning before eating. Fasting hypoglycemia may also occur later in the day, particularly if meals are missed or delayed. An important subset of this group is nocturnal hypoglycemia. In general, the patient should have been without food for at least 6 h to define the condition as fasting hypoglycemia [6].

Fasting hypoglycemia may be due to the use of drugs. Overdose of hypoglycemic agents are an obvious consideration here. But salicylates, sulfa drugs, pentamidine, and quinine may also be responsible [7]. Fasting hypoglycemia can also be seen in ethanolism and in critical illnesses, particularly sepsis [8]. Hypoglycemia is also associated with certain inborn errors of metabolism, such as the Maple syrup urine and glycogen storage diseases [1].

Fasting hypoglycemia can also be due to hepatic disorders involving glycogen storage and enzymes of the counterregulatory mechanisms. The body relies on glycogen to quickly correct hypoglycemia. Inadequate glycogen storage severely limits this capability. Glycogen depletion occurs with starvation, acute hepatic necrosis, advanced cirrhosis, and advanced hepatic tumor infiltration [7].

After glycogen stores are depleted, the body depends on systems that produce glucose from alternative sources (amino acids, lactate, glycerol). The systems are slower to initiate because they require nuclear gene transcription. But once initiated, they can provide a long-term source for glucose production. The inability to complete the processes of gluconeogenesis through such conditions as fructose bisphosphatase deficiency will produce hypoglycemia after the hepatic glycogen stores run out [7].

Other endocrine conditions outside the liver can cause hypoglycemia related to failure of primary counterregulatory signaling. These include diseases of the pituitary and adrenal glands with deficiencies of growth hormone, adrenocorticotrophic hormone, cortisol, and epinephrine [1].

A rare but important cause of fasting hypoglycemia is the nonphysiologic secretion of excess insulin or insulin-like factors. This is typically associated with insulin-producing islet cell and/or extrapancreatic tumors [7].

A small number of post-RYGB patients with hypoglycemia and neuroglycopenia have been found to have preexisting insulinoma [5]. These cases may be suspected because they present with severe fasting hypoglycemia shortly after surgery. As will be further discussed below, this presentation is distinct from that of the reactive or postprandial hypoglycemia syndrome commonly discussed after RYGB. The cases with insulinoma occur earlier in the postoperative course and present with fasting rather than reactive hypoglycemia.

Dietary therapy may be effective for improving symptoms in patients with fasting hypoglycemia [6]. Eating frequently is preferred, with a balance of complex carbohydrates and protein. If dietary therapy is inadequate, medical care for patients with fasting hypoglycemia may include intravenous glucose infusion, or octreotide administration, which may be effective in suppressing endogenous insulin secretion [9].

Because exercise increases glucose uptake through its effects on the GLUT4 transporter, patients with fasting hypoglycemia should avoid significant exercise activity [6]. The definitive treatment for fasting hypoglycemia caused by endogenous insulin hypersecretion is surgical resection of the overproducing insulin-secreting cells. Outcomes are generally good for resection of both benign and malignant islet-cell adenomas [10].

REACTIVE HYPOGLYCEMIA

Reactive hypoglycemia occurs in a timed sequence after a meal. This is particularly true if the meal contains a large quantity of carbohydrates. Reactive hypoglycemia may present as soon as 30 min and as long as 5 h after eating. But it is typically noted at 2–3 h postprandially [6].

Reactive hypoglycemia is much more common than fasting hypoglycemia. It is often seen in patients with type 2 diabetes mellitus, insulin resistance, gastrointestinal dysfunction, or hormonal deficiencies [6]. A definitive diagnosis may be elusive. Therefore, it is not uncommon to classify patients as having idiopathic reactive hypoglycemia [1].

A careful study of glucose and insulin dynamics should disclose an alteration in insulin secretion in patients with symptoms of reactive hypoglycemia. In most patients, overt hyperinsulinism can be documented. Increased insulin sensitivity is a less likely but possible cause [1]. Consuming excessive quantities of refined carbohydrate is often the trigger to hyperinsulinism [6].

Confirmation of reactive hypoglycemia can be documented with measurements of blood glucose during a postprandial symptomatic episode. In our practice, we utilize a 3-h oral glucose tolerance test for this purpose. Onset of symptoms usually occurs within a few hours after the ingestion of the glucose test solution.

Because the exaggerated insulin response is provoked by the elevation of blood glucose, control of glucose intake is an essential component of therapy. Dietary intervention for patients with reactive hypoglycemia can be thought of as the polar opposite to that of fasting hypoglycemia. Instead of frequent consumption of carbohydrates, a restriction of carbohydrate is necessary. Increasing the dietary intake of protein and fiber content may also be helpful [6]. Patients should avoid simple sugars and refined starches completely.

In contradistinction to those with fasting hypoglycemia, the majority of patients with reactive hypoglycemia see an improvement of their symptoms with the initiation of a routine exercise program [6]. This is because the increased glucose uptake induced by exercise at the GLUT4 transporter has the effect of decreasing insulin resistance [2]. This, in turn, reduces insulin hypersecretion in response to a meal.

Medical therapy is generally not indicated in the common form of reactive hypoglycemia. However, some authors have recommended the use of insulin sensitizing therapies such as metformin or pioglitazone [6]. Nutritional supplementation with cinnamon, chromium, and alpha lipoic acid may also be beneficial [11].

ASYMPTOMATIC POSTBARIATRIC HYPOGLYCEMIA

Nearly all patients who have undergone a RYGB will experience some degree of postoperative hypoglycemia as part of the "dumping syndrome." The dumping syndrome is an expected result of the surgical diversion of nutrient flow into the distal gut. It is categorized by symptoms of abdominal pain, bloating, and diarrhea. It is also often associated with vasomotor symptoms such as flushing, diaphoresis, weakness, hypotension, and tachycardia [12].

The dumping syndrome is induced after the consumption of refined carbohydrates. Because of the anatomical change created by the operation, these carbohydrates present rapidly to the distal gut [12]. The presence of glucose, disaccharides, and other refined carbohydrates exerts an osmotic effect in the bowel, causing water to rush into the lumen. This distends the lumen of the bowel, creating a sense of fullness and bloating.

As the simple sugars are acted upon by the lumenal enzymes of digestion, a rapid rise in blood glucose occurs. Insulin levels increase sharply in response to the carbohydrate load. A brief, severe drop in plasma glucose follows [12]. Counterregulatory hormones are then released to defend against the low blood sugar.

Counterregulatory hormone release is thought to be partially responsible for the vasomotor symptoms, which accompany the dumping syndrome. However, because of its short duration, dumping syndrome-associated hypoglycemia is not usually considered an etiology of significant neuroglycopenia [12,13].

In fact, the majority of RYGB patients seem to be unaware of their dumping syndrome-associated hypoglycemia. In the clinic, we are often surprised by how well our postoperative RYGB patients tolerate even severe levels of hypoglycemia (<40). Many are completely asymptomatic. Some have mild symptoms that they only realize as hypoglycemia-related when they experience the symptoms during glucose challenge testing in the laboratory.

Others have reported similar observations. Halperin et al. [14] showed that 50% of completely asymptomatic RYGB individuals had an interstitial glucose below 70 mg/dL, and 33% had a value below 60 mg/dL (as low as 40 mg/dL) following a mixed meal tolerance test (MMTT). Vidal et al. [15] reported that one third of asymptomatic RYGB patients developed hypoglycemia after MMTT. One eighth of these patients had a glucose <50 mg/dL [15]. Goldfine et al. [16] studied glucose response to a liquid mixed meal in patients with no hypoglycemic symptoms after GB surgery. Three of the nine subjects (33%) developed asymptomatic hypoglycemia [16].

Given that an increase in accidental death rates has been reported after GB, it has been speculated that a contributing factor to such accidents may be asymptomatic hypoglycemia [17]. It is unclear why similar glucose concentrations in some patients produce symptoms while others do not. An individual's susceptibility to neuroglycopenia may vary after GB, and further study is warranted.

Cryer [18] recently discussed the lack of hypoglycemia awareness on the basis of hypoglycemia-associated autonomic failure (HAAF). He points out that "hypoglycemia attenuates defenses (including increased epinephrine secretion and symptomatic defenses) against subsequent hypoglycemia in nondiabetic persons and patients with type 1 diabetes" [18]. Therefore, it is possible that recurrent hypoglycemia from dumping syndrome might cause defective glucose counterregulation. This could produce hypoglycemia unawareness. Within this construct, the issue for the RYGB patient may not be so much the degree of hypoglycemia but the range of responses to it. Some patients are clearly completely oblivious to hypoglycemia, while others are acutely sensitive to it.

SYMPTOMATIC NEUROGLYCOPENIC HYPOGLYCEMIA AFTER RYGB

Severe, symptomatic hyperinsulinemic hypoglycemia was first reported as a postoperative complication of GB in 2005 [19]. From its first description, this condition appeared to be very different from the common cases of hypoglycemia seen in relation to the dumping syndrome. As we began to evaluate patients in our own clinic for this condition, a pattern emerged that permitted us to differentiate it from the more common hypoglycemia associated with dumping syndrome.

In order to clarify the terminology, we have elected to separate our patients on the basis of whether or not they have a presentation of symptomatic neuroglycopenic hypoglycemia (SNH). For the purposes of this review, we will designate this severe form of postoperative hypoglycemia as SNH-GB. This is to distinguish it from other forms of postoperative hypoglycemia.

SNH-GB is almost never the cause of fasting hypoglycemia. A postoperative GB patient with fasting hypoglycemia should be considered for other conditions including insulinoma. Furthermore, SNH-GB does not generally appear in the immediate postoperative period. It usually seems to require months or even years after surgery to develop, whereas cases of insulinoma after GB may appear in the immediate postoperative period.

Unlike the hypoglycemia seen in connection with the dumping syndrome, SNH-GB is believed to be quite uncommon. Marsk et al. [20] reviewed the incidence of hypoglycemia after GB in Sweden using a nationwide cohort of 5040 patients. They analyzed the rates of hospitalization for hypoglycemia, confusion, syncope, epilepsy, and seizures. The median time from surgery to symptoms was 2.7 years. The risk for hypoglycemia and related diagnoses was less than twofold to sevenfold higher after GB patients. But the absolute risk was low at 0.2% [21].

Our clinical experience also supports a low incidence of SNH-GB. Our metabolic center has cared for more than 10,000 RYGB patients over the last 20 years. But we have less than 20 patients with SNH-GB.

SNH-GB is believed to be the result of endogenous hyperinsulinemia. Unlike patients with insulinoma, the hyperinsulinism in these cases is not present in the fasting state. Instead, the excess insulin is a physiologic, albeit exaggerated, response to food ingestion. Neuroglycopenia in these patients occurs in a timed sequence after meals. It is more exaggerated after carbohydrate intake [5].

A likely mechanism for SNH-GB is pancreatic islet beta-cell overperformance and secretion. The site of dysregulation is uncertain. It may be the result of enhanced glucose sensing by the beta-cell via the GLUT 2 transporter [2]. It is also possible that these patients have a mutation in their pancreatic glucokinase, which renders them overly sensitive to glucose levels. Either of these two conditions is expected to result in exaggerated insulin secretion in response to a glucose challenge. On the other hand, excessive insulin synthesis and secretion through transcription factors and release signaling may be taking place. The role of enterohormone beta-cell signaling has also been explored [22]. It may be that multiple mechanisms exist and that patients develop the condition from one or more mechanisms simultaneously.

It is also possible that mechanisms more typically seen with fasting hypoglycemia are at work in SNH-GB. These include glycogen depletion, malnutrition, or alterations in counterregulatory hormones. A fascinating aspect of this area is the role of decreased levels of ghrelin after RYGB. Ghrelin has recently been shown to increase glucose levels in starvation via its effect on growth hormone release. Therefore, the absence of ghrelin in a postoperative RYGB patient would be expected to contribute to some degree to hypoglycemia.

The anatomical reconstruction of the gastrointestinal system is responsible for hormonal changes that are favorable to the process of weight loss. In addition, these alterations have a normalizing effect on the patient's metabolism. The most widely studied changes include alterations in glucagon-like peptide1 (GLP1), glucosedependent insulinotropic polypeptide (GIP), peptide YY (PYY) levels, ghrelin, and leptin [23–25]. Some of these hormonal changes are also expected to favorably alter beta-cell function.

Incretins, especially GLP1, have been shown to be responsible for augmentation of insulin release after glucose consumption (the incretin effect). Many authors believe that this phenomenon is partially responsible for the early remission of type 2 diabetes as seen after RYGB [26,27]. The same incretin-related, exaggerated insulin response could explain the development of SNH-GB. Evidence for this possibility is found in a study by Goldfine et al. They demonstrated that neuroglycopenic patients have higher postoperative GIP and GLP-1 levels than RYGB without neuroglycopenia.

According to Campos et al. [28], the exaggerated levels of GIP and GLP-1 after RYGB generally decline after approximately 1 year in most cases. This coincides with the substantial weight loss and the improved insulin sensitivity that accompanies it [28]. In patients with SNH-GB, it is possible that elevated levels of GIP and GLP-1 persist longer than in RYGB patients without SNH [29].

Table 18.1 illustrates the characteristics of patients with SNH-GB that have been treated at our metabolic center.

TABLE 18.1
Symptoms and Severity of Hypoglycemia in SNH-GB Patients Treated at Our Metabolic Center

Age	Gender	Pre-op BMI	Post-op BMI	Time Post-op (year)[a]	Clinical Description	Timing (h)	Glucose (mg/dL)	Stage (I–III)[b]
38	F	55.5	32.4	0.9	Presyncope, confusion	2	22	I
22	F	47.0	32.3	2.1	Presyncope, blurred vision	Nonfasting	8	III
26	F	35.8	22.1	0.8	Presyncope, muscle weakness, memory loss	2	41	II
41	F	47.4	33.7	2.5	Altered mental status	Nonfasting	42	II
68	F	44.3	33.1	5	Diaphoresis, fatigue, tremors	Nonfasting	50	I
36	F	54.0	38.2	10	Hunger, carbohydrate cravings	1, 1.5, 2	45, 58, 65	I
29	F	59.1	40.1	2	Presyncope, fatigue	Fasting	68	II
64	F	44.0	31.1	0.5	Presyncope, tremors, fatigue	3	80	I
49	M	61.1	40.0	10	Asymptomatic	1.5, 2	54, 68	I
31	F	36.8	29.0	11	Asymptomatic	1.5, 2	30, 54	I
40	F	53.2	34.0	6	Asymptomatic	1.5, 2	21, 65	I
48	M	50.1	25.9	0.5	Nausea, fatigue, headaches	1.5	60	I
55	M	44.1	29.0	3	Presyncope, lightheadedness	2	52	I
53	F	50.0	22.4	1	Asymptomatic	2	40	I
22	F	65.0	34.7	2	Loss of consciousness	Nonfasting (CGM)	11, 14, 17, 43	I

[a] First neuroglycopenic episode.
[b] Our grading system will be discussed in the section titled Treatment Modalities.

PATHOPHYSIOLOGIC MECHANISMS

In Service et al.'s [10] initial description of hyperinsulinemic hypoglycemia, they described six GB patients 6 months to 8 years after surgery who suffered from refractory postprandial neuroglyco-penia. All had endogenous hyperinsulinemic hypoglycemia. One patient had evidence of an insulinoma. Selective arterial calcium-stimulation testing was positive in all six.

These patients underwent gradient-guided, partial pancreatic resection. The pancreatic pathology was consistent with nesidioblastosis. The findings included enlarged islets, hypertrophic beta-cells accompanied by multilobulated islets, enlarged and hyperchromatic beta-cell nuclei (Figure 18.1), and ductulo-insular complexes (Figure 18.2). All patients recovered after surgery [30–35].

Shortly after the report by Service et al. in the *New England Journal of Medicine*, Patti et al. [19] reported three patients with severe postprandial hypoglycemia and hyperinsulinemia. The patients

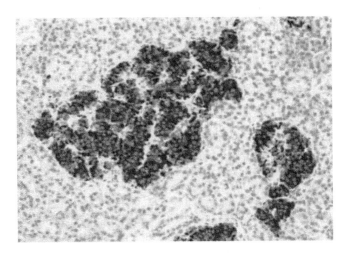

FIGURE 18.1   (**See color insert.**) The middle of the figure contains an enlarged islet from a patient with immunohistochemical staining for insulin. The islet appears approximately three times larger than the normal-sized islet in the lower right-hand corner of the figure. (From Service GJ et al., *N Engl J Med* 2005;353(3):249–54. With permission.)

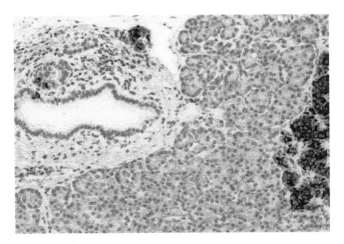

FIGURE 18.2   Pancreatic ducts shown with evidence of nesidioblastosis (insulin-positive cells). A portion of an enlarged islet with immunohistochemical staining for insulin is on the right. (From Service GJ et al., *N Engl J Med* 2005;353(3):249–54. With permission.)

were unresponsive to dietary and pharmaceutical intervention. In one patient, reversal of GB was attempted but was ineffective in reversing the hypoglycemia. All three patients ultimately underwent partial pancreatectomy for control of neuroglycopenia. In one patient, even this step was insufficient and total pancreatectomy was eventually performed. The pancreatic pathology of all patients revealed diffuse islet hyperplasia and expansion of beta-cell mass (Figure 18.3). In one of these cases, nesidioblastosis was reported as the pathological diagnosis.

Nesidioblastosis post-RYGB is considered a weight loss-independent effect of diabetes resolution in association with increased insulin release. The acquired form of nesidioblastosis may be due to the increase in levels of incretin hormones, which have been shown to have a trophic effect on pancreatic beta-cell mass in rodent models [36–38]. GLP1 induces the expression of the transcription factor pancreatic–duodenum homeobox1 (PDX1), which regulates islet growth [39]. Other explanations include overexpression of insulin-like growth factors, which may contribute to the islet-cell replication and nesidioblastosis [35].

Some authors argue that nesidioblastosis is not the cause of SNH-GB. It is possible that the hyperinsulinism observed results purely from hyperfunctioning beta-cells persisting from prolonged preoperative obesity [40,41]. Several of the patients with post-RYGB SNH who underwent partial pancreatectomy did not have histologic criteria for nesidioblastosis [42,43]. Thus, it remains unknown whether some patients have a predilection to developing nesidioblastosis or acquire nesidioblastosis post-surgery due to genetic or obesity-related effects [44]. Further research is needed to elucidate the specific causes.

Singh and Vella [45] proposed three pathophysiological mechanisms for SNH-GB: expansion of beta-cell mass, enhanced beta-cell function, and causes not related to the beta-cell. But they concluded that the mechanism "is most likely a combination of anatomic, hormonal, metabolic changes or an unrecognized genetic predisposition" [45].

With regard to the expansion of beta-cell mass, Singh and Vella cite the report of Service et al. as well as that of Patti et al. The latter also found islet hyperplasia in patients with hyperinsulinemic hypoglycemia after GB surgery. Patti et al. suggested that islet hypertrophy may be a characteristic of obesity and that hypoglycemia could be the result of unopposed action of the hyperplastic islets in the face of reduced postoperative caloric intake.

But Singh and Vella point out that this does not explain the lag time between the surgery and development of SNH-GB. They conclude that, "there is insufficient evidence to implicate a beta-cell

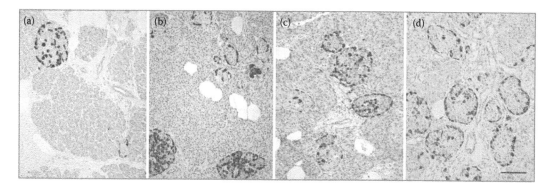

FIGURE 18.3   (a) Normal endocrine and exocrine pancreas enhanced with immunohistochemical staining for glucagon (*black*). (b) Patient 1. Islet hyperplasia seen by immunohistochemical staining for glucagon (*black*). (c) Patient 2. Islet hyperplasia seen by immunohistochemical staining for glucagon (*black*). Individual islets have a normal organization for humans but are in atypical clusters surrounding ductal profiles. Islets (*center*) are seen in close proximity to ductules that have glucagon-positive cells in their epithelium. (d) Patient 3. Islet hyperplasia seen by immunohistochemical staining for glucagon (*black*). Magnification bar (panel d) represents 100 μm. (From Patti ME et al., *Diabetologia* 2005;48(11):2236–40. With permission.)

anatomical pathology for hyperinsulinemic hypoglycemia in gastric bypass patients. The link between the two, if it exists, is best considered multifactorial and not mediated by a single factor" [45].

CLINICAL AND LABORATORY EVALUATION OF SNH AFTER RYGB

The evaluation of SNH-GB begins with a careful history and review of the laboratory data. As has already been discussed, a primary consideration is whether the episodes are fasting or postprandial in nature. Therefore, it is important to look for any fasting hypoglycemia patterns. This includes the possibility of nocturnal hypoglycemia, as this may also be a sign of fasting hyperinsulinemia. Such patients may require hospitalization to evaluate them for overnight hypoglycemia.

One of our most complex cases, for example, is a woman whose hypoglycemia almost always presents overnight. She failed medical management and required overnight home dextrose infusion to stabilize her.

An assessment of the patient's general health, weight stability, and hepatic and renal function should be obtained. The history should also focus on questions regarding the possibility of adrenal insufficiency, such as hyperpigmentation and orthostatic hypotension. One should also eliminate other causes of hypoglycemia such as excess alcohol consumption and hypoglycemic medications. Finally, it is also important to obtain a family history of hypoglycemia and to eliminate a pattern of multiple endocrine neoplasia (MEN) among family members.

The laboratory evaluation begins with the documentation of hypoglycemia by a venous laboratory sample at the time of symptoms. An accurate measurement of the degree of hypoglycemia is essential and should not rely on methodology such as that found in handheld finger-stick devices. However, devices such as the continuous glucose monitoring system (CGMS) may be of value to detect trends of glucose responses.

The classical criteria for the diagnosis of hypoglycemia are based upon Whipple's triad: (1) symptoms of hypoglycemia, (2) low plasma glucose at the time of symptoms, and (3) relief of symptoms with the correction of the low glucose [5]. In our experience, this is difficult to achieve by routine analysis, and we prefer to perform provocative testing in the laboratory.

We routinely employ a low-level (50 g), 2-h glucose tolerance test on our post-RYGB patients with symptoms of hypoglycemia. Plasma glucose is obtained every 30 min along with corresponding levels of plasma insulin. The patients are requested to record any and all symptoms during the provocative testing. They are also instructed to bring a low glycemic high-protein snack to the testing center to be consumed after completion of the study. Similarly, they are further instructed to record whether consumption of the snack resolved any symptoms presented during the test.

In addition to the glucose tolerance test, fasting C-peptide, and proinsulin levels, sulfonylurea screen and anti-insulin antibodies are recommended. We generally also perform an evaluation of pituitary and adrenal function in these individuals. For those in whom laboratory data suggest fasting insulin hypersecretion, anatomic evaluation is recommended utilizing advanced imaging techniques.

The findings of signs, symptoms, or both with a plasma glucose of less than 55 mg/dL, insulin of at least 3.0 uIU/mL, C-peptide of at least 0.6 ng/mL, and proinsulin of at least 5.0 pmol/L are indicative of endogenous fasting hyperinsulinism. Beta-hydroxybutyrate levels should be very low, 2.7 mmol/L or less. A plasma glucose response of at least 25 mg/dL after intravenous glucagon administration also points to hyperinsulinism [5].

TREATMENT MODALITIES

Cases of SNH-GB can present with symptoms such as loss of consciousness, confusion, presyncope, and seizures. Dietary control of symptoms is always initially preferred. Medical and surgical approaches also exist. We have proposed a simple method to designate SNH-GB patients into three subsets, grades I–III. Grade I patients generally respond to aggressive dietary intervention. Grade II patients require some form of medical therapy, whereas grade III patients generally require intravenous glucose maintenance and should be referred for corrective surgery.

Our gradation method is based on the treatment response, not the degree of hypoglycemia. We have documented cases of very severe hypoglycemia in each grade of SNH. We suspect that the difference in response to various treatment modalities is based on the underlying pathophysiology. The use of a grading system like the one we employ permits a progression of therapy based on the patients' requirements. This ensures that the least invasive modalities are applied in each case.

All patients should start therapy with a strict low-carbohydrate high-protein diet. If any carbohydrates are included at all, they should have a very low glycemic index. Meal timing is another useful consideration. Repeated intake of low glycemic carbohydrates (<10 g effective CHO) and high protein (>10 g high-quality protein) every 2 to 3 h may also be of value to promote euglycemia.

The patient should be instructed to avoid alcohol and limit caffeine consumption. For safety purposes, they should receive a handheld glucometer during their evaluation and be instructed on its use. Capillary blood sugar should be measured before activities that could place the patient at risk for accident or physical harm in the event of hypoglycemia. This includes such activities as driving, using power tools, ladders, etc. Because of its effect on glucose uptake, blood sugar should be measured before and after exercise. It should also be checked at bedtime and during the night, particularly if the patient experiences severe waking headaches, vivid dreams, nocturnal sweating, etc.

Family members should receive instruction on glucagon injection use, and the patient should be given a medical ID bracelet to identify the hypoglycemic condition to first responders.

We feel that the use of alpha glycoside inhibitors, such as acarbose, should be included as first-line therapy in all patients with SNH. These drugs slow the digestion of dietary starch so that glucose levels stabilize after meals. Thus, they can be considered as an augmentation of dietary therapy.

Grade I SNH patients will generally respond favorably to such diet-based therapy. Those who do not should be classified as grade II or grade III SNH cases.

Grade II patients should be considered for pharmaceutical therapy aimed at reducing hyperinsulinism. Calcium channel blockers (i.e., nifedipine or verapamil) decrease insulin release by affecting the calcium ion response at the beta-cell level [42].

Octreotide is an octapeptide with pharmacologic properties mimicking those of the natural hormone somatostatin. It has been used with varying degrees of success in nesidioblastosis to help decrease insulin hypersecretion. Diazoxide, when taken orally, is used in the treatment of hypoglycemia. It works by preventing release of insulin from the pancreas.

Patients who do not respond to either dietary or pharmaceutical approaches must be considered to have grade III SNH, which will require some form of surgical therapy. Often these patients must be initiated on parenteral intravenous dextrose infusion to maintain glycemia until surgery can be performed. In some cases, full total parenteral nutrition (TPN) therapy may be necessary. Another alternative is the placement of a gastrostomy feeding tube into the remnant stomach. This would permit administration of tube feeding formulas to the native stomach and duodenum, possibly normalizing glucose uptake and insulin response.

All patients with grade III SNH should undergo a surgical evaluation aimed at assessing the technical possibility of RYGB reversal. Although this is the logical step, it is not always possible because of the surgical anatomy or other clinical issues. In some cases, insurance qualification has been difficult to obtain.

But if surgical reversal is feasible, it should be presented to the patient with a thorough consideration of the risks and benefits. Patients who have been morbidly obese are often reluctant to reverse their weight loss surgery. However, given the life-threatening nature of their hypoglycemia, and the inability to control it with dietary or medical means, surgical reversal must be given its due consideration.

In some cases, the possibility of conversion to a sleeve gastrectomy or placement of an adjustable gastric band after reversal of RYGB has allowed patients to maintain their weight loss from the original surgery while still benefiting from the effects of resolved hypoglycemia. After reversal, especially with conversion to a sleeve gastrectomy, it is initially crucial to implement a low-carbohydrate diet in order to promote decreased insulin secretion [13].

At least one patient was reported to have hyperinsulinemic hypoglycemia after RYGB reversal [19]. In such severe cases, pancreatic resection, ranging from partial to total, may be necessary.

SUMMARY

In this chapter, we have provided an overview of the issues related to hypoglycemia after RYGB. We have reviewed the relevant literature and outlined current controversies as to the pathogenesis of this condition. Finally, we have presented recommendations for the evaluation and management of these cases based on our extensive experience.

ACKNOWLEDGMENTS

The authors acknowledge the assistance of Adel B. Mazanderani and Zachary Simon Rothkopf in the preparation of this manuscript.

REFERENCES

1. Sherwin RS, Felig P. Hypoglycemia. In: Felig P, Baxter JD, Broadus AE, Frohman LA, editors. *Endocrinology and Metabolism*. New York: McGraw-Hill, 1987, pp. 1179–201.
2. Gould GW, Holman GD. The glucose transporter family: Structure, function and tissue-specific expression. *Biochem J* 1993;295:329–41.
3. Brodows RG, Ensinck JW, Campbell RG. Mechanism of plasma cyclic AMP response to hypoglycemia in man. *Metabolism* 1976;25(6):659–63.
4. Jones TW, Borg WP, Borg MA, Boulware SD, McCarthy G, Silver D, Tamborlane WV, Sherwin RS. Resistance to neuroglycopenia: An adaptive response during intensive insulin treatment of diabetes. *J Clin Endocrinol Metab* 1997;82(6):1713–8.
5. Cryer PE, Axelrod L, Grossman AB, Heller SR, Montori VM, Seaquist ER, Service FJ. Evaluation and management of adult hypoglycemic disorders: An endocrine society clinical practice guideline. *J Clin Endocrinol Metab* 2009;94(3):709–28.
6. Hamdy O. Hypoglycemia: Practice essentials. Medscape Reference: Drugs, Diseases and Procedures, 2013 (cited 2013 August). Available from: http://emedicine.medscape.com/article/122122-overview#showall.
7. Cryer PE. The barrier of hypoglycemia in diabetes. *Diabetes* 2008;57(12):3169–76.
8. van der Crabben SN, Blümer RM, Stegenga ME, Ackermans MT, Endert E, Tanck MW, Serlie MJ, van der Poll T, Sauerwein HP. Early endotoxemia increases peripheral and hepatic insulin sensitivity in healthy humans. *J Clin Endocrinol Metab* 2009;94(2):463–8.
9. Vezzosi D, Bennet A, Rochaix P, Courbon F, Selves J, Pradere B, Buscail L, Susini C, Caron P. Octreotide in insulinoma patients: Efficacy on hypoglycemia, relationships with octreoscan scintigraphy and immunostaining with anti-sst2A and anti-sst5 antibodies. *Euro J Endocrinol* 2005;152: 757–76.
10. Service GJ, Thompson GB, Service FJ, Andrews JC, Collazo-Clavell ML, Lloyd R. Hyperinsulinemic hypoglycemia with nesidioblastosis after gastric-bypass surgery. *N Engl J Med* 2005;353(3):249–54.
11. Anderson RA. Chromium and polyphenols from cinnamon improve insulin sensitivity. *Proc Nutr Soc* 2008;67(1):48–53.
12. Tack J, Arts J, Caenepeel P, De Wulf D, Bisschops R. Pathophysiology, diagnosis and management of postoperative dumping syndrome. *Nat Rev Gastroenterol Hepatol* 2009;6:583–90.
13. Cui Y, Elahi D, Andersen DK. Advances in the etiology and management of hyperinsulinemic hypoglycemia after Roux-en-Y gastric bypass. *Gastrointest Surg* 2011;15(10):1879–88.
14. Halperin F, Patti ME, Skow M, Bajwa M, Goldfine AB. Continuous glucose monitoring for evaluation of glycemic excursions after gastric bypass. *J Obes* 2011;2011:869536.
15. Vidal J, Nicolau J, Romero F, Casamitjana R, Momblan D, Conget I, Morínigo R, Lacy AM. Long-term effects of Roux-en-Y gastric bypass surgery on plasma glucagon-like peptide-1 and islet function in morbidly obese subjects. *J Clin Endocrinol Metab* 2009;94(3):884–91.

16. Goldfine AB, Mun EC, Devine E, Bernier R, BazHecht M, Jones DB, Schneider BE, Holst JJ, Patti ME. Patients with neuroglycopenia after gastric bypass surgery have exaggerated incretin and insulin secretory responses to a mixed meal. *J Clin Endocrinol Metab* 2007;92:4678–85.

17. Adams TD, Gress RE, Smith SC, Halverson RC, Simper SC, Rosamond WD, Lamonte MJ, Stroup AM, Hunt SC. Long-term mortality after gastric bypass surgery. *N Engl J Med* 2007;357(8):753–61.

18. Cryer PE. Mechanisms of hypoglycemia-associated autonomic failure in diabetes. *N Engl J Med* 2013;369:362–72.

19. Patti ME, McMahon G, Mun EC, Bitton A, Holst JJ, Goldsmith J, Hanto DW, Caller M, Arky R, Nose V, Bonner-Weir S, Goldfine AB. Severe hypoglycaemia post-gastric bypass requiring partial pancreatectomy: Evidence for inappropriate insulin secretion and pancreatic isle hyperplasia. *Diabetologia* 2005;48(11):2236–40.

20. Marsk R, Jonas E, Rasmussen F, Näslund E. Nationwide cohort study of post-gastric bypass hypoglycaemia including 5,040 patients undergoing surgery for obesity in 1986–2006 in Sweden. *Diabetologia* 2010;53(11):2307–11.

21. Foster-Schubert KE. Hypoglycemia complicating bariatric surgery: Incidence and mechanisms. *Curr Opin Endocrinol Diabetes Obes* 2011;18(2):129–33.

22. Lautz D, Halperin F, Goebel-Fabbri A, Goldfine AB. The great debate: Medicine or surgery. What is best for the patient with type 2 diabetes? *Diabetes Care* 2011;34(3):763–70.

23. Hage MP, Safadi B, Salti I, Nasrallah M. Role of gut-related peptides and other hormones in the amelioration of type 2 diabetes after roux-en-y gastric bypass surgery. *ISRN Endocrinol* 2012;2012:504756.

24. Pournaras DJ, le Roux CW. Obesity, gut hormones, and bariatric surgery. *World J Surg* 2009;33:1983–8.

25. Karra E, Yousseif A, Batterham RL. Mechanisms facilitating weight loss and resolution of type 2 diabetes following bariatric surgery. *Trends Endocrinol Metab* 2010;21:337–44.

26. Cummings DE, Overduin J, Foster-Schubert KE. Gastric bypass for obesity: Mechanisms of weight loss and diabetes resolution. *J Clin Endocrinol Metab* 2004;89:2608–15.

27. Van Gaal LF, De Block CEM. Bariatric surgery to treat type 2 diabetes: What is the recent evidence? *Cur Opin Endocrinol Diabetes Obes* 2012;19:352–8.

28. Campos GM, Rabl C, Peeva S, Ciovica R, Rao M, Schwarz JM, Havel P, Schambelan M, Mulligan K. Improvement in peripheral glucose uptake after gastric bypass surgery is observed only after substantial weight loss has occurred and correlates with the magnitude of weight lost. *J Gastrointest Surg* 2010;14:15–23.

29. Bose M, Oliván B, Teixeira J, Pi-Sunyer FX, Laferrère B. Do incretins play a role in the remission of type 2 diabetes after gastric bypass surgery: What are the evidence? *Obes Surg* 2009;19:217–29.

30. Anlauf M, Wieben D, Perren A, Sipos B, Komminoth P, Raffel A, Kruse ML, Fottner C, Knoefel WT, Mönig H, Heitz PU, Klöppel G. Persistent hyperinsulinemic hypoglycemia in 15 adults with diffuse nesidioblastosis: Diagnostic criteria, incidence, and characterization of β-cell changes. *Am J Surg Path* 2005;29:524–9.

31. Hong R, Choy DY, Lim SC. Hyperinsulinemic hypoglycemia due to diffuse nesidioblastosis in adults: A case report. *World J Gastroenterol* 2008;14:140–4.

32. Kloppel G, Anlauf M, Raffel A, Perren A, Knoefel WT. Adult diffuse nesidioblastosis: Genetically or environmentally induced? *Human Pathol* 2008;39:3–8.

33. McElroy MK, Lowy A, Weidner M. Case report: Focal nesidioblastosis ("nesidioblastoma") in an adult. *Human Pathol* 2010;41:447–51.

34. Raffel A, Krausch MM, Anlauf M, Wieben D, Braunstein S, Klöppel G, Röher HD, Knoefel WT. Diffuse nesidioblastosis as a cause of hyperinsulinemic hypoglycemia in adults: A diagnostic and therapeutic challenge. *Surgery* 2007;141:179–83.

35. Rumilla KM, Erickson LA, Service FJ, Vella A, Thompson GB, Grant CS, Lloyd RV. Hyperinsulinemic hypoglycemia with nesidioblastosis: Histologic features and growth factor expression. *Mod Pathol* 2009;22:239–45.

36. Drucker DJ. Glucagon-like peptides: Regulators of cell proliferation, differentiation, and apoptosis. *Mol Endocrinol* 2003;17:161–71.

37. Hadjiyanni I, Baggio LL, Poussier P, Drucker DJ. Exendin-4 modulates diabetes onset in non obese diabetic mice. *Endocrinology* 2008;149:1338–49.

38. Perfetti R, Zhou J, Doyle ME, Egan JM. Glucagon-like peptide-1 induces cell proliferation and pancreatic-duodenum homeobox1 expression and increases endocrine cell mass in the pancreas of old, glucose-intolerant rats. *Endocrinology* 2000;141:4600–5.

39. Habener J, Stoffer D, Elahi D, Hani EH, Froguel P. Role of homeodomain transcription factor IPF 1 in the pathogenesis of diabetes mellitus. *Front Diabetes* 2000;15:197–205.

40. Meier JJ, Butler AE, Galasso R, Butler PC. Hyperinsulinemic hypoglycemia after gastric bypass surgery is not accompanied by islet hyperplasia or increased beta-cell turnover. *Diabetes Care* 2006;29:1554–9.

41. Patti ME, McMahon G, Mun EC, Bitton A, Holst JJ, Goldsmith J, Hanto DW, Callery M, Arky R, Nose V, Bonner-Weir S, Goldfine AB. Severe hypoglycaemia postgastric bypass requiring partial pancreatectomy: Evidence for inappropriate insulin secretion and pancreatic islet hyperplasia. *Diabetologia* 2005;48:2236–40. Comment from: Meier JJ, Nauck MA, Butler PC (2005).

42. Zagury L, Moreira RO, Guedes EP, Coutinho WF, Appolinario JC. Insulinoma misdiagnosed as dumping syndrome after bariatric surgery. *Obes Surg* 2004;14:120–3.

43. Abellan P, Camara R, Merino-Torres JF, Perez-Lazaro A, del Olmo MI, Ponce JL, Rayon JM, Pinon F. Severe hypoglycemia after gastric bypass surgery for morbid obesity. *Diabetes Res Clin Pract* 2008;79:e7–9.

44. Goldfine AB, Mun E, Patti ME. Hyperinsulinemic hypoglycemia following gastric bypass surgery for obesity. *Curr Opin Endocrinol Diabetes* 2006;13:419–24.

45. Singh E, Vella A. Hypoglycemia after gastric bypass surgery. *Diabetes Spect* 2012;25(4):217–21.

19 Micronutrient-Deficient Encephalopathy after Bariatric Surgery

Olga A. Melzer and Michael M. Rothkopf

CONTENTS

INTRODUCTION

With the rising epidemic of obesity in the United States, bariatric surgery has become a valuable option to achieve sustained weight loss and decrease the burden of metabolic comorbidities, such as diabetes and hyperlipidemia. It is recommended for patients with BMI > 40 kg/m^2 and BMI > 35 kg/m^2 with comorbidities related to obesity [1]. More than 100,000 weight loss procedures are performed annually in the United States [2]. Advancements in the surgical techniques resulted in the lowering of overall mortality rates in the immediate postoperative period [3]. However, as postoperative time elapses, the risks of nutritional deficiencies increase, especially in patients without close metabolic monitoring.

Neurologic complications of bariatric surgery have become increasingly recognized [4–6], with micronutrient-deficient encephalopathy (MDE) being the most disturbing of the group. This chapter will review the encephalopathy syndromes due to micronutrient deficiencies after bariatric surgery. Although patients with malabsorptive procedures are more likely to develop nutritional deficiencies, severe abnormalities were also seen in patients after purely restrictive surgeries. Thiamine deficiency is the most common etiology of MDE. However, other deficiencies can result in cerebral dysfunction and should not be overlooked. These conditions highlight the importance of close lifelong metabolic monitoring of patients after weight loss procedures.

In this chapter, we will review the published case reports of MDE following weight loss surgery. We will detail the original authors' description of each case. We will also describe the published large case study series of MDE after bariatric surgery. We will then proceed to summarize the prior literature reviews on the subject. We will describe our prior data analysis of the available literature and a comparison of encephalopathy types detected. Recommendations for postoperative bariatric metabolic monitoring will be suggested.

PUBLISHED CASE REPORTS

In 1981, Ayub et al. [7] described seven patients with metabolic encephalopathy after jejunoileostomy. The patients presented with episodic confusion, lethargy, slurred speech, and unsteadiness. The symptoms developed long after the procedure from 8 to 54 months. The episodes lasted from 2 hours to 4 days with spontaneous resolution. Although blurred vision was reported, nystagmus was not uniformly found. Only one patient responded to vitamin B complex supplementation. The etiologic mechanism was not identified.

In the same year, Reynolds et al. [8] reported three cases of metabolic encephalopathy after jejunoileostomy. Each patient presented at 1 year, 6 years, and 3 years after the surgery. Memory loss, speech difficulties, speech arrests, and paraphasia were common symptoms. Patients had normal liver function tests and levels of copper and zinc, and had no abnormal CT head findings. One patient had a thiamine level done, which was normal. All patients had resolution of their symptoms after procedure reversal with restoration of absorption. The cause of this reversible dementia was not determined.

In September of 1981, Rothrock and Smith [9] reported a case of metabolic encephalopathy occurring in a morbidly obese 33-year-old female. She presented with confusion, ophthalmoplegia, and ataxia 2 months after gastric stapling. The patient reported 3 weeks of protracted vomiting. Wernicke's encephalopathy (WE) was suspected on clinical presentation, and she was treated with parenteral thiamine. Her condition improved except for persistent gait problems. Thiamine deficiency was not confirmed.

In 1982, Haid et al. [10] reported two cases of metabolic encephalopathy after gastric plication for morbid obesity. Their first case was a 33-year-old female who presented with confusion, nystagmus, and ataxia. Her surgery was 15 weeks prior to the onset of symptoms. She reported protracted vomiting and minimal food intake for 10 weeks before development of her symptoms. She received multivitamins but no additional thiamine supplementation. She continued to deteriorate, became febrile, became comatose, was intubated, and died of septic shock. On autopsy, destructive lesions were found in the tectal area, mammillary bodies, and periventricular white matter.

Haid's second case was a 32-year-old female who presented with memory loss, ophthalmoplegia, and ataxia 10 weeks after surgery. She also reported protracted vomiting and minimal food intake for 4 weeks. She was diagnosed with Wernicke's syndrome based on her clinical presentation. She responded to parenteral thiamine with only mild persistent ataxia. Thiamine deficiency was not confirmed.

Milius et al. [11] described a case of metabolic encephalopathy occurring after gastric partitioning. The patient was a morbidly obese 32-year-old female who developed memory loss, nystagmus, decreased deep tendon reflexes, and ataxia approximately 3 months after the surgery. She responded to parenteral thiamine and multivitamins with only minimal residual memory deficit. Thiamine deficiency was not confirmed.

In response to the Haid publication, MacLean [12] reported a case of metabolic encephalopathy in a letter to the editor of *JAMA*. The patient was a morbidly obese 24-year-old female, who had gastric plication done approximately 4 months prior to the presentation. She developed headaches, organic brain syndrome, paretic gaze nystagmus, and ataxia after several weeks of recurrent vomiting. A CT of the head and cerebrospinal fluid (CSF) examination were both normal. The patient was given thiamine and responded with only minimal residual encephalopathy. Thiamine deficiency was not confirmed.

In 1983, Sassaris et al. [13] reported four cases of neuropsychiatric syndromes after gastric partitioning for morbid obesity, two of whom had metabolic encephalopathy. The first was a 40-year-old female who developed confusion, nystagmus, gait disturbance, and decreased deep tendon reflexes 2 months after surgery. She reported persistent vomiting prior to the presentation. She was treated with parenteral thiamine and trace elements. She partially improved but had residual gait problems and memory loss. Thiamine deficiency was not confirmed.

Sassaris et al.'s second case was a 30-year-old female who presented with memory problems, gait disturbance, and decreased deep tendon reflexes 2 months after surgery. She was treated with parenteral thiamine and nutritional support based on her clinical presentation. She recovered with some residual memory deficits. Thiamine deficiency was not confirmed.

In 1984, Fawcett et al. [14] described a case of metabolic encephalopathy occurring after gastric partitioning. The patient was a morbidly obese 45-year-old female who presented with confusion, ophthalmoplegia, decreased deep tendon reflexes, and ataxia approximately 1 month after surgery. The patient improved with thiamine and had no residual deficits. Thiamine deficiency was not confirmed.

Villar and Ranne [15] reported two cases of Wernicke's syndrome after gastric partitioning. Their first patient presented with ophthalmoplegia and ataxia approximately 1 month after surgery. The second developed nystagmus, ataxia, and loss of touch in all four extremities 8 months after surgery. Both patients reported protracted vomiting before the presentation. The second patient was reported to be lethargic. The first patient had a normal thiamine level. The second patient had a low thiamine level but normal red blood cell transketolase activity. Both patients responded to parenteral thiamine with only mild residual ataxia.

Despite having normal laboratory workup, the patients had a clinical presentation consistent with WE. The authors suggested that genetic defects at the level of thiamine-requiring enzymes may predispose those individuals to WE in the absence of severe thiamine deficiency. For example, they pointed out that magnesium deficiency impairs the utilization of thiamine and might exacerbate the effect of a mild thiamine deficiency.

In the same paper, Villar and Ranne reported on thiamine and red blood cell transketolase activity in 15 patients before and after gastric partitioning for morbid obesity. Thiamine and red blood cell transketolase activity dropped to low normal levels at 6 weeks after the surgery and recovered at 1 year.

In January 1985, Oczkowski and Kertesz [16] reported a case of WE after gastroplasty for morbid obesity. The patient was a 25-year-old female who presented with horizontal and vertical gaze paretic nystagmus, ophthalmoplegia, hypoesthesias, and ataxia. Her symptoms developed 14 weeks after the surgery. She reported a 4-week history of protracted vomiting and minimal food intake. She had no cognitive changes. CT and MRI of the head and CSF examinations were normal. The patient was treated with thiamine and had only nystagmus as a residual symptom. Thiamine deficiency was not confirmed.

In July 1985 Paulson et al. [17] reported six cases of metabolic encephalopathy after gastric partitioning for morbid obesity. The patients presented with confusion, psychosis, or coma between 1 and 4 months after the surgery. One had ophthalmoplegia, two had nystagmus, but the other three had no eye movement disorder. The response to thiamine was incomplete in these patients, although there was sufficient improvement in four to allow for a presumptive diagnosis of WE. Thiamine deficiency was not confirmed.

Two of the cases were felt to be due to an unknown cause. It is interesting to note that one of these patients had dysarthria as a presenting sign.

In 1985, Somer et al. [18] reported a case of metabolic encephalopathy after gastric plication. The patient was a morbidly obese 39-year-old male who developed memory loss, nystagmus, quadriparesis, and absent deep tendon reflexes 3 months postoperatively. CT of the head was normal. Folate and cyanocobalamin levels were low, but the red blood cell transketolase activity was in the high normal range. He was treated with total parenteral nutrition (TPN) and additional parenteral thiamine, folate, and carnitine with a partial improvement. Thiamine deficiency was not confirmed.

In 1987, Abarbanel et al. [3] analyzed neurologic complications among 500 bariatric surgery patients (457 Roux-en-Y gastric bypass; 43 gastroplasty). Only two patients had metabolic encephalopathy and responded to thiamine. The first patient, a 39-year-old female, had mild memory disturbance and nystagmus. Her symptoms resolved completely after parenteral thiamine. The second patient, a 26-year-old female, presented with confusion, ophthalmoplegia, and retinal hemorrhages. An electroencephalogram (EEG) showed diffuse slowing. CT of the head was normal. Her confusion and nystagmus improved gradually after parenteral thiamine; however, her polyneuropathy persisted. Thiamine deficiency was not confirmed in either of the cases.

In the same year, Kramer and Locke [19] described a case of metabolic encephalopathy 2 months after Roux-en-Y gastric bypass and gastric stapling for obesity. The patient was a 24-year-old female who presented with encephalopathy, nystagmus, blurred optic disk margins, and peripapillary hemorrhages. She had been taking multivitamins daily. Thiamine levels were not available. She had a normal CT of the head. She became febrile and semicomatose, and developed complete ophthalmoplegia. She was placed on a ventilator and was given TPN, antibiotics, and parenteral thiamine. Her ophthalmoplegia and mental status improved, but she had persistent Korsakoff's psychosis. Sixteen months later, she committed suicide. Postmortem examination of the brain revealed atrophic mammillary bodies and infarction at the superior aspect of the third ventricle. Cystic infarcts were also noted in the periventricular locations.

In 1988, Albina et al. [20] described a case of metabolic encephalopathy following vertical band gastroplasty. The patient was a morbidly obese 28-year-old male, who presented with a new onset seizure disorder, leg weakness, and nystagmus, 4 months after the surgery. He developed ophthalmopathy 2 months later. He responded to a course of TPN and enteral feeding. Thiamine deficiency was not confirmed.

In 1993, Primavera et al. [21] examined their database of 1663 patients who underwent biliopancreatic diversion for morbid obesity. Three of those patients, a 28-year-old female, a 55-year-old male, and a 34-year-old male, developed metabolic encephalopathy 2–5 months after surgery. All of the patients had mental status abnormalities, ophthalmoplegia, and unsteady gait. One patient recovered completely after thiamine administration, and the other two patients had residual deficits. Thiamine deficiency was not confirmed.

In 1996, Seehra et al. [22] described two cases of metabolic encephalopathy following vertical banded gastroplasty for morbid obesity. The first patient was a 55-year-old female who presented with confusion, nystagmus, and depressed deep tendon reflexes 4 months after surgery. She reported persistent vomiting 2 months before her symptoms developed. The patient responded to parenteral thiamine. Thiamine deficiency was not confirmed.

The second patient was a 40-year-old female who presented with confusion, disorientation, ophthalmopathy, and ataxia 5 months after surgery. She reported having protracted vomiting 2 months earlier, at which time the band was removed. The patient responded to parenteral multivitamins. Thiamine deficiency was not confirmed.

In 1997, Christodoulakis et al. [23] described a case of WE after vertical banded gastroplasty. The patient was a morbidly obese 25-year-old female who presented with ophthalmoplegia, paresthesia, and depressed deep tendon reflexes 4 months after surgery. She had no mental status changes. CT and MRI of the head and CSF examinations were normal. The patient responded well to parenteral thiamine. Thiamine deficiency was not confirmed.

In 1998, Grace et al. [24] described a case of metabolic encephalopathy after Roux-en-Y gastric bypass surgery. The patient was a morbidly obese 46-year-old male who presented with confusion and ataxia, 13 years after the surgery. He was reported to consume a large amount of alcohol. He had low levels of vitamin E, vitamin C, thiamine, riboflavin, pantothenic acid, pyridoxine, cyanocobalamin, selenium, zinc, copper, and magnesium. He responded to parenteral thiamine and a complex regimen of oral micronutrients.

In 1999, our group [25] reported a case of metabolic encephalopathy 20 years post-jejunoileostomy. The patient was a 61-year-old male who presented with episodic mental confusion, slurred speech, hemiparesis, and dysmetria. He was admitted for evaluation of a suspected acute stroke. CT of the head, cerebral angiogram, and MRI of the brain were normal. Laboratory data revealed low iron, magnesium, potassium, and cyanocobalamin. He had an anion gap of 21. Serum retinol level was extremely low at 2 µg/dL (normal range = 30–100). The 25-OH vitamin D was nondetectable. He responded to TPN and aggressive micronutrient repletion with resolution of his symptoms. He was followed closely for 11 years and given additional replacement therapy based on his laboratory findings. His neurologic symptoms never recurred.

There were four publications in 2000 of patients with metabolic encephalopathy following surgery for morbid obesity.

Kushner [26] described a case of metabolic encephalopathy after Roux-en-Y gastric bypass. The patient was a morbidly obese 48-year-old female who presented with memory loss, difficulty ambulating, and excessive weight loss 14 months after the surgery. She was treated empirically with parenteral thiamine followed by enteral nutrition and had a complete recovery. Thiamine deficiency was not confirmed.

Cirignotta et al. [27] described a case of metabolic encephalopathy after vertical banded gastroplasty. The patient was a morbidly obese 36-year-old female who presented with confusion, ophthalmopathy, quadriparesis, and absent deep tendon reflexes 3 months after the surgery. She had a history of bulimia. A cerebral MRI showed increased signal intensity in the periaqueductal gray matter, mammillary bodies, and dorsomedial thalamic nucleus. The patient responded well to parenteral thiamine.

Bozbora et al. [28] described the first case of metabolic encephalopathy after adjustable gastric banding. The patient was a 28-year-old female who presented with confusion and ataxia 6 weeks after the surgery. She reported episodes of recurrent vomiting. A cerebral MRI was normal. She was treated with parenteral thiamine based on clinical presentation and experienced a complete recovery. Thiamine deficiency was not confirmed.

Salas-Salvado et al. [29] described two cases of Wernicke's syndrome following surgery for morbid obesity. The first patient presented with ophthalmoptosis and ataxia 1 month after Roux-en-Y gastric bypass. She had undergone gastric banding 2 years earlier. She responded to parenteral thiamine and multivitamins. Thiamine deficiency was not confirmed.

Salas-Salvado et al.'s second case was a 31-year-old female who presented with severe vomiting 1 year after gastroplasty and gastrojejunal bypass. Bandelette stenosis was found and the band was surgically removed. She developed seizures, confusion, nystagmus, and ataxia in the postoperative period. CT of the brain was negative. Red blood cell transketolase activity was abnormal. She responded to parenteral thiamine and had a complete recovery.

In 2001, Toth and Voll [30] described a case of metabolic encephalopathy after banded gastroplasty for morbid obesity. The patient was a 35-year-old morbidly obese female who presented with disorientation, memory loss, nystagmus, asterixis, and ataxia 4 months after the surgery. She had a history of bulimia. CT of the brain was negative. A cerebral MRI showed increased signal intensity in the medial thalamic nuclei. The patient responded to parenteral thiamine, folate, and multivitamins with only residual nystagmus.

In 2002, Chaves et al. [31] reported four patients with neurological complications following Roux-en-Y gastric bypass for morbid obesity. An additional case in their series was a patient who had received an intragastric balloon for supermorbid obesity. Only one patient presented with metabolic encephalopathy. The average onset of symptoms was 2.4 months after surgery. All patients had persistent nausea and vomiting. The patients responded to thiamine and multivitamins with slow resolution of symptoms. Thiamine deficiency was not confirmed.

In 2003, Sola et al. [32] described a case of metabolic encephalopathy after laparoscopic Swedish adjustable gastric banding. The patient was a 24-year-old morbidly obese male who developed persistent nausea 3 months postoperatively. He was admitted and supported with intravenous therapy without multivitamins. He underwent band removal and developed ophthalmoplegia, decreased deep tendon reflexes, and ataxia. He responded to parenteral thiamine with resolution of his symptoms. Thiamine deficiency was not confirmed.

There were three publications in 2003 of patients with metabolic encephalopathy following surgery for morbid obesity.

Vanderperren et al. [33] reported a case of metabolic encephalopathy and respiratory failure after vertical banded gastroplasty. The patient was a 33-year-old morbidly obese female who presented with altered mental status, ophthalmopathy, lower extremity weakness, and decreased deep tendon reflexes 3 months after the surgery. The brain MRI showed an increased T2 signal in the thalamic area, around the third and fourth ventricle, and the periaqueductal midbrain. Red blood cell transketolase activity was decreased. Thiamine therapy was initiated with prompt clinical response.

Watson et al. [34] reported a case of metabolic encephalopathy after gastroplasty. The patient was a 26-year-old morbidly obese female who presented with confusion, ophthalmopathy, and ataxia 3 months after the surgery. MRI of the brain showed hyperintensity in the periaqueductal gray region. The patient responded to thiamine, with only residual nystagmus and difficulty with short-term memory.

Houdent et al. [35] reported a case of metabolic encephalopathy after gastroplasty. The patient was a 41-year-old morbidly obese male who presented with obtundation, memory loss, and nystagmus 4 months after the surgery. The thiamine level was low. The patient responded to thiamine.

There were three publications in 2004 of patients with metabolic encephalopathy following surgery for morbid obesity.

Loh et al. [36] reported a case of metabolic encephalopathy after Roux-en-Y gastric bypass. The patient was a 50-year-old morbidly obese male who presented with confusion, ophthalmopathy, and ataxia 2 months after the surgery. MRI of the brain showed gadolinium enhancement of the mammillary bodies and hyperintensity in the dorsal medial thalamus and periaqueductal gray region. The patient responded to thiamine, with only residual nystagmus and difficulty with short-term recall.

Escalona et al. [37] reported a case of metabolic encephalopathy after Roux-en-Y gastric bypass. The patient was a 35-year-old morbidly obese female who presented with cognitive impairment, dysarthria, nystagmus, ophthalmoplegia, and ataxia 1 month after the surgery. The patient responded to thiamine. Thiamine deficiency was not confirmed.

Nautiyal et al. [38] reported a case of metabolic encephalopathy after Roux-en-Y gastric bypass. The patient was a 46-year-old morbidly obese female who presented with nystagmus, lower extremity weakness, diminished deep tendon reflexes, and ataxia 3 months after the surgery. The initial brain MRI showed an increased T2 signal in the right putamen and caudate nucleus. The serum thiamine level was low. The patient responded to thiamine therapy.

There were three publications in 2005 of patients with metabolic encephalopathy following surgery for morbid obesity.

Fandino et al. [39] reported a case of metabolic encephalopathy after Roux-en-Y gastric bypass. The patient was a 43-year-old morbidly obese male who presented with confusion, diminished deep tendon reflexes, and ataxia 2 months after the surgery. The thiamine level was reduced. The patient responded to thiamine and multivitamins.

Parsons et al. [40] reported a case of metabolic encephalopathy after Roux-en-Y gastric bypass. The patient was a 24-year-old morbidly obese female who presented with respiratory failure, encephalopathy, weakness, visual disturbance, and ataxia 4 months after the surgery. MRI showed brainstem and thalamic abnormalities. She responded to thiamine.

Foster et al. [41] reported a case of metabolic encephalopathy after Roux-en-Y gastric bypass. The patient was a 35-year-old morbidly obese female who presented with confusion, ophthalmoplegia, diminished deep tendon reflexes, and ataxia 4 months after the surgery. The MRI showed hyperintensity at the floor of the fourth ventricle, medial thalami, and periaqueductal gray matter. The patient clinically responded to thiamine.

There were four publications in 2006 of patients with metabolic encephalopathy following surgery for morbid obesity.

Worden and Allen [42] reported a case of metabolic encephalopathy after Roux-en-Y gastric bypass. The patient was a 32-year-old morbidly obese female who presented with confusion, nystagmus, diminished deep tendon reflexes, and amnesia 4 months after the surgery. She responded to parenteral thiamine and TPN. Thiamine deficiency was not confirmed.

Al-Fahad et al. [43] reported a case of metabolic encephalopathy after Roux-en-Y gastric bypass. The patient was a 29-year-old morbidly obese female who presented with memory loss, ophthalmoplegia, diminished deep tendon reflexes, and quadriplegia 1 month after the surgery. She responded to parenteral thiamine. Thiamine deficiency was not confirmed.

Sanchez-Crespo and Parker [44] reported a case of metabolic encephalopathy after Roux-en-Y gastric bypass. The patient was a 30-year-old morbidly obese female who presented with confusion, nystagmus, ataxia, and quadriplegia 18 months after the surgery. She responded to parenteral thiamine.

Rothkopf [45] reported a 59-year-old female with metabolic encephalopathy, 35 years status post-jejunoileostomy. She developed episodic vertigo, confusion, slurred speech, expressive aphasia, and ataxia. There was no evidence of ophthalmoplegia. Acute cerebrovascular pathology was ruled out with imaging studies. Laboratory data revealed low levels of iron, magnesium, potassium, and vitamin B12. Several vitamin levels were extremely low, including vitamin A, vitamin E alpha, pyridoxine, and vitamin K1. The patient was started on TPN and aggressive micronutrient repletion with resolution of her symptoms.

There were two publications in 2007 of patients with metabolic encephalopathy following surgery for morbid obesity.

Juhasz-Pocsine et al. [46] described 26 patients with neurologic complications after bariatric surgery and reviewed the previous literature. Two of their patients, both female, had metabolic encephalopathy. Neither had a history of vomiting, but both had experienced profound weight loss. They presented 4 weeks after the surgery with confusion, ataxia, and diminished deep tendon reflexes but no ophthalmoplegia or nystagmus. They responded to parenteral nutritional support including thiamine with recovery of mental status; however, weakness and ataxia were persistent. The patients had no specific laboratory or imaging abnormalities that were reported by the authors. One of the patients had a normal thiamine level.

Makarewicz et al. [47] reported a case of WE after sleeve gastrectomy. The patient was a 38-year-old morbidly obese female who presented with confusion, hypokineses, nystagmus, diplopia with impaired eye movements, and peripheral neuropathy approximately 2 weeks after the surgery. She reported having uncontrolled vomiting. MRI of the brain was normal. She was treated with intravenous thiamine, wide spectrum multivitamins, mineral preparation, and TPN with resolution of eye symptoms and residual slight dementia. Thiamine deficiency was not confirmed.

There were two publications in 2008 of patients with metabolic encephalopathy following surgery for morbid obesity.

Bhardwaj et al. [48] reported a case of WE after Roux-en-Y gastric bypass. The patient was a 46-year-old female who presented with ataxia, blurred vision, vertigo, and intractable vomiting 3 months after the surgery. CT scan of the brain was normal. An EEG revealed epileptiform waves in occipital lobes, and she was started on valproic acid for possible seizures. After initiation of intravenous dextrose solution, she became progressively somnolent and had to be intubated. An MRI of the brain showed increased T2 signal in the mammillary bodies, medial thalamus, and extending inferiorly into the periaqueductal gray matter. She was treated with intravenous thiamine; however, she had incomplete recovery and remained ventilator-dependent at 6 weeks follow-up.

Rothkopf [49] reported a case of metabolic encephalopathy in a 48-year-old female 5 years after Roux-en-Y gastric bypass. The patient presented with a 3-month history of episodic vertigo, confusion, dysarthria, and ataxia. There was no evidence of nystagmus or ophthalmoplegia. CVA was ruled out with normal cerebral vascular imaging studies. Her labs showed low levels of vitamin C, biotin, and vitamin B6. Her symptoms resolved after several days of aggressive multivitamin supplementation.

In 2009, Velasco et al. [50] reported a case of WE after vertical banded gastroplasty. The patient was a 35-year-old male who presented 4 years after the surgery with blurred vision, gait instability with ataxia, and memory loss to recent events. He reported frequent vomiting and no multivitamin intake. MRI of the brain showed bilateral symmetric hyperintense signal in the mammillary bodies. Blood thiamine concentration was unobtainable at their institution. The patient was treated with intramuscular thiamine with slow resolution of his symptoms.

There were two publications in 2010 of patients with metabolic encephalopathy following surgery for morbid obesity.

Iannelli et al. [51] reported a case of WE after Roux-en-Y gastric bypass. Their patient was a 27-year-old female who presented 10 months after the surgery with a history of persistent vomiting and initially had no neurological signs. She was started on intravenous dextrose solution and in 5 days developed diplopia, nystagmus, quadriplegia, urinary incontinence, and memory loss to recent events. MRI of the brain revealed multiple ranges of subcortical edema in the occipital regions. She was treated with intravenous thiamine and had a complete recovery. Thiamine deficiency was not confirmed.

Ba and Siddiqi [52] reported a case of WE after Roux-en-Y procedure. The patient was a 47-year-old female who presented with tremor, generalized weakness, blurred vision, nystagmus, short-term memory loss, and disorientation 2 months after the surgery. She reported episodes of protracted vomiting. MRI of the brain was unremarkable. She was treated with intravenous thiamine and multivitamins with rapid resolution of her confusion and visual symptoms. Resting tremor persisted and later responded to levodopa. Thiamine deficiency was not confirmed.

There were four publications in 2011 of patients with metabolic encephalopathy following surgery for morbid obesity.

Jeong et al. [53] reported a case of WE after sleeve gastrectomy. The patient was a 24-year-old male who presented with difficulty walking, dysmetria, weakness, dysarthria, diplopia, and nystagmus 7 months after the surgery. His surgery was complicated by persistent anastomotic leak, and TPN was administered for 60 days without supplemental multivitamins or thiamine. MRI of the brain was normal. Blood thiamine level was reduced. The patient was treated with intravenous thiamine with gradual improvement of his symptoms.

Btaiche et al. [54] reported a case of metabolic encephalopathy after duodenal switch. The patient was a 58-year-old male who presented with severe fatigue, confusion, progressive neuropathies, and ataxia approximately 9 years after the surgery. MRI of the brain showed diffuse white matter disease. Blood work showed pancytopenia and multiple micronutrient deficiencies, including copper, zinc, vitamin A, vitamin E, and 25-hydroxyvitamin D. The authors attributed his symptoms to severe copper deficiency. The patient was treated with intravenous and oral copper and had gradual improvement of his symptoms with residual ataxia. It is unclear if he received a replacement of other micronutrients.

Rothkopf et al. [55] reported a case of WE after Roux-en-Y gastric bypass. The patient was a 52-year-old female who presented with a 3-week history of memory loss, gait disturbance, and ophthalmoplegia. She began to develop her symptoms approximately 1 year after the surgery. MRI of the brain was normal. The patient was treated with high-dose thiamine therapy with complete resolution of her symptoms. Thiamine deficiency was not confirmed. WE may respond to high-dose thiamine therapy even after a prolonged presentation. This patient most likely had persistent cytotoxic edema rather than demyelination even after 4 weeks of symptoms.

In the same year, Dennard et al. [56] described a case of non-Wernicke's cerebral dysfunction after laparoscopic adjustable gastric banding (LAGB). A 27-year-old female presented with a 2-year history of progressive fatigue, lightheadedness, dizziness, falling, vertigo, paresthesia, and dysarthria. MRI and EEG were unremarkable. She was 4 years s/p LAGB with a 250-lb. weight loss. She was noncompliant with the metabolic monitoring protocol and was not taking vitamin supplements as prescribed. She was admitted to the hospital because of severe syncope. She walked with a cane. Vitamin levels were obtained during the admission, and she was started on aggressive IV multivitamin and trace element replacement. Her workup revealed low levels of vitamin A, vitamin D, vitamin E, vitamin B6, and carnitine. Thiamine, niacin, cyanocobalamin, tocopherol, iron, and copper levels were normal. She was given replacement dosages of vitamins A, D, and B6 and carnitine while hospitalized and for 3 months thereafter. The patient experienced a full recovery and returned to normal activity.

There were seven publications in 2012 of patients with metabolic encephalopathy following surgery for morbid obesity.

Scarano et al. [57] reported a case of WE after sleeve gastrectomy. The patient was a 27-year-old female who presented with generalized fatigue, diplopia, hearing impairment, forgetfulness, balance disturbance, and distal muscle weakness 3 months after the surgery. She reported episodes of vomiting. MRI of the brain showed bilateral hyperintensities of the thalamus, periaqueductal gray matter, mammillary body, caudate nucleus, and striatum. Urinary thiamine level was low. She was started on intravenous thiamine therapy along with vitamin B12 and folate supplementation with progressive improvement in her status.

Sharabi and Bisharat [58] reported a case of WE after sleeve gastrectomy. The patient was a 43-year-old female who presented with generalized weakness, confusion, nystagmus, and diplopia 3 months after the surgery. She reported recurrent episodes of vomiting and poor oral intake. CT of the brain was normal. She was started on intravenous thiamine immediately. Her condition deteriorated and she required mechanical ventilation. Thiamine and vitamin B6 levels were low. Her neurological status was slowly improving. She was readmitted after 12 weeks of rehabilitation with septic shock and died of multiorgan failure.

Jethava and Dasanu [59] reported a case of WE after Roux-en-Y gastric bypass surgery. The patient was a 44-year-old female who presented with disorientation, memory deficits, nystagmus, difficulty following commands, ataxia, and hearing loss 1 1/2 months after the surgery. She reported persistent vomiting. MRI of the brain showed abnormal symmetric intraparenchymal signal in the thalami bilaterally. The blood thiamine level was low. She was treated with parenteral thiamine with partial resolution of her symptoms.

Kuhn et al. [60] reported a case of WE after combined gastroplasty with gastric banding for severe obesity. The patient was a 40-year-old female who presented with nystagmus, generalized muscle weakness, memory deficits, and ideomotor apraxia 3 months after the surgery. She reported a history of recurrent vomiting, and her diet was without vitamin supplementation. MRI of the brain showed high signal intensity lesions in the dorsomedial thalami, both hypothalami, mammillary bodies, mesencephalic tectum, and the periaqueductal gray region. She was started on intravenous thiamine with slow improvement in her symptoms. At 2 months follow-up, she had residual cerebellar gait syndrome and nystagmus.

Merola et al. [61] published a case of WE after Roux-en-Y gastric bypass as a clinical problem-solving case in the *New England Journal of Medicine*. The patient was a 31-year-old female who presented with an 8-month history of abdominal pain and vomiting 5 years after her surgery. She was started on intravenous fluid with dextrose and had an abrupt development of ataxia, oculomotor dysfunction, and encephalopathy. MRI of the brain showed enhancements and enlargement of the mammillary bodies. Whole blood thiamine was low. She also had deficiencies of folate, copper, zinc, and 25-hydroxyvitamin D. She was given intravenous thiamine and other micronutrients with improvement of her symptoms.

Moize et al. [62] reported a case of WE after sleeve gastrectomy. The patient was a 35-year-old female who presented with generalized weakness, ataxia, nystagmus, and ophthalmoplegia 3 1/2 months after the surgery. She reported frequent episodes of vomiting. Brain MRI showed hyperintense signals in the medial thalami, mammillary bodies, periaqueductal gray matter, and periventricular region of the third ventricle. Plasma thiamine level was low. She was treated with intravenous thiamine with resolution of her symptoms.

Becker et al. [63] reported a case of dry beriberi and WE after gastric lap band surgery. The patient was a 35-year-old woman who presented with somnolence, ophthalmoplegia, nystagmus, short-term memory loss, and generalized weakness 4 months after the surgery. She reported protracted vomiting prior to development of her symptoms. MRI showed bilateral high signal abnormalities in the thalami and hypothalamus and possibly the mammillary bodies. Thiamine, folate, and copper levels were low. She was treated with thiamine and multivitamins with improvement of her symptoms.

In 2013, Beh et al. [64] published a case of WE after gastric band procedure. The patient was a 48-year-old female who presented with progressive gait instability, leg paresthesia and weakness, nystagmus, and diminished reflexes 6 years after the surgery. She reported nearly daily vomiting episodes and excessive consumption of alcohol. MRI of the brain revealed hyperintensities of the mammillary bodies. Serum thiamine and folate were low. She was started on intravenous thiamine with complete resolution of her symptoms.

PUBLISHED RECORD REVIEWS OF NEUROLOGIC COMPLICATIONS AFTER WEIGHT LOSS SURGERY

As noted above, Abarbanel et al. [3] examined records of 500 patients who had bariatric surgery at their institution from 1979 to 1984. Twenty-three patients (4.6%) had neurologic complications. WE was found in two patients (0.4%). The authors noted that prolonged vomiting was a risk factor for WE in bariatric patients. Some patients had no clinical symptoms while following a low-carbohydrate diet. The use of intravenous dextrose infusions was a common precipitating factor. Parenteral thiamine was recommended for all bariatric patients who present with vomiting.

Thaisetthawatkul et al. [65] performed a retrospective analysis of 435 patients who underwent bariatric surgery at the Mayo Clinic from 1985 to 2001. They reported that 16% of bariatric surgery patients had neurological complications including mononeuropathies, polyneuropathies, and radiculoplexopathies. However, no encephalopathy cases were described.

Koffman et al. [66] reported metabolic encephalopathy in 30 patients (0.3%) after reviewing 9996 cases, 27 of whom had thiamine deficiency. The authors pointed out the implications of other micronutrient deficiencies in development of neurologic complications.

As noted above, Juhasz-Pocsine et al. [46] described 26 patients with neurologic conditions after bariatric surgery encountered in their tertiary medical center. Encephalopathy was described in two patients. Myelopathy was the most frequent problem. All patients had multiple nutritional deficiencies; however, they did not show dramatic improvement with correction.

LITERATURE REVIEWS

Several literature reviews have been published on the neurologic complications of bariatric surgery. In 2004, Berger [67] reported an incidence between 5% and 10% and described neurologic manifestations ranging from peripheral neuropathy to encephalopathy. It is clear that "no part of the neuraxis is exempt" from the micronutrient deficiencies of bariatric surgery.

In 2007, Singh and Kumar [68] performed a specific review of the development of WE after various types of bariatric surgery. They analyzed 32 previously published cases. Protracted vomiting was frequently seen in those patients.

In 2008, Aasheim [69] performed a literature search and identified 84 cases of WE. Most patients developed symptoms within 6 months after bariatric surgery. Frequent vomiting and intravenous glucose administration without thiamine were identified as risk factors. Aasheim also reported the follow-up results and showed that incomplete recovery was seen in 49% of patients, with residual memory deficits and ataxia.

In response to the systematic review by Aasheim, Sechi [70] published a Letter to the Editor pointing out the disturbingly high percentage of treatment failures. He stated that these could be attributed to delayed diagnosis, insufficient thiamine dose, and abnormalities in thiamine-dependent enzyme function. He also commented on the possibility of concomitant deficiencies of other micronutrients, such as vitamin B12, calcium, vitamin D, vitamin A, folic acid, iron, zinc, and magnesium.

DISCUSSION

We identified 81 published cases of micronutrient-deficient metabolic encephalopathy in patients after bariatric surgery. Overall, this is an uncommon neurological complication with reported incidence of 0.5%. Sixty-three of these cases are patients with confirmed or likely WE. The diagnosis was established based on either a classic clinical presentation with the triad of confusion, ataxia, and ophthalmopathy, positive objective laboratory/imaging data, or a response to thiamine supplementation.

However, 18 of the published cases could not be considered to be compatible with WE. They differed significantly from Wernicke's in terms of clinical symptoms, laboratory workup, or imaging studies. In fact, since many did not have a global cerebral dysfunction, some would argue that these cases did not even fall within the specific terminology of encephalopathy. Therefore, the term "micronutrient-responsive cerebral dysfunction" (MRCD) may be preferred. We believe that a careful analysis of the literature reveals that a subset of bariatric patients exists who are suffering from an alternate syndrome of MRCD other than Wernicke's.

CONFIRMED CASES OF WE

In our survey, 26 out of 81 patients can be classified as confirmed cases of WE, based on clinical presentation and objective confirmatory data. Objective data included laboratory findings of low serum thiamine, low urine thiamine, abnormal red blood cell transketolase activity, specific MRI brain findings, and autopsy results.

Eleven of the confirmed cases had the classic triad of confusion, ataxia, and ophthalmoplegia. Fifteen had two out of three symptoms, usually lacking ataxia (in nine patients). However, in several of those patients, gait abnormalities could not be tested. Four of the confirmed cases required ventilatory support.

Most of the patients with confirmed WE reported severe vomiting prior to the development of neurologic symptoms. Nineteen patients presented within 4 months after a bariatric procedure. Such a short latency period suggests depleted thiamine stores at baseline, which was further exacerbated by vomiting. Patients may not develop symptoms while they maintain a low-carbohydrate diet, which is generally advised in the early postoperative period. Carbohydrate intake, and particularly intravenous dextrose infusion, increases the requirement for thiamine and may have provoked WE in some of the patients.

CLINICALLY SUSPECTED CASES OF WE

Thirty-seven out of 81 patients had probable WE without objective confirmation. Eleven had the classic triad of confusion, ataxia, and ophthalmoplegia. Twenty-one cases had two of the three features, usually lacking ataxia (18 patients). All except five patients had ocular symptoms. Just as with cases of confirmed WE, most patients reported protracted vomiting prior to presentation. The latency period was short as well, within 4 months of surgery.

Some patients had a normal brain MRI. Thiamine levels were not done in the majority of cases. Villar and Ranne's case had a normal thiamine level despite classic symptoms of WE. Decreased affinity of enzymes to thiamine or defects in thiamine transport could have accounted for this discrepancy [71]. All patients showed a clinical response to thiamine supplementation.

Table 19.1 provides summary of both confirmed and suspected WE cases.

TABLE 19.1

Confirmed and Suspected WE Cases after Bariatric Surgery

Authors	Year	Surgery	Latency (months)	Age	Gender	Clinical Signs	Objective Confirmation	Clinical Confirmation
Ayub et al.	1981	Jejunoileostomy	54.0	35	M	Confusion, unsteadiness, slurred speech		Response to B complex
Rothrock	1982	Gastric stapling	2.0	35	F	Confusion, ophthalmoplegia, ataxia		Thiamine response
Haid et al.	1982	Gastric plication	3.0	33	F	Lethargy, nystagmus, ataxia, diminished DTRs	Autopsy	
Haid et al.	1982	Gastric plication	2.0	32	F	Memory loss, nystagmus, ophthalmoplegia, ataxia		Thiamine response
Milius et al.	1982	Gastric partitioning	3.0	32	F	Memory loss, nystagmus, diminished DTRs, ataxia		Thiamine response
Maclean	1982	Gastric plication	4.0	24	F	Organic brain syndrome, nystagmus, ataxia		Thiamine response
Sassaris et al.	1983	Gastric partitioning	2.0	40	F	Confusion, nystagmus, gait disturbance, diminished DTRs		Thiamine response
Sassaris et al.	1983	Gastric partitioning	2.0	30	F	Memory loss, gait disturbance, diminished DTRs		Thiamine response
Fawcett et al.	1984	Gastric partitioning	1.0	45	F	Confusion, ophthalmoplegia, diminished DTRs, ataxia		Thiamine response
Villar and Ranne	1984	Gastric partitioning	1.0	33	F	Ophthalmoplegia, ataxia		Thiamine response
Villar and Ranne	1984	Gastric partitioning	8.0	23	F	Nystagmus, paresthesia, ataxia	Thiamine level	
Oczkowski and Kertesz	1985	Gastroplasty	3.0	25	F	Nystagmus, ophthalmoplegia, hypoesthesia, ataxia		Thiamine response
Paulson et al.	1985	Gastric partitioning	3.0	30	M	Encephalopathy, confusion, psychosis, diminished DTRs, weakness, nystagmus		Partial thiamine response
Paulson et al.	1985	Gastric partitioning	2.0	53	F	Encephalopathy, confusion, psychosis, diminished DTRs, weakness, ophthalmoplegia		Partial thiamine response
Paulson et al.	1985	Gastric partitioning	4.0	42	F	Encephalopathy, confusion, psychosis, diminished DTRs, weakness		Partial thiamine response
Paulson et al.	1985	Gastric partitioning	0.6	20	F	Encephalopathy, conf, psychosis, diminished DTRs, weakness		Partial thiamine response
Somer et al.	1985	Gastric plication	3.0	39	M	Memory loss, nystagmus, quadriparesis, diminished DTRs		Thiamine, TPN response

Study	Year	Procedure		Age	Sex	Signs/Symptoms	Diagnosis	Response
Abarbanel et al.	1987	RYGB	12.0	39	F	Memory disturbance, nystagmus		Thiamine response
Abarbanel et al.	1987	RYGB	3.0	26	F	Confusion, ophthalmoplegia, retinal hemorrhage		Thiamine response
Kramer and Locke	1987	RYGB	2.0	24	F	Encephalopathy, nystagmus, blurred optic disk, perivascular hemorrhage	Autopsy	Response to TPN
Albina et al.	1988	VBG	4.0	28	M	Seizure, leg weakness, nystagmus, ophthalmoplegia		Thiamine response
Primavera et al.	1993	Biliopancreatic diversion	2.0	28	F	Mental status changes, ophthalmoplegia, unsteadiness		Thiamine response
Primavera et al.	1993	Biliopancreatic diversion	5.0	34	M	Mental status changes, ophthalmoplegia, unsteadiness		Thiamine response
Primavera et al.	1993	Biliopancreatic diversion	3.0	56	M	Mental status changes, ophthalmoplegia, unsteadiness		Thiamine response
Seehra et al.	1996	VBG	4.0	55	F	Confusion, nystagmus, diminished DTRs		Thiamine response
Seehra et al.	1996	VBG	5.0	40	F	Confusion, ophthalmoplegia		Thiamine response
Christodoulakis et al.	1997	VBG	4.0	25	F	Ophthalmoplegia, paresthesia, diminished DTRs		Thiamine response
Grace et al.	1998	RYGB	96.0	46	M	Confusion, ataxia	Thiamine level	
Kushner	2000	RYGB	14.0	48	F	Memory loss, difficulty ambulating		Thiamine response
Cirignotta et al.	2000	VBG	3.0	36	F	Confusion, ophthalmoplegia, quadriparesis, diminished DTRs	MRI	
Bozbora et al.	2000	AGB	1.5	28	F	Confusion, ataxia		Thiamine response
Salas-Salvado et al.	2000	RYGB	1.0	32	F	Ophthalmoplegia, ataxia		Thiamine response
Salas-Salvado et al.	2000	Gastroplasty and gastrojejunal bypass	12.0	31	F	Confusion, nystagmus, ataxia	Red blood cell transketolase	
Toth and Voll	2001	Banded gastroplasty	4.0	35	F	Disorientation, memory loss, nystagmus, asterixis, ataxia	MRI	
Chaves et al.	2002	RYGB	2.4	24	M	Encephalopathy, ophthalmoplegia, ataxia		Thiamine response
Sola et al.	2003	Swedish adjustable gastric banding	3.0	24	M	Nystagmus, diminished DTRs		Thiamine response
Vanderperren et al.	2003	VBG	3.0	33	F	Mental status changes, ophthalmoplegia, diminished DTRs	MRI	

(continued)

TABLE 19.1 (Continued)
Confirmed and Suspected WE Cases after Bariatric Surgery

Authors	Year	Surgery	Latency (months)	Age	Gender	Clinical Signs	Objective Confirmation	Clinical Confirmation
Watson et al.	2003	Gastroplasty	3.0	26	F	Ophthalmoplegia, ataxia	MRI	
Houdent et al.	2003	Gastroplasty	4.0	41	M	Memory disturbance, nystagmus	Thiamine level	
Loh et al.	2004	RYGB	2.0	50	M	Confusion, ophthalmoplegia, ataxia	MRI	
Escalona et al.	2004	RYGB	1.0	35	F	Cognitive impairment, dysarthria, nystagmus, ophthalmoplegia, ataxia		Thiamine response
Nautiyal et al.	2004	RYGB	3.0	46	F	Nystagmus, leg weakness, diminished DTRs, ataxia	MRI, thiamine level	
Fandino et al.	2005	RYGB	2.0	43	M	Confusion, diminished DTRs, ataxia		
Parsons et al.	2005	RYGB	4.0	24	F	Respiratory failure, encephalopathy, weakness, visual disturbance, ataxia	Thiamine level	
Foster et al.	2005	RYGB	4.0	35	F	Confusion, ophthalmoplegia, diminished DTRs, ataxia	MRI	
Worden	2006	RYGB	4.0	32	F	Confusion, nystagmus, diminished DTRs, amnesia		Thiamine response
Al-Fahad et al.	2006	RYGB	1.0	29	F	Memory loss, ophthalmoplegia, diminished DTRs, quadriplegia		Thiamine response
Sanchez-Crespo and Parker	2006	RYGB	18.0	30	F	Confusion, nystagmus, ataxia, quadriplegia		Thiamine response
Makarewicz et al.	2007	Sleeve gastrectomy	0.5	38	F	Confusion, hypokineses, nystagmus, diplopia, peripheral neuropathy		Thiamine and TPN response
Bhardwaj et al.	2008	RYGB	3.0	46	F	Ataxia, blurred vision, vertigo	MRI	Thiamine response
Velasco et al.	2009	VBG	48.0	35	M	Blurred vision, ataxia, memory loss	MRI	Thiamine response

Iannelli et al.	2010	RYGB	10.0	27	F	Diplopia, nystagmus, quadriplegia, urinary incontinence, memory loss		Thiamine response
Ba and Siddiqi	2010	RYGB	2.0	47	F	Tremor, weakness, blurred vision, nystagmus, memory loss, disorientation		Thiamine response
Jeong et al.	2011	Sleeve gastrectomy	7.0	24	M	Ataxia, dysmetria, weakness, dysarthria, diplopia, nystagmus	Blood thiamine level	Thiamine response
Rothkopf et al.	2011	RYGB	12.0	52	F	Memory loss, gait disturbance, ophthalmoplegia		Thiamine response
Scarano et al.	2012	Sleeve gastrectomy	3.0	27	F	Generalized fatigue, diplopia, hearing impairment, forgetfulness, balance disturbance	MRI, urinary thiamine level	Thiamine response
Sharabi and Bisharat	2012	Sleeve gastrectomy	3.0	43	F	Generalized weakness, confusion, nystagmus, diplopia	Blood thiamine level	Thiamine response
Jethava and Dasanu	2012	RYGB	1.5	44	F	Disorientation, memory deficits, nystagmus, ataxia, hearing loss	MRI, blood thiamine level	Thiamine response
Kuhn et al.	2012	Gastroplasty with gastric banding	3.0	40	F	Nystagmus, generalized weakness, memory deficits, ideomotor apraxia	MRI	Thiamine response
Merola et al.	2012	RYGB	60.0	31	F	Ataxia, oculomotor dysfunction, encephalopathy	MRI, blood thiamine level	Thiamine response
Moize et al.	2012	Sleeve gastrectomy	3.5	35	F	Generalized weakness, ataxia, nystagmus, ophthalmoplegia	MRI, plasma thiamine level	Thiamine response
Becker et al.	2012	AGB	4.0	25	F	Somnolence, difficulty walking, nystagmus, ophthalmoplegia, memory loss	MRI, thiamine level	Thiamine response
Beh et al.	2013	AGB	72.0	48	F	Gait instability, leg paresthesias, weakness, nystagmus, diminished DTR	MRI, serum thiamine level	Thiamine response

Note: AGB, adjustable gastric banding; DTRs, deep tendon reflexes; MRI, magnetic resonance imaging; RYGB, Roux-en-Y gastric bypass; TPN, total parenteral nutrition; VBG, vertical banded gastroplasty. Summary: 63 cases—36 restrictive, 23 combined, 4 malabsorptive; 50 women, 13 men; average latency 8.9 months; average age 34.8 years.

CLINICAL FEATURES AND PATHOPHYSIOLOGY OF WE AFTER BARIATRIC SURGERY

The diagnosis of WE is usually based on clinical grounds with the classic triad of confusion, ophthalmoplegia, and ataxia. However, only 30% of patients present with all three of the classic features [69]. Nystagmus and/or ophthalmopathy is usually found in the majority of patients, and confusion is the second most common symptom of the three [49]. Most patients present within the first 6 months after bariatric surgery. Gastric bypass or other restrictive procedures had been performed in most of the cases. Protracted vomiting was seen in many patients before the development of symptoms. In some cases, intravenous administration of glucose without thiamine was the precipitating factor.

The diagnosis can be confirmed by the presence of laboratory, imaging, or pathology data, consistent with thiamine deficiency. In the absence of objective testing, a therapeutic trial of thiamine administration with resolution of symptoms is a valid approach. Laboratory diagnosis can be based on either blood thiamine concentrations or by measuring the red blood cell transketolase activity.

Among imaging studies, brain MRI is considered the most valuable method to confirm diagnosis of WE. MRI studies typically show an increased T2 signal in the paraventricular regions of the thalamus, the hypothalamus, mammillary bodies, the periaqueductal region, the floor of the fourth ventricle, and midline cerebellum. On histological examination, multiple, small areas of hemorrhage with some spongiosis is seen mainly in the periaqueductal gray matter, the mammillary bodies, and medial thalamus.

Thiamine is a simple compound composed of pyrimidine and thiazole rings linked by a methylene bridge. The phosphorylated form of thiamine is a coenzyme in major cellular biochemical reactions, such as the alpha-ketoglutarate–dehydrogenase complex and the pyruvate–dehydrogenase complex in the tricarboxylic acid cycle, and transketolase in the pentose–phosphate pathway [72]. The total body thiamine store is 30–100 mg and can be depleted in as little as 18 days [71]. Thiamine deficiency may occur from inadequate intake, increased metabolic demands from high carbohydrate intake, and malabsorption.

Thiamine deficiency inactivates those enzymes and leads to a decrease in glucose utilization and ATP production. The transketolase reaction is involved in redox equilibrium, nucleic acid synthesis, and maintenance of membrane phospholipid integrity. Thiamine is also important in the conversion of glutamate to gamma aminobutyric acid. Glutamate accumulation may increase free radicals and neuronal excitotoxicity.

The biochemical changes of thiamine deficiency result in severe impairment of cellular functions, accumulation of lactate, acidosis, DNA fragmentation, and cytotoxic edema. Despite the extent of neuronal injury, many changes are reversible with prompt intravenous thiamine administration. However, delay in thiamine repletion may cause irreversible structural damage and residual neurologic deficits.

Magnesium is a cofactor that has a crucial role in the proper function of many enzymes, including transketolase and conversion of thiamine into thiamine pyrophosphate. Magnesium deficiency may be responsible for impairment of thiamine function with seemingly normal thiamine blood levels.

A genetic predisposition to WE was also proposed [15], with symptoms of WE occurring in the absence of abnormal blood levels of thiamine. Decreased affinity of transketolase for thiamine pyrophosphate and defects in thiamine transport systems could be contributing factors.

WE is considered a medical emergency, and thiamine should be administered based on clinical suspicion without awaiting diagnostic confirmation. Intravenous thiamine 500 mg every 8 h for 2–3 days followed by 250 mg thiamine until clinical improvement ceases should be given [73]. Smaller doses are not recommended and may not improve neurologic symptoms.

MRCD OTHER THAN WERNICKE'S

Although thiamine deficiency is the most common cause of MDE after bariatric surgery, cerebral dysfunction can result from other deficiencies and must not be overlooked.

Eighteen of 81 published MDE reports after bariatric surgery appeared to represent a syndrome distinctly different from WE. None of these patients had nystagmus or ophthalmoplegia. Many patients had episodic events rather than continuous symptoms. Dysarthria was commonly seen. The latency period was longer than that for the WE cases (>6 months after bariatric surgery), and protracted vomiting was not a common feature. Most patients had malabsorptive or combined weight loss procedures. The patients either had normal thiamine levels or did not respond to thiamine therapy. We have labeled these cases as *non-Wernicke's MRCD* occurring after bariatric surgery.

We previously performed a statistical analysis between published non-Wernicke's MRCD patients and those with either confirmed or suspected WE after bariatric surgery [74]. The presence or absence of each finding was analyzed using the chi-square test or Fisher's exact test. Continuous data, such as age and latency time, were reported as the mean ± standard deviation and were analyzed using the Student's t test. A stepwise multivariate regression analysis was performed with retention of the univariate variables at $P < .12$ for consideration in the final model. The statistics were conducted using the Statistical Package for Social Sciences, version 14 (SPSS, Chicago, IL). A P value of $< .05$ was considered statistically significant.

We found significant differences between the groups based on the case reports of vertigo ($P = .016$), ophthalmoplegia ($P < .001$), nystagmus ($P = .02$), and dysarthria ($P < .001$). The presentation tended to be affected by the type of surgical procedure, in that patients with malabsorptive surgery appeared to be more likely to develop a non-WE presentation ($P = .001$). When the analysis was limited to patients with confirmed WE, ophthalmoplegia ($P = .015$), nystagmus ($P = .049$), dysarthria ($P = .001$), and ataxia ($P = .032$) were significant factors. A multivariate regression model for all WE versus non-WE produced an R^2 value of .657 ($P < .001$) for the prediction of non-WE versus WE. This was true when the combined findings of the presence of dysarthria (standardized coefficient beta = −.447), the absence of ophthalmoplegia (standardized coefficient beta = .457), and the absence of nystagmus (standardized coefficient beta = .461) were identified. When the regression assessment was limited to confirmed WE relative to non-WE, the R^2 value was .547 ($P < .001$), and similar coefficients were noted: dysarthria (standardized coefficient beta = −.473), absence of ophthalmoplegia (standardized coefficient beta = .397), and absence of nystagmus (standardized coefficient beta = .349).

Therefore, we believe that these case reports represent a unique form of MRCD, which occurs in patients with a remote history of bariatric surgery. Patients presented with episodic neurologic impairment with mental confusion, slurred speech, and ataxia, mimicking cerebral ischemia, but without evidence of cerebrovascular disease. We believe that prolonged and severe depletion of multiple micronutrients, such as vitamins A, D, E, and B12 and copper, is the cause of these manifestations of cerebral dysfunction. Patients improved with aggressive micronutrient supplementation or with reversal of their malabsorptive procedure.

D-Lactic acidosis and hepatic failure have also been reported to cause metabolic encephalopathy after bariatric surgery. Those conditions have been ruled out in the presented cases. Thiamine deficiency would not be compatible with episodic manifestation of symptoms, as uncorrected deficiency would lead to cytotoxic edema, which would cause persistent symptoms without correction of the thiamine status.

Urea cycle abnormality was described recently as an alternative cause of metabolic encephalopathy after bariatric surgery. The first patient was reported by Hu et al. [75] in 2007. Their patient was a 29-year-old female who presented with intermittent encephalopathy associated with recurrent hyperammonemia, 6 months after bariatric surgery. Although she had low levels of copper and zinc, her symptoms correlated closely with elevation of ammonia level. Functional enzymatic assay showed markedly reduced ornithine transcarbamylase activity. The patient improved with protein-restricted diet and lactulose. This condition will be described in detail in the Chapter 20 on Hyperammonemic Encephalopathy after Roux-en-Y Gastric Bypass Surgery.

Table 19.2 provides a summary of the published MRCD cases other than WE after bariatric surgery.

TABLE 19.2

MRCD Cases Other than WE after Bariatric Surgery

Author	Year	Surgery	Latency (months)	Age	Gender	Clinical Signs Reported by Authors
Ayub et al.	1981	Jejunoileostomy	14.0	28	F	Episodic confusion, lethargy, slurred speech, unsteadiness
Ayub et al.	1981	Jejunoileostomy	13.0	52	F	Disorient, weakness
Ayub et al.	1981	Jejunoileostomy	8.0	36	M	Confusion, unsteadiness
Ayub et al.	1981	Jejunoileostomy	44.0	48	M	Somnolence
Ayub et al.	1981	Jejunoileostomy	220	27	F	Unsteadiness, weakness
Ayub et al.	1981	Jejunoileostomy	12.0	34	F	Confusion, unsteadiness, slurred speech
Reynolds et al.	1981	Jejunoileostomy	12.0	42	M	Memory loss, confabulation, paraphasia, speech arrests
Reynolds et al.	1981	Jejunoileostomy	68.0	52	F	Memory loss, paraphasia, speech arrests
Reynolds et al.	1981	Jejunoileostomy	31.0	32	F	Vertigo, weakness, speech difficultly
Paulson et al.	1985	Gastric partitioning	2.0	37	F	Encephalopathy, confusion, psychosis, diminished DTRs, weakness
Paulson et al.	1985	Gastric partitioning	1.5	26	F	Unsteadiness, confusion, psychosis, diminished DTRs, weakness, nystagmus
Rothkopf et al.	1999	Jejunoileostomy	240.0	61	M	Confusion, slurred speech, hemiparesis, dysmetria
Rothkopf	2006	Jejunoileostomy	420.0	59	F	Episodic vertigo, confusion, slurred speech, expressive aphasia, ataxia
Juhasz-Pocsine	2006	RYGB	1.0	24	F	Confusion, ataxia, diminished DTRs
Juhasz-Pocsine	2006	RYGB	1.0	31	F	Confusion, ataxia, diminished DTRs
Rothkopf	2008	RYGB	60.0	48	F	Episodic vertigo, confusion, dysarthria, ataxia
Btaiche et al.	2011	Duodenal switch	108.0	58	M	Severe fatigue, confusion, neuropathy, ataxia
Dennard et al.	2011	AGB	48.0	27	F	Dysarthria, paresthesia, vertigo, falls, dizziness, progressive fatigue

Note: AGB, adjustable gastric banding; DTRs, deep tendon reflexes; RYGB, Roux-en-Y gastric bypass. Summary: 18 cases—11 malabsorptive, 4 combined, and 3 restrictive; 13 women, 5 men; average latency 72.4 months; average age 40 years.

Theoretical Pathophysiology of Non-Wernicke's MRCD

Deficiencies of almost all vitamins and trace elements have been reported in bariatric patients. A number of these could potentially serve as the etiology for cerebral dysfunction. Principal among these are the fat-soluble vitamin deficiencies including vitamins A and E. Vitamin B12 deficiency could also be implicated. Among trace element deficiencies, copper deficiency would be the most likely contributor.

Vitamin A deficiency is commonly seen in bariatric patients. The term "vitamin A" refers to a subgroup of retinoids that have the biological activity of all-trans-retinol. Malabsorptive procedures typically result in more pronounced vitamin A deficiency. A follow-up study of patients who underwent biliopancreatic diversion and duodenal switch showed that the incidence of vitamin A deficiency was 52% after 1 year and 69% at 4 years [76]. Jorgensen et al. [77] showed that 95% of patients with jejunoileostomy had low levels of carotene at 15 years of follow-up.

Vision, cell communication, mucin production, embryogenesis, cell differentiation, and growth are some of many biological functions of vitamin A. Retinoids act as transcription factors, modulating messenger RNA formation in cell nuclei through receptors for retinoic acid (RAR) and its 9-cis isomer (RXR) with three subtypes (alpha, beta, and gamma).

The most well-known manifestation of vitamin A deficiency is xerophthalmia with impaired dark adaptation (night blindness) [78,79]. Vitamin A was also shown to have important role in the higher central nervous system function, although this is not traditionally discussed. Misner et al. [80] described retinoid signaling in synaptic plasticity. Cocco et al. [81] linked vitamin A to hippocampal function, related to learning and memory. Etchamendy et al. [82] reported selective memory impairment in vitamin A deficiency.

Corcoran et al. [83] demonstrated accumulation of amyloid beta in the cerebral blood vessels of vitamin A-deficient rats, similar to the pathology seen in patients with Alzheimer's disease. Other animal data support an important role of vitamin A in brain function. Captive lions develop vitamin A deficiency if not fed properly. They exhibit stargazing, ataxia, convulsions, and elevation of intracranial pressures. Supplementation of vitamin A reverses this condition [84,85].

Based on these reports, we can suspect that long-standing vitamin A deficiency in bariatric patients may contribute to the development of MRCD. Our clinical experience also supports this notion, as there was a correlation of patients' symptoms with vitamin A levels. Furthermore, there was a clinical response of the condition to vitamin A replacement.

Vitamin E refers to a group of molecules that exhibit the antioxidant activity of alpha-tocopherol. At least eight different molecules (tocopherols and tocotrienols) have alpha-tocopherol activity. Vitamin E is a potent free radical scavenger that stops propagation of lipid peroxidation in the cell membranes and plasma lipoproteins. Low levels of vitamin E have been reported in bariatric patients.

Nervous tissue, and particularly large-caliber myelinated axons, may be affected by vitamin E deficiency. Axonal degeneration may develop, followed by demyelination. Sokol [86] reviewed neurologic manifestations of vitamin E deficiency and compared the clinical features based on the underlying cause. The patients demonstrated hyporeflexia, cerebellar ataxia, loss of vibratory sense, loss of position sense, ophthalmoplegia, pigmented retinopathy, muscle weakness, and dysarthria. These symptoms bear a real similarity to the symptoms of patients reported with non-Wernicke's MRCD.

Vitamin B12 or cyanocobalamin is one of the most commonly identified deficiencies in bariatric patients. The reported incidence ranges from 30% to 70%, depending on the type of procedure performed, length of follow-up, and the routine use of nutritional supplements [5]. Our experience is that the severity of B12 deficiency in this population exceeds that commonly seen in other groups (i.e., the elderly). Repletion of vitamin B12 status in the bariatric patient may require repeated parenteral therapy and careful follow-up.

Absorption of vitamin B12 is a complex process and involves initial liberation of food protein-bound B12 in the stomach, transport of R-protein-bound B12 to the small intestine, binding with intrinsic factor under action of pancreatic proteases, and final absorption of IF–cyanocobalamin complex in the terminal ileum. Disruption of this process at any level can result in malabsorption of vitamin B12.

Methylcobalamin, an active form of cyanocobalamin, is an important cofactor in many methylation reactions, such as conversion of homocysteine to methionine, which is an important step in DNA synthesis. Other critical methylation reactions in the nervous system are dependent on vitamin B12-mediated methionine production. Neurological manifestations of vitamin B12 deficiency are broad. The most commonly described syndrome is subacute combined degeneration of the spinal cord, presenting with impaired perception of vibration and proprioception, spastic paresis, and extensor plantar response. Autonomic dysfunction is commonly seen. Alterations in higher brain function include dementia, psychosis, mood, and personality changes [87].

Once again, some of these symptoms are reminiscent of those reported in the published cases that we have labeled as non-Wernicke's MRCD. Therefore, it is possible that B12 deficiency plays a role in this syndrome.

Copper is a trace metal and a cofactor in a diverse variety of biochemical pathways, including but not limited to cytochrome-c oxidase in ATP synthesis, peptidylglycine monooxygenase in bioactive peptide synthesis and alpha-amidation of neuropeptides, phenylalanine hydroxylase in phenylalanine oxidation to tyrosine, and superoxide dismutase in free radical scavenging [54].

Although the incidence of copper deficiency in bariatric patients is rare, it is most likely being underdiagnosed in this population [5]. After recognizing it in a number of our patients, we have added copper levels to our routine annual postbariatric laboratory workup.

The clinical manifestations of copper deficiency mimic that of vitamin B12 deficiency and present as pancytopenia and neurologic dysfunction. Peripheral neuropathy, myelopathy, spastic gait, ataxia, optic neuropathy, encephalopathy, central nervous system demyelination, and polyradiculopathy can be seen. There have been cases of copper deficiency inducing reversible MRI findings [88].

Because of the symptom complex observed with copper deficiency, we feel it is important to consider it as part of the pathophysiologic mechanism of non-Wernicke's MRCD.

RECOMMENDATIONS

This chapter underscores the importance of close metabolic follow-up after bariatric surgery. Many patients have preoperative micronutrient deficiencies, which could be further exacerbated by weight loss surgery. Obtaining micronutrient levels and correcting deficiencies before the surgery, as well as semiannual metabolic monitoring after the surgery, should be the standard of practice.

The vitamin panel should include vitamin A, 25-OH vitamin D, alpha- and gamma-tocopherol, vitamin K1, thiamine, riboflavin, pyridoxine, biotin, folate, and cyanocobalamin. The mineral panel should include iron, iron saturation, ferritin, zinc, and copper. Routine laboratory workup should include complete blood count, comprehensive metabolic panel, magnesium, phosphorus, and urinalysis.

Previously, such monitoring was not recommended beyond 1 year after the surgery [67,68].

However, recognition of severe micronutrient deficiencies in patients long after surgery led to recent changes in these guidelines [49,89]. Such monitoring is particularly important for patients with malabsorptive procedures such as duodenal switch or combined procedures such as the Roux-en-Y gastric bypass. The level of deficiency may be quite severe, and patients may require parenteral micronutrient administration to correct the deficiencies.

It is important to recognize that even adequate stores of thiamine can be depleted in a few weeks without regular, ongoing intake. Furthermore, vomiting may rapidly accelerate depletion of total body thiamine. Bariatric patients should be considered at high risk for thiamine deficiency because of their intolerance of food and vitamin supplements, especially in the early postoperative period. Vomiting due to the process of adjusting to the new gastrointestinal anatomy is common. Therefore, the administration of parenteral thiamine is a valid precaution for all bariatric patients in the immediate postoperative period. Any bariatric patient who returns to the hospital because of vomiting or dehydration should be administered with intravenous thiamine as part of their admission medications.

Postoperative bariatric patients who present with a cerebral dysfunction that is not compatible with WE may be suffering from non-Wernicke's MRCD. In this case, aggressive repletion of a broader range of micronutrients will likely be needed for correction of symptoms. These should include vitamins A, D, E, and B12 and copper. Other deficiency states, such as carnitine or pyridoxine, may be present. D-Lactic acidosis and urea cycle disorders should also be considered.

SUMMARY

Eighty-one cases of MDE have been reviewed. The reported incidence is 0.5% and quite less common than peripheral neuropathy. Several review papers have been published on neurologic complications after bariatric surgery and the role of micronutrient deficiencies is being increasingly recognized.

The postoperative bariatric patient is at risk for thiamine deficiency. WE is the underlying cause in the majority of bariatric MDE cases. Patients usually present within 6 months after the surgery, and protracted vomiting frequently precedes the development of symptoms. One or more of the classic triad is generally present (confusion, ataxia, and ophthalmoplegia). Objective confirmation by means of laboratory or imaging studies may not be available. However, a response to thiamine administration can be considered as a clinical confirmation of WE in most cases. WE is a medical emergency, and the administration of thiamine should not be delayed for diagnostic testing. Failure to act quickly and aggressively may have serious long-term consequences.

About 25% of cases of postoperative bariatric MDE are not consistent with WE on their presentation. These patients generally present long after the bariatric surgery. Most of these cases will occur after procedures that contain an element of intestinal malabsorption. However, there have been three cases of non-Wernicke's MRCD occurring after purely restrictive procedures (gastric partitioning and banding). Vomiting is not a common feature of non-Wernicke's MRCD. Patients may display episodic symptoms, often mimicking those of a cerebrovascular accident. For reasons that are unclear at this time, dysarthria is often reported. We believe that this is a separate entity of metabolic encephalopathy secondary to a combination of multiple micronutrient abnormalities. Patients improved with either aggressive micronutrient supplementation or the reversal of their weight loss procedure and restoration of normal gastrointestinal anatomy.

The metabolic physician should be well aware of the signs and symptoms of WE. Every effort should be made to prevent its development. But if it does occur, it must be recognized and treated rapidly. A delay in therapy may have serious and prolonged consequences. The recent recognition of a non-Wernicke's MRCD points to another important category of neurologic disease that the metabolic physician should be prepared to recognize. In this latter case, aggressive repletion of the suspected micronutrient deficiencies will likely be needed for correction of symptoms. Other deficiency states, D-lactic acidosis, and urea cycle disorders should also be considered.

REFERENCES

1. NIH Conference Consensus Development Conference Panel. Gastrointestinal surgery for severe obesity. *Ann Intern Med.* 1991;115:956–961.
2. Steinbrook R. Surgery for severe obesity. *N Engl J Med.* 2004;350:1075–1079.
3. Abarbanel JM, Berginer VM, Osimani A, Solomon H, Charuzi I. Neurologic complications after gastric restriction surgery for morbid obesity. *Neurology.* 1987;37:196–200.
4. Kazemi A, Frazier T, Cave M. Micronutrient-related neurologic complications following bariatric surgery. *Curr Gastroenterol Rep.* 2010;12:288–295.
5. Becker D, Balcer L, Galetta S. The neurological complications of nutritional deficiency following bariatric surgery. *J Obes.* 2012;2012:608534.
6. Frantz D. Neurologic complications of bariatric surgery: Involvement of central, peripheral, and enteric nervous systems. *Curr Gastroenterol Rep.* 2012;14:367–372.
7. Ayub A, Faloon WW, Heinig RE. Encephalopathy following jejunoileostomy. *JAMA.* 1981;246:970–973.
8. Reynolds AF, Villar HV, Kasniak AW. Jejunoileal bypass: A reversible cause of dementia. *Neurosurgery.* 1981;9:153–156.
9. Rothrock JF, Smith MS. Wernicke's disease complicating surgical therapy for morbid obesity. *J Clin Neuroophthalmol.* 1981;1:195–199.
10. Haid RW, Gutmann L, Crosby TW. Wernicke–Korsakoff encephalopathy after gastric plication. *JAMA.* 1982;247:2566–2567.

11. Milius G, Rose S, Owen DR, Schenken JR. Probable acute thiamine deficiency secondary to gastric partition for morbid obesity. *Nebr Med J.* 1982;67:147–150.

12. MacLean JB. Wernicke's encephalopathy after gastric plication. *JAMA.* 1982;248:1311.

13. Sassaris M, Meka R, Miletello G, Nance C, Hunter FM. Neuropsychiatric syndromes after gastric partition. *Am J Gastroenterol.* 1983;78:321–323.

14. Fawcett S, Young GB, Holliday RL. Wernicke's encephalopathy after gastric partitioning for morbid obesity. *Can J Surg.* 1984;27:169–170.

15. Villar HV, Ranne RD. Neurologic deficit following gastric partitioning: Possible role of thiamine. *J Parenter Enteral Nutr.* 1984;8:575–578.

16. Oczkowski WJ, Kertesz A. Wernicke's encephalopathy after gastroplasty for morbid obesity. *Neurology.* 1985;35:99–101.

17. Paulson GW, Martin EW, Mojzisik C, Carey LC. Neurologic complications of gastric partitioning. *Arch Neurol.* 1985;42:675–677.

18. Somer H, Bergstrom L, Mustajoki P, Rovamo L. Morbid obesity, gastric plication and a severe neurological deficit. *Acta Med Scand.* 1985;217:575–576.

19. Kramer LD, Locke GE. Wernicke's encephalopathy. Complication of gastric plication. *J Clin Gastroenterol.* 1987;9:549–552.

20. Albina JE, Stone WM, Bates M, Felder ME. Catastrophic weight loss after vertical banded gastroplasty: Malnutrition and neurologic alterations. *J Parenter Enteral Nutr.* 1988;12:619–620.

21. Primavera A, Brusa G, Novello P, Schenone A, Gianetta E, Marinari G, Cuneo S, Scopinaro N. Wernicke–Korsakoff encephalopathy following biliopancreatic diversion. *Obes Surg.* 1993;3:175–177.

22. Seehra H, MacDermott N, Lascelles RG, Taylor TV. Wernicke's encephalopathy after vertical banded gastroplasty for morbid obesity. *Br Med J.* 1996;312:434.

23. Christodoulakis M, Maris T, Plaitakis A, Melissas J. Wernicke's encephalopathy after vertical banded gastroplasty for morbid obesity. *Eur J Surg.* 1997;163:473–474.

24. Grace DM, Alfieri MA, Leung FY. Alcohol and poor compliance as factors in Wernicke's encephalopathy diagnosed 13 years after gastric bypass. *Can J Surg.* 1998;41:389–392.

25. Rothkopf MM, Kuntz GR, Haverstick LP. Severe vitamin A deficiency masquerading as TIA is a late complication of intestinal bypass surgery. Abstract 110. Report on the 40th Annual Meeting, American College of Nutrition, 1999. *J Am Coll Nutr.* 1999;18(5):550.

26. Kushner R. Managing the obese patient after bariatric surgery: A case report of severe malnutrition and review of the literature. *J Parenter Enteral Nutr.* 2000;24:126–132.

27. Cirignotta F, Manconi M, Mondini S, Buzzi G, Ambrosetto P. Wernicke–Korsakoff encephalopathy and polyneuropathy after gastroplasty for morbid obesity: Report of a case. *Arch Neurol.* 2000;57:1356–1359.

28. Bozbora A, Coskun H, Ozarmagan S, Erbil Y, Ozbey N, Orham Y. A rare complication of adjustable gastric banding: Wernicke's encephalopathy. *Obes Surg.* 2000;10:274–275.

29. Salas-Salvado J, Garcia-Lorda P, Cuatrecasas G, Bonada A, Formiguera X, Del Castillo D, Hernandez M, Olive JM. Wernicke's syndrome after bariatric surgery. *Clin Nutr.* 2000;19:371–373.

30. Toth C, Voll C. Wernicke's encephalopathy following gastroplasty for morbid obesity. *Can J Neurol Sci.* 2001;28:89–92.

31. Chaves LC, Faintuch J, Kahwage S, Alencar FA. A cluster of polyneuropathy and Wernicke–Korsakoff syndrome in a bariatric unit. *Obes Surg.* 2002;12:328–334.

32. Sola E, Morillas C, Garzon S, Ferrer JM, Martin J, Hernandez-Mijares A. Rapid onset of Wernicke's encephalopathy following gastric restrictive surgery. *Obes Surg.* 2003;13:661–662.

33. Vanderperren B, Rizzo M, Van Calster L, Van den Bergh P, Hantson P. Difficult weaning from mechanical ventilation following Wernicke's syndrome developing after gastroplasty. *Intensive Care Med.* 2003; 29:1854.

34. Watson WD, Verma A, Lenart MJ, Quast TM, Gauerke SJ, McKenna GJ. MRI in acute Wernicke's encephalopathy. *Neurology.* 2003;61:527.

35. Houdent C, Verger N, Courtois H, Ahtoy P, Tenieren P. Syndrome de Gayet-Wernicke après gastroplastie pour obésité. *Rev Med Intern.* 2003;24:476–481.

36. Loh Y, Watson WD, Verma A, Chang ST, Stocker DJ, Labutta RJ. Acute Wernicke's encephalopathy following bariatric surgery: Clinical course and MRI correlation. *Obes Surg.* 2004;14:129–132.

37. Escalona A, Perez G, Leon F, Volaric C, Mellado P, Ibanez L, Guzman S. Wernicke's encephalopathy after Roux-en-Y gastric bypass. *Obes Surg.* 2004;14:1135–1137.

38. Nautiyal A, Singh S, Alaimo DJ. Wernicke encephalopathy—An emerging trend after bariatric surgery. *Am J Med.* 2004;117:804–805.

39. Fandino JN, Benchimol AK, Fandino LN, Barroso FL, Coutinho WF, Appolinario JC. Eating avoidance disorder and Wernicke Korsakoff syndrome following gastric bypass: An under-diagnosed association. *Obes Surg.* 2005;15:1207–1210.

40. Parsons JP, Marsh CB, Mastronarde JG. Wernicke's encephalopathy in a patient after gastric bypass surgery. *Chest.* 2005;128:453S–454S.

41. Foster D, Falah M, Kadom N, Mandler R. Wernicke encephalopathy after bariatric surgery: Losing more than just weight. *Neurology.* 2005;65:1987.

42. Worden RW, Allen HM. Wernicke's encephalopathy after gastric bypass that masqueraded as acute psychosis: A case report. *Curr Surg.* 2005;63:114–116.

43. Al-Fahad T, Ismael A, Soliman MO, Khoursheed M. Very early onset of Wernicke's encephalopathy after gastric bypass. *Obes Surg.* 2006;16:671–672.

44. Sanchez-Crespo NE, Parker M. Wernicke's encephalopathy: A tragic complication of gastric bypass. *J Hosp Med.* 2006;1(suppl 2):72.

45. Rothkopf MM. Reversible neurologic dysfunction caused by severe vitamin deficiency after malabsorptive bariatric surgery. *Surg Obes Relat Dis.* 2006;2:656–660.

46. Juhasz-Pocsine K, Rudnicki SA, Archer RL, Harik SI. Neurologic complications of gastric bypass surgery for morbid obesity. *Neurology.* 2007;68:1843–1850.

47. Makarewicz W, Kaska L, Kobiela J, Stefaniak T, Krajewski J, Stankiewicz M, Wujtewicz MA, Lachinski AJ, Sledzinski Z. Wernicke's syndrome after sleeve gastrectomy. *Obes Surg.* 2007;17(5):704–706.

48. Bhardwaj A, Watanabe M, Shah JR. A 46-yr-old woman with ataxia and blurred vision 3 months after bariatric surgery. *Am J Gastroenterol.* 2008;103(6):1575–1577.

49. Rothkopf MM. Micronutrient encephalopathy after bariatric surgery. In: Parsons WV, Taylor CM, editors. *New Research on Morbid Obesity.* Hauppauge, NY, Nova Science Publishers, 2008, pp. 185–204.

50. Velasco MV, Casanova I, Sanches-Pernaute A, Perez-Aguirre E, Torres A, Puerta J, Cabrerizo L, Rubio MA. Unusual late-onset Wernicke's encephalopathy following vertical banded gastroplasty. *Obes Surg.* 2009;19:937–940.

51. Iannelli A, Addeo P, Novellas S, Gugenheim J. Wernicke's encephalopathy after laparoscopic Roux-en-Y gastric bypass: A misdiagnosed complication. *Obes Surg.* 2010;20:1594–1596.

52. Ba F, Siddiqi ZA. Neurologic complications of bariatric surgery. *Rev Neurol Dis.* 2010;7(4):119–124.

53. Jeong HJ, Park JW, Kim YJ, Lee YG, Jang YW, Seo JW. Wernicke's encephalopathy after sleeve gastrectomy for morbid obesity. *Ann Rehabil Med.* 2011;35:583–586.

54. Btaiche IF, Yeh AY, Wu IJ, Khalidi N. Neurologic dysfunction and pancytopenia secondary to acquired copper deficiency following duodenal switch: Case report and review of the literature. *Nutr Clin Pract.* 2011;26:583–592.

55. Rothkopf MM, Haverstick LP, Nusbaum MJ, Scanlan D. Resolution of prolonged Wernicke's encephalopathy (WE) after bariatric surgery. 52nd Annual Meeting American College of Nutrition, November 2011.

56. Dennard D, Rothkopf MM, Haverstick LP. Micronutrient responsive cerebral dysfunction (MRCD) after laparoscopic adjustable gastric banding (LABG). 52nd Annual Meeting American College of Nutrition, November 2011.

57. Scarano V, Milone M, Di Minno MND, Panariello G, Bertogliatti S, Terracciano M, Orlando V, Florio C, Leongito M, Lupoli R, Milone F, Musella M. Late micronutrient deficiency and neurological dysfunction after laparoscopic sleeve gastrectomy: A case report. *Eur J Clin Nutr.* 2012;66:645–647.

58. Sharabi A, Bisharat N. Wernicke's encephalopathy after sleeve gastrectomy. *IMAJ.* 2012;14:708–709.

59. Jethava A, Dasanu CA. Acute Wernicke's encephalopathy and sensorineural hearing loss complicating bariatric surgery. *Conn Med.* 2012;76(10):603–605.

60. Kuhn AL, Hertel F, Boulanger T, Diederich NJ. Vitamin B1 in the treatment of Wernicke's encephalopathy due to hyperemesis after gastroplasty. *J Clin Neurosci.* 2012;19:1303–1305.

61. Merola JF, Ghoroghchian PP, Samuels MA, Levy BD, Loscalzo J. Clinical problem-solving. At a loss. *N Engl J Med.* 2012;367:67–72.

62. Moize V, Ibarzabal A, Dalmau BS, Flores L, Andreu A, Lacy A, Vidal J. Nystagmus: An uncommon neurological manifestation of thiamine deficiency as a serious complication of sleeve gastrectomy. *Nutr Clin Pract.* 2012;27:788–792.

63. Becker DA, Ingala EE, Martinez-Lage M, Price RS, Galetta SL. Dry beriberi and Wernicke's encephalopathy following gastric lap band surgery. *J Clin Neurosci.* 2012;19:1050–1052.

64. Beh SC, Frohman TC, Frohman EM. Isolated mammillary body involvement on MRI in Wernicke's encephalopathy. *J Neurol Sci.* 2013;334:172–175.

65. Thaisetthawatkul P, Collazo-Clavell ML, Sarr MG, Norell JE, Dyck PJ. A controlled study of peripheral neuropathy after bariatric surgery. *Neurology*. 2004;63:1462–1470.

66. Koffman BM, Greenfield LJ, Ali II, Pirzada NA. Neurologic complications after surgery for obesity. *Muscle Nerve*. 2006;33:166–176.

67. Berger JR. The neurological complications of bariatric surgery. *Arch Neurol*. 2004;61:1185–1189.

68. Singh S, Kumar A. Wernicke encephalopathy after obesity surgery. *Neurology*. 2007;68:807–811.

69. Aasheim ET. Wernicke encephalopathy after bariatric surgery. A systematic review. *Ann Surg*. 2008; 248:714–720.

70. Sechi GP. Peculiarities of Wernicke's encephalopathy after bariatric surgery. *Ann Surg*. 2009;249(6): 1066–1067.

71. Sechi GP, Serra A. Wernicke's encephalopathy: New clinical settings and recent advances in diagnosis and management. *Lancet Neurol*. 2007;6:442–455.

72. Pearce JMS. Wernicke-Korsakoff Encephalopathy. *Eur Neurol*. 2008;59:101–104.

73. Sechi GP. Prognosis and therapy of Wernicke's encephalopathy after obesity surgery. *Am J Gastroenterol*. 2008;103:3219.

74. Rothkopf MM, Sobelman JS, Mathis AS, Haverstick LP, Nusbaum MJ. Micronutrient-responsive cerebral dysfunction other than Wernicke's encephalopathy after malabsorptive surgery. *Surg Obes Relat Dis*. 2010;6:171–180.

75. Hu WT, Kantarci OH, Merritt JL 2nd, McGrann P, Dyck PJ, Lucchinetti CF, Tippmann-Peikert M. Ornithine transcarbamylase deficiency presenting as encephalopathy during adulthood following bariatric surgery. *Arch Neurol*. 2007;64:126–128.

76. Slater GH, Ren CJ, Siegel N, Williams T, Barr D, Wolfe B, Dolan K, Fielding GA. Serum fat-soluble vitamin deficiency and abnormal calcium metabolism after malabsorptive bariatric surgery. *J Gastrointest Surg*. 2004;8(1):48–55.

77. Jorgensen S, Olesen M, Gudman-Hoyer E. A review of 20 years of jejunoileal bypass. *Scand J Gastroenterol*. 1997;32(4):334–339.

78. Yarborough GW, Wilson FA, Feman S, Charles S, Chytil F, O'Leary JP. Retinopathy following jejuno-ileal bypass surgery: Report of a case. *Int J Obes*. 1982;6(3):253–258.

79. Chae T, Foroozan R. Vitamin A deficiency in patients with a remote history of intestinal surgery. *Br J Ophthalmol*. 2006;90:955–956.

80. Misner DL, Jacobs S, Shimizu Y, de Urquiza AM, Solomin L, Perlmann T, De Luca LM, Stevens CF, Evans RM. Vitamin A deprivation results in reversible loss of hippocampal long-term synaptic plasticity. *Proc Natl Acad Sci USA*. 2001;98(20):11714–11719.

81. Cocco S, Diaz G, Stancampiano R, Diana A, Carta M, Curreli R, Sarais L, Fadda F. Vitamin A deficiency produces spatial learning and memory impairment in rats. *Neuroscience*. 2002;115(2):475–482.

82. Etchamendy N, Enderlin V, Marighetto A, Pallet V, Higueret P, Jaffard R. Vitamin A deficiency and relational memory deficit in adult mice: Relationships with changes in brain retinoid signalling. *Behav Brain Res*. 2003;145(1–2):37–49.

83. Corcoran JP, So PL, Maden M. Disruption of the retinoid signalling pathway causes a deposition of amyloid beta in the adult rat brain. *Eur J Neurosci*. 2004;20(4):896–902.

84. Bartsch RC, Imes GD, Smit JPJ. Vitamin A deficiency in the captive African lion cub Panthera Leo. *Onderstepoort J Vet Res*. 1975;42(2):43–54.

85. Hartley MP, Kirberger RM, Haagenson M, Sweers L. Diagnosis of suspected hypovitaminosis A using magnetic resonance imaging in African lions (Panthera Leo). *J S Afr Vet Assoc*. 2005;76(3):132–137.

86. Sokol RJ. Vitamin E deficiency and neurologic disease. *Annu Rev Nutr*. 1988;8:351–373.

87. Cole M. Neurological manifestation of vitamin B12 deficiency. In: Goetz C, Aminoff M, editors. *Handbook of Clinical Neurology*, Vol. 26. *Systemic Diseases*. Part II. Amsterdam, Elsevier Science BV, 1998, pp. 367–405.

88. Kumar N, Ahlskog JE, Klein CJ, Port JD. Imaging features of copper deficiency myelopathy: A study of 25 cases. *Neuroradiology*. 2006;48(2):78–83.

89. Valentino D, Sriram K, Shankar P. Update on micronutrients in bariatric surgery. *Curr Opin Clin Nutr Metab Care*. 2011;14:635–641.

20 Hyperammonemic Encephalopathy after Roux-en-Y Gastric Bypass Surgery

Andrew Z. Fenves and Oleg A. Shchelochkov

CONTENTS

Roux-en-Y gastric bypass (RYGB) surgery has become the most common weight loss procedure performed in the United States [1]. This surgery involves the creation of a small gastric pouch and an anastomosis to a Roux limb of jejunum that bypasses 75 to 150 cm of small bowel, thus restricting food intake and limiting nutritive absorption [2].

There are many potential medical and surgical complications of this procedure. Some patients develop short bowel syndrome following this surgery. Other medical complications include hypoglycemia, micronutrient deficiencies, vitamin deficiencies, fat malabsorption, oxalate renal stones, and the late development of malnutrition.

A variety of neurological complications have been described as well, which include optic neuropathy, myelopathy, polyradiculoneuropathy, polyneuropathy, and encephalopathy, which will be the focus of this chapter [3]. A recent systematic review of serious neurologic complications following RYGB identified 58 patients who presented with symptoms of encephalopathy [3]. In many of these patients, symptoms were ascribed to Wernicke encephalopathy caused by acquired thiamine deficiency. However, low vitamin B1 could not be documented in all of the patients [3], thus suggesting that additional causes of encephalopathy may exist.

More recently, case reports [4–6] and one case series [7] described RYGB females with severe encephalopathy due to hyperammonemia. A common feature unifying these patients was the lack of appreciable chronic or acute liver damage. Indeed, in several patients who died of hyperammonemic coma, autopsy or prior liver biopsy revealed no features of cirrhosis.

This observation prompted us to consider the possibility of an inherited urea cycle abnormality as the underlying cause of hyperammonemia in these patients. Since all of the described patients were women, we hypothesized that unrecognized partial ornithine transcarbamylase (OTC) deficiency, an X-linked disorder uncovered by metabolic stress, could underlie some of these cases of RYGB-related hyperammonemic episodes. Consistent with this hypothesis is the report by Hu et al. [4], who described a RYGB patient with functional enzymatic analysis of OTC on the fresh-frozen liver tissue revealing less than 1% of the expected activity.

Between years 2008 and 2012, we have identified or become aware of several more patients with the above-described constellation of clinical findings, namely, women with symptomatic hyperammonemic encephalopathy after RYGB surgery in the absence of cirrhosis. To illustrate the typical features present in these patients, we describe several illustrative cases (the cases are numbered in the same order as in the subsequent tables).

CASE REVIEWS

Case 5

A 26-year-old Caucasian woman presented with confusion and generalized weakness. On admission, she was found to have hypotension and hypoglycemia. She had RYGB surgery 17 months prior to her presentation. Outpatient medications included folic acid, triamterene-hydrochlorothiazide, and pantoprazole. Her physical examination was notable for hypotension and anasarca.

Laboratory evaluation was remarkable for a peak ammonia level of 486 μmol/L and serum albumin of 1.3 g/dL. Imaging studies included an abdominal CT scan notable only for a fatty liver. The patient was treated with oral neomycin and levocarnitine, wide spectrum intravenous antibiotics for presumed sepsis, and total parenteral nutrition. Despite aggressive therapy, her confusion never resolved; she developed cerebral edema and seizures and ultimately expired. Autopsy revealed no evidence of cirrhosis.

Case 9

A 52-year-old Caucasian woman was admitted for evaluation and management of altered mental status. She had RYGB surgery 1 year prior to admission. Other medical problems included a long history of hypertension, end-stage renal failure requiring chronic outpatient hemodialysis three times a week, and a previous episode of deep venous thrombosis. Outpatient medication included amlodipine, carvedilol, lisinopril, folic acid, and famotidine.

Admission laboratory values were notable for a plasma ammonia level of 165 μmol/L, glucose of 33 mg/dL, elevated serum creatinine, and blood urea nitrogen. The patient was treated with oral lactulose and hemodialysis. Her encephalopathy slowly cleared over 1 week. She had a transjugular liver biopsy that revealed mild to moderate steatohepatitis and stage 2 fibrosis. Her mental status ultimately returned to her baseline, and she was discharged to a nursing home.

Case 11

A 46-year-old Caucasian woman presented with altered mental status. She had a previous RYGB surgery for obesity (exact date uncertain). The patient's comorbidities included seizures treated with levetiracetam, hypothyroidism treated with levothyroxine, bipolar disorder treated with duloxetine, peripheral vascular disease, right above-the-knee amputation, chronic obstructive pulmonary disease, history of systolic heart failure, and a previous pulmonary embolism.

On admission, she was unconscious, required intubation, and had an ammonia level of 450 μmol/L. Laboratory data were remarkable for a serum albumin of 1.8 g/dL, hematocrit of 29%, and an undetectable valproic acid level in blood. She was treated with oral lactulose and intravenous sodium benzoate. Her encephalopathy did not improve, and after taking into consideration the woman's multiple comorbid conditions, the patient transitioned to palliative care and expired 10 days after admission.

CASE 14

A 44-year-old African-American woman was admitted with confusion. She had a RYGB surgery 10 years prior to admission and underwent a revision 4 years after the initial surgery. Her plasma ammonia level on admission was 108 µmol/L, which then peaked at 243 µmol/L.

The patient was intubated on the day of admission. She had mild hypoglycemia with a blood sugar of 64 mg/dL, and her serum albumin was 1.7 g/dL. The patient's encephalopathy was refractory to treatment with intravenous sodium benzoate and oral lactulose. She received tube feedings for nutritional support. The patient developed progressive cerebral edema and seizures and expired. Autopsy revealed steatohepatitis but no evidence for cirrhosis.

CASE 15

A 41-year-old Latin American woman had RYGB surgery performed 16 months prior to presentation. She had a complex postsurgical course complicated by partial small bowel obstruction and poor wound healing. She developed chronic abdominal pain and lost about 70 kg in the months following surgery. She presented with generalized weakness and confusion.

Physical examination was notable for mild icterus. Admission laboratory data revealed a serum ammonia level of 99 µmol/L, albumin of 1.4 g/dL, total bilirubin of 3.1 g/dL, AST of 64 U/L, and hemoglobin of 9.3 g/dL. She was treated with oral lactulose with rapid improvement in her mental status. A liver biopsy revealed macrovesicular steatosis and moderate steatohepatitis, but no cirrhosis. She was discharged home with a normal mental status.

CASE 16

A 69-year-old woman underwent RYGB surgery 16 months prior to hospitalization. She lost 50 kg and developed episodes of confusion 12 months after surgery. During the hospitalization, her serum ammonia levels ranged between 181 and 201 µmol/L. Other labs during her hospital stay were notable for low serum zinc, copper, carnitine, and vitamin A levels. Her vitamin B_1, B_2, B_6, and B_{12} levels were measured in the normal range. Insulin levels were elevated during fasting.

Although an inherited disorder of ureagenesis was suspected, enzymatic analysis on fresh liver samples revealed an apparent normal OTC activity. The liver biopsy histology was notable for steatosis and a mild inflammatory infiltrate. The patient was treated with a low-protein diet, lactulose, neomycin, intravenous arginine, a 10% dextrose intravenous infusion, carnitine, zinc, copper, and biotin. The patient improved with an ammonia level falling to 33 µmol/L, and she was discharged from the hospital.

CHARACTERIZATION OF THE RYGB-RELATED HYPERAMMONEMIC ENCEPHALOPATHY

We summarized epidemiological characteristics, laboratory findings, and, whenever available, biopsy and autopsy results for all 16 women identified either clinically by our group or through a review of the literature (Tables 20.1 and 20.2). We note that all of the patients identified to date on the ground of their overlapping clinical features have been females. Their ages ranged from 26 to 69 years with the mean of 45 years. The time between the RYGB and the first reported hyperammonemic episode ranged between 1 month and 11 years.

In every patient, the gastric bypass achieves its clinical goal by leading to significant weight loss. Most of the patients had normal alanine aminotransferase (ALT), with few patients showing minimal elevations ranging from 62 to 66 U/L. Two patients also had mild elevations of serum bilirubin, 3.5 and 3.6 mg/dl, respectively, while the rest had normal values.

Ten of the 16 patients had at least one documented hypoglycemic episode. Baseline insulin levels were measured in three individuals, which were normal in two and elevated in the other. Zinc levels

TABLE 20.1

Clinical Data on 16 Patients Currently Recognized as Having Hyperammonemic Encephalopathy after RYGB Surgery

	Reference	Age (years)	Sex	Years since Bypass	Outcome	Hypoglycemia during Hospitalization
1	Hu	29	F	0.1	Survived	NA
2	Limketkai	35	F	6	Survived	No
3	Fenves	50	F	1.4	Deceased	Yes
4	Fenves	48	F	0.3	Deceased	Yes
5	Fenves	26	F	1.4	Deceased	Yes
6	Fenves	58	F	28	Deceased	Yes
7	Fenves	41	F	6	Deceased	Yes
8	BUMC 1	54	F	NA	Deceased	No
9	BUMC 2	52	F	1	Survived	Yes
10	BUMC 3	49	F	11	Survived	Yes
11	BUMC 4	46	F	NA	Deceased	No
12	Kentucky	39	F	2	Survived	NA
13	BUMC 5	38	F	4.4	Survived	Yes
14	Temple, TX	44	F	10	Deceased	Yes
15	BUMC 6	41	F	0.5	Survived	Yes
16	Morristown, NJ	69	F	1.3	Survived	NA

were reported to be low in 8 of 10 patients. Another notable feature that appears to be uniform in these cases is the severe hypoalbuminemia. All of the patients had marked hypoalbuminemia ranging from 0.8 to 2.5 g/dL (mean 1.7 g/dL).

Collectively, low serum albumin, zinc, and glucose levels reflect either malnutrition, synthetic liver dysfunction, or a combination of the two. The latter seems less likely as the patients' other laboratory tests assessing hepatic synthetic function such as a prothrombin time and bilirubin were not markedly abnormal. Neither did we find evidence of uniform cirrhosis. Indeed, 11 patients in this cohort either underwent a liver biopsy during their hospitalization or had autopsy results. Three of these subjects had mild to stage 2 fibrosis, whereas the others had steatosis, mild inflammation, or both.

The peak ammonia levels varied widely, ranging from 76 to 486 μmol/L. Interestingly in a few patients, the elevations did not exceed 100 μmol/L. Whenever measured, plasma glutamine, considered a surrogate marker of the long-term ammonia control, was either elevated or high normal in all subjects. Citrulline level was decreased in three of five measurements, suggesting either a proximal urea cycle defect or dietarily driven depletion of the urea cycle intermediate metabolites.

None of the patients had characteristic biochemical features of the distal urea cycle disorders, such as elevated citrulline, argininosuccinate, or arginine. An amino acid pattern of high plasma glutamine and low plasma citrulline can be seen in patients affected by OTC deficiency (see Figure 20.1). Orotic acid, a diagnostic marker for urea cycle disorders proximal to carbamoyl transcarbamylase deficiency, was measured in six patients and found elevated in five, again suggestive of the partial OTC deficiency in these patients (normal range 0.4 to 1.2 mmol/mol creatine; the mean level in our six patients was 3.4 mmol/mol).

Collectively, these findings prompted confirmatory genetic investigation in several of the described patients. Interestingly, sequencing of OTC in six patients failed to reveal known deleterious mutations. In three patients, fresh liver tissue was obtained by biopsy, and OTC enzymatic activity was measured. Two patients had very low activity, but the third patient had apparently normal enzymatic activity.

TABLE 20.2

Laboratory and Histologic Data on 16 Patients Currently Recognized as Having Hyperammonemic Encephalopathy after RYGB Surgery

	Reference	Albumin[a] (g/dL)	ALT[a] (U/L)	Bilirubin[a] (mg/dL)	Peak Ammonia Level (μmol/L)	Liver Biopsy Results	Zinc Level (μg/dL)	Urine Orotic Acid (mmol/mol creatine)	Glutamine (μmol/L)	Citrulline (μmol/L)	OTC Activity in Liver Tissue
1	Hu	2.1	44	NA	92	No cirrhosis	30	3.2	2018	17	<1%
2	Limketkai	1.6	26	1	342	No cirrhosis	NA	NA	nl	NA	NA
3	Fenves	2	43	1	138	NA	NA	NA	NA	NA	NA
4	Fenves	2	58	5	86	No cirrhosis	NA	NA	NA	NA	NA
5	Fenves	1.3	26	0.8	486	No cirrhosis	NA	NA	NA	NA	NA
6	Fenves	1.5	66	1.6	76	NA	NA	NA	NA	NA	NA
7	Fenves	2.1	29	7	68	No cirrhosis	NA	NA	NA	NA	NA
8	BUMC 1	0.8	34	1.1	205	NA	19	NA	1824	NA	15%
9	BUMC 2	1.1	39	1.7	171	Fibrosis stage 2	58	NA	1004	33	NA
10	BUMC 3	1.5	49	0.5	96	NA	23	NA	NA	NA	NA
11	BUMC 4	1.7	36	0.5	450	NA	35	3.6	NA	NA	NA
12	Kentucky	1.9	62	3.6	300	No cirrhosis	31	8	3210	11	NA
13	BUMC 5	1.4	43	1.3	157	No cirrhosis	25	1.8	905	NA	NA
14	Temple, TX	1.7	62	1.4	243	Minimal fibrosis	86	nl	1700	NA	NA
15	BUMC 6	1.8	38	3.5	99	Fibrosis stage 2	41	2.7	858	13	NA
16	Morristown, NJ	2.5	41	0.7	201	Steatosis; mild fibrosis	41	0.9	811	40	nl

Note: ALT, alanine aminotransferase; BUMC, Baylor University Medical Center; NA, not available; nl, normal.

[a] Values at time of hospital admission.

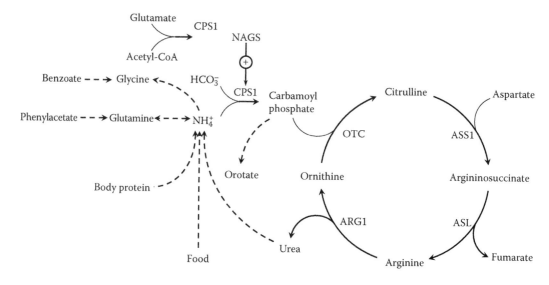

FIGURE 20.1 Clinical aspects of the urea cycle. Urea cycle is the primary metabolic pathway in humans that facilitates the disposal of nitrogenous waste. Urea, the primary vehicle of sequestered ammonia under normal physiological conditions, contains two atoms of nitrogen, one derived from ammonia channeled through carbamoyl phosphate and another from an amino group of aspartate supplied primarily by reactions of transamination. Although liver is the only human organ where physiologically meaningful ureagenesis can take place, other organs express some urea cycle enzyme. In particular, OTC is expressed in enterocytes facilitating synthesis of citrulline in the gut, and ASL is expressed in the kidney facilitating synthesis of arginine from citrulline delivered there via blood. All urea cycle disorders are autosomal recessive conditions, except for OTC deficiency, which is an X-linked condition. Nitrogenous waste in the form of ammonia is derived from several sources including food, urealytic activity of bacteria in the gut, natural and catabolic protein turnover, reactions of deamination and transamination of amino acids, and other nitrogen-containing compounds. The amount and ratio of nitrogen sources feeding into ammonia change constantly in response to various physiological stimuli such as nutritional status or illness. Urea cycle defects result in the blocking of the nitrogen flux through the pathway, thus stimulating synthesis of glutamine, a nonessential amino acid, which contains two amino groups. Partial OTC deficiency, the focus of this paper, results in elevation of ammonia, elevation of glutamine, decreased citrulline, and channeling of excess carbamoyl phosphate into the synthesis of pyrimidines, such as orotate. Nitrogen scavenger sodium phenylacetate and its precursor sodium phenylbutyrate sequester nitrogen by conjugating with glutamine and forming a water-soluble phenylacetylglutamine, which can be removed via kidneys. Sodium benzoate undergoes conjugation with glycine forming water-soluble hippuric acid, which can also serve as an effective ammonia sink. Abbreviations: NAGS, N-acetyl glutamate synthetase; CPS1, carbamoyl phosphate synthetase 1; OTC, ornithine transcarbamylase; ASS1, argininosuccinate synthetase; ASL, argininosuccinate lyase; ARG1, arginase 1.

One of the striking features of this RYGB-related hyperammonemia is the high mortality rate, up to 50% in our cohort. It is notable that in the more recent cases, patients had generally better outcomes. This can be due to a better awareness of this condition and more aggressive therapeutic interventions.

Patients that survived were treated with different modalities, including oral lactulose, oral neomycin, intravenous arginine infusion, oral levocarnitine, oral zinc supplements, and many with total parenteral nutrition. Unfortunately, it is not obvious which, if any, of these therapies was primarily responsible for better outcomes.

POSSIBLE MECHANISMS OF THE RYGB-RELATED HYPERAMMONEMIA

The mechanisms leading to this clinical syndrome require further elucidation. In patients whose biochemical profile was characterized by hyperammonemia, elevated glutamine, and low citrulline, proximal urea cycle disorders, such as partial OTC deficiency or mild CPS1 deficiency, should be considered. Partial OTC deficiency in heterozygous females may remain asymptomatic until patients become acutely or chronically challenged by sufficient physiological stress.

Our survey of possible mechanisms of the RYGB-related hyperammonemia suggests the existence of at least three possible contributing factors. First, a significant reduction in the nutritive intake following the RYGB procedure predisposes to a catabolic state leading to protein breakdown in the peripheral tissues. Protein breakdown is usually followed by reactions of deamination and transamination of freed amino acids fueling hyperammonemia.

Glutamine, a nonessential amino acid, which can be synthesized de novo in humans, harbors two amino groups and thus can serve as a temporary storage or buffer of ammoniac nitrogen. For this reason, glutamine is often considered a surrogate marker of the intermediate- and long-term ammonia control. However, the glutamine buffer has limited capacity to be an effective ammonia sink over a wide range of physiological conditions and therefore cannot prevent the development of hyperammonemia altogether.

Second, the role of nutritional deficiency should be considered and addressed in the diagnosis and management of RYGB-related hyperammonemic encephalopathy. Zinc deficiency can interfere with OTC function [8]. However, not all examined cases exhibited zinc deficiency. Hypoglycemia, another marker of catabolism, can further exacerbate hyperammonemia feeding into the vicious cycle of protein breakdown. Therefore, administration of large amounts of IV dextrose with or without IV insulin is often considered the cornerstone of hyperammonemia treatment as it can promote anabolism and sequestration of nitrogen in the protein in the muscle tissue.

Finally, one cannot ignore the unique anatomy of the Roux-en-Y anastomosis, which typically requires creation of a blind gastric and duodenal pouch. We cannot exclude the role of bacterial overgrowth with secondary increased urealytic activity in the blind proximal gastric and duodenal segment contributing to the increased ammonia production and its recirculation via the portal vein.

Also, we considered the unique role of intestinal enterocytes in the synthesis of citrulline—the key urea cycle intermediate forming the backbone of urea synthesis reaction. Citrulline is primarily synthesized in enterocytes. It is then transported by the blood stream to the kidneys and other organs, where arginine—another key metabolite in the urea cycle—is synthesized. It is not clear at this point whether Roux-en-Y anastomosis is able to interrupt this citrulline–arginine interorgan exchange sufficient to become a clinically relevant contributor to hyperammonemia.

CLINICAL AND DIAGNOSTIC CONSIDERATIONS

OTC deficiency is the most common form of urea cycle disorder [9]. OTC mutations are not picked up by sequencing in up to 10% to 20% of patients with clinical and biochemical features of OTC deficiency [10]. This fact can explain why some of the patients presented in this manuscript had no identifiable mutations despite their clinical presentation suggesting otherwise.

Shchelochkov et al. [11] demonstrated that an additional ~10% of cases of OTC deficiency can be identified on the OTC copy number analysis. Therefore, copy number analysis of OTC is usually considered as the second-tier test, when OTC sequencing fails to identify a deleterious mutation. Although, the focus of this publication was OTC deficiency, other urea cycle disorders should be considered if the diagnosis is not apparent.

A combination of plasma amino acid analysis, urinary orotic acid measurement, and molecular diagnostic methods is usually successful in reaching the final genetic diagnosis in most cases. Valproate-induced hyperammonemia should also be considered in patients treated for comorbid conditions such as seizures and bipolar disorder.

In some patients, the molecular diagnosis may remain elusive despite significant diagnostic efforts. In these cases, a physician may have to resort to liver biopsy and direct enzymatic assay to resolve the diagnosis. We recommend exercising caution when interpreting "normal" OTC activity in females with biochemical features of partial OTC deficiency.

Random X chromosome inactivation in females may result in a mosaic, "patchy" pattern of inactivation of X chromosome in the liver parenchyma. Therefore, a single core may not be sufficient to survey the global OTC activity in the entire liver.

Although the molecular nature of hyperammonemic episodes following RYGB requires further clarification, we would like to outline several broad treatment strategies, which clinicians can employ in the management of patients.

Establishment of hyperalimentation using IV dextrose (glucose infusion rate of 6–8 mg/kg/min) is often accompanied by IV insulin to maintain euglycemia. The use of IV lipids is usually necessary to achieve appropriate caloric intake. Careful management of protein intake to avoid both nitrogen overload and prolonged protein deprivation status can prove to be life-saving treatment modalities.

The use of oral citrulline, IV arginine, and nitrogen scavengers (sodium benzoate, sodium phenylacetate, sodium phenylbutyrate) have been described in detail elsewhere [12] and should be given strong consideration in patients without cirrhosis. In some patients, hemodialysis and hemofiltration may be necessary to lower and prevent rebounding of the ammonia levels. In cases when urea cycle disorder is proven or strongly suspected, prevention of future episodes of decompensation may require modification of the protein intake, supplementation with citrulline, arginine, and oral nitrogen scavengers.

Finally, our experience suggests that prompt diagnosis and management of RYGB-related hyperammonemia can pose a significant diagnostic challenge. Therefore, physicians involved in the assessment of candidates for RYGB should consider obtaining plasma ammonia, amino acid analysis, and urinary orotic acid as part of the routine preoperative workup.

In summary, we describe a unique and likely underrecognized clinical and biochemical syndrome of RYGB-related hyperammonemic encephalopathy characterized by high mortality. Although all of the patients recognized by us to date have been females, we suggest that health care providers maintain a high index of suspicion for a urea cycle disorder in males when they present with overlapping clinical findings. Our clinical experience suggests that prompt recognition of mild forms of urea cycle disorder uncovered by a physiological stress and institution of interventions described above not only can be life-saving for the index patients but can also lead to the recognition of urea cycle disorders in their relatives.

ACKNOWLEDGMENTS

We thank Dr. Sandesh C Nagamani from Baylor College of Medicine for his thoughtful comments and suggestions to improve the manuscript.

REFERENCES

1. Samuel I, Mason EE, Renquist KE et al. Bariatric surgery trends: An 18-year report from the International Bariatric Surgery registry. *Am J Surg*. 2006; 192: 657–662.
2. Elder KA, Wolfe BM. Bariatric surgery: A review of procedures and outcomes. *Gastroenterology*. 2007; 132: 2253–2271.
3. Juhasz-Pocsine K, Rudnicki SA, Archer RL, Harik SI. Neurologic complications of gastric bypass surgery for morbid obesity. *Neurology*. 2007; 68: 1843–1850.
4. Hu WT, Kantarci OH, Merritt LJ, McGrann P et al. Ornithine transcarbamylase deficiency presenting as encephalopathy during adulthood following bariatric surgery. *Arch Neurol*. 2007; 64: 126–128.
5. Limketkai BN, Zucker SD. Hyperammonemic encephalopathy caused by carnitine deficiency. *J Gen Intern Med*. 2007; 23 (2): 210–213.
6. Goodin KM, Pantalos D, Platky K, Gowans G et al. Asymptomatic carrier of ornithine transcarbamylase deficiency unmasked by bariatric surgery. Abstract presented as a poster. Annual Clinical Genetics Meeting, University of Louisville, Louisville, KY, 2010.
7. Fenves A, Boland CR, Lepe R, Rivera-Torres P et al. Fatal hyperammonemic encephalopathy after gastric bypass surgery. *Am J Med*. 2008; 121 (1): e1–e2.

8. Aquilio E, Spagnoli R, Riggio D, Seri S. Effects of zinc on hepatic ornithine transcarbamylase (OTC) activity. *J Trace Elem Electrolytes Health Dis.* 1993; 7: 240–241.

9. Brusilow S, Horwich A. Urea cycle enzymes. In: Scriver C, Sly W, Valle D, Childs B, Kinzler K, Vogelstein B, eds. *The Metabolic and Molecular Basis of Inherited Disease*, 8th edition. New York: McGraw-Hill; 2000: 1909–1963.

10. Yamaguchi S, Brailey LL, Morizono H et al. Mutations and polymorphisms in the human ornithine transcarbamylase (OTC) gene. *Hum Mutat.* 2006; 27: 626–632.

11. Shchelochkov OA, Li FY, Geraghty MT, Gallagher RC et al. High-frequency detection of deletions and variable rearrangements at the ornithine transcarbamylase (OTC) locus by oligonucleotide array CGH. *Mol Genet Metab.* 2009; 96 (3): 97–105.

12. Lichter-Konecki U, Caldovic L, Morizono H, Simpson K. Ornithine carbamoyltransferase deficiency, OTC deficiency. GeneReviews; 2013. TM-NCBI Bookshelf. Available at http://www.ncbi.nlm.nih.gov /books/NBK154378.

Section III

Diseases of Undernutrition and Absorption

21 Bedside Diagnosis of Malnutrition

Arthur D. Heller

CONTENTS

And this I know, moreover, that to the human body it makes a great difference if the bread be fine or coarse, of wheat with or without the hull…baked or raw…Whoever pays no attention to these things, or paying attention, does not comprehend them, how can he understand the diseases which befall a man? For, by every one of these things a man is affected and changed this way or that, and the whole of his life is subjected to them, whether in health, convalescence, or disease. Nothing else then can be more important or more necessary to know, than these things.

Hippocrates
On Ancient Medicine

INTRODUCTION

Mention malnutrition and the mental picture is of the undernourished: starving babies with bloated stomachs in some Third World backwater or skid-row alcoholics suffering from deficiency diseases that have long been largely eradicated in the United States [1,2]. Although that archetype may be true, it is inadequate, incomplete, and inaccurate. Significant numbers of hospitalized patients are undernourished, with relatively simple means to identify them [3,4]. In addition, as we have seen in this country, and increasingly in much of the developed world, it is the overfed, typically obese or overweight, that can impact health resources of the individual and society as much or more than the underfed [5]. In Hippocrates' *Aphorisms*, he states that "Excess of food produces disease, and at the same time, points out the remedy" (Section 1, Aphorism 17). He later states, "Those who are by nature very corpulent, expire more suddenly than those who have a spare habit" (Book 2, Aphorism 44). Indeed, both are undernourished.

Although the central role of nutrition in clinical medicine has been recognized for millennia, physician awareness remains inadequate [6–8]. The state of nutrition education in US medical schools was reviewed by the National Academy of Sciences in 1985 [7]. Their report noted the inadequacies of the training in preclinical and clinical years.

Attempts to remedy the shortcomings have occurred over the ensuing years, including the Physical Diagnosis—Nutritional Aspects manual produced in 1988 by the New York–New Jersey Regional Center for Clinical Nutrition Education at The New York Academy of Medicine (NYAM; 8), as well as the online educational tool, Nutrition in Medicine Project from the University of North Carolina at Chapel Hill [9]. Updated evaluations of the state of nutrition education in medical schools still assess the situation as "precarious" [6]. As stated in the NYAM manual, the clinical instruction of nutrition with emphasis on "diagnosis and care is almost non-existent as a required subject in United States medical schools" [8]. Indeed, it is rarely done in physical diagnosis courses.

This chapter is intended to stimulate an appreciation among students, as well as experienced clinicians, that awareness of nutritional status needs to be integrated into the routine evaluation of every patient. It is important to recognize nutritional issues that are due to underlying disorders, as well as to be aware of those nutritional issues that contribute to abnormal organ function. It is also important to realize that an intrinsic role of the physician is to formulate a plan (with the assistance of other professionals if needed) to treat these nutritional issues [10]. One can maintain a basic approach to the patient with emphasis on history, physical findings, and supportive laboratory data to elicit this information [3,4]. Example case studies will be presented to illustrate the salient points. Images collected from the author's clinical experience are also provided.

THE PHYSICIAN'S ROLE IN DIAGNOSING MALNUTRITION

Physical diagnosis is an *essential* aspect of a physician's job description. With the coming dramatic changes and looming price constraints in medical care in this country, savvy bedside diagnosis and care have become even more important. Whatever direction medical care in the United States takes in the foreseeable future, with medical homes and team approaches, it is still the physician who is central and the leader of the team. Careful bedside diagnosis is cost-effective by reducing unneeded, expensive tests, as well as minimizing the complications that these may cause [11].

Numerous studies have shown that medical and surgical diagnoses can be made in the majority of cases by means of careful history and physical examination. As an added benefit, the doctor–patient relationship is strengthened [12]. These studies also noted that supporting basic laboratory and radiologic studies assist generally to *confirm* the cogent bedside diagnosis, not to *make* the diagnosis [11,13–15]. It is the uncommon diagnosis that is made by high-tech testing alone.

Unfortunately, bedside diagnostic skills, in general, have been deemphasized in medical education at the undergraduate and postgraduate levels [16]. Even exemplary approaches to improved teaching the "lost art" of physical diagnosis, such as the Stanford 25 [17], do not specifically approach the nutritional aspects. Most of the reference texts used in American medical schools for the physical diagnosis course, such as those by Bates [18], DeGowin [19], Berg and Worzala [20], and Orient [21], mention little specifically about nutrition.

Various aspects of clinical nutrition deserve physician attention. Nutrition has the power to impact all aspects of health, from birth to death, in health, convalescence, or disease (as well as development, pregnancy, and lactation). These quantitative nutrient needs have been addressed for the healthy US population by the National Research Council. Periodically reviewed and updated, based on ongoing research, these are published as the recommended dietary allowances and recommended dietary intakes [22].

Most physicians have some appreciation of the chronic influence and long-term effects of dietary intake on the establishment and progression of diseases such as obesity, coronary artery disease, osteoporosis, and cancer. Patients often have a more enthusiastic than educated interest in nutrition than we do, as individual physicians or as a profession. The seemingly never-ending stream of "miracle diets," "secrets your doctor won't tell you" attests to this. It is up to us, as reference sources of reliable information, to maintain at least the factual background and to address these issues to the limits of reasonable data.

More closely aligned with the role of the physician (and surgeon) is the awareness of the interaction of disease processes and the therapies we provide on the nutritional condition of our patients. We should have insight into the effects that nutritional status has on manifestations of disease, as well as on response to treatment. This is relevant for the bedside diagnosis in various aspects of malnutrition.

Familiarity with nutrition support methods and personnel should be a part of every physician's approach to patients. Referral to and utilization of registered dieticians (RDs), as well as physician specialists in nutrition support, to assist and optimize nutritional therapies is strongly encouraged. Indeed, the Joint Commission on Accreditation of Healthcare Organizations [23] recommendations for nutritional and functional screening for hospital inpatients require evaluation within 24 h of admission "when applicable to the patient's condition." Screening for primary care may be performed at the first visit or later as appropriate [23].

Many teaching hospitals have a nutrition support team to handle the complex nutrition cases, i.e., those that may require the high-technology techniques of total parenteral nutrition. However, these teams are by no means universal. Every hospital will have RDs available to assist in the evaluation and treatment of nutrition issues in patients with less severe issues and less intensive therapies. The team incorporates the input of nutrition-oriented physicians (team leaders), clinical dieticians, nutrition-oriented nurse clinicians, and parenteral nutrition-trained pharmacists. Each member has strengths that he/she brings to the team. The physician uses his/her training and insight in evaluating a patient, makes a diagnosis, and presents a treatment plan (a nutrition prescription) to the dietician, who converts this into a practical food and dietary regimen for the patient. The dietician assesses day to day compliance with the plan and serves as the go-to intermediary for patients on specialized diets or tube feedings. The pharmacists and nurse clinicians play a vital role especially in the management of parenteral nutrition patients.

POPULATIONS AT RISK

Sufficient nutrition is required for appropriate reproduction, growth, maintenance, and repair of the organism. Anything that impedes ingestion, absorption, or utilization of the more than 40 known nutrients for a sustained duration has a detrimental effect on the well-being and health of the individual. This manifests in its various stages as primary undernutrition or as due to other causes (secondary undernutrition).

Primary undernutrition occurs in those who do not take in adequate nutrients due to poverty, social isolation, food shortages, famine, faddism, or preferences that lead to an unbalanced and inadequate diet. Hunger and poverty have decreased in this country in the last century. With that, overt clinical deficiency disease, such as scurvy, beriberi, pellagra, night blindness, and rickets has declined over the past decades. However, with the Great Recession, poverty rates have increased. With increasing poverty goes an increasing population at risk for subclinical or overt disease. This population can include the elderly and those who are economically distressed: groups that more obviously appear at risk.

Primary undernutrition may also include those that have chosen to exclude foods for a variety of reasons: ethical, religious, or according to purported benefits or detriments. Restricted diets can lead to imbalance and deficiency ("A regimen too strict and unsubstantial is always dangerous in chronic diseases, and even in those which are acute, when it does not agree with the patient. Again, as the diet pushed to an extreme degree of severity is pernicious, so repletion carried to the utmost degree is dangerous likewise." Hippocrates. *Aphorisms, Section 1, Number 4*. Trans. Thomas Coar, 1822. Valpy, London.).

Secondary malnutrition can occur due to the effects of a disease process on ingestion, absorption, or metabolism/utilization of nutrients. The list of diseases causing this is extensive. The astute clinician will recognize patients at risk as those with chronic gastrointestinal diseases such as pancreatic insufficiency, untreated celiac disease, inflammatory bowel diseases, and those with chronic liver, kidney, lung, neurologic, cardiac, neoplastic, and endocrine diseases. Patients who have had bariatric surgery are a newer and often under-recognized addition to this group. Others including those with poor dentition, depression, anxiety, and eating disorders should also be included.

Any patient undergoing acutely stressful physiologic circumstances, such as trauma, infection, long bone fracture, or burns, will be at increased nutritional risk, even if they were well nourished beforehand. Indeed, there are patients whose medical or social conditions render them chronically at risk and will need long-term, even lifetime, monitoring. The physician should recognize the ongoing issue and obtain assistance from family members, social services, and dieticians when possible ("The physician must not only do that which is immediately his, but engage the patient, their attendants, and all the externals for the benefit of the patient." Hippocrates, *Aphorisms*. Section 1, Number 1). Medications we prescribe, not uncommonly, may cause nausea or decrease appetite and therefore decrease intake; other medications might increase appetite and intake [24].

It is worth mentioning a group of patients at increased nutritional risk because their primary treatments have lengthened their lives at a cost. This varied group can include patients who have undergone radiation therapy, affecting various parts of the GI tract (including the mouth), and/or chemotherapy for cancers, or extensive bowel surgery, for any reason, or are maintained on dialysis for chronic renal failure. It may include patients who have survived strokes. These patients are at chronic risk for malnutrition. All require ongoing monitoring. Some of them may require short-term or long-term supplementation, including intensive nutrition support, such as enteral or parenteral therapy.

Other nutrition support cases may be more problematic. How best to assess and treat patients with dementia? There is no simple or generalized answer. Rehabilitation measures need to be individualized [25]. The number of percutaneous endoscopic gastrostomies (PEGs) has increased to over 200,000/year. A significant percentage (10–15%) occurs in moderately to severely demented individuals with controversial, if not dubious, benefits [25–28].

Bariatric surgical procedures have remarkably increased, with over 200,000 such procedures performed annually in the United States. Those procedures that combine malabsorption with restriction, e.g., gastric bypass, and sleeve gastrectomy with biliopancreatic diversion (with or without a duodenal switch) in particular, have created a subgroup of individuals that are persistently at nutritional risk for deficiencies; this group requires lifetime monitoring and vigilance [29,30].

STAGES OF DEFICIENCY

Deficiency of nutrients manifests in stages. The initial abnormal biochemical events occur at a pace determined by the stage of development and metabolic rate, e.g., children and those under stress are more susceptible. A number of additional factors can impact the state of nutrition. Body stores of a nutrient, its biologic half-life, and genetic factors may affect the rate of use of a nutrient from depots. Host factors involved include age, sex, genetic variability, presence of disease, and other physiologic stress factors. Underlying disease processes can affect consumption of the tissue stores. Environmental factors include those that affect availability of nutrients, their consumption, and requirements. Nutrient factors affecting nutritional status, include chemical structure, factors that interfere with absorption and availability, as well as the effect of imbalances on utilization.

The abnormal biochemical events can often be noted by decreased blood levels, which may reflect tissue levels for many nutrients, e.g., serum vitamin levels and the urinary excretion of magnesium. Many nutrients behave as enzyme cofactors. With progressive depletion of a nutrient, progressive decline in enzyme and receptor activity entails. This leads to altered cellular biochemistry.

This, in turn, can lead to clinical signs and symptoms of deficiency. Deficiency states can be confirmed in the clinical stages, and often in earlier, subclinical, stages with appropriate laboratory testing to support clinical judgment.

ESSENTIAL NUTRIENTS

Everything in balance is sound advice, particularly in things nutritional. There are over 40 nutrients that are essential to humans [8]. They are indispensable to maintain health. We do not produce them; thus, we rely on dietary intake for them. Primary among these are the eight amino acids that are essential in adults: leucine, isoleucine, valine, threonine, phenylalanine, methionine, lysine, and tryptophan. Histidine becomes essential for adults with kidney failure, and in healthy children, along with arginine (perhaps also taurine). Carnitine and cysteine may be essential in chronic liver disease and renal disease.

Two fatty acids (linoleic and linolenic) are essential nutrients. In addition, four fat-soluble vitamins ([A], [D], [E], and [K]) and nine water-soluble vitamins (thiamine [B1], riboflavin [B2], niacin [B3], pyridoxine [B6], pantothenic acid [B5], biotin [B7], folic acid [B9], cobalamin [B12], and ascorbic acid [C]) are essential. Finally, there are seven essential macrominerals (Na, K, Cl, Ca, Mg, phosphate, and sulfate) and six or more essential trace elements (iron, zinc, copper, iodine, chromium, and selenium).

Of course, adequate intake of nonessential amino acids, carbohydrates, and fats are needed to provide enough calories for cell maintenance, repair, and growth. Furthermore, dietary fiber of various types provide bulk, aid digestion, and act as prebiotics providing nutrients for the bowel flora (microbiome), providing potential effects and benefits that are being actively studied.

PRESENTATION OF PROTEIN CALORIE MALNUTRITION

The clinician is most likely to see the effects of malnutrition presenting as of protein-calorie malnutrition: deficiency of protein and/or calories. Often, associated deficiencies of micronutrients can be seen as well. Over time, and with progression, clinical effects of malnutrition manifest, leading to increased morbidity and mortality.

As caloric intake becomes inadequate, one will see weight loss. The body's energy stores (fat and glycogen) become progressively depleted. Even in a lean individual, there are typically ample reserves of fat calories and a small store of carbohydrates (liver and muscle glycogen) available to handle short-term calorie deprivation, e.g., skipping a meal. However, there is no reserve of protein in the body. Protein is present for structure (e.g., muscle fiber, collagen, cell membranes, etc.) or function (enzymes, transport proteins, hormones).

In *simple starvation* without additional physiologic stress (i.e., infection, trauma, burns, etc.), there will be an initial obligatory protein loss to provide the substrate for gluconeogenesis. Simple starvation leads to a decreased metabolic rate as a protective mechanism. In addition, over time (usually about a week), the metabolism shifts to increase fat and ketone utilization as a means of decreasing catabolism and sparing protein content.

As the patient body stores of glycogen, fat, and protein depots are utilized, there will be weight loss. Decreased somatic protein (muscle mass) and visceral proteins (albumin, clotting factors, enzymes, immune products, etc.) ensue. Obligate fluid and sodium retention leads to edema formation. This process results in fatigue and bed rest.

This, in turn, lead to more muscle wasting and increased thrombotic risk. Prolonged bed rest and poor wound healing increase the risk for decubitus ulcers. Protein loss leads to respiratory muscle weakness, which leads to reduced clearance of secretions and increased risk for atelectasis and pneumonia. Decreased immune function increases the risk for a variety of infections. Depleted protein stores can adversely affect bowel and cardiac function. Commonly irritability and apathy occur as the malnutrition progresses.

Things are very different with additional physiologic stress. Infection, trauma, or fever increases metabolism to varying degrees referred to as the stress ("fight or flight") response. It follows that the greater the number and intensity of stressful factors, the worse the effect nutritionally. Patients with trauma, superimposed infection, and especially those with burns greatly magnify the losses induced by simple starvation.

Stress metabolism causes an obligatory increase in hormones such as corticosteroids, catecholamines, and growth hormone. This leads to insulin resistance, which causes carbohydrate intolerance, and leads to a decrease in anabolism and an increase in catabolism. An increased metabolic rate occurs, with compensatory increased deiodination of thyroxine leading to the "euthyroid sick syndrome." The increased stress causes increased production (or decreased clearance) of "acute phase reactants," such as C-reactive protein (CRP), ferritin, globulins, cytokines, and tumor necrosis factor. This further depletes somatic protein depots in muscle. Increased muscle breakdown leads to an increased nitrogen wasting and urea excretion via the kidney. The increase in nitrogen excretion can be measured as an indicator of stress metabolism. An increase in the secretion of aldosterone and antidiuretic hormone (ADH) may lead to fluid retention.

Protein energy malnutrition presents in three general forms: balanced protein-calorie deficiency ("marasmus"), protein deficiency ("kwashiorkor"-like), and mixed, e.g., the marasmic patient who gets acutely sick and loses more protein. Traditionally, these conditions have been described worldwide in children, in the midst of poverty, famine, and commonly (infectious) diarrheal disease. One might expect this in Third World nations, but it can be seen here in the United States, especially in the hospitalized population. As an example, the typical patient with advanced anorexia nervosa exemplifies the "marasmic" phenotype—loss of body fat, decreased muscle mass, but maintenance of visceral protein, e.g., albumin. Such patients typically restrict calories but relatively maintain protein intake. The patient with advanced cirrhosis (loss of protein synthetic function), protein losing enteropathy (excessive protein loss), recurrent pleural effusions, or ascites (3rd spacing of protein) manifests as the "kwashiorkor-like," with edema, swollen belly (ascites), loss of muscle mass, and loss of visceral protein.

Sarcopenia, the loss of muscle mass, is common in the elderly. If long term, without other symptoms, it may not denote any real problem. A chronically thin individual may still be healthy. On the other hand, decreased oral intake, as well as a chronic increase in protein loss (catabolism) can cause loss of muscle mass. When extensive, or protracted over time, it may present as *cachexia*.

Cachexia is more than simply *involuntary* weight loss. Cachexia includes a systemic inflammatory component. Involuntary weight loss of 5% or more over the last 12 months may suggest the diagnosis. Generally the weight loss is associated with an underlying disease. Cachectic patients typically are fatigued, have poor appetite, and have low muscle mass. Decreased muscle strength can be tested by checking grip strength or having the patient stand up from a sitting position. In addition, any one of the following laboratory values is needed for the diagnosis: a CRP (> 5 mg/L), IL-6 (> 4 pg/mL), Hgb < 12 gm/dL, or albumin < 3.2 gm/dL. A normocytic, normochromic anemia as seen in "the anemia of chronic (inflammatory) disease" is a common marker for malnutrition.

Currently, in the United States, primary *vitamin deficiency diseases*, such as classically described symptomatic scurvy (vitamin C, ascorbic acid deficiency), beriberi (vitamin B1, thiamine deficiency), rickets/osteomalacia (vitamin D deficiency), pellagra (niacin deficiency), and night blindness as a result of vitamin A deficiency, are rarely encountered. However, these may be seen in the hospitalized, institutionalized, nursing home population. Others at risk include those with chronic marginal intake, alcohol abusers, cirrhotics, eating-disorder patients, bariatric surgery patients, shut-ins, prisoners, and immigrants from endemic regions of deficiencies.

Common causes of secondary undernutrition include a variety of *malabsorptive syndromes*, such as tropical and nontropical sprue (gluten enteropathy, celiac sprue); extensive inflammatory bowel disease of the small intestine; and parasitic diseases, e.g., tapeworms, hookworms, strongyloidiasis, cryptosporidiosis, extensive giardiasis; pancreatic insufficiency due to chronic pancreatitis (most often seen in chronic alcohol abusers), cystic fibrosis, and chronic liver disease, pancreatic tumors, infections, e.g., HIV. Chronic infection with *Clostridium difficile* is an emerging entity associated with undernutrition, although not specifically a malabsorptive condition.

Anorexia, or loss of appetite, can occur in a variety of conditions including cancer, depression, hypothyroidism, acute or chronic infection or inflammation, and trauma. *Anorexia nervosa* is a separate, specific disorder commonly associated with significant undernutrition. Organ failure, e.g., renal, liver, gut, and heart failure, can lead to altered requirements, as well as altered intake, resulting in undernutrition. Less commonly, chronic respiratory failure can lead to profound weight loss, at least in part from decreased intake. Drug abuse, ranging from stimulants, like cocaine and methamphetamine, to depressants, like heroin, benzodiazepines, and alcohol, can lead to decreased intake and/or altered metabolism, which ultimately yields undernutrition.

Patients may develop *sitophobia* (fear of eating) because of the association of eating with painful or problem symptoms, like nausea or diarrhea. Conditions such as ulcer disease, chronic mesenteric ischemia (intestinal angina), Crohn's disease with strictures or fistulas, or tumors may have low-level symptoms that become intolerable with eating. Patients adapt by minimizing their intake, resulting in weight loss. However, unlike anorexia, the appetite may remain intact.

Finally, one should not forget the effects of iatrogenic undernutrition. Physicians, and our treatments, can be a potent cause of significant undernutrition. The medications we give patients to treat one problem, e.g., cancer chemotherapy, may have undesirable effects, such as nausea, vomiting, diarrhea, and anorexia, as well as possible malabsorption or excess loss. Surgical manipulation of the gut, e.g., resection, loss of the ileocecal valve, and bariatric, gastric, and pancreatic surgery, can all have ongoing and profound effects on nutritional status. Radiation therapy to the head and neck, chest, abdomen, or pelvis can have varying detrimental effects on oral intake, tolerance, and absorption of nutrients.

NUTRITIONAL ASSESSMENT: PATIENT HISTORY

Nutritional assessment is an integral, but often overlooked, aspect of physician evaluation of a patient. Just as in any other system-oriented evaluation, the patient history needs to be obtained with insight that will help to direct the physical exam. The bedside approach helps to elicit enough information to answer the clinical question if the patient is at increased risk to develop or have malnutrition [4]. This requires asking enough of the right questions regarding diet, past and present health conditions, medications, activities, and social setting. The physical exam should include observation of those elements that relate to nutritional status and allow the clinician to distill an overall view and assessment. Of note, most nutritional deficiencies occur as part of a clinical syndrome rather than in isolation. Moreover, most physical signs of deficiency are nonspecific.

The initial screening questions are as follows: Have you lost weight without trying?; Are you eating less because of poor appetite? Further screening can be easily accomplished in the elderly population using the Mini Nutrition Assessment Short-Form, which is a validated tool for evaluating elderly patients [31]. The assessment takes only a few minutes to perform. The components include (1) food intake decline over the past 3 months; (2) weight loss over the past 3 months; (3) Is the patient mobile; (4) psychologic stress/acute stress in the past 3 months; (5) neuropsychological problems (depression and/or dementia); (6) body mass index (BMI); and (7) calf circumference (if BMI is unattainable).

Unintentional weight loss in the elderly can often be related to "the 9 D's": disease, dementia, depression, dysphagia, dysgeusia (taste disorders due to a variety of causes), dentition, diarrhea, drug side effects, and dysfunction [32].

If the patient is deemed to be at nutritional risk, the next step is to delineate the type, cause, and degree of malnutrition. The latter is particularly important because of the need to code the patient's nutritional status appropriately in the medical record. Different ICD-9 codes exist for mild, moderate, and severe malnutrition. Try to delineate the affected nutrients, i.e., calories, protein, fats, vitamins, minerals, and trace elements, alone or more commonly in combination. Outline the duration of malnutrition, separating it into acute, subacute, or chronic.

The astute clinician learns to use various historical and clinical clues to determine which of their patients are at risk for various clinical conditions. Assessing for malnutrition is no different in this regard. Remember, nutritionally, those patients who have increased requirements due to pregnancy, lactation, growth and development, infection (acute or chronic), recovery from (emergency) surgery are at increased risk.

Dietary aspects interact in the biopsychosocial model of health and disease. Biologic (medical) factors include the patient's presenting complaint and illness as well as any recent or past history of surgery. Chronic illnesses and disorders that may influence nutritional risk include allergies, anemia, cardiac disease, hyperlipidemia, diabetes mellitus, hypertension, cancer, obesity, emphysema, chronic bronchiectasis, pulmonary fibrosis, chronic infections such as parasites, tuberculosis, HIV, chronic liver or renal disease, malabsorption and maldigestion, pancreatic disease, autoimmune and rheumatic diseases, and psychiatric disorders such as depression.

It is useful to know a patient's obstacles to eating. This can be as banal as a mouth full of poorly fitting dentures or teeth that require dental work. Dysphagia (difficulty swallowing) can be oral, oral-pharyngeal, or esophageal. Causes can include neurologic disorders, including strokes, pseudobulbar palsies, myasthenia gravis, Parkinson's disease, tumors of the head and neck, mediastinum or esophagus, eosinophilic esophagitis, as well as motor disturbances, including achalasia. Odynophagia (painful swallowing) can be due to infections such as herpes, Candida, cytomegalovirus (especially in the immunocompromised patient), esophagitis due to gastroesophageal reflux disease (GERD), "pill esophagitis," or tumors. Chronic nausea or vomiting, chronic heartburn, gastroesophageal reflux, abdominal pain, constipation or diarrhea, and dyspnea due to a variety of cardiopulmonary causes can all impair food intake.

Medications such as chemotherapeutic agents, corticosteroids, and diuretics can increase risk for a variety of nutritional deficiencies. Prescribed and over-the-counter medications, alcohol, recreational drugs, and tobacco can affect intake or conditions related to nutritional risk. High-dose vitamin/mineral supplements, and herbals can also affect appetite and cause nausea, pain, constipation, or diarrhea.

The family history can be useful to know (e.g., autoimmune diseases, hemochromatosis). Social history information regarding a patient's living situation is important. For example, do they work, live alone, live with family or significant others or companions? Do they have access to fresh and/or nutritious food? What is their daily eating schedule and eating pattern (meals, snacks, skipped meals, etc.)? Knowledge of other factors such as financial means, physical ability to obtain food or cook, and level of physical activity (not simply "exercise") is helpful.

Asking questions about who in the household does the shopping and food preparation can be insightful. Physician-prescribed limitations or self-imposed dietary restrictions due to religious/ethical reasons or undertaken in the pursuit of "a healthy diet" are all important factors that may contribute to dietary imbalance and malnutrition. Fluctuations in weight acutely and over time can be helpful clues. Involuntary weight loss of 10% or more over the prior 6 months is worrisome and denotes a patient at nutritional risk, regardless of measurements of serum proteins.

NUTRITIONAL ASSESSMENT: PHYSICAL EXAMINATION

You could learn a lot by watching.

Yogi Berra

The physical exam is best performed in a systematic way. Many physical signs associated with malnutrition are nonspecific for a variety of reasons. Most diagnosed deficiencies are not in their advanced states; many deficiencies may manifest similar findings. This may be due to a common pathway of phenotypic expression of biochemical derangements, as well as other disease manifestations. For example, ascites may be seen with profound protein depletion (hypoalbuminemia), as well as congestive heart failure, nephrosis, cirrhosis, malignancy, other chronic liver diseases, etc. All of those conditions will have additional effects on the patient's nutritional status.

The initial sense of a patient's well-being starts with the overall appearance of the patient. "Well developed" means that they have had adequate prior nutrition to allow for normal growth and development; "well nourished" refers to current nutrition status. Not all thin patients are cachectic. Some may be chronically thin and very well nourished as opposed to others who have lost weight due to negative caloric balance. Likewise, an overweight patient may have evidence of calorie excess, but still may have protein depletion and hypoalbuminemia.

Useful tools and calculations in the bedside evaluation of patients exist. The "ideal body weight" (IBW) derives from tables and data developed by the Metropolitan Life Insurance Company in 1942–1943. These data have been updated periodically. The term "ideal" is no longer generally used but derived from weight for height data related to lowest mortality rates for age and sex. This varies with frame size, as measured by elbow breadth and wrist circumference. Practically speaking, a simple formula commonly used at the bedside is as follows: for a patient with medium frame size, the baseline weight at height 5 ft. is 106 lbs. for a male and 100 lbs. for a female. In males, for every inch over 5 ft., add 6 lbs. For females, add 5 lbs. per inch above 5 ft. There is a variation of 10% for small and large frame size.

BMI is a commonly used marker for overweight, obesity, and underweight. It is derived from weight (kg)/height (cm^2), as described in the 1800s by Quetelet [33,34]. A significant limitation of this calculation is that there is no discrimination for fat as opposed to muscle, i.e., a muscular well-trained athlete may have the same BMI as the sedentary "couch potato" watching the athlete in a sporting event on television. Even though they may have the same BMI, they will not have the same health consequences of the extra weight.

It is helpful to compare the patient's current or actual weight to their usual weight, as well as to the "ideal" weight. Mild to moderate weight deficiency is within 80–90% of "ideal" (not necessarily usual), and less than 80% of "ideal" is more severe deficiency. Not every patient who has lost weight, especially if the loss has been voluntary, is at increased health risk.

Anthropomorphics, the measurement of skinfold thickness and arm circumference, are useful bedside markers to give a sense of nutritional status, but are infrequently learned by students and even more infrequently performed by physicians. That is unfortunate because such a simple measurement can be quite useful. One need only do enough formal measurements to develop a sense of normal, overweight/obesity, and undernutrition. A finger pinch at the waist and triceps of the nondominant arm can be helpful. Waist circumference (WC) (measured at the uppermost border of the iliac crest) and BMI can give a reasonably quick and accurate marker for obesity-associated health risks. With practice, the clinician can get at least a rough estimate of adiposity and sense of somatic protein content (there is no storage form of protein).

The WC should be measured with the patient standing and the snug, but not tight, tape measurement at the midpoint between the ribs and iliac crest. The WC cutoff for men is 40 in. (102 cm) and for women 35 in. (88 cm). The cutoff for South Asians, Chinese, Japanese, and ethnic Central and South Americans is lower. For men in this demographic, it is 35 in. (90 cm) and for women it is 31 in. (80 cm).

One reads reports of patient examinations with sections abbreviated as "WNL—within normal limits." In point of fact, this often actually means "WNL—we never looked." With the advent of computerized imaging, the physical examination is regrettably becoming a lost art. But these skills are still essential to the metabolic physician. Despite the technological advances, there is still no better way to assess nutritional status than with our eyes, ears, and hands.

The following is an extensive, but not all-inclusive, listing of various abnormal physical findings that may be associated with nutritional abnormalities. It would be prudent for the astute clinician to at least consider these as nutritional problems in the differential diagnosis [10].

1. Hair
   Easily pluckable, sparse: seen with protein (commonly) and less commonly biotin deficiency (rare in the absence of total parenteral nutrition); telogen effluvium occurring after pregnancy or medical or surgical illness.
   Dull, listless: protein deficiency; hypothyroidism can present with similar findings as might overprocessed hair (bleached, etc.).
   Flag sign: protein/calorie deficiency. A change in coloration from black to red or brown can temporally relate to the onset of the deficiency; can be confused with cosmetic "grow-outs."
   Lanugo: fine, downy hair on trunk, face, arms—commonly seen with protein/calorie deficiency; common in anorexia nervosa.
2. Skin
   Xerosis: dry skin, seen with essential fatty acid deficiency
   Petechiae: often with perifollicular hemorrhages—seen with scurvy (vitamin C deficiency), also with vitamin A toxicity; multiple medical conditions affecting platelets, clotting
   Ecchymoses: deficiency of vitamin K (common), C (uncommon); if occurs on one hand, consider bulimia
   Hyperkeratosis especially in sun-exposed areas: niacin deficiency (pellagra)
   Hyperpigmentation: iron overload (hemochromatosis); can also be seen with adrenal insufficiency (Addison's disease), Cushing's disease (hypercortisolism), porphyria, and Peutz–Jegher's syndrome, among other conditions
   Follicular keratosis (with keratin plugging of follicles): vitamin A deficiency, essential fatty acid deficiency; may also be seen with keratosis pilaris, genetic abnormalities, lupus
   Flaky paint dermatitis: associated desquamation; seen with protein/calorie deficiency, paucity of subcutaneous fat, excessive wrinkling
   Purpura: vitamin K deficiency (commonly), vitamin C deficiency (uncommonly); can be seen with a variety of medications—warfarin, aspirin, platelet inhibitors, chemotherapy; seen with chronic liver, renal disease, autoimmune disorders such as lupus, others
   Pallor: deficiency of iron, folate, vitamin B12, copper (with anemia); may also be seen with anemia of chronic (inflammatory) disease, marrow disorders, chronic liver, renal disease
   Decreased skin turgor: dehydration
   Edema: hypoalbuminemia seen with protein deficiency; may be seen in multiple medical illnesses, stress reactions, postoperatively, thiamine deficiency—"wet beriberi"; high-output heart failure; generally rare, N.B. gastric bypass patients with vomiting, hyperemesis gravidarum, alcoholics, bulimics
   Bruising/ecchymoses: deficiency of vitamin K, C, iron—multiple causes, including acute and chronic liver disease, chronic renal disease, marrow disorders, medications including aspirin, antiplatelet drugs, fish oil, and some herbal supplements, e.g., gingko biloba, evening primrose oil
   Decubitus ulcers (pressure sores, bedsores): protein/calorie malnutrition; often other factors including shear, wetness, immobility

Seborrheic dermatitis: essential fatty acid, riboflavin (B2), pyridoxine (B6), zinc, biotin, niacin deficiency; often not associated with nutritional deficiency

Dermatitis: scrotal, vulvar—riboflavin, zinc deficiency; can be confused with tineal or monilial dermatitis; acral—zinc, niacin, essential fatty acid deficiency; nasolabial—pyridoxine (B6) deficiency

Delayed wound healing: protein/calorie, zinc, ascorbic acid deficiency

Ichthyosis: vitamin A deficiency

Xanthomas: hyperlipidemia; palmar xanthomas seen with primary biliary cirrhosis

3. Nails

Spoon shaped (koilonychia): iron deficiency

Brittle, ridged (vertical): nonspecific; occasionally with vitamin A deficiency

Thin, peelable: protein/calorie deficiency; may be seen with overactive thyroid

White speckling: rarely zinc deficiency; more commonly trauma

Splinter hemorrhages: vitamin C deficiency; more commonly trauma, bacterial endocarditis, (especially if associated with Janeway lesions, Osler's nodes, Roth spots, change in murmur, etc.)

Horizontal ridging (Beau's lines): protein/calorie zinc, biotin deficiency; effects of acute catabolic stress, e.g., infection, heart attack, surgery

Leukonychia striata (Aldrich–Mees and Muehrcke's lines): white lines (not ridges)—associated with hypoalbuminemia, multiple causes including renal failure

White nails, leukonychia (Terry's nails): due to decreased blood supply to nail bed; seen in iron deficiency, malnutrition, kidney, heart failure, diabetes, cirrhosis

4. Eyes

Xanthelasma: hyperlipidemia; can be seen with primary biliary cirrhosis; hereditary, without lipid abnormalities.

Ophthalmoplegia: thiamine deficiency (Wernicke's syndrome); N.B. gastric bypass patients with vomiting, bulimics, pernicious vomiting of pregnancy, alcoholics (medical urgency); can be seen with a variety of neurologic disorders, including multiple sclerosis.

Dry conjunctiva (with or without Bitot's spots—conjunctival thickening): vitamin A deficiency, often associated with decreased night vision. Dry eyes can be seen with other conditions including sicca syndrome, Sjogren's syndrome, and other autoimmune disorders.

Papilledema: vitamin A, D toxicity; multiple neurologic causes including pseudo-tumor cerebri (commonly associated with obesity), space-occupying lesions.

5. Lips

Cheilosis (thinning of vermillion border of lips): iron, niacin, pyridoxine, riboflavin, protein deficiency

Angular stomatitis, fissures: iron, B complex, protein/calorie deficiency; can be seen with poor fitting or lack of dentures, neurologic disorders such as Parkinson's disease, fungal or bacterial overgrowth, excessive moisture

6. Teeth

Thinning of enamel (especially molar or lingual aspect of incisors): bulimia; also seen with GERD

Caries: absent fluoride (solely bottled water intake); also poor oral hygiene, methamphetamine use, sicca syndrome, Sjogren's syndrome, bulimia, GERD

White/mottled enamel: excess fluoride

7. Gums

Spongy, swollen, bleeding: ascorbic acid deficiency; can also be seen with infection, malignancy/leukemia, reaction to medications including diphenylhydantoin, and calcium channel blockers

8. Tongue

Large, tender, beefy red, furrowed: niacin, iodine deficiency; can also be seen in amyloidosis, hypothyroidism, Down's syndrome—macroglossia, without tenderness

Atrophic glossitis: loss of lingual papillae—B complex, folate, B12, iron, protein/calorie deficiency

9. Salivary glands

Parotid enlargement: "chipmunk cheeks," seen in bulimics; acute onset, unilateral—stone, infection, rarely tumor

10. Heart

Enlarged, rapid rate, high-output failure: ("wet beriberi") thiamine deficiency, N.B. gastric bypass patients with vomiting; "thyroid storm."

Low output heart failure: acute refeeding syndrome, phosphate depletion syndrome; selenium deficiency (cardiomyopathy); more common causes of low output failure include atherosclerotic cardiovascular disease, occasionally hypothyroidism, amyloidosis, and iron overload disease.

Arrhythmia, sudden death: low magnesium, phosphate depletion, low potassium, vitamin C and B1 deficiency, as well as causes listed above.

11. Abdomen

Ascites: hypoalbuminemia—protein/calorie deficiency; multitude of medical illnesses, including chronic liver disease, fulminant liver failure, Budd–Chiari syndrome, malignancy, congestive heart failure, infection.

Hepatomegaly (steatosis): fatty liver; often associated with obesity, alcohol excess, diabetes, hyperlipidemia/metabolic syndrome, high glucose TPN; may be seen with drug reaction. Other causes of hepatomegaly including cardiac, infiltrative-sarcoid, amyloid, tumor.

Scaphoid abdomen: calorie deficiency (marasmus); wasting diseases, including malignancy, chronic infection, overactive thyroid; when extreme, and associated with catabolic stress—cachexia.

12. Bones

Pain: vitamin D, calcium, phosphorus, vitamin C deficiency; vitamin A toxicity; can also be seen with Paget's disease of bone, pituitary adenomas, neoplasms—primary or more commonly metastatic, hematological abnormalities including multiple myeloma, myelodysplasia, sickle cell crisis (often associated with zinc depletion)

Deformities of epiphyses: vitamin C ("scorbutic rosary" costochondral region), vitamin D deficiency ("rachitic rosary")

Demineralization: calcium, vitamin D deficiency, osteoporosis; can be seen in response to hyperthyroid (or excess thyroid replacement), alcohol abuse, smoking, family history, parathyroid disease, amenorrhea (primary or secondary), chronic pancreatic, renal, liver, or gastrointestinal disease, medications

Hyperostosis: vitamin A toxicity

13. Extremities

Muscle wasting: protein/energy deficiency—seen most often in temporal area; also check shoulder girdle; interosseous wasting seen also in diabetes (neuropathy), rheumatoid arthritis (with decreased grip strength)

Edema: protein deficiency; thiamine deficiency; multiple medical illnesses, including heart failure, acute and chronic kidney injury, acute and chronic liver disease, local vascular issues, lymphedema, thyroid disease, postoperative effects

Muscle twitching or tremor: pyridoxine deficiency; hypomagnesemia, hypocalcemia (Chvostek's sign, Trousseau's sign, carpal pedal spasm), hypokalemia, hypophosphatemia, myoedema; may be seen in upper motor neuron disease

Muscle spasm or cramps: hyponatremia, hypokalemia, hypocalcemia, hypomagnesemia, as well as total body depletion; iron deficiency; selenium deficiency

Muscle weakness: see above; also protein/calorie deficiency

Muscle pain: vitamin A toxicity, vitamin D deficiency, biotin, selenium deficiency; also in various myositis conditions, statin use (questionably related to Co Q10/ubiquinone depletion)

14. Neurological

Altered mental status/personality changes: vitamin B12 deficiency, niacin, magnesium deficiency; may also be seen in liver failure; kidney failure; hypothyroid/hyperthyroid; drug/medication toxicity or side effect; alterations in serum sodium, calcium; adrenal disease; mass lesions of brain including hematomas, neoplasms; pseudotumor cerebri (associated with obesity, can be seen with vitamin A or D toxicity, certain medications such as corticosteroids), normopressure hydrocephalus (associated with gait, incontinence changes); rarely with statin use for hyperlipidemia

Diplopia, ophthalmoplegia: associated with confabulation—thiamine deficiency (Wernicke's encephalopathy—acute urgency); N.B. gastric bypass patients, bulimics, pernicious vomiting of pregnancy

Dementia: vitamin B12 deficiency, chronic thiamine deficiency (Korsakoff's syndrome); hypothyroid, syphilis

Depression, lethargy: protein/calorie deficiency; alterations in serum electrolytes; vitamin B12 deficiency; multiple medical illnesses

Seizures: deficiency of pyridoxine, thiamine; hypoglycemia; hypophosphatemia; hypocalcemia; hypomagnesemia; hyponatremia; alcohol withdrawal (often associated with above, especially hypomagnesemia); trauma, stroke, malignancy (primary or metastatic), infection, lupus

Paresthesias: circumoral and peripheral—hypomagnesemia, hypocalcemia; hyperventilation with alterations in serum levels; hypophosphatemia; vitamin B12 deficiency; pyridoxine deficiency or toxicity; vitamin E deficiency; neurologic conditions

Decreased reflexes: hypercalcemia, hypermagnesemia, low thiamine; commonly in hypothyroid, neurologic conditions

Increased reflexes: hypocalcemia, hypomagnesemia; hyperthyroidism

Dysequilibrium, decreased vibration sense, frequent falls, decreased position sense: vitamin B12 deficiency (also copper?; rarely seen manifesting with optic neuritis as well); other neurological causes

15. Other findings

Oxalate kidney stones: vitamin D deficiency/toxicity, excess vitamin C intake

Uric acid stones: ileostomy; gout

Anemia: iron, folate, vitamin B12, vitamin B6, copper, vitamin E deficiency; chronic disease; inflammatory, liver, kidney; marrow issues

Delayed wound healing: protein, protein/calorie deficiency, zinc deficiency, vitamin deficiency (severe scurvy)

Diarrhea: can be caused by excessive magnesium, vitamin C intake, niacin deficiency, folate depletion, variety of infectious, inflammatory, hormonal conditions; associated with some medications; chronic diarrhea—can be associated with protein/calorie depletion, low stores of zinc, niacin, magnesium, electrolyte abnormalities, iron deficiency (celiac sprue)

SELECTED CLINICAL IMAGES

Below are some clinical images (Figures 21.1 to 21.22).

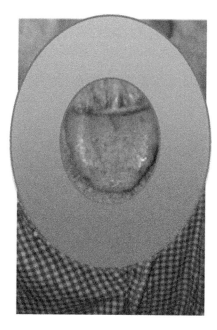

FIGURE 21.1   Telangiectasias of tongue in a patient with hereditary hemorrhagic telangiectasias (Osler–Weber–Rendu syndrome), presented with chronic iron deficiency and occult blood in stool.

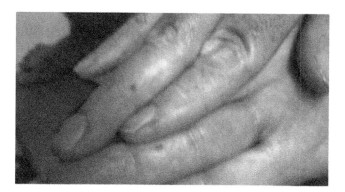

FIGURE 21.2   Telangiectasias of fingers in a patient with hereditary hemorrhagic telangiectasias (Osler–Weber–Rendu syndrome), presented with chronic iron deficiency and occult blood in stool.

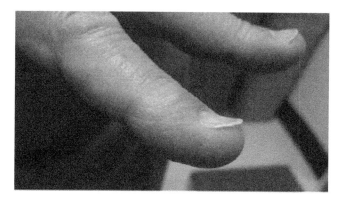

FIGURE 21.3   Koilonychia (spoon nails) in a patient with chronic iron deficiency.

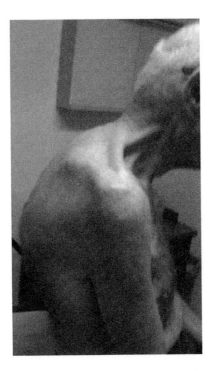

FIGURE 21.4 Atrophy of shoulder girdle in a patient with chronic (undiagnosed, untreated) Crohn's disease of small bowel, COPD. The patient had osteoporosis and vitamin B12, vitamin D, and severe iron deficiencies. Notice increased kyphosis.

(a) 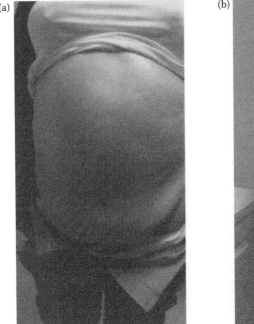 (b)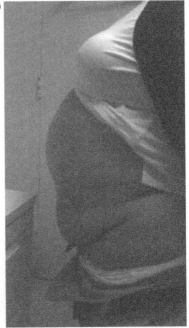

FIGURE 21.5 Panniculus adiposus ("fatty apron") in a morbidly obese woman, with associated metabolic syndrome: hypertension, hyperglycemia, and hyperlipidemia (low HDL, high LDL, and triglycerides). Notice the hepatomegaly due to steatosis, "fatty liver," which can also be associated with steatohepatitis and progression to cirrhosis. (a) Frontal view. (b) Lateral view.

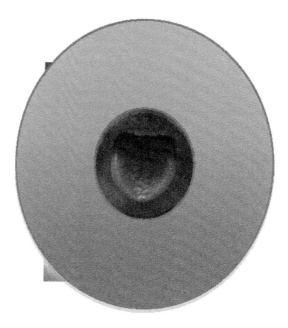

FIGURE 21.6 Atrophic glossitis in a patient with profound iron deficiency, due to inflammatory bowel disease (severe ulcerative colitis). The patient also had folate deficiency (dietary lack), vitamin B12 deficiency, marasmus, and protein–calorie deficiency.

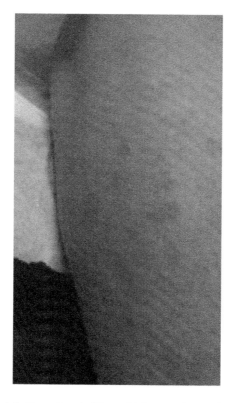

FIGURE 21.7 Psoriaform rash in the patient in Figure 21.6, started on antitumor necrosis factor therapy.

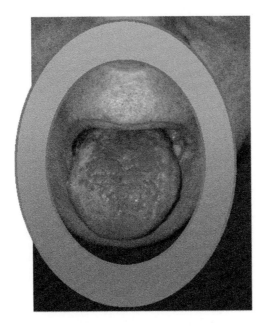

FIGURE 21.8 **(See color insert.)** Atrophic glossitis and cheilitis in a patient with multiple B vitamin deficiencies. This patient had systemic sclerosis. Notice the malar erythema and telangiectasias.

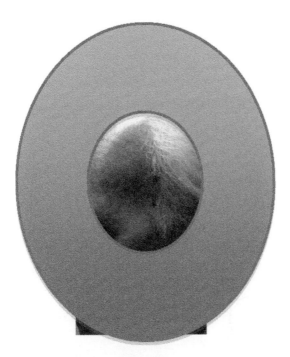

FIGURE 21.9 Temporal wasting in a patient with dementia.

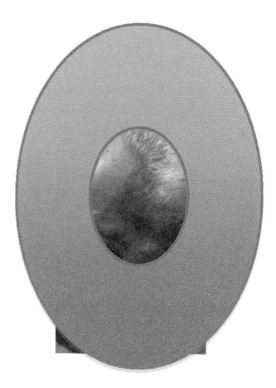

FIGURE 21.10   Temporal wasting in a patient with malabsorption and metastatic cancer.

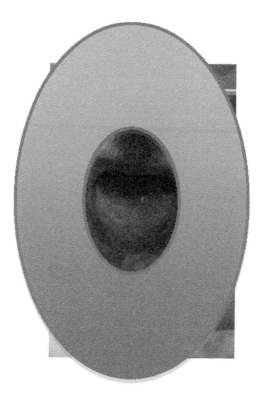

FIGURE 21.11   Atrophic glossitis in a patient with malabsorption and cancer (pictured in Figure 21.10). The patient had vitamin D and multiple B vitamin deficiencies.

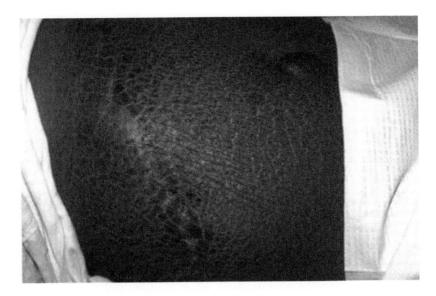

FIGURE 21.12   Ichthyosis in a cirrhotic patient with vitamin A deficiency. Notice the cholecystectomy scar, ascites, and umbilical hernia.

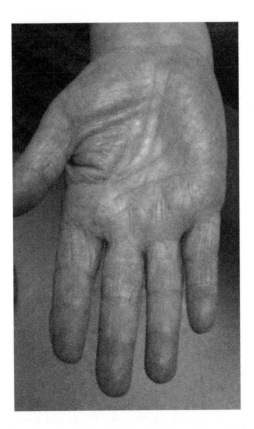

FIGURE 21.13   Palmar erythema in a cirrhotic patient who had protein-calorie and protein deficiency. ALT level was quite low due to vitamin B6 deficiency. Alkaline phosphatase level was low due to zinc depletion.

(a)

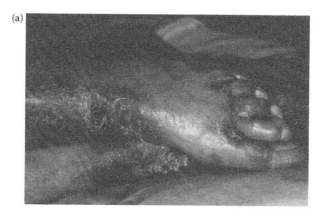

(b)

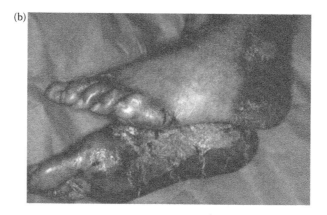

FIGURE 21.14 Severe rash of zinc deficiency in a patient with panmalabsorption due to tropical sprue. (a) Dorsal view. (b) Lateral view.

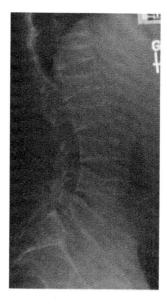

FIGURE 21.15 Severe osteoporosis and osteomalacia in a 25-year-old man maintained on TPN for 9 years, after rupture of a mesenteric aneurysm (due to Ehlers–Danlos syndrome), which led to short bowel syndrome. Notice severe loss of bone height and compression fractures.

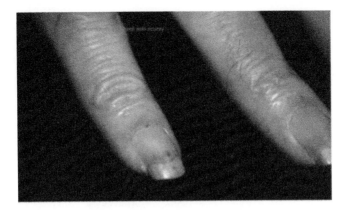

FIGURE 21.16 Splinter hemorrhages in a patient with scurvy. Depressed alcoholic who ate only canned soup and whiskey for 3 months. The patient was found on the floor of the apartment; had gastrointestinal bleeding.

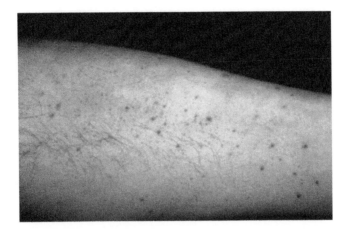

FIGURE 21.17 Perifollicular hemorrhages in the patient in Figure 21.16 with scurvy.

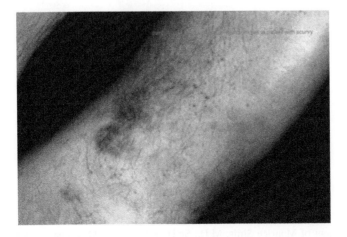

FIGURE 21.18 Ecchymosis and perifollicular hemorrhages in the patient in Figure 21.16 with scurvy.

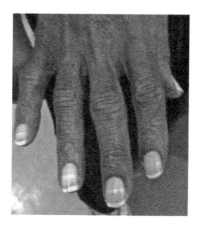

FIGURE 21.19 Aldrich–Mees' lines (leukonychia striata) in a patient with congestive hepatopathy; hospitalized 2–3 months prior to photo with atrial fibrillation, congestive heart failure; received pacemaker. Seen with hypoalbuminemia. Beau's lines are transverse ridges in nail matrix; Muehrcke's lines are vascular and do not grow out with nail.

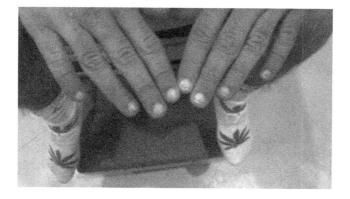

FIGURE 21.20 Terry's nails (leukonychia) in a vegan patient with chronic diarrhea, sitophobia, and abdominal pain.

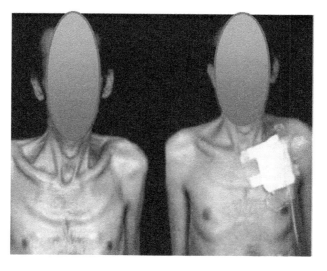

FIGURE 21.21 Patient of Maurice Shils, M.D., Sc.D., referred for TPN, due to severe radiation enteritis. Same patient 6 weeks later. (Credit to Dr. Shils. With permission.)

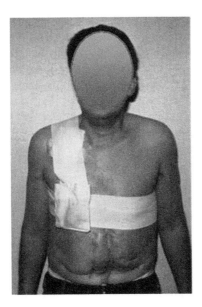

FIGURE 21.22 Same patient of Dr. Shils, 6 years later, maintained solely on home TPN. Notice venting gastrostomy. Calories in formula were reduced after this time. The patient was maintained on home TPN for over 18 years, in good health, able to work full time. (Credit to Dr. Shils. With permission.)

NUTRITIONAL ASSESSMENT: THE LAB

A variety of laboratory tests can assist in confirming the clinical nutritional diagnoses. The complete blood count (CBC) is extremely useful, inexpensive, and easily obtainable. True anemia (low hemoglobin and low RBC count) can be nutritional in nature. Some inherited abnormalities of hemoglobin (thalassemias) can have small cells, with a low hemoglobin/hematocrit. But these conditions have a normal RBC count. Although a patient with thalassemia ("Mediterranean anemia") can also develop an additional nutritional anemia, it would be a change from the baseline CBC values.

Anemia is the end stage of iron deficiency. As iron stores become depleted, red cells become smaller (microcytic, low mean corpuscular volume [MCV]), paler (hypochromic, low mean corpuscular hemoglobin [MCH]), and more variable in size (anisocytosis, increased random distribution width [RDW]). There can also be misshapen cells seen (poikilocytosis). All this often occurs before a decrease in the number of red cells and low hemoglobin/hematocrit (percentage of plasma as red blood cells).

There is a lack of "raw material" for the bone marrow "factory" to make the finished product—red blood cells. As a result, the "factory" produces "irregulars." Looking at the peripheral smear of blood can give the diagnosis. Iron studies, including serum iron, total iron binding capacity (normally about 15–30%), and ferritin (iron storage protein), can confirm the diagnosis. Iron deficiency is about the only disorder that causes a low serum ferritin. Serum ferritin is an "acute phase reactant protein," which can increase in the setting of inflammation or infection. This might give a falsely elevated value, which in some circumstances might limit its use in diagnosing iron deficiency. Questionable cases may require bone marrow evaluation of iron stores to make the diagnosis.

Elevated ferritin levels, associated with iron/binding saturation > 50%, can be seen in iron overload, whether inherited (hemochromatosis), secondary to excess intake of alcohol, supplements, or other inflammatory conditions. Inappropriate iron therapy for patients with thalassemia can be a cause of iatrogenic iron overload.

Vitamin B12 and folic acid deficiency can cause "megaloblastic," macrocytic anemias by a different mechanism than iron deficiency. In these conditions, there is a defect in DNA synthesis in rapidly dividing cells. Red blood cells are large and oval-shaped (macro-ovalocytes, high MCV) as opposed to large red blood cells that can be seen in liver, thyroid, and some other diseases. Characteristic changes are seen in neutrophil (polymorphonuclear [PMN]) white blood cells when viewed under the microscope.

Normally there are three to four nuclear segments seen. In B12 and folic acid deficiencies, PMNs have increased segmentations. More than five 5-lobed PMNs or one 6-lobed PMN make the diagnosis. Platelet count, size, and shape may also be affected. The diagnosis can be confirmed by vitamin B12 and folic acid blood levels. Low normal values may be seen in true deficiency. The more sensitive tests are methylmalonic acid (abnormal in B12 deficiency) and homocysteine (abnormal in both). These tests can be considered as confirmatory. The appropriate patient can be started on empiric therapy once the tests are obtained, pending results.

Biochemical testing can be very useful but can sometimes be confounding. For example, serum values for albumin are commonly used as a marker for protein nutrition status. However, albumin levels can vary with fluid status and physiologic stress. Albumin values can fall dramatically after surgery due to the obligatory fluid retention. Liver disease impedes production of albumin. Some kidney diseases, e.g., glomerulonephritis and nephrotic syndrome, and inflammatory protein-losing gastrointestinal diseases can increase losses.

The serum half-life of albumin is relatively long (18 days), so that changes in nutritional status after starting nutritional rehabilitation can take weeks to confirm. Pre-albumin and retinol binding proteins both have shorter serum half-life (about 2–3 days); thus, they may be better suited to confirm recent changes in nutritional status. As with serum albumin levels, these likewise can be affected by fluid status and stress. Elevations in globulin levels can be seen in inflammatory conditions, among others, including autoimmune disease and multiple myeloma.

Lactate dehydrogenase (LDH) is an enzyme found diffusely in tissues. Elevated LDH values can be seen in megaloblastic anemias (B12 and folic acid deficiency) due to "ineffective erythropoiesis" and premature cell breakdown, as well as multiple other causes.

Increases in alkaline phosphatase values can reflect obstruction to the flow of bile at the intracellular or extracellular level and thus can be seen with bile duct disease, fatty liver, or other liver disease. It may also reflect an increase in bone turnover, as in times of rapid growth, in vitamin D deficiency, as well as in Paget's disease of the bone and a variety of primary sarcomas or metastatic cancers to the bone. 5' nucleotidase or gamma glutamyl transpeptidase (GGTP) levels are increased with biliary/liver causes of elevated alkaline phosphatase, but not in bone causes. This can be very useful in differentiation. Alkaline phosphatase is a zinc-dependent enzyme. Abnormally or unexpectedly low values can be seen in zinc deficiency.

Transaminases, AST (SGOT), and ALT (SGPT) are markers of liver injury and inflammation. Inflammatory conditions of the liver generally increase ALT greater than AST. Alcoholic hepatitis characteristically has the reverse pattern (ALT < AST). Patients with alcoholic hepatitis are routinely deficient in vitamin B6. ALT is more vitamin B6-dependent than is AST; thus, it increases less.

Blood levels of sodium, potassium, magnesium, and calcium may not reflect true body stores of these critical minerals. For example, low serum sodium may occur in a patient with edema and total body sodium excess. Likewise, potassium and magnesium are largely stored within cells, so blood levels may not reflect the true status. A better assessment of the electrolyte status involves urinary measurements of the specific electrolytes and osmoles. But this subject is beyond the scope of this chapter.

Calcium is a bulk mineral, largely stored in the bone. Calcium levels in the blood are closely regulated by parathyroid hormone, calcitonin, and vitamin D. Normal blood levels can be maintained by means of dietary intake or from storage depots like the spine or hips. Therefore, one cannot generally get a sense of calcium nutrition status from blood testing. Bone densitometry, either by dual photon scanning (DEXA) or CT scanning, can give a much better assessment of calcium stores in the bone.

Osteoporosis involves weak, brittle bone with insufficient calcified bone matrix present. This increases risk for fracture. It may or may not coexist with vitamin D deficiency (rickets in children, osteomalacia in adults), which makes for soft, uncalcified bone matrix. It is important to remember that one cannot adequately treat osteoporosis with any of the available medications without first treating an associated vitamin D deficiency. Moreover, adequate calcium in the bone does not necessarily equal strong bone. Therapeutic fluoride, for example, will cause dense bone and improved density on DEXA scans. However, the bone is brittle due to abnormal internal architecture.

See the clinical cases at the end of the chapter for additional examples of laboratory evaluation of vitamin and mineral status.

CALORIE AND PROTEIN REQUIREMENTS

A patient's energy needs would be equal to the basal metabolic rate (BMR) + diet-induced thermogenesis (DIT) + physical activity. Numerous factors may affect the equation. The work of digestion (DIT) spends roughly 7–10% of calories. The postabsorptive state alters the BMR because of the work of digestion and metabolism of the ingested nutrients. Some patients, e.g., anorectics, may complain of feeling warm after eating for this very reason. Likewise, an individual who has been chilled outdoors may feel less cold by eating, even if the food itself is not hot. This effect is also referred to as the "thermic effect of food" (TEF) and the "specific dynamic action" (SDA) of food.

Fever can raise the BMR by 7% for every degree Fahrenheit or 13% for every degree centigrade. Infection has variable effects on BMR. It can increase energy expenditure over a wide range, from minimally up to an increase of 60%. In severe infection, or sepsis, there is sufficient metabolic derangement to induce a stress state, with an associated increase in nitrogen excretion.

Malnutrition and (acute) fasting can decrease the metabolic rate over time to as low as 75% of baseline. Trauma and infection will increase BMR in proportion to the trauma and stress. For example, major burn injuries can increase BMR by up to 80%. Elective surgery may have minimal effect on BMR, but emergency surgery may increase the BMR significantly.

Lastly, basal energy needs are affected by activity and calories spent. BMR calculations are based on a patient at bed rest. Ambulatory but relatively sedentary patients may use an additional 400–800 kcal over baseline. Light activity may add 800–1200 kcal, moderate activity may add 1200–1800 kcal, and vigorous, heavy activity may add 1800–4500 kcal. Be aware that most patients overestimate their degree of activity and underestimate their portion size and caloric intake.

A simple, bedside "thumb nail" approximation of energy expenditure (calorie needs) for the "normal" weight person is roughly 25–27 kcal/kg if inactive, 30–33 kcal/kg if moderately active, and 35 kcal/kg if very active. This can be increased by 5 kcal/kg in the underweight patient and decreased by 5 kcal/kg in the overweight or elderly patient.

Most clinicians do not have access to a metabolic cart. This device is used to measure resting metabolic rate (resting energy expenditure [REE]) at the bedside. The REE represents the minimal energy expenditure of an awake individual at rest in a quiet room, in the postabsorptive state. Where this equipment is available, additional and more accurate approximations of energy expenditure can be obtained. Further, the metabolic cart permits the development of derivations to estimate specific nutritional utilization of carbohydrates, proteins, and fats.

Protein needs are based on maintenance requirements for structure and function, plus 30% increase to account for individual variation, plus an additional 30% allotment for variation in protein quality. In general, 0.8 g/kg of body weight/day is more than adequate for the majority of well-nourished people. However, protein balance can be achieved up to a point, if inadequate calories are taken in. This has been utilized in a variety of weight reduction regimens. Protein needs are maintained with weight loss. Patients who are depleted or undergoing hypercatabolic stress may have increased protein needs, up to 2.0–2.5 gm/kg/day. Likewise, growing children and pregnant or lactating women have increased protein needs. These recommendations are derived from the guidelines of the National Research Council (Recommended Dietary Allowance), which is intended to cover the needs of 96% of normal, healthy people in the United States.

ILLUSTRATIVE CASES

CASE 1

CM, age 42, white male, an inpatient on the psychiatry service, consulted to evaluate cachexia, severe enough to interfere with psychiatric treatment; called to consider PEG feeding.

The patient had a history of an eating disorder (restrictive, exercise abuse), food faddism, tobacco and alcohol abuse, chronic hepatitis C (complicated by idiopathic thrombocytopenic purpura), and osteoporotic spine fracture. He refused treatment for hepatitis C and oral supplements.

The patient's weight was 61.7 kg (up to 67.5 kg while in hospital due to edema). The patient was chronically ill appearing, afebrile and cachectic, with generalized wasting. He was unable to sit up due to generalized weakness. He was alert and oriented to person and place, but not to time. Hair was dry and lifeless, but not pluckable. Skin was dry, scaly, and anicteric, with acral dermatitis, and he has white nails. Neck was supple, without palpable adenopathy, masses, or thyromegaly. Back was nontender; grade 2–3 sacral decubitus ulcer was noted. Lungs had dullness at bilateral bases. Heart exam was normal. Abdomen was distended, soft, nontender, without ascites, organomegaly, and masses. Rectal exam revealed formed, heme negative stool; prostate was normal. Extremity exam revealed anasarca, genital edema, left heel decubitus ulcer, and no clubbing. Neurological exam revealed slowed effect; cranial nerves 2–12 were normal; motor strength 2–3/5; +1 deep tendon reflexes bilaterally; Babinski responses were absent.

Laboratory data revealed the following: normocytic, normochromic anemia; low platelet count; normal white blood count; mild transaminase elevations (ALT > AST); albumin 1.8 (nl 3.5–4.5); pre-albumin 6 (nl 8–16); absent proteinuria; 25 OH vitamin D 14 (nl 30–55); HIV (–); hep C viral load (+). Assessment: profound malnutrition—mixed marasmus (protein/calorie) and kwashiorkor-like (protein depletion). Differential diagnosis included the following: eating disorder; chronic hepatitis (although normal INR and bilirubin argue against cirrhosis); protein loss (although the absence of proteinuria argues against nephrotic syndrome, and the absence of diarrhea argues against a protein losing enteropathy); malabsorption from, e.g., celiac sprue, or a net secretory state associated with hypoalbuminemia; chronic wound (decubitus ulcers); possible zinc deficiency (acral dermatitis in setting of malnutrition and chronic wound); possible essential fatty acid deficiency (scaly rash); vitamin D deficiency in the setting of liver disease, starvation, and a history of fracture; high risk for vitamin B deficiencies.

Oral intake was inadequate. The patient refused oral supplements and physical therapy. The psychiatry service was unable to use needed drugs due to the cachexia. Multiple conferences which included hospital administration and ethics committee occurred. The patient was deemed incompetent by the court and at risk to himself. This enabled tube feeding by nasoenteric feeding tube of an intact protein, polymeric formula; oral feeding; supplementing, and treating demonstrated deficiencies, and monitoring the patient until such time as he could be managed in a specialized inpatient eating disorder unit.

It is an old insight that refeeding such patients needs to be undertaken slowly to prevent the refeeding syndrome associated with hypomagnesemia, hypokalemia, and hypophosphatemia, which yields low cellular ATP, which leads to cell lysis, edema, and congestive heart failure.

Refeeding was started slowly with no more than 25 cal/kg initially, close follow-up, and repletion of electrolytes, magnesium, and phosphate. The patient was managed at an inpatient eating disorder unit for several months. The feeding tube was able to be removed after 2 weeks, once the patient recovered enough to take adequate oral intake to allow for optimal psychiatric treatment, i.e., talk therapy and drug therapy. PEG tube was avoided.

CASE 2

L.O., a 40-year-old man, presents with profound fatigue, daytime somnolence, and depression. He had a complex medical history, including meningitis as a teen and head trauma at age 12. At age 30, he had gastric bypass surgery (restrictive/malabsorptive) complicated by persistent vomiting, thrombophlebitis of the left leg, and an anastomotic leak. He underwent the first of several operations, complicated by infection and/or wound breakdown. He required implantation of an intrathecal pump for pain meds. Aside from his pain doctor, he saw no physicians and was not compliant with diet, supplements, or use of CPAP machine for sleep apnea.

The patient's wife noted that he "wasn't himself" for the past week; he was "listless, and confused," and more irritable than usual. He complained of achy numbness in his legs, was too weak for his usual activities, and was unable to work. He had abdominal and back pain; oral intake had been poor for a few weeks, although he was drinking liquids. There was no fever; he was passing stool and urine without difficulty. He had interrupted sleep. There were no recent falls.

On physical examination, height was 68 in., weight 216 lbs. (presurgical weight was 266 lbs.). Vital signs were stable: heart rate 86, regular; respirations 14, unlabored; blood pressure 110/68 in both arms, without orthostatic changes. He was alert and oriented, but sluggish and easily distracted. He had difficulty filling in the details of his medical history. His exam was noteworthy for conjunctival pallor and pale creases in the palms; normal cardiac and pulmonary exams; obese, scarred abdomen with normal bowel sounds, absent succussion splash, 16-cm-sized liver; brown stool, without occult blood; and normal back exam, including straight leg raise tests. Neurological exam showed decreased extraocular movements, decreased sensation to light touch in the legs, decreased deep tendon reflexes diffusely, down-going plantar responses, proximal muscle weakness in the legs, trace pretibial edema, tenderness to palpation over the tibias, and a slightly broad-based gait, with decreased vibration sensation in the feet.

Initial bedside assessment included possible drug overdosing (due to his intrathecal medications) and seizures. However, acute changes in mental status and neurological exam in any patient with gastric bypass surgery who reports poor intake must include nutritional causes as well. Patient was tested for, and empirically treated for, thiamine deficiency with parenteral and high-dose oral thiamine (100 mg/day) while awaiting test results (which confirmed deficiency). Partial improvement in sensory exam, memory, and eye movements (Wernicke's encephalopathy) occurred. Thiamine deficiency was a causative factor for the decreased sensation and weakness in the legs, as well as mental status changes.

In addition, the history of fatigue, listlessness, weakness, poor job performance, consistent with symptomatic anemia (Hgb 7.5 gm/dL), and pale conjunctiva would be seen with anemia. Pale creases in the palms signaled a more profound anemia (Hgb 7.5). Anemia in bariatric surgery patients is often due to multiple factors such as deficiency of iron, B12, folate, and less commonly copper. This patient had a profound iron deficiency, as well as vitamin B12 deficiency. He was started on parenteral B12 therapy (1000 μg/week for 8 weeks) and switched to high-dose oral therapy (2 mg/day) after B12 stores were filled. The patient was unable to tolerate oral iron; thus, he was given parenteral infusions, with significant clinical improvement, and resolution of anemia.

This patient also had dramatic vitamin D deficiency (25 OH D level 6.2 [N 30–150]), symptomatic with muscle and bone aches. After treatment with high-dose vitamin D2 (50,000 IU/week × 8 doses), his bone pain resolved. He has since been maintained on oral vitamin D3 (1200 IU/day) with good result.

Mental status and cognitive changes improved but continued. Further evaluation confirmed a seizure disorder. Improvement occurred with drug treatment and CPAP use for sleep apnea.

CASE 3

Chief complaint: H.C., a 76-year-old white woman, presents with increasing leg swelling and weakness of 6 weeks duration; 28 pound weight loss over the past year, despite a "voracious" appetite.

There was no nausea, vomiting, swallowing difficulties, heartburn, abdominal pain, or gross blood loss. However, there was bloating. Stools were loose until starting on oral iron months ago. She complained of bone pain but not back pain. Last GYN exam was decades ago. Prior evaluation included CT of abdomen and pelvis and upper GI series—with unknown results. Past medical history (PMH): hysterectomy; vitamin B12 use in the past. Medications: iron sulfate, dipyridamole, calcium carbonate. No known drug allergies. Sister died from "cancer of intestines associated with ileitis." The patient was married, homemaker; no travel, coffee, tobacco, alcohol use. ROS: As above. General weakness, without tingling, paresthesias, clumsiness. No bruising, bleeding.

PE: Chronically ill, cachectic woman in no acute distress. Wt: 71 lbs., Ht: 55", RR: 12, unlabored, HR 84 regular, BP 90/60 left arm sitting, standing. Skin: dry, flaky, slightly decreased turgor; nails normal. HEENT: conjunctival pallor; no lid or globe lag; tongue papillated; teeth in poor repair. Nodes: none palpable. Lungs clear to percussion and auscultation. Cardiac exam: regular rate, rhythm, PMI normal, not displaced; no murmurs, gallops, rubs. Back: nontender, exaggerated kyphosis. Abdomen: scaphoid; active bowel sounds; no bruits, succussion splash; soft; no organomegaly; no tenderness; no masses. Pelvic: atrophic introitus, vaginal vaults; equivocal tenderness, fullness in right adnexa. Rectal: unremarkable; stool brown, formed, heme positive. Extremities: generalized wasting/atrophy. 2+–3+ pretibial edema; myoedema. Neurological exam was normal including cognition, cranial nerves, cerebellar, tone, sensation, vibration and proprioception, deep tendon, and plantar reflexes; motor strength 2+–3+ bilaterally.

At the bedside, this was a profoundly malnourished, chronically ill appearing woman. Clinically, she was anemic, had combined protein-calorie deficiency, and likely other deficiencies, e.g., myoedema as a sign of phosphate depletion. Chronic loose stools could increase risk for magnesium depletion and zinc depletion. Bone pain could be from malignancy and vitamin D deficiency. Dry, flaky skin could be due to essential fatty acid deficiency, vitamin A deficiency, and zinc depletion. She did not have cardiac failure. Possible causes included malignancy-GYN and/or gastrointestinal, localized and/or metastatic (although the "voracious" appetite argued against this). Chronic loose stools could be seen with infection/parasite/*C. difficile* colitis/malabsorption due to celiac disease, bacterial overgrowth of small bowel, pancreatic disease, inflammatory bowel disease, malignancy, e.g., tumor of neuroendocrine origin. She refused hospitalization or invasive testing.

Initial lab data revealed microcytic, hypochromic anemia (Hgb 8.6, MCV 68); absolute lymphopenia; low phosphate; elevated alkaline phosphatase; mildly elevated transaminases; high LDH; low albumin, normal globulin; low magnesium, iron stores; markedly low lipids; mild increase in INR; and normal "cancer antigens." Additional lab tests included vitamin B12 (361), with elevated methylmalonic acid; low serum and RBC folate; low vitamin A; low beta carotene; low 25 OH vitamin D (5.0); low normal serum zinc; and normal serum selenium.

Assessment confirmed multiple deficiencies and a single organism bladder infection (going against, e.g., a fistula from bowel to bladder). Low beta carotene and folate could be due to inadequate intake. Low folate goes against small bowel bacterial overgrowth. Low carotene, vitamin A, and increased INR (evaluation for vitamin K status) are consistent with fat malabsorption. Cause of the malnutrition still to be confirmed.

Previously obtained radiology studies: upper GI series revealed three duodenal diverticula, normal mucosal pattern; CT scan revealed cholelithiasis, "abdominal cysts," but no evidence of malignancy. Further evaluation included markedly abnormal D-xylose test, consistent with significant jejunal mucosal abnormality and malabsorption; markedly abnormal anti-gliadin antibody (IgA), and anti-endomysial antibody, consistent with celiac sprue. The patient refused any invasive evaluation.

Initial treatment included ciprofloxacin for the bladder infection (which would likely have a favorable effect on small bowel bacterial overgrowth due to intestinal diverticula): strict gluten-free diet, reviewed with a dietician; supplementation with a polymeric, protein supplement; supplemental folic acid (5 mg/day), vitamin B12 (1000 µg/week × 8 weeks, then monthly), vitamin D2 (50,000 IU/week);

iron sulfate (324 mg tid), vitamin A (5000 IU/day), vitamin K (5 mg/day), vitamin E (400 IU/day), and multivitamin/mineral supplement.

The patient responded with improved bowel habit, increased vigor, strength, and well-being, loss of edema, and with weight gain to a maximum 85 lbs. With poor compliance, the patient noted prompt symptom recurrence and weight loss. The patient was switched to an intact protein, polymeric supplement. Follow-up labs revealed normalization of iron, vitamins A, D, K, and Zn and anemia. Serum protein status improved but remained marginal in setting of frequent poor compliance with gluten-free diet. Follow-up DEXA scan confirmed very severe osteoporosis; the patient deferred any treatment.

The spectrum of nutritional problems in celiac sprue is extensive, leading to a variety of the many manifestations of the disease. The autoimmune reaction to gliadin and related proteins leads to inflammatory changes in the small bowel mucosa. Initial changes occur spottily in the upper small bowel, but with time can become much more extensive, leading to loss of absorptive surface area and a net secretory environment. This will lead to impaired amino acid and peptide absorption, impaired disaccharide hydrolysis, and malabsorption of fat. Consequences can include anemia due to iron, folic acid, vitamin B12, and copper deficiency; deficiencies of pyridoxine (B6), ascorbic acid, possible deficiencies of thiamine, riboflavin, niacin, pantothenic acid; and deficiencies of fat-soluble vitamins A, D, E, and K. Mineral deficiencies affecting calcium and magnesium are common. Trace metal deficiencies affecting zinc and copper occur.

CONCLUSION

In summary, awareness of nutritional aspects of medical care is an age-old insight that remains relevant today, confirmed by years of empirical and clinical research. The most effective clinician will use all the available tools at his/her disposal, including skilled use of history, effective observation in the physical exam, and appropriate use of additional technology. Such an approach can improve practitioners' relationships with patients, their own clinical skills, improve student and trainee education, decrease unnecessary costs, and improved patient outcome.

REFERENCES

1. A.D.A.M. Medical Encyclopedia. A.D.A.M., Atlanta, GA, 2013. Available at http://www.adameducation.com.
2. World Food Programme. Available at http://www.wfp.org/hunger/malnutrition, 2009.
3. White JV et al. Consensus statement of the Academy of Nutrition and Dietetics/American Society for Parenteral and Enteral Nutrition: Characteristics recommended for the identification and documentation of adult malnutrition (undernutrition). *J Acad Nutr Diet* 2012; 112 (11): 1899, 275–283.
4. Anthony PS. Nutrition screening tools for hospitalized patients. *Nutr Clin Pract* 2008; 23 (4): 373–382.
5. Organization for Economic Cooperation and Development. Available at http://www.oecd.org/health/healthsystems, 2013.
6. Adams KM, Kohlmeir M, Zeisel SH. Nutrition education in U.S. medical schools: Latest update of a national survey. *Acad Med* 2010; 85 (9): 1537–1542.
7. Committee on Nutrition in Medical Education. Food and Nutrition Board National Research Council. *Nutrition Education*. National Academies Press, Washington, D.C., 1985.
8. Shils ME, Lowell BC, Deen D. *Physical Diagnosis-Nutritional Aspects: A Manual for Instructors and Students*. The Regional Center for Clinical Nutrition Education at The New York Academy of Medicine, The New York Academy of Medicine, New York, 1993.
9. Nutrition in Medicine. Available at http://www.NutritioninMedicine.net, 2013.
10. Ross AC et al. eds. *Modern Nutrition in Health and Disease*, 11th edition. Lippincott, Williams & Wilkins, Baltimore, MD, 2014.
11. Paley L et al. Utility of clinical examination in the diagnosis of emergency department patients admitted to the department of medicine of an academic hospital. *Arch Int Med* 2011; 171 (15): 1393–1140.
12. Goodman R. Commentary: Health care technology and medical education: Putting physical diagnosis in its proper place. *Acad Med* 2010; 85 (6): 945–946.

13. Reilly BM. Physical examination in the care of medical inpatients: An observational study. *Lancet* 2003; 362 (9390): 1100–1105.

14. Sandler G. The importance of the history in the medical clinic and the cost of unnecessary test. *Am Heart J* 1980; 100 (6 Pt 1): 928–931.

15. van Dijk N et al. High diagnostic yield and accuracy of history, physical examination, and ECG in patients with transient loss of consciousness in FAST: The fainting assessment study. *J Cardiovasc Electrophysiol* 2008; 19 (1): 48–55.

16. Max J. The lost art of the physical exam. Available at http://yalemedicine.yale.edu/winter2009/features /feature/51079, 2009.

17. Verghese A. Stanford initiative in bedside medicine. Available at http://medicine.stanford.edu/education /stanford_25.html, 2014.

18. Bates B. *A Guide to Physical Examination and History Taking*, 7th edition. J.B. Lippincott Co., Philadelphia, PA, 1999.

19. DeGowin RL. *DeGowin's Diagnostic Examination*, 7th edition. McGraw-Hill, New York, 1999.

20. Berg D, Worzala K. *Atlas of Adult Physical Diagnosis*. Lippincott Williams & Wilkins, Baltimore, MD, 2006.

21. Orient JM. *Sapira's The Art & Science of Bedside Diagnosis*, 4th edition. Williams & Wilkins, Baltimore, MD, 2009.

22. Dietary reference intakes National Academy of Sciences. Institute of Medicine. Food and Nutrition Board. Available at http://fnic.nal.usda.gov/dietary-guidance/dietary-reference-intakes/dri-tables, 2010.

23. Available at http://www.jointcommission.org/standards_information/jcfaqdetails.aspx?, 2013.

24. McCabe BJ, Frankel EH, Wolfe JJ, eds. *Handbook of Food-Drug Interactions*. CRC Press, Boca Raton, FL, 2003.

25. Volkerta YN et al. ESPN guidelines on enteral nutrition. *Clin Nutr* 2006; 25: 330–360.

26. Mediratta P et al. Trends in percutaneous endoscopic gastrostomy placement in the elderly from 1993 to 2003. *Am J Alzheimers Dis Other Demen.* 2012; 27 (8): 609–613.

27. Shaikh AK et al. Revisiting the use of percutaneous endoscopic gastrostomy tubes in patients with advanced dementia. *Palliat Care Res Treat* 2009; 3: 1–2.

28. Regnard C et al. Gastrostomies in dementia: Bad practice or bad evidence? *Age Aging* 2010; 39 (3): 282–284.

29. Poitou Bernert C et al. Nutritional deficiency after gastric bypass: Diagnosis, prevention and treatment. *Diabetes Metab* 2007; 33 (1): 13–24.

30. Ziegler O et al. Medical follow up after bariatric surgery: Nutritional and drug issues general recommendations for the prevention and treatment of nutritional deficiencies. *Diabetes Metab* 2009; 35: 544–557.

31. Kaiser MJ et al. Validation of the Mini Nutritional Assessment-short form (MNA-SF): A practical tool for identification of nutritional status. *J Nutr Health Aging* 2009; 13 (9): 782–788.

32. McMinn J et al. Clinical review: Investigation and management of unintentional weight loss in older adults. *BMJ* 2011; 342: d1742.

33. Quetelet A. Nouveaux Memoire de l'Academie Royale des Sciences et Bellees Lettres de Bruxelles, 1832; Recherches sur le poids de l'homme aux Different Ages.

34. Quetelet A. *A Treatise on Man and the Development of his Faculties*. Burt Franklin, NY, originally published 1842. Reprinted in 1968.

35. DuBois D, DuBois EF. Clinical calorimetry tenth paper a formula to estimate the approximate surface area if height and weight are known. *Arch Int Med* 1916; 17: 863–871.

36. Keys A et al. Indices of relative weight and obesity. *J Chronic Dis* 1972; 25 (6–7): 329–343.

22 Nutritional Support
Enteral and Parenteral Nutrition

Stanley J. Dudrick, Lisa P. Haverstick,
and Michael M. Rothkopf

CONTENTS

INTRODUCTION

It would not be appropriate to write a book on metabolic medicine and surgery without including a chapter on nutritional support of hospitalized patients. This therapy is one of the transformative modalities that have defined the specialty. The complexity of the required formulas and the potential for metabolic complications created a need for specialists who were willing to take on the challenge of caring for patients requiring specialized nutritional support. Furthermore, the development of individualized home enteral and parenteral nutrition methods and techniques for patients requiring long-term ambulatory nutrition support has become a major daily activity for practitioners in the field.

The modern history of nutritional support begins in the mid-twentieth century with research by Dr. Rose, Dr. Rhoads, Dr. Wretlind, Dr. Elman, Dr. Allen, and Dr. Moore, among others, on providing intravenous nutrition via peripheral veins. However, technological and technical hurdles impeded the emergence of a practical, efficacious form of total parenteral nutrition (TPN) [1–11].

In 1968, Dr. Stanley Dudrick and his colleagues at the University of Pennsylvania pioneered the use of central venous TPN, crystallizing the prior concepts and efforts into a practical reality [12–17]. This momentous accomplishment was built on a history that spanned nearly 350 years beginning with William Harvey's published description of the circulation of blood in 1628. Sydney Ringer designed a solution of sodium, potassium, and calcium salts for perfusing frog hearts in 1882. Alexis Hartmann modified this formula in 1932 by adding lactate. The widespread acceptance of Ringer's lactate heralded the era of modern IV fluid administration [18].

Dudrick's breakthrough hinged on the development of safe, practical access to the superior vena cava (SVC) for efficacious long-term infusion of nutrient substrates. The dilutional effect of the high blood flow through this large-diameter vessel permitted the administration of hypertonic solutions, which were necessary to provide nutrient requirements within limitations of water tolerances. Documented proof of this approach was a watershed event, opening the doors to a flood of rapid developments that were necessary to advance the seminal concept to a clinically accepted therapeutic adjunct and primary modality.

In a parallel timeline, scientific studies of nutrition led to the recognition of the protein-sparing effect of glucose during fasting and the specifics of essential and nonessential amino acid requirements [1,3,19–29]. An understanding of essential vitamins, trace elements, and other micronutrients was also emerging. The concepts of nitrogen balance, nutritional assessment, resting, and stress metabolism completed the theoretical framework for the diagnosis, understanding, and treatment of malnutrition [1,3,19–29].

Enteral feeding formulas also benefited from subsequent scientific advancements, resulting in development and standardization of infusion principles and practices and disease-specific formulations. As a result, a trend has emerged toward greater use of enteral feeding and the use of TPN only when absolutely necessary [30,31]. An understated important contribution of TPN is that it demonstrated beyond a doubt the relevance and value of optimal parenteral nutritional support in the most severely malnourished and critically ill patients, thus paving the way for promoting advances in oral and enteral nutrition support technology and applications, and improving outcomes in a wide variety of clinical situations by a larger number and broader base of practitioners.

PATIENT SELECTION

Patients who are not able to eat, or whose intakes are inadequate to meet their metabolic requirements, are candidates for some form of specialized nutritional support. Nutritional status will generally deteriorate when intake is reduced in combination with injury, stress, or illness. Because a malnourished patient is at higher risk for complications, it is a clinical imperative to address the nutritional risk and make every effort to reduce it.

In a normally nourished individual, the institution of specialized nutritional support is not ordinarily an emergency. Nutritionally replete patients can usually withstand 24–48 h without nutrition before the onset of metabolic adaptation to starvation (see Chapter 1). The goal in these patients is to prevent endogenous protein from the lean tissues, especially muscle, from being sacrificed and catabolized to form glucose by providing basal energy requirements via the infusion of 400–600 g of isotonic dextrose intravenously. This concept is referred to as "nitrogen sparing."

In a patient who is already malnourished on admission, the primary goal is nutritional repletion. This cannot be a rapid process. In general, it is estimated to take two to three times longer to achieve repletion of protein and energy stores as it did to deplete them. It is also important to realize that provision of excessive nutrition or rapid nutrient administration will not replete the patient faster. Such well-intentioned, but injudicious, overfeeding may cause untoward, even lethal, metabolic consequences [2,3,19,20].

The stress of illness creates greater metabolic needs and increases the likelihood that lean body mass (LBM) will be depleted rapidly and extensively. This also mandates that the metabolic and nutritional requirements will be higher in the critically ill, such as those having sustained trauma, burns, and sepsis, and the catabolic effects of their stress may be impossible to overcome. The nutritional goal in these patients is suppression of the catabolic rate to the greatest extent possible, while simultaneously trying to provide required nutrients without overfeeding [32–39].

The highest risk case is a patient who is both malnourished and suffering from a critical illness. The patient is already depleted, and the stress of illness will undoubtedly add further to the loss of LBM. Nutritional repletion will not be likely to occur during the acute phase of a patient's critical illness. Nutritional maintenance may be the only achievable goal at this point and should be pursued judiciously to the maximal extent possible and practical. This translates to an attempt to keep up meticulously with the daily metabolic needs [32–39]. The heightened requirements of the patient for energy and protein should be estimated and delivered, and any existing micronutrient deficiencies should also be identified and restored [40,41]. The full recovery of the patient's nutritional status will generally not be achieved until well into the recuperative phase of the illness.

An estimate of the patient's stress level will be a factor in determining the need for the aggressiveness of nutritional support. Ideally, one could assess the degree of stress metabolism through the use of metabolic gas analysis and calorimetry, but if this is unavailable, indirect measures of stress such as circulating biomarkers (i.e., CRP and IL-6) may suffice.

A full nutritional assessment should be performed to determine the patient's macronutrient and micronutrient status (detail on the bedside diagnosis of malnutrition is found in Chapter 21). A nutritional prescription would then be outlined to define the goals of treatment. Adjustments in therapy will be necessary as data return to the chart and as the clinical status and biochemical homeostasis evolve.

Some patients can be fed with calorie, protein, and micronutrient supplements to complement their spontaneous dietary intake. An ongoing daily assessment of oral intake should be performed by the staff to determine the adequacy of intake and documented in the medical record.

For those who cannot eat, the use of enteral nutrition via a nasogastric, nasojejunal, gastrostomy, or jejunostomy tube should be attempted. Enteral nutrition follows the nutritional prescription with a goal based on the estimated calorie and protein requirements. The tube feeding should be started slowly, the concentration increased incrementally first, and then the infusion can be advanced to the goal rate and volume as tolerated. Careful monitoring for intolerance and complications is mandatory.

There are special situations in which either oral intake or enteral feeding is taking place, but the quantity of nutritional intake is inadequate for meeting the patient's nutritional requirements. In this setting, a component of TPN (such as the amino acids) should be added as needed as a supplemental modality.

If oral or tube feeding is impossible or not tolerated, TPN must be considered. TPN can be thought of as a "lifeboat" or "stop-gap" measure to prevent loss of nutritional status. As in the lifeboat analogy, one never chooses to use it if a more judicious option exists. But, by the same token, it is clearly indicated if the only alternative is further deterioration and the risk of associated complications.

The consequences of malnutrition on the patient's wound healing, recovery from illness, and length of hospital stay have been well documented [29]. Therefore, few would disagree with the need to prevent and treat malnutrition, but the preferred methodology for achieving these goals remains controversial. A dichotomy exists between metabolic practitioners and those in nonmetabolic specialties as to when to utilize TPN. Similarly, there is an obvious difference in how these clinicians view the safety and efficacy of TPN. Moreover, there is no single methodology that can be uniformly applied rationally in all clinical situations, with the expectation of optimal safety and efficacy.

The ongoing debate regarding the use of enteral versus parenteral nutrition for the nutritional management of hospitalized patients is beyond the scope of this chapter. However, it is important to realize the many limitations in interpreting both sides of the issue [39,42].

The science is complex, involving a wide range of therapy options available to a heterogeneous mixture of patients with different diagnoses and acuity levels. Furthermore, a patient's condition may change in the course of study, creating uncontrollable variables among the study groups. These conundrums are shared by many other types of studies in critically ill patients. The data may be further compromised by the fact that the provision of nutrients is often based only on an estimate of patient needs. There are few studies in which calorie and protein needs have been directly measured. Therefore, the provision of nutrients could have been mismatched for the precise metabolic requirements.

This is not to suggest that enteral feeding is not an important preferable option. Providing nutrients via the gastrointestinal (GI) tract stimulates physiologic gut hormone production, which may have whole body effects. We are also in the midst of a new understanding regarding the importance of maintaining a healthy bowel flora, which may help the immune system and prevent other diseases [30,31]. Enteral nutrition can have a crucial role in these processes.

Nonetheless, there are some patients for whom the enteral route is not the most appropriate access to achieve the goals of therapy. A malnourished, stressed patient with a dysfunctional gut must be considered a candidate for TPN. In these situations, it would be counterproductive to delay adequate rational parenteral nutritional support when attempts at enteral feeding are likely to fail.

TPN INDICATIONS

A reasonable place to start the discussion about which patients are likely to require TPN rather than enteral feeding would be with a malnourished patient who has undergone extensive GI surgery. The return to normal GI function may not occur for 7–10 days. Earlier attempts at oral or enteral feedings may induce vomiting, aspiration, ileus, or other untoward complications [43,44].

The primary indication for early TPN consideration is the short bowel syndrome (SBS). This is especially true in the immediate postoperative period before the bowel has had time to adapt. These patients can have major electrolyte and fluid disturbances due to excessive GI losses. They may require TPN for prolonged periods of time until reasonably effective bowel adaptation occurs [43–45]. Enterocytes eventually undergo a period of hyperplasia, which makes it possible for the remaining bowel to assume much of the previously normal absorptive capacity. The presence of specialized nutrients in the intestinal lumen may help to facilitate this process. TPN should generally be continued until adequate gut function can be assured. Patients who have less than 5 ft of residual small bowel beyond the ligament of Treitz are sometimes unable to adapt entirely successfully and may require long-term TPN.

Patients with bowel obstruction, either partial or complete, are obvious candidates for TPN. This is especially true in patients for whom surgery is not an option and placement of an effective feeding tube distal to the obstruction is not possible. Patients with chronic intestinal pseudo-obstruction may also require TPN.

TPN can be useful in managing gastric outlet obstruction (GOO) from either a benign or malignant disease process that prevents the emptying of the stomach contents into the small intestine, and effective feeding distal to the site is not feasible. The standard approach to a patient with GOO is the insertion of a nasogastric tube (NGT) for several days to decompress the size of the stomach. If the obstruction is due to scarring from an ulcer, then surgery may be required. If the obstruction is due to edema, surgery may be avoided with gastric decompression alone. Depending on the length of time needed for gastric decompression, it may be necessary for the patient to be started on parenteral nutrition until oral intake can be resumed.

In a patient with acute pancreatitis, the degree of severity of the disease, along with the nutritional status of the patient, will be the determining factors in the decision of when to initiate nutritional support. Serum lipids must be closely monitored in order to avoid hypertriglyceridemia. Use of parenteral nutrition in a patient with mild, acute, or relapsing pancreatitis of short duration remains controversial, and enteral nutrition has been used successfully in most of this subgroup of pancreatitis patients safely and efficaciously by skilled nutrition practitioners [46].

GI tract fistulas, which can form due to disease, surgery, or trauma, have long been recognized as indications for the use of parenteral nutrition. Malnutrition due to the inability to feed the patient enterally, electrolyte disturbances, and sepsis all contribute to the increased mortality associated with enterocutaneous fistulas. Optimization of the patient's nutritional status and advances that have been made in wound care and abdominal reconstructive surgical techniques have decreased mortality rates. Putting the GI tract "at rest," with the use of medications such as octreotide to decrease pancreatic and other GI tract secretions, nasogastric suction, prompt use of antibiotics to control infection, and maintenance of nutrition and hydration status have all contributed to improved outcomes for this patient population. This is especially important in a patient in whom it is not possible to place a feeding tube distal to the fistula or in patients with high output fistulas (usually more than 500 mL/day) [43,44].

TPN can be quite effective in ameliorating hyperemesis gravidarum with persistent nausea and vomiting. Studies have demonstrated that the nutritional status of the mother plays a significant role in determining fetal outcome [47]. Neural tube defects and congenital anomalies have been identified with malnutrition in the first trimester of pregnancy, whereas low birth weight, small for gestational age infants, and an underdeveloped central nervous system have been associated with malnutrition in the last half of pregnancy [47–49].

Radiation enteritis is a complication of cancer treatment that results in damage to the cells that line the small or large intestine in patients who have undergone radiation treatments in the abdominal or pelvic area. It can cause swelling, inflammation, and other distortions of the enterocytes, which can lead to malabsorption. Patients may experience diarrhea, weight loss, and loss of appetite. Dietary modification is the first line of treatment, along with the use of antidiarrheal agents. If prolonged or severe, diarrhea can lead to the need for either short- or long-term parenteral nutrition in order to maintain the nutrition and hydration status of the patient as the bowel regains its normal healthy status and function.

Patients with inflammatory bowel disease, such as Crohn's disease or ulcerative colitis, frequently experience weight loss, especially the former. There is a high incidence of malnutrition in patients who are diagnosed with inflammatory bowel disease. Surgical resection of the diseased bowel, or the need for bowel rest in order to avoid surgery, is an indication for short-term use of parenteral nutrition. Parenteral nutrition may also be indicated for a patient who is unresponsive to standard medical therapy [50].

Malabsorption is defined as defective or inadequate absorption of nutrients from the alimentary tract. It may be caused by infective agents, structural defects of the GI tract, alterations of the GI tract as a result of a surgical procedure, mucosal abnormalities, enzyme deficiencies, digestive failure, and/or systemic diseases affecting the GI tract.

Steatorrhea due to the presence of excess fat in the stool may be the result of either impaired fat digestion or fat absorption. The most common causes of steatorrhea include malabsorption, pancreatic insufficiency, pancreatitis, pancreatic cancer, SBS, and cystic fibrosis.

Intestinal dysmotility, as a result of abnormal intestinal contractions required to move food through the digestive tract, may require TPN for adequate nutrition support. Included in this category is chronic intestinal pseudo-obstruction, which presents as a functional blockage without an occluding lesion. Parenteral nutrition may be indicated if the condition is unresponsive to prokinetic medications, although these medications are less effective in the small intestine than in the stomach.

Patients who are unable to meet their nutritional requirements via voluntary oral intake and who refuse to have a feeding tube inserted may be candidates for the temporary use of parenteral nutrition until they are able to resume their usual dietary intake. Patients with a prior history of ascites or cirrhosis may also require parenteral nutrition because the risk of inserting a feeding gastrostomy may far outweigh the potential benefits to the patient.

Surgical resection of a portion of the GI tract to remove a malignant tumor may render the patient a temporary candidate for parenteral nutrition. Loss of structure means loss of function and often indicates the subsequent need for supplemental or TPN until use of the remaining GI tract is possible and adequate for meeting nutrient requirements [43,44].

Chylous ascites, caused by the accumulation of lymphatic fluid in the abdominal cavity, is a potential indication for the use of TPN. Chylothorax, due to leakage of lymphatic fluid into the pleural cavity, usually caused by lymphoma or trauma, or as a result of thoracic surgery, is another indication for the use of parenteral nutrition. This is especially true in a patient in whom fat-free enteral feedings fail to reduce chylous output significantly, or when the losses are great enough to produce hypoalbuminemia [51].

RELATIVE TPN CONTRAINDICATIONS

Even in the conditions outlined above, TPN may be contraindicated at times. This is particularly true in patients with septicemia, or hepatic or renal failure. It should also be used cautiously in any patient with evidence of allergy to a TPN component, such as to the egg-derived emulsifier in lipid emulsion.

As a general rule, we prefer to avoid intravenous infusion in patients with persistent bacteremia. Septicemia is a major potential complication of TPN. In the patient who is already bacteremic, the concern is that the nutrient infusion may worsen or, at the very least, prolong the bacteremia. If this occurs, it may be due to hyperglycemia secondary to providing glucose above physiologic utilization. If TPN must be given to a septic patient, glucose levels must be assiduously controlled and maintained in the euglycemic range [52,53].

TPN has the potential to cause liver damage. A small number of patients who were dependent on long-term TPN developed liver failure and have required orthotopic liver transplant. Although the mechanism of TPN-related transaminitis is unclear, most practitioners would hesitate to continue TPN administration when the liver enzymes are significantly increasing. Therefore, we ordinarily consider standard TPN contraindicated in a patient with advancing liver failure.

The administration of amino acids is a driving factor in the production of ammonia. Since excessive ammonia can be toxic in humans, the liver must either shuttle it to the kidneys or metabolize it to urea. The urea cycle enzymes exist in the hepatic mitochondria and cytosol. With hepatic cellular dysfunction, this important process is impaired, and the risk for developing hyperammonemia is increased. As liver failure worsens, blood ammonia concentration may reach toxic levels. The added burden of processing the amino acid-derived ammonia may worsen the condition of the already compromised hepatocytes and place the patient in further danger. Therefore, the use of standard TPN may be contraindicated in preexisting liver failure, and special high branched chain amino acid TPN formulations may be indicated or helpful in providing nutrition support to these critically ill patients.

Patients with end-stage liver failure often experience severe hypoglycemia due to lack of gluconeogenesis once glycogen stores in the liver are depleted. These patients require a constant infusion of dextrose to prevent hypoglycemia. The inability to support gluconeogenesis also indicates that the liver may be unable to metabolize other nutrients as well, and provision of nutritional support to these patients may increase metabolic stress levels. Until and unless the patient undergoes liver transplantation, the most appropriate nutritional support regimen may be the parenteral provision of dextrose and appropriate vitamins and minerals continuously while maintaining euglycemia [54–60].

The kidneys are responsible for excretion of nitrogenous waste and regulation of fluid, electrolyte, and acid–base balance. They also perform metabolic processes such as the production of renin and erythropoietin, and converting vitamin D from food or the skin into the biologically active metabolic substrate. When the kidneys are unable to perform these activities due to loss of functioning nephrons, accumulation of metabolic waste products occurs, and dialysis may be necessary to restore homeostasis.

Nutritional support for a patient with acute renal failure is focused on minimizing the hypercatabolic and hypermetabolic response to the injury, which caused the decline in renal function. Protein, carbohydrate, and lipid metabolism are all altered in a patient with acute renal failure, and protein, electrolytes, and fluids must be carefully balanced during this time. Indications for, and contraindications to, the use of nutritional support in a patient with acute renal failure should follow the same guidelines used in initiating nutritional support in other critically ill patients [61].

In patients with chronic renal failure, the type of renal replacement therapy that the patient is receiving can have a significant impact on the ability of the practitioner to provide adequate nutritional support. The etiology of the underlying chronic kidney disease also must be evaluated, especially in a patient with diabetes in order to achieve optimal glycemic control. Parenteral nutrition should be reserved for use in critically ill or metabolically stressed patients who are unable to meet their nutritional requirements via oral intake or the use of enteral supplementation.

Intradialytic parenteral nutrition (IDPN) has been used with some success in malnourished patients who have failed to respond to oral or enteral supplementation. IDPN involves the infusion of a concentrated nutrient solution via the venous drip chamber of the dialysis tubing. The amount of fluid that can be delivered is determined by the length of the dialysis treatment (usually 4 hours) and is intermittent in nature since the patient is not dialyzed daily. IDPN is not recommended as the sole means of nutritional support but rather as a supplemental starvation deterrent.

Use of lipid emulsions may be contraindicated in both adult and pediatric patients who are allergic to eggs. Depending on the type of lipid emulsion used, it may also be necessary to screen the patient for a soy allergy. The use of corn-derived dextrose may pose a potential problem for those patients who are allergic to corn and corn products. The amino acid components of the formula are rarely allergenic for patients requiring parenteral nutrition.

VENOUS ACCESS

Once the decision has been made to initiate parenteral nutrition, the next step is to choose the access route for administration of TPN. TPN can be administered via the peripheral or central route. In either case, a dedicated TPN line is strongly mandated.

PERIPHERAL ACCESS

The easiest way to begin TPN is through a peripheral vein. The peripheral veins in the upper extremities are preferred as those of the lower extremities are associated with an increased risk of thromboembolism. A peripheral IV access is obviously the easiest and least costly to place. It is also the easiest to replace or remove, and as a result of ease of removal and low threshold for removal, and usually shorter duration in situ, has the lowest incidence of catheter-related infections. Peripheral

TPN may be appropriate for short-term therapy, usually 2 weeks or less. The most common complications associated with the use of peripheral intravenous access are infiltration, occlusion, phlebitis, catheter embolism, and hematoma [62–65].

The peripheral veins are exquisitely sensitive to the osmolarity of the components of the solution infused. This generally mandates that the solutions should contain less than 10% dextrose and 5% amino acids. It is a good practice for metabolic consultants to calculate the osmolarity of the TPN solution and ascertain that the solution is appropriate for the venous access (see Components of TPN Solutions) [63].

Infusions with a final osmolarity of less than 600 mOsm can ordinarily be tolerated peripherally for 1–2 days. Since peripheral IV sites are usually changed after 48 hours, therapy can sometimes be sequentially continued for several days. As the osmolarity of the TPN solution increases, the length of time that the infusion is tolerated decreases. TPN solutions having an osmolarity of more than 900 mOsm should be considered above the tolerance level for safe, rational peripheral administration in most patients [62].

Peripheral TPN can provide sufficient protein, electrolytes, vitamins, and trace elements for some selected patients, but the ability to support the total caloric requirements, especially in a stressed individual, will be compromised by a peripheral formula. In addition, the peripheral route cannot be utilized optimally if patients require fluid restriction, such as those with cardiac, renal, or hepatic failure.

Similarly, peripheral intravenous access may be inappropriate if the patient has major electrolyte imbalances and requires aggressive specific replacement of the components. Infusion of TPN admixtures that contain large amounts of electrolytes, particularly potassium, may be deleterious to peripheral veins. Patients with major water balance problems, such as SIADH, may also be inappropriate candidates for peripheral TPN.

CENTRAL VENOUS ACCESS

In 1929, Forssmann reported the first successful central venous catheter (CVC) access in humans by advancing a #4 French catheter 35 cm from the left antecubital fossa into his own vena cava. He later conceived the role of central venous access for drug administration, blood sampling, and cardiac pressure monitoring. He subsequently shared the 1956 Nobel Prize in Medicine with Cournand and Richards who had studied the catheterization and physiology of the cardiovascular system at Columbia University. However, it was not until the development of flexible, plastic, radio-opaque catheters that CVCs became a practical reality for these functions [65–77].

In 1952, Aubaniac [65] described the technique of subclavian venipuncture for CVC access. This demonstrated for the first time a method to access the SVC directly and to administer blood and fluids rapidly for resuscitation. Clinicians also adopted the use of single lumen CVCs inserted by this route for cardiac pressure monitoring. The Seldinger technique, originally designed for arteriography in 1953, pioneered a method of guidewire placement and advancement as an obturator for the catheter that reduced insertion risk. In 1966, Dudrick realized that subclavian CVC access could provide an infusion technique with sufficient dilution to compensate for the administration of hypertonic glucose and other nutrient solutions and developed techniques, practices, and principles for safe insertion and long-term maintenance of central venous feeding catheters [12,16]. Today, CVC access remains the preferred route for the administration of TPN and other hypertonic or thrombogenic solutions [65–77].

The single lumen, percutaneously placed CVC was, initially, the standard device for administering TPN. CVCs placed via the infraclavicular, supraclavicular, or internal jugular (IJ) approach were widely used for this purpose throughout the 1970s and 1980s. Subcutaneous tunneling of these catheters (also demonstrated by Dudrick) allowed for their long-term safe and secure use. Shortly afterward, Hickman and Broviac developed Silastic™, Dacron™-cuffed catheters, which were specifically designed to be tunneled and intended for long-term TPN therapy.

Technological advances in catheter materials greatly improved and allowed CVCs to be more radio-opaque, less flimsy, and less thrombogenic. A number of approaches have also been made to produce catheters less likely to promote adherence and growth of bacteria. Soft, flexible, minimally irritating materials have also permitted a return to the antecubital route for less technically demanding CVC placement. The development of multilumen catheters in the late 1980s further advanced the progression to the current standards for long-term CVC placement and TPN infusion [65–77].

CENTRAL VENOUS POSITIONING

A CVC is defined by the position of the catheter tip, not the point of its entry into the vascular system. After insertion and advancement under sterile conditions, the distal tip should lie in the lower SVC or proximal right atrium. This is the so-called "Zone A position" [73], which is ideal for dilution of a hyperosmolar solution. The infusate is diluted by the rapid, high-volume blood flow of the SVC, which is approximately 2000 mL/min [69]. This position is also high enough to minimize the catheter-related risks of perforation of the right atrium, damage to the tricuspid valve, or the induction of arrhythmias.

Catheters may also be used for TPN when the tip is in the upper SVC (the "Zone B position") [73]. This area has a similar blood flow and dilution capacity to Zone A. However, it has the disadvantage of lying in a vessel with a thinner wall, which has a higher risk of erosion. The tip of Zone B catheters may also abut the vessel wall, making blood aspiration more difficult.

Catheters whose tips are in the brachiocephalic vein are considered to be in the "Zone C position" [73]. This is generally not preferred but can be utilized if the TPN osmolarity is reduced and if other better options for CVC tip placement are not feasible. The risks of thrombosis and thromboembolism are higher in this location.

The most common sites of access for percutaneous insertion are the subclavian and IJ veins. The clinical condition of the patient must be taken into consideration when deciding where to obtain central venous access. For example, patients with tracheostomies, fistulas, recent wounds, skin drainage, or burns to the chest may not be appropriate candidates for the use of percutaneous subclavian catheterization because of the increased risk of infection at the insertion site.

The patients' anatomy also plays an important role in the insertion site. Patients with short, thick necks are difficult candidates for IJ CVCs. Patients with previous fractures of the clavicle or those with pectus excavatum or kyphosis may have a higher risk of pneumothorax with a subclavian approach.

Cut-down access can be accomplished via the cephalic or basilic veins. The use of a cut-down approach imparts a significant degree of safety, as the vein is directly visualized and can be cannulated with complete control. However, this practice is becoming a lost art. It requires patience and technical skill and is time-consuming. Most clinicians have abandoned the cut-down for central line placement in favor of more technologically advanced percutaneous options.

Perhaps the most significant development in the area of CVC placement is the use of an ultrasound-guided insertion method. This technique permits the operator to visualize the anatomic location of the target vein and the surrounding structures. The scout needle can be safely inserted into the vein beneath the sterile ultrasound probe. The Seldinger guide wire technique can then be applied to complete the catheter insertion, and fluoroscopy or chest radiography can confirm appropriate catheter pathway and tip placement.

CVCs may directly exit the skin at the insertion site or be tunneled under the skin to provide a safer, more stable, and permanent platform. Such tunneled catheters can be maintained for long-term use such as home parenteral nutrition therapy.

CVCs can be single, double, or multiluminal in design. The availability of additional CVC lumens allows for separate channels to be dedicated for TPN infusion, antibiotic or other pharmacologic or supplemental fluid administration, and blood withdrawal.

PERIPHERALLY INSERTED CENTRAL CATHETER LINES

Today, many of the catheters used for TPN are peripherally inserted central catheter (PICC) lines. These are inserted via a peripheral arm vein, often the antecubital vein. They are soft and flexible, and generally made from silicone rubber or other biocompatible materials. The catheter is advanced with a stiffening wire guide within the lumen. An approximation of surface anatomy is taken with a measuring tape. The distance from the antecubital region to the sternal notch is measured. The catheter length to be inserted is then sized to match the measurement.

After the target vein has been cannulated, the PICC is advanced through the insertion cannula ("through the needle approach"). Markings along the outside of the PICC allow the operator to estimate the length of catheter that has been inserted. Once the PICC has been sufficiently advanced to the length previously measured, the tip should lie within the region of the SVC. A chest x-ray is mandatory to confirm appropriate ideal placement position prior to initiating TPN.

PICC lines are available in single, double, or triple lumen designs. As was noted in the discussion on CVC design, multiluminal catheters permit the designation of a dedicated channel for TPN while permitting access for other intravenous therapies and blood withdrawal. However, the small external diameter of the PICC line (generally <4 French) dictates that the extra lumens will be small. Therefore, the utility of PICC lines for blood withdrawal may be limited.

PICC lines have several advantages over traditional CVC catheters. They may be placed at the bedside, reducing the need for the operating room or special procedures. They can generally be inserted by a trained IV nurse or technician. Both of these factors have resulted in a decreased cost of CVC insertion and an increased likelihood of TPN utilization.

Another important advantage of the PICC line is its ease of removal. All TPN catheters theoretically will eventually become contaminated and require replacement. In a patient requiring long-term TPN, it is only a matter of time before the indwelling catheter becomes infected. Therefore, the clinician must always factor in the likely need to remove and replace the venous access device eventually. A Hickman catheter or an infusion port will require surgical removal. The PICC line can be readily removed at the bedside, or in the emergency room or outpatient office, while taking precautions to avoid air embolism or hemorrhage.

SPECIALIZED TPN CATHETERS

Broviac first described the use of a silicone rubber (Silastic™) atrial catheter for prolonged parenteral alimentation in 1973 [75]. This catheter was small in external diameter and intended originally for use in pediatrics. Hickman later enlarged, simplified, and modified the catheter primarily for use for adults. Both catheters were intended to be tunneled under the skin and included a Dacron™ cuff placed subcutaneously to help anchor the catheter and to aid in maintaining sterility.

These catheters became extensively used for TPN and later for oncologic and other intravenous therapies. The manufacturers of these catheters eventually added extra lumen options, and the Hickman and Broviac catheter lumens must be flushed with heparin and clamped when not in use.

The Groshong catheter is similar to the Broviac and Hickman catheters in that it is cuffed and intended to be tunneled (although nontunneled options exist). But the Groshong catheter tip ends in a slit valve. The intention of this design feature was to obviate regurgitation of blood into an open-ended CVC and to minimize the need for catheter clamps and heparinization. The valve opens outward during infusion therapy and inward during blood withdrawal in response to pressure differentials. The valve remains closed during pressure neutrality when the catheter is not being used for infusion or for obtaining blood specimens.

Implanted ports (such as the Port A Cath™) can also be used for infusing TPN. These devices are implanted beneath the skin and can be accessed intermittently via a special Huber-point needle. When the device is not in use, the port can be flushed, and the needle removed, disconnecting the CVC and patient from the external environment, thus minimizing infection risk and maximizing patient freedom of mobility between intermittent infusion periods. Patients can even shower or swim when these implanted ports are completely disconnected from infusion lines and needles.

All central venous lines require that strict attention be paid to their maintenance. The direct access that they provide from the external environment to the venous system is accompanied by the empirically increased potential risk of infection. Care must be taken by the patient and/or their care-givers to ensure that sterile technique is used meticulously and conscientiously every time the system is accessed. The saline and heparin used to flush the infusion line must be completely removed before blood draws if samples of undiluted blood are to be obtained for studies. TPN should be stopped prior to blood draws, and sufficient blood should be withdrawn and discarded to clear the catheter to avoid contaminating the blood sample with the TPN solution.

Most practitioners consider the use of transparent, bio-occlusive dressings to be a standard of care for CVC insertion sites. However, the literature remains mixed on such issues as to the type of dressing, the use of antiseptic impregnated dressings, and the frequency of dressing changes for optimal use and results. Institutional Infection Committee Practices and Procedures should be followed, data collected, and modifications made as indicated.

CHALLENGE OF INITIATING TPN IN SEVERELY MALNOURISHED INDIVIDUALS

It is best to initiate nutritional support therapy judiciously in patients who have been nil per os (NPO), receiving nothing by mouth, for more than 5 days to avoid the risk of refeeding syndrome, Wernicke's syndrome, or beriberi [77–83]. The provision of glucose to a starving individual results in insulin release. The insulin-mediated uptake of glucose causes cellular uptake of phosphorus and potassium. Magnesium use is increased in its role as a cofactor in the Na^+/K^+ cellular pump. Thiamine utilization is increased as glucose is metabolized. Knowledge of, and strict attention to, these facts is essential to avoid potentially tragic complications and to provide concomitant judicious nutrition support.

The malnourished patient should be considered depleted in volume, total body phosphorus, potassium, and magnesium, plus likely to be thiamine deficient. Therefore, we prefer to initiate nutritional support with a mixture of saline, electrolytes, multivitamins, and thiamine in profoundly malnourished individuals.

REFEEDING SYNDROME

This metabolic imbalance was first recognized when starving prisoners of war and concentration camps were liberated and given regular rations. Some of these individuals unfortunately succumbed to electrolyte cellular shifts induced by the sudden enthusiastic reintroduction of copious nutrients to a severely depleted body cell mass, which proved to be well-intentioned but ill-advised.

In modern times, the refeeding syndrome is almost entirely seen in severely malnourished patients who are given high dextrose-containing TPN formulas without adequate preparation or caution. Patients at increased risk for developing refeeding syndrome include those who are more likely to be depleted of major electrolytes because of prolonged fasting or severe losses through vomiting or diarrhea. Some of the patients commonly seen include those with primary or metastatic cancer involving the GI tract, complicated abdominal surgery, anorexia nervosa, and elderly nursing home residents.

The metabolic mechanism is related to the movement of electrolytes between the intracellular and extracellular spaces during the rapidly changing metabolic states. Total body electrolyte stores, serum electrolyte levels, plasma pH balance, and the cellular uptake of glucose all factor in the pathogenesis of this dangerous iatrogenic syndrome.

Malnutrition is characterized by a whole body cell mass depletion of major intracellular ions, including phosphorus, potassium, and magnesium. During the starvation state, the serum concentrations of these electrolytes are also generally low, and total body water is constricted. Furthermore, a confounding factor in interpreting clinical data may relate to the mild metabolic acidosis of starvation, which may induce misleading laboratory results.

As parenteral glucose is provided, its cellular uptake and metabolism pulls phosphorus, potassium, and magnesium from the extracellular space into the cells. If the extracellular levels are already depleted, the marginal serum levels of these electrolytes will fall rapidly. The clinical manifestations of the refeeding syndrome will occur once the extracellular electrolyte levels become too low to support their usual metabolic roles.

A component of the cellular shift also relates to the change in pH induced by refeeding. Ordinary starvation is a ketogenic state. The release of ketone bodies is a defense mechanism intended to suppress gluconeogenesis and spare somatic protein. Ketones such as beta hydroxybutyrate and acetoacetate are acidic, and their presence in starvation induces a mild metabolic acidosis. The metabolic acidosis further induces a cellular shift of intracellular ions into the extracellular space. The reversal of starvation ketosis ameliorates the acidemia, raising the plasma pH and reversing the ion shift back into the cells. In an already depleted patient, the result may be a critically low level of essential electrolytes.

Phosphate is the major intracellular anion, and it plays an essential role in energy provision through the cellular and mitochondrial production of ATP. As phosphate is taken up by tissues recovering from starvation, serum levels fall rapidly. As a result, muscle weakness occurs, and rhabdomyolysis may further complicate the situation.

The high energy requirements of the respiratory muscles render them particularly sensitive to hypophosphatemia. The clinical effect of this biochemical deficiency may be manifested as respiratory failure. In a patient already on ventilator support, hypophosphatemia may result in a failure to be able to wean the patient. Cardiac failure, hypotension, and arrhythmias are also seen in hypophosphatemia, as are seizures, coma, and sudden death.

Potassium is the major intracellular cation. The total body store of potassium is approximately 2000 mEq, only a fraction of which is in the vascular (extracellular) space. The depletion of total body potassium (TBK) results in moderate to severe hypokalemia. This disrupts muscle function, leading to weakness, myalgia, and cramps. As the condition worsens, flaccid paralysis, hyporeflexia, and rhabdomyolysis can ensue. Respiratory depression can result from the severe impairment of diaphragmatic and accessory respiratory muscle function.

Electrocardiogram (EKG) changes are among the most prominent and serious effects of hypokalemia. Diminished T waves, ST depression, and the presence of U-waves can be observed. Less commonly, a wide PR interval and atrioventricular block have been seen. Ventricular tachycardia (VT), ventricular fibrillation (VF), and even cardiac arrest can also occur. Electromechanical dissociation is another important lethal complication, as the small, depleted heart is acutely challenged by higher blood flow, volume, and pressure demands before it has had sufficient time and substrate for the myocardium itself to recover from the period of prolonged starvation and atrophy.

The total body content of magnesium is between 20 and 30 g, half of which is found in bone. Hypomagnesemia affects electrochemical processes in the cardiac and nervous system. The cardiac manifestations are the most feared results of this disturbance. EKG changes, a prolonged QT interval, VT, VF, and Torsades de pointes can be seen. Hyperactive deep tendon reflexes, a positive Chvostek sign, tremors, delirium, and convulsions are among the neurological manifestations. Prudent and judicious nutritional rehabilitation and restoration of the starved patient will appropriately avoid the potentially lethal refeeding syndrome [78–81].

WERNICKE'S SYNDROME

Wernicke's syndrome is a condition related to refeeding syndrome but caused by thiamine deficiency rather than by electrolyte imbalance. The body has a relatively small pool of available thiamine. Even a well-nourished patient has only enough stored thiamine available for about 1 month before depletion.

Patients in danger of Wernicke's syndrome have a similar risk profile to those with refeeding syndrome in that they may both be severely malnourished secondary to a significant period of limited intake. But a mildly undernourished patient with protracted vomiting can be at risk for Wernicke's syndrome out of proportion to their nutritional status. Severe vomiting can deplete thiamine stores in a matter of days. This explains, in part, the occurrence of Wernicke's syndrome in patients having bulimia or who have undergone recent bariatric surgery.

Patients with a history of ethanolism are at particular risk for Wernicke's syndrome because of deranged absorption, metabolism, and storage of thiamine. In addition, magnesium-deficient patients have a heightened risk of Wernicke's syndrome because magnesium is a cofactor in thiamine-requiring enzyme systems.

Thiamine deficiency results in cytotoxic edema, proliferation of pleomorphic microglia, demyelination, apoptosis, and cell death. The entire neuroaxis is susceptible, but the periaqueductal gray matter, mammillary bodies, medial thalamus, and superior vermis of the cerebellum are particularly sensitive areas. The symptoms of ataxia, confusion, and ophthalmoplegia are considered the classic triad, but many other symptoms and signs, including peripheral neuropathies, can occur [82,83].

As in the refeeding syndrome, patients who are thiamine-deficient and receive dextrose-containing TPN may accelerate and accentuate the manifestations of Wernicke's syndrome. If this is not recognized and treated promptly, permanent injury and disability can occur.

Beriberi

A form of thiamine deficiency can present as beriberi in TPN patients who are deprived of sufficient thiamine. This has been reported recently, in part, because of manufacturing shortages, which have necessitated giving TPN without the usual multivitamins. Beriberi can also be seen when initiating thiamine-free TPN in severely malnourished patients.

Beriberi has two subtypes, referred to as dry and wet beriberi. Dry beriberi is similar to Wernicke's syndrome in that it manifests primarily in the nervous system but generally presents as peripheral neuropathy rather than as encephalopathy. Wet beriberi refers to the cardiac manifestations of thiamine deficiency, including heart failure, vasodilation, and edema.

TPN Admixture

TPN is a comprehensive means of providing all of the body's nutrients via the intravenous route. It includes the provision of nutrients necessary for maintenance of nutrition and hydration, growth and development, repletion of nutritional deficiencies, as well as recovery from critical illness and major surgical procedures.

In practical terms, TPN is a solution composed of amino acids, dextrose, electrolytes, vitamins, and trace elements that is either infused separately or combined with a lipid emulsion, usually into the SVC. When all components are mixed into one bag, it is often referred to as a total nutrient admixture (TNA) [84].

A TPN admixture consists of seven main components consisting of water, macronutrients, and micronutrients. The macronutrients are composed of glucose, amino acids, and lipids. The amino acid base solution generally contains a mixture of 15 essential and nonessential amino acids. The fat emulsion contains a mixture of five fatty acids, egg phospholipids, and glycerol.

The micronutrients include vitamins, electrolytes, and trace elements. There are generally 12 separate vitamins contained within the multivitamin component of TPN (vitamins A, D, E, K, B_1, B_2, B_3, B_5, B_7, B_9, B_{12}, and C). There are usually seven separate major electrolytes within the electrolyte additive component (sodium, potassium, phosphate, magnesium, calcium, chloride, and acetate). Similarly, there are generally four separate trace elements (copper, zinc, chromium, and manganese) contained within the trace element additive component. Additional nutrients, such as selenium, may be added separately to these standard components. Pharmaceuticals, such as insulin and H2 blockers, may also be added to the formula. Therefore, the finished TPN admixture can have as many as 50 separate components, defining TPN as one of the most complex therapies administered to any patient.

COMPONENTS OF TPN SOLUTIONS

DEXTROSE

Pharmaceutical-grade dextrose (d-glucose) is produced by the hydrolysis of cornstarch. It is manufactured as hydrous (monohydrate; bound to a molecule of water) and anhydrous forms. Because of the presence of the added water molecule, hydrous dextrose has a caloric equivalent of 3.4 kcal/g, rather than the 4 kcal/g of anhydrous dextrose. Hydrous dextrose is the standard energy component in TPN solutions. It is available in concentrations ranging from 2.5% to 70%. The 70% concentration is most commonly used for compounding a TPN solution in order to minimize the water volume of the formulation. Sterile water is then added to balance the volume and osmolarity as desired. Dextrose is the major source of exogenous energy provided in the nutrient admixture and provides the body cell mass with metabolic fuel to generate ATP. It is also administered to control gluconeogenesis and ketone production, and for the suppression of catabolism.

Based on the early work of Gamble [24] and Harris and Benedict [41], the basal caloric goals for providing metabolic fuel as glucose can be met by providing between 100 and 200 g/day. For the average individual, the daily glucose requirement can be estimated at 3 g/kg of ideal body weight (IBW) per day. In a 70-kg male, this translates to roughly 210 g/day. Glucose is rarely required above this level unless the patient is in a severely stressed metabolic state and yet can metabolize it.

The glucose output from the hepatic veins in normal individuals is about 2 mg/kg/min [27]. In a 70-kg male, this approximates 201 g of glucose per day, which is consistent with the 3 g/kg/day estimate noted above. Since TPN is an artificial means of providing posthepatic vein nutrient levels, the glucose infusion rate should mimic this physiologic situation under normal metabolic conditions.

Metabolic needs may increase the glucose requirement, and accordingly, an increase in the glucose infusion rate may be clinically warranted. However, most authors recommend not exceeding 6 mg/kg/min, which would equate to a maximum of 360 mg/kg/h. In a 70-kg male, this would equal 604 total grams of exogenous glucose per day, which is about the maximum level of glucose utilization by the body cell mass [12–17].

Dudrick's initial experiments and much of the early work in TPN utilized an average glucose intake of about 500 g/day in depleted adult, complex surgical patients. But later trends in less critically ill or injured patients aimed for a lower intake, closer to their lesser physiologic requirements. Excess glucose delivery carries a metabolic risk. It increases CO_2 production, which may be a factor in the ability to wean a patient from the ventilator. An excessive glucose load, accompanied by hyperinsulinemia, may induce fatty liver disease. Furthermore, recent studies on ICU morbidity and length of stay have linked ill-advised iatrogenic hyperglycemia as a factor in poor outcomes [51,52]. These untoward outcomes are obviated by rational, judicious, proficient use of TPN.

As much as we attempt to avoid hyperglycemia with TPN, we must also monitor patients meticulously to avoid hypoglycemia. Hypoglycemic events are also known to impact ICU survival. The risk of hypoglycemia may be the result of adding insulin to the TPN formula in a diabetic patient or a patient with stress-induced insulin resistance. Intravenous insulin has a half-life of 30 min. If the TPN is interrupted, the insulin can persist in the circulation beyond the availability of the glucose (with its shorter half-life) to match it. Therefore, our preference is to give low doses of insulin in the TPN and cover the remainder of the precise insulin requirement with a sliding scale as indicated or desired to maintain euglycemia. Eventually, nutrient delivery and insulin delivery pumps and servo-controlled mechanisms will be crafted and used routinely for the safe, efficacious, euglycemic infusion of TPN.

Lipids

Fatty acids can be utilized as metabolic fuel by many organ systems, the notable exceptions being the red blood cells (RBCs) and the central nervous system (CNS). Essential fatty acids and fat soluble vitamins play other important roles in human metabolism.

Although the importance of providing a source of exogenous lipids has long been recognized, early production attempts of lipid substrate were unsuccessful [85–94]. The first commercial lipid products (Yanol™, Lipophysan™, Lipomul™, and Infonutrol™) proved to be toxic and were withdrawn from the market [9].

Dr. Arvid Wretlind and colleagues, working at the Karolinska Institute in Sweden, realized that if fat emulsion was to be safe for intravenous administration, it would necessarily mimic the natural mechanisms by which fat is transported within the body. This led them to conceptualize the development of a highly emulsified soybean oil product composed of fat globules 0.5–1.0 μm in size (Intralipid™) instead of the wide range of 1.0- to 10.0-μm particles in the previous emulsions [10,87]. Other intravenous fat emulsions (IVFEs) have also been developed by competing organizations, but Intralipid™ has remained the dominant IVFE.

Intralipid™ particles are composed of triglycerides emulsified by egg yolk phospholipids. The emulsification process yields a particle that is similar in size (0.5 μm) and consistency to those of a native postprandial chylomicron [91]. Remarkably, it soon became apparent that this "artificial chylomicron" mimicked the behavior of the natural chylomicrons as well. The Intralipid™ particle could activate lipoprotein lipase and stimulate fatty acid uptake by the adipocyte and other tissues [92]. However, unlike natural chylomicrons, the soybean oil emulsion particles are not bound to proteins and are phagocytized by the cells of the reticuloendothelial system as if they were foreign bodies, and the fatty acids are then released for use by other cells for energy production, for storage as fat, or for other cellular functions.

This led to the use of IVFEs as a standard component of TPN. The replacement of some of the nonprotein calories as lipids allowed for a reduction in the provision of calories in the form of glucose. This, in turn, reduced the risks of hyperglycemia associated with high dextrose formulas. Intravenous nutrition could now become a more balanced formula delivering more physiologic levels of the macronutrients—protein, carbohydrate, and fat.

IVFEs are available in concentrations of 10%, 20%, and 30% (Table 22.1). They were initially designed to be administered separately from the dextrose and amino acid solutions through a peripheral or central vein. This was due to the fact that lipids initially could not be provided in plastic bags and required specialized tubing for administration. In the late 1980s, technical advances in intravenous plastic bag and tubing materials permitted the mixture of lipids within the TPN solution, creating the concept of the TNA.

Plant-derived triglycerides are the source of fatty acids in IVFE. Both soy and safflower oil have been utilized in the past, but currently, only soybean oil-based IVFEs are available in the United States. Soybean oil is a mixture of neutral triglycerides, with mainly unsaturated fatty acids. Their

TABLE 22.1

Composition of Lipid Emulsions

Content/1000 mL	10% Intralipid	20% Intralipid	30% Intralipid
Soya oil	100 g	200 g	300 g
Egg lecithin	12 g	12 g	12 g
Glycerol	22 g	22 g	16.7 g
Sodium hydroxide	To pH 6.0–9.0	To pH 6.0–9.0	To pH 6.0–9.0
Water	QS to 1000 mL	QS to 1000 mL	QS to 1000 mL
Osmolality	300	350	310
Energy content	1.1 kcal/mL	2.0 kcal/mL	3.0 kcal/mL

components are linoleic (44–62%), oleic (19–30%), palmitic (7–14%), linolenic (4–11%), and stearic (1.4–5.6%).

Investigational IVFE products include a mixture of medium-chain triglycerides, having a carbon chain length of 6–12, and long-chain triglycerides. Olive oil has been used experimentally, as has fish oil and borage oil. The latter two have been considered good sources for omega-3 fatty acids.

Egg yolk phospholipid is used as an emulsifier at a concentration of 1.2%. Therefore, caution must be exercised in their use in patients with egg allergy. The phospholipids are extracted from egg yolk powder and purified. A virus removal and inactivation step ensures sterility. Fatty acids of mainly 16–20 carbon chain length dominate within egg yolk phospholipids. The final emulsion is forced through a dialyzing membrane, which allows only fat globules 0.5 μm in size or smaller to pass through the micropores, thus standardizing the lipid particle size and increasing its stability, utilization, transport, and safety.

IVFEs are emulsions. There is nothing dissolved in the water, and they would have an effective osmolarity of zero. However, infusions of low osmolarity products carry the risk of producing hemolysis. Therefore, the addition of soluble nutrients such as glycerol ensures that the lipid emulsion is isotonic. With the presence of egg yolk phospholipids and glycerol, the caloric value of lipid emulsions is slightly higher than that of the triglyceride alone. For example, 100 mL of 20% Intralipid contains 20 g of soybean oil, 1.2 g of lecithin, and 2.2 g of glycerol. The caloric equivalents are 180 kcal from soy, 10.8 kcal from lecithin, and 8.8 kcal from the glycerol. This yields a total of 199.6 kcal per 100 mL (roughly 2 kcal/mL). In the case of 10% Intralipid, the product contains 10 g of soybean oil, but the same 1.2 g of lecithin and 2.2 g of glycerol. Therefore, the caloric equivalents are 90 kcal from soy, 10.8 kcal from lecithin, and 8.8 kcal from the glycerol. This yields a total of 109.6 kcal per 100 mL (roughly 1.1 kcal/mL). IVFEs also contain a small amount of vitamin K_1 and vitamin E.

Much investigational work is underway to improve IVFEs by increasing the use of fish oil to provide omega-3 fatty acids in addition to the omega-6 fatty acids in currently available products. It is theorized that the parenteral nutrition associated liver disease (PNALD) seen in some adults and in premature infants will be avoided in the future by modification of the currently used fat emulsions with structured lipids and omega-3 fatty acids [94].

PROTEIN

The development of a safe, effective form of intravenous protein for use in nutritional support has its origins in the 1930s and 1940s. Whipple and colleagues began experiments using plasma protein infusions in animals. Rose had validated the concept of "essential amino acids" and detailed the requirements for amino acid administration. Protein hydrolysates from fibrin [11] and, later, casein [10] led to the first commercial intravenous protein products, called Aminosol™ in both the United States and Sweden, but derived from different protein sources (fibrin source for United States and casein source for Sweden).

Intravenous crystalline amino acids were introduced experimentally by Bansi in 1964. Wretlind created a more complete version in the late 1960s, essentially replacing his initial protein hydrolysate product with the new crystalline amino acid formula. After a few evolutionary changes to adjust the amino acid content, crystalline amino acid solutions became the standard substrates for intravenous protein delivery. Standard crystalline amino acid solutions are a mixture of essential and nonessential amino acids. They are generally referred to as "mixed amino acids" and come in a range of concentrations from 3% to 20%. The most commonly utilized are 8.5%, 10%, or 15% concentrations. Modified formulations are available for special clinical conditions (renal failure, liver failure, pulmonary, stress metabolism) (Table 22.2).

Eight essential amino acids (lysine, leucine, isoleucine, valine, methionine, phenylalanine, threonine, and tryptophan) and seven nonessentials (alanine, arginine, histidine, proline, serine, tyrosine, and glycine) are found in most commercial adult amino acid products. Cysteine and taurine are also found in some preparations. Most pediatric amino acid formulations also include cysteine and taurine, as well as aspartate and glutamate. These amino acids are considered "essential" in infants and some children.

TABLE 22.2
Commercially Available Amino Acid Solutions

Concentrations (%)

Standard Adult Amino Acid Solutions

Aminosyn	3.5, 8.5, 10, 15
Clinisol	15
Prosol	20
Freamine III	10
Travasol	10

Hepatic Failure Amino Acid Solutions

Hepatamine	8
Hepatasol	8

Renal Failure Amino Acid Solutions

Nephramine	5.4
Aminosyn RF	5.2

Stress Metabolism Amino Acid Solutions

Freamine HBC	6.9
Aminosyn HBC	6.9

Glutamine is highly unstable in solution and is, therefore, not practical for use in commercial formulations. Moreover, it can be produced in the body from other amino acids. However, it can be added separately to TPN if desired by the pharmacist immediately prior to infusion or can be provided in the form of a dipeptide (L-alanyl-L-glutamine) to satisfy those who believe that it is a conditionally essential amino acid in some clinical situations. The dipeptide is not approved for use in TPN in the United States by the FDA but is used throughout most of the rest of the world. Its "essentiality" remains controversial.

The provision of protein within the TPN admixture is intended to support nitrogen balance rather than energy balance. Nonetheless, one cannot ignore the fact that a significant percentage of the amino acids provided will ultimately be utilized as fuel via gluconeogenesis. The amount of protein converted to energy depends on many variables, including the degree of stress metabolism, the quantity and quality of nonprotein calories available, and the amount, variety, and ratios of amino acids given [95–98].

Each amino acid has its own unique caloric value. This ranges from a low of 2.875 kcal/g for aspartic acid to a high of 6.723 kcal/g for phenylalanine. The mean energy content of amino acids is 4.781 [95]. Since the various commercial forms of amino acid solutions have different mixtures of amino acids, they also have a slight variability in energy content. However, as a general rule, most clinicians estimate the caloric equivalent of amino acid solutions at 4 kcal/g.

Parenthetically, it is interesting to note that despite the obvious variability in the content of amino acids in the many available solutions, they all appear to be comparably effective in achieving the goals of TPN when admixed with all of the other required nutrients. This appears to be analogous to the multiple sources of "complete" proteins that are available to us in the variety of protein-containing foods and mixtures that we ingest in our diets (meat, fish, dairy products, eggs, beans, plants, etc.).

ELECTROLYTES

As was mentioned in the section on Refeeding Syndrome, electrolyte depletion occurs as a consequence of malnutrition. Total body stores of sodium, potassium, calcium, magnesium, phosphate,

TABLE 22.3
Electrolyte Content of GI Fluids

Source	Volume (mL/day)	Sodium (mEq/L)	Potassium (mEq/L)	Chloride (mEq/L)	Bicarbonate (mEq/L)
Saliva	500–2000	10–60	20–30	10–40	20–30
Gastric	2000–2500	30–100	4–15	50–250	0
Small bowel	2000–3000	70–150	3–8	70–120	10–30
Bile	500–1000	135–145	5–10	40–110	30–50
Pancreas	600–800	120–140	5–8	60–100	30–140

Source: Adapted from Madsen H, Frankel EH, *Practical Gastroenterology*, 40:46–68, 2006.

chloride, and bicarbonate may be abnormal. Replacement of these critical nutrients is a major goal of nutritional support, both to correct deficiencies and to support synthesis and anabolism.

The intracellular and extracellular spaces have an inverse relationship in terms of their major electrolytes. Potassium, calcium, and magnesium are the major intracellular cations, whereas phosphate is the major intracellular anion. In the extracellular space, sodium and chloride, plus acetate, maintain these isoelectric relationships.

Both intracellular and extracellular electrolyte balance must be achieved. There is a delicate interplay between the intracellular and extracellular compartments involving the movement of cations and anions. Careful attention must be paid in normalizing both compartments in order to achieve homeostasis and metabolic balance.

In addition to their roles in membrane kinetics, enzymatic cofactors, and electrochemical gradients, electrolytes play an important part in the acid–base balance of fluids and tissues. The metabolic physician must also consider both electrolyte balance and acid–base balance when prescribing balanced nutritional support.

The astute clinician must also be aware of electrolyte losses occurring simultaneously with nutritional repletion. For example, a patient with bowel obstruction and a NGT draining gastric contents is losing a great deal of fluid and electrolytes. Both salivary and gastric fluids are being drained via the NGT. Each of these components has its own unique electrolyte profile (Table 22.3). The losses of these components should be factored into the comprehensive replacement prescription of TPN for the patient.

In another example, a patient with an enterocutaneous fistula could be losing small bowel, biliary, and pancreatic secretions. These components have their own unique electrolyte profiles, and attention must be paid to the replacement of these losses in the process of restoring metabolic and nutritional balance.

Furthermore, losses from different areas of the GI tract due to NG suction, vomiting, fistulas, or diarrhea will also alter acid–base balance. Loss of gastric secretions will increase hydrogen ion and chloride losses resulting in metabolic alkalosis. Losses from the lower GI tract and the kidneys will increase bicarbonate losses resulting in hyperchloremic metabolic acidosis. The metabolic physician should be prepared to alter the TPN formula to compensate for these situations while simultaneously meeting nutritional requirements [43,99,100].

RECOMMENDED RANGE OF ELECTROLYTES FOR TPN

From a practical perspective, the quantities of electrolytes added to the TPN formula generally conform to a standard set of ranges. For completeness, the usual concentrations per liter of TPN and total anticipated daily requirements are listed in Table 22.4. Keep in mind that these requirements are based on normal physiology without taking into account excessive losses or preexisting derangements.

TABLE 22.4

Recommended Range of Electrolytes for TPN

Electrolyte	Range	Requirement
Sodium	0–200 mEq	1–2 mEq/kg/day
Potassium	0–240 mEq	0.5–2 mEq/kg/day
Phosphate	0–60 mM	20–40 mM/day
Magnesium	0–48 mEq	4–20 mEq/day
Calcium	0–25 mEq	4–15 mEq/day
Chloride	Variable	Variable
Acetate	Variable	Variable

In the case of sodium administration, quantities ranging from 0 to 200 mEq per liter are given the TPN formula. The total sodium requirements are within the range of 1–2 mEq/kg/day, but sodium replacement will vary depending on the clinical condition. Patients with congestive heart failure or those with ascites may not tolerate a high sodium intake because of its volume expansion capacity, and sodium must be reduced in the formulation. Alternatively, hyponatremia is commonly seen during TPN administration when inadequate sodium is provided. The sodium additive can be given as sodium chloride, sodium acetate, or sodium phosphate. The choice of sodium salt will depend on the other electrolyte and acid–base balance requirements.

Potassium is also available in a variety of different salts, including potassium chloride, potassium acetate, and potassium phosphate. However, potassium administration must be carefully regulated because of the risk of inducing arrhythmia during rapid infusion. In general, we prefer not to exceed 10 mEq/h in a peripheral line or 20 mEq/h in a central venous line. Daily requirement of potassium is in the range of 0.5–2 mEq/kg/day. Potassium requirements are increased with nasogastric suction, vomiting, diarrheal losses, and medications such as diuretics. On the other hand, potassium requirements are decreased in patients with renal insufficiency and reduced potassium excretion.

As was noted above, both sodium and potassium are available in the phosphate salt form. Therefore, the phosphate requirement needs to be factored into the sodium and potassium requirements. Roughly 20–40 mmol of phosphate is typically required per day, although some patients require as much as 60 mmol/day.

Magnesium requirements range from 4 to 20 mEq/day, but as much as 48 mEq can be given daily. Magnesium for TPN administration is available as either the sulfate or chloride salt.

Calcium requirements range from 4 to 15 mEq/day. TPN formulas rarely contain more than 20 mEq of calcium, except for use in patients with severe hypocalcemia. Calcium for TPN administration is available as either the gluconate or chloride salt.

As noted above, chloride and acetate are utilized as anions within the TPN electrolyte milieu as needed, based upon the acid–base balance.

VITAMINS

As TPN developed into an established therapy, the need for complete vitamin support became obvious. However, in the early days after the invention and clinical application of TPN, and its acceptance by the medical community, few options for intravenous multivitamins existed. The only existing product, Multiple Vitamin Infusion, United States Pharmacopeia (MVI, USP), lacked biotin, folate, and B_{12}. Therefore, physicians ordering TPN had to add these nutrients separately [101].

The American Medical Association sponsored an ad hoc committee to determine the optimum vitamin replacement therapy for adult and pediatric patients receiving TPN at the request of its Council on Nutrition. This "Nutrition Advisory Group" defined the formulations for multivitamins in TPN in 1976. Their recommendations were transmitted to the FDA and approved in 1978. They

TABLE 22.5
Composition of Adult MVI

Composition of Adult MVI	Dose
Vitamin A	3300 IU
Vitamin D	5 mg
Vitamin E	10 IU
Vitamin K	150 mcg
Ascorbic acid	200 mg
Thiamine (B1)	6 mg
Riboflavin (B2)	3.6 mg
Niacin (B3)	40 mg
Pyridoxine (B6)	6 mg
Pantothenic acid	15 mg
Cyanocobalamin (B12)	5 mcg
Folic acid	600 mcg
Biotin	60 mcg

have been used ever since then with little modification. These recommendations provided the basis for the formulation of MVI—12™ and equivalent commercially available products (Table 22.5).

Virtually all TPN pharmacies make use of this formulation as the basis for vitamin replacement during parenteral nutrition. Some practitioners use a double dose of multivitamin in anticipation of deficiency states. Our practice is to measure vitamin levels at the initiation of a TPN course and then add additional vitamin components if deficiencies are detected.

A disturbing development recently has been the intermittent paucity or lack of availability of vitamins and other micronutrient components for inclusion in TPN. These are allegedly due to manufacturing difficulties and the lack of adequate suppliers. This has left the current practitioner facing a series of shortages in almost every area of TPN delivery.

TRACE ELEMENTS

As with the development of a standardized multivitamins formula, the AMA Nutrition Advisory Group proposed standards and guidelines for the use of trace element formulations in TPN. These were published in 1979 and have been broadly accepted [102] (Table 22.6). However, a number of different trace element formulations exist that go beyond the standards recommended initially by the committee. These have some modified quantities of trace elements or provide for the addition of trace elements that were not included originally. An example of this is the inclusion of selenium within the formulation, especially in foreign countries.

Most practitioners rely on the TPN pharmacies to select the particular trace element formulations for use in their parenteral nutrition formulas. As with the multivitamin preparations, some

TABLE 22.6
Trace Elements Used in TPN

Trace Elements	Amount Recommended
Chromium	10–15 mcg
Copper	0.3–0.5 mg
Manganese	60–100 mcg
Selenium	20–60 mcg
Zinc	2.5–5.0 mg

practitioners use a double dose of trace elements in anticipation of deficiency states. Again, our practice is to measure micronutrient levels at the initiation of a TPN course and then add additional trace element components as indicated if deficiencies are detected.

One of the most common deficiencies observed is zinc. Zinc is involved in more than 200 enzymatic functions in the body. It is found in high quantity within the pancreatic secretions, perhaps because of its role as a zymogen activator. Therefore, increased amounts are required in patients with colonic disorders, severe diarrhea, and with small bowel losses, such as those that occur with enterocutaneous fistula [43,44].

Copper deficiency is a rare development but an important one to recognize. Copper is needed for hematopoiesis and for hormone regulation and energy production. It may manifest clinically as a peripheral neuropathy or gait disturbance.

OSMOLARITY

As was discussed in the section on Central Venous Access, the final osmolarity of the TPN admixture will determine its tolerability in a peripheral vein. Peripheral TPN with an osmolarity below 600 mOsm is generally well tolerated for a few days. Since peripheral intravenous access catheters are generally changed every 48–72 h, this can be practical for up to 2 weeks. However, this only applies if a patient has good peripheral access and does not require volume restriction.

As osmolarity of the final mixture rises to between 600 and 900 mOsm, tolerability via peripheral venous access declines. A final TPN osmolarity above 900 mOsm generally demands a central line for administration.

Therefore, it becomes incumbent upon the metabolic physician to be aware of the osmolarity of the TPN formula ordered. Each component has its own approximate osmolarity as shown in Table 22.7. For precision, it may be necessary to refer to a table or a calculator program, but for simplicity, one can estimate the osmolarity on the basis of the macronutrients in the formulation.

Dextrose has an approximate osmolarity of 5 mOsm/g. Amino acid solutions have approximately twice the osmolarity of dextrose, or 10 mOsm/g. Lipid emulsions are isotonic and have an osmolarity of 0.28 mOsm/mL.

To estimate the osmolarity of the TPN formula, start by multiplying the grams of dextrose X 5 and add the grams of amino acid X 10. If lipid emulsion is being used, multiply the volume of lipid emulsion X 0.28. Add the multiplied values of the macronutrient osmolarities together and divide

TABLE 22.7
Calculating Osmolarity of TPN Solution

Additive	mOsm/Unit
Dextrose	5 mOsm/g
Amino acids	10 mOsm/g
Lipid	0.28 mOsm/g
Calcium gluconate	0.662 mOsm/mEq
Magnesium sulfate	1 mOsm/mEq
Sodium chloride	2 mOsm/mEq
Sodium acetate	2 mOsm/mEq
Sodium phosphate	4 mOsm/mM
Potassium chloride	2 mOsm/mEq
Potassium acetate	2 mOsm/mEq
Potassium phosphate	2.47 mOsm/mM
MVI concentrate	4.11 mOsm/dose
MTE concentrate	0.36 mOsm/mL

by the total volume (in liters) of the TPN formula. This will yield a rough estimate of the final solute concentration of the formula.

TPN formulas containing large quantities of electrolytes, particularly sodium and potassium, will have higher osmolarity. As a rule, sodium and potassium salts have an osmolarity of about 2 mOsm/mEq. The phosphate salts are notable exceptions, with potassium phosphate having an osmolarity of about 2.5 mOsm/mmol and sodium phosphate about 4 mOsm/mmol. The remaining micronutrients generally play a minor role in the osmolarity of the TPN [62,63].

WRITING THE TPN ORDER

The first step in writing the TPN order is to estimate the patient's energy requirements. Several different formulas can be used for estimating the caloric needs of the patient. Of these, the Harris Benedict equation remains the most commonly used:

$$\text{Males: BMR (kcal/day)} = 66.47 + (13.75 \times \text{weight in kg}) + (5.0 \times \text{height in cm})$$
$$- (6.76 \times \text{age in years})$$

$$\text{Females: BMR (kcal/day)} = 665.1 + (9.56 \times \text{weight in kg}) + (1.85 \times \text{height in cm})$$
$$- (4.68 \times \text{age in years})$$

To convert height in inches to centimeters: multiply height in inches by 2.54. For example, 5'7" becomes 67 × 2.54 or 170 cm.

As a rough estimate, we prefer a range of caloric intake based on the patient's IBW. In obese individuals, we use the adjusted body weight [(maximum weight − IBW)/4 + IBW] instead of IBW alone.

The calorie range will vary depending on whether the patient requires maintenance or repletion. We typically use a range of 25–30 kcal/kg for maintenance. For patients who require nutritional repletion, a higher range of 35–40 kcal/kg is utilized initially. Patients with stress metabolism may require even more, but must be closely monitored. For more detail on assessing nutritional requirements, please see Chapter 21.

Indirect calorimetry may provide a more accurate assessment of the patient's energy requirements. This technique uses oxygen consumption and CO_2 production data obtained from a closed system measuring respiratory gases. However, the equipment required to perform the test may not be readily available, or it may be inappropriate for use in certain patient populations (i.e., the intubated patient).

Once caloric needs have been established, fluid requirements are determined. The clinical status of the patient will also influence this requirement, but, in general, the use of 1 mL/kcal is a reasonable starting point. Additional fluid can be added to replace GI losses. Decreased amounts may be indicated and appropriate for the patient with hepatic, renal, or cardiac failure.

Next, determine the protein needs based on body weight. A range of 1.0–2.0 g/kg is generally used. Available laboratory studies, the degree of malnutrition, and the clinical condition of the patient may alter these requirements.

Once the caloric and protein needs have been estimated, the TPN formula can be concocted. One method in common use is to separate the protein calories from the total caloric requirement and then to provide a portion of the nonprotein calories as dextrose, with the remainder provided as fat. In this scenario, one simply multiplies the grams of protein by 4 to determine protein calories and subtracts this value from total caloric requirement. Three fourths of the remaining calories are provided as dextrose, and the remaining one fourth are provided as lipid emulsion.

Another method bases the glucose and lipid intake on physiologic requirements. In this scenario, the glucose requirement is estimated at approximately 3–5 g per kilogram body weight per day. The lipid requirements are estimated at 0.4–0.8 g per kilogram body weight per day.

Both methods should result in a similar initial prescription for the macronutrients. Our practice is to give only 50% of estimated caloric needs in the initial TPN infusion to avoid refeeding syndrome,

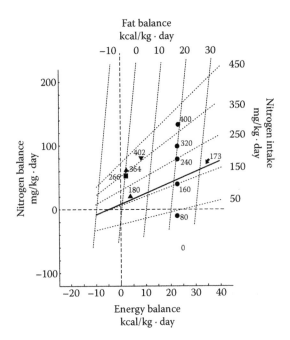

FIGURE 22.1 Relationship between nitrogen and energy balance. (From Shaw SN et al., *Am J Clin Nutr,* 37:930–940, 1983.)

and then advance to goal cautiously. This "TPN initiation formula" can also help to determine the tolerance of the patient to therapy.

Calculate the TPN micronutrient components based on the clinical condition and laboratory data as noted above. Add a standard dose of TPN multivitamins and trace elements. It may be necessary to supplement the standard vitamin and trace elements based on laboratory data.

Insulin and H2 blockers may be added as necessary. However, most medications are not compatible with the TPN formula. In the early days of therapy, heparin was routinely added to TPN. This is no longer considered necessary, although some practitioners still add heparin for peripheral TPN.

Regardless of the method used to calculate the initial formula, adjustments will be required based on the patient's clinical response and biochemical indices. An important factor may be the need to increase protein intake in order to achieve nitrogen balance. A relationship exists between nitrogen and energy balance such that increasing amounts of caloric intake may permit increases in nitrogen retention (Figure 22.1) [103].

COMPLICATIONS

TPN is a complex therapy provided to some of the most critically ill hospitalized patients. Complications can and do occur, but steps can be taken to help minimize their incidence and severity. Complications are usually divided into those that are related to insertion of the catheter and those that are related to long-term therapy, and they can be subdivided further into three categories: mechanical, metabolic, and infectious.

MECHANICAL COMPLICATIONS

Mechanical complications are usually related to the venous access device. This underscores the need to match the device carefully to the needs of the patient. For example, do not choose to have a catheter placed in the subclavian vein in a patient who has a draining head/neck wound, or a PICC line for a patient with a shunt for hemodialysis in the same arm, etc. (Table 22.8).

TABLE 22.8

Mechanical Complications Associated with TPN

Complication	Cause	Treatment/Prevention
Pneumothorax	Insertion by inexperienced personnel	Insertion by experienced personnel or in interventional radiology
Catheter embolism	Sheared catheter from pulling catheter back through the needle used for insertion	Don't withdraw catheter through needle
Sepsis	Not using aseptic technique for catheter insertion Poor catheter care	Use aseptic technique for all aspects of catheter care
Thrombosis	Hyperosmolar solution Coagulation defects Injury to vein	Use central line for hyperosmolar solutions Screen patients for coagulopathies Experienced personnel to insert central line
Air embolism	Air entering line	Proper positioning of patient during insertion and dressing changes
Occlusion	Incorrect technique used to flush line	Follow protocol for flushing catheter

Pneumothorax is the most common complication associated with subclavian central venous catheterization, and occurrence rates are similar (2–5%) for both IJ and subclavian vein approaches. Pneumothorax, or a collapsed lung, occurs when air leaks into the space between the lung and the chest wall, causing the lung to collapse. Common symptoms include chest pain, hypoxemia, and shortness of breath. Pneumothorax can lead to cardiac arrest, respiratory failure, or shock if not treated promptly. It can be readily diagnosed by chest x-ray. In some cases, insertion of a chest tube is necessary to reinflate the lung.

Hydrothorax is the accumulation of serous fluid in the chest cavity. This complication may occur in a patient with ascites due to cirrhosis of the liver.

Catheter-related embolism refers to the accumulation of fibrin or platelets on the venous access device and subsequent embolization of this "sleeve." This may be related to the thrombogenicity of the physical-chemical components of the catheter.

Infiltration refers to the leakage of fluid and or medication into the tissue surrounding the IV catheter. It is usually caused by incorrect placement of the catheter or migration of the catheter due to frequent or excessive movement at or near the insertion site. Signs and symptoms may include swelling, tenderness, pain, or burning at the site. The elderly are more prone to this condition due to the fragility of their blood vessels in comparison with younger patients. If IV infiltration occurs, it is necessary to remove the catheter and elevate the injured limb if possible. Therapy should be restarted at a site distant from the original site, preferably contralaterally.

Occlusion refers to a blockage in the catheter that prevents the IV solution from being infused. There are many causes of catheter occlusion, and most are easily prevented or treated. The site of placement of the IV line is important. If it is situated in an area of frequent movement, the catheter may become occluded. The line may "kink" if the patient puts pressure on the line by falling asleep on the arm in which the catheter is inserted. The catheter may become occluded if the flow rate of the solution is too slow, or if the infusion is completed or interrupted and the infusion of the solution is not restored promptly, or if the line is not flushed properly. Care must be taken when flushing the catheter. If the line is difficult to flush, there may be a blockage in the catheter due to blood clot or a chemical precipitate. Trying to "force flush" may damage or rupture the catheter and render it useless or dangerously compromised. Nursing protocols must be carefully followed in the hospital or home setting to prevent occlusion of the venous access device. Thrombolytic agents can be used to clear the occlusion. If the occlusion is thought to be lipid based, the use of a sterile 70% alcohol solution may be used. Antibiotics are sometimes added to the catheter after manipulation to minimize the risk of secondary bacterial contamination during thrombolytic attempts.

Thrombosis refers to the formation of a blood clot within a blood vessel that obstructs the flow of blood through the vessel. It may be caused by inflammation or injury to the lining of the blood vessel, atherosclerosis, high levels of lipids in the blood, coagulation defects, etc. Anticoagulant therapy with Coumadin may be initiated, but removal of the catheter may be required [104–107].

METABOLIC COMPLICATIONS

Providing a complex therapy to the most critically ill patient population portends that metabolic complications can, and do, occur on a regular basis. Preventing these complications is the goal of the specialist who is managing the patient's care. Having a good understanding of the metabolic response to injury and its effects on nutrient metabolism is key to preventing and treating these complications.

Metabolic complications can be avoided or minimized if the patient is closely monitored and an appropriate formula is used. Use of a low dextrose formula and starting slowly and cautiously can reduce the risk of hyperglycemia. It may be necessary initially to hydrate the patient adequately, including adding MVI, and then to advance the formula gradually, especially in the severely malnourished patient. Overfeeding the patient will not restore their nutritional status faster and can cause the problems previously discussed. Provision of small amounts of enteral feeding can prevent the gut atrophy, which can result from prolonged use of TPN and NPO. It may also help to prevent the hepatic dysfunction, which can occur with long-term use of TPN without concomitant small GI "trophic" feedings.

Metabolic complications can be divided into the following categories: fluid and electrolyte disturbances, abnormal glucose metabolism, hypertriglyceridemia, hepatic dysfunction, essential fatty acid deficiency (EFAD), metabolic bone disease, GI atrophy, and gastric hyperacidity (Table 22.9).

FLUID AND ELECTROLYTE DISTURBANCES

Before starting parenteral nutrition, it is important that the patient is hemodynamically stable. Central venous access enables the clinician to provide large volumes of fluid if necessary, but the nutrient composition of the formula that is used must be carefully tailored to the requirements of the individual patient.

A patient with renal, hepatic, or cardiac dysfunction will most likely require some volume restriction of the formula. There are various methods for determining fluid requirements, and an in depth discussion of this topic is beyond the scope of this chapter. But providing either 30–35 mL/kg/day or 1 mL/kcal/day are to frequently used starting volume guidelines. When calculating the daily fluid allotment, it is important to consider all sources of fluid that the patient is receiving concomitant with TPN. Infusions of antibiotics and other medications intravenously concomitantly with TPN, together with "keep open" intravenous infusions, can cause serious water overload if not monitored and controlled closely.

Abnormalities in sodium, potassium, magnesium, calcium, phosphorus, and chloride levels can be due to the underlying medical condition, which is contributing to the need for parenteral nutrition support. Frequent laboratory assessments may be necessary at the start of therapy to correct/prevent abnormalities. However, once the patient is stable on the nutrition support regimen, the need for laboratory assessments decreases.

ABNORMAL GLUCOSE METABOLISM

TPN is usually administered to hospitalized patients continuously over a 24-h period. Thus, the patient is never "fasting" for laboratory studies even though they may be NPO. Hyperglycemia is usually defined as a glucose > 200 mg/dL. However, especially in the critically ill ICU patient, strict glycemic control is the goal, and maintaining the blood sugar < 150 mg/dL is preferred. It may be necessary either to decrease the carbohydrate content of the solution (and, therefore, the calorie

TABLE 22.9

Metabolic Complications of TPN

Complication	Cause	Treatment/Prevention
Hypervolemia	Renal, hepatic, or cardiac dysfunction	Hemodynamically stable prior to initiation of therapy
	Provision of excess fluid	Check I&O daily
Hypovolemia	Excess fluid losses	Hemodynamically stable prior to initiation of therapy
		Monitor I&O daily
Hypernatremia	Provision of excess sodium	Decrease sodium intake
	Excess fluid losses	Monitor I&O
Hyponatremia	Inadequate sodium intake	Increase sodium in TPN
	Fluid overload	Monitor I&O—decrease fluid volume
	Hyperglycemia	Glycemic control
Hyperkalemia	Renal failure	Reduce potassium content of TPN
	Provision of excess potassium	Check medication profile
	Lab error	
Hypokalemia	Excess potassium losses	Replace losses
	Inadequate potassium intake	Increase potassium content of TPN
Hypercalcemia	Hyperparathyroidism	Treat underlying condition
	Neoplasms	Decrease calcium content of TPN formula
Hypocalcemia	Hypoalbuminemia	Correct for hypoalbuminemia
	Inadequate intake	Increase calcium in TPN
	Hypomagnesemia, hyperphosphatemia	Check electrolyte levels and correct appropriately
	Vitamin D deficiency	Replete nutrient deficiencies
	Pancreatitis	Treat underlying disease process
Hypermagnesemia	Renal failure	Reduce magnesium in TPN
	Excess magnesium provision	
Hypomagnesemia	Refeeding syndrome	Correct deficiencies
	Increased losses	Increase magnesium in TPN
Hyperphosphatemia	Renal failure	Reduce phosphate content of TPN
	Provision of excess phosphate	
Hypophosphatemia	Refeeding syndrome	Correct deficiencies
	Sepsis, vomiting, malabsorption	Treat underlying causes
Hyperglycemia	Diabetes mellitus	Insulin as needed
	Provision of excess glucose from TPN and other IV sources	Reduce dextrose provided in all infusates to restore blood glucose to physiological levels
	Sepsis	Treat infection
Hypoglycemia	Abrupt discontinuation of TPN	Taper TPN prior to stopping infusion
	Excess insulin	Decrease insulin
Hypertriglyceridemia	Provision of excess lipid	Decrease lipid content of TPN
	Sepsis, MSOF	Treat underlying condition

intake) or to add or increase insulin in the solution. A reasonable starting point is 0.1 unit of insulin for each gram of dextrose in the formulation. Maintain the low dextrose formula until glycemic control is achieved. Once stabilized, the dextrose and thus the caloric content of the solution can be increased. Hyperglycemia in a patient who formerly was in good glycemic control may signal the incipient or early development of sepsis.

HYPERTRIGLYCERIDEMIA, EFAD, AND HEPATIC DYSFUNCTION

Abnormal lipid metabolism can occur because of the metabolic response to stress and illness. It may be necessary to eliminate the lipid component in a patient with a documented egg allergy, a patient with preexisting hypertriglyceridemia, and a morbidly obese patient, if limiting caloric intake is the goal of therapy. Lipid should never exceed 60% of the total calorie intake, and 30–40% of the total caloric ration as fat, or less, is usually sufficient. The lipid rations should be limited to 1 g/kg/day or less.

In a patient with elevated liver enzymes, providing a small amount of lipid every other day may be sufficient for preventing the development of EFAD and still meet calorie goals. In a patient with a documented carnitine deficiency, the addition of carnitine to the regimen may help to improve lipid metabolism and clearance.

The etiology of hepatic dysfunction associated with parenteral nutrition is multifactorial. Components of the TPN solution may be associated with the development of hepatic dysfunction, and/or deficiencies or imbalances in the TPN solution may be responsible for abnormal hepatocyte function. Inflammation related to omega-6 fatty acids in the lipid emulsion has been implicated in the hepatic disorders. Continued investigation to determine etiology and mechanisms, and prevention and therapy of PNALD, are indicated and are likely to resolve this problem in the near future (Table 22.10).

Repeated catheter infections and secondary sepsis can also contribute to abnormal liver enzymes, especially in the patient on long-term parenteral nutrition support [43,104–107].

METABOLIC BONE DISEASE

Metabolic bone disease, characterized by pain in the long bones and weight-bearing joints, along with decreased rates of bone formation, is not usually associated with short-term use of parenteral nutrition. It is more frequently encountered in the patient on long-term nutritional support, and there are many factors to consider in its etiology.

Aluminum content of the solution is less of a factor since the manufacturers of TPN components are required by the FDA to label the amount of aluminum expected to be in the product at the time of expiration. Provision of excess amino acids remains an issue. In order to avoid this complication, it is often recommended to keep the amino acid content of the formula at 1 g/kg/day. The change in 1981 from casein hydrolysate as the primary protein source to the use of crystalline amino acids is also credited with helping to resolve this issue by helping to reduce exposure over time to high concentrations of aluminum. Reduction in the aluminum content of the formula and a decrease in the amount of protein provided also helped to contribute to reductions in urinary calcium losses, improved vitamin D status, and thus improved bone histology.

Inadequate calcium, phosphorus, magnesium, copper, and vitamin D have all been implicated in the etiology of metabolic bone disease. Lack of weight bearing exercise, alcohol abuse, and

TABLE 22.10
Long-Term Complications of TPN Therapy

Complication	Cause	Treatment/Prevention
Abnormal liver enzymes	Provision of excess calories	Decrease calories in TPN
	Provision of excess dextrose	Decrease dextrose
	Continuous TPN infusion	Cycle TPN
	Carnitine deficiency	Correct deficiency
	Sepsis	Treat underlying infection
	Lack of enteral stimulation	Provide "trophic" feedings
Metabolic bone disease	See section on Metabolic Bone Disease	Treat underlying cause
GI atrophy	Lack of enteral stimulation	Use GI tract whenever possible
Sepsis	Catheter care protocol not strictly followed	Reinforce proper technique
		Surveillance blood cultures
		Treat symptoms promptly

smoking also contribute to the development of metabolic bone disease, as well as hyperparathyroid-ism, chronic acidosis, inflammation, and estrogen deficiency. Heparin, methotrexate, cyclosporine, warfarin, and phenytoin may all increase calcium losses, and >10 mg/day of corticosteroids can cause osteopenia and hypercalciuria. Continuous 24-h infusion of TPN may actually decrease uri-nary calcium losses. However, in the long-term homecare patient, 24-h infusion rather than a cycled infusion is often not preferred for quality of life reasons.

Optimally, treatment of metabolic bone disease would involve limiting the aluminum content or eliminating it completely from the TPN solution components provided by the manufacturers. However, this has been difficult to achieve. Providing adequate amounts of nutrients is recognized as important for bone health (calcium, phosphorus, copper, magnesium, and vitamin D). Limiting the use and/or dosage of medications that are recognized as having a negative effect on bone health is also indicated [108,109].

GI ATROPHY

"If you don't use it, you lose it." This especially applies aptly to the intestinal functions of the patient on parenteral nutrition. Placing the gut at rest may be necessary in the initial phase of recovery from various surgical procedures, and in a patient with acute pancreatitis who is severely malnourished, but not for long term. Provision of some enteral stimulation can aid in bowel recovery after massive resection. The amount of nutrition that is required to be provided via the enteral route for optimal trophic effects still remains an area of intense investigation. However, it appears that very minimal amounts of oral or enteral intake will suffice to prevent GI atrophy and to stimulate bile flow.

GASTRIC HYPERACIDITY

Prolonged use of parenteral nutrition, in the absence of enteral feedings, can lead to gastric hyper-acidity. Gastric hyperacidity can contribute to increased diarrhea, dehydration, electrolyte abnor-malities, peptic ulcers, and gastritis. The addition of an H2 blocker to the TPN solution can reduce gastric hyperacidity and reduce the incidence of these complications.

INFECTIOUS COMPLICATIONS

Infectious CVC complications require immediate attention. A fever spike and/or redness or swell-ing of the catheter insertion site are clear indications for corrective action. Blood cultures, both peripheral and through the infusion line, are mandated. Empiric antibiotics may be started and then adjusted specifically based on culture results. In some cases, it may be necessary to remove the line, wait until cultures revert to negative, and replace the venous access at another site. Strict catheter care protocols must be established and followed assiduously to prevent central venous line infec-tions, as some patients have limited sites that can be used for infusion therapy. This is especially important for a patient who will require long-term therapy or lifetime therapy [110,111]. There is absolutely no alternative to meticulous, conscientious, competent adherence to the established prin-ciples of asepsis and antisepsis in preventing infectious complications. They have been shown to be minimized to a level of 1% or less by multiple nutrition/metabolic support teams, and this must be the goal of all who use TPN as the potent life-saving technique that it was designed to be.

SUMMARY

Similar to the broad field of medicine, nutrition support is an amalgam of art and science. Both areas of endeavor had their origins in curiosity; empirical observations; theoretical concepts; innova-tions; experiments; philosophy; ideals; and the practical application or translation of newly acquired knowledge and/or experience to clinical use. This had formed the basis of the practice of medicine for millennia, and advances had been made slowly and tediously for hundreds of years until the late nineteenth and early twentieth centuries, when discovery, creativity, science, and technology virtually exploded, and has continued to advance geometrically. Furthermore, this phenomenal increase in knowledge, technology, and expertise is likely to continue in the foreseeable future and to have a significant influence on the application of nutrition support to the practice of medicine, maintenance of health, and achievement of optimal clinical and human performance and outcomes. However, in the future, it is expected that all new ideas, concepts, proposals, or adjuncts related to improving the quality of health care in general and nutrition support specifically will be accompanied by considerable doubt, skepticism, criticism, prejudice, controversies, challenges, and resistance to change. Therefore, the scientific method must continue to be applied consistently, diligently, fairly, dispassionately, honestly, morally, and ethically to allow evaluation of as many aspects of problems, solutions, and situations as possible in order to achieve optimal evaluation, interpretation, and useful applications.

Those of us interested in providing optimal nutrition support to all of our patients know that it is imperative that knowledge, judgment, proficiency, and competency must prevail in choosing the best nutrient constituents of a feeding regimen and in deciding how these formulations might best be provided for the maximal benefit and safety of patients under virtually any condition or adverse situation. Not to have knowledge, experience, or proficiency with every tool in our clinical armamentarium detracts from our education and training; our trust, competence, and professionalism; and our morals, ethics, and obligations. Above all, the practice of optimal nutrition support should not be adversely influenced by self-ambition, self-interest, prejudice, financial gain, stature, or other distractions. Practitioners who always treat their patients with enteral nutrition and those who always treat their patients with parenteral nutrition are both likely to be practicing less than optimal nutrition support. The judicious use of the most appropriate feeding modality or combination in every conceivable clinical situation requires extensive experience, judgment, proficiency, wisdom, and equanimity. It is incumbent upon practitioners of nutrition support to appraise a given clinical situation comprehensively, to identify and define the goals of nutrition support, and to choose and use the most appropriate nutrition support proficiently in the comprehensive management of a patient. All of the members of the health care profession must direct our efforts, talents, and resources to perfecting nutrition support to the point that we all could nourish our patients by the most efficacious methods and techniques possible to provide substrates sufficient in quality and quantity to support and allow the maximum number of cells in the body cell mass to perform optimally the functions for which they were designed. We owe it to our patients and profession to do so. Mastering the information, knowledge, technology, data, skills, judgment, and wisdom presented in this outstanding volume will undoubtedly be an invaluable asset in achieving this challenging and honorable goal.

ACKNOWLEDGMENTS

The authors thank Zachary Simon Rothkopf for his editorial assistance in preparation of the manuscript.

REFERENCES

1. Rose WC. The amino acid requirements of adult man. *Nutr Abstr Rev* 1957;27:631–647.
2. Elwyn DH. Protein metabolism and requirements in the critically ill patient. *Crit Care Clin* 1987;3:57–69.
3. Elwyn D. Nutritional requirements of adult surgical patients. *Crit Care Med* 1980;8:9–20.
4. Rhoads JE, Riegel C, Koop CE et al. The problem of nutrition in patients with gastric lesions requiring surgery. *Western J Surg Gynec Obstet* 1943;51:229–233.
5. Rhoads JE, Alexander CE. Nutritional problems of surgical patients. *Ann NY Acad Sci* 1955;63:268–275.
6. Rhoads JE. The history of nutrition. In: *Manual of Surgical Nutrition*. Ballinger WF, Collins JA, Drucker WR et al. (eds). WB Saunders, Philadelphia, PA, 1975:1–9.
7. Wretlind A. Development of fat emulsions. *JPEN J Parenter Enteral Nutr* 1981;5:230–235.

8. Vinnars E, Hammerqvist L. 25th Annual Arvid Wretlind's lecture. Silver anniversary, 25 years with ESPEN, the history of nutrition. *Clin Nutr* 2004;23:955–962.

9. Edgren B, Wretlind A. The theoretical background of the intravenous nutrition with fat emulsions. *Nutr Dieta Eur Rev Nutr Diet* 1963;13:364–386.

10. Wretlind A. Complete intravenous nutrition: Theoretical and experimental background. *Nutr Metab* 1972;14(suppl):1–57.

11. Elman R. Parenteral replacement of protein with the amino-acids of hydrolyzed casein. *Ann Surg* 1940;112:594–602.

12. Dudrick SJ, Wilmore DW, Vars HM et al. Long-term total parenteral nutrition with growth, development, and positive nitrogen balance. *Surgery* 1968;64:134–142.

13. Dudrick SJ. Early developments and clinical applications of total parenteral nutrition. *JPEN J Parenter Enteral Nutr* 2003;27:291–299.

14. Dudrick SJ. History of parenteral nutrition. *J Am Coll Nutr* 2009;28:243–251.

15. Dudrick SJ, Rhoads JE. New horizons for intravenous feeding. *JAMA* 1971;215:939–949.

16. Dudrick SJ, Wilmore DW, Vars HM. Long-term total parenteral nutrition with growth in puppies and positive nitrogen balance in patients. *Surg Forum* 1967;18:356–357.

17. Dudrick SJ, Wilmore DW, Vars HM, Rhoads JE. Can intravenous feeding as the sole means of nutrition support growth in the child and restore weight loss in an adult? An affirmative answer. *Ann Surg* 1969;169:974–984.

18. Moore B. In memory of Sidney Ringer (1835–1910) some account of the fundamental discoveries of the great pioneer of bio-chemistry of crystalloids in living cells. *Biochem J.* 1911;5:i.b3–xix.

19. Long CL. Energy and protein needs in the critically ill patient. *Cont Surg* 1980;16:29–42.

20. Hoffer LJ, Bistrian BR. Appropriate protein provision in critical illness: A systematic narrative review. *Am J Clin Nutr* 2012;96:591–600.

21. Weller LA, Calloway DH, Margen S. Nitrogen balance of men fed amino acid mixtures based on Rose's requirements, egg white protein and serum free amino acid patterns. *J Nutr* 1971;101:1499–1508.

22. Irwin ME, Hegsted SM. A conspectus of research in amino acid requirements in man. *J Nutr* 1971;101:539–545.

23. Premji SS, Soraisham AS, Chessell L, Sauve R. Dietary protein requirements for pre-term infants in the neonatal period: Past, present, and future. In: *Protein Research Progress.* Boscoe AB, Listow CR (eds). Nova Science Publishers, New York, 2008.

24. Gamble JL. Physiological information gained from studies on the life raft ration. *Nutr Rev* 1989;47:199–201.

25. Cuthbertson DP. Post-shock metabolic response. *Lancet* 1942;239:433–437.

26. Frankenfeld D. Energy expenditure and protein requirements after traumatic injury. *Nutr Clin Pract* 2006;21:430–437.

27. Wolfe R, Odonnell T, Stone M et al. Investigation of factors determining the optimal glucose infusion rate in total parenteral nutrition. *Metabolism* 1980;29:892–900.

28. Cahill JF Jr. Starvation in man. *N Engl J Med* 1970;282:669–675.

29. Blackburn GL, Bistrian BR, Maini BS, Schlamm HT, Smith MF. Nutritional and metabolic assessment of the hospitalized patient. *JPEN J Parenter Enteral Nutr* 1977;1:11–22.

30. Fukatsu K, Kudsk KA. Nutrition and gut immunity. *Surg Clin North Am* 2011;91:755–770.

31. Moore FA, Feliciano DV, Andrassy RJ et al. Early enteral feeding, compared with parenteral, reduces postoperative septic complications: The results of a meta-analysis. *Ann Surg* 1992;216:172–183.

32. Pullicino E, Elia M. Mechanisms of nutritional repletion during total parenteral nutrition. *Gut* 1989;30:69–70.

33. Burke PA, Young LS, Bistrian BR. Metabolic vs nutrition support: A hypothesis. *JPEN J Parenter Enteral Nutr* 2010;34:546–548.

34. Ziegler TR. Parenteral nutrition in the critically ill patient. *N Engl J Med* 2009;361:1088–1097.

35. McClave SA, Martindale RG, Vanek VW et al. Guidelines for the provision and assessment of nutrition support therapy in the adult critically ill patient: Society of Critical Care Medicine (SCCM) and American Society for Parenteral and Enteral Nutrition (A.S.P.E.N.). *JPEN J Parenter Enteral Nutr* 2009;33:277–316.

36. Wilmore DW. Catabolic illness: Strategies for enhancing recovery. *N Engl J Med* 1991;325:695–702.

37. Singer P, Berger MM, Van den Berghe G et al. ESPEN guidelines on parenteral nutrition: Intensive care. *Clin Nutr* 2009;28:387–400.

38. Bartlett RH, Dechert RE. Nutrition in critical care. *Surg Clin North Am* 2011;91:595–607.

39. Lowry SF. The route of feeding influences injury responses. *J Trauma* 1990;30:S10–S15.

40. Roza AM, Shizgal HM. The Harris Benedict equation reevaulated: Resting energy requirements and the body cell mass. *Am J Clin Nutr* 1984;40:168–182.
41. Harris JA, Benedict FG. *Biometric Studies of Basal Metabolism in Man*. Publication no. 279. Carnegie Institute of Washington, DC, 1919.
42. Jeejeebhoy KN. Total parenteral nutrition: Potion or poison? *Am J Clin Nutr* 2001;74:160–163.
43. Rolandelli RH, Siegel BK. Nutritional support nutritional management of hospitalized patients. In: *ACS Surgery: Principles and Practice*, 8th Edition. Souba WW, Fink MP, Jurkovich GJ et al. (eds). WebMD Professional Publishing, New York, 2008.
44. Rees Parrish C, Krenitsky J, Willcutts K, Radigan AE. Chapter 27 gastrointestinal disease. In: *The A.S.P.E.N. Nutrition Support Core Curriculum: A Case Based Approach—The Adult Patient*. Gottschlich M (ed in chief). American Society for Parenteral and Enteral Nutrition, Silver Spring, MD, 2007.
45. Rees Parrish C. The clinician's guide to short bowel syndrome. *Pract Gastroenterol* 2005;31:67–106.
46. Gianotti L, Meier R, Lobo DN et al. ESPEN guideline on parenteral nutrition: Pancreas. *Clin Nutr* 2009;28:428–435.
47. Cimbilik C, Paauw JD, Davis AT. Pregnancy and lactation. In: *The ASPEN Nutrition Support Core Curriculum: A Case Based Approach—The Adult Patient*. Gottschlich M (ed in chief). American Society for Parenteral and Enteral Nutrition, Silver Spring, MD, 2007.
48. Levine MG, Esser D. Total parenteral nutrition for the treatment of severe hyperemesis gravidarum: Maternal nutritional effects and fetal outcome. *Obstet Gynecol* 1988;72:102–107.
49. Paauw JD, Bierling S, Cook C, Davis AT. Hyperemesis gravidarum and fetal outcome. *JPEN J Parenter Enteral Nutr* 2005;29:93–96.
50. Christie PM, Hill GL. Effect of intravenous nutrition on nutrition and function in acute attacks of inflammatory bowel disease. *Gastroenterology* 1990;99:730–736.
51. Mc Cray S, Rees Parrish C. Nutritional management of chyle leaks: An update. *Pract Gastroenterol* 2011;94:12–32.
52. Van den Berghe G, Wouters PJ, Bouillon R et al. Intensive insulin therapy in critically ill patients. *N Engl J Med* 2001;345:1357–1359.
53. Lewis KS, Kane-Gill SL, Bobek MB, Dasta JF. Intensive insulin therapy for critically ill patients. *Ann Pharmacother* 2004;38:1243–1251.
54. Lee V. Liver dysfunction associated with parenteral nutrition: What are the options? *Pract Gastroenterol* 2006;45:49–68.
55. Plauth M, Cabre E, Campillo B et al. ESPEN guidelines on parenteral nutrition: Hepatology. Comprehensive European clinical practice guidelines on parenteral nutrition support in patients with hepatic dysfunction. *Clin Nutr* 2009;28:436–444.
56. Freund HR. Abnormalities of liver function and hepatic damage associated with total parenteral nutrition. *Nutrition* 1991;7:1–5.
57. Sax HC, Bower RH. Hepatic complications of total parenteral nutrition. *JPEN J Parenter Enteral Nutr* 1989;12:615–618.
58. Jeejeebhoy KN. Hepatic manifestations of total parenteral nutrition: Need for prospective investigation. *Hepatology* 1988;8:428–429.
59. Baker AL, Rosenberg IH. Hepatic complications of total parenteral nutrition. *Am J Med* 1987;82:489–497.
60. Quigley EMM, Marsh MN, Shaffer JL, Markin RS. Hepatobiliary complications of total parenteral nutrition. *Gastroenterology* 1993;84:1012–1019.
61. Cano NJM, Aparico M, Brunori G et al. ESPEN guidelines on parenteral nutrition: Adult renal failure. *Clin Nutr* 2009;28:401–414.
62. Kuwahara T, Asanami S, Kubo S. Experimental infusion phlebitis: Tolerance osmolality of peripheral venous endothelial cells. *Nutrition* 1998;14:496–501.
63. Adapted from information gathered from calculating osmolarity of an IV admixture viewed on http://www.rx kinetics.com/iv_osmolarity.html.
64. Gazitua R, Wilson K, Bistrian BR et al. Factors determining peripheral vein tolerance to amino acid infusions. *Arch Surg* 1979;114:897–900.
65. Aubaniac R. A new route for venous injection or puncture: The subclavicular route, subclavian vein, brachiocephalic trunk. *Sem Hosp* 1952;28:3445–3447.
66. Patrick SP, Tijunelis MA, Johnson S, Herbert ME. Supraclavicular subclavian vein catheterization: The forgotten central line. *West J Emerg Med* 2009;10:110–114.
67. Daily PO, Griepp RB, Shumway NE. Percutaneous internal jugular vein cannulation. *Arch Surg* 1970;101:534–536.

68. Padberg FT, Ruggiero J, Blackburn GL, Bistrian BR. Central venous catheterizations for parenteral nutrition. *Ann Surg* 1982;193:264–270.

69. Krzywda EA, Andris DA, Edmiston CE et al. Parenteral access devices. In Gottschlich MM: *The Science and Practice of Nutrition Support: A Case-Based Core Curriculum.* Dubuque, IA: Kendall/Hunt Publishing Dubuque, IA, 2001:230.

70. Galloway S, Bodenham A. Long term central venous access. *Br J Anesth* 2004;92:722–734.

71. Hollmann W, Forssman W. Eberswalde, the 1956 Nobel Prize for medicine. *Eur J Med Res* 2006;11:406–408.

72. Sansivero GE. Venous anatomy and physiology: Considerations for vascular access device placement and function. *J Intravenous Nurs* 1998;21:S107–S114.

73. Fletcher SJ, Bodenham AR. Editorial II Safe placement of central venous catheters: Where should the tip of the catheter lie? *Br J Anesth* 2000;2:188–191.

74. Schummer W, Saks Y, Schummer C. Towards optimal central venous catheter tip position. In Vincent JL: *Yearbook of Intensive Care and Emergency Medicine*, Springer, Berlin 2008;581–590.

75. Broviac JW, Cole JJ, Scribner BH. A silicone rubber atrial catheter for prolonged parenteral alimentation. *Surg Gynecol Obstet* 1973;136(4):602–606.

76. Bodenham AR, Simcock L. Complications of central venous access. In: *Central Venous Catheters.* Hamilton H, Bodenham AR (eds). Wiley-Blackwell, Oxford, UK, 2009.

77. Dudrick SJ, Macfadden BV, Van Buren CT et al. Parenteral hyperalimentation: Metabolic problems and solutions. *Ann Surg* 1972;176:259–264.

78. Crook MA, Hally V, Panteli JV. The importance of the refeeding syndrome. *Nutrition* 2001;17:632–637.

79. Marinella MA. The refeeding syndrome and hypophosphataemia. *Nutr Rev* 2003;61(9):320–323.

80. Solomon SM, Kirby DF. The refeeding syndrome: A review. *JPEN J Parenter Enteral Nutr* 1990;14:90–97.

81. Brook MJ, Melnik G. The refeeding syndrome: An approach to understanding its complications and preventing it occurrence. *Pharmacotherapy* 1995;15(6):713–726.

82. Rothkopf MM, Sobelman JS, Mathis AS et al. Micronutrient-responsive cerebral dysfunction other than Wernicke's encephalopathy after malabsorptive surgery. *Surg Obes Relat Dis* 2010;6:171–180.

83. Velez RJ, Myers B, Guber MS. Severe acute metabolic acidosis (acute beriberi): An avoidable complication of total parenteral nutrition. *JPEN J Parenter Enteral Nutr* 1985;9:216–219.

84. Driscoll DF. Total nutrient admixtures: Theory and practice. *Nutr Clin Pract* 1995;10:114–119.

85. Waitzburg DL, Torrinhas RS, Jacintho TM. New parenteral lipid emulsions for clinical use. *JPEN J Parenter Enteral Nutr* 2006;30:351–367.

86. Wanten GJS, Calder PC. Immune modulation by parenteral lipid emulsions. *Am J Clin Nutr* 2007;85:1171–1184.

87. Wretlind A. Current status of intralipid and other fat emulsions. In: *Fat Emulsions in Parenteral Nutrition.* Meng HC, Wilmore DW (eds). American Medical Association, Chicago, 1976:109–122.

88. Ferezou J, Bach AC. Structure and metabolic fate of triacylglycerol and phospholipid-rich particles of commercial parenteral fat emulsions. *Nutrition* 1999;15:44–50.

89. Hallberg D. Elimination of exogenous lipids from the bloodstream: An experimental methodological study in dogs and man. *Acta Physiol Scand* 1965;254(suppl):1–24.

90. Iriyamak K. Lipid for parenteral use: Development and future perspectives. *Nutrition* 1994;10(suppl):521–522.

91. Product information Fresenius Kabi Australia Intralipid. File name IntP1070510, Fresenius Kabi Australia Pty Limited, Pymble, New South Wales, Australia, 2010:1–9.

92. Taskinen MP, Tulikoura I, Nikkila EA, Ehnholm C. Effect of parenteral hyperalimentation on serum lipoproteins and on lipoprotein lipase activity of adipose tissue and skeletal muscle. *Eur J Clin Invest* 1981;11:317–323.

93. Mirtallo JM, Dasta JF, Kleinschmidt KC, Varon J. State of the art review: Intravenous fat emulsions: Current applications, safety profile and clinical implications. *Ann Pharmacother* 2010;44:699–700.

94. Dudrick SJ. A 45 year obsession and passionate pursuit of optimal nutrition support: Puppies, pediatrics, surgery, geriatrics, home TPN, A.S.P.E.N., etc. In: *A.S.P.E.N. Anthology of Jonathan E. Rhoads Lectures, 1978–2008.* American Society for Parenteral and Enteral Nutrition, Silver Spring, MD, 2009;284–299.

95. May ME, Hill JO. Energy content of diets of variable amino acid composition. *Am J Clin Nutr* 1990;52:770–776.

96. Yarandi SS, Zhao VM, Hebbar G, Ziegler TR. Amino acid composition in parenteral nutrition: What is the evidence? *Curr Opin Clin Nutr Metab Care* 2011;14:75–82.

97. Heird WC, Dell RB, Driscoll JM et al. Metabolic acidosis resulting from intravenous alimentation mixtures containing synthetic amino acids. *N Engl J Med* 1972;287:943–948.

98. Shizgal HM, Spanier AH, Kurtz RS. Effect of parenteral nutrition on body composition in the critically ill patient. *Am J Surg* 1976;131:156–161.

99. Gennari FJ, Weise WJ. Acid-base disturbances in gastrointestinal disease. *Clin J Am Soc Nephrol* 2008;3:1861–1868.

100. Madsen H, Frankel EH. The hitchhiker's guide to parenteral nutrition management for adult patients. *Pract Gastroenterol* 2006;40:46–68.

101. American Medical Association Department of Foods and Nutrition. Multivitamin preparations for parenteral use: A statement by the nutrition advisory group. *JPEN J Parenter Enteral Nutr* 1979;3:258–262.

102. American Medical Association Department of Foods and Nutrition. Guidelines for essential trace element preparations for parenteral use. A statement by an expert panel. *JAMA* 1979;241:2051–2054.

103. Shaw SN, Elwyn DH, Askanazi J et al. Effects of increasing nitrogen intake on nitrogen balance and energy expenditure in nutritionally depleted adult patients receiving parenteral nutrition. *Am J Clin Nutr* 1983;37:930–940.

104. Ghabril MS, Aranda-Michel J, Scolapio JS. Metabolic and catheter complications of parenteral nutrition. *Curr Gastroenterol Rep* 2004;6:327–334.

105. McGee DC, Gould MK. Preventing complications of central venous catheterization. *N Engl J Med* 2003;348:1123–1133.

106. Pittiruti M, Hamilton H, Biffi R, MacFie J, Pertkiewicz M. ESPEN Guidelines on parenteral nutrition: Central venous catheters (access, care, diagnosis and therapy of complications). *Clin Nutr* 2009;28:365–377.

107. Wolfe BM, Ryder MA, Nishikawa RA et al. Complications of parenteral nutrition. *Am J Surg* 1986;152:93–99.

108. Seidner DL. Parenteral nutrition associated metabolic bone disease. *J Parenter Enterl Nutr* 2002;26(5 suppl):S37–S42.

109. Buchman AL, Moukarzel A. Metabolic bone disease associated with total parenteral nutrition. *Clin Nutr* 2000;9:217–231.

110. Trautner B, Darouiche RO. Catheter-associated infections: Pathogenesis affects prevention. *Arch Intern Med* 2004;164:842–850.

111. Ogrady NP, Alexander M, Burns LA et al. Guidelines for the prevention of intravascular catheter related infections. *Clin Infect Dis* 2011;52:e162–e193.

23 Metabolic Effects of Omega-3 Fatty Acids

Beverly B. Teter

CONTENTS

INTRODUCTION

Dietary fats have been reported to be connected with several diseases since the early 1960s. These included coronary heart disease, obesity, and several others. Most of these connections were hypotheses based on finding certain lipids at the "site" of the "crime" and assuming that they caused the "crime." In some cases, there was some epidemiological evidence that certain types of lipids were found to be associated with certain observed diseases. In other instances, they were found to be beneficial. One of the best known theories became known as the "Diet/Heart Hypothesis" and was widely accepted by the medical profession in spite of objections by some well-respected researchers and practitioners.

During the ensuing years, there have been numerous studies conducted with careful designs and sound statistics, and slow progress has been made, which indicates that many of the early concepts are not entirely accurate. Analytical assays have been refined, imaging techniques and metabolic assays as well as genetic information and surgical techniques have improved, and we are now able to begin to understand the disease processes more fully. The omega-3 fatty acids (FAs) have received a lot of attention in recent years, so their metabolism is better understood.

BACKGROUND ON OMEGA-3 FAs

The omega-3 FAs are one of two groups of FAs that are unique in that they cannot be made *de novo* in the human body and in many other mammals. This is why cats and dogs are obligatory carnivores. Humans and many mammals are not able to insert a double bond in the FA chain in either the n-6 or n-3 position. These positions are at the omega end of the FA chain. The omega end is the end where the last $-CH_3$ group resides on the FA carbon chain. The n-3 FAs have a double bond three carbons in from the end and, the n-6 FAs have a double bond six carbons from the end. All other double bonds they may have are closer to the carboxyl end. Modifications of the carbon number (chain length) all occur at the carboxyl end of the carbon chain where the carboxyl group ($-C = O_2H$) is attached. Thus, once an n-3 or n-6 FA is made by a plant or sea animal, that position is fixed and the FA will always have the n-3 or n-6 bond unless oxidized away. If the FA starts out as an 18:2 n-6 or 18:3 n-3 FA, it can be elongated and desaturated to become a longer chain polyunsaturated FA

449

Source	Family	First FA	Desaturase	Product	Elongation
			(form C=C)		(add 2 C's)
Diet or Oleic acid	n–9	Δ9–18:1 + Δ6 desat →	6,9 –18:2 →	8,11–20:2 → Synthesis

Desaturase	Elongation	Desaturase
(form C=C)	(add 2 C's)	(add 2 C's)
Δ5 desat → 5,8,11–20:3* →	7,10,13–22:3	Δ4 desat → 4,7,10,13 – 22:4

*Evidence of EFA deficiency.

Source	Family	First FA	Desaturase	Product	Elongation
			(form C=C)		(add 2 C's)
Diet only	n–6	Δ9,12 – 18:2 + Δ6 desat →	6,9,12 – 18:3 →	8,11,14 – 20:3 +
		Linoleic acid		γ–Linoleic

Desaturase	Elongation	Elongation	Desaturase
(form C=C)	(add 2 C's)	(add 2 C's)	(form C=C)
Δ5 desat → 5,8,11,14 – 20:4 →	7,10,13,16 – 22:4 +	Δ4 →	4,7,10,13,16 – 22:5
Arachidonic acid*		Docosapentaenoic acid	

*Major fatty acid of membranes and prostaglandin precursor for PG E_2 and $F_{2\alpha}$.

Source	Family	First FA	Desaturase	Product	Elongation
			(form C=C)		(add 2 C's)
Diet only	n–3	9,12,15 – 18:3 + Δ6desat →	6,9,12,15 – 18:4 →	8,11,14,17 – 20:4 →
		α-Linoleic acid		

Desaturase	Elongation	Elongation	Desaturase
(form C=C)	(add 2 C's)	(add 2 C's)	(form C=C)
Δ5 desat → 5,8,11,14,17 – 20:5* →	7,10,13,16,19 – 22:5+	Δ4 desat →	4,7,10,13,16,19 – 22:6

*Precursor to Prostaglandins E_3 and $F_{3\alpha}$. Also characteristic of nervous tissues.

FIGURE 23.1 Metabolism of the three major fatty acid families in humans and their end products.

(PUFA) such as docosahexanoic acid (DHA, $C_{22}H_{32}O_2$) with six double bonds or eicosapentaenoic acid (EPA, $C_{20}H_{30}O_2$) with five double bonds, etc. These very long chain FAs are abundant in the brain and nervous tissues, retina, male reproductive tissues, and cell membranes as part of the phospholipids. Double bonds can be added by humans and most mammals at the delta-9 position by an enzyme called "delta-9 desaturase" as the carbon chain is elongated, thus allowing the formation of DHA and EPA from shorter chain n-3 and n-6 FAs in the diet. Cats cannot meet their physiological need for arachidonic acid (20:4 n-6) due to low delta-6 desaturase activity necessary for the transformation. Humans cannot make essential FAs (EFAs) either. Thus, the diet must supply the need and both linoleic (LA) and α-linolenic (αLN acid) are essential FAs in the diet. Figure 23.1 shows pathways for some of these reactions.

SHORT HISTORY OF OMEGA-3 FAs

Two classic papers by Burr and Burr[1,2] established the need for certain FAs in the diet of animals and humans. Almost 40 years later, Dr. Holman[3] published a paper describing essential FA deficiency. Later, Eskimos were reported to have prolonged bleeding times and less platelet aggregation associated with high levels of EPA in their platelets.[4] This led to speculation that omega-3 FA may be protective for heart disease and atherosclerosis. Another epidemiological report[5] demonstrated that the Inuit Eskimos in Greenland had significantly lower death rates from cardiovascular disease (CVD) than did the Danish population despite similar cholesterol levels. The Inuit diet is high in omega-3s due to the high intake of fat from whales, seals, and fish, whose diets are rich in omega three fatty acids. Subsequently, EFA deficiencies were identified in infants on a low-fat diet deficient in PUFA and in adults and children on parenteral alimentation low in, or devoid of, fat for long periods of time. Supplementation led to improvements in the EFA deficiency symptoms.[5] One symptom observed in humans and lab animals is skin lesions. There are reports that vitamin E can help control some of these effects. The old method for determining EFA deficiency was to measure water intake of the test animals compared to controls. Water was lost from the "weeping" lesions. A recent study in mice[6] determined that a diet high in vitamin E and omega-3 FAs reduced ulcerative dermatitis in C57Bl/6J mice compared to the usual mouse chow diet. This strain is subject to skin lesions as they age. The skin lipids also were altered by the diet.

WHERE DO ESSENTIAL FAs COME FROM?

Two FAs are absolutely essential since they cannot be made by humans. They are linoleic acid (LA, 18:2n-6) and α-linolenic acid (α-LN, 18:3n-3). These FAs and their derivatives are precursors for downstream products such as prostaglandins, thromboxanes, and prostacyclins. These downstream compounds have potent effects throughout the body. The omega-3 and omega-6 FAs compete for the same enzymes to make their derivatives. Humans need about 1% to 2% of their calories as linoleic acid (18:2n-6), and the ratio of n-6 to n-3 FAs should be about 3:1. Most plants and plant oils are rich in n-6 PUFAs with very little to none of the n-3. The US diet is deficient in omega-3 oils from food sources (Table 23.1). Our cows are fed with corn in their diets, which is rich in omega-6. Our meat and poultry sources are fed with corn and grains in their finishing diets; even the farmed fish have corn and other grains instead of the krill and fish, which make up their natural diets. When this is considered and added to the competition for the n-6 and n-3 FAs to use the same enzyme

TABLE 23.1
FA Content of Some Common Diet Oils

Oil or Fat	SCFA	LCFA	PUFA ω6	PUFA ω3	%S	%M	%P
Saturated Oils %							
Coconut	62	36	2	–	92	6	2
Palm kernel	56	26	2	–	83	15	2
Butter fat	13	79	2	1	63	31	3
Cocoa butter	–	96	3	–	62	35	3
Beef tallow	–	93	3	1	46	47	4
Lard	–	90	10	–	42	48	10
Monounsaturated Oils %							
Olive	–	88	10	1	17	72	11
Canola	–	68	32	10	6	62	32
Peanut	–	66	32	–	14	50	32
Polyunsaturated Oils %							
Safflower	22	78	78	–	9	13	78
Sunflower	–	32	68	1	12	19	69
Soybean	–	39	54	7	15	24	61
Corn	–	41	58	1	13	28	59
Cottonseed	–	46	54	1	26	20	55

Notes: SCFA: short-chain FA; LCFA: long-chain FAs; PUFA: polyunsaturated FA; S: saturated; M: monounsaturated; P: polyunsaturated.

systems, it is no wonder that we tend to be marginally supplied with enough omega-3 derivatives for good health. In addition, the omega-6 FA derivatives are mostly inflammatory, and the omega-3 FA derivatives produce mostly anti-inflammatory derivatives.

The EFAs are "essential" due to the many roles they play in maintaining good health. They have a structural role in all membranes of the cells in the body. Their presence increases the fluidity of the cellular membranes of which they are structural components of the phospholipids, which can moderate the activity of transfer of nutrients into and out of the cells and subcellular organelles. They act as precursors for the eicosanoids, such as prostaglandins and leukotrienes, which are involved in inflammation and its control, as mentioned above, and with maintaining the skin barrier. Arachidonic acid [AA, 20:4 (n-6)] regulates epidermal proliferation via prostaglandin E_2.

Deficiency symptoms may appear a few weeks or months after dietary intake becomes inadequate or absorption may be limited due to surgery or intestinal inability to absorb the EFAs. Recovery is usually within several weeks after supplementation. The omega-3s and omega-6s are very subject to oxidation. Supplements should be stored in dark containers at cool room temperatures to avoid oxidation, which will lead to a "fishy" smell. Oxidized FAs can lead to inflammation of the involved tissues.

Animal fats are good sources of the preformed longer chain EFAs, especially the cold water fish oils, but vegetable oils have only the precursor FAs—AA and αLN. Vitamin E is a good antioxidant to protect the oxidation of the EFAs especially when the diet is supplemented with large doses of EFA. The longer the chain length and the more double bonds in the molecule, the more easily it is oxidized. An excess amount of EFA and the derivatives are not needed for good health, but adequate amounts are required. The ratio of ω6:ω3 is important and should be about 3:1 in a healthy diet. As can be observed from Table 23.1, this ratio would be hard to achieve eating only vegetable oils. Only butter fat and beef tallow (beef fat) are in the close range. Flaxseed oil is rich in ω3 but is not abundant in our food supply. Walnuts are uniquely rich in ALA with 47.5 g/100 g ALA. Cold water fish are the richest supply of ω3 FAs. Warm water fish do not have them to the same extent if at all. These long-chain FAs act as antifreeze for the cold water environment that the fish live in. It keeps their cell membranes fluid so that they can function. Fish from warmer seas do not need them.

Before the required labeling of *trans* FAs (tFA), most of the PUFAs were chemically hydrogenated and the EFAs were lost. The commercially hydrogenated oils first lose the PUFAs—trienes and dienes—while the tFA containing monoenes increased. Saturates did not change to any great extent since they were totally saturated. This left the monoenes to increase. This was just what was needed for the food industry since the melting point could be raised enough that margarine could be formed into a "stick"-like butter and had similar melting points. Likewise, shortening could be created with higher melting points for baking or frying. The loss of the PUFAs conferred a higher melting point and also a higher flash point for deep fat frying. The higher melting point made the product solid at room temperature and appropriate for baking pastries and cakes, for margarine, etc. The problem with this process is that almost all the EFAs were destroyed, and the additional monoenes produced had the *trans* configuration, which is unhealthy. The consumption of tFA has been associated with heart disease and other illnesses.[7] Although tFA content of some foods has been substantially reduced, packaged foods that contain less than 0.5 g/serving may declare "0" grams even if it is 0.49 g/serving. Since the serving sizes have been reduced in many cases, if a person were to eat several servings, he or she could consume a substantial amount of tFA. One aspect of the label requirements is that the source of the tFA is not required to be labeled. The isomer distribution of *chemically* made tFA isomers is very different than those naturally made by the enzymes in the rumen organisms of the cows and other ruminants producing milk. These reactions as well as the ones in human bodies are enzyme directed so that the double bonds are only introduced in certain positions. Commercially produced tFA are the product of a catalyst, heat, time, and pressure, and the isomer distribution is random depending on the thermodynamics involved (Figure 23.2). The isomers produced in mammals have beneficial effects that are lost in fat-free milk products. Some are still

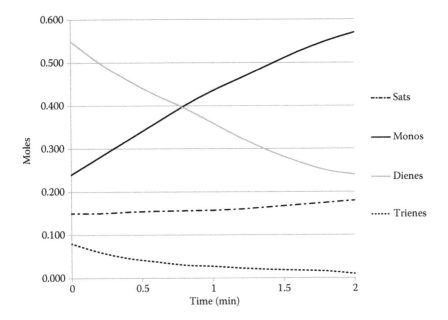

FIGURE 23.2 Kinetics of hydrogenation.

present in the animal body fat but to a much lesser degree. The isomer called 9c,11t-linoleic acid (9c,11tCLA; 9c,11t conjugated linoleic acid) has been shown by Dr. Ip[8] (IP) to be very anticarcinogenic and is present in cow milk. Furthermore, humans can make it from the 11t-octadecanoic (t11-18:1) acid also found in cow milk. His studies showed dramatic differences in mice fed with the 9c,11t-CLA isomer when challenged with a carcinogen. The mice on the CLA diet developed fewer and smaller mammary tumors. If the dam was on the diet during pregnancy and lactation and the pups were weaned to the CLA diet, they got the least tumors compared to the ones only receiving it at one of these times. These isomers are *not* in fat-free dairy products since they are milk fat components.

DIETARY INTAKE OF OMEGA-3 FAs

A recent paper[9] concluded that "Daily ingestion of 56 g of walnuts improves endothelial function in overweight adults with visceral adiposity." Forty-six overweight adults were randomly assigned to an *ad libitum* diet—with or without 56 g of walnuts daily—for 8 weeks and then switched to the opposite diet after a 4-week washout period. The flow-mediated vasodilatation of the brachial artery improved, as well as the secondary measurements of serum lipids and blood pressure, and anthropometric measures were maintained. In another study, a meta-analysis showed that walnut-supplemented diets decreased LDL-C and total cholesterol compared to controls.[10]

CURRENT APPROACHES TO EFA MAINTENANCE

Given the low levels of omega-3 FAs in the dietary oils of most of the food consumed in the United States and the very high levels of omega-6 FAs in the diet, the daily intake of omega-3 FAs needs to be closely monitored. The recommendations to lower the fat intake in the diet have also contributed to decreasing the EFA intake to levels that are probably too low for many people, and the ratio of ω6:ω3 is not adequate unless they are careful to choose omega-3-rich foods several times a week. Most consumers are not even aware of the requirement for the essential FAs. To compound the problem, the diets being recommended are high in carbohydrates because they are low in fat. The three main components in the US diet are carbohydrate, protein, and fat. Since the protein intake has remained about the same since 1900, about 20% of energy, if either carbohydrate or fat increases the other component will a priori will decrease to maintain equal calories. Starting in childhood, the diet is high in grains, sugars, breads, etc. and low in fat and often low in meats that provide some of the fat. Fortunately, the baby formulae are now fortified with omega-3s, but that is only for a short time before weaning. The extensive growth of the brain and nervous system in neonates and young children requires a large amount of EFA to develop properly. Fat is the major component of the white matter of the brain and is a major component of the myelin. The brain contains 25% of the lipid weight as cholesterol. The myelin covering the neurons in the brain contains about 70% of that cholesterol. The central nervous system synapses require free cholesterol to work properly. The rest of the body is composed of about 2% cholesterol, which is used for steroid and sex hormone synthesis, as well as the basis for vitamin D synthesis in the skin when exposed to ultraviolet light and synthesis of bile salts to aid digestion. It is possible that many infants are not getting the building blocks they need for optimal development, such as neonates from the commercial foods they are given. Nursed infants probably get more EFAs from the mother and also cholesterol in the milk, which is not present in most infant foods. Fortunately, most baby formulae now are fortified with omega-3s to some extent, but when weaned, it is uncertain if they are consuming enough omega-3 for optimal development of the brain, eyes, and other tissues. Until they are eating table food, they do not consume much cholesterol, so they have to make all of it that they need. Their small livers may not be able to provide enough for good growth and brain development.

A recent study (DHA Oxford learning and Behaviour [DOLAB] study) linked low omega-3 blood levels with behavior and cognitive deficits.[11] This new study from the United Kingdom examined 493 healthy children aged 7 to 9 years old who had low scores on their reading tests. Blood content of EFA was determined by a finger stick sample prior to the start of treatment. Reading and working memory were tested by standardized tests, and behavior was rated by parents and teachers. The lower DHA levels were associated with poorer reading skills ($p \leq 0.042$) and working memory performance ($p \leq 0.001$) as well as higher levels of parent rated oppositional behavior and emotional liability ($p \leq 0.0001$). Supplementation with 600 mg DHA daily for 16 weeks improved the reading skills and the behavior of the children with the lowest 20% of reading scores.

A study[12] of attention deficit/hyperactivity disorder in 233 children (ADHD) 7 to 12 years old living in Australia noted improvement in the treatment groups receiving PUFA or PUFA+ MVM (multivitamins + mineral) supplement during the first 15 weeks, but no improvement was seen in the placebo group until they were placed on PUFA for 15 additional weeks. There was improvement in the tests of ability to switch and control attention in the PUFA groups compared to control ($p = 0.002$). The placebo group improved from weeks 16 to 30 after being given PUFA. During the second 15 weeks, the PUFA groups continued to improve in attention control and significantly in vocabulary. There was no additional benefit from the vitamin/mineral additions.

A research paper from the National Institutes of Health in the United States has estimated the EFA content of the US food supply for 1909 and 1999.[13] Due to a 1000-fold increase in the consumption of soybean oil, the 18:2n-6 consumption has risen from 2.79% to 7.21% energy ($p < 0.000001$) since 1909. This represents a 2.6-fold increase. Conversely, the availability of the n-3 FA, ALA, increased from 0.39% to 0.72% of energy—a 1.8-fold increase. The ratio of ω6:ω3 in 1909 was about 7.2:1 and today is about 10:1 if the estimates are based on the nutrient content in 1999. If the nutrient content was based on the 1909 model, then the LA/ALA ratio increased from 6.4 in 1909 to 10.0 in 1999. The calculations based on 1909 consumption data declines appeared in all the EFAs (AA, EPA, and DHA). The authors' conclusion was that consumption of LA has substantially increased since 1909 due to increased consumption of soy oil in the diet during the last 100 years.

Recently, many research papers have been published that indicate a strong association of inflammation and vascular diseases. This may be the missing link between the omega-3 dietary effects reported for many years and a rationale for their efficacy. It has been reported[14] that ethyl esters of the omega-3 FAs given to one group of weight loss subjects made the blood vessels more elastic (20%) compared to the control group receiving olive oil. The study group was small (25 total), but the results suggest that a larger scale study may be of value. The test group received 4 g/day of omega-3 ethyl esters for 12 weeks along with the weight-reducing diet. The supplement contained 46% EPA and 38% DHA. At the end of the first 15 weeks, the 13 subjects who took the omega-3 oils showed significant improvements in systolic blood pressure, heart rate, and triglyceride levels compared to the diet-only group. The omega-3 group showed significant improvement in arterial elasticity.

Mental stress is known to have detrimental effects on the cardiovascular system. The type A personality is a known risk factor for CVD. Subjects given 9 g/day of a fish oil supplement containing 1.6 g EPA and 1.1 g DHA displayed reduced increases in heart rate and muscle sympathetic nerve activity related to mental stress. The authors[15] recruited 67 people with normal blood pressure and submitted them to a 5-min stress protocol at the beginning of the study and 8 weeks later. They were assigned either a fish oil supplement or placebo, which was olive oil. The authors commented that "These findings support and extend the growing evidence that fish oil may have positive health benefits regarding neural cardiovascular control in humans."

DHA and EPA may differ in their effects depending on the gender of the patient. A double-blinded, randomized placebo-controlled trial was conducted on 94 healthy men and women.[16] Either an EPA-rich (1000 mg EPA/200 mg DHA) or DHA-rich (200 mg EPA/1000 mg DHA) supplement was given for 4 weeks. At baseline and at the end of 4 weeks, the parameters measured were platelet aggregation, thromboxane B$_2$ (TX)B$_2$, P-selectin (P-sel), von Willebrand factor (vWF), and plasminogen activator inhibitor-1. In both men and women, the EPA and DHA reduced platelet aggregation relative to placebo (-11.8%, $p = 0.013$ and -14.8%, $p = 0.001$, respectively). The subgroup analysis indicated that, in men only, the EPA reduced platelet aggregation by -18.4% vs. placebo ($p = 0.005$), and in women only, the DHA reduced platelet aggregation -18.9% compared to placebo ($p = 0.001$). There were significant interactions for sex × treatment observed on hemostatic markers and uptake of n-3 PUFAs.

Inflammation is becoming a biomarker for vascular and other diseases such as chronic obstructive lung disease, peripheral artery occlusive disease, and diabetes. Hess and Hegele[17] suggest that improving antioxidant defenses in diabetic patients may prevent against vascular complications. An issue of the *Canadian Journal of Cardiology* (vol. 28) is devoted to inflammation and biomarkers in vascular disease.

The observed increases in inflammatory medical conditions could be a reflection of the increased ratio of omega-6 FAs present in the diet and tissues during the lifespan of most people alive today. The downstream products of the metabolism of the omega-6 FAs are predominately inflammatory in nature and are thought to be involved with initiating several conditions, such as atherosclerosis[18] via the inflammasome, which activates the caspase-activating complex that leads the release of interleukin, IL-1-β, synthesis by the activated macrophages, endothelial cells, and smooth muscle cells. The interleukin cascade has been linked to other inflammatory conditions such as psoriasis, gout, inflammatory arthritis, inflammatory bowel disease, type 2 diabetes, and atherosclerosis.[18] This connection with inflammation may be the main effect of statin drug action—reducing inflammation and not the reduction of cholesterol. To achieve the reduction in inflammation, only a small amount of statin is effective. Since type 2 diabetes and metabolic syndrome are considered to be inflammatory conditions, this may be their connection with CVD. The cholesterol-rich "scab" that forms to isolate the vascular inflammation may just be an "innocent bystander." Adequate intake of the long-chain essential FAs in appropriate ratios will likely prevent and/or mediate many of the chronic and acute metabolic conditions that plague many people today. Lowering the excessively high carbohydrate intake (proinflammatory), holding the protein levels constant, and consuming animal fat and high EFA oils and nuts could go a long way to correcting EFA deficiency in the US diet.

A word of caution: "If some is good a whole lot may not be better." The EFAs are very easily oxidized if not stored properly. For oils, that means to store in the dark at a cool temperature. If it smells like "old fish," do not eat it. The same can happen in our bodies if the intake is beyond what we can use. These as well as all fats and carbohydrate can be used for energy. In the process of creating energy, they are "burned," i.e., oxidized, and in the process, reactive oxygen species (ROS) can be formed. The saturated and monounsaturated fats are better energy sources due to their stability in storage, and they actually produce more energy.

The omega-3 FAs play a critical role in maintaining mental and physical health. Their intake is inadequate in a large portion of our population. Changes in the diet during the last hundred years have decreased their intake to "deficiency" levels in most people. Simple diet changes or supplementation can probably correct this problem.

REFERENCES

1. Burr, G.O., M.M. Burr. A new deficiency disease produced by the rigid exclusion of fat from the diet. *J. Biol. Chem.* 82:345–367, 1929.
2. Burr, G.O., M.M. Burr. On the nature and role of the fatty acids essential in nutrition. *J. Biol. Chem.* 86:587–621, 1930.
3. Holman, R.T. Essential fatty acid deficiency. *Prog. Chem. Fat Other Lipids* 9:279–348, 1968.
4. Dryerburg, J., H.O. Bang. Haemostatic function and platelet polyunsaturated fatty acids in Eskimos. *Lancet* 2:433–435, 1979.
5. Bautista, M.C., M.M. Engler. The Mediterranean diet: Is it cardio protective? *Prog. Cardiovasc. Nurs.* 20(2):70–76, 2005.
6. Barnard, D.E., M.F. Starost, B.B. Teter, J. Sampugna, B. Morse, C. Foltz. Dietary effects on the development of ulcerative dermatitis in C57BL/6J mice. NCAB AALAS National Meeting, Ellicott City, MD, September 21, 2005.
7. Mensink, R.P., M.B. Katan. Effect of dietary trans fatty acids on high-density and low-density lipoprotein cholesterol levels in healthy subjects. *New Engl. J. Med.* 323:439–445, 1990.
8. Ip, C., C. Jiang, H.J. Thompson, J.A. Scimeca. Retention of conjugated linoleic acid in the mammary gland is associated with tumor inhibition during the post-initiation phase of carcinogenesis. *Carcinogenesis* 18:755–759, 1997.
9. Katz, D.L., A. Davidhi, V. Ma, Y. Kavak, L. Bifulco, V.Y. Njike. Effects of walnuts on endothelial function in overweight adults with visceral obesity: A randomized, control crossover trial. *J. Am. Coll. Nutr.* 37(6):415–423, 2012.
10. Banel, K., F.B. Hu. Effects of walnut consumption on blood lipids and other cardiovascular risk factors: A meta-analysis and systematic review. *Am. J. Clin. Nutr.* 90:56–63, 2009.
11. Montgomery, P., J.R. Burton, R.P. Sewell, T.F. Spreckelsen, A.J. Richardson. Low blood long chain omega-3 fatty acids in UD children are associated with poor cognitive performance and behavior: A cross-sectional analysis from the DOLAB study. *PLOS One* 8(6):e66697, 2013.
12. Sinn, N., J. Bryan, C. Wilson. Cognitive effects of polyunsaturated fatty acids in children with attention deficit hyperactivity disorder symptoms: A randomized controlled trial. *J. Dev. Behav. Pediatr.* 28(2):82–91, 2007.
13. Blasbalg, T.L., J.R. Hibbein, C.E. Ramsden, S.F. Majchrzak, R.R. Rawlings. Changes in consumption of omega-3 and omega-6 fatty acids in the United States during the 20th century. *Am. J. Clin. Nutr.* 93:950–962, 2011.
14. Wong, A.T.Y., D.C. Chan, P.H.R. Barrett, L.A. Adams, G.F. Watts. Supplementation with n3 fatty acid ethyl esters increases large and small artery elasticity in obese adults on a weight loss diet. *J. Nutr.* 143(4):437–441, 2013.
15. Carter, J.R., C.E. Schwartz, H. Yang, M.J. Joyner. Fish oil and neurovascular reactivity to mental stress in humans. *Am. J. Physiol. Regul. Integr. Comp. Physiol.* 304(7):R523–R530, 2013.
16. Phang, M., L.F. Lincz, M.L. Garg. Eicosapentaenoic and docosahexaenoic acid supplementations reduce platelet aggregation and hemostatic markers differentially in men and women. *J. Nutr.* 143:457–463, 2013.
17. Hess, D.A., R.A. Hegele. Linking diabetes with oxidative stress, adipokines, and impaired endothelial precursor cell function. *Can. J. Cardiol.* 28:629–630, 2012.
18. Verma, S., M. Gupta, P.M. Ridler. Therapeutic targeting of inflammation in atherosclerosis: We are getting closer. *Can. J. Cardiol.* 28:619–622, 2012.

24 Nutrition and Immunity of the Gut

Kenneth A. Kudsk and Joseph F. Pierre

CONTENTS

INTRODUCTION AND CLINICAL BACKGROUND

Parenteral nutrition was introduced as an important adjunct in the care of critically ill patients who were unable to take an oral diet adequate to meet nutritional and metabolic needs. Initial clinical studies by investigators at that time focused on the effect of parenteral feeding on several parameters of systemic immunity including total lymphocyte count, *in vitro* blastogenesis of circulating peripheral lymphocytes, and delayed cutaneous hypersensitivity responses to antigens. The first experiments that generated subsequent work investigating nutrition and gut immunity started in a laboratory of Dr. George Sheldon in the late 1970s. These studies examined the effect of malnutrition on susceptibility to intraperitoneal sepsis using hemoglobin and *Escherichia coli* in a rat model. Peterson et al. [1] demonstrated that well-nourished animals survived the septic challenge approximately 70% of the time. Animals administered a nutrient-poor agar orally for 2 weeks lost approximately 20% of their weight, resulting in a 10% survival to the septic challenge. Refeeding malnourished animals with chow prior to the septic challenge resulted in a survival rate comparable to the well-nourished mice, but surprisingly, two groups of animals fed adequate amounts of parenteral nutrients—either with or without fat—sustained a near-100% mortality after the septic insult (Figure 24.1). While it was speculated that the parenteral formula might be lacking some nutrients essential for the rat, there were a confounding variables; the enterally fed animals received a solid chow diet, while the parenterally fed animals received a liquid diet of glucose and amino acids. A subsequent experiment randomized previously malnourished animals to chow or to pair feeding with parenteral nutrition administered orally or intravenously [2]. The result demonstrated no deficiencies with the parenteral formula itself; animals that received nutrition via the gastrointestinal tract survived like well-nourished animals, whereas the animals that received the same formula intravenously survived like malnourished animals. This experiment was repeated in well-nourished animals with identical results [3].

Subsequently, several clinical investigators examined the effect of route of nutrition in trauma patients requiring celiotomy in whom a feeding tube has been placed into the jejunum at the time

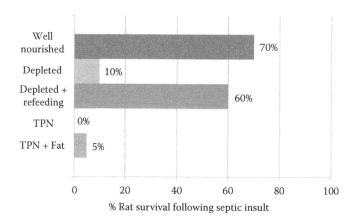

FIGURE 24.1 Effect of nutrition manipulation upon septic survival. Survival of malnourished rats to an infectious challenge with *E. coli* after dietary manipulation. Protein depletion significantly reduces septic survival compared to well-nourished animals. Refeeding improved the survival of protein-depleted rats. Parenteral feeding either with or without fat failed to improve survival.

of abdominal surgery. Patients were randomized to enteral feeding, to nothing, or to parenteral nutrition depending on the study [4]. In an initial study of moderately injured patients randomized to either enteral nutrition or starvation, the enterally fed patients sustained a significantly lower incidence of infection than the unfed patients. This study was repeated with moderately injured patients randomized to parenteral or enteral nutrition with similar results [5]. A subsequent study included both moderately and severely injured patients, all of whom had feeding jejunostomies placed at the time of abdominal surgery for their injuries [6]. The patients were randomized to be fed via the jejunostomy with an isotonic diet or fed parenterally with an isocaloric, isonitrogenous formula within 24 h of injury. As a group, the enterally fed patients sustained significantly fewer infections: Pneumonia occurred in 31% of the parenterally fed patients but only 11.8% of the enterally fed patients. Similarly, abscesses developed in 17.8% of parenterally fed patients but only 3.9% of patients fed enterally. But the magnitude and severity of injury affected these results. Using an

TABLE 24.1

Infectious Risk in Moderately and Severely Injured Trauma Patients on Enteral or Parenteral Nutrition

	All Injured Patients	
	Enteral	Parenteral
Pneumonia	11.8%	31%*
Intra-abdominal Abscess	1.9%	13.3%*
	Severely Injured Only	
	Enteral	Parenteral
Pneumonia	18%	56%*
Intra-abdominal Abscess	9%	33%*

Note: Parenteral nutrition results in significantly greater risk of pneumonia and intra-abdominal abscess compared with enteral feeding in both moderately and severely injured trauma patients.

*P < .05 vs. enteral.

injury severity score system that evaluates total body injury to the head, chest, abdomen, skeletal system, and soft tissue as well as a second system that evaluates the degree and severity of intra-abdominal injuries, patients were classified into less severely and more severely injured by the two scoring systems. The more severely injured patients receiving parenteral feeding sustained a 56% incidence of pneumonia compared to 18% in the enterally fed group. The incidence of intra-abdominal abscess was 33% in the parenterally fed group versus 9% in enterally fed group (Table 24.1). All of these differences were significant. The question of why this happened subsequently led to the study of nutrition and gut immunity. The basic principle generated by these experiments was that if nutrition support, and enteral feeding in particular, really alters susceptibility to infection, there should be a reason, it should be measurable, and it should be testable in clinical populations.

BACTERIA/HOST HOMEOSTASIS

The number of bacteria in the human gastrointestinal tract outnumbers the total number of cells in the human body by at least a ratio of 10:1. These bacteria contain an accumulative genetic diversity that is 300 times greater than our own [7,8]. Under normal conditions, there exists a symbiosis between the bacteria within the gut and the host that results in favorable conditions for both. Gut bacteria have important roles in host digestion, immune stimulation and maintenance, and synthesis of short-chain fatty acids and vitamins that help maintain host homeostasis [8]. However, as the human body responds to injury and stress with changes in metabolism, hormone secretion, systemic perfusion, and other factors, the environment for bacteria in the intestinal tract also changes, and the bacteria also respond to their stress. The work of Alverdy and his colleagues [9,10] shows that in a nonhostile environment, bacterial virulence genes remain downregulated; however, the addition of stressors results in an upregulation of these genes. One effect of these genes generates the formation of adherence appendages on the surface of the bacteria, which increases their ability to attach to mucosal cells and renders them more toxic to the host. The stressors of this host–microbe interaction are varied and include various forms of standard intensive care unit (ICU) care such as antibiotics, administration of vasoactive drugs, blockade of gastric acid production, opiate administration reducing gut motility, parenteral nutrition, and gut "starvation" due to lack of enteral feeding [11]. Alverdy's laboratory showed that bacteria harvested from animals that have undergone surgical stress after a hepatectomy have increased messenger RNA (mRNA) expression of exotoxin A and PA-1 lectin/adhesin, which were shown experimentally to play key roles in gut-derived sepsis [12].

MUCOSAL IMMUNITY

The body defends against these more virulent bacteria by maintaining normal antibacterial defenses. These defenses can be roughly categorized into two different categories, adaptive and innate mucosal immunity. Adaptive mucosal immunity is represented by cells within the lamina propria of the lung and intestine, which produce and secretory immunoglobulin A (sIgA) for transport across the mucosa into the lumen. This sIgA is the integral effector molecule of the adaptive immune system; it is specifically structured in a dimeric form to attach to both specific and nonspecific antigens expressed on the luminal bacteria, a process called opsonization, which restricts the bacterial ability to attach to the mucosa. Preventing attachment precludes bacterial invasion and epithelial stress. Innate mucosal immunity is a teleologically older system, which produces molecules that slows the growth of and/or lyses bacteria using antimicrobial peptides and proteins produced by Paneth cells. Such antimicrobial peptides include the defensins, secretory phospholipase A_2 (sPLA$_2$), lysozyme, and RegIIIγ [13]. Another important component of innate mucosal immunity are mucin glycoproteins produced by intestinal goblet cells, which constitute the mucous layer that covers and protects the intestinal epithelial surface [14]. Over the past two decades, these two systems—adaptive and innate mucosal immunity—and their response to the route and type of nutrition have been the focus of several laboratories.

ADAPTIVE MUCOSAL IMMUNITY

Under normal circumstances, approximately 80% of the lymphocytes circulating in the bloodstream are destined for the mucosal immune system and are identifiable by their expression of two integrins, L-selectin and $\alpha_4\beta_7$ [15]. Naive T and B cells are attracted to mucosal addressin adhesion molecule-1 (MAdCAM-1) expressed on the high endothelial venules of the Peyer's patches in the small intestine, and chemokines direct the migration of the cells into this structure [16]. Within the Peyer's patches, the cells become sensitized to antigens transported from the gut lumen through M cells that cover the luminal surface of Peyer's patches. After processing of the antigens by dendritic cells and macrophages within the Peyer's patches, the T and B cells are sensitized to the antigens and migrate through mesenteric lymph nodes into the thoracic duct and bloodstream for distribution into the lamina propria of the respiratory and gastrointestinal tract. The B lymphocytes subsequently mature into plasma cells under the appropriate cytokine influence, producing immunoglobulin A (IgA) specific for the bacterial antigens to which the cell has been sensitized. The T cells produce a balance of IgA-inhibiting Th1-type cytokines and IgA-stimulating Th2-type cytokines, which regulate IgA production by plasma cells. The steps beginning with Peyer's patch detection of luminal antigen, diffuse distribution to diverse mucosal sites, and the subsequent release of IgA at mucosal surfaces constitute the common mucosal immune hypothesis (Figure 24.2).

This system is dependent on gut stimulation with nutrition—or lack of enteral stimulation—and has been studied by altering the route and type of nutrition in a murine model. The mouse was chosen because of its similarity to the human mucosal immune system. Humans secrete 85–90% of the IgA directly from the lamina propria into the lumen of the gastrointestinal tract using a specific transport protein, polymeric immunoglobulin receptor (pIgR). While rats release most of their IgA into the portal vein to the liver with release into the gastrointestinal tract via the biliary system, the mouse system functions similarly to that of humans, with direct transport of most IgA under the direction of similar cytokine signals. In our work [17], chow is considered the normal positive control where the gut-associated lymphoid tissue (GALT) system is functioning under normal conditions. The negative

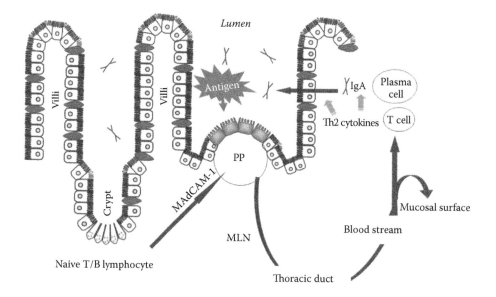

FIGURE 24.2 An overview of the common mucosal immune hypothesis. Luminal antigen is sampled at the Peyer's patch (PP) by naive lymphocytes that subsequently undergo maturation and proliferation in the mesenteric lymph nodes (MLNs), exit the thoracic duct, and home back to mucosal surfaces. In the intestinal lamina propria, IgA-producing B cells (plasma cells) and Th2 lymphocyte cytokines support the release of IgA across the epithelium.

control is administration of parenteral (intravenous) nutrition (IV-TPN) containing amino acids, dextrose, electrolytes, vitamins, and minerals, which produces no enteral nutrient stimulation to the gastrointestinal tract but prevents the development of lethal malnutrition in this murine model. To examine the effect of route of nutrition, animals are administered the same parenteral formula into the stomach (intragastric [IG-TPN]) to control for the route of nutrition, while a final group receives a more complex enteral liquid diet (CED) similar to formulas that are administered to patients clinically. This CED contains proteins, complex carbohydrates, as well as fat. Each of the diets is administered in a quantity adequate to meet the metabolic and nutritional needs of the mice. These four groups allow a comparison of IV-TPN with IG-TPN, which controls for the route of nutrition and the comparison between IG-TPN and CED, which controls for complexity of diet. Both IG-TPN and the CED are formulated to be isonitrogenous and isocaloric. The major difference between the chow and CED animals is the complexity of chow and the intermittency of eating with chow rather than the continuous feeding of the CED into the stomach. Consistently, the results of these comparisons demonstrate that the degree of enteral stimulation affects the integrity of GALT, with the effects of chow > CED > IG-TPN > IV-TPN. Unfortunately, a fasting control is not possible, since the changes in mucosal immunity usually occur within 3–4 days and fasted animals expire from severe malnutrition within this period of time. Thus, parenteral nutrition allows us to study the effect of eating and of enteral formulas on the mucosal immune system without the confounding variable of malnutrition.

The administration of parenteral nutrition significantly reduces the T and B lymphocyte mass within the Peyer's patches of the gut, the lamina propria of the small intestine, and the lung [16,18]. Reductions in T and B lymphocytes within Peyer's patches occur within 24 h, reaching a nadir of 40% of normal by the fourth to the fifth day [19] (Figure 24.3). Animals fed parenterally for 5 days and then allowed to chow experience a return of T and B cell numbers to normal within 48 h in these sites. Similar observations of these cell changes have been documented in patients undergoing resection of the GI tact in operations that included part of the distal small intestine. In work by Okamoto et al. [20], the numbers of T cells present in the lamina propria of small intestine specimens obtained from patients fed preoperatively with parenteral nutrition were significantly fewer than in patients fed orally up to the time of surgery. In the murine model, the overall effect was a significant reduction in the luminal levels of sIgA within the gastrointestinal tract or the respiratory tract (Figure 24.4).

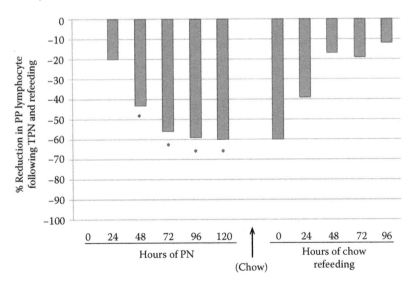

FIGURE 24.3 Peyer's patch lymphocyte counts following parenteral nutrition (PN) and chow refeeding. The percentage of Peyer's patch lymphocytes is significantly reduced following 48 h of PN, and levels reach a nadir at 40% of chow levels. Reintroducing chow reverses this effect within 48 h. $^*P < .05$ versus chow.

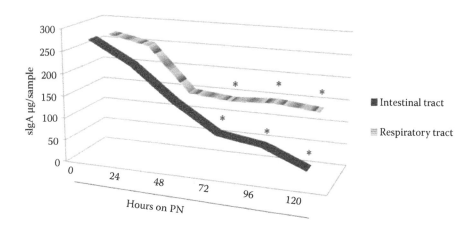

FIGURE 24.4   PN decreases intestinal and respiratory tract secretory IgA. IgA levels in intestinal (solid) and respiratory (striped) tract washes drop over time if animals are fed PN with no enteral stimulation. *$P < .05$ versus chow.

Mucosal address in cell adhesion molecule-1 (MadCAM-1) expression appears to be an important factor in the reduced T and B lymphocyte mass during lack of enteral stimulation during parenteral feeding. Cell migration into the Peyer's patches occurs through the interaction of L-selectin and $\alpha_4\beta_7$ expressed on the naive T and B lymphocytes, with the MAdCAM-1 expressed on the high endothelial venules of the Peyer's patches. Experimentally, administration of blocking antibodies against $\alpha_4\beta_7$, L-selectin, or MadCAM-1 reduces the lymphocyte numbers within the Peyer's patches by approximately 60% to the same level of parenterally fed animals [17,21,22]. Quantification of MadCAM-1 expression in the Peyer's patches of parenterally fed mice confirms an almost immediate decrease in MadCAM-1 expression in the Peyer's patches, which reaches a nadir by 48 h [22]. MadCAM-1 expression rapidly recovers to normal levels within 12 h after reinstituting enteral feeding.

In addition to B-cell reduction, there are proportional decreases in T cells. T cells control B-cell production of IgA through cytokine production and secretion. Under normal conditions, the T cells produce a balance of cytokines in favor of the IgA-stimulating Th2 cytokines, which include interleukin (IL)-4, IL-5, IL-6, and IL-10. Animals receiving no enteral stimulation experience significant drops in IL-4 and IL-10, reducing the cytokine stimulation for IgA production by the plasma cells [23,24]. Through both the reduction in total T and B cell lymphocyte mass and the altered Th2 cytokine levels, an overall reduction in the production and levels of sIgA in both the lung and the respiratory tract is achieved.

IgA transport by the mucosa also is compromised. After production and release of IgA by plasma cells, the IgA attaches to pIgR expressed on the basal surface of the epithelial cells. The IgA–pIgR complex is transported across the cell and released into the lumen. During release, a small piece of the pIgR (secretory component) remains attached to IgA molecule, identifying it as sIgA. The levels of intestinal pIgR are proportionate to the degree of enteral stimulation, with the highest levels expressed with chow feeding, lower levels in CED animals, a further reduction with IG-PN, and the lowest levels expressed in animals fed parenterally [25]. Since one molecule of pIgR is used for each IgA molecule transported to the lumen, the overall reduction in pIgR contributes to impaired transport of IgA and lower levels of sIgA for acquired mucosal immunity.

These lower sIgA levels do result in functional consequences to the animal. The impairments in mucosal protection were confirmed through two basic experiments. In the first, animals were administered the H1N1 virus intranasally [26]. This virus generates an IgA-mediated defense in the mice. Naive animals exposed to this virus shed the virus from the nasal passages for approximately 10 days. Newly generated H1N1- specific sIgA then sterilizes the nasal passages and induces immunity so that subsequent administration of the virus results in rapid neutralization and elimination of the virus from the nasal passages. In our experiments, mice previously immunized to the virus were randomized to chow, CED, or parenteral nutrition and reinnoculated with the virus after 5 days of feeding with the experimental diet. While the chow and CED cleared the virus properly, 50% of animals fed parenterally had continued viral shedding 40 h following the second viral dose, demonstrating the loss of established immunity to this virus in those mice (Figure 24.5). Feeding chow to parenterally fed mice regenerated the immunity quickly to demonstrate that function, but not immunologic memory, was lost following the period of parenteral feeding. In a second experiment [27], animals were administered an otherwise lethal dose of *Pseudomonas* into the trachea after randomization to the various diets, and mortality was recorded. Nonimmune animals die 90% of the time with this *Pseudomonas* challenge. However, prior nasal immunization with *Pseudomonas* antigens contained in liposomes reduces mortality to 10%. After immunizing animals with the *Pseudomonas* antigen/liposome mixture to establish immunity, animals were randomized to the three diets. While mortality remained low after chow or CED, almost 90% parenterally fed animals died (Figure 24.6). These two experiments demonstrated that a functional loss of IgA-mediated immunity occurs with a lack of enteral stimulation, which is reversible by feeding via the gut. Immunologic memory, however, remains intact.

While this experimental work provides an cogent explanation for the lowered incidence of pneumonia and intra-abdominal abscess formation in severely injured trauma patients fed enterally, a direct cause-and-effect relationship between the alterations in human mucosal immunity and those infections still has not been established. In attempts to establish this relationship in trauma patients, sequential bronchoalveolar lavage (BAL) specimens were obtained from trauma patients injured severely enough to warrant intubation for at least 7 days following their trauma [28]. BAL specimens

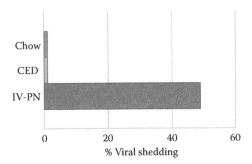

FIGURE 24.5 Route and type of nutrition influence viral shedding. In a model of continued viral infection and shedding, enterally fed mice receiving chow or a CED maintained normal immunity, while 50% of animals receiving intravenous parenteral nutrition (IV-PN) lost immunity.

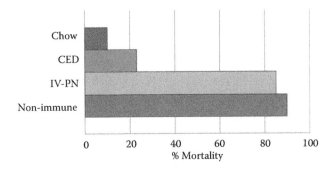

FIGURE 24.6 Mortality 48 h after *Pseudomonas* pneumonia challenge. Survival after intratracheal Ps is increased by previous immunization and reduces mortality from 90% in nonimmune animals to 10% in immunized chow-fed mice. Feeding animals a CED after immunization also improves survival, but animals fed parenterally (IV-PN) lose all immunity.

were obtained within 18–36 h of injury after obtaining informed consent. BAL specimens were also obtained immediately after intubation of patients undergoing elective surgeries such as inguinal hernia repair or laparoscopic cholecystectomy to quantify baseline levels of epithelial lining fluid (ELF) and respiratory IgA levels. Urea nitrogen levels were measured in blood and BAL specimens to determine the amount of ELF returned in the 60 mL used for the BAL washings. The ELF, amount of IgA in the ELF, and total IgA were calculated and compared between the elective surgery patients and the trauma patients. Trauma increased the volume of ELF, the concentration of IgA in the ELF, and total IgA within the BAL to levels that were higher than in specimens obtained from patients undergoing elective surgery immediately after intubation. These clinical data were reproduced in our mouse model. Just as in the human response to injury, airway IgA levels increased significantly in animals after injury. This response appeared to be TNF driven since TNF blockade completely eliminated the increase after the injury [29]. Interestingly, animals fed parenterally for 5 days that were exposed to the same surgical stress failed to generate any IgA increase after injury.

In summary, it appears that acquired immunity is significantly depressed when the gastrointestinal tract is not fed or stimulated via enteral nutrition. There are significant reductions in T and B lymphocytes throughout the mucosal immune system, a deterioration in IgA-simulating Th2-type cytokines, a loss of established IgA-mediated immunity, and an inability to respond to injury with normal increases in luminal IgA levels.

INNATE MUCOSAL IMMUNITY

The innate immune system of the intestine is an ancient teleological defensive system that is conserved across a broad range of species, signifying its fundamental importance in host defense against microbes. The hallmark of innate defense systems is the release of non-antigen-specific molecules that defend the intestinal surface by impacting the growth and composition of gut microbes. Two important sources of this immune function within the intestinal epithelium are specialized secreting cell types, the Paneth and goblet cells (Figure 24.7). Paneth cells are located at the base of the intestinal crypts of Lieberkuhn [13], where they produce and release a host of antimicrobial peptides and proteins such as lysozymes, defensins, and sPLA$_2$ into the crypt and lumen [30]. These

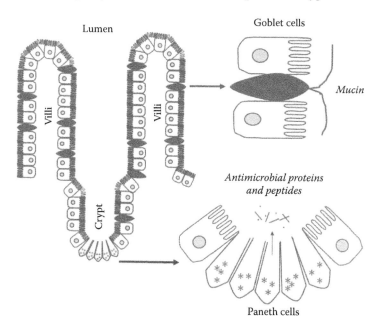

FIGURE 24.7   Overview of intestinal Paneth and goblet cell distribution.

molecules help maintain a sterile environment near the rapidly differentiating epithelial stem cells within the crypts, and their loss is implicated in intestinal inflammation [31]. Phospholipase A_2 (PLA_2) is a family of lipolytic enzymes consisting of more than 30 different isoforms in the body. The secretory forms ($sPLA_2$) consist of 10 calcium-dependent enzymes that play various roles in systemic inflammation and defense [32]. The $sPLA_2$ group IIA isoform has been shown to prime neutrophils within the intestinal tissue that have attached to the gut vascular endothelium lining in response to expression of intercellular adhesion molecule-1 (ICAM-1) following injury [33,34]. The $sPLA_2$-IIA isoform is also secreted into the gut lumen by the Paneth cells, where it is bactericidal against gram-positive and several gram-negative bacterial species. Due to cationic state, it is drawn to negatively charged bacterial membranes, where it cleaves fatty acids from phospholipids, reducing bacterial growth and viability [13,35]. The amount of $sPLA_2$-IIA detected in the small intestinal lumen of mice depends upon the degree of enteral stimulation [36]. While parenteral feeding results in a significant reduction in intestinal $sPLA_2$-IIA activity within the luminal fluid compared to chow-fed mice, the administration of either the parenteral feeding solution into the stomach or CED enterally significantly increases $sPLA_2$-IIA activity toward normal chow levels (Figure 24.8). The observed changes in luminal levels of $sPLA_2$-IIA are consistent with changes in Paneth cell expression, where parenteral feeding results in less $sPLA_2$-IIA in the intracellular granules [37]. When intestinal secretions are tested for antibacterial effectiveness, the bactericidal activity of intestinal secretions obtained from parenterally fed animals is significantly depressed compared to the other groups. When $sPLA_2$-IIA activity is blocked using a specific inhibitor, some but not all of the bactericidal activity is lost from intestinal secretions, confirming the importance of both $sPLA_2$-IIA as well as the other secreted antibacterial Paneth cell molecules [37]. Further investigations into the role of Paneth cells and the other antimicrobial molecules in innate mucosal immune defense systems are currently underway.

The other important specialized secreting epithelial cell of the intestine is the goblet cell, which is predominantly responsible for production and secretion of mucin glycoproteins, in addition to other molecules that protect and repair the epithelium [14]. Unlike the Paneth cells, which remain at the base of the intestinal crypts, the goblet cells migrate up the intestinal villi over the course of 3 to 5 days before sloughing off into the intestinal lumen. During this migration, goblet cell secretion of mucin glycoproteins forms the mucous layering that covers and protects the epithelial surface. Functionally, mucous creates a viscoelastic layer that allows the smooth passage of food during peristalsis. From an immunological standpoint, mucins are anionically charged and allow the localization and concentration of the cationic antimicrobial Paneth cell compounds and sIgA at the

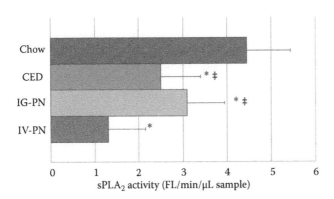

FIGURE 24.8 $sPLA_2$ activity in the small intestinal lumen is influenced by route and type of nutrition. Compared with chow, administration of a CED containing complex carbohydrates and fats via gastrostomy, administration of parenteral nutrition via gastrostomy (IG-PN), or administration of parenteral nutrition intravenously (IV-PN) significantly reduces $sPLA_2$ activity within the small bowel lumen. The level of $sPLA_2$ activity in IV-PN is also significantly lower than CED or IG-PN. *$P < .05$ versus chow; ‡$P < .05$ versus IV-PN.

epithelial surface to limit bacterial interaction [38]. Mucins also maintain gut homeostasis through their role as a nutrient source to endogenous bacteria. Certain commensal bacteria metabolize the mucin glycoprotein sugar structures, encouraging nonpathogenic bacteria to grow in closer proximity to the host and physically limit colonization of that micro-niche by opportunistic pathogens [8]. The most abundant mucin in the intestine is Mucin (MUC) 2. Animal knockout experiments demonstrate that the loss of MUC2 results is severe spontaneous colitis that can be lethal upon bacterial challenge [39,40]. We recently demonstrated that the administration of parenteral nutrition or intragastric elemental nutrition reduces the luminal concentration of MUC2 [41,42], demonstrating that this aspect of innate mucosal immunity is also reduced.

SURROGATES OF ENTERAL FEEDING WHEN THE GUT CANNOT BE FED

Unfortunately, enteral access cannot be obtained in some critically ill patients. In others, access may be present, but enteral feeding is not possible due to intestinal atony, enterocutaneous fistulas, or severe hemodynamic instability. Clinically, it would be valuable if clinicians could exogenously normalize the defects in mucosal immunity in these patients by supplementing the parenteral formula with a GALT-stimulating agent. One family of agents potentially capable of performing this function is the neuropeptides released by the enteric nervous system [43]. Experimentally, these peptides directly affect mucosal immunity. One specific example is gastrin-releasing peptide, studied experimentally using its analog, bombesin (BBS) [44]. Administration of this gastrointestinal neuropeptide stimulates release of other gut hormones, including gastrin, cholecystokinin, neurotensin, and others. In the experimental models, subcutaneous or intravenous injections of BBS three times a day into parenterally fed mice significantly increases the T and B cells within the GALT to the level of chow-fed animals as well as levels of intestinal and respiratory IgA. BBS administration increases innate immunity by stimulating expression of antimicrobial compounds in Paneth cell granules but does not appear to stimulate their release, since $sPLA_2$-IIA levels remain low within the gastrointestinal tract fluid. Interestingly, BBS administration completely reverses the defect in bacterial [45] and viral [46] immunity documented in mice fed only parenteral nutrition.

SUMMARY

Lack of enteral stimulation from enteral feeding significantly impairs gut mucosal immunity, leading to reduction in the number of cells entering the mucosal immune system as well as the number of T and B cells within the effector sites of the lamina propria of the lung and gastrointestinal tract. Alterations in cytokines together with these T and B cell reductions reduce IgA production and release, resulting in impairment of loss of established IgA-mediated defenses. The lack of enteral nutrition also negatively impacts innate immunity, impairing the release and production of molecules designed to destroy bacteria and provide mucosal defense.

ACKNOWLEDGMENTS

This research is supported by National Institutes of Health (NIH) grant no. R01 GM 53439.

This project was supported by award no. I01BX001672 from the Biomedical Laboratory Research & Development service of the Veterans Affairs (VA) Office of Research and Development.

The contents of this article do not represent the views of the VA or the United States government.

REFERENCES

1. Petersen SR, Kudsk KA, Carpenter G, Sheldon GE. Malnutrition and immunocompetence: Increased mortality following an infectious challenge during hyperalimentation. *J Trauma* 1981;**21**:528–33.
2. Kudsk KA, Carpenter G, Petersen S, Sheldon GF. Effect of enteral and parenteral feeding in malnourished rats with E. coli-hemoglobin adjuvant peritonitis. *J Surg Res* 1981;**31**:105–10.

3. Kudsk KA, Stone JM, Carpenter G, Sheldon GF. Enteral and parenteral feeding influences mortality after hemoglobin-E. coli peritonitis in normal rats. *J Trauma* 1983;**23**:605–9.
4. Moore E, Jones T. Benefits of immediate jejunostomy feeding after major abdominal trauma–A prospective, randomized study. *J Trauma* 1986;**26**:874–81.
5. Moore F, Moore E, Jones T, McCroskey B, Peterson V. TEN versus TPN following major abdominal trauma–reduced septic morbidity. *J Trauma* 1989;**29**:916–22; discussion 922–3.
6. Kudsk KA, Croce MA, Fabian TC, Minard G, Tolley EA, Poret HA et al. Enteral versus parenteral feeding. Effects on septic morbidity after blunt and penetrating abdominal trauma. *Ann Surg* 1992;**215**:503–11; discussion 511–3.
7. Guarner F. [Role of intestinal flora in health and disease]. *Nutr Hosp* 2007;**22 Suppl 2**:14–9.
8. Pflughoeft KJ, Versalovic J. Human microbiome in health and disease. *Annu Rev Pathol* 2012;**7**:99–122.
9. Alverdy J, Stern E. Effect of immunonutrition on virulence strategies in bacteria. *Nutrition* 1998;**14**:580–4.
10. Alverdy JC, Laughlin RS, Wu L. Influence of the critically ill state on host-pathogen interactions within the intestine: Gut-derived sepsis redefined. *Crit Care Med* 2003;**31**:598–607.
11. Morowitz MJ, Carlisle EM, Alverdy JC. Contributions of intestinal bacteria to nutrition and metabolism in the critically ill. *Surg Clin North Am* 2011;**91**:771–85, viii.
12. Wu LR, Zaborina O, Zaborin A, Chang EB, Musch M, Holbrook C, Turner JR, Alverdy JC. Surgical injury and metabolic stress enhance the virulence of the human opportunistic pathogen Pseudomonas aeruginosa. *Surg Infect* (Larchmt) 2005;**6**:185–95.
13. Porter EM, Bevins CL, Ghosh D, Ganz T. The multifaceted Paneth cell. *Cell Mol Life Sci* 2002;**59**:156–70.
14. McGuckin MA, Lindén SK, Sutton P, Florin TH. Mucin dynamics and enteric pathogens. *Nat Rev Microbiol* 2011;**9**:265–78.
15. Reese SR, Kudsk KA, Genton L, Ikeda S. l-selectin and alpha4beta7 integrin, but not ICAM-1, regulate lymphocyte distribution in gut-associated lymphoid tissue of mice. *Surgery* 2005;**137**:209–15.
16. Li J, Kudsk KA, Gocinski B, Dent D, Glezer J, Langkamp-Henken B. Effects of parenteral and enteral nutrition on gut-associated lymphoid tissue. *J Trauma* 1995;**39**:44–51; discussion 51–2.
17. Kudsk KA. Jonathan E Rhoads lecture: Of mice and men... and a few hundred rats. *JPEN J Parenter Enteral Nutr* 2008;**32**:460–73.
18. Hermsen J, Gomez F, Sano Y, Kang W, Maeshima Y, Kudsk K. Parenteral feeding depletes pulmonary lymphocyte populations. *JPEN J Parenter Enteral Nutr* 2009;**33**:535–40.
19. King BK, Li J, Kudsk KA. A temporal study of TPN-induced changes in gut-associated lymphoid tissue and mucosal immunity. *Arch Surg* 1997;**132**:1303–9.
20. Okamoto K, Fukatsu K, Ueno C, Shinto E, Hashiguchi Y, Nagayoshi H et al. T lymphocyte numbers in human gut associated lymphoid tissue are reduced without enteral nutrition. *JPEN J Parenter Enteral Nutr* 2005;**29**:56–8.
21. Ikeda S, Kudsk K, Fukatsu K, Johnson C, Le T, Reese S et al. Enteral feeding preserves mucosal immunity despite in vivo MAdCAM-1 blockade of lymphocyte homing. *Ann Surg* 2003;**237**:677–85; discussion 685.
22. Zarzaur BL, Fukatsu K, Johnson CJ, Eng E, Kudsk KA. A temporal study of diet induced changes in Peyer's patch Mad-CAM-1 expression. *Surg Forum* 2001:194–6.
23. Wu Y, Kudsk KA, DeWitt RC, Tolley EA, Li J. Route and type of nutrition influence IgA-mediating intestinal cytokines. *Ann Surg* 1999;**229**:662–7; discussion 667–8.
24. Fukatsu K, Kudsk K, Zarzaur B, Wu Y, Hanna M, DeWitt R. TPN decreases IL-4 and IL-10 mRNA expression in lipopolysaccharide stimulated intestinal lamina propria cells but glutamine supplementation preserves the expression. *Shock* 2001;**15**:318–22.
25. Sano Y, Gomez F, Kang W, Lan J, Maeshima Y, Hermsen J et al. Intestinal polymeric immunoglobulin receptor is affected by type and route of nutrition. *JPEN J Parenter Enteral Nutr* 2007;**31**:351–6; discussion 356–7.
26. Kudsk K, Li J, Renegar K. Loss of upper respiratory tract immunity with parenteral feeding. *Ann Surg* 1996;**223**:629–35; discussion 635–8.
27. King B, Kudsk K, Li J, Wu Y, Renegar K. Route and type of nutrition influence mucosal immunity to bacterial pneumonia. *Ann Surg* 1999;**229**:272–8.
28. Kudsk K, Hermsen J, Genton L, Faucher L, Gomez F. Injury stimulates an innate respiratory immunoglobulin a immune response in humans. *J Trauma* 2008;**64**:316-23; discussion 323–5.
29. Hermsen J, Sano Y, Gomez F, Maeshima Y, Kang W, Kudsk K. Parenteral nutrition inhibits tumor necrosis factor-alpha-mediated IgA response to injury. *Surg Infect* (Larchmt) 2008;**9**:33–40.
30. Elphick DA, Mahida YR. Paneth cells: Their role in innate immunity and inflammatory disease. *Gut* 2005;**54**:1802–9.

31. Simms LA, Doecke JD, Walsh MD, Huang N, Fowler EV, Radford-Smith GL. Reduced alpha-defensin expression is associated with inflammation and not NOD2 mutation status in ileal Crohn's disease. *Gut* 2008;**57**:903–10.

32. Koduri RS, Grönroos JO, Laine VJ, Le Calvez C, Lambeau G, Nevalainen TJ et al. Bactericidal properties of human and murine groups I, II, V, X, and XII secreted phospholipases A(2). *J Biol Chem* 2002;**277**:5849–57.

33. Partrick DA, Moore EE, Silliman CC, Barnett CC, Kuypers FA. Secretory phospholipase A2 activity correlates with postinjury multiple organ failure. *Crit Care Med* 2001;**29**:989–93.

34. Gago LA, Moore EE, Partrick DA, Sauaia A, Davis CM, Toal TR et al. Secretory phospholipase A2 cleavage of intravasated bone marrow primes human neutrophils. *J Trauma* 1998;**44**:660–4.

35. Beers SA, Buckland AG, Koduri RS, Cho W, Gelb MH, Wilton DC. The antibacterial properties of secreted phospholipases A2: A major physiological role for the group IIA enzyme that depends on the very high pI of the enzyme to allow penetration of the bacterial cell wall. *J Biol Chem* 2002;**277**:1788–93.

36. Pierre JF, Heneghan AF, Tsao FH, Sano Y, Jonker MA, Omata J et al. Route and type of nutrition and surgical stress influence secretory phospholipase A2 secretion of the murine small intestine. *JPEN J Parenter Enteral Nutr* 2011;**35**:748–56.

37. Omata J, Pierre JF, Heneghan AF, Tsao FH, Sano Y, Jonker MA et al. Parenteral nutrition suppresses the bactericidal response of the small intestine. *Surgery* 2013;**153**:17–24.

38. Meyer-Hoffert U, Hornef MW, Henriques-Normark B, Axelsson LG, Midtvedt T, Putsep K et al. Secreted enteric antimicrobial activity localises to the mucus surface layer. *Gut* 2008;**57**:764–71.

39. Bergstrom KS, Kissoon-Singh V, Gibson DL, Ma C, Montero M, Sham HP et al. Muc2 protects against lethal infectious colitis by disassociating pathogenic and commensal bacteria from the colonic mucosa. *PLoS Pathog* 2010;**6**:e1000902.

40. Van der Sluis M, De Koning BA, De Bruijn AC, Velcich A, Meijerink JP, Van Goudoever JB et al. Muc2-deficient mice spontaneously develop colitis, indicating that MUC2 is critical for colonic protection. *Gastroenterology* 2006;**131**:117–29.

41. Pierre JF, Heneghan AF, Feliciano RP, Shanmuganayagam D, Roenneburg DA, Krueger CG et al. Cranberry proanthocyanidins improve the gut mucous layer morphology and function in mice receiving elemental enteral nutrition. *JPEN J Parenter Enteral Nutr* 2013;**37**:401–9.

42. Heneghan A, Pierre J, Gosain A, Kudsk K. IL-25 stimulation of parenteral nutrition (PN) restores Innate immune molecules. *Annals of Surgery* 2014;**259**:394–400.

43. Genton L, Kudsk KA. Interactions between the enteric nervous system and the immune system: Role of neuropeptides and nutrition. *Am J Surg* 2003;**186**:253–8.

44. Li J, Kudsk K, Hamidian M, Gocinski B. Bombesin affects mucosal immunity and gut-associated lymphoid tissue in intravenously fed mice. *Arch Surg* 1995;**130**:1164–9; discussion 1169–70.

45. DeWitt R, Wu Y, Renegar K, King B, Li J, Kudsk K. Bombesin recovers gut-associated lymphoid tissue and preserves immunity to bacterial pneumonia in mice receiving total parenteral nutrition. *Ann Surg* 2000;**231**:1–8.

46. Janu P, Li J, Renegar K, Kudsk K. Recovery of gut-associated lymphoid tissue and upper respiratory tract immunity after parenteral nutrition. *Ann Surg* 1997;**225**:707–15; discussion 715–7.

25 Nutrition Therapy for Inflammatory Bowel Disease

Leo Galland

CONTENTS

Nutrition may impact on the course and influence treatment of inflammatory bowel disease (IBD) in four ways:

1. Symptoms of IBD may cause patients to alter their diets, restricting nutritious foods like fruits and vegetables, producing nutrient deficits.
2. Intestinal inflammation may cause malabsorption or nutrient losses, producing frank malnutrition.
3. Nutritional deficiencies may interfere with tissue repair or immune regulation, aggravating the clinical course of IBD.
4. Dietary patterns, nutrient deficits, or nutrient excess may contribute to the development of IBD in people at risk.

Clinical, laboratory, and epidemiologic studies (described in sections Nutritional Epidemiology of IBD, Malnutrition in IBD, and Nutritional Therapies) indicate roles for all four mechanisms in patients with Crohn's disease or ulcerative colitis (UC).

PATHOPHYSIOLOGY

UC is characterized by superficial inflammation that originates in the mucosal epithelium, is confined to the colon, and is continuous, always including the mucosa of the terminal rectum and spreading proximally without skip areas. Crohn's disease, in contrast, can affect any part of the alimentary canal from mouth to anus, is often discontinuous with patches of inflammation separated by patches of noninflamed bowel, and is frequently transmural. The pathophysiology that underlies these distinctive anatomic abnormalities is complex, with new paradigms being generated every few years.

UC can be viewed as a metabolic disorder of the colonic epithelium caused by impaired utilization of its chief source of energy, butyric acid. A four-carbon fatty acid produced by colonic microbial fermentation, butyrate supplies about 70% of energy requirements of the colonic mucosa[1] and has direct anti-inflammatory effects, interfering with signaling of NF-κB, a transcription factor that is pivotal for activating genes involved in the inflammatory cascade.[2] There is a marked decrease of butyrate oxidation in colonic biopsies of patients with UC, producing a state of mucosal starvation, which may account for the superficial colitis characteristic of that disorder. Indian researchers demonstrated an 84% reduction in the activity of a mitochondrial enzyme, acetoacetylCoA thiolase, which catalyzes the final step in mitochondrial butyrate metabolism.[3] This defect appears to be the result of oxidative stress because it can be fully corrected in vitro by addition of reducing agents and can be induced in normal mucosa by the addition of hydrogen peroxide. It is not seen in mucosal specimens from patients with Crohn's disease, but only in those with UC.

A second metabolic disturbance specific for UC is impaired secretion of phosphatidylcholine (PC). A component of cell membranes, PC is secreted into the intestinal mucus barrier, where it downregulates signaling of the inflammatory cytokine tumor necrosis factor-alpha (TNF-α).[4] PC concentration in ileal and colonic mucus of patients with UC is about one sixth the concentration found in healthy controls or patients with Crohn's disease, suggesting that this deficit may play a specific pathogenetic role in UC.[5] PC secretion is similarly reduced in the right colon of patients with left-sided colitis, indicating that the defect is not merely a result of inflammation. Because PC protects against oxidative stress,[6] it is possible that deficient intestinal PC secretion permits a progressive increase in oxidative stress along the length of the colon, with the threshold for mitochondrial damage being reached first near the anal verge, hence the propensity for UC to begin in the terminal rectum and spread toward the cecum.

Crohn's disease, in contrast, may be viewed as an immune deficiency disorder, with defective innate immunity encouraging the hyperactive T-lymphocyte activation characteristic of Crohn's.[7] Identification of nucleotide-binding oligomerization domain-containing protein 2 (NOD2) as a susceptibility gene for Crohn's disease stimulated initial interest in the role of innate immunity in Crohn's. Subsequently, numerous other genes that regulate innate immune responses have emerged as Crohn's susceptibility genes.[8] Many researchers now believe that defects in innate immunity and autophagy interfere with elimination of antigens that penetrate the gut mucosa beyond the epithelial monolayer, promoting activation of the adaptive immune system, which creates transmural inflammation.[9] This view is consistent with the propensity for Crohn's to involve the small intestine, the organ in which most of the body's lymphocytes reside, and the random location and patchy nature of Crohn's lesions, which may be occurring at sites of antigen penetration.

No single concept, however well it explains the pathology, can account for the clinical diversity of IBD as it affects individual patients. Clinical presentation, natural history, and response to treatment vary greatly among patients with the same diagnosis. Most researchers agree that development of IBD requires four separate components: the input of multiple genetic variations, alterations in the intestinal microflora, acquired aberrations of innate and adaptive immune responses, and global changes in environment and hygiene. None of these components can by itself trigger or maintain IBD, so that a combination of various factors is needed to bring about Crohn's disease or UC in individual patients. This model implies that different and diverse mechanisms underlie IBD in different patients and that each patient may have a distinctive illness with his or her own clinical manifestations and a personalized response to therapy.[10]

The number of genes found to be associated with IBD continually increases. A study from the Wellcome Trust published in late 2012 identified 163 distinct genetic loci associated with IBD; 30 were specific for Crohn's disease, 23 were specific for UC, and 110 were shared by both conditions. The genes involved regulate innate and acquired immune responses, microbial pattern recognition receptors, autophagy, T-helper-17 lymphocyte differentiation, and the integrity of the intestinal mucosal barrier.[11] Most are low-risk genes, and the interacting effects of multiple predisposing genetic anomalies are likely to account for the varied clinical presentations seen among patients with IBD.[12]

There is a bidirectional relationship between gut microbes and inflammation in IBD. Normal gut flora can act as triggers for the inflammatory response and are believed to play a central role in IBD pathogenesis.[13] In both Crohn's disease and UC, an increased number of surface-adherent and intracellular bacteria have been observed in mucosal biopsies.[14,15] Recent research indicates that these alterations in gut flora may be the result of inflammation, even if they contribute to its perpetuation. Induction of ileal inflammation in mice by various unrelated triggers, for example, causes an increase in levels of adherent and invasive Proteobacteria (*Escherichia coli* in particular) and a decline in bacterial diversity, which is the most consistent microbiologic finding in patients with IBD.[16] This effect may be caused by the accumulation of nitrates in inflamed tissue, a result of upregulated synthesis of nitric oxide.[17]

IBD is also associated with an increase in sulfate-reducing bacteria in the colon.[18] Sulfate reduction converts dietary sulfur into hydrogen sulfide (H_2S) and organic sulfides, which in turn interfere with mucosal uptake of luminal butyrate.[19] Patients with UC demonstrate impaired removal of H_2S by the enzyme thiosulfate sulfurtransferase (TST), an effect due largely to inflammation.[20] Sulfides in turn enhance nitric oxide synthesis,[21] contributing to the vicious cycle of mucosal inflammation and bacterial dysbiosis that drives IBD.

Patients with UC and Crohn's disease share immunological abnormalities that are common among patients with other types of autoimmune disorders, including upregulation of TH17+ lymphocytes and the proinflammatory cytokines TNF-α and interleukins-1, -6, and -23 (IL-1, IL-6, and IL-23), accompanied by downregulation of regulatory T cells and the anti-inflammatory cytokine IL-1 receptor antagonist (IL-1Ra).[22–25] The immune response underlying the pathology of Crohn's disease, as in other granulomatous diseases, is driven by lymphocytes with a type 1 helper T cell (TH1) phenotype and their cytokines: IL-2 and interferon-gamma (γ-IFN). The lymphocytes that organize the inflammatory response in UC demonstrate an atypical type 2 helper T cell (TH2) phenotype, with IL-5 as a distinctive cytokine mediator.[26]

A provocative and unexplained difference between Crohn's disease and UC is the effect of cigarette smoking, which increases the risk and decreases therapeutic responsiveness of patients with Crohn's but has the opposite effect in patients with colitis.[27]

NUTRITIONAL EPIDEMIOLOGY OF IBD

Attempts to identify a role of diet in the etiology of IBD are hampered by difficulty in describing a true pre-illness diet, because gastrointestinal symptoms may precede the diagnosis of IBD by several years, and gastrointestinal symptoms cause people to make dietary changes. The reported inverse association between fruit and fiber consumption and the development of Crohn's disease or the apparent protective effect of vegetable consumption on development of UC[28] may result from the bias introduced by retrospective population-based analysis. Prospective studies overcome this limitation, but there are very few and they have all been conducted with middle-aged European adults, who may not be representative of other ethnic or age groups. In the European Investigation into Cancer (EPIC) study, high consumption of vegetable oils rich in linoleic acid (18:2n6) increased the risk of incident UC.[29] Individuals who subsequently developed UC had higher levels of arachidonic acid (20:4n6), a metabolite of linoleic acid, in fat biopsies at baseline than did controls.[30] In contrast, dietary omega-3 fatty acids, especially docosahexaenoic acid (DHA, 22:6n3), were shown to exert a preventive effect on subsequent development of UC.[31] In the E3N study, higher intake of animal protein was associated with a significant increase in the risk of developing UC, but the risk for developing Crohn's disease, although increased, failed to reach statistical significance.[32]

An Italian case control study of newly diagnosed IBD patients that attempted to control for previous changes in dietary habits found a marked increase in the incidence of UC with margarine consumption (odds ratios of 11.8 and 21.37 for moderate or high margarine use) and a smaller but significant association between consumption of meat or cheese and Crohn's disease.[33] Fish appeared to have a protective effect, as it did in a study of children with new onset Crohn's disease.[34]

Japan has experienced the appearance and increase of IBD in association with cultural and nutritional Westernization. A nationwide Japanese study found an increased incidence of Crohn's disease to be associated with an increased consumption of omega-6–rich vegetable oils and animal protein.[35] When Japanese patients with Crohn's disease in remission adopted a traditional Japanese diet by avoiding sweets, bread, margarine, cheese, and snack foods and limiting meat and fish, their clinical relapse rate was only 6% after 2 years.[36] These patients remained on maintenance medication, so the effect cannot be attributed to diet alone.

High linoleic acid consumption may predispose to intestinal inflammation through its conversion to arachidonic acid, the precursor of most inflammatory prostaglandins and leukotrienes. High protein consumption may increase intestinal inflammation by supplying excess dietary sulfur, increasing colonic sulfide synthesis.[37]

Vitamin D promotes innate immunity by enhancing production of antimicrobial factors like cathelicidins and defensins that guard the epithelial surface of the gastrointestinal tract.[38] Induction of cathelicidin and beta-defensin activity is impaired in patients with Crohn's disease.[39] Researchers conducting the Harvard Nurses' Health Study constructed and validated a formula based on diet, supplementation, age, weight, and sun exposure that accurately predicted plasma levels of 25-OH cholecalciferol. An increase in predicted plasma vitamin D level from 22.3 ng/mL (mean of the lowest quartile) to 32.2 ng/mL (highest quartile mean) was associated with a 46% reduction in risk of incident Crohn's disease during two decades of follow-up.[40] No other micronutrient has yet been shown to influence risk of developing IBD when studied prospectively,[41] although nutritional deficits are common effects of IBD that may predispose to complications of IBD.

MALNUTRITION IN IBD

Malnutrition is a major reversible complication of IBD.

The mechanisms of malnutrition include anorexia resulting from the systemic effects of IL-1, a catabolic state induced by TNF-α, malabsorption due to disease or surgical resection, nutrient losses through the inflamed and ulcerated gut, small bowel bacterial overgrowth resulting from strictures or fistulas, and the side effects of drug therapy.[42]

Inflammation increases oxidative stress in the bowel mucosa and decreases levels of antioxidants.[43]

Nutritional deficiencies described in mucosal biopsies of patients with IBD include vitamin C,[44] zinc, copper, and the zinc- and copper-dependent enzyme, superoxide dismutase (Cu–Zn SOD).[45]

Plasma levels of vitamins A and E are lower, and plasma levels of the oxidative stress marker, 8-hydroxy-deoxyguanosine (8-OHdG), are higher in IBD patients than in controls.[46] Compared to controls, children and adults with IBD have lower blood levels of zinc and selenium, mineral cofactors of antioxidant enzymes,[47–49] and adults with UC may show lower levels of beta-carotene, magnesium, selenium, and zinc.[50]

Micronutrient deficits may favor self-perpetuation of IBD by causing defects in the mechanisms of tissue repair.[51] Micronutrient deficiencies may also contribute to important complications of IBD, including growth retardation (zinc), anemia (iron, folate, vitamin B12), bone disease (calcium, vitamin D, and possibly vitamin K), hypercoagulability (folate, vitamins B6 and B12, which together regulate blood levels of homocysteine), impaired wound healing (zinc, vitamins A and C), and colorectal cancer risk (folate and possibly vitamin D and calcium).[52–54] Among patients with UC, homocysteine levels greater than 15 μmol/L are associated with a significant increase in the risk of developing colon cancer. If plasma folate is normal, cancer risk increases by 250%; if folate is low, risk increases by 1700%.[55]

NUTRITIONAL THERAPIES

There is no single diet or set of supplements that is right for every patient with Crohn's disease or UC. In this author's experience, any intervention, even if supported by clinical trial data, may cause exacerbation of IBD in an individual patient. Each patient should serve as his or her own control, with symptoms, signs, and laboratory parameters followed closely. The evidence-based information presented below is at best a guide to help practitioners apply therapeutic options to individual patients. The only thing that matters is what works for this patient.

ENTERAL FEEDING

Defined formula diets, either elemental or polymeric, are successful in improving nutritional status of patients with IBD and preventing complications of surgery.[56]

In Crohn's disease, but not in UC, enteral feeding of defined formula diets as primary therapy has been shown to induce remission of active disease in 30% to 80% of patients.[51,52] Although enteral feeding is most commonly used in pediatric patients, because of growth-enhancing and steroid-sparing effects,[57] it is equally effective in adults[58] and appears to have a direct anti-inflammatory effect on the bowel mucosa.[59]

Theories to explain the anti-inflammatory effect of enteral feeding in CD include alteration in intestinal microbial flora,[60] diminution of intestinal synthesis of inflammatory mediators, and non-specific nutritional repletion or provision of important micronutrients to heal the diseased intestine.[51,52] Decreased dietary antigen uptake, an early concept, is not a likely mechanism; polymeric diets, composed of whole protein, are as effective as elemental diets, in which nitrogen is supplied as free amino acids.[61,62] There are conflicting results concerning the effect of supplemental food on the response to enteral feedings.[63,64]

Part of the benefit derived from enteral feeding may reflect dietary fat content.[51,52] Those liquid diets that are most effective in inducing remission of active Crohn's disease are either very low in fat or supply one third of their dietary fat in the form of medium-chain triglycerides (MCT) from coconut oil.[65,66] Addition of long-chain triglycerides derived from vegetable oils attenuates benefit,[67] whereas diets enriched with MCT oil are as effective as very low fat diets.[68] MCT oil may have a direct anti-inflammatory effect, modulating expression of adhesion molecules and cytokines.[51] The potential role of omega-3 fats in treatment of IBD is discussed in Supplements.

Many clinicians believe that patients treated early in the course of CD are more likely to respond than those with longstanding disease,[52] and small studies indicate that remission may be more likely in patients with ileal involvement than colonic involvement only[69] and with perforating/fistulating disease than with more superficial disease.[70] The main disadvantage to enteral feedings is poor compliance due to lack of palatability and the high rate of relapse (over 60%) following their discontinuation. The use of exclusion diets (discussed below) may significantly extend the benefit of enteral feeding regimens.

EXCLUSION DIETS

Exclusion diets eliminate specific symptom-producing foods and have been used to maintain remission of IBD. Although self-reported food intolerance is common among patients with IBD,[71] most of the data from controlled studies have been gathered from patients with Crohn's disease. In the East Anglia Multicentre Controlled Trial, 84% of patients with active Crohn's disease entered clinical remission after 2 weeks of a liquid elemental diet,[72] which produced a significant decrease in erythrocyte sedimentation rate (ESR) and C-reactive protein (CRP) and an increase in serum albumen. Patients were then randomized to receive treatment with prednisolone or treatment with a specific food exclusion diet without medication. To determine which foods each patient needed to avoid, a structured series of dietary challenges was conducted. Patients would introduce foods of their choice one at a time. Any food that appeared to provoke symptoms was excluded from further consumption; foods that did not provoke symptoms were included in a maintenance diet. At 6 months, 70% of patients treated with diet were still in remission, compared with 34% of patients being treated with prednisolone. After 2 years, 38% of patients treated with specific food exclusion were still in remission without medication, compared to 21% of steroid-treated patients. In previous uncontrolled studies, some of the same authors had used a diet consisting of one or two meats (usually lamb or chicken), one starch (usually rice or potatoes), one fruit, and one vegetable instead of the elemental diet in order to induce remission (later named the LOFFLEX Diet). Structured food challenges were then used to construct a maintenance diet free of symptom-provoking foods. Compliance with the specific food elimination diet was associated with a rate of relapse under 10% per year.[73] Individual foods found most likely to provoke symptoms in this study were wheat, cow's milk and its derivatives, cruciferous vegetables, corn, yeast, tomatoes, citrus fruit, and eggs.

Sensitivity to yeast may play an important role in Crohn's disease. Intestinal epithelial lymphocytes of Crohn's patients are abnormally sensitive to antigens derived from *Candida albicans*.[74] A large proportion of Crohn's patients develop antibodies to baker's and brewer's yeast, *Saccharomyces cerevisiae* (ASCA).[75] Lymphocytes of ASCA-positive patients proliferate after stimulation with mannan, a lectin common to most types of yeast. For these patients, lymphocyte proliferation is associated with increased production of TNF-α.[76] A small placebo-controlled study found that patients with stable, chronic Crohn's disease experienced a significant reduction in the Crohn's disease activity index (CDAI) during 30 days of dietary yeast elimination and a return to baseline disease activity when capsules of *S. cerevisiae* were added to their diets.[77]

An observational study of patients with UC suggested that dietary practices based upon food avoidance did not appear to modify the risk of relapse,[78] but a small experimental study from South Africa found that diarrhea, rectal bleeding, and the appearance of the colon on sigmoidoscopy improved significantly more for patients receiving a diet that systematically eliminated symptom-provoking foods than for those assigned to only monitor their diets.[79] The potential value of this study is reduced by the small number of patients and the maintenance of remission despite return to an unrestricted diet after 6 months. Earlier reports from dietary trials led to an estimate that 15–20% of patients with UC have specific food intolerance that affects severity of illness, with cow's milk protein being the leading offender.[80]

THE SPECIFIC CARBOHYDRATE DIET

The specific carbohydrate diet (www.scd.org) is a food-based approach to enteral nutrition for patients with IBD for which there are many anecdotal reports of long-term remission without medication.[81] Its alleged mechanism of action is improvement of nutritional status and alteration in ileocecal flora by the proper choice of nutritious carbohydrate sources.[82] It is far more effective for patients with Crohn's disease than UC (Elaine Gottschall, personal communication, 1994). In practice, the diet consists of meat, poultry, fish, eggs, most vegetables and fruits, nut flours, aged cheese, homemade yogurt, and honey. Forbidden foods include all cereal grains and their derivatives (including sweeteners other than honey), legumes, potatoes, lactose-containing dairy products, and sucrose. Early observational studies found that high sucrose intake predisposed to Crohn's disease[83–86] and that control of disease was enhanced by its avoidance.[87]

I have used the specific carbohydrate diet as primary treatment for patients with Crohn's disease for over 20 years, observing an overall response rate of 55%, unrelated to duration of illness but being most effective in those with ileitis or perianal fistulae.[88] Improvement occurred in symptoms and laboratory parameters, such as serum albumen and ESR, and permitted decreased use of glucocorticoids.

DIET FOR UC

Nutritional approaches to treatment of UC have examined the therapeutic potential of short-chain fatty acids (SCFA), butyric acid in particular.[52] Not only do SCFA nourish the colonic epithelium, but they also lower intraluminal pH, favoring growth of Lactobacilli and Bifidobacteria (considered to be beneficial organisms, or probiotics) and inhibiting the growth of Clostridia, Bacteroides, and *Escherichia coli*, potential pathogens. In addition to serving as the preferred energy substrate for colonic epithelial cells, butyrate has a true anti-inflammatory effect, preventing activation of the proinflammatory nuclear transcription factor, nuclear factor kappa B (NF-κB).[89] When added to 5-ASA enemas, butyrate (80 mmol/L) induces remission in ulcerative proctitis that is resistant to combined 5-ASA/hydrocortisone enemas.[90] Because butyrate is normally produced by bacterial fermentation of indigestible carbohydrate in the colon, studies have examined the effect of fiber supplementation on the course of UC. These studies are described below in Prebiotics.

Patients with UC are not deficient in butyrate, but as described above appear unable to utilize it, perhaps because organic sulfides produced by their enteric flora inhibit the epithelial effects of butyrate.[91,92] Protein consumption is a major determinant of sulfide production in the human colon.[93] Higher intake of protein, especially from animal sources, is associated with an increased risk of developing UC.[32] For patients with UC in remission, the risk of relapse is directly influenced by higher consumption of protein, especially meat protein, and by total dietary sulfur and sulfates.[94] An interesting effect of 5-ASA derivatives, drugs proven to help prevent relapse of colitis, is inhibition of sulfide production by gut bacteria, with sulfasalazine having the strongest effect.[95] Levels of sulfate-reducing bacteria, required for production of sulfides from dietary sulfate, are higher in fresh fecal samples of UC patients with active pouchitis than in patients with normal ileoanal pouches or in postcolectomy patients with familial polyposis who have ileoanal pouches.[96]

Based on these findings, a reasonable if unproven dietary approach to help patients with UC achieve or maintain remission would be high in fiber and omega-3 fatty acids, and low in meat, eggs, dairy fat, and vegetable oils.

SUPPLEMENTS

Nutritional supplements may be used to correct or prevent the deficiencies that are common among patients with IBD or to achieve an anti-inflammatory effect.

FOLATES

5-ASA derivatives, sulfasalazine in particular, impair folate transport.[97] Reduction of folate levels in patients with IBD is associated with hyperhomocysteinemia,[98] a risk factor for deep vein thrombosis,[99] an extraintestinal complication of IBD. Coadministration of folic acid with 5-ASA derivatives prevents folate depletion and has been shown to reduce the incidence of colon cancer in patients with UC.[100,101] One study found that a high dose of folic acid (15 mg/day) reversed sulfasalazine-induced pancytopenia in two patients.[102]

VITAMIN B12

Because vitamin B12 absorption may be impaired by ileal inflammation and by small bowel bacterial overgrowth, deficiency of vitamin B12 has long been described as a potential complication of Crohn's disease.[103] Although frank vitamin B12 deficiency is unusual, lower vitamin B12 levels are associated with increased serum homocysteine in patients with Crohn's disease.[104] Ischemic strokes in a woman with Crohn's disease were associated with vitamin B12-reversible hyperhomocysteinemia.[105] A single dose of 1000 µg of cobalamin by injection corrects the megaloblastic anemia associated with Crohn's disease.[106]

VITAMIN B6

Median vitamin B6 levels are significantly lower in patients with IBD than controls; low levels are associated with active inflammation and hyperhomocysteinemia.[107] Although some homocysteine is removed by folate-B12-dependent remethylation, the bulk of homocysteine is converted to cystathionine in a reaction catalyzed by vitamin B6. Ischemic stroke and high-grade carotid obstruction in a young woman with Crohn's disease were attributed to hyperhomocysteinemia, vitamin B6 deficiency, and a heterozygous methylene–tetrahydrofolate reductase gene mutation. The authors believed that vitamin B6 deficiency was the principal cause of hyperhomocysteinemia in this patient.[108]

VITAMINS E AND C

Blood levels of vitamins E and C are often reduced in patients with IBD.[109] Administration of alpha-tocopherol 800 IU per day and vitamin C 1000 mg per day to patients with stable, active Crohn's disease decreased markers of oxidative stress but had no effect on the CDAI.[110] A small study of patients with ulcerative proctitis demonstrated significant improvement after 2 weeks of vitamin E administered as a rectal suppository.[111]

VITAMIN A

Although levels of carotenoids[112] and retinol[113] are diminished in patients with active Crohn's disease, low levels appear to be related not to malabsorption but to inflammation[114,115] and a reduction in circulating retinol binding protein.[116] Supplementation with vitamin A at doses of 100,000 to 150,000 IU per day had no effect on symptoms or CDAI.[117,118]

Vitamin D

Reduced blood levels of 25-OH cholecalciferol, the major vitamin D metabolite, are common in patients with Crohn's disease and are related to malnutrition and lack of sun exposure.[119,120] Reduced vitamin D status in Crohn's patients is associated with reduced circulating IL-10, an anti-inflammatory cytokine, without a reduction in proinflammatory cytokines like TNF-α.[121] Administration of 1200 IU of vitamin D3 daily for 12 months reduced the risk of relapse in patients with inactive Crohn's disease by over 50%.[122] Administration of vitamin D, 1000 IU per day for 1 year, prevented bone loss in patients with active disease.[123] The major causes of bone loss in IBD, however, are the effects of inflammatory cytokines and glucocorticoid therapy,[124] not vitamin D status. Calcitriol (1,25-dihydroxycholecalciferol), the most active metabolite of vitamin D, may actually be increased in patients with IBD because activated intestinal macrophages increase its synthesis; elevated calcitriol is associated with increased risk of osteoporosis and may serve as a marker of disease activity.[125] Hypercalcemia is a rare complication of excess calcitriol, and serum calcium should be monitored in patients with IBD receiving vitamin D supplements.[126]

Vitamin K

Biochemical evidence of vitamin K deficiency has been found in patients with ileitis and in patients with colitis treated with sulfasalazine or antibiotics.[127] Serum vitamin K levels in Crohn's patients are significantly decreased compared with normal controls and are associated with increased levels of undercarboxylated osteocalcin, indicating a low vitamin K status in bone,[128] which is inversely related to lumbar spine bone density.[129] Furthermore, the rate of bone resorption in Crohn's disease is inversely correlated with vitamin K status, suggesting that vitamin K deficiency might be another etiological factor for osteopenia of IBD.[130] Optimal dose of vitamin K for correction of deficiency is not known. Patients with active disease may not absorb oral vitamin K, even at high dosage.[131]

Calcium

Although calcium supplementation is recommended for maintaining bone density in patients with IBD, especially those receiving glucocorticoids, calcium supplementation (1000 mg/day) with 250 IU of vitamin D per day conferred no significant benefit to bone density at 1 year in patients with corticosteroid-dependent IBD and osteoporosis.[132] Nonetheless, calcium supplementation should be given to patients with low dietary calcium intake. In experimental animals, low dietary calcium increases severity of IBD.[133]

Zinc

Low plasma zinc is common in patients with Crohn's disease and may be associated with clinical manifestations such as acrodermatitis, decreased activity of zinc-dependent enzymes like thymulin and metallothionein, reduction in muscle zinc concentration, and poor taste acuity.[52-54] Zinc absorption is impaired and fecal zinc losses are inappropriately high.[134] Zinc-deficient adolescents with Crohn's disease grow and mature more normally when zinc deficiency is treated. Anecdotally, correction of zinc deficiency as a specific intervention has been associated with global clinical improvement, suggesting that zinc replacement may have beneficial effects on disease activity.[135] A small study of patients in remission from Crohn's disease found that high-dose supplementation with zinc sulfate, 110 mg three times a day for 8 weeks, significantly decreased small intestinal permeability for a period of 12 months.[136] In patients with active disease, zinc sulfate, 200 mg/day (but not 60 mg/day), significantly increased plasma zinc and thymulin activity.[137]

SELENIUM

Low selenium levels in patients with Crohn's disease are associated with increased levels of TNF-α and decreased levels of the antioxidant enzyme, glutathione peroxidase (GSHPx).[138] Although selenium supplementation raises plasma selenium to the level of a control population, it did not significantly increase activity of GSHPx.[139] Patients with small bowel resection are at risk for severe selenium deficiency; monitoring of selenium status and selenium supplementation has been recommended for this group in particular.[140] Patients on enteral feeding with liquid formula diets experience decreased selenium concentrations proportional to duration of feeding, suggesting that additional selenium supplementation is also needed by them.[141]

MAGNESIUM

Magnesium deficiency is a potential complication of IBD, a result of decreased oral intake, malabsorption, and increased intestinal losses due to diarrhea. Urinary magnesium is a better predictor of magnesium status than serum magnesium in this setting.[142] Reduced urinary magnesium excretion is a significant risk factor for urolithiasis, one of the extraintestinal manifestations of IBD.[143] For patients with IBD, the urinary ratio of magnesium and citrate to calcium is a better predictor of lithogenic potential than urinary oxalate excretion.[144] Supplementation with magnesium citrate may decrease urinary stone formation, but diarrhea is a dose-related, limiting side effect.

CHROMIUM

Glucocorticoid therapy increases urinary chromium excretion and chromium picolinate, 600 μg/ day, can reverse steroid-induced diabetes in humans, with a decrease in mean blood glucose from 250 to 150 mg/dL. Chromium supplementation may be of benefit for patients receiving glucocorticoids who manifest impaired glucose tolerance.[145]

IRON

Anemia occurs in about 30% of patients with IBD.[146] Its causes include iron deficiency due to blood loss, cytokine-induced suppression of erythropoiesis, and side effects of medication. Some authors have speculated that iron deficiency actually increases the IFN-γ response in TH-1-driven inflammation and may contribute to aggravation of Crohn's disease.[147] Most clinicians, however, avoid oral iron supplements, believing they can increase oxidative stress in the gut, because very high dose iron supplementation consistently aggravates experimental colitis in rodents.[148] The doses used in rodent studies, however, are orders-of-magnitude greater than the doses given to patients. The relative risks and benefits of oral iron supplementation for patients with IBD are uncertain.

FISH OILS

Biochemical studies indicate that 25% of patients with IBD show evidence of essential fatty acid deficiency.[149] In experimental animals, fish oil feeding ameliorates the intestinal mucosal injury produced by methotrexate.[150] In tissue culture, omega-3 fatty acids stimulate wound healing of intestinal epithelial cells.[151] As mentioned above,[31] high dietary intake of omega-3 fatty acids is associated with reduced incidence of UC. For patients with active colitis, a fish oil preparation supplying 3200 mg of eicosapentaenoic acid (EPA) and 2400 mg of DHA per day decreased symptoms and lowered the levels of leukotriene B4 (LTB4) in rectal dialysates, with improvement demonstrated after 12 weeks of therapy.[152] A similar preparation improved histological score and symptoms of patients with proctocolitis.[153] At a dose of 4200 mg of omega-3 fatty acids per day, fish oils were shown to reduce dose requirements for anti-inflammatory drug therapy of UC.[154] At a dose of 5100 mg of omega-3 fatty acids per day, fish oils combined with 5-ASA derivatives prevented early relapse of UC better than 5-ASA derivatives plus placebo, but fish oils alone did not maintain remission.[155] In all studies of colitis, the fish oil preparations consisted of triacylglycerols. In vitro, fish oil has a more pronounced anti-inflammatory effect on tissue culture of colonic specimens from patients with UC than of those with Crohn's colitis.[156] Controlled trials of omega-3 therapy for Crohn's disease have been generally disappointing,[157] although an early study from Italy using a delayed-release preparation supplying free EPA (1800 mg/day) and free DHA (800 mg/day) was much more effective than placebo in preventing relapse of Crohn's disease in patients not taking 5-ASA derivatives.[158] The main side effect of fish oils is diarrhea.

GLUTAMINE

Glutamine appears to have a special role in restoring normal small bowel permeability and immune function. Patients with intestinal mucosal injury secondary to chemotherapy or radiation benefit from glutamine supplementation with less villous atrophy increased mucosal healing and decreased passage of endotoxin through the gut wall.[159] Although nutritional practitioners often advocate glutamine therapy for treatment of IBD, controlled studies have shown no benefit from glutamine supplementation at doses as high as 20 g/day in patients with Crohn's disease.[160,161] Glutamine excess aggravates experimental colitis in rodents[162] and increases oxidative stress[163] and may be contraindicated in humans with colitis.

N-ACETYLGLUCOSAMINE

N-Acetylglucosamine (NAG) is a substrate for synthesis of glycosaminoglycans, glycoproteins that protect the bowel mucosa from toxic damage. Synthesis of NAG by N-acetylation of glucosamine is impaired in patients with IBD.[164] In explants of bowel tissue from patients, incorporation of added NAG was depressed in patients with inactive UC, increasing to control levels in those with active colitis, probably indicating response of gut tissue to inflammation.[165] In a pilot study, NAG (3 to 6 g/day for more than 2 years) given orally to children with refractory IBD produced symptomatic improvement in the majority of patients and an improvement in histopathology.[166] In children with distal colitis or proctitis, the same dose of NAG was administered by enema with similar effects.

N-ACETYLCYSTEINE

N-Acetylcysteine (NAC) is needed for synthesis of glutathione, has antioxidant and anti-inflammatory effects, and has been shown to ameliorate experimental colitis. In a small, short-term clinical trial, NAC (800 mg/day) when added to mesalamine therapy of patients with active UC produced a significant improvement in clinical response compared to mesalamine plus placebo.[167]

PHOSPHATIDYLCHOLINE

A clinical trial of delayed-release PC 500 mg four times a day allowed 80% of patients with steroid-dependent UC to withdraw from steroids without disease exacerbation; response rate in the placebo arm was only 10%.[168] In other placebo-controlled studies by the same group, 6000 mg/day of delayed release PC added to 5-ASA inhibitors effected significant reductions in clinical, endoscopic, and histologic disease activity and improvement in quality of life when compared to placebo.[169] Response to delayed-release PC takes a median of 5 weeks and occurs at doses as low as 1000 mg/day.[170]

MELATONIN

Although some researchers have advocated melatonin as a therapy for IBD and a controlled study showed possible benefit of 5 mg/day in sustaining remission of UC,[171] melatonin is a potent inducer of TH1 lymphocytes and aggravation of both UC and Crohn's disease with melatonin supplementation has been reported.[172–174]

PROBIOTICS

Probiotic therapy of IBD is attracting considerable attention because of the recognition that alteration of intestinal microflora may modulate intestinal immune responses[175] and microbes may act as triggers for inflammation in patients with IBD.[176]

Because of the large number of probiotic preparations available, this section will only discuss those preparations that are commercially available in the United States and that have been studied in clinical trials of patients with IBD. More data exist for their benefits in UC than in Crohn's disease.

VSL-3 is a proprietary mixture of *Lactobacillus acidophilus, L. bulgaricus, L. casei, L. plantarum, Bifidobacterium brevis, B. infantis, B. longum*, and *Streptococcus salivarius* ssp *thermophilus*, supplied in sachets containing 900 billion colony-forming units (CFU) each. When added to therapy with the 5-ASA derivative balsalazide, VSL-3 (one sachet twice a day) induced faster remission of active UC than balsalazide or mesalamine alone.[177] Induction of remission with VSL-3 alone has been attained in 42%[178] to 54%[179] of adults with mild to moderate UC. VSL-3 also prevents relapse of pouchitis (postcolectomy inflammation of the ileal pouch),[180] with two sachets once a day producing remission rates far better than placebo over a 1-year period.[181] A clinical trial in children receiving steroid and mesalamine induction therapy for UC found that VSL-3 when compared to placebo increased the rate of remission induction from 36.4% to 92.8% and reduced the rate of relapse within 12 months from 73.3% to 21.4%.[182] A possible problem with VSL-3 is poor compliance among patients not participating in clinical trials, perhaps due to the cost or inconvenience of administration.[183]

Lactobacillus GG

Lactobacillus rhamnosus var. GG at a dose of 10 to 20 billion CFU per day was found to prevent onset of pouchitis in patients with ileal pouch-anal anastomosis during the first 3 years after surgery in a placebo-controlled trial.[184] *Lactobacillus* GG has been ineffective in inducing or maintaining remission of patients with Crohn's disease[185] or in preventing relapse of Crohn's disease after surgical resection.[186]

Saccharomyces boulardii

This plant-derived yeast demonstrates multiple anti-inflammatory effects when administered to laboratory animals, including interference with the activity of NFκB, a critical promoter of inflammatory cytokine transcription, and promotion of peroxisome proliferator-activated receptor-gamma (PPAR-γ) activity, which protects the gut mucosa from inflammation.[187] *S. boulardii* has shown benefit in both UC and Crohn's disease. The addition of *S. boulardii* (250 mg three times a day) to maintenance mesalamine therapy of patients with chronic, active UC was associated with induction of remission within 4 weeks in 17 out of 25 patients.[188] This trial was uncontrolled. In a placebo-controlled trial, the same dose was given to patients with stable, active Crohn's disease and mild to moderate diarrhea. *S. boulardii* reduced the frequency of diarrhea and the CDAI when given over a 10-week period, with benefits apparent within 2 weeks.[189] When added to mesalamine therapy of patients with Crohn's disease in remission, *S. boulardii* (1000 mg/day) reduced the frequency of relapse from 37% to 6.25% during 6 months, when compared to mesalamine alone[190] and produced a decrease in the pathological elevation of small intestinal permeability.[191]

Although *S. boulardii* is considered nonpathogenic, case reports of *S. boulardii fungemia* have been described in critically ill or immunocompromised patients exposed to *S. boulardii*. At least 18 reports of this complication have been published, including one in which airborne spread of *S. boulardii* occurred in an intensive care unit.[192]

PREBIOTICS

Prebiotics are nondigestible food ingredients that stimulate the growth or modify the metabolic activity of intestinal bacterial species that have the potential to improve the health of their human host. Criteria associated with the notion that a food ingredient should be classified as a prebiotic are that it remains undigested and unabsorbed as it passes through the upper part of the gastrointestinal tract and is a selective substrate for the growth of specific strains of beneficial bacteria (usually *Lactobacilli* or *Bifidobacteria*), rather than for all colonic bacteria. Prebiotic food ingredients include bran, psyllium husk, resistant (high amylose) starch, inulin (a polymer of fructofuranose), lactulose, and various natural or synthetic oligosaccharides, which consist of short-chain complexes of sucrose, galactose, fructose, glucose, maltose, or xylose. The best-known effect of prebiotics is to increase fecal water content, relieving constipation. Bacterial fermentation of prebiotics yields short-chain fatty acids like butyrate. Fructooligosaccharides (FOS) have been shown to alter fecal biomarkers (pH and the concentration of bacterial enzymes like nitroreductase and beta-glucuronidase) in a direction that may convey protection against the development of colon cancer[193] and to reduce fecal concentration of hydrogen sulfide in healthy volunteers,[194] an effect that might decrease colonic inflammation in patients with UC. Several studies have in fact suggested benefits of various prebiotics for the treatment of UC.

Oat bran, 60 g/day (supplying 20 g of dietary fiber), increased fecal butyrate by 36% in patients with UC and diminished abdominal pain.[195] A dietary supplement containing fish oil and two types of indigestible carbohydrate, FOS and xanthum gum, allowed reduction of glucocorticoid dosage when compared to a placebo, in patients with steroid-dependent UC.[196] A Japanese germinated barley foodstuff (GBF) containing hemicellulose-rich fiber, at a dose of 20 to 30 g/day, increased stool butyrate concentration,[197] decreased the clinical activity index of patients with active UC,[198] and prolonged remission in patients with inactive UC.[199] Wheat grass juice, 100 mL twice daily for 1 month, tested in a small placebo-controlled trial of patients with distal UC,[200] produced a significant reduction in rectal bleeding, abdominal pain, and disease activity as measured by sigmoidoscopy.

SYNBIOTICS

Synbiotics are combinations of probiotics and prebiotics. A mixture of *Bifidobacterium longum* and inulin-derived FOS administered for 1 month as monotherapy to patients with UC produced improvement in sigmoidoscopic appearance, histology, and several biochemical indices of tissue inflammation when compared to a placebo control.[201] A Japanese study found that the administration of *B. longum* 20 billion CFU/day with psyllium powder 8 g/day for 4 weeks to patients with UC reduced CRP by 76% and improved the quality of life, whereas neither agent alone was effective.[202]

BOVINE COLOSTRUM

Colostrum is the first milk produced after birth and is particularly rich in immunoglobulins, antimicrobial peptides (e.g., lactoferrin and lactoperoxidase), and other bioactive molecules, including growth factors. Peptide growth factors in colostrum might provide novel treatment options for a variety of gastrointestinal conditions.[203] Colostrum enemas, 100 mL of a 10% solution, administered twice a day by patients with distal UC, proved superior to a control enema in promoting healing; all patients were also taking a fixed dose of mesalamine.[204] Studies of oral colostrum in IBD have not been reported, but 125 mL three times a day fed to healthy human volunteers was shown to prevent the increase in intestinal permeability produced by indomethacin,[205] suggesting that peptide growth factors survive passage through the stomach and upper small bowel.

DEHYDROEPIANDROSTERONE

Dehydroepiandrosterone (DHEA) is the steroid hormone produced in greatest quantity by the human adrenal cortex, circulating primarily in the sulfated form, DHEA-S. DHEA inhibits activation of NF-κB, which is activated in inflammatory lesions. Patients with IBD have lower levels of DHEA-S in serum and intestinal tissue than controls,[206] partially associated with prior treatment with glucocorticoids.[207] In men with IBD, low DHEA-S is associated with increased risk of osteoporosis.[208] In a pilot study, 6 of 7 patients with refractory Crohn's disease and 8 of 13 patients with refractory UC responded to DHEA (200 mg/day for 56 days) with decrease in the clinical activity index.[209] A case report demonstrated benefit of the same dose of DHEA in a woman with severe refractory pouchitis, with relapse occurring 8 weeks after discontinuation of DHEA.[210]

PHYTOCHEMICALS

Plants contain numerous substances with pharmacologic activity that may be useful in the treatment of inflammation. The notion of anti-inflammatory foods is an important component of the functional foods concept.[211] Various plant food extracts have been studied as potential anti-inflammatory drugs in laboratory models of IBD,[212] but only two have been tested in human clinical trials: curcumin and mastic gum as of this writing.

CURCUMIN

A complex of flavonoids derived from the spice turmeric (Curcuma longum), curcumin has potent anti-inflammatory effects in vitro.[213,214] Despite its poor solubility, stability, and systemic bioavailability, curcumin has shown benefits in two small clinical trials of patients with CD and UC. In a placebo-controlled trial of UC patients in remission, curcumin 1000 mg twice a day was administered with meals for 6 months along with maintenance sulfasalazine or mesalamine. The relapse rate in the curcumin group was 4.65% compared to 20.51% in the placebo group. At 12 months, however, the difference between curcumin and placebo failed to reach statistical significance.[215] In an uncontrolled study, four of five patients with CD demonstrated reduction of the sedimentation rate and CDAI, and four of five patients with ulcerative proctitis were able to reduce concomitant medication dosage while taking a pure curcumin preparation.[216] A study of patients with colorectal cancer demonstrated that a dose of 3600 mg/day of curcumin orally yielded only trace levels in peripheral blood but reached a pharmacologically active concentration in neoplastic and normal colonic mucosa, inhibiting a key step in carcinogenesis.[217] Because IBD is a major risk factor for colon cancer, this finding makes curcumin an attractive therapeutic agent.

PASTICCIA LENTISCUS RESIN (MASTIC GUM)

In the Mediterranean region, mastic gum has a long history of use as a food and herbal remedy for gastrointestinal complaints. A pilot study of 10 patients with mild to moderate active CD given 2220 mg/day of mastic gum over 4 weeks demonstrated reduction in the CDAI and circulating levels of CRP and IL-6,[218] associated with a reduction in TNF-α production by peripheral blood mononuclear cells.[219]

REFERENCES

1. De Preter V, Geboes KP, Bulteel V, Vandermeulen G. Kinetics of butyrate metabolism in the normal colon and in ulcerative colitis: The effects of substrate concentration and carnitine on the β-oxidation pathway. *Aliment Pharmacol Ther.* 2011;34(5):526–532.
2. Segain JP, Raingeard de la Blétière D, Bourreille A et al. Butyrate inhibits inflammatory responses through NFkappaB inhibition: Implications for Crohn's disease. *Gut.* 2000;47(3):397–403.

3. Santhanam S, Venkatraman A, Ramakrishna BS. Impairment of mitochondrial acetoacetyl CoA thiolase activity in the colonic mucosa of patients with ulcerative colitis. *Gut.* 2007;56(11):1543–1549.

4. Treede I, Braun A, Jeliaskova P, Giese T, Füllekrug J, Griffiths G, Stremmel W, Ehehalt R. TNF-alpha-induced up-regulation of pro-inflammatory cytokines is reduced by phosphatidylcholine in intestinal epithelial cells. *BMC Gastroenterol.* 2009;9:53.

5. Braun A, Treede I, Gotthardt D, Tietje A, Zahn A, Ruhwald R, Schoenfeld U, Welsch T, Kienle P, Erben G, Lehmann WD, Fuellekrug J, Stremmel W, Ehehalt R. Alterations of phospholipid concentration and species composition of the intestinal mucus barrier in ulcerative colitis: A clue to pathogenesis. *Inflamm Bowel Dis.* 2009;15(11):1705–1720.

6. Lee HS, Kim BK, Nam Y et al. Protective role of phosphatidylcholine against cisplatin-induced renal toxicity and oxidative stress in rats. *Food Chem Toxicol.* 2013;58:388–393.

7. Yamamoto-Furusho JK, Korzenik JR. Crohn's disease: Innate immunodeficiency? *World J Gastroenterol.* 2006;12(42):6751–6755.

8. Gersemann M, Wehkamp J, Stange EF. Innate immune dysfunction in inflammatory bowel disease. *J Intern Med.* 2012;271(5):421–428.

9. Parkes M. Evidence from genetics for a role of autophagy and innate immunity in IBD pathogenesis. *Dig Dis.* 2012;30(4):330–333.

10. Schirbel A, Fiocchi C. Inflammatory bowel disease: Established and evolving considerations on its etiopathogenesis and therapy. *J Dig Dis.* 2010;11(5):266–276.

11. Joskins L, Ripke S, Weersma RK et al. Host-microbe interactions have shaped the genetic architecture of inflammatory bowel disease. *Nature.* 2012;491(7422):119–124.

12. Ananthakrishnan AN, Xavier RJ. How does genotype influence disease phenotype in inflammatory bowel disease? *Inflamm Bowel Dis.* 2013;19(9):2021–2030.

13. Podolsky DK. Inflammatory bowel disease. *N Eng J Med.* 2002;347:417–429.

14. Darfeuille-Michaud A, Neut C, Barnich N et al. Presence of adherent Escherichia coli strains in ileal mucosa of patients with Crohn's disease. *Gastroenterology.* 1998;115:1405–1413.

15. Swidinski A, Vladhoff A, Pernthaler A et al. Mucosal flares in inflammatory bowel disease. *Gastroenterology.* 2002;122:44–54.

16. Craven M, Egan CE, Dowd SE et al. Inflammation drives dysbiosis and bacterial invasion in murine models of ileal Crohn's disease. *PLoS One.* 2012;7(7):e41594.

17. Winter SE, Winter MG, Xavier NM et al. Host-derived nitrate boosts growth of *E. coli* in the inflamed gut. *Science.* 2013;339:708–711.

18. Jia W, Whitehead RN, Griffiths L, Dawson C et al. Diversity and distribution of sulphate-reducing bacteria in human faeces from healthy subjects and patients with inflammatory bowel disease. *FEMS Immunol Med Microbiol.* 2012;65(1):55–68.

19. Rowan FE, Docherty NG, Coffey JC, O'Connell PR. Sulphate-reducing bacteria and hydrogen sulphide in the aetiology of ulcerative colitis. *Br J Surg.* 2009;96(2):151–158.

20. De Preter V, Arijs I, Windey K et al. Decreased mucosal sulfide detoxification is related to an impaired butyrate oxidation in ulcerative colitis. *Inflamm Bowel Dis.* 2012;18(12):2371–2380.

21. Roediger WE, Babidge WJ. Nitric oxide effect on colonocyte metabolism: Co-action of sulfides and peroxide. *Mol Cell Biochem.* 2000;206(1–2):159–167.

22. MacDonald TT, DiSabatino A, Gordon JN. Immunopathogenesis of Crohn's disease. *JPEN J Parenter Enteral Nutr.* 2005;29(4):S118–S125.

23. Dionne S, D'Agata ID, Hiscott J et al. Colonic explant production of IL-1 and its receptor antagonist in imbalanced in inflammatory bowel disease. *Clin Exper Immunol.* 1998;112:381–387.

24. Eastaff-Leung N, Mabarrack N, Barbour A, Cummins A, Barry S. Foxp3(+) regulatory T cells, Th17 effect or cells, and cytokine environment in inflammatory bowel disease. *J Clin Immunol.* 2010;30(1):80–89.

25. De Nitto D, Sarra M, Cupi ML, Pallone F, Monteleone G. Targeting IL-23 and Th17-cytokines in inflammatory bowel diseases. *Curr Pharm Des.* 2010;16(33):3656–3660.

26. Fuss IJ, Neurath M, Boirivant M et al. Disparate CD4+ lamina propria (LP) lymphokine secretion profiles in inflammatory bowel disease: Crohn's disease LP cells manifest increased secretion of IFN-gamma, whereas ulcerative colitis LP cells manifest increased secretion of IL-5. *J Immunol.* 1996;157:1261–1270.

27. Cosnes J. Smoking, physical activity, nutrition and lifestyle: Environmental factors and their impact on IBD. *Dig Dis.* 2010;28(3):411–417.

28. Hou JK, Abraham B, El-Serang H. Dietary intake and risk of developing inflammatory bowel disease: A systematic review of the literature. *Am J Gastroenterol.* 2011;106:563–573.

29. IBD in EPIC Study Investigators, Tjonneland A, Overvad K, Bergmann MM, Nagel G, Linseisen J, Hallmans G, Palmqvist R, Sjodin H, Hagglund G, Berglund G, Lindgren S, Grip O, Palli D, Day NE, Khaw KT, Bingham S, Riboli E, Kennedy H, Hart A. Linoleic acid, a dietary n-6 polyunsaturated fatty acid, and the aetiology of ulcerative colitis: A nested case-control study within a European prospective cohort study. *Gut.* 2009;58(12):1606–1611.

30. de Silva PS, Olsen A, Christensen J, Schmidt EB, Overvaad K, Tjonneland A, Hart AR. An association between dietary arachidonic acid, measured in adipose tissue, and ulcerative colitis. *Gastroenterology.* 2010;139(6):1912–1917.

31. John S, Luben R, Shrestha SS, Welch A, Khaw KT, Hart AR. Dietary n-3 polyunsaturated fatty acids and the aetiology of ulcerative colitis: A UK prospective cohort study. *Eur J Gastroenterol Hepatol.* 2010;22(5):602–606.

32. Jantchou P, Morois S, Clavel-Chapelon F et al. Animal protein intake and risk of inflammatory bowel disease: The E3N prospective study. *Am J Gastroenterol.* 2010;105:2195–2201.

33. Maconi G, Ardizzone S, Cucino C et al. Pre-illness changes in dietary habits and diet as a risk factor for inflammatory bowel disease: A case-control study. *World J Gastroenterol.* 2010;16(34):4297–4304.

34. Amre DK, D'Souza S, Morgan K et al. Imbalances in dietary consumption of fatty acids, vegetables, and fruits are associated with risk for Crohn's disease in children. *Am J Gastroenterol.* 2007;102:2016–2025.

35. Shoda R, Matsueda K, Yamato S et al. Epidemiologic analysis of Crohn disease in Japan: Increased dietary intake of n-6 polyunsaturated fatty acids and animal protein relates to the increased incidence of Crohn disease in Japan. *Am J Clin Nutr.* 1996;63:741–745.

36. Chiba M, Abe T, Tsuda H et al. Lifestyle-related disease in Crohn's disease: Relapse prevention by a semi-vegetarian diet. *World J Gastroenterol.* 2010;16(20):2484–2495.

37. Magee EA, Richardson CJ, Hughes R, Cummings JH. Contribution of dietary protein to sulfide production in the large intestine: An in vitro and a controlled feeding study in humans. *Am J Clin Nutr.* 2000;72(6):1488–1494.

38. Hewison M. Vitamin D and the immune system: New perspectives on an old theme. *Endocrinol Metab Clin North Am.* 2010;39:365–379.

39. Wehkamp J, Schmid M, Stange EF. Defensins other antimicrobial peptides in inflammatory bowel disease. *Curr Opin Gastroenterol.* 2007;23:370–378.

40. Ananthakrishnan AN, Khalili H, Higuchi LM et al. Higher predicted vitamin D status is associated with reduced risk of Crohn's disease. *Gastroenterology.* 2012;142(3):482–489.

41. Andersen V, Olsen A, Carbonnel F et al. Diet and risk of inflammatory bowel disease. *Dig Liver Dis* 2012;44:185–194.

42. Gassull MA. Nutrition and inflammatory bowel disease: Its relation to pathophysiology, outcome and therapy. *Dig Dis.* 2003;21:220–227.

43. Simmonds NJ, Rampton SD. Inflammatory bowel disease—A radical view. *Gut.* 1993;34:865–868.

44. Buffinton GD, Doe WF. Altered ascorbic acid status in the mucosa from inflammatory bowel disease patients. *Free Radic Res.* 1995;22(2):131–143.

45. Lih-Brody L, Powell SR, Collier KP et al. Increased oxidative stress and decreased antioxidant defenses in mucosa of inflammatory bowel disease. *Dig Dis Sci.* 1996;41:2078–2086.

46. D'Odorico A, Bortolan S, Cardin R, D'Inca R, Martines D, Ferronato A, Sturniolo GC. Reduced plasma antioxidant concentrations and increased oxidative DNA damage in inflammatory bowel disease. *Scand J Gastroenterol.* 2001;36(12):1289–1294.

47. Ojuawo A, Keith L. The serum concentrations of zinc, copper and selenium in children with inflammatory bowel disease. *Cent Afr J Med.* 2002;48(9–10):116–119.

48. Hendricks KM, Walker WA. Zinc deficiency in inflammatory bowel disease. *Nutr Rev.* 1988;46:401–408.

49. Hinks LJ, Inwards KD, Lloyd B, Clayton B. Reduced concentrations of selenium in mild Crohn's disease. *J Clin Pathol.* 1988;41:198–201.

50. Geerling BJ, Badart-Smook A, Stockbrugger RW, Brummer RJ. Comprehensive nutritional status in recently diagnosed patients with inflammatory bowel disease compared with population controls. *Eur J Clin Nutr.* 2000;54(6):514–521.

51. Gassull MA. Review article: The role of nutrition in the treatment of inflammatory bowel disease. *Aliment Pharmacol Ther.* 2004;20 Suppl 4:79–83.

52. Gassull MA. Nutrition and inflammatory bowel disease: Its relation to pathophysiology, outcome and therapy. *Dig Dis.* 2003;21:220–227.

53. Hwang C, Ross V, Mahadevan U. Micronutrient deficiencies in inflammatory bowel disease: From A to zinc. *Inflamm Bowel Dis.* 2012;18(10):1961–1981.

54. Waśko-Czopnik D, Paradowski L. The influence of deficiencies of essential trace elements and vitamins on the course of Crohn's disease. *Adv Clin Exp Med*. 2012;21(1):5–11.

55. Phelip JM, Ducros V, Faucheron JL et al. Association of hyperhomocysteinemia and folate deficiency with colon tumors in patients with inflammatory bowel disease. *Inflamm Bowel Dis*. 2008;14(2):242–248.

56. Guagnozzi D, González-Castillo S, Olveira A, Lucendo AJ. Nutritional treatment in inflammatory bowel disease. An update. *Rev Esp Enferm Dig*. 2012;104(9):479–488.

57. Griffiths AM. Enteral nutrition in the management of Crohn's disease. *JPEN J Parenter Enteral Nutr*. 2005;29:S108–S117.

58. Dray X, Marteau P. The use of enteral nutrition in the management of Crohn's disease in adults. *JPEN J Parenter Enteral Nutr*. 2005;29(4 Suppl):S166–S169.

59. Sanderson IR, Croft NM. The anti-inflammatory effects of enteral nutrition. *JPEN J Parenter Enteral Nutr*. 2005;29(4 Suppl):S134–S138.

60. Lionetti P, Callegari ML, Ferrari S, Cavicchi MC, Pozzi E, de Martino M, Morelli L. Enteral nutrition and microflora in pediatric Crohn's disease. *JPEN J Parenter Enteral Nutr*. 2005;29(4 Suppl):S173–S175.

61. Verma S, Brown S, Kirkwood B, Giaffer MH. Polymeric versus elemental diet as primary treatment in active Crohn's disease: A randomized, double-blind trial. *Am J Gastroenterol*. 2000;95(3):735–739.

62. Zachos M, Tondeur M, Griffiths AM. Enteral nutritional therapy for inducing remission of Crohn's disease. *Cochrane Database Syst Rev*. 2001;(3):CD000542.

63. Greenberg GR, Fleming CR, Jeejeebhoy KN et al. Controlled trial of bowel rest and nutritional support in the management of Crohn's disease. *Gut*. 1988;29:1309–1315.

64. Johnson T, Macdonald S, Hill SM, Thomas A, Murphy MS. Treatment of active Crohn's disease in children using partial enteral nutrition with liquid formula: A randomised controlled trial. *Gut*. 2006;55(3):356–361.

65. Gonzalez-Huix F, de Leon R, Fernandez-Bañares F, Esteve M, Cabré E, Acero D, Abad-Lacruz A, Figa M, Guilera M, Planas R, Gassull MA. Polymeric enteral diets as primary treatment of active Crohn's disease: A prospective steroid-controlled trial. *Gut*. 1993;34:778–782.

66. Middleton SJ, Rucker JT, Kirby GA, Riordan AM, Hunter JO. Long-chain triglycerides reduce the efficacy of enteral feeds in patients with active Crohn's disease. *Clin Nutr*. 1995;14:229–236.

67. Bamba T, Shimoyama T, Sasaki M, Tsujikawa T, Fukuda Y, Koganei K, Hibi T, Iwao Y, Munakata A, Fukuda S, Matsumoto T, Oshitani N, Hiwatashi N, Oriuchi T, Kitahora T, Utsunomiya T, Saitoh Y, Suzuki Y, Nakajima M. Dietary fat attenuates the benefits of an elemental diet in active Crohn's disease: A randomized, controlled trial. *Eur J Gastroenterol Hepatol*. 2003;15(2):151–157.

68. Sakurai T, Matsui T, Yal T et al. Short-term efficacy of enteral nutrition in the treatment of active Crohn's disease: A randomized-controlled trial comparing nutrient formulas. *JPEN J Parenter Enteral Nutr*. 2002;26:98–103.

69. Afzal NA, Davies S, Paintin M, Arnaud-Battandier F, Walker-Smith JA, Murch S, Heuschkel R, Fell J. Colonic Crohn's disease in children does not respond well to treatment with enteral nutrition if the ileum is not involved. *Dig Dis Sci*. 2005; 50(8):1471–1475.

70. Ikeuchi H, Yamamura T, Nakano H, Kosaka T, Shimoyama T, Fukuda Y. Efficacy of nutritional therapy for perforating and non-perforating Crohn's disease. *Hepatogastroenterology*. 2004;51(58):1050–1052.

71. Ballegaard M, Bjergstrom A, Brondum S et al. Self reported food intolerance in chronic inflammatory bowel disease. *Scand J Gastroenterol*. 1997;32:569–571.

72. Riordan AM, Hunter JO, Cowan RE et al. Treatment of active Crohn's disease by exclusion diet: East Anglian multicentre controlled trial. *Lancet*. 1993;342:1131–1134.

73. Alun Jones V, Workman E, Freeman AH. Crohn's disease: Maintenance of remission by diet. *Lancet*. 1985;ii:177–180.

74. Pirzer U, Schonhaar A, Fleischer B et al. Reactivity of infiltrating T lymphocytes with microbial antigens in Crohn's disease. *Lancet*. 1991;338:1238–1239.

75. Barnes RMR, Allan S, Taylor-Robinson CH et al. Serum antibodies reactive with Saccharomyces cerevisiae in inflammatory bowel disease: Is IgA antibody a marker for Crohn's disease? *Int Arch Allergy Appl Immunol*. 1990;92:9–15.

76. Konrad A, Rutten C, Flogerzi B, Styner M, Goke B, Seibold F. Immune sensitization to yeast antigens in ASCA-positive patients with Crohn's disease. *Inflamm Bowel Dis*. 2004;10(2):97–105.

77. Barclay GR, McKenzie H, Pennington J, Parratt D, Pennington CR. The effect of dietary yeast on the activity of stable chronic Crohn's disease. *Scand J Gastroenterol*. 1992;27(3):196–200.

78. Jowett SL, Seal CJ, Phillips E, Gregory W, Barton JR, Welfare MR. Dietary beliefs of people with ulcerative colitis and their effect on relapse and nutrient intake. *Clin Nutr*. 2004;23(2):161–170.

79. Candy S, Borok G, Wright JP et al. The value of an elimination diet in the management of patients with ulcerative colitis. *S Afr Med J.* 1995;85:1176–1179.
80. Wright R, Truelove SC. A controlled trial of various diets in ulcerative colitis. *Br Med J.* 1965;2:138–141.
81. Nieves R, Jackson RT. Specific carbohydrate diet in treatment of inflammatory bowel disease. *Tennessee Med.* 2004;97:407.
82. Gottschall E. *Breaking the Vicious Cycle.* Kirkton Press, Kirkton, Ontario, 1994.
83. Matsui T, Mitsuo I, Fujishima M et al. Increased sugar consumption in Japanese patients with Crohn's disease. *Gastroenterol Jpn.* 1990;25:271.
84. Martini GA, Brandes JW. Increased consumption of refined carbohydrates in patients with Crohn's disease. *Klin Wochens.* 1976;54:367–371.
85. Thurnton JR, Emmett PM, Heaton KW. Diet and Crohn's disease: Characteristics of the pre-illness diet. *Br Med J.* 1979;2:762–764.
86. Mayberry JF, Rhodfes J, Newcombe RC. Increased sugar consumption in Crohn's disease. *Digestion.* 1980;20:323–326.
87. Heaton KW, Thornton JR, Emmett PM. Treatment of Crohn's disease with an unrefined-carbohydrate, fiber-rich diet. *Br Med J.* 1979;2:764–766.
88. Galland L. Nutritional therapy for Crohn's disease: Disease modifying and medication sparing. *Altern Ther.* 1999;5:94–95.
89. Inan MS, Rasoulpour RJ, Yin L, Hubbard AK, Rosenberg DW, Giardina C. The luminal short-chain fatty acid butyrate modulates NF-kappaB activity in a human colonic epithelial cell line. *Gastroenterology.* 2000;118:724–734.
90. Vernia P, Annese V, Bresci G, d'Albasio G, D'Inca R, Giaccari S, Ingrosso M, Mansi C, Riegler G, Valpiani D, Caprilli R; Gruppo Italiano per lo Studio del Colon and del Retto. Topical butyrate improves efficacy of 5-ASA in refractory distal ulcerative colitis: Results of a multicentre trial. *Eur J Clin Invest.* 2003;33(3):244–248.
91. Roediger WE, Duncan A, Kapaniris O, Millard S. Reducing sulfur compounds of the colon impair colonocyte nutrition: Implications for ulcerative colitis. *Gastroenterology.* 1993;104(3):802–809.
92. Roediger WE, Moore J, Babidge W. Colonic sulfide in pathogenesis and treatment of ulcerative colitis. *Dig Dis Sci.* 1997;42(8):1571–1579.
93. Magee EA, Richardson CJ, Hughes R, Cummings JH. Contribution of dietary protein to sulfide production in the large intestine: An in vitro and a controlled feeding study in humans. *Am J Clin Nutr.* 2000;72(6):1488–1494.
94. Jowett SL, Seal CJ, Pearce MS, Phillips E, Gregory W, Barton JR, Welfare MR. Influence of dietary factors on the clinical course of ulcerative colitis: A prospective cohort study. *Gut.* 2004;53(10): 1479–1484.
95. Edmond LM, Hopkins MJ, Magee EA, Cummings JH. The effect of 5-aminosalicylic acid-containing drugs on sulfide production by sulfate-reducing and amino acid-fermenting bacteria. *Inflamm Bowel Dis.* 2003;9(1):10–17.
96. Ohge H, Furne JK, Springfield J, Rothenberger DA, Madoff RD, Levitt MD. Association between fecal hydrogen sulfide production and pouchitis. *Dis Colon Rectum.* 2005;48(3):469–475.
97. Mason JB. Folate, colitis, dysplasia, and cancer. *Nutr Rev.* 1989;47(10):314–317.
98. Chowers Y, Sela BA, Holland R et al. Increased levels of homocysteine in patients with Crohn's disease are related to folate levels. *Am J Gastroenterol.* 2000;95:3498–3502.
99. Den Heijer M, Koster T, Blom HJ et al. Hyperhomocysteinemia as a risk factor for deep-vein thrombosis. *N Engl J Med.* 1996;334:759–762.
100. Lashner BA, Provencher KS, Seidner DL, Knesebeck A, Brzezinski A et al. Effect of folate supplementation on the incidence of dysplasia and cancer in chronic ulcerative colitis. A case-control study. *Gastroenterology.* 1989;97:255–259.
101. Diculescu M, Ciocirlan M, Ciocirlan M, Pitigoi D, Becheanu G, Croitoru A, Spanache S et al. Folic acid and sulfasalazine for colorectal carcinoma chemoprevention in patients with ulcerative colitis: The old and new evidence. *Rom J Gastroenterol.* 2003;12:283–286.
102. Logan EC, Williamson LM, Ryrie DR. Sulphasalazine associated pancytopenia may be caused by acute folate deficiency. *Gut.* 1986;27:868–872.
103. Beeken WL. Remediable defects in Crohn disease. *Arch Int Med.* 1975;135:686–690.
104. Romagnuolo J, Fedorak RN, Dias VC. Hyperhomocysteinemia and inflammatory bowel disease: Prevalence and predictors in a cross-sectional study. *Am J Gastroenterol.* 2001;96:2143–2149.
105. Penix LP. Ischemic strokes secondary to vitamin B12 deficiency-induced hyperhomocystinemia. *Neurology.* 1998;51(2):622–624.

106. Abe S, Wakabayashi Y, Hirose S. Megaloblastic anemia associated with diffuse intestinal Crohn's disease. *Rinsho Ketsueki*. 1989;30(1):51–55.
107. Saibeni S, Cattaneo M, Vecchi M et al. Low vitamin B6 plasma levels, a risk factor for thrombosis, in inflammatory bowel disease: Role of inflammation and correlation with acute phase reactants. *Am J Gastroenterol*. 2003;98:112–117.
108. Younes-Mhenni S, Derex L, Berruyer M, Nighoghossian N, Philippeau F, Salzmann M, Trouillas P. Large-artery stroke in a young patient with Crohn's disease. Role of vitamin B6 deficiency-induced hyperhomocysteinemia. *J Neurol Sci*. 2004;221(1–2):113–115.
109. Fernandez-Banares F, Abad-Lacruz A, Xiol X, Gine JJ, Dolz C, Cabre E, Esteve M, Gonzalez-Huix F, Gassull MA. Vitamin status in patients with inflammatory bowel disease. *Am J Gastroenterol*. 1989;84(7):744–748.
110. Aghdassi E, Wendland E, Steinhard H et al. Antioxidant vitamin supplementation in Crohn's disease decreases oxidative stress: A randomized controlled trial. *Am J Gastroenterol*. 2003;98:348–353.
111. Mirbagheri SA, Nezami BG, Assa S, Hajimahmoodi M. Rectal administration of d-alpha tocopherol for active ulcerative colitis: A preliminary report. *World J Gastroenterol*. 2008;14(39):5990–5995.
112. Rumi G Jr, Szabo I, Vincze A, Matus Z, Toth G, Mozsik G. Decrease of serum carotenoids in Crohn's disease. *J Physiol Paris*. 2000;94(2):159–161.
113. Bousvaros A, Zurakowski D, Duggan C, Law T, Rifai N, Goldberg NE, Leichtner AM. Vitamins A and E serum levels in children and young adults with inflammatory bowel disease: Effect of disease activity. *J Pediatr Gastroenterol Nutr*. 1998;26(2):129–135.
114. Reimund JM, Arondel Y, Escalin G, Finck G, Baumann R, Duclos B. Immune activation and nutritional status in adult Crohn's disease patients. *Dig Liver Dis*. 2005;37(6):424–431.
115. Sampietro GM, Cristaldi M, Cervato G, Maconi G, Danelli P, Cervellione R, Rovati M, Porro GB, Cestaro B, Taschieri AM. Oxidative stress, vitamin A and vitamin E behaviour in patients submitted to conservative surgery for complicated Crohn's disease. *Dig Liver Dis*. 2002;34(10):696–701.
116. Janczewska I, Bartnik W, Butruk E, Tomecki R, Kazik E, Ostrowski J. Metabolism of vitamin A in inflammatory bowel disease. *Hepatogastroenterology*. 1991;38(5):391–395.
117. Wright JP, Mee AS, Parfitt A, Marks IN, Burns DG, Sherman M, Tigler-Wybrandi N, Isaacs S. Vitamin A therapy in patients with Crohn's disease. *Gastroenterology*. 1985;88(2):512–514.
118. Norrby S, Sjodahl R, Tagesson C. Ineffectiveness of vitamin A therapy in severe Crohn's disease. *Acta Chir Scand*. 1985;151(5):465–468.
119. Harries AD, Brown R, Heatley RV, Williams LA, Woodhead S, Rhodes J. Vitamin D status in Crohn's disease: Association with nutrition and disease activity. *Gut*. 1985;26(11):1197–1203.
120. Vogelsang H, Ferenci P, Woloszczuk W, Resch H, Herold C, Frotz S, Gangl A. Bone disease in vitamin D-deficient patients with Crohn's disease. *Dig Dis Sci*. 1989;34(7):1094–1099.
121. Kelly P, Suibhne TN, O'Morain C, O'Sullivan M. Vitamin D status and cytokine levels in patients with Crohn's disease. *Int J Vitam Nutr Res*. 2011;81(4):205–210.
122. Jørgensen SP, Agnholt J, Glerup H, Lyhne S, Villadsen GE, Hvas CL, Bartels LE, Kelsen J, Christensen LA, Dahlerup JF. Clinical trial: Vitamin D3 treatment in Crohn's disease—A randomized double-blind placebo-controlled study. *Aliment Pharmacol Ther*. 2010;32(3):377–383.
123. Vogelsang H, Ferenci P, Resch H, Kiss A, Gangl A. Prevention of bone mineral loss in patients with Crohn's disease by long-term oral vitamin D supplementation. *Eur J Gastroenterol Hepatol*. 1995;7(7):609–614.
124. Trebble TM, Wootton SA, Stroud MA, Mullee MA, Calder PC, Fine DR, Moniz C, Arden NK. Laboratory markers predict bone loss in Crohn's disease: Relationship to blood mononuclear cell function and nutritional status. *Aliment Pharmacol Ther*. 2004;19(10):1063–1071.
125. Abreu MT, Kantorovich V, Vasiliauskas EA, Gruntmanis U, Matuk R, Daigle K, Chen S, Zehnder D, Lin YC, Yang H, Hewison M, Adams JS. Measurement of vitamin D levels in inflammatory bowel disease patients reveals a subset of Crohn's disease patients with elevated 1,25-dihydroxyvitamin D and low bone mineral density. *Gut*. 2004;53(8):1129–1136.
126. Tuohy KA, Steinman TI. Hypercalcemia due to excess 1,25-dihydroxyvitamin D in Crohn's disease. *Am J Kidney Dis*. 2005;45(1):e3–e6.
127. Krasinski SD, Russell RM, Furie BC, Kruger SF, Jacques PF, Furie B. The prevalence of vitamin K deficiency in chronic gastrointestinal disorders. *Am J Clin Nutr*. 1985;41(3):639–643.
128. Nakajima S, Iijima H, Egawa S et al. Association of vitamin K deficiency with bone metabolism and clinical disease activity in inflammatory bowel disease. *Nutrition*. 2011;27(10):1023–1028.
129. Schoon EJ, Muller MC, Vermeer C, Schurgers LJ, Brummer RJ, Stockbrugger RW. Low serum and bone vitamin K status in patients with longstanding Crohn's disease: Another pathogenetic factor of osteoporosis in Crohn's disease? *Gut*. 2001;48(4):473–477.

130. Duggan P, O'Brien M, Kiely M, McCarthy J, Shanahan F, Cashman KD. Vitamin K status in patients with Crohn's disease and relationship to bone turnover. *Am J Gastroenterol*. 2004;99(11):2178–2185.
131. Fugate SE, Ramsey AM. Resistance to oral vitamin K for reversal of overanticoagulation during Crohn's disease relapse. *J Thromb Thrombolysis*. 2004;17(3):219–223.
132. Bernstein CN, Seeger LL, Anton PA, Artinian L, Geffrey S, Goodman W, Belin TR, Shanahan F. A randomized, placebo-controlled trial of calcium supplementation for decreased bone density in corticosteroid-using patients with inflammatory bowel disease: A pilot study. *Aliment Pharmacol Ther*. 1996;10(5):777–786.
133. Cantorna MT, Zhu Y, Froicu M, Wittke A. Vitamin D status, 1,25-dihydroxyvitamin D3, and the immune system. *Am J Clin Nutr*. 2004;80(6 Suppl):1717S–1720S.
134. Griffin IJ, Kim SC, Hicks PD, Liang LK, Abrams SA. Zinc metabolism in adolescents with Crohn's disease. *Pediatr Res*. 2004;56(2):235–239.
135. Hendricks KM, Walker WA. Zinc deficiency in inflammatory bowel disease. *Nutr Rev*. 1988;46:401–408.
136. Sturniolo GC, Di Leo V, Ferronato A, D'Odorico A, D'Inca R. Zinc supplementation tightens "leaky gut" in Crohn's disease. *Inflamm Bowel Dis*. 2001;7(2):94–98.
137. Brignola C, Belloli C, De Simone G, Evangelisti A, Parente R, Mancini R, Iannone P, Mocheggiani E, Fabris N, Morini MC et al. Zinc supplementation restores plasma concentrations of zinc and thymulin in patients with Crohn's disease. *Aliment Pharmacol Ther*. 1993;7(3):275–280.
138. Reimund JM, Hirth C, Koehl C, Baumann R, Duclos B. Antioxidant and immune status in active Crohn's disease. A possible relationship. *Clin Nutr*. 2000;19(1):43–48.
139. Geerling BJ, Badart-Smook A, van Deursen C, van Houwelingen AC, Russel MG, Stockbrugger RW, Brummer RJ. Nutritional supplementation with N-3 fatty acids and antioxidants in patients with Crohn's disease in remission: Effects on antioxidant status and fatty acid profile. *Inflamm Bowel Dis*. 2000;6(2):77–84.
140. Rannem T, Ladefoged K, Hylander E, Hegnhoj J, Jarnum S. Selenium status in patients with Crohn's disease. *Am J Clin Nutr*. 1992;56(5):933–937.
141. Kuroki F, Matsumoto T, Iida M. Selenium is depleted in Crohn's disease on enteral nutrition. *Dig Dis*. 2003;21(3):266–270.
142. Galland L. Magnesium and inflammatory bowel disease. *Magnesium*. 1988;7(2):78–83.
143. Bohles H, Beifuss OJ, Brandl U, Pichl J, Akcetin Z, Demling L. Urinary factors of kidney stone formation in patients with Crohn's disease. *Klin Wochenschr*. 1988;66(3):87–91.
144. McConnell N, Campbell S, Gillanders I, Rolton H, Danesh B. Risk factors for developing renal stones in inflammatory bowel disease. *BJU Int*. 2002;89(9):835–841.
145. Ravina A, Slezak L, Mirsky N, Bryden NA, Anderson RA et al. Reversal of corticosteroid-induced diabetes mellitus with supplemental chromium. *Diabet Med*. 1999;16:164–167.
146. Gasche C, Lomer MC, Cavill I, Weiss G. Iron, anaemia, and inflammatory bowel diseases. *Gut*. 2004;53(8):1190–1197.
147. Oldenburg B, Koningsberger JC, Van Berge Henegouwen GP et al. Iron and inflammatory bowel disease. *Aliment Pharmacol Ther*. 2001;15:429–438.
148. Oldenburg B, Koningsberger JC, Van Berge Henegouwen GP, Van Asbeck BS, Marx JJ. Iron and inflammatory bowel disease. *Aliment Pharmacol Ther*. 2001;15(4):429–438.
149. Siguel EN, Lerman RH. Prevalence of essential fatty acid deficiency in patients with chronic gastrointestinal disorders. *Metabolism*. 1996;45:12–23.
150. Vanderhoof JA, Blackwood DJ, Mohammadpour H, Park JH. Effect of dietary menhaden oil on normal growth and development and on ameliorating mucosal injury in rats. *Am J Clin Nutr*. 1991;54(2):346–350.
151. Ruthig DJ, Meckling-Gill KA. Both (n-3) and (n-6) fatty acids stimulate wound healing in the rat intestinal epithelial cell line, IEC-6. *J Nutr*. 1999;129:1791–1798.
152. Stenson WF, Cort D, Rodgers J et al. Dietary supplementation with fish oil in ulcerative colitis. *Ann Int Med*. 1992;116:609–615.
153. Almallah YZ, Ewen SW, El-Tahir A, Mowat NA, Brunt PW, Sinclair TS, Heys SD, Eremin O et al. Distal proctocolitis and n-3 polyunsaturated fatty acids (n-3 PUFAs): The mucosal effect in situ. *J Clin Immunol*. 2000;20:68–76.
154. Aslan A, Triadafilopoulos G. Fish oil fatty acid supplementation in active ulcerative colitis: A double-blind, placebo-controlled, crossover study. *Am J Gastroenterol*. 1992;87:432–437.
155. Loeschke K, Ueberschaer B, Pietsch A, Gruber E, Ewe K, Wiebecke B, Heldwein W, Lorenz R et al. n-3 Fatty acids retard early relapse in ulcerative colitis in remission. *Dig Dis Sci*. 1996;41:2087–2094.

156. Meister D, Ghosh S. Effect of fish oil enriched enteral diet on inflammatory bowel disease tissues in organ culture: Differential effects on ulcerative colitis and Crohn's disease. *World J Gastroenterol.* 2005;11(47):7466–7472.

157. Turner D, Zlotkin SH, Shah PS, Griffiths AM. Omega 3 fatty acids (fish oil) for maintenance of remission in Crohn's disease. *Cochrane Database Syst Rev.* 2009;(1):CD006320.

158. Belluzzi A, Brignola C, Campieri M et al. Effect of an enteric coated fish-oil preparation on relapses in Crohn's disease. *N Engl J Med.* 1996;334:1557–1560.

159. van der Hulst RR et al. Glutamine and the preservation of gut integrity. *Lancet.* 1993;341(8857):1363–1365.

160. Akobeng AK, Miller V, Stanton J, Elbadri AM, Thomas AG. Double-blind randomized controlled trial of glutamine-enriched polymeric diet in the treatment of active Crohn's disease. *J Pediatr Gastroenterol Nutr.* 2000;30(1):78–84.

161. Den Hond E, Hiele M, Peeters M, Ghoos Y, Rutgeerts P. Effect of long-term oral glutamine supplements on small intestinal permeability in patients with Crohn's disease. *JPEN J Parenter Enteral Nutr.* 1999;23(1):7–11.

162. Shinozaki M, Saito H, Muto T. Excess glutamine exacerbates trinitrobenzenesulfonic acid-induced colitis in rats. *Dis Colon Rectum.* 1997;40(10 Suppl):S59–S63.

163. Sido B, Seel C, Hochlehnert A, Breitkreutz R, Dröge W. Low intestinal glutamine level and low glutaminase activity in Crohn's disease: A rational for glutamine supplementation? *Dig Dis Sci.* 2006;51(12):2170–2179.

164. Burton AF, Anderson FH. Decreased incorporation of 14C-glucosamine relative to 3H-N-acetyl glucosamine in the intestinal mucosa of patients with inflammatory bowel disease. *Am J Gastroenterol.* 1983;78:19–22.

165. Ryder SD, Raouf AH, Parker N, Walker RJ, Rhodes JM et al. Abnormal mucosal glycoprotein synthesis in inflammatory bowel diseases is not related to cigarette smoking. *Digestion.* 1995;56:370–376.

166. Salvatore S, Heuschkel R, Tomlin S, Davies SE, Edwards S, Walker-Smith JA, French I, Murch SH et al. A pilot study of N-acetyl glucosamine, a nutritional substrate for glycosaminoglycan synthesis, in paediatric chronic inflammatory bowel disease. *Aliment Pharmacol Ther.* 2000;14:1567–1579.

167. Guijarro LG, Mate J, Gisbert JP, Perez-Calle JL, Marin-Jimenez I, Arriaza E, Olleros T, Delgado M, Castillejo MS, Prieto-Merino D, Gonzalez Lara V, Pena AS. N-acetyl-L-cysteine combined with mesalamine in the treatment of ulcerative colitis: Randomized, placebo-controlled pilot study. *World J Gastroenterol.* 2008;14(18):2851–2857.

168. Stremmel W, Ehehalt R, Autschbach F, Karner M. Phosphatidylcholine for steroid-refractory chronic ulcerative colitis: A randomized trial. *Ann Intern Med.* 2007;147(9):603–610.

169. Stremmel W, Merle U, Zahn A, Autschbach F, Hinz U, Ehehalt R. Retarded release phosphatidylcholine benefits patients with chronic active ulcerative colitis. *Gut.* 2005;54(7):966–971.

170. Stremmel W, Braun A, Hanemann A, Ehehalt R, Autschbach F, Karner M. Delayed release phosphatidylcholine in chronic-active ulcerative colitis: A randomized, double-blinded, dose finding study. *J Clin Gastroenterol.* 2010;44(5):e101–e107.

171. Chojnacki C, Wisniewska-Jarosinska M, Walecka-Kapica E et al. Evaluation of melatonin effectiveness in the adjuvant treatment of ulcerative colitis. *J Physiol Pharmacol.* 2011;62(3):327–334.

172. Sánchez-Barceló EJ, Mediavilla MD, Tan DX, Reiter R. Clinical uses of melatonin: Evaluation of human trials. *J Curr Med Chem.* 2010;17(19):2070–2095.

173. Calvo JR, Guerrero JM, Osuna C, Molinero P, Carrillo-Vico A. Melatonin triggers Crohn's disease symptoms. *J Pineal Res.* 2002;32(4):277–278.

174. Maldonado MD, Calvo JR. Melatonin usage in ulcerative colitis: A case report. *J Pineal Res.* 2008;45(3):339–340.

175. O'Sullivan GC, Kelly P, O'Halloran S, Collins C, Collins JK, Dunne C, Shanahan F. Probiotics: An emerging therapy. *Curr Pharm Des.* 2005;11(1):3–10.

176. Baker PI, Love DR, Ferguson LR. Role of gut microbiota in Crohn's disease. *Expert Rev Gastroenterol Hepatol.* 2009;3(5):535–546.

177. Tursi A, Brandimarte G, Giorgetti GM, Forti G, Modeo ME, Gigliobianco A. Low-dose balsalazide plus a high-potency probiotic preparation is more effective than balsalazide alone or mesalazine in the treatment of acute mild-to-moderate ulcerative colitis. *Med Sci Monit.* 2004;10(11):PI126–PI131.

178. Sood A, Midha V, Makharia GK, Ahuja V, Singal D, Goswami P, Tandon RK. The probiotic preparation, VSL#3 induces remission in patients with mild-to-moderately active ulcerative colitis. *Clin Gastroenterol Hepatol.* 2009;7(11):1202–1209, 1209.

179. Bibiloni R, Fedorak RN, Tannock GW, Madsen KL, Gionchetti P, Campieri M, De Simone C, Sartor RB. VSL#3 probiotic-mixture induces remission in patients with active ulcerative colitis. *Am J Gastroenterol.* 2005;100(7):1539–1546.

180. Gionchetti P, Rizzello F, Venturi A et al. Oral bacteriotherapy as maintenance treatment in patients with chronic pouchitis: A double-blind placebo controlled trial. *Gastroenterology.* 2000;119:305–309.

181. Mimura T, Rizzello F, Helwig U, Poggioli G, Schreiber S, Talbot IC, Nicholls RJ, Gionchetti P, Campieri M, Kamm MA. Once daily high dose probiotic therapy (VSL#3) for maintaining remission in recurrent or refractory pouchitis. *Gut.* 2004;53(1):108–114.

182. Miele E, Pascarella F, Giannetti E, Quaglietta L, Baldassano RN, Staiano A. Effect of a probiotic preparation (VSL#3) on induction and maintenance of remission in children with ulcerative colitis *Am J Gastroenterol.* 2009;104(2):437–443.

183. Shen B, Brzezinski A, Fazio VW, Remzi FH, Achkar JP, Bennett AE, Sherman K, Lashner BA. Maintenance therapy with a probiotic in antibiotic-dependent pouchitis: Experience in clinical practice. *Aliment Pharmacol Ther.* 2005;22(8):721–728.

184. Gosselink MP, Schouten WR, van Lieshout LM, Hop WC, Laman JD, Ruseler-van Embden JG. Delay of the first onset of pouchitis by oral intake of the probiotic strain Lactobacillus rhamnosus GG. *Dis Colon Rectum.* 2004;47(6):876–884.

185. Schultz M, Timmer A, Herfarth HH, Sartor RB, Vanderhoof JA, Rath HC. Lactobacillus GG in inducing and maintaining remission of Crohn's disease. *BMC Gastroenterol.* 2004;4(1):5.

186. Prantera C, Scribano ML, Falasco G, Andreoli A, Luzi C. Ineffectiveness of probiotics in preventing recurrence after curative resection for Crohn's disease: A randomised controlled trial with Lactobacillus GG. *Gut.* 2002;51(3):405–409.

187. Pothoulakis C. Review article: Anti-inflammatory mechanisms of action of Saccharomyces boulardii. *Aliment Pharmacol Ther.* 2009;30(8):826–833.

188. Guslandi M, Giollo P, Testoni PA. A pilot trial of Saccharomyces boulardii in ulcerative colitis. *Eur J Gastroenterol Hepatol.* 2003;15(6):697–698.

189. Plein K, Hotz J. Therapeutic effects of Saccharomyces boulardii on mild residual symptoms in a stable phase of Crohn's disease with special respect to chronic diarrhea—A pilot study. *Z Gastroenterol.* 1993;31(2):129–134.

190. Guslandi M, Mezzi G, Sorghi M, Testoni PA. Saccharomyces boulardii in maintenance treatment of Crohn's disease. *Dig Dis Sci.* 2000;45(7):1462–1464.

191. Garcia Vilela E, De Lourdes De Abreu Ferrari M, Oswaldo Da Gama Torres H, Guerra Pinto A, Carolina Carneiro Aguirre A, Paiva Martins F, Marcos Andrade Goulart E, Sales Da Cunha A. Scand Influence of Saccharomyces boulardii on the intestinal permeability of patients with Crohn's disease in remission. *J Gastroenterol.* 2008;43(7):842–848.

192. Cassone M, Serra P, Mondello F, Girolamo A, Scafetti S, Pistella E, Venditti M et al. Outbreak of Saccharomyces boulardii subtype boulardii fungaemia in patients neighboring those treated with a probiotic preparation of the organism. *J Clin Microbiol.* 2003;41:5340–5343.

193. Galland L. Functional foods: Health effects and clinical applications, in *Encyclopedia of Human Nutrition*, 2nd edition. John Wiley & Sons, London, 2005, pp. 360–366.

194. Lewis S, Brazier J, Beard D, Nazem N, Proctor D. Effects of metronidazole and oligofructose on faecal concentrations of sulphate-reducing bacteria and their activity in human volunteers. *Scand J Gastroenterol.* 2005;40(11):1296–1303.

195. Hallert C, Bjorck I, Nyman M, Pousette A, Granno C, Svensson H. Increasing fecal butyrate in ulcerative colitis patients by diet: Controlled pilot study. *Inflamm Bowel Dis.* 2003;9(2):116–121.

196. Seidner DL, Lashner BA, Brzezinski A, Banks PL, Goldblum J, Fiocchi C, Katz J, Lichtenstein GR, Anton PA, Kam LY, Garleb KA, Demichele SJ. An oral supplement enriched with fish oil, soluble fiber, and antioxidants for corticosteroid sparing in ulcerative colitis: A randomized, controlled trial. *Clin Gastroenterol Hepatol.* 2005;3(4):358–369.

197. Bamba T, Kanauchi O, Andoh A, Fujiyama Y. A new prebiotic from germinated barley for nutraceutical treatment of ulcerative colitis. *J Gastroenterol Hepatol.* 2002;17(8):818–824.

198. Kanauchi O, Mitsuyama K, Homma T, Takahama K, Fujiyama Y, Andoh A, Araki Y, Suga T, Hibi T, Naganuma M, Asakura H, Nakano H, Shimoyama T, Hida N, Haruma K, Koga H, Sata M, Tomiyasu N, Toyonaga A, Fukuda M, Kojima A, Bamba T. Treatment of ulcerative colitis patients by long-term administration of germinated barley foodstuff: Multi-center open trial. *Int J Mol Med.* 2003;12(5):701–704.

199. Hanai H, Kanauchi O, Mitsuyama K, Andoh A, Takeuchi K, Takayuki I, Araki Y, Fujiyama Y, Toyonaga A, Sata M, Kojima A, Fukuda M, Bamba T. Germinated barley foodstuff prolongs remission in patients with ulcerative colitis. *Int J Mol Med.* 2004;13(5):643–647.

200. Ben-Ayre E, Goldin E, Wengrower E et al. Wheat grass juice in the treatment of active distal alternative colitis. *Scand J Gastroenterol*. 2002;37:444–449.
201. Furrie E, Macfarlane S, Kennedy A, Cummings JH, Walsh SV, O'Neil DA, Macfarlane GT Synbiotic therapy (Bifidobacterium longum/Synergy 1) initiates resolution of inflammation in patients with active ulcerative colitis: A randomised controlled pilot trial. *Gut*. 2005;54(2):242–249.
202. Fujimori S, Gudis K, Mitsui K, Seo T, Yonezawa M, Tanaka S, Tatsuguchi A, Sakamoto C. A randomized controlled trial on the efficacy of synbiotic versus probiotic or prebiotic treatment to improve the quality of life in patients with ulcerative colitis. *Nutrition*. 2009;25(5):520–525.
203. Playford RJ, Macdonald CE, Johnson WS. Colostrum and milk-derived peptide growth factors for the treatment of gastrointestinal disorders. *Am J Clin Nutr*. 2000;72(1):5–14.
204. Khan Z, Macdonald C, Wicks AC, Holt MP, Floyd D, Ghosh S, Wright NA, Playford RJ et al. Use of the 'nutriceutical', bovine colostrum, for the treatment of distal colitis: Results from an initial study. *Aliment Pharmacol Ther*. 2002;16:1917–1922.
205. Playford RJ, MacDonald CE, Calnan DP, Floyd DN, Podas T, Johnson W, Wicks AC, Bashir O, Marchbank T. Co-administration of the health food supplement, bovine colostrum, reduces the acute non-steroidal anti-inflammatory drug-induced increase in intestinal permeability. *Clin Sci (Lond)*. 2001;100(6):627–633.
206. de la Torre B, Hedman M, Befrits R et al. Blood and tissue dehydroepiandrosterone sulphate levels and their relationship to chronic inflammatory bowel disease. *Clin Exp Rheumatol*. 1998;16:579–582.
207. Straub RH, Vogl D, Gross V, Lang B, Scholmerich J, Andus T et al. Association of humoral markers of inflammation and dehydroepiandrosterone sulfate or cortisol serum levels in patients with chronic inflammatory bowel disease. *Am J Gastroenterol*. 1998;93:2197–2202.
208. Szathmari M, Vasarhelyi B, Treszl A, Tulassay T, Tulassay Z et al. Association of dehydroepiandros-terone sulfate and testosterone deficiency with bone turnover in men with inflammatory bowel disease. *Int J Colorectal Dis*. 2002;17:63–66.
209. Andus T, Klebl F, Rogler G, Bregenzer N, Scholmerich J, Straub RH et al. Patients with refractory Crohn's disease or ulcerative colitis respond to dehydroepiandrosterone: A pilot study. *Aliment Pharmacol Ther*. 2003;17:409–414.
210. Klebl FH, Bregenzer N, Rogler G, Straub RH, Scholmerich J, Andus T. Treatment of pouchitis with dehydroepiandrosterone (DHEA)—A case report. *Z Gastroenterol*. 2003;41(11):1087–1090.
211. Galland L. Functional foods: Health effects and clinical applications, in *Encyclopedia of Human Nutrition*, 3rd edition, edited by Benjamin Caballero, Lindsay Allen and Andrew Prentiss. Academic Press, London, 2013, pp. 366–371.
212. Singh UP, Singh NP, Busbee B et al. Alternative medicines as emerging therapies for inflammatory bowel diseases. *Int Rev Immunol*. 2012;31(1):66–84.
213. Epstein J, Docena G, MacDonald TT, Sanderson IR. Curcumin suppresses p38 mitogen-activated protein kinase activation, reduces IL-1beta and matrix metalloproteinase-3 and enhances IL-10 in the mucosa of children and adults with inflammatory bowel disease *Br J Nutr*. 2010;103(6):824–832.
214. Youn HS, Saitoh SI, Miyake K, Hwang DH. Inhibition of homodimerization of Toll-like receptor 4 by curcumin. *Biochem Pharmacol*. 2006;72(1):62–69.
215. Hanai H, Iida T, Takeuchi K et al. Curcumin maintenance therapy for ulcerative colitis: Randomized, multicenter, double-blind, placebo-controlled trial. *Clin Gastroenterol Hepatol*. 2006;4(12):1502–1506.
216. Holt PR, Katz S, Kirshoff R. Curcumin therapy in inflammatory bowel disease: A pilot study. *Dig Dis Sci*. 2005;50(11):2191–2193.
217. Garcea G, Berry DP, Jones DJ, Singh R, Dennison AR, Farmer PB, Sharma RA, Steward WP, Gescher AJ. Consumption of the putative chemopreventive agent curcumin by cancer patients: Assessment of cur-cumin levels in the colorectum and their pharmacodynamic consequences. *Cancer Epidemiol Biomarkers Prev*. 2005;14(1):120–125.
218. Kaliora AC, Stathopoulou MG, Triantafillidis JK, Dedoussis GV, Andrikopoulos NK. Chios mastic treat-ment of patients with active Crohn's disease. *World J Gastroenterol*. 2007;13(5):748–753.
219. Kaliora AC, Stathopoulou MG, Triantafillidis JK, Dedoussis GV, Andrikopoulos NK. Alterations in the function of circulating mononuclear cells derived from patients with Crohn's disease treated with mastic. *World J Gastroenterol*. 2007;13(45):6031–6036.

26 Nutritional Management of Short Bowel Syndrome in the Adult with Crohn's Disease

Melvyn Grovit, Kathie Grovit Ferbas, and Alfred E. Slonim

CONTENTS

INTRODUCTION

Short bowel syndrome (SBS) is a multisystemic disorder, which can occur as an outcome of trauma, volvulus, necrotizing enterocolitis, vascular occlusion, neoplastic diseases, congenital disorders, and inflammatory bowel diseases (IBD), Crohn's disease (CD), and ulcerative colitis (UC). While each of the aforementioned may necessitate surgical intervention resulting in SBS, we focus here on SBS following surgical intervention in the CD patient. This chapter will discuss the pathophysiological consequences and management considerations of SBS, and will also introduce novel complimentary nutrition and nutraceutical applications relevant to CD that allow for a significantly higher adaptive function. The principal author (MG) has lived the life cycle of SBS for 51 years, commencing at age 26. This was the result of multiple resections owing to extensive CD, which began in his early teenage years. Surgical intervention was of necessity, as the extent of the disease became life threatening. It is interesting to consider how different this course might have been, given what we now know about the importance of diet and nutritional supplementation in the management of CD. In reading this chapter, it is critical to bear in mind that the underlying genetic and epigenetic factors that precipitate development of CD remain, despite surgical interventions resulting in SBS. As such, it is essential for clinicians to remember that these are patients with <200 cm of small bowel who *also* have a chronic inflammatory disease.

Approximately 10% of the estimated 1 million Americans with IBD develop their disease before 17 years of age. Recent epidemiological studies indicate an increase in the incidence of juvenile-onset IBD, which has been particularly true for CD.[1] The incidence of juvenile CD is estimated at 5 per 100,000 children per year, and juvenile CD demonstrates some clear differences from adult-onset CD.[2,3] For instance, juvenile-onset CD is characterized by a higher proportion of incidence in males, an increased prevalence of jejunoileitis, and a more frequent requirement for second-line immunosuppressant and monoclonal antibody therapeutics. Moreover, most moderate–severe juvenile patients are in a constant catabolic state, resulting in poor weight gain and growth failure, primarily due to anorexia and malabsorption. Most juvenile patients suffer weight loss or have lack of weight gain, whereas 40–45% also demonstrate growth failure. An association between impaired growth and low IGF-I levels is well recognized in children with CD.[4] However, growth hormone (GH) production is normal in such children, which suggests that resistance to the effects of GH is present. Early studies emphasized the role of undernutrition in the suppression of insulin-like growth factor-I (IGF-I) production. Both protein and caloric intake regulate IGF-I production, either by decreasing GH receptor density or through postreceptor mechanisms. Growth impairment in CD is a measure of disease severity, and restoration of growth is an indicator of successful treatment. Overall, these features suggest that juvenile-onset CD is a more severe phenotype than adult-onset CD.

In an attempt to avoid disease progression, patients (adult and juvenile) are treated with anti-inflammatory, immunomodulatory, and monoclonal antibody (mAb) therapeutics that frequently produce short-term remissions, but rarely succeed in reversal of growth failure.[5] Of relevance, attenuation and loss of efficacy over time secondary to the induction of antidrug antibodies (Abs) are significant issues in the use of many of these drugs. For example, trials have demonstrated 60% induction of antidrug Abs in response to treatment with today's most commonly used mAb, infliximab (Janssen Biotech).[6] Furthermore, enthusiasm for these new pharmaceutical agents is tempered by their potential short-term and long-term toxicity.[7] These are immunosuppressive dominant therapeutics, many of which carry black box warnings that almost always cause unintended consequences that will need to be managed and, ideally, be resolved.

Recalcitrant CD, with the need for emergent surgical intervention, can result in an increased incidence and prevalence of SBS. Importantly, by the age of 30, the risk of having undergone an extensive intestinal resection was reported in one study to be 48% in the juvenile-onset group versus 14% in the adult-onset group.[3] Regardless of the precipitating cause, once there is extensive resection of bowel with functional loss of intestinal surface area, patients suffer from diarrhea, malabsorption, pan macronutrient and micronutrient deficiencies, and weight loss. The management of SBS requires long-term medical and nutritional intervention, and may also necessitate additional surgery, in order to achieve homeostasis.[8] As a corollary, we now have the knowledge and many of the tools to consider nonsurgical interventions much earlier in order to decrease the necessity for, or the severity of, unavoidable surgeries in CD and other IBDs.

There is a variable period of gastrointestinal tract (GIT) adaptation following surgery, and the rate of recovery depends upon the location and extent of the surgery, the presence or absence of the ileocecal valve, the presence of concomitant disease, and the status of the colon and the residual functioning bowel.[9] It is critical that, following surgery, efforts must be directed to enhancing bowel adaptation and stabilizing immune function. With appropriate enteral feeding, enhancement of bowel adaptation occurs as a function of time, generally within 1 year of surgery.[10]

GENETICS, MICROBIOTA AND THE INTESTINAL IMMUNE SYSTEM

Irrespective of cause, SBS presents numerous challenges owing to the activity and periodic overgrowth of the intestinal microbiota, which results in ensuing malabsorption, metabolic and neurological decompensation, and immune dysregulation. The human microbiome consists of commensal bacteria, archaea, eukaryotes, and viruses,[11] but the overwhelming preponderance of organisms are bacteria, and they outnumber our own cells by a ratio of 10:1. Diversity estimates suggest an exponentially large number of genes associated with the microbiome as compared with the human genome.[12] Advances in sequencing and bioinformatics have made it possible to study the microbiome in the absence of laboratory culture, thereby obviating the introduction of fitness bias in sampling. This capability has expanded our ability to study the role of the human microbiota in both healthy and pathogenic states,[12–14] and it may now be possible to identify the role of the microbiota in immune function and its role in maintenance of health and in the development of disease.[15] Moreover, it holds the possibility that manipulation of the microbiome in the near future may open the door for dramatic changes in the treatment and prevention of inflammatory conditions of the GIT, as well as of the many other organ systems influenced by the GIT.

By far, the largest microbial community resides in the distal gut. Estimates from sequencing studies suggest the presence of up to 4000 microbial species in the GITs of healthy Western individuals comprising approximately 800,000 microbial genes.[16] The level of microbial diversity may be even higher in persons living in developing countries.[17] Many of these taxa are involved with housekeeping processes such as ATP synthesis and glycolysis, along with those more typically associated with functions of the GIT, including metabolism of complex sugars and vitamin processing.[12,18] Analyses of GI microbiota suggest that normal microbiota are more similar in monozygotic twins, and that microbiomes from family members appear to be more similar in nature than those of unrelated individuals. These trends appear to remain in place as familial and physical distance is attained.[17] It is not clear, however, what role genetics versus environment plays in these findings.

Interestingly, the human fetus develops within what is believed to be an essentially sterile environment, acquiring a microbiome that ultimately reaches 10^{14} total and diverse bacteria at equilibrium within 1–3 years of life.[19,20] Founder populations acquired at birth have been reported to differ, depending upon mode of delivery. As such, children delivered vaginally primarily acquire the maternal *Lactobacillus* and *Prevotella* species[21] encountered in the birth canal, whereas children born by C-section acquire skin-associated bacterial populations, including *Staphylococcus*, *Corynebacterium*, and *Propionibacterium* spp. from the host of individuals with whom these neonates are in contact. This early dichotomy may play a role in downstream pathogenic processes, as it has been reported that children born via C-section have a higher risk for a number of atopic diseases than children delivered vaginally.[22–24] These original exposures have powerful epigenetic consequences. Nonetheless, it is not hard to envision a time in the near future where the neonatal microbiome will be routinely profiled and adjusted to preclude development of a host of pathologies.

How then do these founder populations evolve into unique and diverse populations throughout the body, and what role does the microbiome play in the development of IBDs? As indicated above, initial populations of gastrointestinal bacteria evolve over the first 36 months of life and are likely influenced by changes in diet, environment, and health status. In fact, diet is likely to be a key determinant of the human microbiome. For instance, in a study of the first 2.5 years of life of a single child, Koenig et al.[25] report that introduction of a fully adult diet resulted in genetic changes within the microbiome associated with polysaccharide digestion and vitamin biosynthesis. Other class changes were observed coincident with changes from breast milk to formula and peas, and a change from formula to cow's milk. Studies of obesity and diabetes in mice and men suggest a preponderance of Firmicutes over Bacteroidetes in the gut.[26] IBDs, such as CD and UC, similarly perturb the microbiome, and the immunobiology of the GIT is inextricably linked to the microbiome.

The most widely held hypothesis on the pathogenesis of IBD is an overly aggressive immune response to a subset of commensal enteric bacteria in genetically susceptible hosts. To this end, it has been shown that macrophages and dendritic cells in the lamina propria are increased in absolute number, the production of proinflammatory cytokines and chemokines is enhanced, and the expression of adhesion molecules and costimulatory molecules is increased.[27,28]

While it is likely that inflammatory responses play a critical role in the pathogenesis of CD, the role of the intestinal microbiota in the development of disease is becoming increasingly apparent. As indicated above, the distal ileum and colon are colonized with extremely complex, metabolically active organisms. Genetic defects in mucosal barrier function lead to the increased presence of microbial antigens that overwhelm normal regulatory mechanisms.[29] It is likely that functional microbial alterations interact with host genetic defects to cause disease. There have been approximately 163 loci in genome-wide association studies (GWAS) with confirmed susceptibility to IBD, and 113 of these IBD loci are shared with other immune-mediated disorders, such as ankylosing spondylitis and psoriasis. A significant amount of evidence is now accumulating and directed toward the interaction of host defense and the dynamics of the intestinal microbiota.[30] Of importance, mutations in pattern recognition receptors including nucleotide-binding oligomerization domain 2/caspase recruitment domain 15 (NOD2/CARD 15) at the *IBD1* locus,[31–34] deleted in malignant brain tumors 1 (DMBT1),[35,36] and TLR4 have been identified in patients with CD. NOD2 belongs to the CED4/APAF1 superfamily of apoptosis regulators. The protein has two caspase recruitment domains (CARD), a nucleotide binding domain, and at its carboxy terminus, a leucine-rich region

(LRR) capable of binding bacterial lipopolysaccharide (LPS). Binding of the LRR to bacterial LPS can induce NF-κB expression in wild-type NOD2, but not in proteins bearing frameshift or missense mutations in the LRR of CD patients.[32] This aberrant NF-κB signaling has been postulated to result in attenuated expression of antibacterial factors via both innate and acquired immune pathways.[37–39] Similarly, DMBT1 has been linked to the suppression of LPS-induced TLR4 mediated NF-κB activation.[40] Together, these findings suggest that aberrant responses to resident flora may be involved in the development of gut lesions in CD.[30] These genetic mutations are likely only the first in a line of anomalies to be identified in CD and other IBD, with more to be discovered through further GWAS in additional populations.[41] Currently these are a set of loosely defined associations, but systems biology holds the promise that a clearer picture will emerge that will identify an era of personalized medical treatment.

PATHOPHYSIOLOGIC MECHANISMS AND APPLIED NUTRITION DIRECTIVES

The intestinal immune system, which is located in the lamina propria, comprises 60–70% of the complete human immune system. Food-derived antigens, commensal microbiota, and invasive pathogens, are continuously presented to the mucosal surface of the intestine, where there is a single layer of cells separating the potentially injurious contents in the bowel lumen from the intestinal immune system. Maintenance of gut mucosal integrity has been shown to be dependent on a number of peptide growth factors, one of which is the trefoil factor family (TFF). The major effect of TFF is elicited by rapid upregulation at sites of injury, where they contribute to early-phase repair and restitution of intestinal epithelia.[42] An in vivo study of transgenic overexpressed GH and wild-type mice, in which colitis was induced by exposure to dextran sodium sulfate (DSS), revealed that GH-enhanced mice achieved more rapid mucosal repair and remission of inflammation than did wild-type mice.[43] Interestingly, while tissue IGF-I levels were similar in both types of mice, the intestinal tissue levels of TF of the GH transgenic mice were significantly higher than the wild-type mice, suggesting that the reparative action of GH was probably mediated by enhancement of intestinal TF secretion. We have similarly hypothesized that administration of recombinant human GH (rhGH), in the presence of high protein nutrition, could repair damaged intestinal epithelium and restore the epithelial barrier in CD patients, thereby decreasing toxic luminal antigens reaching the mucosal immune system. In order to test this hypothesis, a 4-month placebo-controlled trial of rhGH in adult CD patients was undertaken, which demonstrated a significant improvement in rhGH-treated patients, manifested by a decrease in CD activity index (CDAI) and a decrease in the use of CD medications.[44] In this study, 13 of the 17 rhGH-treated patients went into remission, over a 4-month period, and all 13 patients remained in remission for at least a further 4 months after discontinuing rhGH. In contrast, there was no change in CDAI in the placebo-treated patients, none of whom went into remission. Similar findings were reported in juvenile CD patients by a randomized control trial of rhGH in 20 juvenile CD patients by Denson et al.[45] We believe this type of an approach justifies further research in CD patients to clarify whether GH may delay or reduce the extent of surgical intervention necessary in these patients. Administration of low-dose GH appears to enhance the beneficial action on intestinal repair of our exclusion diet and nutraceutical therapy in both juvenile and adult CD patients. How long GH therapy is necessary is not completely clear. We usually administer GH for 1–2 years in juvenile patients, where it is additionally beneficial for catch-up growth. In adult patients, we have administered GH, with subsequent colonoscopy evidence of epithelial repair of the distal ileum within 6–12 months, after which GH is discontinued. Our experience with the use of GH in SBS is limited to a few single cases, and in those patients, the response appeared to be less apparent. This may be due to the fact that parts of the ileum have been surgically removed, which is where GH appears to have its maximal reparative action.

Nonetheless, the onslaught of mucosal injury often results in the need for surgical intervention. The anatomical reduction of the microenvironment in SBS is such that the microbial content now proliferates in a significantly reduced area with less absorptive surface. In addition, the absence of the ileocecal valve permits proximal migration of anaerobic bacteria. The combination of these two factors throws the patient into a catastrophic state of dysregulation, which can result in anaerobic bacterial overgrowth and subsequent deconjugation of bile salts, leading to malabsorption, particularly of fat and fat-soluble vitamins and, secondarily, of minerals. It is, therefore, challenging to maintain the integrity of the remaining intestinal barrier construct, protect against harmful pathogens, and yet be able to provide tolerance to commensal bacteria and self-antigens.[46]

The adult small bowel ranges from 350 to 600 cm in length, and the adult colon is approximately 150 cm in length. A residual bowel of <200 cm in length is generally defined as SBS. But it is more than a reduction in length that is in play here. The absorptive surface area of a healthy small intestine is 250 m^2 or roughly the size of a tennis court. Losing one third to one half of that surface area is an almost overwhelming insult to the human body. Each section of the bowel has specific functions, and surgical resections will adversely affect those functions to varying degrees. In CD, it is not unusual to have multiple resections involving several regions of bowel, which can result in an outcome of mixed decompensations, such as rapid transit time, increased secretory activity, and pan-malabsorption of macronutrients, including protein, carbohydrates, fat, calcium, magnesium, and micronutrients such as iron, manganese, zinc, fluid, and electrolytes. Hepatopancreatobiliary abnormalities can occur over time as well as nephrolithiasis due to hyperoxaluria and disturbances in renal tubular management of citrate and magnesium.[47]

Given the enormous loss of absorptive surface, parenteral nutrition is most advisable during the immediate postoperative period. Subsequent management includes the provision of enteral feeding to facilitate bowel adaptation and introduction of measures to affect an increase in intestinal transit time. We have found it useful initially to take 500 mg of activated charcoal capsules 15 min before meals three times a day (t.i.d.) and 30 mg of codeine sulfate following meals t.i.d. Activated charcoal before meals and codeine taken after meals seem to provide a more comfortable change in transit time. Other antimotility agents, such as loperamide and diphenoxylate with atropine, and other opiates, such as paregoric and tincture of opium, may be of value, and their efficacy should be evaluated on a case-by-case basis. At this point, it is essential that sufficient vitamins and minerals are supplemented so as to compensate for any competing adsorption by activated charcoal. As bowel adaptation improves over time, it is possible to eliminate or reduce the quantity and frequency of charcoal and codeine administration. Activated charcoal also has the property of adsorbing bile salts in the setting of choleretic diarrhea.

Small quantities of apple pectin, 125 mg one to three times daily, can increase transit time and facilitate functional improvement of enterocytes and colonocytes.[48] Pectin is a soluble fiber that is transformed into butyrate by the bacteria of the microbiome,[49–51] which has been shown to have healing properties of colonocytes.[52] Another alternate strategy that has shown to be beneficial is the addition of peptides and amino acids in the form of Seacure (Proper Nutrition).[53] The use of 1000 mg Seacure 20 min before meals (a.c.) t.i.d. for approximately 30 days has been shown to significantly increase transit time and decrease the number of daily bowel movements. After 30 days, it is usually advisable to incrementally reduce the dose of Seacure, beginning with the lunchtime feeding, in order to optimize comfort and bowel function. Seacure appears to delay peristaltic activity quite effectively when administered according to the aforementioned dosage plan.

Glutamine is a nonessential amino acid that is the principle fuel of enterocytes and colonocytes, rendering it useful in the early stages of villous adaptation.[54] In SBS, there is also considerable loss of sodium in the bowel effluent, and glutamine may improve fluid and electrolyte absorption by facilitating sodium transport.[10] In our patients, we have found that 750 mg of glutamine twice a day (b.i.d.) between meals has been useful in delaying transit time. Digestion and absorption must optimally occur more rapidly in order to compensate for the rapid transit time. To that end, we have utilized plant-derived digestive enzymes (Maximizer, R-Garden) that are unaffected by the pH in the GIT and have shown to be of significant benefit. The dosage is one to four capsules, depending upon meal size, taken during the course of the meal.

Altering the inflammatory activity of source essential fatty acids in the intestinal tract should be thoughtfully considered. The GIT is normally in a state of inflammation, but the nature and balance are complex. Not all inflammation is equal, and there are a number of diseases where pathologies are the direct result of overactive or underactive inflammatory processes (reviewed in ref. 55). In our experience, many of the difficulties encountered in the field stem from a failure of therapists to recognize this basic immunologic distinction. We have found that an exclusion diet is supportive of this goal. In fact, the first step in successful management of the SBS patient is dietary exclusion. This is not only essential physiologically, but it has the added benefit of empowering the patient—excluding foods is perhaps the one thing that the patient can directly control. To this end, diminishing the intake of n-6 linoleic acid by excluding corn, soy, all grains except rice, grain-fed meats, and peanuts gradually limits the proinflammatory 2-series prostaglandins and 4-series leukotrienes/lipoxins, which occur during the desaturation and elongation of linoleic acid.[56] In contrast, increasing the alpha-linolenic acid content of the diet by including flax, canola, green vegetables, seafood, and fish oils gradually increases the D-series resolvins, protectins, and maresins, which promote an anti-inflammatory effect from the long-chain synthesis of n-3 polyunsaturated fatty acid.[56] Grain exclusion is of particular importance in the setting of CD, as patients with CD typically have antibodies (Abs) to α-mannose residues in cell wall mannans of *Saccharomyces cerevisiae*, or baker's yeast, and the presence of these Abs appears to track with disease severity.[57–59]

Exclusion of all milk products is also essential in IBDs. We have repeatedly seen a dramatically rapid and favorable clinical response within 4–5 days by complete restriction of all dairy. Whether there is a defect in the innate immune system or a cellular immune response leading to an increased absorption of antigenic milk proteins is not clear. What is clear is that it is not just lactose intolerance that is problematic, and in all of our patients, there is a prompt, consistent, and reproducible improvement in clinical symptomology by withholding all dairy products. Almond milk without added carrageenan (see below for a discussion of carrageenan) and rice milk are suitable substitutes for dairy and are readily available for consumers. Augmentation of higher quality protein can be accomplished with additional egg white protein. Rice-based amino acid chelated calcium (Miller Pharmacal) 280 mg t.i.d. after meals is also useful as a calcium supplement with improved absorption.[60]

Proximate living to a southern equatorial region appears to be inversely related to the increased incidence and frequency of CD suggesting a possible role for vitamin D in immune function, and vitamin D deficiency occurs frequently in IBD and SBS.[30] Vitamin D is an extremely important modulator of gene expression in immune function, and it has been shown that there is an inverse relationship between 25-hydroxycholecalciferol and disease activity in CD.[61] Gene expression analyses have confirmed that there are significant nonskeletal health benefits with respect to vitamin D sufficiency. In a recent study by Hossein-Nezhad et al.[62] 291 genes were identified with vitamin D activity, and their biologic functions were observed to be associated with 160 pathways associated with autoimmune diseases, infectious diseases, cardiovascular disease, and cancer. It has been our observation that CD and SBS patients are frequently deficient in vitamin D, and that their requirement is greater than the RDA range as currently recommended. It is our practice to determine optimal dose of vitamin D by establishing baseline levels without any supplement for several days prior to the test, and then to repeat the test in 3–4 months following administration of vitamin D_3 in the range of 2000–5000 IU/day. In some instances of SBS, it may be necessary to advise 10,000 IU for 5 days per week and 5000 IU for 2 days per week until a 25-hydroxycholecalciferol above 40 ng/mL is achieved. Thereafter, a daily dose of 2000–5000 IU of vitamin D_3 can be instituted for maintenance. Follow-up blood studies for 25-hydroxycholecalciferol are advisable every 3–4 months until the target value is achieved and maintained. In our experience, CD and SBS are conditions requiring greater vitamin D sufficiency rather than a low normal value, i.e., 32 ng/mL.

Water-soluble B-complex vitamins and vitamin C should be supplemented daily, particularly if there is significant jejunal resection. We have utilized a complete B-complex in the 25-mg dose range once daily and vitamin C at 250 mg twice daily in our patient population. As vitamin B_{12} is absorbed in the ileum, resections of the ileum will require lifetime supplementation of 1000 µg either by the intramuscular route monthly or as a daily 5000-mg microsublingual supplementation with confirmation of absorption by periodic follow-up laboratory evaluation. Deficiencies of the fat-soluble vitamins A, D, E, and K do occur and should be supplemented daily, as fat malabsorption can be significant in SBS and CD. Periodic follow-up reevaluation of fat-soluble vitamin blood levels is advisable.[1]

Bacterial overgrowth is a recurring issue in SBS and is preferably managed with antibiotics and probiotics. In our experience, ciprofloxacin and/or metronidazole are the antibiotics of choice. MG (author) has utilized a plan for antibiosis that has been effective for over 25 years: ciprofloxacin 500 mg b.i.d. for 3 days only, taken at the beginning of each cycle of bacterial overgrowth. Until such time as the technology and scientific knowledge allow for individual probiotic regimens to be devised, we have found that Lactobacillus GG (Culturelle) without inulin twice weekly on a regular basis is a satisfactory dose. This plan has increased the time interval between episodes of bacterial overgrowth to an 8-week cycle limiting the frequency and need for microbial reduction. D-lactic acid encephalopathy can occur with bacterial overgrowth, and the aforementioned plan is a viable management strategy.[63]

In our clinical experience, elimination of all carrageenan is also an essential nutrition directive in this setting. High molecular weight (>100 kDa) carrageenan (CGN), a sulfated polysaccharide extracted from red algae (*Rhodophyceae*), has become ubiquitous in the food chain since the proliferation of low-fat food products. It is used as a thickener and an emulsifying agent that imparts a fat-like texture to foods, and it is estimated that the average human consumption of carrageenan is approximately 250 mg/day.[64] Acid treatment triggers CGN hydrolysis to the lower molecular weight (<50 kDa) poligeenan and/or degraded CGN (dCGN). These low molecular weight CGN derivatives are routinely used to generate animal models of IBD,[65–70] and it has been postulated that similar hydrolysis of food-grade high molecular weight CGN can occur during gastric digestion.[71,72] While the EU has banned the use of CGN in infant formula, US policy promotes its use in infant formula as an emulsifying agent to produce a more uniform product (reviewed in refs. 73 and 74). Although the safety of CGN in human food supply remains a contentious issue,[73,74] Tobacman has reported the harmful proinflammatory effects of carrageenan in vitro and in vivo using both low molecular weight and native high molecular weight CGN.[64,73,75–81] Among the most salient findings of these studies are data supporting CGN-mediated inflammation and apoptosis via increased activation of TNF-α, which in turn stimulates an inflammatory cascade by upregulating the noncanonical pathway of NF-κB, the nuclear transcription factor for inflammation.[77,80,81] This is significant not only in the promotion of inflammation but also potentially in limiting the effectiveness of TNF-α biological response modifiers (BRMs). Similarly, End et al.[36] report that CGN may directly impact DMBT1-mediated innate mucosal immune functions and/or homeostatic processes.

Hepatic steatosis, cholestasis, cholelithiasis, and hepatic fibrosis are common conditions occurring, particularly in the setting of parenteral nutrition. Early enteral feeding and judicious use of medium-chain triglycerides, omega-3 fatty acid supplementation, and ursodeoxycholic acid may be used to advantage in managing cholestasis.[82] Curcumin, one of the principal therapeutic substances in the spice turmeric, has anticholestatic, anti-inflammatory, and antifibrotic activity.[63,83–86] However, its activity in cholangiopathies is unknown. It has, however, demonstrated a favorable effect upon activating PPARγ in cholangiocytes in vitro and inhibition of ERK1/2 signaling in portal myofibroblasts in the mouse model.[85] We have leveraged simple approaches such as 500 mg curcumin 95 (Jarrow) two to three times daily mid-meal to reduce the inflammatory potential of some foods and microparticles added to food during processing. NF-κB is the genetic nuclear transcription factor for regulating the inflammatory response. It is well documented in the literature that curcumin's anti-inflammatory activity intervenes in the upregulation of NF-κB by modulating the magnitude of cytoplasmic translocation of NF-κB into the nuclear locus. In addition, curcumin downregulates proinflammatory cytokines and enzymes, such as cyclooxygenase 2, 5-lipoxygenase, and TNF-α, which are involved in neoplastic, cardiovascular, neurodegenerative, pulmonary, and metabolic disorders.[84,86,87] In addition, over time, curcumin has the functional property of increasing transit time by slowing peristaltic activity. In some instances, such as in choleretic diarrhea, 500 mg once daily with Seacure 1000 mg 20 min before meals will provide a balance of benefit. Cholestyramine is also of use in the setting of choleric diarrhea.[63]

Importantly, it is not only the GI system that is perturbed in the setting of SBS. It is at this point when one enters the realm of daily management of a patient. Every action has a reaction, and the consequences may be disproportional to the smallest dietary decision. It is our opinion that a certified clinical nutrition specialist should be a critical member of the management team. Documented calcium oxalate nephrolithiasis is common and can be managed by the use of per-oral amino acid chelated magnesium, 50–75 mg b.i.d., and magnesium citrate, 200–400 mg t.i.d. (22–44 mg magnesium and 178–356 mg citrate), each form titrated until urinary excretion of citrate and magnesium is within effective inhibitory levels.[88] If adequate attention is given to increasing transit time, careful titration of magnesium and citrate should not result in increased bowel frequency. All other factors influencing stone formation, such as 24-h urinary calcium, oxalate, phosphorus, sodium, potassium, uric acid, pH, and volume, should be assessed to address stone-forming and crystal-inhibiting elements. It is also advisable to take a calcium carbonate supplement, such as 280 mg of chelated amino acid rice-based calcium (Miller Pharmacal) t.i.d. with meals to bind oxalate locally in the bowel. In addition to being a reliable calcium source as indicated above, this will also facilitate an increase in bowel transit time. Calcium oxalate formed in the bowel is a large molecule and not easily absorbed, whereas free oxalate in the bowel is readily absorbed and then binds with calcium in the renal system to form calcium oxalate calculi. As such, provision of exogenous calcium can serve to bind up excess oxalate thereby decreasing the risk of formation of calcium oxalate renal calculi.

Hepatopancreatobiliary abnormalities in the setting of malabsorption secondary to SBS and/or CD can occur owing to deficiencies of protein, essential fatty acids, choline, and vitamin E absorption, relapsing intestinal bacterial overgrowth and decreased effectiveness of pancreatic enzyme activity due to gastric hypersecretion. IBD, particularly UC, is a significant risk factor for primary sclerosing cholangitis (PSC). While it does occur in CD, it is much less common than in UC. One should have an index of suspicion with a reported elevated alkaline phosphatase as this may be the only laboratory indicator of PSC.[89]

There are several food selection and preparation issues causing increased diarrhea in SBS beside bowel length, and they are extremely important in this setting. Any food high in water-insoluble fiber, such as wheat bran, will result in shorter transit time and create more diarrhea. Foods, such as eggplant, mushrooms, and celery will also result in added bowel dysfunction and could promote the development of a fiber bezoar. Fat intake should be kept low in order to limit choleric diarrhea. High sugar content and hypertonic fluids can result in osmotic diarrhea and therefore should be limited in content and dilute in form. A most common cause of this is increased intake of foods and beverages with high content of high fructose corn syrup. Drinking the majority of fluids *between* meals rather than at meals will avoid a dumping syndrome, which interferes with maximal digestion and absorption of nutrients and also promotes diarrhea.

Vegetables should and can be included in the diet of an individual with SBS. An appropriate way to eat vegetables is to steam them until soft so that the fiber content is greatly reduced. Boiling is never a recommended method as essential water-soluble vitamins will be lost during cooking. If this is unsatisfactory in any given patient, one should consider pureeing after steaming or try juice extraction of even raw vegetables, but in normal portion sizes *only*. For instance, if a single carrot and a handful of lettuce comprise a salad, then this is what should go into the juicer. If pureeing, one can add back small portions of the water in which the vegetables were steamed to retain the heat-stable nutrients that may be lost during steaming. Frequent small feedings are generally more advisable than the traditional three meals daily. Fruits are best-cooked, pureed, and eaten in small quantities. Over time, with thoughtful eating of nutrient dense foods throughout the lifecycle, one can achieve comfort and homeostasis living with the SBS.

CONCLUSION

The surface area of the normal human GIT is enormous, approaching approximately 400 m² in size. The GIT is colonized by an extensive array of bacteria, yeast, and viruses, all of which are separated from the blood by a single layer of columnar epithelium. Moreover, the GIT is the largest immuno-logic organ in the body. By design, the GIT exists in a constant state of physiologic inflammation. Inflammation is, however, a double-edged sword. On one hand, we need inflammatory processes to protect against disease. On the other hand, there are an ever-growing number of pathogenic condi-tions that arise due to an inability to keep the inflammatory process in check. Genetic and epigenetic factors often converge to disrupt this delicate balance, resulting, among other things, in an array of IBDs. CD is one such multifactorial IBD with potentially life-threatening consequences. Severely decompensated CD can, and often does, necessitate repeated bowel resections that ultimately lead to the development of SBS. Patients with SBS routinely lose over one third of the surface area of their GIT. As such, living as a patient with SBS requires a sophisticated global understanding of the perturbed and complex human physiology that seriously impacts daily living and adversely affects quality of life.

Over an 11-year period, we have demonstrated that there are multimodal applied nutrition direc-tives that can favorably alter the outcome of living with CD and SBS. Our experience with the exclusion diet and nutraceutical interventions described in this chapter have led us to recognize that these nutrition-based principles are critical for the survival of patients living with SBS. Moreover, we hypothesize that early interventions can result in a significant reduction in size and number of necessary bowel resections. In other words, it is our contention that the guidance laid out here has a role both in management of postsurgical SBS and in potentially decreasing the need for surgical interventions precipitating SBS.

We have repeatedly seen many of the postsurgical interventions outlined here, primarily the elimination of dairy, corn, all grains (except rice), carrageenan, and other proinflammatory foods (such as soy and peanuts) that promote healing of the GIT. It is our belief that we have treated a number of patients over the years for which this intervention may have obviated the need for addi-tional surgeries. We know too much to make it acceptable any longer to advise patients to "eat what you like as long as it does not bother you." This doctrine has, in the past, inadvertently led to many unintended consequences. It is clearly inconsistent with the newly evolving paradigm of promoting a scientifically personalized approach to the management of health and modulation of disease.

REFERENCES

1. Chouraki, V. et al. The changing pattern of Crohn's disease incidence in northern France: A continuing increase in the 10- to 19-year-old age bracket (1988–2007). *Alimentary Pharmacology & Therapeutics* **33**, 1133–1142 (2011).
2. Kugathasan, S. et al. Epidemiologic and clinical characteristics of children with newly diagnosed inflam-matory bowel disease in Wisconsin: A statewide population-based study. *The Journal of Pediatrics* **143**, 525–531 (2003).
3. Sauer, C.G. & Kugathasan, S. Pediatric inflammatory bowel disease: Highlighting pediatric differences in IBD. *Gastroenterology Clinics of North America* **38**, 611–628 (2009).
4. Walters, T.D. & Griffiths, A.M. Mechanisms of growth impairment in pediatric Crohn's disease. *Nature Reviews Gastroenterology & Hepatology* **6**, 513–523 (2009).
5. Pfefferkorn, M. et al. Growth abnormalities persist in newly diagnosed children with Crohn disease despite current treatment paradigms. *Journal of Pediatric Gastroenterology and Nutrition* **48**, 168–174 (2009).
6. Baert, F. et al. Influence of immunogenicity on the long-term efficacy of infliximab in Crohn's disease. *The New England Journal of Medicine* **348**, 601–608 (2003).
7. Donovan, M., Lunney, K., Carter-Pokras, O. & Cross, R.K. Prescribing patterns and awareness of adverse effects of infliximab: A health survey of gastroenterologists. *Digestive Diseases and Sciences* **52**, 1798–1805 (2007).
8. Ukleja, A., Scolapio, J.S. & Buchman, A.L. Nutritional management of short bowel syndrome. *Seminars in Gastrointestinal Disease* **13**, 161–168 (2002).
9. Solhaug, J.H. & Tvete, S. Adaptive changes in the small intestine following bypass operation for obesity. A radiological and histological study. *Scandinavian Journal of Gastroenterology* **13**, 401–408 (1978).

10. Sundaram, A., Koutkia, P. & Apovian, C.M. Nutritional management of short bowel syndrome in adults. *Journal of Clinical Gastroenterology* **34**, 207–220 (2002).
11. Turnbaugh, P.J. et al. The human microbiome project. *Nature* **449**, 804–810 (2007).
12. Qin, J. et al. A human gut microbial gene catalogue established by metagenomic sequencing. *Nature* **464**, 59–65 (2010).
13. Ley, R.E., Turnbaugh, P.J., Klein, S. & Gordon, J.I. Microbial ecology: Human gut microbes associated with obesity. *Nature* **444**, 1022–1023 (2006).
14. Gill, S.R. et al. Metagenomic analysis of the human distal gut microbiome. *Science* **312**, 1355–1359 (2006).
15. Jeffery, I.B. & O'Toole, P.W. Diet-microbiota interactions and their implications for healthy living. *Nutrients* **5**, 234–252 (2013).
16. Human Microbiome Project Consortium. A framework for human microbiome research. *Nature* **486**, 215–221 (2012).
17. Yatsunenko, T. et al. Human gut microbiome viewed across age and geography. *Nature* **486**, 222–227 (2012).
18. Arumugam, M. et al. Enterotypes of the human gut microbiome. *Nature* **473**, 174–180 (2011).
19. Adlerberth, I. & Wold, A.E. Establishment of the gut microbiota in Western infants. *Acta Paediatrica* **98**, 229–238 (2009).
20. Vael, C., Verhulst, S.L., Nelen, V., Goossens, H. & Desager, K.N. Intestinal microflora and body mass index during the first three years of life: An observational study. *Gut Pathogens* **3**, 8 (2011).
21. Dominguez-Bello, M.G., Blaser, M.J., Ley, R.E. & Knight, R. Development of the human gastrointestinal microbiota and insights from high-throughput sequencing. *Gastroenterology* **140**, 1713–1719 (2011).
22. Adlerberth, I. et al. Gut microbiota and development of atopic eczema in 3 European birth cohorts. *The Journal of Allergy and Clinical Immunology* **120**, 343–350 (2007).
23. Bisgaard, H. et al. Reduced diversity of the intestinal microbiota during infancy is associated with increased risk of allergic disease at school age. *The Journal of Allergy and Clinical Immunology* **128**, 646–652, e641–e645 (2011).
24. van Nimwegen, F.A. et al. Mode and place of delivery, gastrointestinal microbiota, and their influence on asthma and atopy. *The Journal of Allergy and Clinical Immunology* **128**, 948–955, e941–e943 (2011).
25. Koenig, J.E. et al. Succession of microbial consortia in the developing infant gut microbiome. *Proceedings of the National Academy of Sciences of the United States of America* **108**, Suppl 1, 4578–4585 (2011).
26. Ley, R.E. Obesity and the human microbiome. *Current Opinion in Gastroenterology* **26**, 5–11 (2010).
27. Sartor, R.B. Mechanisms of disease: Pathogenesis of Crohn's disease and ulcerative colitis. *Nature Clinical Practice Gastroenterology & Hepatology* **3**, 390–407 (2006).
28. Sartor, R.B. Key questions to guide a better understanding of host–commensal microbiota interactions in intestinal inflammation. *Mucosal Immunology* **4**, 127–132 (2011).
29. Shanahan, F. The colonic microbiota and colonic disease. *Current Gastroenterology Reports* **14**, 446–452 (2012).
30. Jostins, L. et al. Host-microbe interactions have shaped the genetic architecture of inflammatory bowel disease. *Nature* **491**, 119–124 (2012).
31. Pascoe, L., Zouali, H., Sahbatou, M. & Hugot, J.-P. Estimating the odds ratios of Crohn disease for the main CARD15/NOD2 mutations using a conditional maximum likelihood method in pedigrees collected via affected family members. *European Journal of Human Genetics* **15**, 864–871 (2007).
32. Hugot, J.P. et al. Association of NOD2 leucine-rich repeat variants with susceptibility to Crohn's disease. *Nature* **411**, 599–603 (2001).
33. Ogura, Y. et al. A frameshift mutation in NOD2 associated with susceptibility to Crohn's disease. *Nature* **411**, 603–606 (2001).
34. Hampe, J. et al. Association between insertion mutation in NOD2 gene and Crohn's disease in German and British populations. *The Lancet* **357**, 1925–1928 (2001).
35. Renner, M. et al. DMBT1 confers mucosal protection in vivo and a deletion variant is associated with Crohn's disease. *Gastroenterology* **133**, 1499–1509 (2007).
36. End, C. et al. DMBT1 functions as pattern-recognition molecule for poly-sulfated and poly-phosphory-lated ligands. *European Journal of Immunology* **39**, 833–842 (2009).
37. Kobayashi, K.S. Nod2-dependent regulation of innate and adaptive immunity in the intestinal tract. *Science* **307**, 731–734 (2005).
38. Maeda, S. Nod2 mutation in Crohn's disease potentiates NF-κB activity and IL-1 processing. *Science* **307**, 734–738 (2005).

39. Strober, W. & Watanabe, T. NOD2, an intracellular innate immune sensor involved in host defense and Crohn's disease. *Mucosal Immunology* **4**, 484–495 (2011).
40. Rosenstiel, P. et al. Regulation of DMBT1 via NOD2 and TLR4 in intestinal epithelial cells modulates bacterial recognition and invasion. *Journal of Immunology (Baltimore, MD: 1950)* **178**, 8203–8211 (2007).
41. Graham, D.B. & Xavier, R.J. From genetics of inflammatory bowel disease towards mechanistic insights. *Trends in Immunology* **34**, 371–378 (2013).
42. Playford, R.J. & Ghosh, S. What is the role of growth factors in IBD? *Inflammatory Bowel Diseases* **14**, Suppl 2, S119–S120 (2008).
43. Williams, K.L. et al. Enhanced survival and mucosal repair after dextran sodium sulfate-induced colitis in transgenic mice that overexpress growth hormone. *Gastroenterology* **120**, 925–937 (2001).
44. Slonim, A.E. et al. A preliminary study of growth hormone therapy for Crohn's disease. *The New England Journal of Medicine* **342**, 1633–1637 (2000).
45. Denson, L.A. et al. A randomized controlled trial of growth hormone in active pediatric Crohn disease. *Journal of Pediatric Gastroenterology and Nutrition* **51**, 130–139 (2010).
46. Rankin, L. et al. The transcription factor T-bet is essential for the development of NKp46(+) innate lymphocytes via the notch pathway. *Nature Immunology* **14**, 877 (2013).
47. Barksdale, E.M. & Stanford, A. The surgical management of short bowel syndrome. *Current Gastroenterology Reports* **4**, 229–237 (2002).
48. Spiller, G.A. et al. Effect of purified cellulose, pectin, and a low-residue diet on fecal volatile fatty acids, transit time, and fecal weight in humans. *The American Journal of Clinical Nutrition* **33**, 754–759 (1980).
49. Koropatkin, N.M., Cameron, E.A. & Martens, E.C. How glycan metabolism shapes the human gut microbiota. *Nature Reviews Microbiology* **10**, 323–335 (2012).
50. Waldecker, M. et al. Histone-deacetylase inhibition and butyrate formation: Fecal slurry incubations with apple pectin and apple juice extracts. *Nutrition* **24**, 366–374 (2008).
51. Willing, B.P., Gill, N. & Finlay, B.B. The role of the immune system in regulating the microbiota. *Gut Microbes* **1**, 213–223 (2010).
52. Velazquez, O.C., Lederer, H.M. & Rombeau, J.L. Butyrate and the colonocyte. Production, absorption, metabolism, and therapeutic implications. *Advances in Experimental Medicine and Biology* **427**, 123–134 (1997).
53. Delfino, A. BPC: A fish protein concentrate for human consumption. In Santos, W. (ed.), *Nutrition and Food Science: Present Knowledge and Utilization*, Vol. 2, 249–267, Plenum Press, New York (1980).
54. Wu, G. Functional amino acids in nutrition and health. *Amino Acids* **45**, 407–411 (2013).
55. Senovilla, L., Galluzzi, L., Zitvogel, L. & Kroemer, G. Immunosurveillance as a regulator of tissue homeostasis. *Trends in Immunology* **34**, 47–481 (2013).
56. Lopez, H.L. Nutritional interventions to prevent and treat osteoarthritis. Part I: Focus on fatty acids and macronutrients. *PM & R: The Journal of Injury, Function, and Rehabilitation* **4**, S145–S154 (2012).
57. Main, J. et al. Antibody to saccharomyces cerevisiae (bakers' yeast) in Crohn's disease. *BMJ (Clinical Research Ed.)* **297**, 1105–1106 (1988).
58. Sendid, B. et al. Specific antibody response to oligomannosidic epitopes in Crohn's disease. *Clinical and Diagnostic Laboratory Immunology* **3**, 219–226 (1996).
59. Walker, L.J. et al. Anti-saccharomyces cerevisiae antibodies (ASCA) in Crohn's disease are associated with disease severity but not NOD2/CARD15 mutations. *Clinical and Experimental Immunology* **135**, 490–496 (2004).
60. Lerner, A., Rossi, T.M., Park, B., Albini, B. & Lebenthal, E. Serum antibodies to cow's milk proteins in pediatric inflammatory bowel disease. Crohn's disease versus ulcerative colitis. *Acta Paediatrica Scandinavica* **78**, 384–389 (1989).
61. Jorgensen, S.P. et al. Active Crohn's disease is associated with low vitamin D levels. *Journal of Crohn's & Colitis* **7**, 407–413 (2013).
62. Hossein-Nezhad, A., Spira, A. & Holick, M.F. Influence of vitamin D status and vitamin D3 supplementation on genome wide expression of white blood cells: A randomized double-blind clinical trial. *PLoS ONE* **8**, e58725 (2013).
63. Slonim, A.E., Grovit, M. & Bulone, L. Effect of exclusion diet with nutraceutical therapy in juvenile Crohn's disease. *Journal of the American College of Nutrition* **28**, 277–285 (2009).
64. Yang, B., Bhattacharyya, S., Linhardt, R. & Tobacman, J. Exposure to common food additive carrageenan leads to reduced sulfatase activity and increase in sulfated glycosaminoglycans in human epithelial cells. *Biochimie* **94**, 1309–1316 (2012).

65. Al-Suhail, A.A., Reid, P.E., Culling, C.F., Dunn, W.L. & Clay, M.G. Studies of the degraded carrageenan-induced colitis of rabbits. I. Changes in the epithelial glycoprotein O-acylated sialic acids associated with ulceration. *The Histochemical Journal* **16**, 543–553 (1984).

66. Oestreicher, P., Nielsen, S.T. & Rainsford, K.D. Inflammatory bowel disease induced by combined bacterial immunization and oral carrageenan in guinea pigs. Model development, histopathology, and effects of sulfasalazine. *Digestive Diseases and Sciences* **36**, 461–470 (1991).

67. Kitano, A. et al. Multifunctional effects of anticomplementary agent K-76 on carrageenan-induced colitis in the rabbit. *Clinical and Experimental Immunology* **94**, 348–353 (1993).

68. Marcus, A.J. Colonic mucosal lymphoid hyperplasia and aphthoid ulcers in Crohn's disease. *Clinical Radiology* **52**, 480–481 (1997).

69. Noa, M. & Mas, R. Effect of D-002 on the pre-ulcerative phase of carrageenan-induced colonic ulceration in the guinea-pig. *The Journal of Pharmacy and Pharmacology* **50**, 549–553 (1998).

70. Benard, C. et al. Degraded carrageenan causing colitis in rats induces TNF secretion and ICAM-1 upregulation in monocytes through NF-κB activation. *PLoS ONE* **5**, e8666 (2010).

71. Ekstrom, L., Kuivinemn, J. & Johanasson, G. Molecular weight distribution and hydrolysis behaviour of carrageenans. *Carbohydrate Research* **116**, 89–94 (1983).

72. Ekstrom, L. Molecular-weight distribution and the behaviour of kappa carrageenan on hydrolysis. *Carbohydrate Research* **135**, 283–289 (1985).

73. Tobacman, J.K., Bhattacharyya, S., Borthakur, A. & Dudeja, P.K. The carrageenan diet: Not recommended. *Science* **321**, 1040–1041 (2008).

74. Cohen, S.M. & Ito, N. Critical review of the toxicological effects of carrageenan and processed eucheuma seaweed on the gastrointestinal tract. *Critical Reviews in Toxicology* **32**, 413–444 (2002).

75. Tobacman, J.K. Review of harmful gastrointestinal effects of carrageenan in animal experiments. *Environmental Health Perspectives* **109**, 983–994 (2001).

76. Yu, G. et al. Structural studies on kappa-carrageenan derived oligosaccharides. *Carbohydrate Research* **337**, 433–440 (2002).

77. Bhattacharyya, S., Dudeja, P. & Tobacman, J. Carrageenan-induced NFκB activation depends on distinct pathways mediated by reactive oxygen species and Hsp27 or by Bcl10. *Biochimica et Biophysica Acta (BBA)—General Subjects* **1780**, 973–982 (2008).

78. Bhattacharyya, S., Borthakur, A., Dudeja, P.K. & Tobacman, J.K. Carrageenan induces cell cycle arrest in human intestinal epithelial cells in vitro. *The Journal of Nutrition* **138**, 469–475 (2008).

79. Bhattacharyya, S. et al. Carrageenan-induced innate immune response is modified by enzymes that hydrolyze distinct galactosidic bonds. *The Journal of Nutritional Biochemistry* **21**, 906–913 (2010).

80. Bhattacharyya, S., Dudeja, P.K. & Tobacman, J.K. Tumor necrosis factor-induced inflammation is increased but apoptosis is inhibited by common food additive carrageenan. *Journal of Biological Chemistry* **285**, 39511–39522 (2010).

81. Borthakur, A. et al. Prolongation of carrageenan-induced inflammation in human colonic epithelial cells by activation of an NFκB-BCL10 loop. *Biochimica et Biophysica Acta (BBA)—Molecular Basis of Disease* **1822**, 1300–1307 (2012).

82. Kelly, D.A. Preventing parenteral nutrition liver disease. *Early Human Development* **86**, 683–687 (2010).

83. Maheshwari, R.K., Singh, A.K., Gaddipati, J. & Srimal, R.C. Multiple biological activities of curcumin: A short review. *Life Sciences* **78**, 2081–2087 (2006).

84. Aggarwal, B.B. & Sung, B. Pharmacological basis for the role of curcumin in chronic diseases: An age-old spice with modern targets. *Trends in Pharmacological Sciences* **30**, 85–94 (2009).

85. Baghdasaryan, A. et al. Curcumin improves sclerosing cholangitis in Mdr2-/- mice by inhibition of cholangiocyte inflammatory response and portal myofibroblast proliferation. *Gut* **59**, 521–530 (2010).

86. Shehzad, A., Rehman, G. & Lee, Y.S. Curcumin in inflammatory diseases. *BioFactors* **39**, 69–77 (2013).

87. Ali, T., Shakir, F. & Morton, J. Curcumin and inflammatory bowel disease: Biological mechanisms and clinical implication. *Digestion* **85**, 249–255 (2012).

88. Rudman, D. et al. Hypocitraturia in patients with gastrointestinal malabsorption. *The New England Journal of Medicine* **303**, 657–661 (1980).

89. Eaton, J.E., Talwalkar, J.A., Lazaridis, K.N., Gores, G.J. & Lindor, K.D. Pathogenesis of primary sclerosing cholangitis and advances in diagnosis and management. *Gastroenterology* **145**, 521–536 (2013).

Section IV

A Nutritional Relationship to Neurological Diseases

27 Neurological Disease of Metabolism

Guha K. Venkatraman

CONTENTS

INTRODUCTION

The purpose of this chapter is to provide a basic introduction to neurometabolic diseases that are present in the newborn or later in life. The term "neurometabolic diseases" encompasses inborn errors of metabolism, disorders of neural function, and genetic disorders of developmental neural topography. This chapter is structured to assist those who care for pediatric or adult patients who are suspected of suffering from metabolic neurological disorders.

I will strive to highlight recognition of symptoms and signs of neurometabolic disease, initiation of appropriate workup, and the ability to collaborate with metabolists and geneticists. Intricate details of biochemical pathophysiology, metabolic management, and genetic diagnosis are beyond the scope of this chapter. Additionally, individual disorders of organic acids, amino acids, the urea cycle, peroxisomal and mitochondrial disorders are not discussed in a detailed manner. These topics deserve detailed discussion for those with expertise in caring for such diseases.

The known neurometabolic diseases can be grouped into at least five categories for the ease of classification, clinical identification, and management. These categories include small molecule diseases, large molecule diseases, other neurogenetic disorders, leukodystrophies, and etiologies of neurodegeneration. Some experts consider hereditary ataxias to be neurometabolic diseases. However, not all of these disorders are involved in or affected by metabolism. Those disorders that continue into adulthood are summarized in Table 27.1, and those that may have adult onset are listed in Table 27.2.

TABLE 27.1
Neurological Disorders of Metabolism That Continue into Adulthood

Disease	Clinical Features
GM1 gangliosidosis	Extrapyramidal signs, vertebral defects, psychosis
GM2 gangliosidosis (Tay Sach's and Sandhoff's disease)	Cerebellar degeneration, lower motor neuron disease, atypical amyotropic lateral sclerosis
Gaucher's disease type III	Atypical amyotropic lateral sclerosis
Fabry's disease	Peripheral neuropathy, renal failure, cardiac abnormalities, myopathy
Metachromatic leukodystrophy	Cognitive function defects, neuropathies and myopathies, leukodystrophy
Krabbe's leukodystrophy	Hemiparesis, leukodystrophy, pes cavus deformity
Niemann–Pick's disease	Ataxia, dysarthria, dysphagia, basal ganglia abnormalities
Arginase deficiency	Disorientation, coma
Citrullinemia	Coma, restlessness
Hartnup's disease	Skin rash, dementia, ataxia
Homocystinuria (classic)	Cerebrovascular disease, displaced intraocular lens, osteoporosis
Homocystinuria (remethylation defect)	Paresthesia, limb weakness, mental retardation
Ornithine transcarbamylase deficiency	Comatose episodes, sleep disorders
Fatty acid oxidation defects	Liver disease, cardiomyopathy, fatigue
Glutaric aciduria	Reye-like syndrome, dystonia
Propionic acidemia	Chorea, basal ganglia defects
X-linked adrenoleukodystrophy	Ataxia, Addison's disease, dementia, peripheral neuropathy
Alexander disease	Megalencephaly, fetal neurodegeneration, dementia, spasticity
mtDNA encoded electron transport disease	NARP, MELAS, MERRF, Kearns–Sayre syndrome, LHON
Nuclear DNA encoded electron transport disease	Myopathy
Mitochondrial myopathy, encephalopathy with lactic acidemia, and stroke-like episodes (MELAS)	Seizures, developmental delay, sensorineural hearing loss ± diabetes mellitus
Urea cycle defects	Postprandial vomiting, coma, confusion
Porphyria	Limb, neck, or chest pain, muscle weakness, abdominal pain, photosensitivity
Wilson's disease	Kayser–Fleischer rings ± liver disease, dysarthria, loss of coordination, pseudobulbar palsy, parkinsonian features
Cerebrotendinous xanthomatosis	Spasticity, cataracts, tendon xanthomas
Niemann–Pick disease type C	Psychomotor retardation leading to dementia ataxia with dystonia, vertical supranuclear ophthalmoplegia
Oculocutaneous albinism	Pale complexion, blue eyes
Refsum's disease	Peripheral neuropathy, retinitis pigmentosa, cerebellar ataxia
Mucolipidosis type I	Sialidosis type I: visual defect with lens or corneal opacity, ataxia, myoclonus, generalized seizures sometimes with nystagmus, ataxia, dementia ± cherry red spot
	Sialidosis type II: myoclonus, blindness, cherry red spot, dysmorphic features, angiokeratoma
Tyrosinemia type II	Cataracts, skin lesions, slight developmental delay
Pyridoxine-dependent seizures	Persistent seizures responsive to pyridoxine
Electron transport chain disorders	Any combination of symptoms

TABLE 27.2
Neurological Disorders of Metabolism That May Start in Adulthood

Disease	Clinical Features
Fabry's disease	Peripheral neuropathy, renal failure, cardiac abnormalities, myopathy
Metachromatic leukodystrophy	Cognitive function defects, neuropathies and myopathies, leukodystrophy
Homocystinuria (classic)	Cerebrovascular disease, displaced intraocular lens, osteoporosis
Tyrosinemia type II	Cataracts, skin lesions, slight developmental delay
5-Oxoprolinuria	Mental impairment, dysarthria, ataxia, intermittent acidosis, hemolytic anemia with febrile illness
Porphyria (all except porphyria cutanea tarda)	Limb, neck, or chest pain, muscle weakness, abdominal pain, photosensitivity
Fatty acid oxidation defects	Liver disease, cardiomyopathy, fatigue
X-linked adrenoleukodystrophy	Ataxia, Addison's disease, dementia, peripheral neuropathy
Alexander disease	Dementia, spasticity
Mitochondrial encephalomyopathy	Mild mental retardation, early dementia, seizure-like episodes, stroke-like episodes, peripheral neuropathy, myopathy
Wilson's disease	Kayser–Fleischer rings ± liver disease, dysarthria, loss of coordination, pseudobulbar palsy, parkinsonian features
Cerebrotendinous xanthomatosis	Spasticity, cataracts, tendon xanthomas
Lafora polyglucosan body disease (also in adolescence)	Myoclonic epilepsy and dementia
Glycogen storage diseases (adult-onset acid maltase deficiency and branched-chain dehydrogenase deficiency)	Myopathy

SMALL MOLECULE DISORDERS

Small molecule diseases are best classified by identifying the underlying dysfunctional food groups. In this category of illnesses, we screen for the metabolites and manage the corresponding nutrient intake. Generally, small molecule diseases affect enzymes in pathways of intermediary metabolism. The etiology of the dysfunction may be nutritional, toxic, or genetic. The desired end product is not formed because of the metabolic derangement. Additionally, the preceding metabolite or its precursors accumulate. These accumulating metabolites (or the breakdown products thereof) may be toxic.[1]

The accumulated metabolites serve as the diagnostic tool. Further, the diagnosis is confirmed by the presence of a deficient or defective enzyme. Treatment entails limiting the presence of accumulated metabolites, supplementing the deficient resulting metabolites, and/or providing the coenzyme/cofactor that catalyzes the enzymatic reaction.[1,2] Small molecule disorders include disorders of sugar metabolism, mitochondria, protein, urea, fat, toxins, and deficiencies. We will explore each of these disorders in considerable detail.

In the neonatal period, small molecule diseases may present with low Apgar scores, marked hypotonia, and/or poor suck, emesis, coma, or Reye-like syndrome, epilepsy, and unexplained jaundice. Intrauterine growth retardation is not common likely due to the protective nature of maternal metabolism. But patients are eventually likely to suffer a combination of developmental delay, mental retardation, movement disorder, or intermittent ataxia to their infantile symptoms of growth retardation, feeding difficulties, or vomiting. They need not develop symptoms as infants. Additionally, individual disorders may have unique characteristics, i.e., refractory hiccups in non-ketotic hyperglycinemia.[1] Important clinical history questions are summarized in Table 27.3.

Diagnostic investigation should begin with ketones, pH, and sugars. Random blood glucose is a must. Blood electrolytes, blood ammonia, liver function test, blood lactate, and uric acid are imperative. A complete blood count, urine organic/amino acid/acylglycine screen, and blood acyl-carnitine profile is necessary. Blood filter paper expanded newborn screen may be utilized where needed. Specific vitamin levels may be appropriate.[1,3,4]

When the patient is dysmorphic or polyploidy of sex chromosomes is suspected, subtelomeric or chromosomal studies should be considered. Urine and serum heavy metal screen can be important where signs of such poisoning exist. Plain x-rays become necessary in diseases with joint or bony involvement. Some examples are adrenal calcifications in Wolman disease, patellar calcification in peroxisomal disease of the newborn, and dysostosis multiplex, which among other things involves beaked vertebrae. Cerebrospinal fluid (CSF) should be sent for cell protein, glucose, Veneral Disease Research Laboratory (VDRL), lactate, amino acids, and neurotransmitter metabolites/neopterin profile if tremors, dystonia, or spasticity.[1,3]

When other studies do not explain seizures or motor signs, 3-methyl tetrahydrofolate receptor (MTHFR-3) mutation can be sought out by checking the MTHFR level in the CSF. Brain imaging, peripheral nerve/muscle study, or electroencephalography must be performed where indicated. In the presence of ammonia, a urea cycle defect must be suspected. A simplified urea cycle is depicted in Figure 27.1.[5] Therefore, a urine orotic acid level is not out of place. If an elevated blood lactate is present, a pyruvate level must be obtained for the lactate/pyruvate ratio. A lactate/pyruvate ratio of 20 or more implies a disorder of early phases of the electron transport chain.[4]

When mitochondria and the urea cycle fail, multiple pathways and tissues are disrupted. The common clinical outcome is cortical and hepatic failure due to lactic acidosis with or without hyper-ammonemia. In older children, this complex takes the form of a "Reye-like syndrome." In the neo-nate, this condition is usually referred to as overwhelming neonatal metabolic coma.[2,3,6]

Urea cycle defects responsible for Reye-like syndrome include ornithine transcarbamylase (OTC) deficiency (X-linked; males > females), argininosuccinic acid synthase deficiency (homozygote and heterozygote), acetyl glutamate synthetase deficiency, citrullinemia, triple H syndrome (hyperorni-thinemia–hyperammonemia–homocitrullinuria), and lysinuric protein intolerance.[2,3]

Organic acidemias include 3-methylcrotonyl CoA carboxylase, glutaric aciduria type 1 (glutaryl CoA dehydrogenase deficiency), methylmalonic aciduria, propionic aciduria, isovaleric acidemia, and biotinidase deficiency.[1,3,4,6]

Disorders of fatty acid oxidation and ketogenesis include medium-chain acyl CoA dehydro-genase deficiency (MCAD), long-chain acyl CoA dehydrogenase deficiency (LCAD), long-chain hydroxyl–acyl CoA dehydrogenase deficiency (LCHAD), short-chain acyl CoA dehydrogenase

---

TABLE 27.3

History Pearls in Small Molecule Diseases

1. Feeding intolerances (protein load intolerance in organic acidemias and urea cycle defects; fruit juices in fructosemia)
2. Voracious sweet eating (fatty acid oxidation disorders)
3. Developmental delay
4. Exact age of onset (i.e., prior episodes)
5. Family history

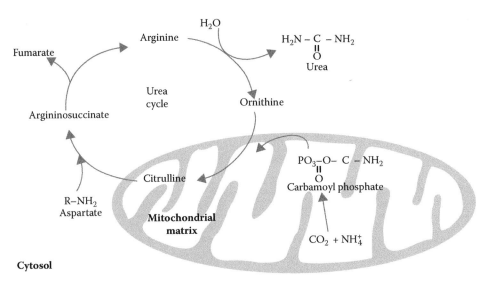

FIGURE 27.1   (**See color insert.**) Simplified urea cycle depicting the key enzymes involved in the pathway. (From http://edoc.hu-berlin.de/dissertationen/xie-jing-2003-12-15/HTML/chapter1.html.)

deficiency (SCAD), multiple acyl CoA dehydrogenase deficiency, and 3-hydroxy-3-methylglutaryl CoA lyase (HMGCoA lyase) deficiency. Carnitine metabolism defects include carnitine palmitoyl transferase I (CPT I) deficiency, CPT II deficiency, CPT translocase deficiency, and 3-ketoacyl CoA thiolase deficiency.[1,3,4,6]

Other disorders include electron transport chain (see Figure 27.2) defects and pyruvate carboxylase deficiency, Wilson's disease, glycogen storage disorders, alpha-1-antitrypsin deficiency, and carbohydrate metabolism disorders. Neonatal jaundice in addition to causing kernicterus may be related to other neurometabolic causes including Crigler–Najjar syndrome, galactosemia, fructosemia, tyrosinemia, organic acidemias, urea cycle defects, hemolysis, neonatal hemochromatosis, Wilson's disease, and alpha-1-antitrypsin deficiency.[1,3,4,6]

Treatment of small molecule diseases entails several systematic steps. The most important step is to avoid catabolism by minimizing fasting, infections, and surgery without dextrose. The next step is to avoid introducing the unmetabolized nutrient. The essential vitamin/cofactor needs to be provided. The missing metabolite should be supplied to bypass the metabolic block. Removal of toxic metabolites (e.g., chelation in Wilson's disease and cathartics in organic acidemias and urea cycle defects in order to minimize unmetabolized toxins such as propionate from intestinal commensals) is important. Toxic drugs need to be avoided when possible (e.g., the use of barbiturates in porphyria). Other aspects include genetic counseling and/or family planning, experimental gene replacement as appropriate, psychosocial interventions, bone marrow transplant (if effective), phototherapy or dialysis when indicated, enzyme replacement, and additional consultation as deemed necessary.[1] Specific treatment options are too detailed and beyond the scope of this chapter.

Pyruvate dehydrogenase/Complex I → CoQ → Complex II → Complex III →
Cytochrome C → Complex IV/V

FIGURE 27.2   Simplified electron transport chain.

DISORDERS OF SUGAR METABOLISM

The common pathogenic mechanism in such disorders is disruption of enzymes involved in the metabolism and utilization of a simple sugar, nicotinamide adenine dinucleotide (NADM)/nicotinamide adenine dinucleotide phosphate (NADPH), phosphocreatine, or adenosine triphosphate (ATP).

1. *Galactosemia*: Galactose-1-phosphate uridyl transferase with several variants. Clinical features include congenital hepatomegaly, jaundice, vomiting, neonatal sepsis, failure to thrive, microcephaly, infantile idiopathic intracranial hypertension, acidosis, thrombocytopenia, hypoglycemia, urinary-reducing substances, renal Fanconi syndrome, seizures, later cataracts, mental retardation, speech dyspraxia, and hypergonadotropic hypogonadism. Salient laboratory findings include urine-reducing substances (galactosuria) and galactitol as well as blood galactose. The underlying etiology is a recessive mutation of 9p13. Treatment includes galactose-free diet, educational assistance, endocrine, and ophthalmologic evaluations. This condition carries a good prognosis with diet and support.[2,3,7]

2. *Fructosemia (hereditary fructose intolerance)*: The enzyme defect is hepatic fructose-1-phosphate aldolase. The symptoms after ingestion of sucrose or fructose include tremor, disorientation, hypoglycemia, and vomiting, without or with convulsions and coma. Chronic growth failure, jaundice, hepatomegaly, proteinuria, and aminoaciduria are also seen. The symptoms are severe in infants but are milder later as individuals develop an aversion to sweet items. Lab findings include fructosuria with or without fructosemia, aminoaciduria, hypophosphatemia, hyperuricemia, and hypokalemia. There are several autosomal dominant and recessive forms of this condition. Treatment includes avoiding sucrose/fructose and IV glucose during crisis. Prognosis is good with strict adherence to dietetic regimen but can be fatal otherwise.[1–3,7]

3. *Glut-1 transporter defect*: The deficient enzyme is the cerebral glut-1 transporter. Clinical features include intractable epilepsy, mental retardation, and other neurological signs. Seizures may be worsened by phenobarbital therapy. Laboratory findings include CSF glucose less than 40 mg/dL. This is an autosomal recessive condition. A ketogenic diet is recommended. The prognosis is good if treated early, otherwise can result in mental impairment.[2,3]

4. *Cerebral creatine defects*: The defective enzyme is guanidine acetate methyltransferase. The clinical features in neonates include the presence of seizures with or without hypotonia. Developmental delay occurs often and an extrapyramidal movement disorder may occur later in life. Hallmark lab findings include very low creatinine in the serum and CSF. MR spectroscopy of the brain should be considered. Urine tests positive for guanidinoacetate. This is also an autosomal recessive condition. Treatment entails usage of creatine monohydrate, which results in improvement of symptoms.[3]

MITOCHONDRIAL DISEASES

Mitochondrial disease is commonly associated with disorders of pyruvate metabolism and the electron transport chain. So these disorders are included in section on disorders of sugar metabolism because pyruvate is the end product of sugar metabolism and the beginning of the electron transport chain. The mitochondrion is involved in more than just energy metabolism, which is estimated to be less than 10% of its functions. The other roles include pyruvate metabolism, beta-oxidation of fatty acids, free radical detoxification, carnitine shuttle, sterol/sex hormone synthesis, citric acid cycle, pyrimidine synthesis (dihydroorotate dehydrogenase involved in orotic aciduria), heme synthesis (via delta-amino levulinic acid synthetase), and even neurotransmitter metabolism. However, in the last two decades, newer techniques have emerged for molecular genetic diagnoses, which have helped identify electron transport chain disorders encoded in the maternally inherited mitochondrial genome.[2,4]

Most mitochondrial diseases are characterized by various degrees of acidosis (lactate and/or pyruvic and other organic/decarboxylic acids), developmental delays, seizures, motor dysfunction, and organ dysfunction including kidney, liver, and blood cells. All such disorders may present in infanthood, but maturity may be required for full manifestation. Some diseases do not present until adulthood.[2,4] The various subcategories of mitochondrial diseases are described as below.

1. Electron transport chain defects of oxidative phosphorylation
    a. Nuclear gene mutations and X-linked gene mutations.
    b. Mitochondrial DNA depletion syndromes and miscellaneous mitochondrial defects include Alper's hepatocerebral degeneration, those caused by deficiencies of thymidine kinase, DNA polymerase gamma A1 or deoxyguanosine kinase, and Menke kinky hair disease (ATPase 7a, Xq12 mutation leading to copper deficiency leading to cytochrome c dysfunction).[4]
    c. Enzyme defects in fatty acid oxidation, which include CoA deficiency, carnitine palmitoyl transferase I, carnitine palmitoyl transferase II, carnitine uptake defect, carnitine depletion, electron transfer flavoprotein (complex III), very long chain acyl or hydroxyl acyl CoA dehydrogenase, long-chain 3-OH-acyl CoA dehydrogenase, medium-chain acyl CoA dehydrogenase, short-chain acyl CoA dehydrogenase, 3-OH-acyl CoA dehydrogenase, Enoyl-CoA hydrolase, and 3-keto thiolase deficiency.[4,8]
    d. Pyruvate metabolism-related enzyme defects include monocarboxylase transferase, pyruvate carboxylase complex, pyruvate dehydrogenase complex, phosphoenolpyruvate carboxykinase, and disorders of carnitine metabolism.[4,8,9]
    e. Enzyme defects in the citric acid cycle include alpha-ketoglutarate dehydrogenase and fumarase.[4,8,9]
    f. Disorders of fatty acid oxidation often present as a short-chain acyl CoA dehydrogenase deficiency as cyclic vomiting, 3-ketothiolase as cyclic vomiting and migraine, medium-chain acyl CoA dehydrogenase deficiency causing seizures with hypoketotic hypoglycemia in the setting of fasting, apparent life-threatening events, and sudden infant death.[4,9]
    g. Long-chain disorders of fatty oxidation present as acute fatty liver with or without rhabdomyolysis. Most can present with cardiomyopathy, retinopathy, Reye-like syndrome, and intermittent lethargy or coma.[4,9]
    h. Disorders of carnitine metabolism can present as rhabdomyolysis, acute fatty liver, myopathy, Reye-like syndrome, developmental delay, and/or clinical symptoms of cramps.[8]
2. Syndromes of dysfunction of oxidative phosphorylation
    a. Alper disease is hepatocerebral degeneration, often caused by mitochondrial depletion associated with defects of DNA polymerase gamma A1 (POLG1), deoxyguanosine kinase, or thymidine phosphorylase.[4,6]
    b. Ataxia caused by POLG1 and PEO1 twinkle C100RF2 nuclear mutations and many mitochondrial deletions.[4,6]
    c. Barth syndrome, as a result of X-linked cardiomyopathy and leucopenia.[4,6]
    d. Cardiomyopathy, which can be hypertrophic, dilated, histiocytoid, or fibroelastosis. Cardiomyopathy can also be caused by mitochondrial mutations, thymidine kinase nuclear mutations causing mitochondrial depletion, and other nuclear gene mutations.[3,4,6]
    e. Childhood diabetes without or with deafness (CPEO).[2,6]
    f. Cytochrome oxidase deficiencies.[6]
       SCO1 nuclear gene: hepatopathy and encephalopathy
       SCO2 nuclear gene: cardiomyopathy and encephalopathy
       COX 10 nuclear gene: proximal renal tubulopathy, encephalopathy, and leukodystrophy
       COX 15 nuclear gene: Leigh syndrome and fatal neonatal cardiomyopathy

g. Deafness without or with aminoglycoside ototoxicity.[6]

h. Diabetes insipidus, mellitus, optic atrophy, and deafness (DIDMOAD) also known as Wolfram syndrome. This is caused by three gene defects.[4,6,8]

i. Dystonia with or without Leber hereditary optic neuropathy (LHON).[4,6]

j. Hackett–Tarlow syndrome is a juvenile myopathy.[4]

k. Hypotonia, epilepsy, autism, and developmental delay commonly known by the acronym HEADD.[10]

l. Kearns–Sayre characterized by chronic progressive external ophthalmoplegia (CPEO) caused by several mitochondrial and nuclear mutations.[4,7]

m. Hearing loss, ataxia, myoclonus (HAM).[4]

n. Leigh's disease characterized by subacute encephalomyelopathy; SURF1 nuclear gene and mitochondrial genome mutations.[4,7]

o. Leber hereditary optic neuropathy (LHON).[1,3,6–9,11]

p. Luft: hypermetabolic uncoupling of oxidative phosphorylation.[9]

q. MELAS: Myopathy, encephalopathy, lactic acidosis, and stroke-like episodes.[1,3,6–9,11]

r. Menke: ATPase 7a, Xq12 mutation leading to copper deficiency and subsequently cytochrome C dysfunction.[6,9,11]

s. Myopathy: nuclear gene thymidine kinase mutation causing mitochondrial depletions and mitochondrial mutations.[3,8,9,11]

t. NARP: neurodegeneration, retinitis pigmentosa, and ataxia.[1,3,6–9,11]

u. MERRF: myoclonus, epilepsy, with ragged red fibers.[1,3,6–9,11]

v. MNGIE: myopathy, neuropathy, gastrointestinal disorder, encephalopathy, nuclear DNA; ECGF1 gene thymidine phosphorylase deficiency; high blood deoxyuridine and thymidine.[3,4,7]

w. Optic atrophy: nuclear gene OPA1; dynamin-related GTPase defect, which is autosomal dominant.[4]

x. Parkinsonism: Leigh mutations; also DNA polymerase gamma A1 (POLG1).[4]

y. Sensory neuropathy: POLG1 and PEO1, twinkle C10ORF2 nuclear mutations, and mitochondrial deletions.[4]

z. Complex I/II, and other mitochondrial mutations.[4,7]

In summary, mitochondrial disorders, whether of electron transport chain or not, usually are multisystem disorders with slow, intermittently accelerated degeneration. Some are slow enough to be virtually static. Metabolic stress may worsen these disorders. In the newborn, oxidative phosphorylation diseases mimic hypoxic/ischemic encephalopathy (HIE). They can also present with hypotonia, seizures, intrauterine growth retardation, cardiomyopathy, lactic acidosis, feeding difficulty/dysphagia, sideroblastic anemia, or hepatopathy.

DISORDERS OF PROTEIN METABOLISM

These can be subdivided as organic acidopathies, urea cycle defects, aminoacidopathies, and disorders of glutathione metabolism. The porphyrias are also classified along with the aforementioned conditions.

Small molecule disorders of protein metabolism that cause abnormal urine organic acids include propionic acidemia (PPA), which involves defective propionyl CoA carboxylase. This condition displays autosomal recessive inheritance. Patients present with recurrent ketosis, acidosis, dehydration, Reye, osteoporosis, and rash. Lab work shows elevated proprionic acid levels, glycine, methylcitrate, tiglylglycine, neutropenia, thrombocytopenia, hyponatremia, and ammonia. Urine may test positive for ketones. Spongiform brain may be observed. Treatment involves restriction of isoleucine, valine, threonine, and methionine, as well as addition of carnitine and metronidazole. Growth hormone supplementation as well as biotin for rash and management of Reye's syndrome is important. The condition carries a better prognosis in adulthood, but neonatal fatality is imminent should prompt treatment not occur.[1-3]

Methylmalonic acidemia (MMA) is caused by eight variations of methylmalonyl CoA mutase mutation. Early clinical features include recurrent hypotonia, ketoacidosis, dehydration, Reye, hepatomegaly, monilia, and growth failure. Later features include osteoporosis, chorea, seizures, ataxia, tremor, and mental impairment. Lab findings include high MMA, glycine, neutropenia, megaloblastic anemia, hypersegmented neutrophils with or without ammonia, cystathione, and homocysteine. "Ketones" may be found in urine. Spongiform brain may develop. The underlying genetics include recessive chromosome 6. Treatment involves B12 supplementation, with or without isoleucine, threonine, methionine, and valine. Alanine, carnitine, metronidazole, growth hormone, and Reye therapy maybe administered as needed. Newborn screening and prompt treatment carry a good prognosis.[2,3,6]

MMA and homocystinuria are caused by disorders of methylmalonyl CoA mutase and methionine synthase. Clinical features included recurrent hypotonia, ketoacidosis, dehydration, Reye, hepatomegaly, growth failure, and candidiasis. Later manifestations include mental impairment, chorea, seizures, ataxia, tremor, and osteoporosis. Salient lab findings include MMA in C and D neutropenia–thrombocytopenia, high glycine, and megaloblastic anemia. Hypersegmented polymorphonuclear cells, urine ketones, with or without ammonia, homocysteine, and cystathione are also seen. In addition, T2 MR basal ganglia lesions can be seen. Genetics include autosomal recessive inheritance. Treatment involves hydroxyl-B12 or methyl B12. Restriction of isoleucine, threonine, valine, and methionine is rarely needed. Alanine, carnitine, and growth hormone substitution may be required. Reye therapy may also be required. Prognosis is poorer than other cobalamin defects.[2,3,6]

Multiple carboxylase deficiency may be caused by a holocarboxylase synthase defect leading to deficiency of proprionyl CoA carboxylase, 3-methyl-crotonyl-CoA, and pyruvate carboxylase. Biotidinase deficiency may be the primary enzyme defect as well. The clinical features include infantile red scaly rash, alopecia, cyclic vomiting, and coma. Reye syndrome may occur. The other manifestations are akin to PPA and MMA. Cobalamin disorders, stupor, hypotonia, hydrocephalus, ataxia, deafness, blindness, and seizures are seen in biotinidase defect. Salient lab findings include elevated lactate, methylcitrate, 3-OH-isovaleric acid, 3-methyl-crotonyl glycine, ammonia, and urine ketones. Abnormal electroencephalogram (EEG) is a common finding. Spongiform brain may be seen. This condition follows an autosomal recessive inheritance pattern. Treatment entails early supplementation of biotin, which produces a dramatic response. Starting prenatal biotin is also helpful. The prognosis is good if the condition is treated early. Late complications include dilated ventricles and deafness. The blindness may be permanent.[2,3,6]

3-Methyl-crotonyl glycinuria is caused by a defect in 3-crotonyl CoA carboxylase. Clinical features may include Reye-like syndrome later in infancy, seizures, developmental delay, growth failure, and coma. Ketoacidosis, hypoglycemia, hyperammonemia, hepatopathy, 3-methyl-crotonyl glycinuria, 3-OH-isovalerate, and low free carnitine are hallmark laboratory findings. This condition shows autosomal recessive inheritance pattern. Treatment entails reduction of protein/leucine intake, carnitine addition, and Reye therapy. This condition may carry a normal prognosis.[2,3,6]

Isovaleryl CoA dehydrogenase defect is the cause of isovaleric acidemia. Clinical features include neonatal Reye, sweaty-feet smell, projectile vomiting, cerebral hemorrhages, intermittent pancreatitis, fatty liver, microcephaly, ataxia, tremor, seizures, and developmental delay. Lab findings are similar to crotonyl glycinuria. But in addition to the metabolic abnormalities seen in that condition, leukopenia and thrombocytopenia may be seen. Urine shows isovalerylglycine, 3-OH-isovalerate, low free carnitine, spongiform brain, and abnormal EEG. This is a recessively inherited autosomal condition. Reye therapy, restriction of dietary leucine, and addition of carnitine/glycine are mainstays. If treated early, the outcome may be normal. However, 50% die in an acute neonatal event.[2,3,6]

Glutaric aciduria I is caused by glutaryl CoA dehydrogenase defect. The clinical features include megalocephaly, acute childhood/infantile encephalitic-like crisis, dystonia, degenerative spasticity, ataxia, dyskinesia, seizures, profuse sweating, and cyclic vomiting. MRI reveals a wide operculum, putamen/caudate hyperintensities, urine glutaric acid, mild fatty liver, spongiform white matter changes, and mild acidosis. This is an autosomal recessive inheritance pattern commonly seen in the Swedish, Ojibway, and the Amish. Treatment consists of lysine/tryptophan restriction, addition of riboflavin/carnitine as well as IV saline/dextrose for cyclic vomiting, and Baclofen. Early treatment usually carries a normal prognosis.[2–4,6]

Type II glutaric aciduria involves a defect in electron transfer flavoprotein or its multiple acyl CoA dehydrogenase. Clinical features include sweat odor, fatal neonatal acidosis, dysmorphic features, myopathy, late-onset hypoglycemic emesis, and lipid storage disorder. Laboratory findings include glutarate, lactate, ethylmalonate, butyrate, adipic acid, methylbutyrate, isobutyrate, and isovalerate. Hypoketotic hypoglycemia, hyperammonemia, urea cycle intermediates in urine, low serum carnitine, and polycystic kidneys are seen. This condition displays an autosomal recessive inheritance pattern. There is currently no known treatment. Individuals often exhibit poor development.[2,3,6]

D-2-Hydroxy-glutaric aciduria is caused by a defect in the corresponding dehydrogenase. Macrocephaly, emesis, hypotonia, seizures, developmental delay, late dystonia, and coarse features are the usual clinical features. Salient laboratory findings include generalized cerebral atrophy, oxoglutaric acids, and D-2-hydroxy-glutaric acid. This is a recessively inherited autosomal condition. Treatment is unknown. The outcome is poor development.[2,3,6]

L-2-Hydroxy-glutaric aciduria is caused by an unknown enzyme defect. Clinical features include moderate delays, ataxia, hypotonia, tremor, seizures, mild spasticity, and neonatal apnea. Laboratory findings include L-2-hydroxyglutaric acid, white matter/caudate hypoplasia, and cerebellar atrophy. Genetics include autosomal recessive inheritance pattern. There is no known treatment. The laboratory must distinguish D from L isomers for diagnosis. Outcome is moderately impaired.[2,3,6,8]

Ethylmalonic aciduria involves a cytochrome oxidase defect. Clinical features include slow neurodegeneration, petechiae, acrocyanosis, hyperreflexia with hypotonia, epicanthal folds, and tortuous retinal vessels. Childhood mortality remains a possibility. Edematous brain and lung is a characteristic feature. Hallmark findings include ethylmalonic, lactic, pyruvic acids, episodic acidosis, and T2 basal ganglia lesions on MRI. Autosomal recessive inheritance pattern is observed. The underlying gene is ETHE1. There is currently no treatment and the prognosis is fatal.[2,3,6]

3-Hydroxy-isobutyric aciduria is a defective oxidation of valine and B-alanine. This condition is characterized by recurrent ketoacidosis, cyclic vomiting, Russell–Silver growth failure, clinodactyly, and hypospadias. Salient lab findings include 3-hydroxy-isobutyric, 2-ethyl-3-hydroxyproprionic, lactic acids, and hypoglycemia. The severe forms are characterized by dysmorphic brains. Genetics are most likely X-linked. Amino acid restriction and addition of growth hormone and carnitine are the mainstays of treatment. This condition carries a good prognosis if treated.[2,3,6]

4-Hydroxy-butyric aciduria is a succinic semialdehyde dehydrogenase defect. Clinical features include mental impairment, hyperkinesis, intermittent lethargy, autism, hypotonia, motor delay, hyporeflexia, ataxia, and seizures. Hallmark lab findings include urine 4-hydroxybutyric acid and cerebral atrophy. The condition displays autosomal recessive inheritance pattern. Treatment includes benzodiazepine and vigabatrin. Outcome includes mild-to-moderate impairment.[1,7]

2-Methyl-3-hydroxybutyric aciduria involves 3-oxothiolase or mitochondrial acetoacetyl CoA thiolase. Clinical features include recurrent severe ketosis and cyclic vomiting. Hallmark lab findings include 2-methyl-3-hydroxy-isobutyric aciduria, hyperglycinemia, hyperglycemia, and MR T2 hyperintensity in the basal ganglia. This is a recessive 11q22 mutation. Treatment includes restriction of isoleucine and carnitine. Vomiting may require IV rehydration. This condition carries a good prognosis if treated.[1,7]

Malonic aciduria may be due to a malonyl CoA decarboxylase defect, but in cases where there are normal malonyl CoA decarboxylase levels, the etiology is unknown. Global delay, growth failure, seizures, candidiasis, myoclonic epilepsy, severe dystonia, and spasticity remain the most prominent clinical features. Laboratory findings include methylmalonic, methylglutaric, malonic, and dicarboxylic/lactic acids, and hyperammonemia without or with hypoglycemia. There is progressive atrophy of the basal ganglia, white matter, and cortex. Genetics are autosomal recessive and rarely X-linked. Treatment includes supportive care during episodes of ketoacidosis. Carnitine and clonazepam are also possible options. Prognosis is generally poor.[1,7]

2-Oxoadipic aciduria is a 2-oxoadipic acid dehydrogenase defect. Clinical features include growth failure, global developmental delay, hypotonia, edema, seizures, ataxia, ichthyosis, and ventricular dilation. Laboratory findings include elevated aminoadipic acids and 2-oxoadipic acid. This condition involves autosomal recessive genetics. Treatment is not known, but lysine restriction has been successful in some cases. Acute acidosis management is important. Prognosis varies.[1,7]

Methylglutaconic aciduria I involves 3-methylglutaconyl CoA hydratase defect. Clinical features include speech delay, global neurological dysfunction, or no symptoms. Hallmark lab findings include fasting hypoglycemia, elevated urine 3-methylglutaconic, 3-methylglutaric, 3-hydroxyisovaleric acids, and acidosis. This is an autosomal recessive condition. Treatment involves restriction of pantothenic acid and restriction of leucine. Patients may potentially be left with mild impairment.[1,2,7]

Type II, also known as Barth syndrome, involves deficient tafazzin, a mitochondrial membrane protein. There is resulting impairment in phospholipid metabolism. Neutropenia, cardiomyopathy, growth failure, lipid myopathy, and recurrent infections are the usual features. Lab findings include 3-methylglutaconic, 3-methylglutaric aciduria, low carnitine, and hypertrophic ventricular fibroelastosis. This condition displays X-linked inheritance involving TAZ1/G4.5 gene, located on chromosome Xq28. Treatment includes restriction of protein, addition of carnitine/cholesterol, and pantothenic acid replacement. Heart transplant may also be needed. This condition can be fatal.

Type III or Costeff syndrome includes a defect in a mitochondrial membrane protein that impairs ATP synthase. Clinical features include neurodegeneration, extrapyramidal signs, spasticity, and mitochondrial cytopathy. Hallmark lab findings include possible acidosis, hypoglycemia, sideroblastic anemia (Pearson aplastic anemia), and markers of disorders of oxidative phosphorylation. Autosomal recessive inheritance or mitochondrial deletions are the basis for this condition. Treatment involves pantothenic acid supplementation and mitochondrial therapies. The prognosis is generally variable.[1,2,7]

Type IV involves unknown mitochondrial dysfunction. Patients have dysmorphic features and cerebral dysfunction. Elevated urine methylglutaconic acid is seen. The underlying genetic basis is unclear. Treatment involves mitochondrial therapies and potential treatment with pantothenic acid. The prognosis tends to be variable.[1,2,7]

UREA CYCLE DEFECTS AND HYPERAMMONEMIA

Orotic aciduria and hyperammonemia are caused by OTC defect. Clinical features include male infantile or childhood Reye-like hyperammonemic crisis, coma, seizures, stroke-like episodes, and affected females. Hallmark laboratory findings include elevated glutamine, alanine, orotic acid, ornithine, low citrulline in fluids, and respiratory alkalosis. This condition displays X-linked dominant inheritance. Treatment includes protein restriction, benzoate, arginine, citrulline, phenylbutyrate/phenylacetate, pyridoxine, folate, IV dextrose, and mannitol; dialysis may be necessary. Glutamine supplementation is also essential. This condition is potentially lethal acutely but treatable.[1,2,7]

Ornithinemia is a carbamyl phosphate synthase defect. Clinical features include neonatal hyperammonemic crisis. Salient findings include elevated ornithine. Low citrulline, arginine, elevated orotic acid, and BUN are also seen. Respiratory alkalosis is a common feature. This condition involves autosomal recessive genetics. Treatment is identical to OTC with N-carbamyl-glutamate. Treatment is successful, but this condition is potentially acutely lethal.[1,2,7]

Citrullinemia and orotic aciduria are defects of arginine-succinate synthase. Neonatal seizures, hyperammonemia without or with Reye-like crisis, recurrent or cyclic vomiting, headache, tremor, seizures, and ataxia can be seen intermittently. Short hair is also seen. Laboratory findings include citrullinemia, orotic acidemia, and argininosuccinate deficiency. This is an autosomal recessive condition. Treatment is the same as for OTC. Upon stabilization, arginine supplementation maintenance therapy is usually sufficient. Protein restriction may be necessary. The condition is treatable but may be acutely lethal. Moderate mental impairment is seen. The 10-year survival rate is 75%.[1,2,7]

Arginino-succinic aciduria is a defect of arginine-succinase lyase. The clinical features are the same as arginine-succinate synthetase deficiency but for the presence of more significant hepatomegaly and trichorrhexis nodosa. High arginine-succinate, alanine, glutamine, and moderate citrulline are the common laboratory findings. This is also an autosomal recessive condition. Treatment and prognosis are identical to arginine-succinate synthetase deficiency.[1,2,7,8]

Argininemia is an arginase defect that presents as spastic quadriplegia, microcephaly, opisthotonos, and seizures. Lab findings include high arginine, cystine, ornithine, lysine, orotic, and arginic acids. This is also an autosomal recessive condition. Treatment includes low arginine diet with addition of lysine, benzoate, and ornithine. Prognosis is good. Triple H syndrome is an ornithine mitochondrial transporter defect. Clinical features include intermittent emesis or Reye syndrome. Lab findings include hyperornithine, homocitrulline, and ammonia. This condition displays autosomal recessive inheritance. Protein restriction and ornithine/lysine addition are treatments. Prognosis is good.[2,3,7,8,11]

Lysinuric protein intolerance is a defect in cationic amino acid transport. Clinical features include growth failure, intermittent emesis, Reye syndrome, or diarrhea. Nephritis, fractures, pulmonary fibrosis, pancreatitis, terminal liver failure, and liponecrosis may occur. Low blood amino acids are seen and urine amino acids are elevated. This is also an autosomal recessive disease. Treatment is protein restriction, amino acid substitution, and methylprednisolone for lungs. Prognosis is guarded.[4,11]

DISORDERS OF PROTEIN METABOLISM THAT CAUSE ABNORMAL URINE AMINO ACIDS

Phenylketonuria is characterized by a defect in phenylalanine hydroxylase and tyrosinase as a secondary defect. Clinical features include blond hair, blue eyes, pale skin, eczema, mousy odor, infantile vomiting, short structure, hyperactivity, mental impairment, seizures, tremor, spasticity, and athetosis. Hallmark lab findings include low tyrosine and high phenylalanine. This condition displays 12 q recessive inheritance. Treatment includes lifelong restriction of phenylalanine. Carnitine may be added. Pregnant patients should be treated to protect fetus. Prognosis is good during treatment.[1–4,7,8]

Hyperphenylalaninemia is a GTP cyclohydrolase or pyruvoyl tetrahydrobiopterin metabolism defect. Microcephaly, growth/mental impairment, hypotonia, mild vomiting, dystonia, parkinsonian rigidity, seizures, and drooling are common features. Lab findings include elevated phenylalanine/prolactin and low tyrosine. This is an autosomal recessive condition. Treatment includes tetrahydrobiopterin and folinic acid. If treated, the prognosis is excellent.[1,2,7,8]

Homocystinuria I is a cystathionine synthase defect. Clinical features included ectopic lens, glaucoma, cataracts, retinal detachment, vascular occlusions, malar flush, osteoporosis, and bony dysplasia. Aortic dilation, behavioral disturbances, and strokes are also seen. Homocysteine and methionine are both high. This is an autosomal recessive condition. Betaine, folate, and pyridoxine substitution are the treatment. Prognosis is fair.[1,2,7,8]

Type II homocystinuria is a N-(5,10)-methylene-tetrahydrofolate reductase defect. Clinical features include vessel disease/strokes, mental delay, psychosis, and infantile spasms. Homocysteine is high and methionine is low or normal. This condition is autosomal recessive. Treatment includes folate or folinic acid and B12. Betaine and pyridoxine will help. The prognosis is variable.[1,2,7,8]

Tyrosinemia type I includes a defect of cytosolic tyrosine aminotransferase of which there are two manifestations: oculocutaneous and Richner–Hanhart syndromes. Clinical features include painful keratitis with inflammation, lacrimation, and painful hands and feet. Mild to severe mental impairment, self-injury, seizures, and hyperactivity may be seen. High tyrosine causes crystallization and keratosis. The underlying mutation is 16q22 recessive. The treatment is restriction of tyrosine and phenylalanine with addition of etretinate. Prognosis is excellent when treated.[1,2,7-9]

Type II tyrosinemia is the hepatorenal form. This is a fumarylacetoacetate hydrolase defect. Clinical features include liver failure, cirrhosis, hepatocellular carcinoma, rickets, cabbage odor, Reye-like crisis (which is rare), and painful peripheral neuropathy. Patients may also develop myopathy, cardiomyopathy, self-injury, seizures, and behavioral disorder. Lab findings include high tyrosine and alpha fetoprotein. Serum succinylacetone is diagnostic. The triad of aminoaciduria, glycosuria, and phosphaturia are shared with Fanconi nephropathy. This is a 15q23 recessive mutation observed in French-Canadians. Treatment includes restriction of phenylalanine and tyrosine. Use of NTBC [2-(2-nitro-4-trifluoromethylbenzoyl)-1,3-cyclohexanedione] reverses liver failure and can thwart river transplant. Prognosis is excellent on NTBC treatment.[1,2,7-9]

Maple syrup urine disease is a branched chain oxoaciduria. This is a branched-chain ketoacid dehydrogenase-4 protein complex E1-alpha, E1-beta, E2, and thiamine/E3. Clinical features include neonatal coma, hydrocephalus that leads to opisthotonos, seizures, delays, and recurrent ataxia. There are also intermediate and intermittent forms. Protein intake triggers the formation of a maple syrup of fluids and earwax. Branched-chain amino and oxoacids are elevated. Brain edema and myelinolysis are frequently seen. Acidosis is not a common finding. Genetics involve recessive mutations of E1-α on 19q13, E1-β on 6p21, E2 on 1p31, and E3 on 7q31. Treatment includes amino acid restriction as well as thiamine addition. Dialysis and exchange transfusion may also be required. IV dextrose and nonbranched-chain amino acids to overcome catabolism are treatments. The prognosis is generally excellent.[1,2,7-9]

Nonketotic hyperglycinemia is a glycine cleavage disorder at the 4-enzyme complex. Features include severe neonatal coma, myoclonus, hiccups, and seizures. Hypotonia is an early feature and spasticity is a late feature. Patients may develop mental stagnation. The severity and progression tend to vary. Laboratory findings include high CSF/plasma glycine ratio (>0.06, normal = 0.02); EEG shows burst-suppression activity. MRI brain shows spongiform white greater than gray matter. This is an autosomal recessive condition. Treatment involves dextromethorphan, pyridoxine, and anticonvulsants. This condition is often fatal to the neonate.[1,2,7-9]

Ornithinemia with gyrate atrophy is an ornithine-5-aminotransferase defect. Clinical features include gyrate atrophy of choroid and retina and mental and renal impairment. Hallmark lab findings include ornithinemia with normal ammonia. This condition involves autosomal recessive inheritance. Treatment involves protein restriction and addition of lysine. The condition carries a variable prognosis.[1,2,7-9]

DISEASES OF GLUTATHIONE METABOLISM

These fall under aminoacidopathies as there is an accumulation of individual amino acids. They usually follow an autosomal mode of inheritance. Full features are usually expressed in adulthood. Pyroglutamic aciduria (5-oxoprolinuria) is caused by glutathione synthetase deficiency. It is associated with mental impairment, dysarthria, ataxia, intermittent acidosis, and hemolytic anemia with febrile illnesses. Diaphragmatic hernias may also be seen. If the condition is limited to red blood cells, the neurological manifestations are not seen. Gamma-glutamylcysteine synthetase deficiency is associated with myopathy, peripheral neuropathy, spinocerebellar degeneration, intermittent hemolytic anemia, and generalized aminoaciduria. Acute psychosis has been observed. Glutathione peroxidase is a selenium-dependent enzyme and is impaired in selenium deficiency. This condition causes a painful skeletal myopathy. The rest of the glutathione-related enzyme deficiencies do not cause neurological manifestations.[1,2,7-9]

Porphyrias are disorders of heme metabolism causing excretion of porphyrins, which at times causes dark urine. They are either erythropoietic or hepatic. Symptoms may be acute, intermittent, or subacute. Neuropsychiatric symptoms may be seen likely from abnormal tryptophan metabolism and increased serotonin. Kluver–Bucy syndrome, weakness, sensory neuropathies, which may resemble Guillain–Barre syndrome, and seizures may be seen. Abdominal symptoms include pain, vomiting, nausea, diarrhea, or constipation. Sometimes, the symptoms are so intense that surgical exploration may be prompted. Some cause a photosensitive rash. Chest pain, tachycardia, and hypertension may be observed. Metabolic, toxic, or infectious stress triggers exacerbations. Bromides are considered safe anticonvulsants as most commonly used anticonvulsants may trigger an attack. Autosomal dominant inheritance pattern makes porphyrias fairly common diseases, and testing of extended family may be a good idea. Secondary porphyria presents as an unexplained laboratory finding. Porphyria cutanea tarda may be the only disorder of infancy, and photosensitive rash is the presenting symptom.[1,2,4,7–9]

SMALL MOLECULE DISEASES OF FAT METABOLISM

These conditions include disorders of fatty acid beta-oxidation and those of cholesterol metabolism. Disorders of fatty acid beta-oxidation are organic acidemias. Poorly metabolized fats produce unusual organic acids (e.g., adipic acid, sebacic acid, suberic acid, octenedioic acid, etc.), which may be toxic. This may lead to deficiency of appropriate fatty acids downstream from the enzyme defect. There may also be energy depletion because as much as 60% of energy needs are met by fat calories. This may force a state of nonketotic hypoglycemia. These are mitochondrial disorders given that beta-oxidation is a mitochondrial process.[1,2,8]

Disorders of cholesterol metabolism cause either excess or deficiency of cholesterol and metabolites or precursors. These conditions may lead to a combination of neuronal cell membrane disruption, fetal cerebral development, and myelin formation disruption. Atheromatous buildup may lead to ischemic complications. All of the above will result in neurological complaints. These disorders range anywhere from familial hyperlipidemia syndromes to cerebrotendinous xanthomatosis.[1] Most of these conditions cause a range of neurological symptoms including psychomotor retardation with/or neuropsychiatric symptoms, ataxia, and seizures. Detailed coverage of these disorders is beyond the scope of this chapter.

DISORDERS OF PURINE AND PYRIMIDINE METABOLISM

These are important causes of developmental delay and spasticity. Some disorders, particularly adenosine deaminase deficiency, do not typically cause neurological symptoms. Lesch–Nyhan syndrome may present in the neonate as hypotonia.[1–4,7] When this condition is left untreated, it may lead to mental retardation, severe spasticity, and self-injury. Dihydropyrimidine dehydrogenase deficiency causes uracil, 5-hydroxymethyluracil, and thymine excretion in the urine, and is associated with hypotonia, microcephaly, seizures, delayed myelination, and mental retardation. Replacement of the underproduced beta alanine is the proposed therapy.[12]

NUTRIENT DEFECTS

These conditions include ataxia from vitamin E deficiency (AVED); zinc deficiency with alopecia, moniliasis, and dermatitis enteropathica; copper deficiency; and X-linked Menke kinky hair disease (Xq12). In addition, one must consider Wilson's disease (copper removal deficiency); taurine deficiency causing myopathy; selenium deficiency causing painful myopathy, cardiomyopathy, and blond hair roots; and selenium excess causing neuropathy. Carnitine deficiency can cause hepatopathy/myopathy. Hartnup disease (tryptophan transport and renal reabsorption defect as well as ataxia), cerebral folate deficiency (movement disorder, neurological delay and seizures), and Hallervorden–Spatz disease (neurodegeneration with brain iron deposition in the bilateral pallidi) also belong in this group. Pyridoxine deficiency, responsiveness, or dependency (ALDH7A1) gene on chromosome 5q may cause α-aminoadipic semialdehyduria and pipecolic acidemia.[2,4,13,14]

TOXINS

Toxins cause their symptoms by blocking enzyme, receptor, or structural protein function. If intermediary enzymes are involved, the symptoms may resemble those of nutritional/vitamin deficiencies. Acetaldehyde, a metabolite of ethanol, impairs pyruvate dehydrogenase, which is part of a thiamine-dependent enzyme complex. Neonatal toxin exposure originates in the maternal circulation and may include drugs of abuse, methyl mercury, or lead rarely. Symptoms are not specific and may include hypotonia or hypertonia with seizures secondary to drug withdrawal.[7] Iatrogenic toxicity is also a source for toxins.

DISEASES-CAUSING HYPOGLYCEMIA

Both large and small molecule diseases cause hypoglycemia. As the glycogen or lipid stores are depleted during a fast, small molecule diseases tend to manifest as hypoglycemia.[1,2,4,7–9]

LARGE MOLECULE DISEASES

A. Diseases characterized by storage of sugars, glycolipids, or glycoproteins
  1. Glycogen storage disorders
  2. N-acetyl galactosaminidase deficiency
  3. Mucopolysaccharidoses
  4. Congenital disorders of glycoprotein synthesis
B. Diseases characterized by accumulation of cholesterol and complex lipids
  1. Intracellular cholesterolosis
  2. Sphingolipidoses
  3. Peroxisomal disorders of long-chain fatty acid metabolism
  4. Mucolipidoses
  5. Neuronal ceroid lipofuscinosis
C. Miscellaneous storage disorders
  1. N-acetylaspartate excess (aspartoacylase deficiency = Canavan disease)
  2. Glutamyl ribose-5-phosphate storage disease (ADP-ribosyl protein lyase deficiency)
  3. Alexander disease

Aldolase deficiency is characterized by myopathy, developmental delay, febrile hemolysis, rhabdomyolysis, and absence of glycogen in muscle. An alternative syndrome described, although there is no known enzyme defect as of yet, is characterized by cardiomyopathy, mental retardation, and autophagic vacuolar myopathy.[4]

Lafora polyglucosan body disease in adolescents and adults is characterized by myoclonic epilepsy and dementia. Muscle biopsy reveals non-lysosomal, round, periodic acid-schiff (PAS)-positive perikaryotic inclusions in the neurons, muscle, liver, and skin. In the neonatal periods, these conditions present as hypoglycemia.[1,3,4,7]

Mucopolysaccharidoses are generally characterized by dysmorphic features, bony dysostosis, visceromegaly, short stature, sometimes primary cerebral dysfunction, and sometimes myelopathies and compressive neuropathies, depending on the specific disorder. All store mucopolysaccharides (glycosaminoglycans) and most are excreted in the urine. They generally follow an autosomal recessive inheritance pattern. Some of these diseases also share chemical and clinical characteristics with lipidoses.[1,2,4,8]

Glutamyl ribose-5-phosphate lysosomal storage disease is caused by ADP-ribosyl protein lyase deficiency and is X-linked. This disease causes infant-onset dementia, progressive neuronal loss, and renal failure. Neonates may have hypotonia and renal impairment.[1,2,4,8]

Congenital disorders of glycoprotein synthesis are caused by defective glycosylation of proteins in the Golgi apparatus. The most common screening test is identification of hypoglycosylated transferrin isoforms (carbohydrate-deficient transferrin) in plasma. Common symptoms include microcephaly, seizures, apnea, and hypotonia from combined myopathy and neuropathy. Cerebellar hypoplasia, olivary gliosis, diarrhea, growth failure, renal/hepatic dysfunction, and mild coagulopathy from factor XI dysfunction can be seen. Fatal neonatal cases with infantile spasms and apnea are known. The conditions are autosomal recessive without known successful treatment. Addition of phosphomannomutase deficiency may reduce diarrhea and aid growth.[9,15]

Other miscellaneous storage diseases include Canavan disease [N-acetylaspartate (NAA) excess from aspartoacylase deficiency] characterized by megalencephaly, hypotonia, optic atrophy, dysphagia, developmental delay with fatal neurodegeneration, and seizures. Brain MRI and head CT reveal watery myelin. Urine and MR brain spectroscopy show increased NAA. Pathology reveals degenerative spongy leukodystrophy. The condition is observed predominantly in the Jewish population and is autosomal recessive. The condition occurs in the juvenile, congenital, and infantile ataxia forms. This is a chromosome 17 p mutation and gene therapy is currently investigational.[2-4,7]

Alexander disease is an autosomal recessive leukodystrophy characterized by megalencephaly and Rosenthal fiber hypertrophied astrocytes adherent to blood vessels in the white matter. This disease is either infantile or newborn, which is more common than the rare juvenile or adult forms. It causes growth retardation secondary to feeding inability, dementia, spasticity, and fetal neurodegeneration. In older presentations, it can resemble multiple sclerosis. This condition is not treatable at present.[2-4,7]

DISEASES OF FAT STORAGE

Peroxisomal diseases are caused by peroxisomal dysfunction. They are both small and large molecule diseases. The result is fluid accumulation of unmetabolized long-chain fatty acids in the plasma. But these metabolites are not stored in fixed intracellular collections, which is the case with other large molecule diseases. The known roles of peroxisome include generation of hydrogen peroxide for biochemical reactions, synthesis of plasmalogens (e.g., phosphatidylethanolamine); beta-oxidation of very long chain and long-chain fatty acids; oxidation of phytanic acid and pipecolic acid; some steps of bile acid formation; and some steps of dicarboxylic acid metabolism.[2-4]

Defects of the peroxisome will result in disruption of other steps of metabolism. So, the best tool is measurement of very long chain and long-chain fatty acids in blood. Further assessment is conducted through analysis of enzymes in skin fibroblasts or through gene tests. Inheritance is usually autosomal recessive with the exception of X-linked adrenoleukodystrophy.[2-4,7]

Peroxisomal disorders present with central and/or peripheral myelin dysfunction (leukodystrophy without or with demyelinating polyneuropathy), sometimes with organ, primarily liver dysfunction. In cases of newborn and infantile presentations, skeletal or other organ dysplasia is common. The most severe forms are neonatal.[2-4,7]

Zellweger cerebrohepatorenal syndrome and neonatal adrenoleukodystrophy are multisystem malformation syndromes of hypomyelination and cortical dysplasia. Renal microcysts and hepatic dysplasia are also seen in these syndromes. Neonatal adrenal leukodystrophy is also characterized by neonatal peripatellar calcifications and chondrodysplasia. Optic pallor is often present and seizures can be severe and intractable.[2-4,7]

Refsum's disease presents with peripheral neuropathy in early adulthood and is characterized by accumulation of phytanic acid. The neonatal form is severe and does not have the same metabolic defect or treatment as the adult form, but presents with elevated phytanic acid. Treatment includes genetic counseling and symptomatic treatment. The prescribed diet contains glyceryl trierucate and trioleate, which are variants of Lorenzo oil. The defective pathways are effectively bypassed by this diet and are known to delay demyelination in asymptomatic patients with X-linked adrenoleukodystrophy genotype.[1-4,6,7]

Adrenal hormone replacement is the treatment for adrenal dysfunction if present. In the neonatal kind as well as Zellweger disease, cholic acid/deoxycholic and docosahexanoic acids may be helpful. Vitamin K supplementation is useful in the setting of severe liver dysfunction. A diet low in phytanic acid and plasmapheresis are the usual treatment. Some peroxisomal disorders are accompanied by pyruvate dehydrogenase dysfunction. Bone marrow transplant is currently being investigated as a treatment in X-linked adrenoleukodystrophy.[2-4,7]

INTRACELLULAR CHOLESTEROLOSIS

Some diseases of cholesterol metabolism can be grouped as small and others large molecule diseases. The conditions that involve extracellular accumulations of cholesterol metabolites are generally classified as small molecule diseases. Examples of these conditions include familial dyslipidemia syndromes, cerebrotendinous xanthomatosis, and mevalonic aciduria. Those conditions that involve intracellular accumulation of cholesterol metabolites are intracellular cholesteroloses.[3,4]

The defective enzymes are lysosomal, and the lipids are stored as large intracellular inclusions. Given that these conditions clinically appear similar to lipidoses, despite the intracellular inclusion being characterized by a small molecule, they are classified as large molecule diseases. These intracellular lipidoses include cholesterol ester storage disease and its severe variants, Wolman disease as well as Niemann–Pick C disease. The clinical features include seizures, organomegaly, movement disorders, and gray dysfunction. Niemann–Pick A and B are disorders of sphingomyelin rather than cholesterol storage. Niemann–Pick C is prevalent in the French Acadian population. Neonatal presentation is quite rare.[4,7]

Glycolipidoses and sphingolipidoses are defects of lysosomal metabolism of sphingolipids causing intralysosomal more than intracytoplasmic accumulation of complex sphingolipids, glycopeptides, and glycolipids. If the accumulation occurs in oligodendrocytes, or Schwann cell, the predominant features are those of a leukodystrophy (spasticity, ataxia, demyelinating dementia, and subsequently demyelinating neuropathy). If the accumulation is in astrocytes or neurons, a poliodystrophy characterized by seizures, movement disorder, axonal neuropathy, and retinal dysfunction ensues. Cellular accumulation does not receive the substance excreted in urine. Cell death is slow due to the accumulation or due to deficiency or toxic effects of metabolites in the affected sphingomyelin formation pathways. Infantile, late childhood, and adult forms are seen. All of these conditions are autosomal recessive except for Fabry's, which is X-linked. Treatment is generally supportive and all are fatal except for Fabry and Secher, which respond to enzyme replacement.[4,7,11,13,16]

All cholesteroloses have similar clinical features except for largely hepatic involvement in Niemann–Pick's and largely splenomegaly in Gaucher's disease. Niemann–Pick and Gaucher diseases produce histologically similar vacuoles and sea blue foamy histiocytes. The stained or accumulated substances are different in each disease. In the case of mucopolysaccharidosis and oligosaccharidoses, abnormal glycosaminoglycans and oligosaccharides can be detected in urine and enzyme testing confirms diagnosis.[1-4,7,13,16]

Sandhoff syndrome and multiple sulfatase deficiency combine features of the above saccharidoses and sphingolipidoses. Gaucher's type 2, Krabbe's globoid cell leukodystrophy, GM-1/2 gangliosidosis, and multiple sulfatase deficiency are present in the neonatal period. Krabbe's disease is characterized by infantile hypertonia, irritability, and high protein in the CSF.[3,4,13,16]

Mucolipidoses are characterized by lysosomal storage and urinary excretion of mucolipid sialyloligosaccharides, sialylglycopeptides, glycolipids, and at times mucopolysaccharides. Clinical features include organomegaly, coarse features, neural/retinal degeneration, and cloudy cornea. Diagnosis is by clinical features, urinary screening, and fibroblast or leukocyte assay. These conditions are autosomal recessive and may present in newborns, and treatment is genetic counseling and symptomatic care.[3,4,13,16]

Neuronal ceroid lipofuscinosis is a lysosomal storage disorder characterized by intractable epilepsy, dementia, retinal blindness, movement disorder, global neurodegeneration, and death. The pathological feature is accumulation of complex osmiophilic inclusions, which were described originally as lipofuscins in light microscopy. Diagnostic tests are characterized by an abnormal electroretinogram and a photomyoclonic response on EEG. There is accumulation of membranous sphingolipid containing structures. There may be mild visceromegaly or coarse features. There is no reliable urinary marker. There are four presentations and the infantile form can present in the newborn with seizures, lack of visual engagement, and hypotonia.[1–4,7,14]

METABOLIC SYNDROME AND ITS RELATIONSHIP TO NEUROLOGICAL DISORDERS

Obesity is a chronic pathological condition and involves accumulation of excess adipose tissue, which increases the risk for multiple morbidities and mortality. It is a major health hazard in the United States, and two thirds of the adult population is overweight or obese. Metabolic syndrome (MetS) is a complex syndrome characterized by increased abdominal fat, insulin resistance, hypertension, and dyslipidemia. Obesity is also a primary risk factor for cardiovascular disease and type II diabetes mellitus. In metabolic syndrome, high-density lipoprotein (HDL) and triglycerides are elevated.[17–21]

In addition to causing insulin resistance, an increase in free fatty acid (FFA) concentrations in normal subjects when compared to levels in obesity also creates oxidative stress and subnormal vascular reactivity. An increase in FFA concentration results in elevation of acetyl CoA/CoA and NaDH/NAD+ ratio in the mitochondria. This process renders pyruvate dehydrogenase inactive leading to an increase in citrate concentrations, which in turn inhibits phosphofructokinase (PFK). This results in increased intracellular concentration of glucose-6-phosphate. Hexokinase II activity decreases as a result, and there is a subsequent increase in intracellular glucose concentration as well as decreased glucose uptake in the periphery.[22,23] The other proposed mechanism entails greater muscle FFA availability or reduced metabolism. This process in turn leads to accumulation of fatty acyl CoA, ceramides, and diacylglycerol. As a consequence, a serine/threonine cascade leading to the phosphorylation of insulin receptors is activated resulting in decreased activation of phosphatidylinositol-3-kinase (PI-3-K). As a result, there is a reduction in subsequent events as well as glucose transport.[17,18,24]

Cytokines and adipokines play a significant role in insulin resistance and hyperinsulinemia. Leptin is involved in energy balance, body weight, and food intake regulation. Leptin is also responsible for inhibition of weight gain and appetite by regulating peptide (decreasing orexigenic and increasing anorexigenic) expression in the hypothalamus. Further, leptin helps decrease muscle and liver intracellular lipid quantity. Lower leptin levels increase energy intake and limit the high energy consumption of the immune system, thyroid function, and reproduction.[21,23–25]

STROKE IN METABOLIC SYNDROME

The association between stroke and metabolic syndrome is increasingly discussed in recent literature with a recent National Health and Nutrition Examination Survey (NHANES) study indicating a strong association between the two entities. Community studies have indicated that there may be sex-dependent risk differentials for metabolic syndrome. One study has reported increased stroke risk in women with metabolic syndrome. Most of these studies have shown impairment of antioxidant systems and increase in lipid peroxidation products in stroke.[26]

Another study has shown less effective nitrous oxide synthase inhibition affecting cerebrovascular blood flow in diabetics. There is an increase in coagulability in diabetics, which may be attributable to increased serum plasminogen activator inhibitor-1 and antithrombin-III levels. C-reactive protein and lipoprotein-associated PLA2 are also elevated and are correlated with increased thrombotic factors and stroke incidence. Platelet hyperreactivity is also implicated. Carotid intima-media thickness also increases in metabolic syndrome resulting in increased stroke risk. High fat and carbohydrate diet results in increased FFA levels in blood and skeletal muscles enhancing oxidative stress, inflammation, and reduced vascular changes. Brain astrocytes and microglia demonstrate increased level of cytokines in metabolic syndrome.[22,27,28]

ALZHEIMER'S DISEASE IN METABOLIC SYNDROME

As is well known, Alzheimer's disease is a neurodegenerative disorder characterized by senile plaques, neurofibrillary tangles, which are aggregates of amyloid-β (Aβ) peptides derived from proteolytic cleavages of amyloid precursor protein (APP), and hyperphosphorylated tau. Interactions between insulin and Aβ as well as insulin excess inhibit degradation of both Aβ40 and Aβ42 (Aβ derivatives). Aβ derivatives avoid insulin degradation in a dose-dependent manner.[29]

Hyperglycemia induces toxic effects of glucose metabolites in the brain and its vasculature, which results in altered synaptic plasticity as well as poor memory and learning.[30] Further, there is an increase in Aβ generation through upregulation of β-secretase activity (β and γ secretases cleave APP to form Aβ). 4-Hydroxynonenal (4-HNE) is a product of oxidative stress and also stimulates upregulation of β-secretases. Additionally, marked abnormalities in insulin and IGF-I and IGF-II signaling mechanisms are observed in the brains of Alzheimer's patients. An entity known as type III diabetes is currently entertained in the literature. This condition selectively involves the brain and has cellular features of both types I and II diabetes. There is some evidence to suggest that insulin signaling imbalances in the brain may lead to Alzheimer's disease. The possible role of antidiabetic drugs is now entertained in the treatment of Alzheimer's disease.[31–35]

Several studies have shown a link between stress, anxiety, and depression and metabolic syndrome. There are several interesting pieces of literature reflecting this correlation. One interesting resource is the article named Psychoneuroimmunology of Depression by Leonard and Myint in the journal *Human Psychopharmacology*.[36]

There are several ongoing studies in regards to metabolic syndrome and its neurological implications. There are several investigational trials that are underway for the treatment of the inborn errors of metabolism highlighted in this chapter. The readers of this chapter as well as the medical community are strongly urged to look for emerging literature in the field of metabolic neurology.

SUMMARY

The disorders of metabolism that carry neurological implications are many and include mitochondrial disorders, disorders of carbohydrate, and protein and lipid metabolism. The majority of these disorders are caused by inborn errors. Although the presentation of such disorders may be complex, key features help the astute clinician with categorization and prompt identification of these conditions leading to proper care, be it therapeutic or supportive, thus prolonging life. Metabolic syndrome is a well-known entity that has posed a notable challenge to today's health care experts, as it is a systemic process affecting multiple organ systems including the nervous system. These disorders affect neurons and associated vasculature causing irreparable damage resulting in both stroke and neurodegenerative disorders. Clinical expertise in the diagnosis of such disorders requires a strong understanding of the underlying biochemical pathways. Ongoing research is bound to be promising in the approaching years.

ACKNOWLEDGMENTS

I sincerely thank my dear wife Dr. Surya Guha, my mother Dr. Sree Venkatraman, and my dear cousin Sandya Iyer for their help in preparation of the format of this chapter.

REFERENCES

1. Enns GM, Steiner RD. Diagnosis and treatment of children with suspected metabolic disease. In: *Pediatrics*. Osborn LM et al., eds. Elsevier, Philadelphia, PA, 2005:1866–1875.
2. Leslie ND. Principles of metabolism. In: *Pediatrics*. Osborn LM et al., eds. Elsevier, Philadelphia, PA, 2005:110–121.
3. Filiano JJ. Neurometabolic disease. In: *Neurology Board Review Guide*. Coffey J, Jenkyn L, eds. Clinical Communications, Greenwich, CT, 1995.
4. Filiano J, Olson A. Neurodegenerative diseases. In: *Pediatrics*. Osborn LM et al., eds. Elsevier, Philadelphia, PA, 2005.
5. Available at http://edoc.hu-berlin.de/dissertationen/xie-jing-2003-12-15/HTML/chapter1.html.
6. Thoene JG, Cocker NP. *Physicians' Guide to Rare Diseases*, 2nd ed. Dowden Publishing, Montvale, NJ, 1995.
7. Lockman LA. Coma. In: *The Practice of Pediatric Neurology*. Swaiman K, ed. CV Mosby, St. Louis, MO, 1982:150.
8. Lyon L, Adams RD, Kolodny EH. *Neurology of Hereditary Metabolic Diseases of Children*, 2nd ed. McGraw-Hill, New York, 1996.
9. Nyhan WL, Ozand PT. *Atlas of Metabolic Diseases*. Chapman & Hall Medical, London, 1998.
10. Filiano JJ, Goldenthal MJ, Rhodes CH, Marin-Garcia J. Mitochondrial dysfunction in patients with hypotonia, epilepsy, autism, and developmental delay: HEADD syndrome. *J Clin Neurol* 2001;17(6):435–439.
11. Rosenberg RN, Prusiner SB, DiMauro S, Barchi RL. *The Molecular and Genetic Basis of Neurological Disease*, 2nd ed. Butterworth-Heinemann, Boston, 1997.
12. Wilson G, Cooley WC. *Preventive Management of Children with Congenital Anomalies and Syndromes*. Cambridge University Press, Cambridge, 2000.
13. Available at http://www.genetests.com.
14. Available at http://www.pubmed.gov/OMIM.
15. Kim S, Westphal V, Srikrishna G, Mehta DP, Peterson S, Filiano J, Karnes PS, Patterson MC, Freeze HH. Dolichol phosphate mannose synthase (DPM1) mutations define congenital disorders of glycosylation Ie (CDG-Ie). *J Clin Invest* 2000;105(2):131–132.
16. Victor M, Ropper AH. *Principles of Neurology*, 7th ed. McGraw-Hill, New York, 2001:983–1049; 1106–1174.
17. Flegal KM, Carroll MD, Ogden CL, Curtin R. Prevalence and trends in obesity among US adults, 1999–2008. *JAMA* 2010;303:235–241.
18. Reaven GM, Laws A. *Insulin Resistance: The Metabolic Syndrome X*. Humana Press, Totowa, NJ, 1999.
19. Grundy SM, Hansen B, Smith SC Jr, Cleeman JI, Kahn RA, American Heart Association. Clinical management of metabolic syndrome report of the American Heart Association/National Heart, Lung, and Blood Institute/American Diabetes Association conference on scientific issues related to management. *Circulation* 2004;109:551–556.
20. Friedman JM. Modern science versus the stigma of obesity. *Nat Med* 2004;10:563–569.
21. Trayhurn P, Hoggard N, Mercer JG, Rayner DV. Leptin: Fundamental aspects. *Int J Obes Relat Metab Disord* 1999;23(Suppl 1):22–28.
22. Nazir FS, Alem M, Small M, Connell JM, Lees KR, Walters MR, Cleland SJ. Blunted response to systemic nitric oxide synthase inhibition in the cerebral circulation of patients with type 2 diabetes. *Diabet Med* 2006;23:398–402.
23. Yu YH, Ginsberg HN. Adipocyte signaling and lipid homeostasis: Sequelae of insulin-resistant adipose tissue. *Circ Res* 2005;96:1042–1052.
24. Shimabukuro M, Koyama K, Chen G, Wang MY, Trieu F, Lee Y, Newgard CB, Unger RH. Direct antidiabetic effect of leptin through triglyceride depletion of tissues. *Proc Natl Acad Sci USA* 1997;94:4637–4641.
25. Flier JS. What's in a name? In search of leptin's physiologic role. *J Clin Endocrinol Metab* 1998;83:1407–1413.
26. Engstrom G, Stavenow L, Hedblad B, Lind P, Eriksson KF, Janzon L, Lindgarde F. Inflammation-sensitive plasma proteins, diabetes, and mortality and incidence of myocardial infarction and stroke: A population based study. *Diabetes* 2003;52:442–447.
27. Tripathy D, Mohanty P, Dhindsa S, Syed T, Ghanim H, Aljada A, Dandona P. Elevation of free fatty acids induces inflammation and impairs vascular reactivity in healthy subjects. *Diabetes* 2003;52(12):2882–2887.

28. Trovati M, Mularoni EM, Burzacca S, Ponziani MC, Massucco P, Mattiello L, Piretto V, Cavalot F, Anfossi G. Impaired insulin-induced platelet antiaggregating effect in obesity and in obese NIDDM patients. *Diabetes* 1995;44:1318–1322.

29. Farooqui AA. *Neurochemical Aspects of Neurotraumatic and Neurodegenerative Diseases.* Springer, New York, 2010.

30. Frisardi V, Solfrizzi V, Capurso C, Imbimbo BP, Vendemiale G, Seripa D, Pilotto A, Panza F. Is insulin resistant brain state a central feature of the metabolic-cognitive syndrome? *J Alzheimers Dis* 2010;21:57–63.

31. De la Monte SM, Wands JR. Alzheimer's disease is type 3 diabetes-evidence reviewed. *J Diabetes Sci Technol* 2008;2:1101–1113.

32. Strader AD, Woods SC. Gastrointestinal hormones and food intake. *Gastroenterology* 2005;128(1): 175–191.

33. Craft S, Reger MA, Baker LD. *Insulin Resistance in Alzheimer's Disease—A Novel Therapeutic Target. Alzheimer's Disease and Related Disorders Annual 5.* Taylor and Francis, London, 2006:111–133.

34. Revill P, Moral M, Prous JR. Impaired insulin signaling and pathogenesis of Alzheimer's disease. *Drug Today* 2006;42:785–790.

35. Whitamer RA. Type 2 diabetes and risk of cognitive impairment and dementia. *Curr Neurol Neurosci Rep* 2007;7:373–380.

36. Leonard BE, Myint A. The psychoneuroimmunology of depression. *Hum Psychopharmacol* 2009; 24(3):165–175.

28 Nutritional Approaches to Epilepsy

Jeffrey M. Politsky and Yelena Karbinovskaya

CONTENTS

INTRODUCTION AND HISTORY OF DIETARY MANAGEMENT OF EPILEPSY

Epilepsy is defined as "any group of syndromes characterized by paroxysmal transient disturbances of brain function that may be manifested as episodic impairment or loss of consciousness, abnormal motor phenomena, psychic or sensory disturbances, or perturbation of the autonomic nervous system due to electrical activity disturbances in the brain."[1] There are about 40 different types of epileptic syndromes and about 200 different types of seizures. Epilepsy as a disease has existed since ancient times, with the Greeks having some of the earliest reports of "the falling sickness." Dietary treatment for epilepsy has also been considered a prominent therapy since the earliest mentions of epilepsy. Many "treatments" were considered for epilepsy, which included a decrease or increase in consumption of certain foods. Hippocrates was one of the first to report fasting as a method to stop a seizure. Aristotle believed that food formed an evaporated material in the veins that would rise upward, turn around, and descend. He believed that if too much evaporated material is carried up into the veins, the veins will swell and compress the respiratory center causing convulsions.[2]

In the early 1900s, two French physicians wrote the first research paper on the significance of fasting in epileptic seizures.[3] They used a "detoxifying" method that involved a low-calorie vegetarian diet and some intervals of fasting and purging. Another physician, Dr. Conklin, in the early 1900s believed that epilepsy was related to the intestines and their ability to digest different amounts and types of foods. He believed that excretion of certain toxins from the intestines could lead to seizure activity. He used this theory to treat his patients with sporadic periods of fasting lasting up to 25 days with only water to drink in the hopes of giving the intestines a complete rest. His methods demonstrated high cure rates particularly in the pediatric population.[4,5] In the 1920s, Dr. Wilder suggested that the benefits of starvation, which produced a ketotic state, could be achieved through a diet that is high in fat and low in carbohydrates. There were several other researchers who supported Wilder's findings. The ketogenic diet could be found as treatment for epilepsy in many textbooks throughout the twentieth century. However, when diphenylhydantoin was discovered in 1938, research was refocused on mechanisms of action of antiepileptic drugs (AEDs) rather than the ketogenic diet. As more AEDs were brought to the market, the use and popularity of the diet decreased. Since then, fewer physicians and dieticians were being trained on the use of diet, and as a result, fewer hospitals were offering it to their patients. In an attempt to reintroduce the diet and make it more palatable, Dr. Huttenlocher introduced the medium triglyceride diet in the 1970s. After the discovery of sodium valproate and its use in the Lennox–Gastaut syndrome, it became clear that using AEDs over the diet was preferred by most patients and families given the time commitment and control necessary for the diet.[6]

In the mid-1990s, there was a resurgence of interest in dietary therapy for epilepsy due to a young boy's success with the diet after numerous AEDs had failed and the media attention that resulted. The media programming created a special presentation on Charlie, a 2 year old, who suffered from epilepsy refractory to many medications. His parents brought him to Johns Hopkins, where he was started on the diet and soon became seizure-free. His parents created "The Charlie Foundation"[7] to raise awareness and use of the diet for other patients, and also for physicians who were not familiar with the diet.[6]

IMPLEMENTATION OF DIETARY THERAPY

The ketogenic diet implemented at Johns Hopkins Hospital in the early 1990s was considered for children aged 1–15 with any type of seizures who could not be controlled with medications or with the use of other methods (i.e., surgery, vagus nerve stimulation). The children had to be admitted to the hospital under the observation of an epilepsy specialist and a trained nutritionist. The original protocol required a 24- to 48-h fasting period in order to accelerate development of the ketotic state. After the initial fasting period, the ketogenic ratio of calories would be introduced. The ratio entailed a 4:1 (fat/protein + carbohydrates) distribution of calories with 1 g/kg/day of protein. The time in the hospital was used to achieve an appropriate ketotic state and to educate the children and caregivers about administrating the diet at home. Additionally, screening was required to rule out any medical contraindications to the diet as well as assess any issues with the diet. More recently, alternative methods of initiating the diet were introduced. These included a greater age range of eligible patients, no fasting period, outpatient initiation, alternative fat/nonfat ratios (3.5:1, 3:1, 2:1, 1:1), and also alternative and more liberal diets such as the modified Atkins diet (MAD), medium-chain triglycerides (MCT), and the low glycemic index treatment (LGIT).[5,8]

PHYSIOLOGY AND MECHANISM OF ACTION OF THE KETOGENIC DIET

Many hypotheses have been proposed to suggest a mechanism of the action of the ketogenic diet and its alternatives. However, the true process is incompletely understood. The ketogenic diet produces many metabolic changes that are meant to mimic a starvation state. The ratio of high fat to protein and low carbohydrates creates changes in glucose, free fatty acids, and ketone levels. One theory suggests that changes in energy metabolism from ketone bodies, including beta-hydroxybutyrate, acetoacetate, and acetone, have an anticonvulsant effect when crossing the blood–brain barrier.[9] Another theory proposes that steady and lowered glucose levels without large fluctuations are at least partially responsible for the anticonvulsant effects.[10,11] Other studies have suggested the importance of γ-aminobutyric acid (GABA) levels involved in decreasing excitability in cells. GABA levels both at baseline and during treatment with the diet correlated with a larger decrease in seizure frequency.[12] While the definite anticonvulsive mechanism of the diet remains elusive, there is significant evidence to demonstrate its efficacy in refractory epilepsy. Overall, the ketogenic diet and its modified alternatives have many effects on the metabolism of the brain, and it has been shown to produce significant anticonvulsive effects that have helped many children and adults decrease seizures in both frequency and duration.

INDICATIONS FOR DIETARY TREATMENT OF EPILEPSY

The ketogenic diet and its alternatives are not typically recommended as first-line therapy for seizure disorders. However, based on recent recommendations, it should be highly indicated in pediatric patients who have unsuccessfully tried two to three anticonvulsant therapies. The diet is a significant lifestyle adjustment for children and is typically considered only after medications have been attempted. However, the diet is considered to have only a small benefit in children who are candidates for epilepsy surgery and/or who have a focal epileptic syndrome. There are some epileptic syndromes or metabolic genetic disorders with seizures in which dietary management should be considered earlier in the course of treatment due to significant documented success. These include myoclonic-astatic epilepsy, infantile spasms, tuberous sclerosis, Rett syndrome, and Dravet syndrome. Myoclonic-astatic epilepsy (Doose syndrome) is an epilepsy syndrome characterized as a primary generalized idiopathic seizure disorder that most prominently includes myoclonic and astatic seizures.[13] The ketogenic diet is one of the most effective therapies for this syndrome with 58% of patients becoming seizure-free and another 35% experiencing a >50% reduction in seizures.[14] Rett syndrome is a neurodevelopmental disorder that is progressive in nature and affects females. Children with this disorder typically develop normally at first and then experience a regression of motor and language skills. Epilepsy is also frequently seen in this disorder.[15] Using the ketogenic diet in the patients showed improvement in seizure control along with some small behavioral and motor improvements.[16] Infantile spasms is a seizure disorder characterized by clusters of spasms by flexor, or extensors of the head, neck, torso, and limbs. There is usually cognitive impairment as well as some additional seizure types.[17] Research has shown that the ketogenic diet significantly (>50%) decreases seizures within 6 months to 2 years of treatment.[18] Tuberous sclerosis is characterized by hamartomas that form in multiple organ systems, including dermatological, renal, and neurologic. Neurologic abnormalities typically include intractable early onset epilepsy and cognitive dysfunction.[19] Kossoff and Thiele[20] found that 92% of children had a >50% decrease in seizures at 6 months and 67% had >90% decrease in seizures. Dravet syndrome is a severe epileptic syndrome that begins in infancy and usually leads to progressive developmental decline. Early diagnosis and seizure control is particularly important in these patients since this will help reduce the impact of cognitive decline.[21] The ketogenic diet is commonly attempted in patients with this syndrome after three to four failed AEDS. One study showed a >75% reduction in seizures in 77% of patients.[22] Other studies have demonstrated similar efficacy.[23] Additionally, the ketogenic diet is considered first-line therapy for pyruvate dehydrogenase deficiency and GLUT-1 deficiency.[9]

INITIATING THE DIET

PRE-DIET

Prior to starting the ketogenic diet or its alternatives, it is important to consult an epilepsy center with experience in administering the diet. The diet has to be supervised by a trained nutritionist. Several evaluations need to occur before the diet is started.

Diary

A patient or caregiver should have a well-documented record of seizures, including frequency, duration, and triggers. A food diary should also be kept for about a month prior to starting the diet.[24]

Contraindications

There are several metabolic conditions that have to be ruled out before starting the ketogenic diet. The conditions include metabolic disorders that, if present, can be significantly debilitating or fatal with the ketogenic diet. These inborn errors of metabolism include primary or acquired carnitine deficiency (any type), β-oxidation defects, pyruvate carboxylase deficiency, organic aciduria, and porphyria.[9,24]

Screening Labs

While it is center-dependent which evaluation labs are performed, the current guidelines set forth in 2009 in a consensus statement by physicians and nutritionists with experience in administering the diet recommend the tests given in Table 28.1.

Other additional labs are performed in some epilepsy centers across the world. These are listed in Table 28.2.

The lab workup is necessary to assess for presence of conditions that could cause difficulties during the diet. The metabolic effects of the diet could precipitate elevations in liver enzymes,

---

TABLE 28.1

Screening Labs

CBC

CMP

Zinc

Selenium

Fasting lipid profile

Serum acylcarnitine profile

UA

Urine Ca^{2+} and Cr

Seizure medication levels

Urine organic acids

Serum amino acids

TABLE 28.2

Additional Labs

Amylase

Lipase

Lactate

Urine ALA and PBG

Renal U/S (if hx of nephrolithiasis)

EEG

MRI

CSF

EKG (if hx of heart disease)

kidney stones, gastro-esophageal reflux disease (GERD), constipation, dehydration, acute pancreatitis, increased bleeding/bruising, aspiration pneumonia, sepsis, growth retardation, and dyslipidemia.[8,9,25,26]

Psychosocial Evaluation

Starting a restrictive diet is a challenge for any individual. Many factors need to be taken into account in order to be well prepared, especially considering the population of patients. In the case of the ketogenic diet and its alternatives, strict adherence is very important. When treating the pediatric population, it is crucial that the caregivers understand the involvement and extent of the diet. They need to be prepared to be exact with the administration of the diet and take into account any allergies and dietary restrictions due to religious beliefs. Along with this, potential behavior issues should be addressed.[9] Additionally, the child should be counseled on the diet as well—with an explanation appropriate for his/her level of understanding. There has been little research looking at the psychosocial effects of the ketogenic diet and its alternatives; however, some small studies suggest a decrease in psychosocial adjustment and an increase in mood problems. Cognitive skills and attention were shown to have slight improvements with the diet.[27] Expectations of the potential effectiveness should be discussed to ensure that the family has a realistic view of the treatment and side effects, necessary trial period for the diet (usually at least 3 months), and medical complications that may arise.[9]

DIET CHOICE

When deciding the appropriate diet for each patient, it is important to consider the day-to-day life of the patient and his/her ability to be compliant. There are four main dietary options that can be offered: ketogenic, MCT, MAD, and LGIT. The details of each diet will be discussed later in this chapter; however, there are several general suggestions when selecting the best diet choice for each patient.

1. Ketogenic diet
   a. Patients who have an all liquid diet, such as infants or enterally fed[9,28]
   b. Patients with pyruvate dehydrogenase deficiency, GLUT-1 deficiency, myoclonic astatic epilepsy[9,28]
   c. Patients who need more structure in the diet[28]
2. MCT
   a. Patients with constipation (due to the laxative effects of MCT oil)[9,29]
   b. Patients who cannot tolerate the amount of fat required by the ketogenic diet[29]

3. MAD
   a. Patients and caregivers unable to handle the time commitment for measuring meals of the ketogenic diet[30]
   b. Patients living far away from a treatment center, who would prefer more outpatient management and less follow-up appointments[30]
   c. Patients needing more freedom in the diet and less limitation on protein, fluid, and calories[9,28]
   d. Adolescents and adults[9,30,28]
4. LGIT
   a. Patients' food preferences requiring more carbohydrates in the diet (40–60 g/day LGIT vs. 10 g/day on ketogenic diet)[31]
   b. Patients and caregivers unable to handle the time commitment for measuring meals of the ketogenic diet
   c. Patients needing more freedom in the diet and less limitation on protein, fluid, and calories[9]
   d. Adolescents and adults

Clinical Case Examples—Which Diet to Choose?

1. Eric is a 7-year-old boy with cerebral palsy and drop seizures occurring daily. He has a gastrostomy tube that has been in place for many years. He has failed two anti-seizure drugs. Eric's parents would like to try dietary therapy. Which diet would be best for him to attempt?

   Eric is a great candidate for the ketogenic diet. Given that he is fed via a G-tube, it will be easy to transition Eric to the diet. He will be switched to Ketocal instead of the formula he is currently receiving and will need to be monitored with blood work and urine ketones.

2. Allie is a 10-year-old girl with intractable absence-type seizures. She has considerable behavioral problems and is a picky eater. Allie has three siblings (two older and one younger). Allie's parents would like to try dietary therapy but are concerned about Allie's behavior and ability to be on such a restrictive diet. Which diet would be best for Allie?

   This case is not as simple as Eric's. Due to the behavioral problems and the fact that there are several other siblings in the house, it may be harder to start Allie on the ketogenic diet. However, some parents report improvements in behavior once the child is on the diet. Just like for every child, it is best to work with the family and figure out what will suit them the best. In this case, if the parents are willing to try, it may be best to attempt the ketogenic diet first and see if it is effective and tolerable. If it is effective but hard to tolerate for Allie, the medical team can change the diet of Allie to MCT or MAD or LGIT. It is important to have good communication with the family and address their concerns as they occur.

3. Tom is a 29-year-old man who has intractable generalized tonic–clonic seizures. He has tried four different medications and a temporal lobe resection, all of which failed to control his seizures. He would like to try dietary therapy. Which diet would be best for Tom to try?

   Since Tom is an adult, the ketogenic diet will likely be too restrictive and cumbersome for him to attempt. It is best for him to try the MAD or LGIT, which allows for more flexibility and food options.

INITIATION

Initiation of any new diet should be done under the care of a physician. The ketogenic diet and its alternatives require an interdisciplinary approach with training in pediatric epilepsy care, including an epileptologist, a dietitian, a registered nurse, a social worker, and a pharmacist.[24]

Ketogenic Diet

Starting the diet usually requires an admission to the hospital for about 4 days. This is done in order to monitor the patient carefully and to provide thorough education to the caregivers. Historically, the diet has been initiated with a period of fasting lasting 24–48 h. The reasoning behind this was to quickly induce ketosis for more rapid seizure control.[12] The fasting period is still used in some centers and also as third- or fourth-line therapy in status epilepticus.[32] However, more recent studies have shown that a fasting period is not needed to initiate the diet, and there is an equal level of efficacy in patients starting with or without an initial fast. Moreover, the group of patients starting the diet with a fasting period typically experiences increased incidence of hypoglycemia, dehydration, acidosis (needing treatment), and weight loss.[33]

The diet can be started gradually with full calories and increasing the KD ratio every day from 1:1 (fat/nonfat), 2:1, 3:1, to 4:1. This approach allows the patient to slowly adjust to the change in dietary lipid content. After the initiation is complete and the caregivers are well educated on how to calculate the diet, the child may be discharged home and followed outpatient with detailed record keeping of seizures, growth, and nutrition status.[9,24]

Medium-Chain Triglycerides

For this alternative diet approach, a hospital admission is typically required for about 4 days. Patients begin on a one third ketogenic shake, which is made up of milk with MCT oil, long-chain triglycerides (LCT), and sugar or protein powder. This shake is given every 2–3 h. During the admission, patients progress to a two thirds ketogenic shake for six feeds. Once this is tolerated, the diet is advanced to full solid foods. Once again, during the hospital admission, caregivers and children are educated about administering the diet. Patients are discharged from the hospital once they are able to tolerate the diet.[34]

MAD and LGIT

Both of these diets are more liberal and can be started on an outpatient basis. The monitoring of a multidisciplinary team is still necessary, but follow-up can be less frequent. MAD limits carbohydrates to 10–20 g/day, whereas LGIT allows only carbohydrates with a low glycemic index (GI) but up to 40–60 g/day.[28]

DIETARY SPECIFICS OF THE KETOGENIC DIET

The classic ketogenic diet uses a ratio of 4:1 (4 g fat/1 g protein + carbohydrates) (Table 28.5). With this ratio, 90% of the calories comes from fat and 10% comes from a protein (6–8%) and carbohydrates combination (~2%).[9] Some children have trouble tolerating such a high amount of fat; in those cases, a ratio of 3:1 may be used. Total calories per day are usually calculated based on the recommended daily allowance (RDA), based on the weight of the child. Level of activity, metabolic rate, and current weight, height, and state of health should all be taken into account when calculating the RDA. Protein quantity is usually calculated at 1 g/kg/day.[5,24]

There are three basic structures of meal plans for the diet[5] (Table 28.3):

- Poultry/fish/meat, vegetable/fruit, fat, whipping cream
- Cheese, fruit/vegetable, fat, whipping cream
- Egg, fruit/vegetable, fat whipping cream

Initially, fluid restriction in the ketogenic diet was thought to increase the effectiveness of seizure control; however, this has since been disproven. Currently, fluid intake is recommended to be at a maintenance level based on the weight of the child[5] (Table 28.4).

The following example is a sample diet plan to help better understand how to calculate the ketogenic diet in terms of calories per day and required breakdown of protein, fat, and carbohydrates.

TABLE 28.3

Example of Ketogenic Meal with a 4:1 Ratio

Food	Grams	Calories	Ratio
Heavy whipping cream	106		
Carrots	9		
Chicken breast	16		
Butter	8		
Total		450 kcal	4:1

Source: Kossoff, EH et al., *Ketogenic Diets: Treatment of Epilepsy and Other Disorders.* 5th ed. Demos, 2011; Miranda, MJ et al., *Epilepsy Research*, 1–8, 2012.

TABLE 28.4

Maintenance Fluids

Weight	Fluid Intake
1–10 kg	100 mL/kg
10–20 kg	1000 mL + 50 mL/kg for each kilogram over the first 10 kg
≥20 kg	1500 mL = 20 mL/kg for each kilogram over the first 20 kg

CALCULATING THE DIET FOR A SAMPLE PATIENT[5]

Jack is a 3-year-old boy who weighs 30 lbs. (13.6 kg). He has been prescribed a 4:1 ketogenic diet. A nutritionist makes the determination that Jack's weight is appropriate—this determination is based on previously mentioned factors.

1. Calories per kilogram
   a. Jack has had a complete medical and dietary assessment, and a nutritionist has set Jack's diet to be 100 kcal/kg. This number is usually based on the RDA and is comparable to the child's current food intake.
2. Total calories
   a. To calculate the total number of calories per day, multiply the weight by number of calories per kg:

$$13.6 \text{ kg} \times 100 \text{ kcal/kg} = 1360 \text{ kcals}$$

3. Dietary unit composition
   a. Dietary units in a 4:1 diet are made up of 4 g of fat to 1 g protein and carbohydrates combined.
   b. Fat has 9 calories per gram ($9 \times 4 = 36$), and protein and carbohydrate each have 4 calories per gram ($4 \times 1 = 4$).
   c. So the 4:1 ratio diet has 40 ($36 + 4$) calories. The calories vary with the ratio (Table 28.5).

Since Jack is on a *4:1* diet ratio, his dietary units will be made up of *40 calories each.*

4. Dietary unit quantity
   a. Divide the *total calories allotted* (1360) by the *number of calories in each dietary unit* (40). This will determine the number of dietary units allowed every day.

$$1360/40 = 34 \text{ dietary units per day}$$

TABLE 28.5
Ratios and Calories

Ratio	Fat Calories	Carbs Plus Protein Calories	Calories Per Dietary Unit
1:1	1 g × 9 kcal/g = 9	1 g × 4 kcal/g = 4	9 + 4 = 13
2:1	2 g × 9 kcal/g = 18	1 g × 4 kcal/g = 4	18 + 4 = 22
3:1	3 g × 9 kcal/g = 27	1 g × 4 kcal/g = 4	27 + 4 = 31
4:1	4 g × 9 kcal/g = 36	1 g × 4 kcal/g = 4	36 + 4 = 40

5. Fat allowance
   a. Multiply the number of dietary units by the units of fat in the ketogenic ratio to get the grams of fat allowance per day.
   b. On Jack's 4:1 diet with 34 dietary units/day, he will have

$$34 \times 4 = 136 \text{ g of fat per day}$$

6. Carbohydrate + protein allowance
   a. Multiply the number of dietary units by the number of units of protein and carbohydrate combined to get the daily allowance.
   b. Jack will have 34 × 1 = 34 g of protein and carbohydrate daily
7. Protein allowance
   a. The nutritionist should determine the optimal protein level during the nutritional assessment. This should, once again, take into account the child's general health, activity, age, growth, etc.
   b. Jack's nutritionist has decided that he will need 1.2 g of protein/kg.
   c. Weight × protein/kg → 13.6 kg × 1.2 g/kg = 16.32 g total protein
8. Carbohydrate allowance
   a. Subtract the total protein from the total protein + carbohydrate.
   b. Jack's carbohydrate allowance will be 34 − 16.32 = 17.68 g of carbohydrate per day.
9. Meal order
   a. Divide the daily protein, carbs, and fat allowances into the desired number of meal and snacks per day (Table 28.6).
   b. Jack's nutritionist decided to give him 3 meals and 2 snacks per day.
10. Liquids
    a. Jack weighs 13.6 kg, so the calculation is 1000 + (3.6 × 50) = 1180 mL fluid per day.
    b. Cream is included as part of the fluid allowance; however if the weather is particularly warm, fluid calculations should be adjusted accordingly.

TABLE 28.6
Meal and Snack Allowances

	Daily	Per Meal	Per Snack
Protein	16.32 g	4.08	2.04
Fat	136 g	34	17
Carbohydrates	17.68 g	4.42	2.21
Calories	1360	340	170

DIETARY SUPPLEMENTS

Despite its therapeutic effect on seizure activity, the ketogenic diet does not provide adequate vitamins and minerals that would normally be found in a regular diet. In fact, only 5 of 24 essential micronutrients exist in the diet. Vitamin D, calcium, phosphorus, most water-soluble vitamins, fiber, linolenic acid, and vitamin K were found to be especially deficient in kids on the diet.[24] As a result, it is very important to supplement the diet with the proper vitamins and minerals. Additionally, the assistance of an experienced pharmacist is necessary to choose supplement with low carbohydrate content.

Due to the poor nutritional profile of the ketogenic diet, every child should be on a multivitamin. There are several brands used that are low in carbohydrate, for example, sugar-free Scooby Doo vitamins (Bayer), Bugs Bunny sugar-free (Bayer), and Nano VM (Solace Nutrition).[5] Calcium and vitamin D levels tend to be low in children with epilepsy even before starting the diet due to the fact that many antiepileptic medications affect their metabolism.[5,24] Thus, when starting the diet, it is critical to supplement both calcium and vitamin D. The Institute of Medicine has recommended some guidelines for appropriate calcium and vitamin D doses by age group.[5]

One of the side effects that can be precipitated by the diet is nephrolithiasis. As a result, some centers now give oral citrates to help alkalinize the urine and make urine calcium soluble. Sometimes children may get a carnitine deficiency during the course of the diet; therefore, many treatment centers will check the carnitine level prior to beginning the diet and monitor throughout the course with supplementation as needed.[5]

SPECIAL CONSIDERATIONS FOR ALL-LIQUID DIETS

All-liquid ketogenic diets (i.e., KetoCal) are usually used for infants and children fed enterally with a gastrostomy or jejunostomy tube. In general, kids on this formula-based diet have great compliance and high efficacy. Also, most formulas already contain all the necessary minerals and vitamins; however, sometimes the amounts are insufficient for the age group and should thus be further supplemented.[5,9]

ALTERNATIVE DIETS (MCT, MAD, LGIT)

MEDIUM-CHAIN TRIGLYCERIDES

The MCT diet was originally developed as an alternative to the ketogenic diet because of its ability to achieve a ketotic state with less fat consumption (70–75% MCT vs. 90% in ketogenic diet). The traditional ketogenic diet is composed of fat sources mostly made up of LCT. In the MCT diet,

---

TABLE 28.7
Example of MCT Meal

Food	Grams	Calories
Salmon (raw)	35	
Potato (boiled)	50	
Double cream	17	
Cheddar cheese	8	
French beans (boiled)	45	
Pear	50	
MCT oil	24	
Total		450 kcal, 45% MCT

Source: Miranda, MJ et al., *Epilepsy Research*, 1–8, 2012.

---

some of the LCT sources of fat are replaced by MCT oil (Table 28.7). MCT is absorbed by being carried directly to the liver and does not require carnitine to transport it. This metabolic difference increases the ability to yield more ketones than LCT.[5]

The effectiveness of the MCT diet has been shown to be equal to the ketogenic diet. MCT oil usually comprises somewhere between 30% and 60% of the fat energy in the diet, depending on how well the patient is able to tolerate the oil. MCT oil can be given to patients in the form of coconut oil, MCT oil, or as an emulsion and should be included with every meal. The MCT diet is a better option for kids who are very particular about their food, teenagers, and patients who have larger appetites. This diet allows patients to be able to eat more food with more vegetables and fruits. In addition, there are fewer common and rare side effects. Typically, the MCT diet is not recommended for patients who are under 1 year old, have chronic diarrhea, are enterally fed, and have aspiration issues.[29,34]

As evidenced by the example in Table 28.7, there is a lot more food allowed in a sample meal of MCT vs. ketogenic diet. The MCT diet typically has the following breakdown: fat (MCT 30–60%, LCT 11–45%), protein (10%), and carbohydrates (15–19%).[28]

Modified Atkins Diet

As compared to the ketogenic, the MAD allows for an almost balanced diet with 60% fat, 30% protein, and 10% carbohydrates. The ratio of fat/nonfat is about 2:1 on this diet.[5,30]

Overall, MAD is much better tolerated than the ketogenic diet. It was also found to be comparably but slightly less effective in controlling seizures (see Figures 28.1 and 28.2[35] for comparison). Much like any diet that significantly limits a major food group, this diet needs to be supplemented with vitamins and minerals, though less so than the ketogenic diet.[30] There are several important factors to consider with the MAD that contribute to making it maximally effective:

1. Strong ketosis is needed for better seizure control. Patients with β-hydroxybutyrate levels >3 mol/L that did not fluctuate significantly were shown to have the best seizure control.[30]
2. Starting the diet with more strict guidelines for carbohydrate intake (<10 g/day) and increasing this amount after a couple of months also demonstrated better seizure control. This stricter induction phase seems to play a role in better ketosis.[30]

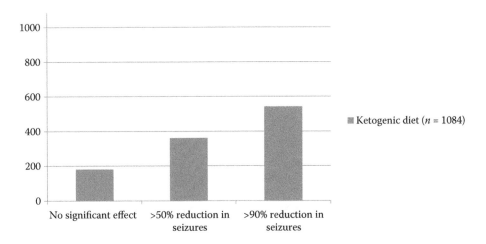

FIGURE 28.1 Ketogenic diet effect on seizures. (From Henderson, CB et al., *J Child Neurol*, 21:193–198, 2006.)

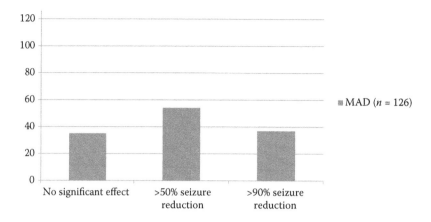

FIGURE 28.2 MAD effect on seizures. (From Henderson, CB et al., *J Child Neurol*, 21:193–198, 2006.)

TABLE 28.8
Example of MAD Meal

Food	Ounces
Turkey breast	3–4
Swiss cheese	2–3
Spinach and mushroom salad	

Source: Miranda, MJ et al., *Epilepsy Research*, 1–8, 2012.

---

3. Following the concept of a stricter induction phase, administering the diet with a ketogenic liquid supplement for the first month yielded faster ketosis and better overall seizure control with reduction in frequency and duration.[36]
4. Patients who do not have an improvement in seizure control on MAD will not have any further efficacy from the ketogenic diet. However, patients who do achieve some improvement with MAD may be able to get even better results if switched to the ketogenic diet.[37]

The MAD tends to be recommended for teenagers, adults, or children who are picky eaters and cannot tolerate the ketogenic diet (Table 28.8). Additionally, starting the MAD does not require an inpatient hospital admission and can be started on an outpatient basis with the help of a multidisciplinary team. For responsible teenagers and adults, it is even possible for the diet to be successfully managed via email.[38]

LOW GLYCEMIC INDEX TREATMENT

The LGIT, like the MAD, is implemented when patients are unable to tolerate the ketogenic diet. The concept behind this diet is that stable glucose levels contribute more to seizure control than ketosis level. The GI estimates how much each gram of carbohydrate in a particular food raises the blood glucose level after the consumption of the food, relative to consumption of glucose. LGIT has a low level ketosis but keeps blood glucose stable by only allowing certain carbohydrates that have a low GI. The GI of certain foods can be changed by adding proteins or fats to the carbohydrates. This will slow the digestion and, as a result, lower the GI. Therefore, LGIT only allows certain carbohydrates to be ingested while on the diet; however, the amount of carbohydrates allowed is higher than the ketogenic or any of its other alternatives (40–60 g/day LGIT vs. 10–20 g MAD vs. less than 10 g KD) (Table 28.9).[5,28]

TABLE 28.9
Example of LGIT Meal

Food	Amount
Low-carb pita pocket	1/2
Roast beef	4 oz.
Cheddar cheese	1 oz.
Horseradish mayo	1/2 tbsp.
Roasted red pepper	1/2 cup
Heavy cream	2 oz.

Source: Kossoff, EH et al., *Ketogenic Diets: Treatment of Epilepsy and Other Disorders*, 5th ed. Demos, 2011.

TABLE 28.10
Examples of Low vs. High GI Foods

Food	GI
Lettuce	10
Peanuts	15
Broccoli	15
Pears	16
Apples	38
Ice cream	61
Mashed potato	70
Waffles	76
Pretzels	83

Source: Kossoff, EH et al., *Ketogenic Diets: Treatment of Epilepsy and Other Disorders*, 5th ed. Demos, 2011.

LGIT allows carbohydrates with a GI < 50 to be consumed with a ratio of about 1:1 (fat/nonfat) (Table 28.10). There is no overall caloric restriction. The proportions of the diet are usually about 60% fat, 20–30% protein, and 10% carbohydrates. Better seizure control on diet has been correlated with lower and more stable glucose levels, not β-hydroxybutyrate levels/ketosis.[10,31,28]

The LGIT, like the MAD, tends to be recommended for teenagers, adults, or children who are picky eaters and cannot tolerate the ketogenic diet. This diet is better tolerated than the ketogenic diet and allows for more food options. LGIT can be started on an outpatient basis, without the necessity for a hospital stay.[5,28]

GENERAL NOTE ON ALTERNATIVE DIETS

While there has been a significant amount of research done on the ketogenic diet and even the MCT diet that has shown its effectiveness, there are fewer studies that have been completed looking at the LGIT and MAD. The studies that have been performed show strong results in efficacy and low side effects. However, more research is needed to comparatively look at the efficacy of the ketogenic diet/MCT vs. LGIT and MAD. See Figure 28.3 for a comparison of ratios in each diet.

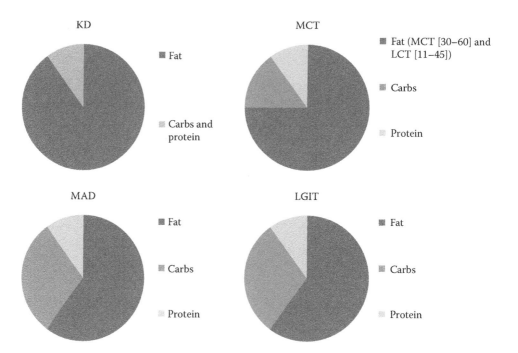

FIGURE 28.3   Ratios for the ketogenic diet vs. alternative diets.

SIDE EFFECTS OF THE KETOGENIC DIET AND ITS ALTERNATIVES

KETOGENIC DIET SIDE EFFECTS

Side effects are important to note and address with any medical treatment. With the ketogenic diet, side effects are usually the main reason for discontinuing the diet. Adverse effect can occur at the beginning of the diet, during the course of it, or after its cessation.

Some centers start the diet with a fasting period of 24–48 h. This can sometimes result in hypoglycemia; however, unless the child is symptomatic or the blood glucose falls below 30 mg/dL, no treatment is necessary. Additionally, when starting the diet, children may become acidotic. If the acidosis becomes symptomatic, it typically presents as vomiting and/or sleepiness. In this situation, treatment is given in the form of IV fluids and sometimes bicarbonate.[5]

Other side effects that may occur at the start of the diet include dehydration (treated with oral fluids or IV fluids in severe cases), vomiting (from the keto shake), and refusal to eat. Vomiting can be treated by having the child take smaller sips and/or starting solid foods faster. Encouraging children to eat can be done by advancing to solid foods quicker or mixing the keto shake into more palatable foods.[5]

Adverse effects while already on the diet include constipation, weight changes, infections, vitamin and mineral deficiency, hypercholesterolemia, lipid abnormalities, carnitine deficiency, and nephrolithiasis.[5,8,24] Each of these adverse effects should be addressed as they arise with appropriate treatment. Nephrolithiasis risk is increased and arises in 1/20 cases.[5] Kidney stones can present nonspecifically with fever, abdominal pain, and poor appetite but can also present with flank pain or blood in the urine. Increased fluid intake in patients who are at risk of developing kidney stones is recommended. Additionally, citrates can be given prophylactically when starting the diet.[5,24]

More severe side effects can also occur while on the diet. Some of these side effects can arise from antiepileptic medications but can be exacerbated with the ketogenic diet. These include acute pancreatitis, hepatitis, hemolytic anemia, Fanconi renal tubular acidosis, cardiomyopathy, increases in liver function testing (LFTs), increased bruising, prolonged QT (measure of time between Q wave and T wave on ECG), and coma.[5,8,11,24]

Since the diet has demonstrated very promising results for seizure control, it has recently been used for longer periods of time than initially intended. As a result, long-term side effects are now seen.[5] Most of the long-term side effects are related to calcium and vitamin D deficiencies. Typically, the most common long-term adverse effects are growth retardation, bone fractures, and nephrolithiasis.[5,26] If a patient is on the diet for over 2 years, it is suggested that they get a dual-energy X-ray absorptiometry (DEXA) scan to assess the condition of their bones.[5] This measure can help guide further management and take appropriate precautions against fractures. Children most at risk for fractures are those who are non-ambulatory, are astatic, have drop seizures, or have frequent generalized convulsions.[5] Growth retardation can also be seen with children on the diet. Typically, once the diet is stopped, these kids will have a "catch-up" of growth.[26] If the diet cannot be stopped due to seizures, then it is possible to transition these patients to the MAD, which will increase the amount of protein in the diet.[5] Some international centers have also tried growth hormone administration with promising results, though no official studies have been performed.[5]

ALTERNATIVE DIETS (MCT, MAD, LGIT) SIDE EFFECTS

The same side effects seen in the ketogenic diet can be seen in its alternatives. However, these effects are much rarer and less serious. The only exception is the MCT diet, which in some studies was found to have more gastrointestinal side effects, particularly abdominal pain and diarrhea. These side effects of the MCT can be reduced by adjusting the ratio of the fat given as MCT oil.[29]

PSYCHOSOCIAL ISSUES AND EFFECTS

As previously discussed, the ketogenic diet (or its alternatives) can have a negative effect on psychosocial adjustment and cause an increase in mood problems.[27] However, some of the psychosocial effects are not negative and can actually improve a patient's quality of life. There has been some evidence that after a few months on the diet, children will have cognitive, attentive, and behavioral improvement even if the seizure control is not significant.[39]

One study looked at the sleep quality of children on the ketogenic diet. The study compared the polysomnographic recordings prior to the diet to the ones taken at 3 months into the diet and then again at 12 months. It was found that children on the diet experienced an increase in REM sleep, decreased daytime sleepiness, and a decrease in the total amount of sleep needed to feel rested. The researchers also found an increase in attention, improved behavior, and an improved overall quality of life.[40]

SAMPLE FOOD IDEAS FOR CARBOHYDRATE ALTERNATIVES

The ketogenic diet and its alternatives can be seen as being extremely restrictive diets that are hard to follow. Children may feel like they are unable to eat anything that "normal" kids can eat, and caregivers may have trouble putting together meals. This section is meant to inspire some creativity to make the diets more palatable and provide a greater variety of food. There are no exact measurements given for recipes, just some general ideas for making keto-friendly meals.

BAKED GOODS

Most baked goods in everyday life require flour. Unfortunately, regular flour is loaded with carbohydrates. There are several great alternative "flours" (Table 28.11) that can be used to make anything from pancakes, muffins, brownies, etc… All baked goods can be sweetened with carbohydrate-free sweetener, which is available in most grocery stores. See Figures 28.4 and 28.5[41] for simple LGIT recipes.

TABLE 28.11
Flour Alternatives

Flour	Serving (g)	Carbohydrates (g)	Protein (g)	Fat (g)
Almond flour	28	6	6	14
Coconut flour	14	8	2	2
Flaxseed meal	13	4	3	4.5

Note: All these products are made by Bob's Red Mill.

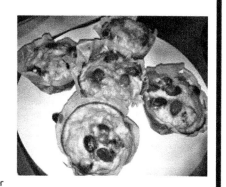

Banana Cranberry Muffins
Makes 6 muffin. 1 serving = 1 muffin.
Carbs per serving: 12.3

Ingredients:
2.5 Bananas (mashed)
½ cup almond flour
2 eggs
3/4 cup unsweetened cranberries
(fresh or frozen not dried)

Instructions:
1. Preheat oven to 375
2. Mix together all ingredients and pour into either greased muffin tin or use muffin paper
3. Bake for 20 min

FIGURE 28.4 LGIT banana cranberry muffins. (From http://BigSpoonOrLittleSpoon.com.)

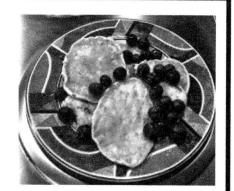

Cottage Cheese Pancakes
Makes about 8-9 small pancakes.
Serving size: About 5 pancakes
Carbs per serving: 11.95

Ingredients:
2 eggs
1 cup cottage cheese
2 tsps of Stevia
1 tbsp of flaxseeds
1/2 cup almond flour
Pinch of baking soda
1 tsp coconut oil

Instructions:
1. Heat a medium sized skillet with a bit of coconut oil
2. Mix all ingredients together in bowl
3. Using a spoon, scoop about 1 tbsp onto the hot skillet, lower heat to low and cover the skillet
4. Cook each pancake about 1-2 min then flip over and cook another 30-45 s

FIGURE 28.5 LGIT cottage cheese pancakes. (From http://BigSpoonOrLittleSpoon.com.)

Pasta, Bread, Rice, and Crackers

For children, especially those living in the United States, carbohydrate-heavy meals like pasta are staples in a diet. It can be very hard to give those up. There are several alternatives that can be used that, when mixed with heavy whipping cream or butter and some vegetables, can create a great keto-friendly meal.

One company that is used by many keto-families is Miracle Noodle.[42] This company makes noodles, rice, pasta, and flour from soluble fiber called glucomannan, which is carbohydrate- and sugar-free. Flavoring these with vegetable and olive oil and adding a source of protein can create great-tasting meals. Additionally, spaghetti squash can be used as an alternative to regular spaghetti. The flours listed above as well as ground macadamia nuts can be used to make crackers. Bread can be made from flax flour mixed with almond flour. Crepes can be made by using sour cream instead of flour and adding egg, butter, and cream and some sort of fruit topping.

Fried Food

There are many kids today who love fast food such as chicken nuggets, french fries, milkshakes, and ice cream, while normally, a parent would not encourage these types of foods for a child's healthy diet. On the ketogenic diet, the modified version of these foods may be a great meal idea. Almond flour mixed with egg can be used to make a light batter for chicken nuggets. Ice cream can be made with heavy whipping cream mixed with unsweetened cocoa and/or fruit and then frozen. This same mixture can be mixed with KetoCal supplement to create something like a milkshake. French fries can be made with zucchini using the same light batter with almond flour and egg.

DIETARY THERAPY FOR EPILEPSY IN ADULTS

Dietary therapy for epilepsy in adults was previously seen as being too restrictive, and as a result, the research on using dietary therapy in adults is sparse. There are a couple of reasons for this. One is the lack of adult epilepsy dietary centers or programs that would help initiate a dietary protocol for adults along with consistent follow-up care. Most dietary epilepsy centers that exist are pediatric. Another reason for the research lacking in adult dietary treatment of epilepsy is the difficulty in changing eating habits. As most people know, going on a diet of any kind is difficult; however, going on the ketogenic diet for a grown adult will not only require an overhaul of food selections but also psychological and social issues. Being on the ketogenic diet significantly limits the options for eating out at restaurants, which can impact an adult's social and personal life. However, with the introduction of KD alternatives, adults are now being offered the dietary treatment option with several smaller studies demonstrating good results.

An article recently published by Kossoff et al.[43] discussed adult dietary therapy from the perspective of transitioning pediatric patients to adult care. The patients mentioned in this article were already on the ketogenic diet or one of its alternatives. Their transition to adult care took place at a newly opened Adult Epilepsy Diet Center (AEDC) in Johns Hopkins Hospital. Some of the issues encountered during the transition were as follows: the need for an adult neurologist trained with dietary therapy and an adult dietitian trained for the ketogenic diet, and addressing adult issues such as independent living, pregnancy, and different nutritional requirements than those for children.[44] These quality-of-life issues are extremely important to address in any patient that is changing their medical care to a new physician. In the case of dietary treatment for epilepsy, a team-based approach is necessary to provide proper support and counseling to the patient.

There are several smaller studies that have shown good results with starting patients on MAD or LGIT on an outpatient basis and providing additional information and follow-up via email. These studies demonstrated promising results for initiating and maintaining dietary therapy in adults with epilepsy, with about 50% of patients benefiting significantly from treatment.[11,44,45]

While no treatment whether pharmacological or dietary is completely benign, MAD and LGIT can certainly present a better option for obese adults looking to lose weight and help seizure control and also in women who are planning a pregnancy.[45] The importance of dietary counseling is crucial for both parents of children with epilepsy and also for adults wanting to try the diet. Resources, recipes, and reliable follow-up with a nutritionist are invaluable for successful implementation of dietary therapy.

CONCLUSION

Dietary therapy for epilepsy goes back thousands of years, with fasting being one of the earliest recorded treatments for stopping seizures. The ketogenic diet came about roughly a century ago as a means to induce a ketotic state to mimic the effects of starvation on the brain. Throughout the century, alternative dietary methods such as MAD, MCT, and LGIT have been introduced and have proved to be equally effective and more palatable. Dietary therapy is now a well-established treatment modality for refractory epilepsy. While originally only implemented in children, dietary therapy has now been adapted for adults as well. Additionally, increasing interest in the implications of the ketogenic diet and its modified alternatives not only has led to a better understanding of the diet but also shows promising research opportunities for numerous other neurological conditions such as brain tumors, Parkinson's disease, Alzheimer's, brain trauma, and many more.

SOURCES FOR MORE INFORMATION INCLUDING RECIPES AND SUPPORT GROUPS

The Charlie Foundation (http://www.charliefoundation.org)
Matthews Friends (http://www.matthewsfriends.org)
The Carson Harris Foundation (http://www.carsonharrisfoundation.org)
Keto Calculator (http://www.ketocalculator.com)
MAD (http://modifiedmom.wordpress.com)
LGIT recipes (http://BigSpoonOrLittleSpoon.com)
Miracle Noodle (http://www.miraclenoodle.com)
No-carb flavoring (http://www.bickfordflavors.com)
Products (http://www.netrition.com)
Northeast Regional Epilepsy Group (http://www.epilepsygroup.com)
Epilepsy Life Links (http://www.epilepsylifelinks.com)

REFERENCES

1. Available at http://www.epilepsyfoundation.org.
2. Temkin, O. *The Falling Sickness*, 2nd edition. Johns Hopkins University Press, Baltimore, MD, 1971.
3. Guelpa, G, Marie, A. La Lutte contre l'epilepsie par la desintoxication et par la reeducation alimentaire. *Rev Ther Medico-Chirurgicale*. 1911;78:8–13.
4. Conklin, HW. Cause and treatment of epilepsy. *J Am Osteopathic Assoc*. 1922;26:11–14.
5. Kossoff, EH, Freeman, JM, Turner, Z, Rubenstein, JE. *Ketogenic Diets: Treatment of Epilepsy and Other Disorders*, 5th edition. Demos, New York, 2011.
6. Wheless, JW. History of the ketogenic diet. *Epilepsia*. 2008;49(Suppl. 8):3–5.
7. The Charlie Foundation. Available at http://www.charliefoundation.org.
8. Kang, HC, Kim, HD. Diet therapy in refractory pediatric epilepsy: Increased efficacy and tolerability. *Epileptic Disord*. 2006;8:309–316.
9. Kossoff, EH, Zupec-Kania, BA, Amark, PE et al. Optimal clinical management of children receiving the ketogenic diet: Recommendations of the International Ketogenic Diet Study Group. *Epilepsia*. 2009;50:304–317.
10. Muzykewicz, DA, Lyczkowski, DA, Memon, N et al. Efficacy, safety, and tolerability of the low glycemic index treatment in pediatric epilepsy. *Epilepsia*. 2009;50:1118–1126.
11. Schwechter, EM, Veliskova, J, Velisek, L. Correlation between extracellular glucose and seizure susceptibility in adult rats. *Ann Neurol*. 2003;53:91–101.

12. Freeman, JM, Vegiotti, P, Lanzi, G et al. The ketogenic diet: From molecular mechanisms to clinical effects. *Epilepsy Res.* 2006;68:145–180.
13. Kelley, SA, Kossoff, EH. Doose syndrome (myoclonic astatic epilepsy): 40 years of progress. *Dev Med Child Neurol.* 2010;52:988–993.
14. Oguni, H, Tanaka, T, Hayashi, K et al. Treatment and long-term prognosis of myoclonic–astatic epilepsy of early childhood. *Neuropediatrics.* 2002;33:122–132.
15. Han, ZA, Jeon, HR, Kim, SW et al. Clinical characteristics of children with Rett syndrome. *Ann Rehabil Med.* 2012;36:334–339.
16. Haas, RH, Rice, MA, Trauner, DA et al. Therapeutic effects of a ketogenic diet in Rett syndrome. *Am J Med Genet Suppl.* 1986;1:225–246.
17. Mytinger, JR, Joshi, S. Pediatric epilepsy research consortium, section on infantile spasms. *J Child Neurol.* 2012;27(10):1289–1294.
18. Hong, AM, Turner, Z, Hamdy, RF et al. Infantile spasms treated with the ketogenic diet: Prospective single-center experiences in 104 consecutive infants. *Epilepsia.* 2010;51:1403–1407.
19. Orlova, KA, Crino, PB. The tuberous sclerosis complex. *Ann NY Acad Sci.* 2010;1184:84–105.
20. Kossoff, EH, Thiele, EA, Pfeifer, HH et al. Tuberous sclerosis complex and the ketogenic diet. *Epilepsia.* 2005;46:1684–1686.
21. Nangia, S, Caraballo, RH, Kang, HC et al. Is the ketogenic diet effective in specific epilepsy syndromes? *Epilepsy Res.* 2012;100:252–257.
22. Caraballo, RH. Non-pharmacological treatments of Dravet syndrome: Focus on the ketogenic diet. *Epilepsia.* 2011;52(Suppl. 2):79–82.
23. Nabbout, R, Copioli, C, Chipaux, M. Ketogenic diet also benefits Dravet syndrome patients receiving stiripentol: A prospective pilot study. *Epilepsia.* 2011;52:e54–e57.
24. Zupec-Kania, BA, Spellman, E. An overview of the ketogenic diet for pediatric epilepsy. *Nutr Clin Pract.* 2008;23:589–596.
25. Berry-Kravis, E, Booth, G, Taylor, A et al. Bruising and the ketogenic diet: Evidence for diet-induced changes in platelet function. *Ann Neurol.* 2001;49:98–103.
26. Williams, S, Basualdo-Hammond, C, Curtis, R et al. Growth retardation in children with epilepsy on the ketogenic diet: A retrospective chart review. *J Am Diet Assoc.* 2002;102:405–407.
27. Lambrechts, DAJE, Bovens, MJM, de la Parra, NM et al. Ketogenic diet effects on cognition, mood and psychosocial adjustment in children. *Acta Neurol Scand.* 2012;10:1–6.
28. Miranda, MJ, Turner, Z, Magrath, G. Alternative diets to the classical ketogenic diet—Can we be more liberal? *Epilepsy Res.* 2012;100(3):278–285.
29. Neal, EG, Chaffe, H, Schwatrz, RH et al. A randomized trial of classical and medium-chain triglyceride ketogenic diets in the treatment of childhood epilepsy. *Epilepsia.* 2009;50:1109–1117.
30. Kang, HC, Lee, HS, You, SJ et al. Use of a modified Atkins diet in intractable childhood epilepsy. *Epilepsia.* 2007;48:182–186.
31. Pfeifer, HH, Thiele, EA. Low-glycemic-index treatment: A liberalized ketogenic diet for treatment of intractable epilepsy. *Neurology.* 2005;65:1810–1812.
32. Shorvon, S, Ferlisi, M. The outcome of therapies in refractory and super-refractory convulsive status epilepticus and recommendations for therapy. *Brain J Neurol.* 2012;135(8):2314–2328.
33. Bergqvist, AGC, Schall, JI, Gallagher, PR et al. Fasting versus gradual initiation of the ketogenic diet: A prospective, randomized clinical trial of efficacy. *Epilepsia.* 2005;46:1810–1819.
34. Liu, YC. Medium-chain triglycerides (MCT) ketogenic therapy. *Epilepsia.* 2008;49:33–36.
35. Henderson, CB, Filloux, FM, Alder, SC, Lyon, JL, Caplin, DA. Efficacy of the ketogenic diet as a treatment option for epilepsy: Meta-analysis. *J Child Neurol.* 2006;21:193–198.
36. Kossoff, EH, Doward, JL, Turner, Z et al. Prospective study of the modified Atkins diet in combination with a ketogenic liquid supplement during the initial month. *J Child Neurol.* 2011;26:147–151.
37. Auvin, S. Should we routinely use modified Atkins diet instead of regular ketogenic diet to treat children with epilepsy? *Seizure.* 2012;21:237–240.
38. Cervenka, MC, Terao, NN, Bosarge, JL et al. E-mail management of the modified Atkins diet for adults with epilepsy is feasible and effective. *Epilepsia.* 2012;53:728–732.
39. Pulsifier, MB, Gordon, JM, Brandt, J et al. Effects of ketogenic diet on development and behavior: Preliminary report of a prospective study. *Dev Med Child Neurol.* 2001;43:301–306.
40. Hallbrook, T, Lundgren, J, Rosen, I. Ketogenic diet improves sleep quality in children with therapy-resistance epilepsy. *Epilepsia.* 2007;48:59–65.
41. Available at http://BigSpoonOrLittleSpoon.com.
42. Available at http://www.miraclenoodle.com.

43. Kossoff, EH, Henry, BJ, Cervenka, MC. Transitioning pediatric patients receiving ketogenic diets for epilepsy into adulthood. *Seizure: Eur J Epilepsy*. 2013;22(6):487–489.
44. Kossoff, EH, Rowley, H, Sinha SR, Vining EP. A prospective study of the modified Atkins diet for intractable epilepsy in adults. *Epilepsia*. 2008;49:316–319.
45. Kossoff, EH, Wang, HS. Dietary therapies for epilepsy. *Biomed J*. 2013;36:2–8.

29 Role of Nutritional Factors in Multiple Sclerosis

Channa Kolb, Sheikh M. Faheem,
and Bianca Weinstock-Guttman

CONTENTS

INTRODUCTION

Multiple sclerosis (MS) is considered an immune-mediated inflammatory disease of the central nervous system (CNS) affecting primarily young adults.[1,2] The cause of MS remains unknown, but its extensively studied epidemiology has highlighted MS as a complex, multifactorial induced disease involving genetic and environmental factors. Data from natural history cohorts show a broad spectrum of disease severities.

MS disease course can be classified into four types: relapsing remitting MS (RRMS), secondary progressive MS (SPMS), primary progressive MS (PPMS), and progressive-relapsing MS (PRMS). In more than 80% of cases, MS follows a relapsing–remitting pattern that involves short-term episodes of neurologic deficits or relapses that recover initially almost completely RRMS being followed by stable or remission periods.

As a natural history, within 10–15 years, 50% of RRMS patients may convert to SPMS stage characterized by a progressive physical and cognitive deterioration and a decrease in the number of relapses. The disease course is considered benign in 10–15% of patients as they do not need an assistive device for walking even after 20 years from disease onset, but often the cognitive status is not included in this assessment.[3–5]

On the other end of the spectrum, there are fulminant forms of MS that lead to severe disability within a few years. The clinical variance may be related to etiology, the underlying pathological features, and often superimposed comorbidities (i.e., dyslipidemia, cardiovascular disease, diabetes).[6] About 10–15% of MS patients experience steadily progressive neurologic deterioration without superimposed relapses PPMS or very rare relapses superimposed on an initial continuous progressive course PRMS.

Inflammation, demyelination, and axon degeneration are the major pathologic mechanisms that cause the signs and symptoms of MS.[7]

As the cause for MS is unknown, a possible dietary influence was often considered as influencing the risk for developing the disease and eventually its disease course. This chapter will provide a short updated literature overview summarizing the possible link between diet, dietary supplements, and MS.

EPIDEMIOLOGY

MS is estimated to affect more than 2.1 million people worldwide.[8] According to the National Multiple Sclerosis Society reported data, approximately 450,000 individuals in the United States are affected by MS. MS can occur in persons of any age[9]; however, it is usually diagnosed between 20 and 45 years. The female-to-male ratio of MS incidence has increased since the mid-twentieth century, from an estimated 1.4 in 1955 to 2.3 in 2000.[10,11] The reason is unknown, but changes in environmental factors in addition to a better and earlier diagnosis are suspected.[12–13]

The prevalence of MS tends to increase with latitude[14,15] (lower rates in tropics and higher rates in northern Europe), but there are many exceptions to this gradient (e.g., low rates among Chinese and Japanese; high rates among Palestinians). MS affects more often Caucasian than African-American (prevalence 2:1) and lower risk for Oriental Asian.

The etiology of MS remains an enigma. The most widely accepted theory supports an interplay between genetic and presumed environmental factors. The complex multifactorial interactions are considered to initiate and promote a protracted autoimmune process that leads to recurrent immune attacks on the CNS followed by secondary chronic microglial activation and neurodegeneration.[16]

A genetic contribution to disease susceptibility is illustrated by familial clustering of MS as a consequence of an increased MS risk (up to 3.5%) among closer biological relatives of patients.[17] However, only 30% of concordant twins develop MS supporting the prerequisite for additional environmental factors to create an appropriate milieu toward the development of the disease.

There is no major single locus of MS risk, but variation in the human leukocyte allele (HLA) region on chromosome 6, particularly the DRB1*1501 allele, is the strongest MS genetic risk loci identified to date. Genome-wide association studies (GWAS) have resulted in the identification of 58 different disease susceptibility.[18] Although the increased disease risk inferred by each individual locus identified by GWAS is small, the nature of the associated genes highlights a primary role for immune dysfunction in MS.

The major players of environmental factors that are hypothesized as risk factors for MS include geographical location (northern and also southern latitude, 40°–60°), low vitamin D level, and smoking.[19,20]

Normal to high vitamin D level is proposed to have a protective role for MS, while a low vitamin D level is proposed as a risk factor for MS. The incidence of the disease is lower in the equatorial regions of the world. Less exposure to sunlight results in lesser vitamin D in populations at temperate latitudes. Vitamin D decreases the production of proinflammatory cytokines and increases the production of anti-inflammatory cytokines. Thus, vitamin D may help in regulating the immune response.[20] A role of Epstein–Barr virus (EBV) infection especially as clinical mononucleosis was identified as additional risk factors of MS.[14]

It is observed that migration from high-risk to low-risk geographical location before the age of 15 years may alter the chances of MS in a person.[19,21]

Another theory often raised for a long time is that diet may influence the risk of developing MS. This concept was based on epidemiological studies that showed higher prevalence of MS cases in geographic locations where diets low in fish and rich in meat and dairy consumption were present.[22,23]

DIETARY INTERVENTIONAL STUDIES IN MS

One of the earliest studies to address the consideration that implementation of a low saturated fat diet supplemented with polyunsaturated fatty acids may influence the course of MS was initiated by Swank.[24] He initiated a nonrandomized trial with the recommendations for consuming a diet low in saturated fat (15–17 g/day) supplemented with cod liver or vegetable oils early on in the disease course. Data obtained from his initial cohort that was followed for up to 35 years popularized the "Swank diet," as it showed a decrease in disability, relapse severity, and mortality in patients that maintained a low saturated fat regimen as compared to patients that did not follow the diet.[24,25] Although the uncontrolled nonrandomized aspect of this trial limits its scientific evidence strength, it did open the door to understanding how diet may influence MS disease progression.

Other investigators pursued the hypothesis that polyunsaturated fat supplementation may benefit MS patients. An analysis of three double-blind, controlled randomized trials with linoleic vs. oleic acid supplementation showed a decrease in progression, relapse severity, and duration in RRMS patients ingesting linoleic acid.[26] A trial comparing consumption of high-dose omega-3 fatty acids (2.8 g DHE +EPA) vs. olive oil showed a trend that favored high-dose omega-3 fatty acids in decreasing MS relapse severity, duration, and frequency. Unfortunately, these results were not statistically significant.[27]

A double-blind randomized trial investigated the effects of fish oil with a low-fat diet (15% fat) compared to consumption of olive oil with the AHA Step I diet (30% fat) on quality-of-life measures in RRMS patients over 1 year. It was thought that the true effects of polyunsaturated fats may have been masked in prior studies due to lack of standardized control of total fat intake. This study combined a low-fat diet in conjunction with polyunsaturated fat consumption in an attempt to augment the latter's effects on quality-of-life measures. This study measured the effects of diet on patients' mental and physical well-being as measured by the Physical Components Summary Scale of the Short Health Status Questionnaire as the primary outcome. Mental Health Inventory and Modified Fatigue Impact Scale in combination with Expanded Disability Status Scale (EDSS) (disability measure) and relapse rate were used as secondary outcomes. The trend favoring the fish oil group in mental and physical well-being was noted at the end of the 6-month time point. The positive trend continued to the end of the study at 1 year, though this was not statistically significant. Improvement in fatigue was noted in the olive oil group at the end of 6 months. Both the fish oil and olive oil groups noted a decrease in relapse rates compared to a year prior with a trend favoring the fish oil over the olive oil group. EDSS seemed to improve slightly in the fish oil group as opposed to a weak decline noted in the olive oil group.[27]

Another larger well-controlled study investigated the effects of omega-3 supplementation on clinical disease and magnetic resonance imaging (MRI) activity in RRMS patients. This trial used 1350 mg of eicosapentaenoic acid and 850 mg of docosahexaenoic acid daily as the omega-3 fatty acid supplementation.

Interferon beta-1a at 44 μg, as one of the best known disease-modifying therapies for MS, was introduced 6 months into the study to see if this would have an additive effect on the clinical and MRI outcomes over 18 additional months. The determinant of the primary outcome measure was the number of gadolinium-enhancing lesions on T1-weighted MRI studies. MRI activity at the end of 9 and 24 months, as well as fatigue, quality of life, disability progression, and relapse rate, was also studied.

This randomized, double-blind, placebo-controlled trial showed no clinical benefit from omega-3 supplementation compared to placebo or in combination with interferon beta-1a. Omega-3 supplementation did not have a positive impact on MRI disease activity. This study provided class I evidence that omega-3 supplementation alone, or in combination with interferon beta-1a, does not show a clinical benefit in RRMS patients.[27]

There are many obstacles to overcome in dietary intervention studies in MS. One of the obstacles is dietary compliance and high attrition rates. Combining a diet low in saturated fat with polyunsaturated fatty acids may confound the true outcome as a diet low in saturated fat alone can show a significant clinical benefit. Olive oil and other types of monounsaturated and polyunsaturated fatty acids may have their own therapeutic anti-inflammatory effects, complicating their use as a placebo agent in dietary trials.[28]

Previous dietary intervention trials mainly focused on polyunsaturated fatty acid supplementation as a therapeutic intervention in MS undermining the role of lipids on the clinical course of this disease. MS is thought to be a neurodegenerative autoimmune proinflammatory disease marked by Th1-cell-mediated destruction of myelin and axons. These autoreactive T cells secrete inflammatory cytokines such as interferon-γ, TNF-α, interleukin-1 (IL-1), and IL-2.[16] Certain lipids and antioxidants may influence the level of destructive inflammation as is observed in other autoimmune diseases such as rheumatoid arthritis, Crohn's disease, psoriasis, and systemic lupus erythematosus.[29]

Lipoprotein-associated phospholipase A2 (Lp-PLA2) is an enzyme known to promote atherogenesis by inducing oxidative stress and inflammation through mediators such as lysophosphatidylcholine (lyso PC) and oxidized non-esterified free fatty acids.[30,31] Oxidative stress and inflammation are also known to contribute to MS pathology raising interest in this enzyme as a possible modulator of the disease course.[32] One recent study showed that plasma mass and activity of Lp-PLA2 were higher in SPMS than in RRMS patients and that the mass and activity of the enzyme were also increased in RRMS vs. healthy control patients. The increase in Lp-PLA2 activity in secondary progressive patients compared to the other groups seems to suggest that the activity of this enzyme may be more involved in the pathogenesis of progression supporting the neurodegenerative aspect of the disease.[33]

There is now an emerging body of circumstantial evidence for a potential role for cholesterol and lipids in MS. In an analysis of 8983 patients from the North American Research Committee on MS (NARCOMS) registry, Marrie et al.[34] found that comorbidities linked to dyslipidemia were associated with an increased risk for MS disability progression. Although dyslipidemia is still perceived as comorbidity with secondary vascular pathology that may worsen the disability in MS, a more direct adverse effect of hypercholesterolemia on underlying immunopathology and neuropathology of MS is a relatively new but plausible consideration.[35]

Recently, our group examined a cohort of high-risk clinically isolated syndrome (CIS) patients (with ≥2 T2 lesions and ≥2 CSF oligoclonal bands) who were followed as part of a prospective, controlled observational study with clinical and MRI measures for 2 years.[36] All of the patients were treated with once-weekly, intramuscular interferon beta-1a. We found that higher serum low-density lipoprotein cholesterol (LDL-C) and total cholesterol were associated with increased risk for developing new and newly enlarging lesion over 2 years. Interestingly, we also found that higher high-density lipoprotein cholesterol (HDL-C) levels were associated with increased levels of vitamin D3 metabolites.[37] These new findings complement an earlier study of MS patients from our group that found that worsening of disability as assessed by the Extended Disability Status Scale and the MS Severity Scale was associated with higher baseline LDL-C and total cholesterol levels.[38]

As previously shown, low vitamin D is considered an environmental trigger, either due to the lack of adequate sunlight or oral intake, as a risk factor for the development and exacerbation of MS.[39] Therefore, vitamin D supplementation became a strong consideration within the current management of MS. Low levels of vitamin D are also associated with brain atrophy and higher disability scores as measured by the expanded disability status scale and the MS severity scale.[40] Another measure of disability in MS, known as the MS severity score, showed an association between disability and low vitamin D_3 levels.[41] Other studies have also confirmed the importance of vitamin D and its association with disability in MS.[42,43] The standard for a safe supplementation of vitamin D was set forth by the Institute of Medicine's consensus report based on bone health measures suggesting a minimum of 400 IU and a maximum of 4000 IU daily. The concerns regarding vitamin D supplementation are related to data linking excessive intake of vitamin D with heart disease and nephrolithiasis. However, as the level varies between individuals with clear seasonal influences, evaluating the levels and supplementing as necessary to obtain normal levels are recommended. The challenge with vitamin D studies is using a sufficiency level of 20 ng/mL, which is based on bone health studies and not based on other illnesses in which vitamin D may be implicated such as autoimmune diseases and malignancies. We suspect that a much higher level of vitamin D than the accepted standard of >30 ng/mL (as most laboratories suggest) may be necessary for the health of MS patients in preventing relapses and progression of disease.[44]

Phytosterols were also evaluated as a possible therapeutic intervention in MS. The structural similarity of phytosterols to cholesterol allows for decreased cholesterol absorption through competitive inhibition.[45] It is also thought that phytosterols may modulate the immune system in a positive way. One study pretreated macrophages obtained from MS patients with a phytosterol derivative, β-sitosterol, and found that this treatment increased Th2-mediated anti-inflammatory activity while concurrently decreasing proinflammatory cytokine activity.[46]

β-Sitosterol is the most common phytosterol in the human diet. Humans are not able to endogenously produce phytosterols, unlike cholesterol, and require large amounts in the diet to produce a small quantity in the serum.[47] Its protective effects have been studied in cardiovascular disease and cancer. β-sitosterol is also known to be a hypolipidemic agent and may exert its effects on inflammation in this matter as well.[48] Statins have also been studied for their possible immuno-modulatory effect on diseases such as MS.[49] One theory is that statins may slow down leukocyte invasion of the CNS by preventing leukocyte adhesion to brain endothelium.[50] In a recent study, β-sitosterol immunomodulatory effects were compared to statins and found to reduce proinflammatory cytokines secreted by peripheral blood cells from MS patients. As such, TNF-α and IL-12 were decreased by 24% and 27–30%, respectively, versus simvastatin that reduced TNF-α and IL-12 by 98% and 48–58%, respectively. However, the anti-inflammatory modulator IL-10 was increased in β-sitosterol–treated cells by 47% compared to 30% increase noted in simvastatin-treated cells. This study suggests that β-sitosterol may be considered as a potential treatment for MS without the side effects noted in statins.[51] β-Sitosterol may also help augment and mimic the effects of vitamin D on the immune system. This study found that β-sitosterol did augment synergistically the positive immune effects of vitamin D on murine macrophages.[52]

Another study investigated the effects of phytosterols on a mouse model version of MS known as experimental autoimmune encephalomyelitis (EAE). Antigenic peptide known as proteolipid protein (PLP) was used to induce EAE, MS-like illness, in the mice. The mice were pre-fed with either the control lab chow or the phytosterol-enriched diet. Phytosterol-fed mice were found to have 55% less disease severity compared to the controls and also experienced a delay of disease onset for an average of 2 days. The analysis of brain tissue showed a decrease in CNS tissue inflammation by 82% and a 48% decrease in demyelination in mice fed with phytosterols. The brain tissue samples from phytosterol-fed mice revealed a 35% decrease in macrophages and a 10% increase in the anti-inflammatory cytokine IL-10. The proinflammatory mediator CCL2 was inhibited by 50%, and the other inflammatory markers such as TNF-α, IL-6, and IFN-γ were decreased in the phytosterol-fed mice. This study suggests that phytosterols may be used in the future as a preventative intervention and possible treatment for MS.[53]

Luteolin, a member of the flavonoids, is a polyphenolic compound known to contain antioxidant and anti-inflammatory properties.[54] It has implications for MS therapeutics in that it has been shown to block myelin basic protein-induced mast cell stimulation of proinflammatory T cells.[55] It has also been shown to decrease proliferation of T cells in EAE models of MS.[56] Luteolin was found to augment the effects of IFN-β on decreasing proinflammatory cytokine production of IL-1β and TNF-α from peripheral blood mononuclear cells obtained from MS patients in one trial. MMP-9 is an integral mediator in increasing the permeability of the blood–brain barrier to autoreactive T cells and cytokines travelling into the CNS. It can also contribute to permanent axonal damage.[57,58] TIMP-1 works to inhibit MMP-9. In this same trial, luteolin alone, and not IFN-β or the combination of the two, was found to decrease MMP-9 and the MMP-9/TIMP-1 ratio. This study showed that luteolin may be used to enhance the effects of IFN-β on decreasing damaging cytokine production involved in the pathogenesis of MS. Luteolin alone also exhibited very potent anti-inflammatory activity.[59]

Quercetin is another flavonoid compound studied for its therapeutic potential in treating autoimmune diseases. It may inhibit MMP-9 and prevent migration of inflammatory T cells into the CNS.[60] This was seen in one study where oral and interperitoneal administration of quercetin was found to decrease infiltration of T cells and macrophages in experimental autoimmune encephalitis (EAE) rats,[61] whereas another study noted a significant decrease in clinical severity and duration of EAE in rats.[62]

One study evaluated the synergistic effects of combining quercetin with IFN-β on inflammatory cytokine production and proliferation of peripheral blood mononuclear cells isolated from MS patients and healthy controls. IL-1β, TNF-α, and the ratio of MMP-9 to TIMP-1 were measured in this study since they represent key mediators responsible for MS pathology. Results of the study revealed that quercetin alone decreased IL-1β and TNF-α significantly. The combination of quercetin with IFN-β further reduced TNF-α and enhanced the effects of IFN-β in reducing MMP-9 levels.[63] This study showed that quercetin may be a potential therapeutic option alone or in combination with IFN-β for MS, although the quantity of quercetin consumption required to achieve serum therapeutic levels may be well above practical oral supplementation alone.[64]

Ginkgo biloba is a popular herbal supplement that contains flavonoids. The flavonoid-containing supplement has antioxidant properties that may help improve cognition in Alzheimer's patients.[65] In addition, Gingko contains terpene lactones, which inhibit platelet activating factor (PAF).[66,67] PAF is a compound that is known to have proinflammatory and prothrombotic effects. It is theoretically believed that *G. biloba* may have a beneficial therapeutic effect in MS. A small study showed that *G. biloba* improved fatigue, overall function, and symptoms during relapses in MS patients.[68,69] A larger placebo-controlled trial did not show any effect on neurological function.[70] *G. biloba* was found to improve MS-related cognitive dysfunction in one small preliminary study. The safety profile of flavonoids as a dietary supplement at this point favors its use as a potential therapeutic treatment for MS.[63,71,72]

Although an increase in armamentarium of disease-modifying therapies became available for treatment of MS, they are only partially beneficial in preventing progression and relapses in MS and often associated with increased side effects. That is why many patients look to take supplements to aid in treating and preventing progression of disease. Sometimes, patients may take supplements to their detriment, not being aware of potentially dangerous side effects of "natural" therapies. For example, commonly used supplements such as supplemental iron were found to be associated with an increased total mortality risk in older women.[73]

One recent study investigated the dietary and herbal supplement pattern of MS patients compared to healthy controls to see if this pattern interacts in a negative way with the current treatments used for MS. This study also looked at the change in dietary and herbal supplement pattern prediagnosis and postdiagnosis of MS. More MS patients reported using dietary supplements compared to healthy controls (82% vs. 60%, $P < .001$). A multivitamin followed by vitamin D followed by calcium with vitamin D were the most common supplements used after the diagnosis of MS. Most MS patients reported taking B-complex, calcium plus vitamin D, vitamin B12, and vitamin D. The healthy controls reported taking more creatine and iron compared to the MS subjects. A significant increase in the number of supplement uses occurred after the MS diagnosis.

Primrose oil followed by cranberry fruit extract were the most commonly used herbal supplements by subjects after they were diagnosed with MS. Primrose oil, cranberry juice extract, and green tea abstract were used at a significantly higher rate after the diagnosis of MS. More healthy control patients reported using echinacea and ephedra compared to the MS subjects as it is known that these supplements may actually enhance the activity immune system and therefore are considered contraindicated for MS. There was no specific herbal supplement that was used more by one group compared to the other.[74] Another study found that nutritional supplement use by MS patients is about 46% with primrose oil and omega-6 source being the most commonly used.[66,75] In southern Washington and Oregon, vitamins C and E were the most common dietary supplements used.[75] A study from Iran found that vitamin B1, vitamin E, and a multivitamin were the most commonly used supplements in that region.[76] Fish oil and vitamins B12, B1, B2, and B6 were the most common supplements used in southern Australia.[77]

It is important to emphasize that some of the herbal supplements may have significant interactions with current medicines commonly used to treat MS. For instance, St. John's wort that is used in about 10.2% of patients may interact with serotonin inhibitor agents and may place patients at risk for serotonin syndrome. This supplement also induces the metabolism of teracycles, benzodiazepines, and cyclophosphamide. Echinacea, which is used by 15.2% of MS patients, can interact with the metabolism of immunosuppressive agents and corticosteroids since it is metabolized through the cytochrome P450 pathway. Red yeast rice, which is similar to lovastatin, may cause myopathy, and any other immunosuppressive drugs should not be used in combination since they may exacerbate that condition.[74]

Increased sodium chloride intake was found recently to induce proinflammatory cytokines such as Th17, TNF-α, and IL-2 in animal models of MS and human cell models. These cytokines as discussed earlier induce inflammation in autoimmune diseases such as MS. More studies would be required to identify what is considered "elevated" or "excessive" sodium intake. In addition, human studies would be required to see if this could be replicated in real life.[78]

CONCLUSION

Increasing scientific evidence points toward a significant role that nutritional factors may play in the pathogenesis and treatment of MS. MS is a proinflammatory autoimmune neurodegenerative disease that is currently being treated with disease-modifying therapies with only a modest efficacy at best and often with a trade toward an increased side effect profile. The studies reviewed in this chapter support significant objective clinical and radiological MRI as well as subjective self-reports being influenced by nutritional and dietary changes. Further research into metabolic and nutritional factors may expand our knowledge into exploring better treatment options and prevention plans for our MS patients.

REFERENCES

1. McFarland HF, Martin R. Multiple sclerosis: A complicated picture of autoimmunity. *Nat Immunol.* 2007;8(9):913–919.
2. D'Hooghe MB, D'Hooghe T, De Keyser J. Female gender and reproductive factors affecting risk, relapses and progression in multiple sclerosis. *Gynecol Obstet Invest.* 2013;75(2):73–84.
3. Confavreux C, Vukusic S, Adeleine P. Early clinical predictors and progression of irreversible disability in multiple sclerosis: An amnesic process. *Brain.* 2003;126:770–782.
4. Weinshenker BG, Bass B, Rice GP et al. The natural history of multiple sclerosis: A geographically based study. *Brain.* 1991;114(Pt 2):1057–1067.
5. Weinshenker BG, Bass B, Rice GP et al. The natural history of multiple sclerosis: A geographically based study. 2. Predictive value of the early clinical course. *Brain: A Journal of Neurology.* 1989;112(Pt 6)(6):1419–1428.
6. Derfuss T. Personalized medicine in multiple sclerosis: Hope or reality? *BMC Medicine.* 2012;10:116.
7. Lucchinetti CF, Popescu BF, Bunyan RF et al. Inflammatory cortical demyelination in early multiple sclerosis. *New Engl J Med.* 2011;365(23):2188–2197.
8. Polman CH, Reingold SC, Banwell B et al. Diagnostic criteria for multiple sclerosis: 2010 revisions to the McDonald criteria. *Ann Neurol.* 2011;69(2):292–302.
9. Houtchens MK, Benedict RH, Killiany R et al. Thalamic atrophy and cognition in multiple sclerosis. *Neurology.* 2007;69(12):1213–1223.
10. Noonan CW, Williamson DM, Henry JP et al. The prevalence of multiple sclerosis in 3 US communities. *Prev Chronic Dis.* 2010;7(1):A12.
11. Alonso A, Hernán MA. Temporal trends in the incidence of multiple sclerosis: A systematic review. *Neurology.* 2008;71(2):129–135.
12. Scalfari A, Neuhaus A, Degenhardt A et al. The natural history of multiple sclerosis, a geographically based study 10: Relapses and long-term disability. *Brain.* 2010;133(7):1914–1929.
13. Marrie RA, Yu N, Blanchard J et al. The rising prevalence and changing age distribution of multiple sclerosis in Manitoba. *Neurology.* 2011;77:1105.
14. Disanto G, Pakpoor J, Morahan JM et al. Epstein-Barr virus, latitude and multiple sclerosis. *Mult Scler.* 2013;19(3):362–365.
15. Risco J, Maldonado H, Luna L et al. Latitudinal prevalence gradient of multiple sclerosis in Latin America. *Mult Scler.* 2011;17(9):1055–1059.
16. Compston A, Coles A. Multiple sclerosis. *Lancet.* 2008;372(9648):1502–1517.

17. Dyment DA, Ebers GC, Sadovnick AD. Genetics of multiple sclerosis. *Lancet Neurol.* 2004;3(2):104–110.
18. International Multiple Sclerosis Genetics Consortium; Wellcome Trust Case Control Consortium et al. Genetic risk and a primary role for cell-mediated immune mechanisms in multiple sclerosis. *Nature.* 2011;476(7359):214–219.
19. Mowry EM. Vitamin D: Evidence for its role as a prognostic factor in multiple sclerosis. *J Neurol Sci.* 2011;311(1–2):19–22.
20. Raghuwanshi A, Joshi SS, Christakos S. Vitamin D and multiple sclerosis. *J Cell Biochem.* 2008;105 (2):338–343.
21. Islam T, Gauderman WJ, Cozen W, Mack TM. Childhood sun exposure influences risk of multiple sclerosis in monozygotic twins. *Neurology.* 2007;69(4):381–388.
22. Swank RL, Lerstad O, Strjaum A, Backer J. Multiple sclerosis in rural Norway: Its geographical and occupational incidence in relation to nutrition. *N Engl J Med.* 1952;246:721–728.
23. Lauer K. The risk of multiple sclerosis in the USA in relation to socio-geographic features: A factor-analytical study. *J Clin Epidemiol.* 1994;47:43–48.
24. Swank RL, Dugan BB. Effect of low saturated fat diet in early and late cases of multiple sclerosis. *Lancet.* 1990;336(8706):37–39.
25. Swank RL, Goodwin J. Review of MS patient survival on a Swank low saturated fat diet. *Nutrition.* 2003;19:161–162.
26. Dworkin RH, Paty DW. Linoleic acid and multiple sclerosis; A reanalysis of three double blind trials. *Neurology.* 1984;34:1441–1445.
27. Bates D. A double-blind controlled trial of long chain n-3 polyunsaturated fatty acids in the treatment of multiple sclerosis. *J Neurol Neurosurg Psych.* 1989;58:18–22.
28. Wiseman SA, Tijburg LB, Van de Put FH. Olive oil phenolics protect LDL and spare vitamin E in the hamster. *Lipids.* 2002;37(11):1053–1057.
29. Robinson RD, Li-Lian X, Knoell CT. Alleviation of autoimmune disease by ω-3 fatty acids, in effects of fatty acids and lipids in health and disease. *World Rev Nutr Diet.* 1994;76:95–102.
30. Nissen S, Tsunoda T, Tuzeu E et al. Effect of recombinant ApoA-I Milano on coronary atherosclerosis in patients with acute coronary syndromes. *JAMA.* 2003;17:2292–2300.
31. Zalewski A, Macphee C. The role of lipoprotein-associated phospholipase A2 in atherosclerosis: Biology, epidemiology, and possible therapeutic target. *Arterioscler Thromb Vasc Biol.* 2005;25:923–931.
32. Lucas M, Sanchez-Solino O, Solano F, Izquierdo G. Interferon beta-1b inhibits reactive oxygen species production in peripheral blood monocytes of patients with relapsing-remitting multiple sclerosis. *Neurochem Int.* 1998;33:101–102.
33. Sternberg Z, Drake A, Sternberg D et al. Lp-PLA2: Inflammatory biomarkers of vascular risk in multiple sclerosis. *J Clin Immunol.* 2012;32(3):497–504.
34. Marrie RA, Rudick R, Horwitz R et al. Vascular comorbidity is associated with more rapid disability progression in multiple sclerosis. *Neurology.* 2010;74(13):1041–1047.
35. Quintana FJ, Yeste A, Weiner HL, Covacu R. Lipids and lipid-reactive antibodies as biomarkers for multiple sclerosis. *J Neuroimmunol.* 2012;248(1–2):53–57.
36. Weinstock-Guttman B, Zivadinov R, Horakova D et al. Lipid profiles are associated with lesion formation over 24 months in interferon-β treated patients following the first demyelinating event. *J Neurol Neurosurg Psychiatry.* 2013;84(11):1186–1191.
37. Weinstock-Guttman B, Zivadinov R, Ramanathan M. Interdependence of vitamin D levels with serum lipid profiles in multiple sclerosis. *J Neurol Sci.* 2011;311(1–2):86–91.
38. Weinstock-Guttman B, Zivadinov R, Mahfooz N et al. Serum lipid profiles are associated with disability and MRI outcomes in multiple sclerosis. *J Neuroinflammation.* 2011;8:127.
39. Ascherio A, Munger KL. Environmental risk factors for multiple sclerosis. Part II: Noninfectious factors. *Ann Neurol.* 2007;61(6):504–513.
40. Weinstock-Guttman B, Zivadinov R, Qu J et al. Vitamin D metabolites are associated with clinical and MRI outcomes in multiple sclerosis patients. *J Neurol Neurosurg Psychiatry.* 2011;82:189–195.
41. Weinstock-Guttman B, Zivadinov R, Ramanathan M. Inter-dependence of vitamin D levels with serum lipid profiles in multiple sclerosis. *J Neurol Sci.* 2011;311:86–91.
42. Smolders J, Menheere P, Kessels A et al. Association of vitamin D metabolite levels with relapse rate and disability in multiple sclerosis. *Mult Scler.* 2008;14(9):1220–1224.
43. Van der Mei IA, Ponsonby AL, Dwyer T et al. Vitamin D levels in people with multiple sclerosis and community controls in Tasmania, Australia. *J Neurol.* 2007;254(5):581–590.
44. Weinstock-Guttman B, Mehta BK, Ramanathan M et al. Vitamin D and multiple sclerosis. *Neurologist.* 2012;18(4):179–183.

45. Moreau RA, Whitaker BD, Hicks KB. Phytosterols, phytostanols, and their conjugates in foods: Structural diversity, quantitative analysis, and health promoting uses. *Prog Lipid Res*. 2002;41(6):457–500.

46. Ostlund RE Jr. Phytosterols and cholesterol metabolism. *Curr Opin Lipidol*. 2004;15(1):37–41.

47. Moghadasian MH. Pharmacological properties of plant sterols in vivo and in vitro observations. *Life Sci*. 2000;67(6):605–615.

48. Chan YM, Varady KA, Lin T et al. Plasma concentrations of plant sterols: Physiology and relationship with coronary heart disease. *Nutr Rev*. 2006;64(9):385–402.

49. Neuhaus O, Archelos JJ, Hartung HP. Statins in multiple sclerosis: A new therapeutic option? *Mult Scler*. 2003;9(5):429–430.

50. Neuhaus O, Strasser-Fuchs S, Fazekas F et al. Statins as immunomodulators: Comparison with interferon beta 1b in MS. *Neurology*. 2002;59(7):990–997.

51. Desai F, Ramanathan M, Fink C et al. Comparison of the immunomodulatory effects of the plant sterol β-sitosterol to simvastatin in peripheral blood cells from multiple sclerosis patients. *Int Immunopharmacol*. 2009;9:153–157.

52. Alappat L, Valerio M, Awad A. Effects of vitamin D and β-sitosterol on immune function of macrophages. *Int Immunopharmacol*. 2010;10:1390–1396.

53. Valerio M, Hong-Biao L, Heffner R et al. Phytosterols ameliorate clinical manifestations and inflammation in experimental autoimmune encephalomyelitis. *Inflamm Res*. 2011;60:457–465.

54. Hodek P, Trefil P, Stiborova M. Flavonoids-potent and versatile biologically active compounds interacting with cytochromes P450. *Chem Biol Interact*. 2002;139:1–21.

55. Theoharides TC, Kempuraj D, Kourelis T, Manola A. Human mast cells stimulate activated T cells: Implications for multiple sclerosis. *Ann NY Acad Sci*. 2008;1144:74–82.

56. Verbeek R, Plomp AC, Van Tol EA, Van Noort JM. The flavones luteolin and apigenin inhibit in vitro antigen-specific proliferation and interferon-gamma production by murine and human autoimmune T cells. *J Altern Complement Med*. 2004;68:621–629.

57. Rosenberg GA. Matrix metalloproteinases and neuroinflammation in multiple sclerosis. *Neuroscientist*. 2002;8(6):586–595.

58. Newman TA, Woolley St, Hughes PM. T-cell- and macrophage-mediated axon damage in the absence of a CNS-specific immune response: Involvement of metalloproteinases. *Brain*. 2001;124(Pt 11):2203–2214.

59. Sternberg Z, Chadha K, Lieberman A et al. Immunomodulatory responses of peripheral blood mononuclear cells from multiple sclerosis patients upon in vitro incubation with the flavonoid luteolin: Additive effects of IFN-β. *J Neuroinflammation*. 2009;6:28.

60. Sellebjerg F, Sorensen TL. Chemokines and matrix metalloproteinase-9 in leukocyte recruitment to the central nervous system. *Brain Res Bull*. 2003;61(3):347–355.

61. Hendriks JJ, Alblas J, Van der Pol SM et al. Flavonoids influence monocytic GTPase activity and are protective in experimental allergic encephalitis. *J Exp Med*. 2004;200(12):1667–1672.

62. Muthian G, Bright JJ. Quercetin, a flavonoid phytoestrogen, ameliorates experimental allergic encephalomyelitis by blocking IL-12 signaling through JAK-STAT pathway in T lymphocyte. *J Clin Immunol*. 2004;24(5):542–552.

63. Sternberg Z, Chadha K, Lieberman A et al. Quercetin and interferon-β modulate immune responses in peripheral blood mononuclear cells isolated from multiple sclerosis patients. *J Neuroimmunol*. 2008;205(1–2):142–147.

64. Goldberg DM, Yan J, Soleas GJ. Absorption of three wine-related polyphenols in three different matrices by healthy subjects. *Clin Biochem*. 2003;36(1):79–87.

65. Weinmann S, Roll S, Schwarzbach C et al. Effects of Ginkgo biloba in dementia: Systematic review and meta-analysis. *BMC Geriatr*. 2010;10:14.

66. Yadav V, Bourdette D. Complementary and alternative medicine: Is there a role in multiple sclerosis? *Curr Neurol Neurosci Rep*. 2006;6(3):259–267.

67. Bent S, Goldberg H, Padula A, Avins AL. Spontaneous bleeding associated with ginkgo biloba: A case report and systematic review of the literature: A case report and systematic review of the literature. *J Gen Intern Med*. 2005;20(7):657–661.

68. Brochet B, Orgogozo JM, Guinot P et al. Pilot study of Ginkgolide B, a PAF-acether specific inhibitor in the treatment of acute outbreaks of multiple sclerosis. *Rev Neurol (Paris)*. 1992;148(4):299–301.

69. Johnson SK, Diamond BJ, Rausch S et al. The effect of Ginkgo biloba on functional measures in multiple sclerosis: A pilot randomized controlled trial. *Explore (NY)*. 2006;2(1):19–24.

70. Brochet B, Guinot P, Orgogozo JM et al. Double blind placebo controlled multicentre study of ginkgolide B in treatment of acute exacerbations of multiple sclerosis. The Ginkgolide Study Group in multiple sclerosis. *J Neurol Neurosurg Psychiatry*. 1995;58(3):360–362.

71. Conquer JA, Maiani G, Azzini E. Supplementation with quercetin markedly increases plasma quercetin concentration without effects on selected risk factors for heart disease in healthy subjects. *Fundam Appl Toxicol*. 1998;128:593–597.

72. Fang J, Zhou Q, Shi XL, Jiang BH. Luteolin inhibits insulin-like growth factor I receptors signaling in prostate cancer cells. *Carcinogenesis*. 2007;28:713–723.

73. Mursu J, Robien K, Harnack LJ et al. Dietary supplements and mortality rate in older women. *Arch Intern Med*. 2011;171(18):1625–1633.

74. O'Connor K, Weinstock-Guttman B, Carl E et al. Patterns of dietary and herbal supplement use by multiple sclerosis patients. *J Neurol*. 2012;259:637–644.

75. Yadav V, Shinto L, Bourdette D. Complementary and alternative medicine for the treatment of multiple sclerosis. *Expert Rev Clin Immunol*. 2010;6(3):381–195.

76. Shirazi M. Dietary supplementation in Iranian multiple sclerosis patients. *J Med Sci*. 2007;7(3):413–417.

77. Leong EM. Complementary and alternative medicines and dietary interventions in multiple sclerosis: What is being used in South Australia and why? *Complement Ther Med*. 2009;17(4):216–223.

78. Kleinewietfeld M, Manzel A, Titze J et al. Sodium chloride drives autoimmune disease by the induction of pathogenic TH17 cells. *Nature*. 2013;496(7446):518–522.

30 Micromineral Considerations in Alzheimer's Dementia

Diana Pollock

CONTENTS

Research on the many contributing factors to the development of Alzheimer's disease (AD) has branched into many paths, in the attempt to hunt down the biochemical bases for pathological biochemical changes in brain tissue that lead to synaptic and neuronal destruction. One path has led to study of aberrant biometal metabolism associated with AD. Metals are intriguing because the pathologic amyloid plaques that build up in AD brains are rich in copper, zinc, and iron (Adlard and Bush 2006). Zinc also plays a major role in inhibitory modulation of the N-methyl-D-aspartate (NMDA) receptor site, as will be detailed in ZnT3: The Major Zinc Transporter. Without adequate zinc (Zn^{2+}), there is incompetent inhibition of NMDA receptors leading to excessive excitatory glutamate activity. This allows too much calcium into cells, leading to neurotoxicity and cell death. NMDA receptor overactivity is thought to play a leading role in the neurodegeneration seen in AD (as well as other neurodegenerative diseases; review in Gardoni and Di Luca 2006).

Zn^{2+} is the only metal that is a cofactor to over 300 enzymes (Rink and Gabriel 2000). Its many roles include stabilizing the structure of proteins and signaling enzymes at all levels of cellular signal transduction and transcription factors (Beyersmann 2002). One zinc-containing protein that will be reviewed in this chapter breaks down pathologic amyloid plaques, whereas another prevents copper-induced formation of toxic amyloid plaques. An important distinction to other transition metal ions such as copper and iron, zinc does not undergo redox reactions due to its filled (d) shell. Zn^{2+} is a biologically essential trace element critical for many DNA synthesis, RNA transcription, oxidative stress, apoptosis, and aging processes (Murakami and Hirano 2008; Prasad 2009).

Synaptic Zn^{2+} constitutes 20–30% of total brain zinc and is most abundant in the hippocampus, especially in the mossy fiber region (Cole et al. 1999; Lee et al. 2002). The hippocampus is also the initial region to be attacked by the ravages of AD. Studies have shown that metals modulate amyloid beta (Aβ) toxicity in neuronal cultures, with Cu^{2+} increasing Aβ toxicity and Zn^{2+} attenuating it (Cardoso et al. 2005). Stoltenberg et al. (2007) studied a transgenic mouse model of AD and found that low dietary Zn^{2+} resulted in a significant increase in plaque volume, despite apparently unaltered Zn^{2+} ion distribution.

Copper toxicity has been hypothesized to be a causative factor in amyloid plaque formation, with excess copper intake occurring from water supply through copper pipes as well as over the counter (OTC) supplements and vitamins. Increasing intake of zinc can decrease the absorption of copper. Zinc should be taken away from food intake to maximize effectiveness on intestinal metallothionein (MT). Intestinal MT is induced by oral administration of zinc, and copper uptake is blocked (Sturniolo et al. 1999). Zinc deficiency, not only in serum but also cerebrospinal fluid and in brain, has been found in the majority of patients with AD (Brewer et al. 2010; Corrigan et al. 1991; Papageorgiou et al. 1990). The likely cause is inadequate intake due to dietary factors. In addition, it may be that adequate absorption of Zn^{2+} requires other cofactors such as vitamins A and D (Potocnik et al. 2006). However, Frederickson et al. (2005) reviewed evidence showing both functional zinc deficiency as well as overload in the brain, implying that Zn^{2+} is abnormally distributed. A number of different methods have been used to measure Zn^{2+} levels, further complicating literature review. Diagnosis of zinc deficiency before serum zinc goes down is difficult, but after serum zinc goes down, it is a good indicator of zinc deficiency. Serum zinc is low in AD.

There has been intensive research on several relevant Zn^{2+} proteins, with ideas on how they may contribute to removal and reduction of toxic processes leading to the pathology of the AD brain. These proteins are ZnT3, which regulates synaptic Zn^{2+}, Neprilysin (NEP), and the metal transporter MT. In addition, Zn^{2+} concentrations influence microtubule assembly, and intracellular deficiency triggered by sequestration in extracellular amyloid plaques may lead to loss of microtubules and formation of neurofibrillary tangles (NFTs).

ZnT3: THE MAJOR ZINC TRANSPORTER

Zn^{2+} ions are hydrophilic and mostly bound to proteins, and cannot enter cells by simple diffusion. The zinc transporter-3 (ZnT3) is essential for loading Zn^{2+} into synaptic vesicles (Cole et al. 1999). ZnT3 is primarily localized to glutamatergic synapses present in regions of the brain that mediate higher cognitive functions (Palmiter et al. 1996). Zn^{2+} modulates the response of postsynaptic receptors at these synapses (Weiss et al. 1993). ZnT3 knockout mice were found to exhibit age-dependent problems with learning, mimicking the age-related pattern of cognitive loss seen with AD. No problems were seen at 6–10 weeks of age, but at 6 months, learning and memory were quite impaired (Adlard et al. 2010). Motor strength and coordination remained normal. It was found that the hippocampal zinc levels dropped in both wild type and the ZnT3 knockout mice (although to a greater degree with the ZnT3 knockout mice). So the decline in zinc with age is not only synaptic zinc associated with the ZnT3. Glutamatergic dysfunction was suggested due to marked reductions seen in several NMDA receptor subtypes (2A and 2B, but not 1). ZnT3 was also found by these authors to decline with age in wild-type mice as well as in humans. ZnT3 levels were decreased by even greater amount in cortex from patients with AD compared to age-matched controls.

The Zn^{2+} released by ZnT3 is also known to mediate parenchymal and cerebrovascular amyloid formation in certain amyloid precursor protein (APP) transgenic mice (Lee et al. 2002). Again, using ZnT3 knockout mice, Deshpande et al. (2009) found that vesicular Zn^{2+} was crucial to localization of Aβ oligomers in excitatory glutamatergic synapses, when artificial stimulation of brain slices triggered neurotransmission. The majority of accumulation took place at the NR2B NMDA receptor (Deshpande et al. 2009). Similar to synaptic Zn^{2+}, Aβ is normally released at presynaptic terminals in an activity-dependent manner (Kamenetz et al. 2003). Neuronal overexcitation may exacerbate continued synaptic release of the Aβ that may then pathologically complex with Cu^{2+} or Zn^{2+}. Zn^{2+} sequestration in Aβ complexes may lead to reduced Zn^{2+} availability at synaptic terminals and subsequent loss of Zn^{2+} modulatory activity at excitatory synapses (Frederickson et al. 2005).

Rachline et al. (2005) further investigated the role of Zn^{2+} as a modulator of the NMDA (glutamate) receptor site. The N-terminal domain of certain NMDA receptor subunits modulates ion channel gating through binding of extracellular allosteric inhibitors. Zn^{2+} is the modulator for NR2A (Paoletti et al. 2000) and was also shown to modulate the NR2B receptor (Rachline et al. 2005). The coexistence of subunit-specific zinc binding sites of high and low affinity on NMDA receptors raises the possibility that Zn^{2+} exerts both tonic and phasic control of membrane excitability.

As stated by Rachline et al. (2005):

Based on the observation that two homologous domains of NMDA receptors form extracellular Zn^{2+} sensors of markedly different sensitivities (nanomolar versus micromolar), it was proposed that Zn^{2+} ions in the CNS could provide a dual control, phasic and tonic, of membrane excitability by binding to low- and high affinity sites on NMDA receptors. The high Zn^{2+} sensitivity of the NR2A N-Terminal Domain (NTD) site might allow ambient Zn^{2+} levels (in the nanomolar range) (Bogden et al. 1977; Palm and Hallmans 1982) to inhibit NR2A-containing receptors tonically, while leaving unaffected receptors with lower Zn^{2+} sensitivities. In contrast, Zn^{2+} released phasically during synaptic activity could reach high levels (>1 μM) and inhibit most NMDA receptors present at the synapse, in particular those containing the NR2B subunit. The tonic Zn^{2+} modulation of NMDA receptors may be involved in setting the level of background activation of NMDA conductances, which are known to participate in the integrative properties of neurons (Sah et al. 1989). The phasic Zn^{2+} modulation may provide an efficient way to prevent the harmful consequences of NMDA receptor overactivation. There are two interesting aspects of this model. First, the relative amount of tonic versus phasic Zn^{2+} modulation would vary both in time and space: in time, because NR2A expression starts only after birth, whereas NR2B expression is abundant during embryonic stages; in space, because the relative expression level of NR2A and NR2B varies not only from one brain region to the other but also from one subcellular compartment to the other, and even from one synapse to the other within a single neuron (Cull-Candy et al. 2001). Second, synaptically released Zn^{2+} could diffuse to extrasynaptic sites or neighboring synapses (Zn^{2+} spillover) (Ueno et al. 2002) and, in this latter case, mediate heterosynaptic modulation of NMDA receptors, particularly of the most Zn^{2+}-sensitive ones (i.e., NR2A containing). This process may allow for experience-dependent Zn^{2+} mediated modulation of synaptic plasticity. Finally, the idea of a dual, tonic and phasic, modulation of NMDA receptors by extracellular Zn^{2+} could extend to other neurotransmitter receptors, in particular to inhibitory GABA A and glycine receptors for which high-affinity (nanomolar) and low-affinity (micromolar) Zn^{2+} binding sites have also been described previously (Smart et al. 2004).

Additional evidence of the importance of proper functioning of the ZnT3 system is shown by analysis of postmortem brains of individuals with neuropathology of AD who were cognitively normal at time of death on neuropsychological testing, compared to those with AD and age-matched controls. Despite the presence of comparable levels of plaques, tangles, Aβ 1-42, and low molecular weight (toxic) Aβ oligomers, there are a subset of people who remain cognitively intact. Phosphorylated CREB (cAMP response element binding protein) is a transcription factor essential for memory function and synaptic plasticity as well as a marker of intact synaptic function. Decrease in this substance is one of the downstream adverse effects seen due to toxic Aβ (Bito and Takemoto-Kimura 2003). In nondemented with AD pathology (NDAN) individuals, the pCREB is preserved. Aβ (in oligomeric form) was not present in the postsynaptic sites of the NDAN hippocampi samples. Zn^{2+} levels were highest in soluble hippocampus fractions from AD brains, but the NDAN samples also contained significantly elevated Zn^{2+} levels compared to controls (Bjorklund et al. 2012).

Increased vesicular Zn^{2+} was found in AD and NDAN samples, along with reduced Zn^{2+} in the soluble fractions from NDAN as compared to AD, which suggests the existence of a compensatory mechanism in NDAN to remove excess Zn^{2+}. Expression of ZnT3 (ZnT3 transports Zn^{2+} into synaptic vesicles) was preserved in NDAN samples at levels similar to the control samples.

NEPRILYSIN: A ZINC METALLOPROTEASE THAT CORRELATES WITH COGNITIVE SCORES

Most of the amyloid degrading enzymes that have been identified fall into the class of zinc metalloproteases, especially the M13 NEP family (Nalivaeva et al. 2012). NEP is one of the seven members of the human M13 family of zinc-dependent endopeptidases.

NEP is a type-II integral membrane protein, known as a zinc metallopeptidase, composed of 750 residues with an active site at its extracellular carboxyl domain. It is capable of degrading monomeric and oligomeric forms of Aβ (El-Amouri et al. 2008). NEP is expressed predominantly in axonal and synaptic membranes (Fukami et al. 2002). The finding that there is decreased NEP in AD must take into account the fact that there is neuronal and synaptic loss associated with this disease. Wang et al. (2010) adjusted for this issue in evaluation of postmortem brains of Alzheimer, mild cognitive impairment, and normal elderly, and found that there was still true relative deficiency in the AD brain. Wang et al. (2010) also showed that Aβ accumulation was universally and significantly inversely correlated with NEP concentration. NEP was also the only protease found to be inversely correlated with cognitive scores as measured by the Mini Mental State Exam (MMSE) and global neuropsychological z-scores.

Earlier experiments by Wang et al. (2009), using cultured neuronal cells, indicated that NEP mRNA, protein, and activity are upregulated by treatment with Aβ. This is what would be expected if NEP is responsible for degradation of abnormal amyloid buildup, and indeed, compensatory increases in NEP were found in clinically normal individuals with cortical amyloid deposits, a process referred to as pathological aging (Wang et al. 2005).

The abnormal deposition of β-amyloid (Aβ) in the brain as amyloid plaques and in blood vessel walls as the signature of AD pathology depends not only on excessive production of these abnormal aggregates but lack of breakdown as well. Aβ is physiologically produced by proteolytic cleavage of APP by the concerted action of β- and γ-secretases, and its pathologic accumulation in AD indicates an imbalance between Aβ biosynthesis and clearance (Eckman and Eckman 2005). NEP appears to be the dominant mechanism whereby Aβ is broken down (Miners et al. 2008). Others have shown that amyloid production does not differ between normal control and Alzheimer patients; it is the lack of clearance of the beta-amyloid that marks the disease process (Mawuenyega et al. 2010).

The presence of NEP inversely correlates with cortical and hippocampal fields most liable to develop amyloid in APP transgenic mice (Fukami et al. 2002).

NEP −/− genetically engineered mice were found to have Aβ accumulation in the brain and in the area of retina where amyloid is expected in age-related macular degeneration (AMD) (Yoshida et al. 2005). Two other Alzheimer mice models of amyloid accumulation were not found to have amyloid accumulate in this part of the retina: one was a familial APP amyloidosis model (Dutescu et al. 2009), and the other was the familial APP mutation plus presenilin 1 (Ding et al. 2008; Liu et al. 2009).

As proof of concept, Spencer et al. (2011) loaded a lentivirus vector with NEP and achieved reduction in amyloid plaque in APP transgenic mice associated with improved cognition. Synaptic density also increased. This experiment is especially exciting because the compound was delivered by intraperitoneal injection instead of directly into the brain or cerebrospinal fluid (CSF). It was still able to breach the blood–brain barrier (BBB) and deliver NEP to widespread areas of the neocortex and hippocampus, areas hardest hit by AD.

ApoE4, a genetic risk isoform for AD, binds to Aβ and prevents Aβ from degradation by NEP. It also promotes aggregation of Aβ (Wang et al. 2010).

In genetically altered apolipoprotein E (ApoE)-deficient mice, immunohistofluorescent staining revealed that the ablation of ApoE led to the reduced expression of ZnT3 protein, in parallel with the reduction of synaptic zinc. So ApoE is another factor affecting Zn^{2+} (Lee et al. 2010).

In 1991, Constantinidis published a hypothesis that amyloid production led to a leaky BBB, which allowed some trace metals to enter in abnormal amounts, displacing zinc in some enzymes. The dysfunction of zinc enzymes affecting DNA metabolism could result in formation of the abnormal NFTs. Glutamate dehydrogenase (another zinc protease) would also be less active, resulting in more active glutamate, and an excess of glutamatergic activity is a known factor in a number of neurodegenerative diseases. Zinc enzymes of neuronal detoxification, namely, superoxide dismutase, carbonic anhydrase, and lactic dehydrogenase, would also be deficient, leading to neuronal toxicity. The window of time between amyloid plaque production and development of NFTs is about 14 months, with the cognitive deficit following the neuronal toxicity from the NFTs. During this time window, treatment of the functional zinc deficiency may restore zinc-containing enzymes and reduce damage to neurons. That might help the supply of NEP so it can do its job of breaking down toxic Aβ, but repairing zinc dysregulation sooner may prevent formation of insoluble amyloid plaques in the first place.

A new hypothesis to explain the connection between Aβ and NFTs was published by Craddock et al. (2012). First they review evidence that microtubules may be where memories are encoded and stored. One important factor in normal microtubule assembly is zinc concentration. At low to moderate levels intracellularly, all is well, but in the presence of high Zn^{2+} levels, the tubulin forms flat sheets instead of cylinders. Tubulin is the constituent protein of microtubules. Dietary Zn^{2+} deficiency results in the impairment of tubulin polymerization into microtubules. When Zn^{2+} is sequestered extracellularly in amyloid plaques, there is less Zn^{2+} available intracellularly. Their experiments showed that depleted intraneuronal Zn^{2+} leads to microtubule destabilization, NFT formation, and neuronal degeneration. This hypothesis links amyloid pathology to intraneuronal lesions and cognitive impairment via microtubules.

Work by Chung et al. (2010) and others highlight the importance of timing to prevent pathologic changes of AD in the brain. MTs are the major copper and zinc-binding proteins within the brain. The MT 1/2 isoforms are essential neuroprotective agents mostly produced by astrocytes, with elevated expression seen as a response to almost any type of brain injury: traumatic, ischemic, chemical, or neurodegenerative (Cardoso et al. 2005; Chung et al. 2004; Trendelenburg et al. 2002). MTs are capable of binding 7 divalent (Zn^{2+}) ions or up to 12 univalent (Cu^+) ions in vivo (Kagi and Kojima 1987). Chung et al. (2010) gives compelling evidence that Zn7MT-2A can prevent toxic aggregation of insoluble Aβ by copper, but cannot deaggregate it after it has already formed. The prevention of toxic aggregates appears to occur by trapping the copper ions in the MT and releasing the zinc, as copper has a higher binding affinity with MT. Zinc then forms soluble (harmless) amyloid complexes. These experiments were performed in cultured cortical neurons. Therefore, if zinc deficiency results in lower than desirable levels of Zn7MT-2A at a time when copper is present, insoluble Aβ aggregates will likely result.

Another issue examined by Chung et al. (2010) was toxicity to the cultured cortical cells by free copper versus copper complexed with amyloid or MT. Only the complexes of copper plus amyloid resulted in toxicity to neurons from redox reactions. Free copper and copper bound to MT did not result in reactive oxygen species and subsequent toxicity. Again, Zn7MT-2A was able to protect the cells from oxidative toxicity from the Cu-Aβ complexes, possibly by a metal swap mechanism.

Regardless of the mechanism, external manipulation of concentrations of certain metals may influence the aberrant chemical milieu that exists during formation of pathogenic amyloid plaque.

In addition, as previously discussed, zinc deficiency becomes more prevalent with aging and even more so in AD.

In transgenic mice engineered to express both amyloid and tau pathology, zinc supplementation appeared to facilitate production of BDNF and dephosphorylation of tau (Corona et al. 2010). Also, when levels of zinc became too high, tau was hyperphosphorylated, but at correct physiologic levels, tau was dephosphorylated.

Previous attempts to supplement zinc at high doses were limited by gastric side effects until Constantinidis (1991) used zinc-aspartate in ten patients with dementia, aged 56–82 (average age 70 years). Oral administration of 150 mg of zinc per day lasted from 3 to 12 months. Three of the ten also received IV zinc, 30 mg every 2 days. The usual daily requirement for zinc is 5–25 mg/day. Assessments were performed before and after treatment by psychometric tests as well as family reports. Two patients, aged 62 and 67, did not improve (solely on oral treatment). The remaining eight patients showed improvements in memory, language, and social contact. After treatment was discontinued, patients showed recurrence of cognitive decline.

Other zinc supplementation studies have been recently reviewed by Loef et al. (2012), and overall results are inconclusive. Some issues of importance involve the relationship of Zn^{2+} and Zn^{2+} protease functions to the local biochemical milieu. Many of the crucial pathological events of AD happen in the neuronal cell membrane. The composition of this membrane appears to ideally contain more polyunsaturated fatty acids (PUFAs) than is normally provided by the average diet of those populations with high incidence of AD. The major PUFA in the neuronal cell membrane is docosahexaenoic acid (DHA) (Svennerholm 1968). High intake of ω-3 PUFAs has been shown to be associated with improved cognition and reduced risk of AD (Morris et al. 2003). Jayasooriya et al. (2005) fed rats a diet either supplemented with, or deficient in, ω-3 fatty acids. The ω-3-deficient rats had increased expression of ZnT3 in the brain that was associated with increased levels of free Zn^{2+} in the hippocampus. The ω-3-deficient rats had decreased plasma levels of Zn^{2+}, and there were no differences in CSF levels. The upregulation of the ZnT3 gene persisted into adult rats even after repletion with ω-3 fatty acids later. So the deleterious effects of insufficient ω-3 PUFAs in early life may be irreversible.

To further investigate the concept of zinc as a therapeutic agent for AD, a double-blind randomized controlled trial was performed at two separate clinical sites in Florida. In addition, the initial portion of this trial compared side effects of a novel form of zinc, zinc cysteine (reaZin), to that of Galzin (zinc acetate), the currently approved form of zinc intended for use in treatment of Wilson's disease. Galzin is notoriously difficult to tolerate due to the gastrointestinal side effects of nausea and vomiting, and is given as multiple doses over the course of the day. reaZin is an orally administered, once a day, sustained release preparation. It contains 150 mg of elemental zinc (as acetate) and 100 mg of L-cysteine hydrochloride as a sustained release tablet. It must be administered away from food to be effective. The two primary hypotheses were (1) that administration of reaZin would result in improved cognition in AD patients after 6 months of treatment, and (2) that reaZin would be much better tolerated than Galzin, currently used to treat Wilson's disease.

The sustained release of reaZin was designed to greatly improve its tolerability as well as to allow once-a-day administration, compared to three times a day, required for Galzin. Tolerability should be increased because the sustained release prevents the immediate release of a large quantity of zinc salt in one location in the stomach, which is irritating to many patients. Tolerability was evaluated in two preliminary studies, which showed that tolerability of reaZin was much better than Galzin.

The primary end points of the double-blind trial of reaZin we carried out on patients with mild AD were as follows: (1) to show a significant increase in serum zinc; (2) to show a significant reduction in serum free copper in the rein-treated group; and (3) to show that reaZin-treated patients had significantly better cognition scores than placebo patients.

Fifty-seven patients enrolled had a diagnosis of mild to moderate AD. Patients were diagnosed by standard clinical, functional, and AD and Related Disorders Association criteria. Mean MMSE scores of the entire group were 25.6 with a range from 29 to 21. Mean age of the entire group was about 76 years, with a range from 53 to 88. The mean serum zinc of the entire group was 73.7 µg/dL. This is very similar to the serum zinc in 30 Albany AD patients we studied. The mean serum zinc in those 30 patients was 76.2 µg/dL, and this was found to be significantly lower than the value of 82.7 µg/dL in 29 age-matched controls. So we can conclude that our 57 patients were, on average, zinc deficient.

The patients were randomly divided into two groups, one to receive 120 mg of zinc as reaZin once daily, and the other to receive matching placebo. The mean ages of the two groups (76.02 years for the treatment group and 76.16 for the placebo group) and the baseline MMSEs (25.68 for treatment and 25.62 for placebo) were nearly identical.

The patients were evaluated at baseline and 3 and 6 months during therapy. Zinc and copper were measured by atomic absorption, and ceruloplasmin was measured enzymatically. Serum-free copper was calculated by subtracting the ceruloplasmin bound copper from the total serum copper. Cognition was evaluated by MMSE, the Alzheimer's Disease Assessment Scale for Cognition (ADAS-Cog), and the Clinical Dementia Rating Scale, Sum of Boxes (CDR-SOB).

Side effects from the zinc were very minimal. Two patients had one complaint of nausea and another had a vomiting episode. Dose of zinc had to be reduced in one patient because the serum ceruloplasmin decreased, which was being monitored to prevent zinc-induced copper deficiency.

Forty-two patients were evaluable, 21 in each group. The primary end point of increasing serum zinc was accomplished. Serum zinc increased to a mean of 152 µg/dL in the treatment group, a very significant ($p = 0.002$) increase compared to baseline. There was no change in the placebo group.

The primary end point of decreasing serum free copper was also accomplished. The treatment group decreased from a mean of 37.0 µg/dL to 30.8 µg/dL, also very significantly ($p = 0.004$) different. There was no change in the placebo group.

All three of the cognition scoring systems were better in the treatment group versus the placebo group, but none reached statistical significance, although CDR-SOB was close at $p = 0.1$. ADAS-Cog had a p value of 0.36 and MMSE was 0.42. A composite cognitive score using the estimated generalized least squares method applied to all three cognitive scoring systems was also used. This global score yielded a p value of 0.15, indicating a strong trend toward cognitive benefit favoring the zinc treatment group.

A later, post hoc, analysis was very rewarding. It was observed that the effect of zinc was to stabilize cognition, while placebo patients were deteriorating. Second, it was observed that older placebo patients were deteriorating consistently and to a greater degree than younger placebo patients which prevented differences from being statistically significant. It was thought that the greater variability in deterioration in the younger placebo patients was preventing the differences from being statistically significant.

With this in mind, an analysis was carried out restricted to older patients, those age 70 and older. In this group, there were 14 zinc-treated patients and 15 placebo patients. The results on cognitive scoring tests were very exciting. On the ADAS-Cog test, a more positive number indicates deterioration, and the placebo group deteriorated a mean of 1.27 points, while the treated group actually improved by −0.76 points. The differences were significant at $p = 0.037$. On the CDR-SOB, a more positive number indicates deterioration, and the placebo group deteriorated 0.87 points, while the zinc-treated group only deteriorated 0.25 points, again a significant difference ($p = 0.032$). With MMSE, a more negative number indicates deterioration, and the placebo group deteriorated −1.0 points, while the treatment group actually improved a mean of 0.58 points, with the difference approaching significance ($p = 0.067$).

We think that these results are very exciting. If confirmed in a larger and longer study, it means we have a treatment that can strongly stabilize cognition in AD, which until now, we have not had. Our results indicate that zinc is effective in stabilizing cognition in AD at all ages, although so far it was only possible to show it statistically in those age 70 and over. Post hoc results are always less convincing than confirmation of pre hoc hypotheses, but in this case, only post hoc analyses were done; thus, the p values are not greatly weakened.

The mechanism of improvement may be restoration of adequate zinc levels to the neuron, because of the importance of zinc in the neuron as earlier discussed, or reduction in free copper levels, since free copper may be damaging to the neuron, or both.

Some possible reasons behind these findings include inadequate sensitivity of the cognitive tests in the patients with mild cognitive impairment, since less evident decline over the rather short 6-month trial period would be expected (Wouters et al. 2012).

As mentioned previously, other factors may be playing a role in the ability of zinc to effectively perform its duties, including adequate PUFAs and proper ApoE function, to name just a few. The possibility of this type of dysregulation may be most difficult of all to sort out in the complex biochemistry relating to AD.

Another possible mechanism would be dysregulation of how copper and other metals are handled by, for example, APP. APP is a cell-surface glycoprotein and part of its structure (the Domain 2 site) is concerned with metal interaction.

In summary, the lack of sufficient Zn^{2+} would limit the availability and function of important zinc proteins described above. ZnT3 appears to modulate the overactive NMDA receptor site through both tonic and phasic mechanisms. NEP is the dominant zinc protease that breaks down Aβ, and to underscore NEP's clinical significance, its concentration inversely correlates with cognitive function scales. It would therefore seem important for those planning drug development targeting amyloid kinetics to have adequate Zn^{2+} present in order for the receptor sites to respond properly. In fact, one may speculate that memantine, a noncompetitive inhibitor at the NMDA receptor site currently in use to treat AD, may be even more effective if adequate zinc is present. Finally, the scaffolding of neuronal structure and movement, and maybe even memory—microtubules—depends on adequate intraneuronal zinc for stabilization and repair.

REFERENCES

Adlard PA, Bush AI (2006) Metals and Alzheimer's disease. *J Alz Dis* 10:145–163.

Adlard PA, Parncutt JM, Finkelstein DI, Bush AI (2010) Cognitive loss in zinc transporter-3 knock-out mice: A phenocopy for the synaptic and memory deficits of Alzheimer's disease? *J Neurosci* 3(5):1631–1636.

Beyersmann D (2002) Homeostasis and cellular functions of zinc. *Mat Wiss U Werkstofftech* 33:764–769.

Bito H, Takemoto-Kimura S (2003) Ca2+/CREB/CBP-dependent gene regulation: A shared mechanism critical in long-term synaptic plasticity and neuronal survival. *Cell Calcium* 34:425–430.

Bjorklund NL, Reese LC, Sadagoparamanujam V-M et al. (2012) Absence of amyloid β oligomers at the post-synapse and regulated synaptic Zn^{2+} in cognitively intact aged individuals with Alzheimer's disease neuropathology. *Molecular Neurodegeneration* 7:23.

Bogden JD, Troiano RA, Joselow MM (1977) Copper, zinc, magnesium and calcium in plasma and cerebrospinal fluid of patients with neurological diseases. *Clin Chem* 23:485–489.

Brewer GJ, Kanzer SH, Zimmerman EA et al. (2010) Subclinical zinc deficiency and Alzheimer's disease and Parkinson's disease. *Am J Alz Dis Other Demen* 25(7):572–575.

Cardoso SM, Rego AC, Rereira C, Oliveira CR (2005) Protective effect of zinc on amyloid beta 25–35 and 1–40 mediated toxicity. *Neurotox Res* 7:273–281.

Chung RS, Adlard PA, Dittman J et al. (2004) Neuron-glia communication: Metallothionein expression is specifically up regulated by astrocytes in response to neuronal injury. *J Neurochem* 88:454–461.

Chung RS, Howells C, Eaton ED et al. (2010) The native copper- and zinc-binding protein metallothionein blocks copper-mediated Aβ aggregation and toxicity in rat cortical neurons. *PLoS ONE* 5(8):e12030.

Cole TB, Wenzel HJ, Kafer KE et al. (1999) Elimination of zinc from synaptic vesicles in the intact mouse brain by disruption of the ZnT3 gene. *Proc Natl Acad Sci USA* 96:1716–1721.

Constantinidis J (1991) Hypothesis regarding amyloid and zinc in the pathogenesis of Alzheimer's disease. *Alz Dis Assoc Disord* 5(1):31–35.

Corona C, Masciopinto F, Silvestri E et al. (2010) Dietary zinc supplementation of 3xTg-AD mice increases BDNF levels and prevents cognitive deficits as well as mitochondrial dysfunction. *Cell Death Dis* 1:e91.

Corrigan FM, Reynolds GB, Ward NI (1991) Reduction of zinc and selenium in brain in Alzheimer's disease. *Trace Elem Med* 8:1–5.

Craddock TJA, Tuszynski JA, Chopra D et al. (2012) The zinc dyshomeostasis hypothesis of Alzheimer's disease. *PLoS One* 7(3):e33552.

Cull-Candy SG, Brickley S, Farrant M (2001) NMDA receptor subunits: Diversity, development and disease. *Curr Opin Neurobiol* 11:327–335.

Deshpande A, Kawai H, Metherate R et al. (2009) A role for synaptic zinc in activity-dependent Abeta oligomer formation and accumulation at excitatory synapses. *J Neurosci* 29:4004–4015.

Ding JD, Lin J, Mace BE, Herrmann R et al. (2008) Targeting age-related macular degeneration with Alzheimer's disease based immunotherapies: Anti-amyloid-beta antibody attenuates pathologies in an age-related macular degeneration mouse model. *Vision Res* 48:339–345.

Dutescu RM, Li J, Crowston QX et al. (2009) Amyloid precursor processing and retinal pathology in mouse models of Alzheimer's disease. *Graefes Arch Clin Exp Ophthalmol* 247:1213–1221.

Eckman EA, Eckman CB (2005) Abeta-degrading enzymes: Modulators of Alzheimer's disease pathogenesis and targets for therapeutic intervention. *Biochem Soc Trans* 33:1101–1105.

El-Amouri SS, Zhu H, Yu J et al. (2008) Neprilysin: An enzyme candidate to slow the progression of Alzheimer's disease. *Am J Pathol* 172:1342–1354.

Frederickson CJ, Koh JY, Bush AI (2005) The neurobiology of zinc in health and disease. *Nat Rev Neurosci* 6:449–462.

Fukami S, Watanabe K, Iwata N et al. (2002) Abeta-degrading endopeptidase, neprilysin, in mouse brain: Synaptic and axonal localization inversely correlating with Abeta pathology. *Neurosci Res* 43:39–56.

Gardoni F, Di Luca M (2006) New targets for pharmacological intervention in the glutamatergic synapse. *Eur J Pharm* 545:2–10.

Jayasooriya AP, Leigh Ackland M, Mathai ML et al. (2005) Perinatal ω-3 polyunsaturated fatty acids supply modifies brain zinc homeostasis during adulthood. *PNAS* 102(20):7133–7138.

Kagi JH, Kojima Y (1987) Chemistry and biochemistry of metallothionein. *Experientia Suppl* 52:25–61.

Kamenetz F, Tomita T, Hsieh H et al. (2003) APP processing and synaptic function. *Neuron* 37:925–937.

Karr JW, Kaupp LJ, Szalai VA (2004) Amyloid-beta binds Cu^{2+} in an mononuclear metal ion binding site. *J Am Chem Soc* 126:13534–13538.

Lee JY, Cho E, Kim TY et al. (2010) Apolipoprotein E ablation decreases vesicular zinc in the brain. *Biometals* 23:1085–1095.

Lee JY, Cole TB, Palmiter RD et al. (2002) Contribution by synaptic zinc to the gender-disparate plaque formation in human Swedish mutant APP transgenic mice. *Proc Natl Acad Sci USA* 99:7705–7710.

Liu B, Rasool S, Yang Z, Glabe CG et al. (2009) Amyloid-peptide vaccinations reduce (beta)-amyloid plaques but exacerbate vascular deposition and inflammation in the retina of Alzheimer's transgenic mice. *Am J Pathol* 175:2099–2110.

Loef M, von Stillfried N, Walach H (2012) Zinc diet & Alzheimer's disease: A systematic review. *Nutritional Neurosci* 15(5):2–12.

Mawuenyega K, Sigurdson W, Ovod V et al. (2010) Decreased clearance of CNS beta-amyloid in Alzheimer's Disease. *Science* 330(6012):1774.

Miners JS, Baig S, Palmer J et al. (2008) Abeta-degrading enzymes in Alzheimer's disease. *Brain Pathol* 18(2):240–252.

Morris MC, Evans DA, Bienias JL et al. (2003) Consumption of fish and n-3 fatty acids and risk of AD. *Arch Neurol* 60:940–946.

Murakami M, Hirano T (2008) Intracellular zinc homeostasis and zinc signaling. *Cancer Sci* 99:1515–1522.

Nalivaeva NN, Beckett C, Belyaev ND, Turner AJ (2012) Are amyloid-degrading enzymes viable therapeutic targets in AD? *J Neurochem* 120(Suppl 1):167–185.

Palm R, Hallmans G (1982) Zinc concentrations in the cerebrospinal fluid of normal adults and patients with neurological diseases. *J Neurol Neurosurg Psychiatry* 45:685–690.

Palmiter RD, Cole TB, Quaife CJ et al. (1996) ZnT-3, a putative transporter of zinc into synaptic vesicles. *Proc Natl Acad Sci USA* 93:14934–14939.

Paoletti P, Perin-Dureau F, Fayyazuddin A et al. (2000) Molecular organization of a zinc binding N-terminal modulatory domain in a NMDA receptor subunit. *Neuron* 28:911–925.

Papageorgiou C, Kapaki E, Vonmvoutakis C et al. (1990) The use of specific methods in CSF and serum for the investigation of neurological disorder. In VI Congress of the International Society of Greek Neuroscientists, Corfu: Book of Abstracts, p. 26.

Potocnik FCV, von Rensburg SJ, Hon D et al. (2006) Oral zinc augmentation with vitamins A and D increases plasma zinc concentration: Implications for burden of disease. *Metab Brain Dis* 21:139–147.

Prasad AS (2009) Zinc: Role in immunity, oxidative stress and chronic inflammation. *Curr Opin Nutr Metab Care* 12:646–652.

Rachline J, Perin-Dureau F, Le Goff A et al. (2005) The micromolar zinc-binding domain on the NMDA receptor subunit NR2B. *J Neurosci* 25(2):308–317.

Rink L, Gabriel P (2000) Zinc and the immune system. *Proc Nutr Soc* 4:541–552.

Sah P, Hestrin S, Nicoll RA (1989) Tonic activation of NMDA receptors by ambient glutamate enhances excitability of neurons. *Science* 246:815–818.

Smart TG, Hosie AM, Miller PS (2004) Zn^{2+} ions: Modulators of excitatory and inhibitory synaptic activity. *Neuroscientist* 10:432–442.

Spencer B, Marr RA, Gindi R et al. (2011) Peripheral delivery of a CNS targeted, metalo-protease reduces Aβ toxicity in a mouse model of Alzheimer's disease. *PLoS One* 6(1):e16575.

Stoltenberg M, Bush AI, Bach G et al. (2007) Amyloid plaques arise from zinc-enriched cortical layers in APP/PS1 transgenic mice and are paradoxically enlarged with dietary zinc deficiency. *Neuroscience* 150:357–369.

Sturniolo GC, Mestriner C, Irato P et al. (1999) Zinc therapy increases duodenal concentrations of metallothionein and iron in Wilson's disease patients. *Am J Gastroent* 94(2):334–338.

Svennerholm L (1968) Distribution and fatty acid composition of phosphoglycerides in normal human brain. *J Lipid Res* 9(5):570–579.

Trendelenburg G, Prass K, Priller J et al. (2002) Serial analysis of gene expression identifies metallothionein-II as a major neuroprotective gene in mouse focal cerebral ischemia. *J Neurosci* 22(14):5879–5888.

Ueno S, Tsukamoto M, Hirano T et al. (2002) Mossy fiber Zn2+ spillover modulates heterosynaptic N-methyl-D-aspartate receptor activity in hippocampal CA3 circuits. *J Cell Biol* 158:215–220.

Wang DS, Lipton RB, Katz MJ et al. (2005) Decreased neprilysin immunoreactivity in Alzheimer disease, but not in pathological aging. *J Neuropathol Exp Neurol* 64:378–385.

Wang L, Clark ME, Crossman DK et al. (2010) Abundant lipid and protein components of drusen. *PLoS One* 5:e10329.

Wang R, Wang S, Malter JS, Wang DS (2009) Effects of HNE modification induced by Abeta on neprilysin expression and activity in SH-SY5Y cells. *J Neurochem* 108:1072–1082.

Weiss JH, Hartley DM, Koh J, Choi DW (1993) AMPA receptor activation potentiates zinc neurotoxicity. *Neuron* 10:43–49.

Wouters H, Appels B, van der Flier WM et al. (2012) Improving the accuracy and precision of cognitive testing in mild dementia. *J Int Neuropsychol Soc* 18(2):314–322.

Yoshida T, Ohno-Matsui K, Ichinose S et al. (2005) The potential role of amyloid beta in the pathogenesis of age-related macular degeneration. *J Clin Invest* 115:2793–2800.

31 Ingestion of Inorganic Copper from Drinking Water and Supplements Is a Major Causal Factor in the Epidemic of Alzheimer's Disease

George J. Brewer and Sukhvir Kaur

CONTENTS

INTRODUCTION

In this chapter, we will develop and review our hypothesis that ingestion of inorganic copper from drinking water and supplement pills is a major causal factor in the epidemic of Alzheimer's disease (AD). To accomplish this, we will discuss the following topics in sequence:

1. The characteristics of the current epidemic of AD including its much higher prevalence in developed countries.
2. The fact that AD was virtually unknown prior to 1900.
3. The fact that neither a lack of elderly people nor failure to recognize AD is explanation for its absence prior to 1900.
4. The rapid increase in prevalence of AD over the last century, plus its higher prevalence in developed countries, makes it clear that an environmental factor/s is/are responsible for the epidemic.

5. Involvement of inorganic copper ingestion in AD was brought to the fore by AD animal model studies in which inclusion of trace amounts of copper (0.12 ppm) in the drinking water had greatly enhanced AD pathology and cognition loss. Supportive of the role of inorganic copper ingestion on cognition loss is a population study in which the concomitant ingestion of inorganic copper by taking copper-containing supplements and a high-fat diet resulted in marked cognition loss.

6. Increased serum-free copper is intimately involved in the pathogenesis of AD.

7. The use of copper plumbing in developed countries coincides temporally with the AD epidemic.

8. We have data that show that enough copper is present in drinking water from about one third of North American households to greatly enhance AD in animal models.

9. Other risk factors for AD such as a high-fat diet, possession of certain hemochromatosis or transferrin alleles, possession of certain ATP7B alleles, possession of the APOE 4 allele, having high homocysteine levels, or having zinc deficiency all can be related to copper toxicity.

10. The role of copper toxicity in AD is supported by direct studies of labile copper in AD brain.

All of these facts bring together a web of evidence supporting a major crucial role of ingestion of inorganic copper in the current AD epidemic. Those who accept our hypothesis at this point can help themselves by

1. Throwing away vitamin/mineral supplements containing copper

2. Having their drinking water tested for copper levels, and if copper levels are over 0.01 ppm, using a device at the tap to lower copper levels or seek an alternate source of drinking water.

CURRENT EPIDEMIC OF AD

As an example of the current high prevalence of AD in developed countries, in the United States, about 10% of people in their 60s, 20% of those in their 70s, and 30% of those in their 80s have AD (Alzheimer's Association 2010). This amounts to about 6 million Americans with the disease. An equal number have mild cognitive impairment (MCI), about 15% of whom convert to AD yearly. MCI, in which memory is impaired but the person is otherwise functional, is believed to usually be a precursor to AD.

This high prevalence is believed to be steadily increasing. In 1980, there were half as many cases of AD in the United States as we would expect at today's rate. The epidemic is largely confined to developed countries. Ferri et al. (2005) have given prevalence figures for AD in various countries of the world, and developed countries, such as those in North America and Europe, have high prevalence, while undeveloped countries such as those in Africa, South America, and India have relatively low prevalence. Japan is an interesting exception, which we will discuss later. It is a developed country but has low prevalence of AD.

Thus, in summary, there is currently a very large and steadily increasing epidemic of a disease that steals the last years of a huge number of elderly, causes great family and caregivers sorrow and lost time, and is hugely expensive to developed nations. In short, it is a monumental health crisis.

AD WAS VIRTUALLY UNKNOWN PRIOR TO 1900

In 1906, Dr. Alois Alzheimer discovered the first case of the disease that now bears his name (Alzheimer 1907). The evidence is good that AD virtually did not exist, or at least was very rare, prior to 1900. This evidence is nicely articulated by Waldman and Lamb (2005) in their book,

Dying for a Hamburger, and they deserve credit for developing the overall concept that AD was rare or nonexistent in earlier times.

Part of that evidence is that cases of AD-type dementia were not reported in the medical literature, and institutional records likewise do not report cases of this type during this period. Better evidence is that very good and very thorough academic writers of the period did not record a disease like AD.

First, Osler (1910), an internist, edited a comprehensive series of books that encompassed all medical knowledge of the time including one large volume on diseases of the brain. A disease like AD was not mentioned. Second, Freud, a psychiatrist, wrote extensively about mental illnesses and did not describe an AD-type dementia, although he discussed the dementia of syphilis in some detail (Strachey et al. 1966). Third, and probably most important, Boyd (1938), a pathologist, wrote a textbook of pathology that was updated several times, the last edition in 1938, and did not describe amyloid plaques and neurofibrillary tangles, the hallmarks of AD brain pathology, in the brains of autopsied patients. The absence of patients with AD pathology will be especially important in the next section, when we discuss and refute explanations that have been used to explain the lack of cases of AD.

REFUTATION OF EXPLANATIONS THAT HAVE BEEN USED TO EXPLAIN THE LACK OF AD CASES IN THE LAST CENTURY

A common explanation is that since age is a major risk factor for AD, there were not many elderly to develop AD in the period before 1900, but now the increasingly advanced age of many people causes an increased prevalence of AD. However, Waldman and Lamb examined this question and showed that in France in 1911, half the populations were living to age 60, the age of risk for AD. We examined the US census figures for 1900 and found that there were 3 million people over age 60, and there should have been over 30,000 cases of AD at today's rate, more than enough to be written about by Osler and Freud and to show AD brain pathology in the autopsy material of Boyd.

A second explanation is that AD was taken as simply the deterioration of normal aging, referred to as senile dementia. This explanation could conceivably explain the clinicians, Osler and Freud, missing AD, although given how thorough these physicians were, it is a little hard to believe. But this explanation does not explain the absence of amyloid plaques and neurofibrillary tangles in the autopsy material of Boyd. The lack of this hallmark AD brain pathology is key evidence that AD did not exist or was very rare before the 1900s.

ENVIRONMENTAL FACTORS ARE RESPONSIBLE FOR THE AD EPIDEMIC

The two facts—that prevalence is increasing rapidly in spite of elderly people being present in the past, plus the increased prevalence occurring in developed countries—can only be explained by the presence of a new causal environmental factor or factors present in the developed countries.

There are many new environmental factors associated with development. A change in diet is one, as affluence leads to more meat in the diet. In fact, Waldman and Lamb named their book *Dying for a Hamburger* because they postulated it was increased beef eating that was responsible for the new AD epidemic. Their hypothesis was that AD was a prion disease caused by eating infected beef. While increased beef eating is associated with the affluence of development, there is no evidence that AD is a prion disease. However, Waldman and Lamb could be on the right track, namely, that changed dietary factors are a partial cause of the AD epidemic. Grant (1997) has shown that AD prevalence is positively correlated with fat in the diet across many countries. Increased fat ingestion is associated with development because it is part of increased meat intake, which of course requires affluence. It is part of our hypothesis that increased fat ingestion from the Western diet is a new environmental factor that is playing a role in the epidemic of AD in developed countries. However, we think there is more to it than that and we will elaborate in the next section.

DATA SUGGESTING INORGANIC COPPER INGESTION COULD BE A MAJOR ENVIRONMENTAL CAUSAL FACTOR IN THE AD EPIDEMIC

An epiphany in our thinking about the cause of the AD epidemic occurred when Sparks and Schreurs published their 2003 paper, which showed that addition of a tiny amount (0.12 ppm) of copper to the drinking water of rabbits in a cholesterol-fed animal model of AD greatly enhanced not only the typical AD brain pathology but also loss of cognition. For reference, the US EPA allows 1.3 ppm of copper, ten times the toxic amount, in human drinking water.

The way in which the discovery of Sparks and Schreurs was made is interesting, in that it shows how scientific discoveries can be made through serendipity and careful investigation. The investigators were puzzled because they could not reproduce their rabbit model findings in Arizona after leaving their West Virginia laboratory. After a time, they realized that in Arizona they were using distilled drinking water, while they used tap water in West Virginia. Careful investigations of the possible causative substances in tap water revealed that there were trace amounts of copper. The finding that trace amounts of copper enhanced AD disease in animal models was confirmed, including in the mouse model (Sparks et al. 2006) and by a second group (Deane et al. 2007). This study shows that copper in drinking water is much more toxic than copper in food. This amount of copper added to food would not be toxic.

Another interesting study was reported by Morris et al. (2006). In this study of Chicago residents, cognition was tracked over time, and ingestion of various nutrients, including minerals, was recorded. It was found that those in the highest quintile of copper intake, who were there because of taking copper supplements, if they also ate a high-fat diet, lost cognition at six times the rate of other groups.

The studies of Sparks and Schreurs and of Morris et al. have in common that the copper ingested is inorganic copper. Copper in food is organic; by that we mean the copper is bound to food proteins. Copper in drinking water or in copper supplement pills is inorganic, that is, it is a simple inorganic salt of copper not bound to anything. Some data we developed several years ago may explain the sharply increased toxicity of inorganic copper compared to organic copper. The organic copper in food is absorbed from the intestine and then passes through the liver, where it is put into safe channels. However, it appears that a portion of ingested inorganic copper bypasses the liver and enters directly into the blood stream, immediately becoming part of and expanding the free copper pool in the blood. The evidence for this is as follows: when we gave an oral dose of copper 64, an inorganic radiolabelled copper salt, within 1–2 h, there was a large peak of radioactivity in the blood, too soon to have been processed by the liver (Hill et al. 1986). We estimate that 15% of the radioactivity appeared in the blood and represented a direct infusion of free copper from ingestion of inorganic copper.

At this point, we should discuss what is meant by the free copper in the blood. Much of the copper measured in the blood is covalently bound in the ceruloplasmin (Cp) molecule and is not available to cause toxicity. The rest of the copper is more loosely bound to albumin and other molecules, is available to cause toxicity, and is called free copper. Free copper is determined by measuring total serum copper and Cp in the same blood sample, and then subtracting the Cp bound copper from the total serum copper. The free copper amount determined will vary depending upon the method of Cp assay. If Cp is measured enzymatically, free copper is about 25–35% of total serum copper. If Cp is measured immunologically, which is the usual clinical assay, free copper is about 10–20% of total serum copper, the difference caused by the immunologic assay picking up and measuring some apo-Cp, or Cp without its coppers. Either assay gives useful information about the free copper pool, as long as the same assay is used consistently, to correlate changes, etc.

The concept is that as the free copper pool gets larger, copper becomes more toxic. This leads ultimately to Wilson's disease, an inherited disease of copper accumulation and copper toxicity (Brewer and Yuzbasiyan-Gurkan 1992). The serum-free copper is greatly expanded in this disease, and successful treatment results in normalizing serum-free copper.

ROLE OF INCREASED SERUM-FREE COPPER IN THE PATHOGENESIS OF AD

This area has been developed in a nice series of studies from Italy by Squitti and her group. First, they have shown that serum-free copper is higher in AD patients than in age-matched controls (Squitti et al. 2005). Second, they have shown that serum-free copper correlates negatively with a measure of cognition, called MMSE (the lower the MMSE score, the poorer the cognition) (Squitti et al. 2006). Third, they have shown that free copper is a predictor of decline over time in MMSE, that is, the higher the serum-free copper, the more rapid the decline (Squitti et al. 2009).

An important question is, why is the serum-free copper increased in AD? We believe an important factor is ingestion of inorganic copper through the two routes we have discussed in this section, from drinking water and from copper supplement pills. However, other mechanisms may be excessive release of copper from Cp in the blood or a partial failure in the mechanism of copper incorporation into Cp in the liver. Both the Squitti group (2005) and our group (Brewer et al. 2010a) have found in AD that there is an increased amount of Cp in the blood lacking some or all of its coppers. The excessive release of copper from Cp in the blood would further elevate free copper. The Squitti groups have shown that there are liver abnormalities in AD, perhaps secondary to copper toxicity (Squitti et al. 2007). It is possible that the incorporation of copper into the Cp molecule in the liver is affected, and that some of this nonincorporated copper appears in the blood as free copper.

Summarizing the key data presented in the previous two sections, the studies of Sparks and Schreurs (2003) show clearly that tiny amounts of inorganic copper in drinking water are sharply more toxic than copper in food, and strongly enhance AD pathology and loss of cognition in a cholesterol-fed AD model. Morris et al. (2006) showed that ingestion of inorganic copper in the form of copper supplement pills causes dramatic loss of cognition if accompanied by a high-fat diet. Data from our group (Hill et al. 1986) show that a portion of ingested inorganic copper bypasses the liver and contributes directly to expanding the free copper pool of the blood. Then, we discussed the work of Squitti et al. (2005, 2006, 2009), which ties an increased serum-free copper in AD intimately with the pathogenesis of the disease.

SPREAD OF COPPER PLUMBING IN THE DEVELOPED COUNTRIES OF THE WORLD CORRELATES TEMPORALLY WITH THE AD EPIDEMIC

We made the case earlier that a new environmental factor has to be responsible for the sudden epidemic of AD in the last half of the 20th century, but only in developed countries.

The studies of Sparks and Schreurs that trace amounts (0.12 ppm) of copper in drinking water could greatly enhance AD pathology and cognition loss in an AD animal model caused us to look no further than human drinking water, given that the EPA allows 1.3 ppm, ten times the toxic amount in the AD animal studies. We soon discovered that the spread of copper plumbing in developed countries correlated time-wise very strongly with the AD epidemic in those countries.

Copper began to be used for household plumbing in the early 1900s to replace iron pipes. Its use was curtailed by World War 1 and then World War 2. In about 1950, copper plumbing took off, and now 80–90% of US homes use copper plumbing, with the rest using plastic. This great burst of use of copper plumbing in developed countries during the latter half of the 20th century coincides well with the great increase in AD in those countries. Japan is an interesting exception. It is a developed country yet has low prevalence of AD (Ueda et al. 1992). It turns out that Japan has shunned the use of copper plumbing, apparently for fear of copper toxicity. Yet, when Japanese migrate to Hawaii, where copper plumbing is used, their prevalence of AD is similar to that in developed countries (White et al. 1996). Of course, other things change as Japanese move to Hawaii, for example, they may eat a different diet. But the prevalence of AD in Japanese in the two countries shows an interesting consistency with the copper hypothesis.

IS ENOUGH COPPER LEACHED FROM COPPER PLUMBING TO CONSTITUTE A RISK IN CAUSING AD?

We have made the case that the spread of copper plumbing in developed countries, except for Japan, coincides with the explosive AD epidemic, except in Japan. This, together with the study of Sparks and Schreurs, which showed that trace amount of copper in drinking water greatly enhanced AD pathology and cognition loss in an AD animal model, supports our hypothesis that ingestion of inorganic copper is a casual factor in AD. However, this hypothesis can only be valid if copper is actually leached from copper plumbing into drinking water in a high-enough concentration to be toxic. So, are there any data on this question?

By coincidence, we have such data. For years we checked the drinking water copper levels of many patients with Wilson's disease who were coming to see us because of the new Wilson's disease treatments that we were developing. Because the disease is one of copper accumulation and copper toxicity, we wanted to limit our patients to no more than 0.01 ppm copper in their drinking water.

As a result of this program, we accumulated copper concentration data in drinking water of 280 North American households, since our patients were from across all of North America. We found that almost a third of the samples had copper levels above the 0.1 ppm shown by Sparks and Schreurs (2003) to cause AD in the animal model (Brewer 2011). About one third of samples were at or below 0.01 ppm level, a level we feel is safe. The other third were in between these levels and represent a drinking water copper concentration area of unknown safety.

Thus, the bottom line is that one third of the drinking water samples were definitely in the area of probable toxicity, and another one third were of unknown safety. There is definitely enough copper in drinking water to support the hypothesis of inorganic copper ingestion from drinking water as a causal factor in the AD epidemic.

VARIOUS RISK FACTORS FOR AD INTERACT WITH COPPER, FURTHER SUPPORTING THE COPPER HYPOTHESIS

There are various known risk factors for AD, and we will discuss these, and their interaction with copper, one at a time. To begin with, a high-fat diet is a probable risk factor for AD. First, Grant has found a high correlation between AD prevalence and fat in the diet. Second, ingestion of a high fat diet is a characteristic of developed countries because of the high intake of meat. Third, ingestion of inorganic copper and a high-fat diet may fit together like hand and glove, copper causing release of oxidant radicals, and the high-fat diet providing the lipid substrates that are oxidized into derivatives that are damaging to the brain (Huang et al. 1999; Nelson and Alkon 2005). Remember that in the Sparks and Schreurs (2003) study, copper in the drinking water caused greatly increased AD-type damage in a cholesterol-fed animal model. In the studies of Morris et al., rapid cognition loss occurred in the highest quintile of copper intake, people being there because of ingestion of inorganic copper in supplement pills, but these people also ate a high-fat diet. Thus, in both studies, copper and lipids worked together to greatly accelerate brain damage. It is our belief that either ingestion of inorganic copper or a high-fat diet is an AD risk factor by itself. But when both are ingested together over a period of time, they are a more major risk factor and responsible for much of the explosive prevalence of AD that produces our AD epidemic.

Possession of the apolipoprotein E4 allele (Apo E4) is a known risk factor for AD (Miyata and Smith 1996). The Apo E2 allele has a protective effect, and the Apo E3 allele appears to be neutral. Apolipoprotein E may function to help remove copper from the brain. Apo E2 has two copper binding sites, Apo E3 has one, and Apo E4 has none. Thus, the effects of these alleles on AD risk may be due to their ability to bind copper and remove it from the brain.

Elevated homocysteine level in the blood is a risk factor for AD, as it is for atherosclerosis (Seshadri et al. 2002). Homocysteine and copper interact to produce oxidant radicals and oxidize low-density lipoprotein (LDL), contributing to the development of AD. Here again is that connection between copper and lipids to produce brain damage.

Having certain ATP7B alleles is proving to be a risk factor for AD (Bucosai et al. 2012). This fits with the copper hypothesis beautifully, because ATP 7B is the Wilson's disease gene. Mutations in this gene produce Wilson's disease, a disease of copper accumulation and copper toxicity. While the alleles found associated with AD have not yet been shown to produce excess copper accumulation, the presumption is that they do result in free copper levels at least slightly above normal.

Certain hemochromatosis alleles (Moalem et al. 2000) and transferrin alleles (Zambenedetti et al. 2003) have both been found to be risk factors for AD. Both of these genes effect iron metabolism and iron levels. Excess iron and excess copper produce toxicity in the same way by increasing generation of oxidant radicals and oxidant stress. Thus, excess iron accumulation would add to the damage caused by excess copper.

Finally, recently zinc deficiency has been found to be a risk factor for AD (Brewer et al. 2010b). Zinc and copper work hand in hand in that zinc, which is redox inert, can replace copper at binding sites where copper was generating oxidant radicals, and thus reduce oxidant stress. In zinc deficiency, this protective effect is reduced or lost.

DIRECT STUDIES OF COPPER TOXICITY IN AD BRAIN

Recent studies have shown that "labile copper" is elevated in the AD brain, and that this elevation is associated with oxidative pathology in AD (James et al. 2011). This work strongly supports a causal role of copper toxicity in AD.

SUMMARY

In this chapter, we have first reviewed two key facts about AD—that it has reached epidemic proportions in developed countries and that the disease was virtually unknown until the early 1900s. These facts strongly indicate that environmental factors are now present in developed countries that are strongly causal of AD. We have developed the hypothesis that the two environmental factors causal of AD are ingestion of inorganic copper and ingestion of a high-fat diet. We point out that the spread of copper plumbing in developed countries coincides very well, temporally, with the epidemic of AD. We show that inorganic copper, such as that in drinking water or in copper supplements, partially bypasses the liver and enters directly into the blood, enlarging the free copper pool. We cite references to AD animal model studies, in which trace amounts of copper in the drinking water (0.12 ppm) greatly enhance the AD disease, and point out that EPA allows 1.3 ppm, ten times the toxic amount, in human drinking water. We add our data that show that a third of household drinking water in North America has copper levels shown to be toxic and cause AD in the animal model, and another third is of unknown safety. And of course, it is well established that the diet in most developed countries has become high in fat. We discuss various risk factors for AD, all of which have a copper connection. Direct studies of exchangeable copper in the AD brain show that it is elevated and associated with oxidative pathology, strongly supporting a causal role for copper toxicity in AD.

In our opinion, the evidence for our hypothesis of inorganic copper as partially causal of AD is rather strong. Fortunately, those who agree can do some simple things to help lower their risk. First, they can throw out all multivitamin/multimineral supplements containing copper, because this copper is also a form of inorganic copper. Those who have a specific need for copper, or for any other mineral such as calcium or iron, should take it as an individual supplement. Second, they can have their drinking water tested for copper. If levels are over 0.01 ppm, they can take steps to reduce their inorganic copper intake from this source. They do not have to remove their copper plumbing. Installation of a device such as reverse osmosis, on the tap used for drinking water, will reduce copper levels nicely. Finally, reducing meat intake will reduce fat intake, as well as the absorption of both copper and iron, both sources of potentially damaging oxidant radicals. Our hypothesis will not be definitely proven or disproven for a long time, and in the meantime, those who take steps to reduce inorganic copper intake may benefit.

REFERENCES

Alzheimer, A. 1907. Über eine eigenartige Erkrankung der Hirnrinde. *Allg Z Psychiatr* 64:146–148.

Alzheimer's Association. 2010. *Alzheimer's Disease Facts and Figures*, 1–74.

Boyd, W. 1938. *A Textbook of Pathology: An Introduction to Medicine*. Philadelphia, PA: Lea and Febiger.

Brewer, G.J. 2011. Issues raised involving the copper hypotheses in the causation of Alzheimer's disease. *Int J Alzheimers Dis* 2011:537528, 1–11.

Brewer, G.J. and V. Yuzbasiyan-Gurkan. 1992. Wilson disease. *Medicine (Baltimore)* 71:139–164.

Brewer, G.J., S.H. Kanzer, E.A. Zimmerman et al. 2010a. Copper and ceruloplasmin abnormalities in Alzheimer disease. *Am J Alzheimers Dis Other Demen* 25:490–497.

Brewer, G.J., S.H. Kanzer, E.A. Zimmerman et al. 2010b. Subclinical zinc deficiency in Alzheimer's disease and Parkinson's disease. *Am J Alzheimers Dis Other Demen* 25:572–575.

Bucossi, S., R. Polimanti, S. Mariani et al. 2012. Association of K832R and R952K SNPs of Wilson's disease gene with Alzheimer's disease. *J Alzheimers Dis* 29:913–919.

Deane, R., A. Sagare, M. Coma et al. 2007. A novel role for copper: Disruption of LRP-dependent brain A beta clearance. Presentation at the Annual Meeting of the Society for Neuroscience. San Diego, CA.

Ferri, C.P., M. Prince, C. Brayne et al. 2005. Global prevalence of dementia: A Delphi consensus study. *Lancet* 366:2112–2117.

Grant, W.B. 1997. Dietary links to Alzheimer's disease. *Alzheimer Dis Rev* 2:42–55.

Hill, G.M., G.J. Brewer, J.E. Juni et al. 1986. Treatment of Wilson's disease with zinc. II. Validation of oral 64copper with copper balance. *Am J Med Sci* 292:344–349.

Huang, X., C.S. Atwood, M.A. Hartshorn et al. 1999. The Aβ peptide of Alzheimer's disease directly produces hydrogen peroxide through metal ion reduction. *Biochemistry* 38:7609–7616.

James, S.A., I. Volitakis, P.A. Adlard et al. 2011. Elevated labile Cu is associated with oxidative pathology in Alzheimer disease. *Free Radic Biol Med* 52:298–302.

Miyata, M. and J.D. Smith. 1996. Apolipoprotein E allele-specific antioxidant activity and effects on cytotoxicity by oxidative insults and beta-amyloid peptides. *Nat Genet* 14:55–61.

Moalem, S., M.E. Percy, D.F. Andrews et al. 2000. Are hereditary hemochromatosis mutations involved in Alzheimer disease? *Am J Med Genet* 93:58–66.

Morris, M.C., D.A. Evans, C.C. Tangney et al. 2006. Dietary copper and high saturated and trans fat intakes associated with cognitive decline. *Arch Neurol* 63:1085–1088.

Nelson, T.J. and D.I. Alkon. 2005. Oxidation of cholesterol by amyloid precursor protein and β-amyloid peptide. *J Biol Chem* 280:7377–7387.

Osler, W. 1910. *Modern Medicine in Theory and Practice*. Philadelphia, PA and New York: Lea and Febiger.

Seshadri, S., A. Beiser, J. Selhub et al. 2002. Plasma homocysteine as a risk factor for dementia and Alzheimer's disease. *NEJM* 346:476–483.

Sparks, D.L. and B.G. Schreurs. 2003. Trace amounts of copper in water induce beta-amyloid plaques and learning deficits in a rabbit model of Alzheimer's disease. *Proc Natl Acad Sci USA* 100:11065–11069.

Sparks, D.L., R. Friedland, S. Petanceska et al. 2006. Trace copper levels in the drinking water, but not zinc or aluminum, influence CNS. Alzheimer-like pathology. *J Nutr Health Aging* 10:247–254.

Squitti, R., G. Barbati, L. Rossi et al. 2006. Excess of nonceruloplasmin serum copper in AD correlates with MMSE, CSF [beta]-amyloid, and htau. *Neurology* 67:76–82.

Squitti, R., F. Bressi, P. Pasqualetti et al. 2009. Longitudinal prognostic value of serum "free" copper in patients with Alzheimer disease. *Neurology* 72:50–55.

Squitti, R., P. Pasqualetti, G. Dal Forno et al. 2005. Excess of serum copper not related to ceruloplasmin in Alzheimer disease. *Neurology* 64:1040–1046.

Squitti, R., M. Ventriglia, G. Barbati et al. 2007. "Free" copper in serum of Alzheimer's disease patients correlates with markers of liver function. *J Neural Transm* 114:1589–1594.

Strachey, J., A. Freud, A. Strachey and A. Tyson. 1966. *24 Volumes Entitled, The Standard Edition of the Complete Psychological Works of Sigmund Freud, Written between 1895 and 1939*. London: The Hogarth Press and the Institute of Psycho-Analysis.

Ueda, K., H. Kawano, Y. Hasuo and M. Fujishima. 1992. Prevalence and etiology of dementia in a Japanese community. *Stroke* 23:798–803.

Waldman, M. and M. Lamb. 2005. *Dying for a Hamburger: Modern Meat Processing and the Epidemic of Alzheimer's Disease*. New York: Thomas Dune Books/St. Martin's Press.

White, L., H. Petrovitch, G.W. Ross et al. 1996. Prevalence of dementia in older Japanese-American men in Hawaii: The Honolulu-Asia Aging Study. *JAMA* 276:955–960.

Zambenedetti, P., G. De Bellis, I. Biunno et al. 2003. Transferrin C2 variant does confer a risk for Alzheimer's disease in Caucasians. *J Alzheimers Dis* 5:423–427.

32 Zinc, Health, and Immunity

Ananda Prasad

CONTENTS

INTRODUCTION

The role of zinc as a growth factor in *Aspergillus niger* was reported for the first time in 1869 [1]. In 1926, zinc was shown to be essential for the growth of the plants and in 1934 for the growth of the rats [2]. In 1963, its essentiality for humans was established [3].

In this chapter, the discovery, the clinical and biochemical features, and the diagnostic aspects of human zinc deficiency will be presented. Also clinical implications of conditioned deficiency of zinc and therapeutic impact of zinc in human health will be discussed.

DISCOVERY OF HUMAN ZINC DEFICIENCY

I was born in India and after my medical degree (MBBS) from Patna University, Bihar, India, I came to the University of Minnesota Medical School in Minneapolis, Minnesota. I was fortunate in that I was accepted by Professor Cecil J. Watson to be trained as a clinical investigator. In this program, not only did I receive clinical training in internal medicine but also I was required to do basic science research leading to a PhD degree. My training under Professor Watson as a clinical investigator was superb and prepared me very well for a career in academic medicine.

After I finished my training in Minnesota, I was contacted by Professor Hobart Reimann, Chief of Medicine at Jefferson Medical College, Philadelphia, Pennsylvania, who was a personal friend of the Shah of Iran, and at the invitation of the Shah, Professor Reimann had accepted to go to Shiraz,

Iran, as a Professor and the Chief of Medicine at the Nemezee Hospital and Shiraz University, Medical School. The Shah wanted Professor Reimann to establish the teaching of medicine, and the curriculum of the medical school was patterned after that of American medical schools. Professor Reimann asked me to join him and help him in teaching medicine to the students and residents of Nemezee Hospital. I was first very reluctant since I had no interest in Iran; however, Professor Reimann was persuasive and I finally ended up in Shiraz in July 1958.

Within 2 weeks of my arrival, an Iranian resident physician presented me a 21-year-old Iranian villager who was exceedingly retarded in growth. He looked like a 10-year-old boy. He had no secondary sexual characteristics, and his genitalia were infantile. Facial skin appeared rough, and his liver and spleen were enlarged. There was no ascites. The patient was very anemic. His hemoglobin was 5 g%, and the anemia was hypochromic–microcytic due to iron deficiency. His dietary intake consisted of half kilogram bread made of unleavened flour and a few vegetables. There was no animal protein intake. He also consumed 1 lb. of clay, which he obtained from a nearby hill. The habit of clay eating was fairly prevalent among the villagers in Shiraz.

This case presented to me several clinical dilemmas. The first one was that he was severely iron deficient but he had no blood loss. Adult males do not become severely iron deficient without blood loss. The second problem was that I could not explain the extreme growth retardation and hypogonadism on the basis of iron deficiency. Iron deficiency in rats, mice, pigs, and elephants causes hypochromic–microcytic anemia, but it does not affect growth or testicular functions. I hypothesized that iron was being made unavailable for absorption because this patient's dietary intake contained high amounts of phosphate. The question was, is it possible that another transitional element may also be affected adversely due to high content of dietary phosphate? After examination of the periodic table, I selected zinc as another element that might have been affected adversely in this patient, inasmuch as zinc deficiency was known to affect the growth of microorganisms, plants, rats, and pigs.

The problem was that this syndrome did not exist in the medical textbooks, and scientists repeatedly published that zinc deficiency in humans may never be seen.

Contrary to the existent dogma, I published a paper entitled, Syndrome of Iron Deficiency Anemia, Hepatosplenomegaly, Hypogonadism, Dwarfism and Geophagia, in *American Journal of Medicine* in 1961 [4] and suggested that, in this syndrome, perhaps deficiency of both iron and zinc existed in order to account for the clinical features I observed. The suggestion that zinc deficiency existed in humans became very controversial but was provocative.

Soon after the publication of this paper, I was contacted by Professor William Darby, Chief of the Department of Biochemistry and Nutrition and professor of medicine at Vanderbilt University, Nashville, Tennessee, to meet him at the US Naval Medical Research unit No. 3 (NAMRU-3) in Cairo, Egypt, in order to test the hypothesis that zinc deficiency in humans existed and accounted for the growth retardation in humans. I met Professor Darby, Captain John Seal of the US Navy, and Dr. Arnold Schaeffer of the National Institutes of Health (NIH) at the US NAMRU-3 in Cairo, Egypt. NAMRU-3 was originally established by President Franklin Delano Roosevelt after the Second World War mainly to study and develop strategies against several infectious diseases, which were serious problems for the US troops. Prior to my visit, the Rockefeller group of scientists had just completed an exhaustive study of typhus fever, and now they had just left to return to Rockefeller Institute.

Professor Darby negotiated with the US Navy to assign us space, funds, and personnel for my zinc project. Dr. Schaeffer also agreed to give us adequate support from NIH. My first ordeal was to set up a suitable technique to measure zinc in plasma, red cells, hair, and urine by the use of dithizone technique. Atomic absorption spectrophotometry was not available, and the dithizone technique was very labor intensive. Before accepting this challenge, I wanted to assure myself that zinc-deficient dwarfs also existed in Egypt. I went around the villages near Cairo with Professor Darby, and I was able to recognize five to six dwarfs clinically in each village I visited. This pleased me immensely and assured me that I will be able to study zinc metabolism in these subjects. Dr. Darby was also astonishingly pleased and became an enthusiastic supporter of this project.

I accepted the position of director of the zinc project and moved to Cairo, Egypt. I was soon joined by Dr. Harold H. Sandstead, Dr. Arthur Schulert from Vanderbilt University, Dr. August Miale from the US Navy, and Dr. Zohair Farid, an Egyptian physician who was assigned to NAMR-3 to work on this project.

We studied extensively zinc metabolism in over 40 dwarfs. The zinc concentrations in plasma, erythrocytes and hair and zinc content of 24-h urine were decreased in comparison to those of the control subjects of similar ages. We also utilized ^{65}Zn and determined plasma zinc turnover rate and 24-h exchangeable zinc pool in these subjects. The plasma zinc turnover rate was increased, and the 24-h exchangeable zinc pool was decreased in the dwarfs in comparison to the control subjects [3]. The liver function tests were unremarkable.

Based on these observations, we concluded that these dwarfs were zinc deficient [3]. We subsequently carried a zinc supplementation study in these subjects. We subdivided the dwarfs into three groups. The first group received 15 mg of elemental zinc as sulfate orally daily, and the second group received 15 mg of elemental iron as sulfate orally daily. Both these groups stayed in NAMRU-3 wards and received a well-balanced nutritionally adequate diet. The third group stayed in their villages.

The subjects who received zinc supplementation remained anemic but grew in height on an average of 5 to 6 in. annually. They grew pubic hair within 12 weeks, and their genitalia became adult-like within 6 months following supplementation [5]. The iron group corrected their anemia within 3 months, but there was no effect on growth or gonads. Thus, our study, for the first time, showed the differential tissue effects of iron and zinc in humans. The subjects who stayed in the villages showed no changes in hemoglobin, growth, or gonads.

In our studies in the Middle East, we observed the following clinical manifestations in the zinc-deficient dwarfs: growth retardation, hypogonadism in males, rough skin, poor appetite, mental lethargy, and intercurrent infections [6]. I never saw a zinc-deficient dwarf who lived beyond the age of 25 years. I was told by the village health workers that they died due to infections such as pneumonia, meningitis, and other bacterial, viral, or parasitic infections. This suggested to me that zinc deficiency most likely affected adversely immune functions. We now know that zinc is a signal molecule for immune cells, and zinc deficiency affects Th1 functions adversely.

The first example of zinc deficiency in the United States was reported by Caggiano et al. [7] in 1969 in a Puerto Rican subject with dwarfism, hypogonadism, hypogammaglobulinemia, giardiasis, strongyloidiasis, and schistosomiasis. Zinc supplementation corrected the growth failure. In 1972, Hambidge et al. [8] reported zinc deficiency in Mexican-American children living in Denver, Colorado.

In terms of parasitic diseases, I would like to point out that in Iran, there were no hookworm or schistosomiasis infestations, but hydatid disease was common. In Egypt, however, both hookworm and schistosomiasis infections were extremely common [4,6]. In our zinc supplementation trial in Egypt, while we treated all patients for hookworm infection, they were not treated for schistosomiasis, and in Iran, we did not treat hydatid disease in our subjects.

SEVERE DEFICIENCY OF ZINC

Barnes and Moynahan [9] reported a 2-year-old girl with severe acrodermatitis enteropathica (AE) who was zinc-deficient and responded to zinc supplementation. AE is a lethal, autosomal, recessive trait that usually affects infants of Italian, Armenian, or Iranian lineage [10]. The disease develops in the early months of life soon after weaning from breast-feeding. The dermatologic manifestations include bullous pustular dermatitis of the extremities and the oral, anal, and genital areas around the orifices, paronychia, and alopecia. Blepharitis, conjunctivitis, photophobia, and corneal opacities are some of the ophthalmic manifestations. Neuropsychiatric signs include irritability, emotional instability, tremors, and occasional cerebellar ataxia; weight loss, growth retardation, and testicular hypofunction are also commonly seen. Congenital malformations of fetuses and infants born of pregnant women with AE have been reported [11].

AE patients have an increased susceptibility to infections. Thymic hypoplasia and absence of germinal centers in lymph nodes are noted. Abnormal chemotaxis and all T cell-mediated abnormalities are corrected by zinc supplementation. Clinical course is characterized by downhill course with failure to thrive and complicated by intercurrent bacterial, fungal, viral, and other opportunistic infections. Gastrointestinal disturbances include severe diarrhea, malabsorption, steatorrhea, and lactose intolerance. The disease is fatal if untreated. Zinc supplementation results in recovery. Daily zinc supplementation may exceed 50–75 mg in order to manage these cases effectively. The therapy must be monitored carefully.

AD gene is localized to a −3.5-cm region on 8 q 24 chromosome. The gene encodes a histidine-rich protein, which is a zinc transporter ZIP-4. IN AE mutations in this gene have been reported [12].

Severe deficiency of zinc has also been reported in patients who received total parenteral nutrition without zinc [13–15]. In the United States, it is mandatory to include zinc in all parenteral fluid solutions.

Severe deficiency of zinc may occur in patients with Wilson's disease who receive penicillamine therapy [16]. Physicians must be aware of this problem in chelation therapy.

NUTRITIONAL DEFICIENCY OF ZINC

Nutritional deficiency of zinc is widespread, and it is our estimate that this may affect nearly 2 billion subjects in the developing world. This is because in these countries, the population mainly consumes unleavened bread, which has high content of an organic phosphate compound phytate. Phytate complexes both iron and zinc; thus, it is very common to see deficiencies of both iron and zinc in these countries. Growth retardation, immune dysfunction, and cognitive impairment are the most serious consequences of zinc deficiency. I never saw a zinc-deficient dwarf older than 25 years of age in the Middle East. The health professionals reported to me that they were dying of bacterial, viral, and parasitic infections. The phytate zinc molar ratio greater than 20 in the diet is very unfavorable for zinc absorption.

In the United States, our studies have shown that nearly 30% of the Mexican-American children living in Brownsville, Texas, may have zinc deficiency [17]. Zinc deficiency has been also observed in the African-American population in the United States. Women of child-bearing age whose zinc requirement is increased (25 mg/day) do not often meet this requirement by dietary means in the United States. We have reported zinc deficiency in 25–30% of well-to-do elderly subjects in the United States [18]. It is, therefore, very important for physicians to be aware of this nutritional deficiency so that the patients are properly advised and managed in clinical practice.

Following our discovery of the importance of zinc for human health, the National Academy of Sciences, Research Council declared zinc as an essential element for humans and established a recommended dietary allowance (RDA) in 1974 [19]. In 1978, the Food and Drug Administration (FDA) made it mandatory to include zinc in the total parenteral nutrition fluids [20].

Based on the above observations, we classified nutritional deficiency of zinc as seen globally as examples of moderate level of deficiency of zinc and zinc deficiency seen in AE, following total parenteral nutrition without zinc and following penicillamine therapy in patients with Wilson's disease as examples of severe deficiency of zinc. The recognition of mild level of zinc deficiency, however, remained problematic and difficult.

MILD DEFICIENCY OF ZINC

We developed an experimental model of zinc deficiency in humans. We induced a mild deficiency of zinc in human volunteers by dietary means [21]. Adult male volunteers were kept on a metabolic ward at the Clinical Research Center of the University of Michigan Medical School Hospital, Ann

Arbor, Michigan. A semipurified diet, which supplied approximately 3–5 mg of zinc daily, was used to induce zinc deficiency [21].

The volunteers were given a well-balanced hospital diet containing animal protein daily for 4 weeks. The average intake of zinc was 12 mg daily consistent with RDA. Following this, they received 3–5 mg zinc daily while consuming soy protein-based experimental diet. This regime was continued for 28 weeks. Following this, the volunteers received two cookies containing 27 mg of zinc supplement for 12 weeks.

Throughout the study, the levels of all essential nutrients including protein, amino acids, vitamins, and minerals (both microelements and macroelements) were kept constant meeting RDA except for zinc. By this technique, we were able to induce a specific mild deficiency of zinc in human volunteers [21].

In this model, as a result of mild deficiency of zinc, we observed decreased serum testosterone level, oligospermia, decreased natural killer cells (NK) cell lytic activity, decreased IL-2 activity of T helper cells, decreased serum thymulin activity, hyperammonemia, hypogeusia, decreased dark adaptation, and decreased lean body mass [22,23]. Thus, our study clearly established that even mild deficiency of zinc in humans affected adversely certain clinical, biochemical, and immunological functions.

MECHANISM OF ZINC ACTION ON GROWTH AND IMMUNE CELLS

Growth is the first limiting effect of zinc deficiency in experimental animals [24], and zinc deficiency decreases circulating insulin-like growth factor-1 (IGF-1) concentration independent of total energy intake [24–27].

Zinc deficiency in humans decreases circulating IGF-1 concentration. IGF-1 receptor possesses tyrosine kinase activity, which must be phosphorylated for activation following which a cascade of phosphorylations occurs within the cell leading to regulation of cell cycle and cell division. Inasmuch as zinc has been shown to inhibit various protein tyrosine phosphatases [28], I hypothesize that zinc is involved in phosphorylation of tyrosine kinase by inhibiting its phosphatases and is thus critical for cell division and growth.

IGF-1 activation leads to stimulation of thymidine uptake in cells [29]. We have reported earlier that in zinc-deficient rats, the activity of deoxythymidine kinase (TK), an enzyme required for conversion of deoxythymidine to deoxythymidine 5′-monophosphate (dTMP), a precursor of thymidine triphosphate (TTP), is significantly decreased in the implanted sponge connective tissue, and this reduced activity of TK decreased DNA, protein, and collagen synthesis in rats [30]. Thus, it appears that zinc has multiple roles on growth. It is required for IGF-1 generation, phosphorylation of IGF-1 receptor, and upregulation of the activity of TK, all of which are involved in cell division and growth.

Zinc is a second messenger for immune cells. The intracellular zinc status is altered by an extracellular stimulus, and this then participates in signaling events [31]. Kitamura et al. [32] have shown that a decrease in intracellular free zinc is critical for lipopolysaccharides (LPS)-mediated CD4+ T cell activation by dendritic cells (DCs). A reduction in intracellular free zinc increases surface expression of major histocompatibility complex (MHC) class II molecules, which is important for the activation of CD4+ T cells by DCs.

LPS stimulation of zinc-sufficient monocytes results in downregulation of inflammatory cytokines such as tumor necrosis factor-alpha (TNF-α), IL-1β, and IL-8 [33,34]. Zinc inhibits the membrane phosphodiesterase (PDE), which increases second messenger guanosine 3′, 5′ cyclic monophosphate (cGMP). This is followed by subsequent suppression of the NF-κB-dependent mRNAs of TNF-α, IL-1β, and other inflammatory cytokines [35–37]. Additionally, zinc induces A-20, which inhibits NF-κB signaling via TNF receptor-associated factor pathways, resulting in downregulation of mRNAs of inflammatory cytokines [37]. Based on these, we propose that zinc is an important anti-inflammatory agent.

Zinc deficiency affects Th1 functions adversely in humans [22]. Serum thymulin activity and generation of Th1 cytokines IL-2 and interferon-γ (IFN-γ) were affected within 8–12 weeks of institution of zinc-deficient diet in humans, whereas plasma zinc decreased after 20–24 weeks of institution of zinc-deficient diet. Th2 cytokines were not affected by zinc deficient diet.

In HUT-78 cells, a human malignant lymphoblastoid cell line of Th0 phenotype, we have also shown that zinc was required for th1 cell differentiation [38].

DIAGNOSIS OF ZINC DEFICIENCY IN HUMANS

Prior to 1965, plasma zinc was assayed by dithizone technique. In 1965, we established for the first time a simple assay of plasma zinc by atomic absorption spectrophotometry [39]. This technique has been used globally ever since to assess the zinc status of human subjects.

Although plasma zinc assay is simple and easily available, it is not a sensitive indicator of zinc deficiency. Falsely high levels are observed if the red cells are hemolyzed during venesection. There is also a diurnal variation in plasma zinc levels.

In patients with acute stress or infection, or following a myocardial infarction, zinc from the plasma pool may redistribute to other compartments, thus making an assessment of zinc status by plasma zinc levels difficult.

Zinc in red cells and hair may be used for assessment of zinc status. However, turnover of zinc in these cells are slow, and thus, measurement of zinc in these tissues does not reflect recent changes in the body zinc status. Measurement of zinc in granulocytes and lymphocytes is more reliable as an indicator of body zinc status as zinc turnover rate in these cells is more rapid [40]. A quantitative assay of lymphocyte ecto-5'-nucleotidase (5'NT) is also a good indicator of zinc status in our experience [41]. Twenty-four hours of urinary zinc excretion is decreased in patients with zinc deficiency. However, in patients with cirrhosis of the liver, chronic alcoholics, patients with sickle cell disease (SCD), and patients with chronic renal disease, there is hyperzincuria in spite of the fact that they are zinc deficient.

Kaji et al. [42] measured zinc clearance following IV injection of zinc sulfate solution (1 μmol/kg) in Japanese children with low stature. An increased zinc clearance was a useful test for diagnosing marginal zinc deficiency in these children.

In our studies in experimental human model of zinc deficiency by using ^{70}Zn stable isotope, we showed that the absorption of zinc was significantly increased as the deficiency progressed; however, the efficiency of zinc absorption was not sustained when the zinc-restricted diet was continued for 6 months. Our studies showed that measurement of endogenous intestinal zinc excretion and urinary excretion, both of which were decreased, was a very useful test for marginal zinc deficiency in humans [43].

In our experimental model of mild human zinc deficiency, decreased serum thymulin activity, decreased production of IL-2, decreased lymphocyte-ecto-5'nucleotidase activity, decreased intestinal endogenous zinc excretion, and decrease in 24-h urinary zinc excretion occurred within 8 weeks of the institution of the zinc-deficient diet containing approximately 5 mg of zinc daily. Plasma zinc decreased after 20 weeks of the deficient diet regimen, and the zinc concentration of lymphocytes and granulocytes decreased after 12 weeks of institution of the zinc-deficient diet.

In our studies, we observed that three enzymes—alkaline phosphatase in the bone, carboxypeptidase in the pancreas, and deoxythymidine kinase in proliferating tissues in experimental animals—were very sensitive to zinc status [44] in that their activities were affected adversely within 3–6 days of the institution of the zinc-deficient diet to the experimental animals. In human studies, the activity of deoxythymidine kinase in proliferating skin collagen and alkaline phosphatase activity in granulocytes were very useful in assessing body zinc status [45].

We observed that a decrease in plasma thymulin activity in zinc-deficient subjects was corrected in vitro by addition of zinc to the plasma, and a decrease in IL-2 mRNA in phytohemagglutinin-p (PHA)-stimulated mononuclear cells (MNCs) by RT-PCR was also corrected by in vitro zinc addition [46]. These tests, therefore, may be very sensitive diagnostic tests for mild zinc deficiency in humans.

CONDITIONED DEFICIENCY OF ZINC

GASTROINTESTINAL DISORDERS AND LIVER DISEASE

Zinc deficiency has been observed in patients with malabsorption syndrome, Crohn's disease, regional ileitis, and steatorrhea [47]. In patients with cirrhosis of the liver, low serum and hepatic zinc and paradoxically hyperzincuria have been reported [48]. Zinc-responsive night blindness in patients with cirrhosis of the liver has been observed.

Zinc deficiency affects urea synthesis; thus, abnormalities related to amino acids and ammonia may induce hepatic coma in patients with cirrhosis of the liver [48]. We have observed elevated levels of plasma ammonia in the experimental model of human zinc-deficient subjects [49]. In zinc-deficient rats, we reported a decrease in ornithine transcarbamoylase activity in the liver and an increase in the plasma ammonia level in zinc-deficient rats [50]. An increased activity of the purine nucleotide enzyme adenosine monophosphate deaminase (AMP-deaminase) as a result of zinc deficiency has also been reported in rats. Thus, it is possible that several factors may account for hyperammonemia in patients with cirrhosis of the liver. Zinc therapy has been reported to be beneficial in subjects with hepatic encephalopathy by some investigators; however, more studies are needed in this area.

I hypothesize that some of the clinical features of cirrhosis of the liver, such as loss of body hair, testicular hypofunction, poor appetite, mental lethargy, difficulty in healing, abnormal cell-mediated immunity, and night blindness, may be due to the secondary zinc-deficient state in this disease.

RENAL DISEASE

Mahajan et al. [51] documented for the first time that patients with chronic renal disease had low zinc concentration in plasma, leucocytes, and hair; increased plasma ammonia levels; and increased activity of plasma ribonuclease. Zinc supplementation studies showed improvement in uremic hypogeusia and uremic gonadal dysfunction [51,52]. The clinicians must rule out zinc deficiency in patients with chronic renal disease and properly treat these subjects with zinc supplementation if they are deficient.

SICKLE CELL DISEASE

Our studies have documented the occurrence of zinc deficiency in adult SCD patients [53–55]. We have related growth retardation, hypogonadism in males, hyperammonemia, abnormal dark adaptation, and cell-mediated immune dysfunction in SCD patients to deficiency of zinc [53–55]. The biochemical evidence of zinc deficiency in SCD patients included decreased levels of zinc in plasma, erythrocytes, and hair; hyperzincuria; and decreased activities of certain zinc-dependent enzymes such as carbonic anhydrase in red cells, alkaline phosphatase in granulocytes, deoxythymidine kinase activity in newly synthesizing collagen connective tissue, and hyperammonemia. Inasmuch as zinc is known to be an inhibitor of ribonuclease (RNase), an increased activity of this enzyme in the plasma of SCD subjects was regarded as an evidence of zinc deficiency. We carried out controlled zinc supplementation studies in SCD patients, and we showed that zinc supplementation resulted in significant improvement in secondary sexual characteristics, normalized plasma ammonia levels, and reversed dark adaptation abnormality [56]. As a result of zinc supplementation, the zinc levels in plasma, red cells, and neutrophils increased, and we observed expected response to supplementation in the activities of various zinc-dependent enzymes [56]. We have also reported a beneficial effect of zinc supplementation on longitudinal growth and body weight in 14- to 18-year-old SCD patients [57]. Zinc deficiency in patients with SCD was associated with impaired delayed-type hypersensitivity reactions (DTH) and decreased NK cell lytic activity, which was corrected by zinc supplementation.

A 3-month placebo-controlled zinc supplementation trial (25 mg elemental zinc as acetate three times a day) in SCD patients showed that the zinc-supplemented group had decreased incidence of infections and increased hemoglobin and hematocrit, plasma zinc, and antioxidant power in comparison to the placebo group [54]. Plasma nitrite and nitrate (NOx), lipid peroxidation products, DNA oxidation products, and soluble vascular cell adhesion molecule-1 (VcAM-1) decreased in the zinc group.

The zinc group showed significant decreases in lipopolysaccharide-induced TNF-α and IL-1β mRNAs and TNF-induced nuclear factor (NF) of κB-DNA binding in MNCs compared with the placebo group. Zinc supplementation also increased the relative levels of IL-2 and IL2Rα mRNAs in PHA-p stimulated MNCs.

In summary, physicians and hematologists must remain alert to the possibility of zinc deficiency in SCD subjects and use properly zinc supplementation if they are deficient in zinc.

THERAPEUTIC IMPACT OF ZINC

ACUTE DIARRHEA IN CHILDREN

Zinc supplementation prevents and is effective in the treatment of acute diarrhea among children under 5 years of age [58,59]. Zinc is now being routinely used for the treatment of acute diarrhea throughout the world as recommended by the World Health Organization (WHO). It has resulted in saving millions of lives.

Diarrhea causes breakdown of absorptive mucosa resulting in poor absorption of nutrients including zinc. Children with low plasma zinc were observed to be more susceptible to diarrhea pathogens, propagating a vicious cycle of zinc deficiency and infection. In 2004, the WHO issued a global recommendation for daily supplementation with 20 mg zinc in children at least 6 months of age and 10 mg of zinc in infants under 6 months of age for 10–14 days upon diarrheal onset for prevention of diarrhea [58,59]. A meta-analysis of routine supplementation for up to 3 months in seven studies providing one to two times RDA elemental zinc five to seven times per week showed an 18% reduction in incidence of diarrhea, a 25% decrease in diarrhea prevalence, and a 33% reduction in persistent diarrhea episodes among zinc group compared to the placebo group [58,59].

ZINC FOR THE COMMON COLD

Common cold is one of the most frequently occurring diseases in the world [60,61]. Annually, adults in the United States may suffer two to four times with common cold, and children may suffer with common cold six to eight times in a year. The morbidity and subsequent financial loss resulting from absenteeism from work is substantial. Previously prescribed treatments have not provided a consistent relief of symptoms.

Eby et al. [62] first showed that zinc gluconate lozenges administered every 2–3 h were effective in decreasing the severity and duration of common cold. This observation, however, remained very controversial for many years.

We tested the efficacy of zinc acetate lozenges in common cold. We carried out a randomized double-blind, placebo-controlled trial in 50 volunteers who were recruited within 24 h of developing symptoms of the common cold [60,61]. Participants took one lozenge containing 12.8 mg zinc (as acetate) or placebo every 2 to 3 h while awake as soon as they developed cold symptoms. Subjective symptom scores for sore throat, nasal discharge, nasal congestion, sneezing, cough, scratchy throat, hoarseness, muscle ache, fever, and headache were recorded daily for 12 days. Plasma zinc and proinflammatory cytokines were assayed on day 1 and after the participants were well. Compared to the placebo group, the zinc group had shorter overall duration of cold symptoms (4.5 vs. 8.1 days, $p < 0.01$), cough (3.1 vs. 6.3 days, $p = 0.01$), and nasal discharge (4.1 vs. 5.8 days, $p = 0.02$). The total severity scores for all symptoms were also decreased in the zinc group significantly ($p < 0.002$).

We carried out another randomized, double-blind, placebo-controlled trial of zinc in 50 ambulatory volunteers within 24 h of developing common cold symptoms [61]. Participants took one lozenge containing 13.3 mg of zinc (as zinc acetate) or placebo every 2–3 h while awake. The subjective scores of clinical symptoms were recorded daily. Plasma zinc, sIL-1ra, sTNF-r1, and sICAM-1 were assayed on days 1 and 5 [61].

The zinc group in comparison to the placebo had a shorter mean duration of cold (4.0 vs. 7.1 days, $p = 0.001$), shorter duration of cough (2.1 vs. 5.0 days, $p < 0.001$), and nasal discharge (3.0 vs. 4.5 days, $p = 0.02$).

Total severity scores were significantly decreased in the zinc group ($p = 0.002$). The mean changes between zinc and placebo groups (before vs. after therapy) showed significant differences in sIL-1ra ($p = 0.033$) and sICAM-1 levels ($p = 0.04$). Both decreased in the zinc group, and the mean changes between the zinc and placebo groups (before vs. after therapy) showed significant difference ($p < 0.001$).

Our investigations suggest that common cold viruses increase oxidative stress, which activates macrophages and monocytes resulting in increased production of both the inflammatory cytokines and the anti-inflammatory product sIL-1ra; thus, a decrease in sIL-ra in the zinc group following treatment suggests that zinc decreased activation of monocytes and macrophages by decreasing oxidative stress. We have previously shown that zinc functions as an antioxidant [61].

Human rhinovirus type 24 "docks" with ICAM-1 on the surface of the somatic cells [61]. Thus, zinc may act as an antiviral agent by reducing ICAM-1 levels. We have previously shown that zinc functions as a downregulator of NF-κB activity, which participates in the gene expression of adhesion molecules such as ICAM-1 [61].

We conclude that zinc acetate lozenges, if used within 24 h of the onset of common cold in proper dosages, are very effective in decreasing the duration and severity of common cold. We suggest that the beneficial effects seen in the zinc group were due to the antioxidant and anti-inflammatory effects of zinc. We also suggest that a decrease in plasma ICAM-1 levels due to zinc therapy may have decreased the docking of the cold viruses on the surface of the somatic cells.

In order to optimize the therapeutic effect of zinc lozenges in common cold, one must pay attention to several issues. The first is that zinc treatment must begin within 24 h of the onset of cold symptoms. Second, the total daily dose of elemental zinc should be greater than 75 mg. Third, the chemical formulation should be optimal such that zinc is properly ionized in the oral cavity at pH 7.4. Zinc acetate and zinc gluconate are proper salts to use.

If citric acid, glycine, tartrate, and other binders are used, zinc is prevented from ionization. Thus, it is critical that solution chemistry of the preparation is proper and optimal.

Physicians also must realize that one cannot treat common cold by prescribing zinc syrup, zinc tablets, or capsules that are swallowed. Zinc lozenges must be used orally to dissolve slowly in the mouth, which will then allow zinc ions to be released, absorbed, and transported to the virally infected oronasal cavities.

ZINC FOR WILSON'S DISEASE

Wilson's disease is an inherited autosomal disorder of copper accumulation. The excretion of liver copper in the bile is decreased. This leads to failure of copper excretion in the stool and to hepatic accumulation of copper. Eventually, copper also accumulates in other organs such as brain, kidneys, and pancreas. Typically, the patients present with liver disease, neurological disease (movement disorder), or psychiatric disturbances in the second to fourth decade of life. The Kayser–Fleischer ring (copper deposit) seen in the cornea is a diagnostic clinical feature of this disorder.

The gene for Wilson's disease has now been identified. The genetic mutation leads to a defective protein ATP7B, which is responsible for a key step in biliary excretion of copper [63–66]. The disease is recessive, and thus, both copies of the ATP7B gene have to be mutated to cause a failure in the biliary excretion of copper. The gene for Wilson's disease codes for a membrane-bound copper-binding adenosine triphosphatase–type protein, which acts as a copper pump, in either the plasma membrane or the intracellular membrane. A large number of mutations in this gene have been reported, thus complicating the development of an easy DNA test for Wilson's disease.

Early diagnosis of Wilson's disease is very important, inasmuch as effective therapy to decrease copper burden may be undertaken and prevent damage to various organs by copper accumulation. Ninety percent of the patients with Wilson's disease have low levels of ceruloplasmin and cerulo plasmin-bound copper. Non-ceruloplasmin-bound copper is elevated in the plasma in patients with Wilson's disease. Measurement of the 24-h urinary copper is a good diagnostic test, inasmuch as it is consistently elevated in the patients. Urinary copper, however, may be elevated in patients with obstructive liver disease also who do not have Wilson's disease. Liver copper is increased in patients with Wilson's disease.

The initial treatment objective is to decrease copper burden. It is also desirable to prevent copper from shifting from one pool to another while de-coppering is being done.

Several years ago, we were using 150-mg elemental zinc in six divided doses for the treatment of SCD patients [65]. We observed that zinc was an effective antisickling agent. At this level of zinc therapy, our treatment resulted in inducing copper deficiency in these patients [67]. This observation led Brewer et al. [63–66] to develop zinc as an effective anticopper drug for Wilson's disease.

Zinc competes with copper for similar binding sites, and oral zinc decreases uptake of copper efficiently [63]. Zinc may also act by induction of intestinal cell metallothionein (MT). MT once induced has high affinity for binding copper and prevents the serosal transfer of copper into the blood [68]. The intestinal cells turn over rapidly and take the complexed copper into the stool for final excretion. Zinc blocks not only food copper but also the copper that is endogenously excreted via salivary, gastric, and other gastrointestinal juices. Thus, zinc is very effective in producing a negative copper balance.

For management of patients with Wilson's disease, we recommend 50 mg of elemental zinc (as acetate) orally three times a day. Zinc is given in a fasting or post-absorptive state. The only side effect is that 10% of the subjects may have gastric discomfort. This is usually avoided if zinc is administered between breakfast and lunch or after dinner before going to bed.

For maintenance therapy, zinc is the drug of choice. Relatively speaking, zinc has no toxicity and is nonteratogenic, and then it can be given to subjects of all ages including pregnant women. Zinc has been approved by the FDA for the treatment of patients with Wilson's disease.

AGE-RELATED MACULAR DEGENERATION

Twenty-five percent of the subjects over 65 years of age may be affected with age-related macular degeneration (AMD), and the late stages of AMD accounts for nearly 50% of legal blindness in the United States [69]. Newsome et al. [70] showed that zinc levels are reduced in eyes of AMD patients and suggested that zinc deficiency may have caused damage to retina by increasing oxidative stress.

The Age-Related Eye Disease Study (AREDS) group, supported by the National Eye Institute, NIH, have conducted a double-masked clinical trial or supplementation in 11 centers in patients with dry-type AMD [71,72]. A total of 3640 participants were enrolled. Their ages ranged from 55 to 80 years, and the average follow-up period was 6.3 years. They were randomly assigned to receive one of the following: (1) antioxidants (vitamin C 500 mg, vitamin E 400 IU, and beta carotene 15 mg); (2) zinc 80 mg as zinc oxide and copper 2 mg as copper oxide to prevent copper deficiency induced by the therapeutic level of zinc; (3) antioxidants plus zinc; and (4) placebo.

The group receiving both antioxidants and zinc reduced the risk of developing advanced AMD by about 25% and vision loss by about 19%. The group taking zinc alone decreased the risk of developing advanced AMD by about 21% and vision loss by 11%. In the group receiving vitamins alone, the risk of advanced AMD was reduced by 17%, and vision loss was decreased by 10%. No significant side effects were noted in subjects receiving zinc [71]. Interestingly, only zinc-supplemented group showed increased longevity [72]. The risk of mortality was reduced by 27% in the AREDS group who received only therapeutic zinc daily. Most ophthalmologists globally are using zinc and multivitamins as supplement for the treatment of dry type of AMD.

ZINC SUPPLEMENTATION IN THE ELDERLY DECREASED INCIDENCE OF INFECTIONS

The daily intake of zinc in the elderly subjects in the Western world, including the United States, is around 8–10 mg, whereas RDA for zinc is 15 mg [18,73]. The elderly subjects usually skip either breakfast or lunch. Many live alone and do not cook a proper meal for themselves. Our study in the Detroit area has shown that nearly 35% of the well-to-do elderly ambulatory subjects may have a deficiency of zinc based on their plasma zinc levels. The third National Health and Nutrition Examination Survey (1988–1994) also reported that elderly persons ≥ 71 years were at the greatest risk of inadequate zinc [74].

Oxidative stress and increased inflammatory cytokines have been recognized as important contributing factors for several chronic diseases attributed to aging, such as atherosclerosis and related cardiovascular disorders, mutagenesis and cancer, neurodegenerative disorders, type 2 diabetes, and Alzheimer's disease. Together, O^{2-}, H_2O_2, and OH radicals are reactive oxygen species (ROS), and excess production of ROS causes oxidative stress. Oxidative stress generates inflammatory cytokines such as TNF-α and IL-1β by activating monocytes and macrophages, and these in turn generate more ROS. Chronic inflammation has been implicated in high cardiovascular mortality in elderly subjects [75].

We have shown before that zinc supplementation to subject's ages 20–50 years decreased oxidative stress markers such as malondehyde (MDA), 4-hydroxyalkenals (HAE), and 8-hydroxydeoxyguanine in the plasma, downregulated the ex vivo generation of TNF-α and IL-1β mRNA in MNCs, and provided protection against TNF-α–induced NF-κB activation in MNCs [36]. We have also shown that in HL-60 cell line (promyelocytic leukemia cell line), which differentiates to the monocyte and macrophage phenotype in response to PMA, zinc upregulated A20 and the finding of A-20 transactivating factor to DNA, which results in the inhibition of NF-κB activation [37].

Inasmuch as zinc deficiency and susceptibility to infections due to cell-mediated immune dysfunctions have been observed in the elderly, we conducted a randomized trial of placebo-controlled zinc supplementation in 50 healthy elderly subjects (55–87 years) of both sexes and all ethnic groups [73]. Exclusion criteria were as follows: life expectancy of less than 8 months, progressive neoplastic disease, severe cardiac dysfunction, significant renal disease, significant liver disease, and subjects who were not competent clinically. Zinc supplementation consisted of 45-mg elemental zinc as gluconate daily for 12 months.

A comparison of the baseline data between the younger subjects (ages 18–54 years, $n = 31$) and the elderly subjects showed that the plasma zinc was lower, and the percentage of cells producing IL-1β and TNF-α and the generated cytokines was significantly higher in the elderly subjects [73]. Intercellular adhesion molecules, vascular endothelial cell adhesion molecules, and plasma E-selectin were significantly higher in the elderly. IL-10 generated by Th2, which regulates negatively IL-2 generation from Th1 cells, was significantly higher in the elderly. The oxidative stress markers were also higher in the elderly [75].

The mean incidence of infections per subject in 12 months was significantly lower in the zinc-supplemented group compared to the placebo group ($p < 0.01$). The reduction in incidences of infection in the zinc-supplemented group was 66% in comparison to the placebo group.

The plasma zinc increased, and ex vivo generation of TNF-α and IL-1β decreased significantly in the zinc group compared to the placebo group [72]. Oxidative stress biomarkers in the plasma decreased significantly in the zinc group in comparison to the placebo group [75].

Zinc supplementation increased PHA-induced IL-2 mRNA in MNCs, following zinc supplementation to subjects who were zinc deficient. Thus, our studies of zinc supplementation in the elderly showed highly significant effects, inasmuch as immune deficiency, oxidative stress, and increased inflammatory cytokines are known to precede many chronic disorders in the elderly [76].

TOXIC EFFECTS OF ZINC SUPPLEMENTATION

We have seen no side effect if the dose of elemental zinc supplementation is less than 50 mg daily. It is safe and nonmutagenic. If the dose is over 50 mg daily, one must monitor serum copper levels. Higher doses of zinc induce copper deficiency in humans. Usually supplementation with 1 mg of copper sulfate daily is sufficient to correct copper deficiency. In some trials, when elemental zinc was high such as in the case of the AMD trial, 2 mg of copper oxide was also given at the same time to prevent copper deficiency. Zinc should be administered either in the fasting state or post-absorptive state at bedtime. In our experience, the best absorbable salts of zinc are zinc acetate and zinc gluconate.

REFERENCES

1. Raulin J. Chemical studies on vegetation. *Ann Sci Nat* (in French). 1869;11:93–99.
2. Todd WR, Elvehjem CA, Hart EB. Zinc in the nutrition of the rat. *Am J Physiol*. 1933;107:146–156.
3. Prasad AS, Miale A, Farid Z, Schulert A, Sandstead HH. Zinc metabolism in patients with the syndrome of iron deficiency anemia, hypogonadism and dwarfism. *J Lab Clin Med*. 1963;61:537–549.
4. Prasad AS, Halsted JA, Nadimi M. Syndrome of iron deficiency anemia, hepatosplenomegaly, hypogonadism, dwarfism, and geophagia. *Am J Med*. 1961;31:532–546.
5. Sandstead HH, Prasad AS, Schulert AR, Farid Z, Miale A Jr, Bassily S, Darby WJ. Human zinc deficiency, endocrine manifestations and response to treatment. *Am J Clin Nutr*. 1967;20:422–442.
6. Prasad AS, Miale A, Farid Z, Sandstead HH, Schulert AR, Darby WJ. Biochemical studies on dwarfism, hypogonadism, and anemia. *AMA Arch Intern Med*. 1963;111:407–428.
7. Caggiano V, Schnitzler R, Strauss W, Baker RK, Carter AC, Josephson AS, Wallach, S. Zinc deficiency in a patient with retarded growth, hypogonadism, hypogammaglobulinemia, and chronic infection. *Am J Med Sci*. 1969;257:305–319.
8. Hambidge KM, Hambidge C, Jacobs M, Brown JD. Low levels of zinc in hair, anorexia, poor growth and hypogeusia in children. *Ped Res*. 1972;6:868–874.
9. Barnes PM, Moynahan EJ. Zinc deficiency in acrodermatitis enteropathica. *Proc R Soc Med*. 1973;66:327–329.
10. Prasad AS. *Biochemistry of Zinc*. Plenum Press, New York, 1993.
11. Cavdar AO, Babacan E, Arcasoy A, Ertein U. Effect of nutrition on serum zinc concentration during pregnancy in Turkish women. *Am J Clin Nutr*. 1980;33:542–544.
12. Wang K, Zhou B, Kuo YM, Zemansky J, Gitschier J. A novel member of a zinc transporter family is defective in acrodermatitis enteropathica. *Am J Hum Genet*. 2002;71:66–73.
13. Kay RG, Tasman-Jones C. Zinc deficiency and intravenous feeding. *Lancet*. 1975;2:605–606.
14. Okada A, Takagi Y, Itakura T, Satani M, Manabe H. Skin lesions during intravenous hyperalimentation: Zinc deficiency. *Surgery*. 1976;80:629–635.
15. Arakawa T, Tamara T, Igarashi Y. Zinc deficiency in two infants during parenteral alimentation for diarrhea. *Am J Clin Nutr*. 1976;29:197–204.
16. Klingberg WG, Prasad AS, Oberleas D. Zinc deficiency following penicillamine therapy. In: *Trace Elements in Human Health and Disease*, Vol. 1, AS Prasad (ed.), Academic Press, New York, 1976, pp. 51–65.
17. Sandstead HH, Prasad AS, Beck FWJ, Kaplan J, Egger NG, Alcock NW, Carroll RM, Ramanujam VMS, Daval HH, Rocco CD, Plotkin RA, Zavaleta AN. Zinc deficiency in Mexican-American children: Influence of zinc and other micronutrients on T cells, cytokines, and anti-inflammatory plasma proteins. *Am J Clin Nutr*. 2008;88(4):1067–1073.
18. Prasad AS, Fitzgerald JT, Hess JW, Kaplan J, Pelen F, Dardenne M. Zinc deficiency in the elderly patients. *Nutrition*. 1993;9:218–224.
19. *Recommended Dietary Allowance*, Eight Revised Edition. National Academy of Sciences Trace Elements Zinc. National Academy of Sciences, Washington DC, 1974, pp. 99–101.
20. Guidelines for Essential Trace Element preparation for parenteral use. A statement by an expert panel. AMA Department of Foods and Nutrition. Expert panel: Shils ME, Burke AW, Greene HL, Jeejeebhoy KN, Prasad AS, Sandstead HH. *JAMA*. 1979;241(19):2051–2054.

21. Prasad AS, Rabbani P, Abbasi A, Bowersox E, Spivey-Fox MR. Experimental zinc deficiency in humans. *Ann Intern Med.* 1978;89:483–490.

22. Beck FWJ, Prasad AS, Kaplan J, Fitzgerald JT, Brewer GJ. Changes in cytokine production and T cell subpopulations in experimentally induced zinc deficient humans. *Am J Physiol Endocrinol Metab.* 1997;272:1002–1007.

23. Prasad AS, Meftah S, Abdallah J, Kaplan J, Brewer GJ, Bach JF, Dardenne M. Serum thymulin in human zinc deficiency. *J Clin Invest.* 1988;82:1202–1210.

24. MacDonald RS. The role of zinc in growth and cell proliferation. *J Nutr.* 2000;130:1500S–1508S.

25. Ohisson C, Bengtsson BA, Isaksson OG, Andreassen TT, Slootweg MC. Growth hormone and bone. *Endrocrinol Rev.* 1998;19:55–79.

26. Cossack ZT. Decline in somatomedin-C, insulin-like growth factor-1, with experimentally induced zinc deficiency in human subjects. *Clin Nutr. (Edinb.).* 1991;10:284–291.

27. Ninh NX, Thissen JP, Maiter D, Adam E, Mulumba N, Ketelsiegers JM. Reduced liver insulin-like growth factor-1 gene expression in young zinc-deprived rats in associated with a decrease in liver growth hormone (GH) receptors and serum GH-binding protein. *J Endocrinol.* 1995;144:449–456.

28. Wilson M, Hogstrand C, Maret W. Picomolar concentrations of free zinc (II) ions regulate receptor protein tyrosine phosphatase beta activity. *J Biol Chem.* 2012;16:9322–9326.

29. MacDonald RS, Wollard-Biddle LC, Browning JD, Thornton WH, O'Dell BL. Zinc deprivation of murine 3T3 cells by use of diethylenetrinitrilopentaacetate impairs DNA synthesis upon stimulation with insulin-like growth factor-1 (IGF-I). *J Nutr.* 1998;128:1600–1605.

30. Prasad AS, Beck FWJ, Endre L, Handschu W, Kukuruga M, Kumar G. Zinc deficiency affects cell cycle and deoxythymidine kinase (TK) gene expression in HUT-78 cells. *J Lab Clin Med.* 1996;128:51–60.

31. Hirano T, Murakami M, Fukada T, Nishida K, Yamasaki S, Suzuki T. Roles of zinc and zinc signaling in immunity: Zinc as an intracellular signaling molecule. *Adv Immun.* 2008;97:149–176.

32. Kitamura H, Morikawa H, Kamon H, Iguchi M, Hojyo S, Fukada T, Yamashita S, Kaisho T, Akiron S, Murakami M, Hirano T. Toll-like receptor-mediated regulation of zinc homeostasis influences dentritic cell function. *Nat Immunol.* 2006;7:971–977.

33. Haase H, Rink L. Signal transduction in monocytes: The role of zinc ions. *Biometals.* 2007;20:579–585.

34. Rosenkranz E, Prasad AS, Rink L. Immunobiology and hematology of zinc. In: *Zinc in Human Health*, L Rink (ed.), IOS Press, Amsterdam, 2011, pp. 195–233.

35. Shankar AH, Prasad AS. Zinc and immune function: The biological basis of altered resistance to infection. *Am J Clin Nutr.* (suppl) 1998;68:447–463.

36. Prasad AS, Bao B, Beck FWJ, Kucuk O, Sarkar FH. Antioxidant effect of zinc in humans. *Free Rad Biol Med.* 2004;37:1182–1190.

37. Prasad AS, Bao B, Beck FWJ, Sarkar FH. Zinc-suppressed inflammatory cytokines by induction of A20-mediated inhibition of nuclear factor-κB. *Nutrition.* 2010;27:816–823.

38. Bao B, Prasad AS, Beck WJ, Bao GW, Singh T, Ali S, Sarkar FH. Intracellular free zinc up-regulates IFN-γ and T-bet essential for Th1 differentiation in Con-A stimulated HUT-78 cells. *BBRC.* 2011;407:703–707.

39. Prasad AS, Oberleas D, Halsted JA. Determination of zinc in biological fluids by atomic absorption spectrophotometry in normal and cirrhotic subjects. *J Lab Clin Med.* 1965;66:508–516.

40. Wang H, Prasad AS, DuMouchelle EA. Zinc in platelets, lymphocytes and granulocytes by flameless atomic absorption spectrophotometry. *J Micronutrient Anal.* 1989;5:181–190.

41. Meftah S, Prasad AS, Lee D-Y, Brewer GJ. Ecto 5′ nucleotidase (5′NT) as a sensitive indicator of human zinc deficiency. *J Lab Clin Med.* 1991;118(4):309–316.

42. Kaji M, Gotoh M, Takagi Y, Masuda H, Kimura Y, Uenoyama Y. Studies to determine the usefulness of the zinc clearance test to diagnose marginal zinc deficiency and the effects of oral zinc supplementation for short children. *J Am Coll Nutr.* 1998;17:388–391.

43. Lee D-Y, Prasad AS, Hydrick-Adair C, Brewer GJ, Johnson PE. Homeostasis of zinc in marginal human zinc deficiency: Role of absorption and endogenous excretion of zinc. *J Lab Clin Med.* 1993;122:549–556.

44. Prasad AS, Oberleas D, Wolf PL, Horwitz JP. Studies on zinc deficiency: Changes in trace elements and enzyme activities in tissues of zinc-deficient rats. *J Clin Invest.* 1967;46:549–557.

45. Prasad AS, Oberleas D. Thymidine kinase activity and incorporation of thymidine into DNA in zinc-deficient tissue. *J Lab Clin Med.* 1974;83:634–639.

46. Prasad AS, Bao B, Beck FWJ, Sarkar FH. Correction of IL-2 gene expression by in vitro zinc addition to MNC from zinc deficient human subjects: A specific test for zinc deficiency in humans. *Trans Res.* 2006;148(6):325–333.

47. MacMahon RA, Parker ML, McKinnon M. Zinc treatment in malabsorption. *Med J Aust.* 1968;2:210–212.

48. Grungreiff K, Reinhold D. Zinc and the liver. In: *Zinc in Human Health*. L Rink (ed.), IOS Press, Amsterdam, 2011, pp. 473–492.
49. Prasad AS, Rabbani P, Warth JA. Effect of zinc on hyperammonemia in sickle cell anemia subjects. *Am J Hematol*. 1979;7:323–327.
50. Rabbani P, Prasad AS. Plasma ammonia and liver ornithine transcarbamoylase activity in zinc-deficient rats. *Am J Physiol*. 1978;235:203–206.
51. Mahajan SK, Prasad AS, Rabbani P, Briggs WA, McDonald FD. Zinc metabolism in uremia. *J Lab Clin Med*. 1979;94:693–698.
52. Mahajan SK, Abbasi AA, Prasad AS, Rabbani P, Briggs WA, McDonald FD. Effect of oral zinc therapy on gonadal function in hemodialysis patients. *Ann Intern Med*. 1982;97:357–361.
53. Prasad AS, Schoomaker EB, Ortega J, Brewer GJ, Oberleas D, Oelshlegel FJ. Zinc deficiency in sickle cell disease. *Clin Chem*. 1975;21:582–587.
54. Bao B, Prasad AS, Beck FWJ, Snell D, Sunega A, Sarkar FH, Doshi N, Fitzgerald JT, Swerdlow P. Zinc supplementation decreased oxidative stress, incidence of infection and generation of inflammatory cytokines in sickle cell disease patients. *Translational Res*. 2008;152:67–80.
55. Prasad AS, Beck FWJ, Kaplan J, Chandrasekar PH, Ortega J, Fitzgerald JT, Swerdlow P. Effect of zinc supplementation on incidence of infections and hospital admissions in sickle cell disease (SCD). *Am J Hematol*. 1999;61(3):194–202.
56. Warth JA, Prasad AS, Zwas F, Frank RN. Abnormal dark adaptation in sickle cell anemia. *J Lab Clin Med*. 1981;98:189–194.
57. Prasad AS, Cossack ZT. Zinc supplementation and growth in sickle cell disease. *Ann Intern Med*. 1984;100:367–371.
58. Sazawal S, Black RE, Bhan MK, Bhandari N, Sinha A, Jalla S. Zinc supplementation in young children with acute diarrhea in India. *N Eng J Med*. 1995;333:839–844.
59. Fisher Walker CL, Lamberti L, Roth D, Black RE. *Zinc in Human Health*, L Rink (ed.). IOS Press, Amsterdam, 2011, pp. 234–253.
60. Prasad AS, Fitzgerald JT, Bao B, Beck WJ, Chandrasekar PH. Duration of symptoms and plasma cytokine levels in patients with the common cold treated with zinc acetate. *Ann Int Med*. 2000;133:245–252.
61. Prasad AS, Beck FWJ, Bao B, Snell D, Fitzgerald T. Duration and severity of symptoms and levels of plasma interleukin-1 receptor antagonist, soluble tumor necrosis factor receptor, and adhesion molecule in patients with common cold treated with zinc acetate. *J Inf Dis*. 2008;197:795–802.
62. Eby GA, Davis DR, Halcomb WW. Reduction in duration of common cold by zinc gluconate lozenges in a double-blind study. *Antimicrob Agents Chemother*. 1984;25:20–24.
63. Brewer GJ, Yuzbasiyan-Gurkan V. Wilson Disease. *Medicine*. 1992;71:139–164.
64. Brewer GJ. Practical recommendations and new therapies for Wilson's disease. *Drugs*. 1995;2:240–249.
65. Brewer GJ, Schoomaker EB, Leichtman DA, Kruckleberg WC, Brewer LF, Myers N. The uses of pharmacologic doses of zinc in the treatment of sickle cell anemia. In: *Zinc Metabolism: Current Aspects in Health and Disease*. GJ Brewer, AS Prasad (eds.), Allan R. Liss, New York, 1977, pp. 241–258.
66. Brewer GJ, Hill GM, Prasad AS, Cossack ZT, Rabbani P. Oral zinc therapy for Wilson's disease. *Ann Intern Med*. 1983;99:314–320.
67. Prasad AS, Brewer GJ, Schoomaker EB, Rabbani P. Hypocupremia induced by zinc therapy in adults. *JAMA*. 1978;240:2166–2168.
68. Hall AC, Young BW, Bremner I. Intestinal metallothionein and the mutual antagonism between copper and zinc in the rat. *J Inorg Biochem*. 1979;11:57–66.
69. Barzegar-Befroet N, Cahyaki S, Fango A, Peto T, Lengeyel I. Zinc and Eye Disease. In: *Zinc and Human Health*. L Rink (ed.), IOS Press, Amsterdam, 2011, pp. 530–553.
70. Newsome DA, Miceli MV, Tats DJ, Alcock NW, Oliver PD. Zinc content of human retinal pigment epithelium decreases with age and macular degeneration but superoxide dismutase activity increases. *J Trace Elem Exper Med*. 1996;8:193–199.
71. Age-Related Eye Disease Study Research Group (AREDS Report No. 8). A randomized, placebo controlled, clinical trial of high-dose supplemented with vitamins C and E, beta-carotene, for age-related macular degeneration and vision loss. *Arch Ophthalmol*. 2001;119:1417–1436.
72. AREDS Report No.13. Association of mortality with ocular disorders and an intervention of high dose antioxidants and zinc in the age-related eye disease study. *Arch Ophthalmol*. 2004;122:716–726.
73. Prasad AS, Beck FWJ, Bao B, Fitzgerald JT, Snell DC, Steinberg JD, Cardozo LJ. Zinc supplementation decreases incidence of infections in the elderly: Effect of zinc on generation of cytokines and oxidative stress. *Am J Clin*. 2007;85:837–844.

74. Briefel RR, Bialostosky K, Kennedy-Stephenson J, McDowell MA, Ervin RB, Wright JD. Zinc intake of US population: Findings from the Third National Health and Nutrition Survey 1988–1994. *J Nutr.* 2000;1367S–1373S.
75. Bao B, Prasad AS, Beck FWJ, Fitzgerald JT, Snell D, Bao GW, Singh T, Cardozo LJ. Zinc decreases C-Reactive protein, lipid peroxidation, and implication of zinc as an atheroprotective agent. *Am J Clin Nutr.* 2010;91:1634–1641.
76. Libby P. Inflammation in atherosclerosis. *Nature.* 2002;420:868–874.

Index

Page numbers followed by f and t indicate figures and tables, respectively.

Printed and bound by CPI Group (UK) Ltd, Croydon, CR0 4YY

18/10/2024

01776249-0016